Note. only 1 CD when issued 23/3/11

Check 2cds are there on issue or return.

SPORTS AND EXERCISE NUTRITION

Second Edition

WILLIAM D. McARDLE
Professor Emeritus, Department of Family, Nutrition, and Exercise Science
Queens College of the City University of New York
Flushing, New York

FRANK I. KATCH (retired, Santa Barbara, CA)
International Research Scholar
Faculty of Health and Sport
Agder University College
Kristiansand, Norway

Instructor and Board Member
Certificate Program in Fitness Instruction
University of California at Los Angeles (UCLA) Extension Los Angeles, CA

Former Professor and Chair of Exercise Science
University of Massachusetts, Amherst

VICTOR L. KATCH
Professor, Department of Movement Science
Division of Kinesiology
Associate Professor, Pediatrics
School of Medicine
University of Michigan
Ann Arbor, Michigan

LIPPINCOTT WILLIAMS & WILKINS
A **Wolters Kluwer** Company
Philadelphia · Baltimore · New York · London
Buenos Aires · Hong Kong · Sydney · Tokyo

Acquisitions Editor: Pete Darcy
Managing Editor: Rebecca Keifer
Marketing Manager: Christen D. Murphy
Production Editor: Paula C. Williams/Sirkka E. H. Bertling
Designer: Risa Clow
Compositor: Maryland Composition
Printer: R.R. Donnelley & Sons—Willard

Library of Congress Cataloging-in-Publication Data

McArdle, William D.
    Sports and exercise nutrition / William D. McArdle, Frank I. Katch, Victor L. Katch.—
2nd ed.
    p. cm.
    Includes bibliographical references and index.
    ISBN 0-7817-4993-X
    1. Athletes—Nutrition.   2. Physical fitness—Nutritional aspects.   3. Exercise—Physiological
aspects. I. Katch, Frank I. II. Katch, Victor L. III. Title.

TX361.A8M38 2004
613.2′024′796—dc22

2004048934

05 06 07 08 09
1 2 3 4 5 6 7 8 9 10

DEDICATION

PREFACE

In the first edition of *Sports & Exercise Nutrition*, we were hopeful that the emergence of "sports nutrition" courses of study would meld with the established field that incorporates the exercise sciences to create the new field of exercise nutrition. To some extent, this has begun to evolve as graduate programs embrace courses that now have a mainstream component that includes the science of human exercise performance. At full maturity, the new field of exercise nutrition will take its deserved place as a respectable academic field of study. The evolution is far from complete, but exercise physiology and nutrition continue to more fully integrate owing to an ever-expanding base of sound research about the nutritional basis for enhanced exercise and sports performance. Interwoven within this fabric are the clear relationships that emerge from this research, particularly regarding sound nutritional practices, regular physical activity, and good health for individuals of all ages. Students of exercise science and nutrition science now demand coursework related to the specifics of exercise nutrition. As qualified faculty members emerge on the college and university level, complete programs of study have replaced the single course offering in this academic field of study.

Organization. The second edition of *Sports and Exercise Nutrition* has undergone a major revision. As with the first edition, we have designed the text for a one-semester course with what we feel is logical sequencing of material. For example, one cannot understand carbohydrate's use during exercise without first reviewing the rudiments of human digestion and then the composition and effect of carbohydrate in the body. Similarly, ergogenic aids, fluid replacement, and "making weight" (all critical topics to sports and exercise nutrition), can best be evaluated after one understands basic bioenergetics, exercise metabolism, energy balance, and temperature regulation. Thus, Section I integrates information about digestion, absorption, and nutrient assimilation. Section II explains how the body extracts energy from ingested nutrients. We stress nutrition's role in energy metabolism: how do nutrients metabolize, and how does training affect nutrient metabolism? This section ends with the measurement and quantification of the energy content of foods, and the energy requirements of diverse physical activities. Section III focuses on aspects of nutrition that optimize both exercise performance and training responsiveness. We also discuss how one makes prudent decisions in the nutrition-fitness marketplace. Section IV describes fundamental mechanisms and adaptations for thermal regulation during heat stress, including strategies for optimizing fluid replacement. Section V consists of two chapters on pharmacologic, chemical, and nutritional ergogenic aids. We integrate the latest findings related to their effectiveness and implications for health and safety. The three chapters in Section VI explain body composition assessment (laboratory and field methods), sport-specific guidelines about body composition and its assessment, energy balance and weight control (making and gaining weight), and the increasing prevalence of disordered eating among diverse groups of athletes and other physically active people.

New to the Second Edition. Components of the entire text have been upgraded to reflect current research findings and updated recommendations related to nutrition and physical activity. Sections and chapters remain similar to the first edition with the exception of Chapter 7, previously titled *Optimal Nutrition for Exercise and Training*. This now consists of two chapters, *Nutritional Recommendations for the Physically Active Person* (Chapter 7) and *Nutritional Considerations for Intense Training and Sports Competition* (Chapter 8). This more effectively focuses on nutritional recommendations for the physically active person (Chapter 7) and the more specific and unique applications for those involved in intense training and sports competition (Chapter 8).

Bonus Interactive CD-ROMs

for **Sports & Exercise Nutrition**, Second Edition

As a bonus for you, Lippincott Williams & Wilkins has added two interactive CD-ROMs to provide you additional tools to help you succeed!

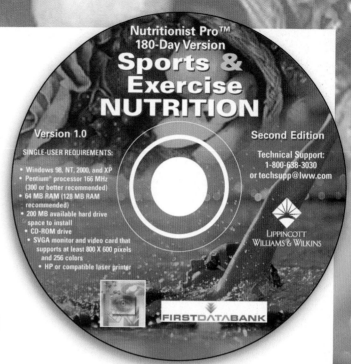

Nutritionist Pro™
180-Day Version
Sports & Exercise NUTRITION

Version 1.0   Second Edition

SINGLE-USER REQUIREMENTS:
- Windows 98, NT, 2000, and XP
- Pentium® processor 166 MHz (300 or better recommended)
- 64 MB RAM (128 MB RAM recommended)
- 200 MB available hard drive space to install
- CD-ROM drive
- SVGA monitor and video card that supports at least 800 X 600 pixels and 256 colors
- HP or compatible laser printer

Technical Support:
1-800-638-3030
or techsupp@lww.com

LIPPINCOTT
WILLIAMS & WILKINS

FIRSTDATABANK

Nutritionist Pro™ Nutritional Analysis Software created by **First DataBank** *(attached to front cover)*	Student Study CD-ROM *(attached to back cover)*

FIRSTDATABANK

This 180-day version of Nutritionist Pro™ combines powerful nutrition analysis functions with the most comprehensive, accurate, and up-to-date nutrition knowledge-base in the world.

Features include:

- Knowledge base—accurate nutrient data, diabetic exchanges, and Food Guide Pyramid servings, plus related information to make your analysis complete.

- Client management—Maintain detailed information on an unlimited number of clients, including assessment data and visit notes.

- Diet analysis—Evaluate diet or food frequencies against specific nutrient requirements.

- Menu analysis—Assess a menu plan by meal, single day or range of days. Compare the analysis to nutrient goals.

- Reports—Rapidly view and print numerous diets, menus, recipes, and reports for clients.

- And more…

This student version is active for 180 days from the first launch of the CD-ROM.

This CD-ROM offers you a quiz tool with approximately 300 multiple choice and true/false quiz questions so you can test your knowledge or prepare for exams. You can choose study mode or test mode and even email your results to your instructor. A comprehensive exam is offered and rationales are given so you can understand the reasoning behind the correct answer.

FOR TECHNICAL SUPPORT,
contact 1-800-638-3030 or
techsupp@lww.com.

LIPPINCOTT
WILLIAMS & WILKINS

A5H400ZZ   CR/KE   1/05

SPORTS AND EXERCISE NUTRITION

Second Edition

Significant Additions and Modifications to the Text Include:

- Inclusion of the latest Dietary Reference Intakes, a radically new and more comprehensive approach to nutritional recommendations in planning and assessing diets for healthy people.
- Use of Dietary Approaches to Stop Hypertension (DASH), an approach that lowers blood pressure in the general population and in people with Stage 1 hypertension to the same extent as pharmacologic therapy, and often more than other lifestyle changes.
- Recommendations of a joint position statement from the American College of Sports Medicine, American Dietetic Association, and Dietitians of Canada about how qualified health, exercise, and nutrition professionals can counsel individuals who engage regularly in physical activity.
- Inclusion of latest information and recommendations from the *Dietary Guidelines for Americans*, the Institute of Medicine, and the American Heart Association concerning diet and lifestyle choices to promote health, support physically active lives, reduce chronic disease risks, and combat the obesity epidemic.
- Presentation of the USDA-designed Healthy Eating Index to monitor changes in diet quality over time. This 100-point analytic tool evaluates how well a person's diet conforms to such recommendations as the *Food Guide Pyramid* and *Dietary Guidelines for Americans* based on dietary balance, moderation, and variety.
- Current epidemiological and clinical findings from the flourishing field of exercise immunology concerning the effects of moderate and strenuous physical activity on immune function, particularly as related to susceptibility to upper respiratory tract infection.
- Discussion of whether additional micronutrient intake, and perhaps carbohydrate ingestion before, during, and after prolonged stressful exercise, boosts normal immune mechanisms to combat infection.
- Analysis of the nutrient composition of commercially prepared liquid and prepackaged nutrition bars, powders, and liquid meals as an alternative approach in precompetition feeding or as supplemental feedings during periods of competition.
- Up-to-date discussion and comparison of energy and nutrient intakes of a large population-based cohort of men and women classified as low, moderate, and high for cardiorespiratory fitness contrasted with nutrient and energy intakes from national dietary recommendations.
- Introduction of the metabolic syndrome, its prevalence, health risks, and criteria for diagnosis.
- Recognizing the diverse demographic backgrounds of individuals in terms of culture and dietary preferences, we also present Mediterranean and Vegetarian Diet Pyramids as well a pyramids applicable to the special needs of children, seniors, and women during pregnancy and lactation.
- Discussion of the Food Guide Pyramid has been expanded to include its usefulness as a model for sound nutrition in menu planning including a sample diet formulated from pyramid recommendations. We also clarify the difference between recommended serving sizes and actual portion sizes typically consumed in the American home and restaurant. Limitations of the pyramid are also discussed.
- Comparison of high-fat diets versus low-fat diets for endurance training and exercise performance.
- Inclusion of the latest data on portion size distortion as reflected by the progressive increase in portion size of such foods as hamburgers, burritos, tacos, French fires, sodas, ice cream, pie, cookies, and salty snacks.
- Evaluation of the macronutrient and energy intakes of men and women over a 30-year period. From 1971 to 2000, women increased caloric intake by 22% while men increased intake by 7%. In 1971 women consumed 1542 kcal on average compared with the year 2000 value of 1887 kcal (+22%), while men increased from 2450 kcal to 2618 kcal (+7%).
- Expanded discussion of potential ergogenic effects of androstenedione and modified versions of this hormone, including the risk of testing positive for the standard marker for the banned anabolic steroid nandrolone.
- Discussion of ergogenic effects and health risks from use of recombinant epoietin (EPO), a synthetic form of the hormone erythropoietin produced by the kidneys to regulate red blood cell production.
- Application of a rapid one-day loading procedure that increases glycogen storage that equals or exceeds values reported using a 2- to 6-day regimen.

- Discussion of gender differences in the response to carbohydrate loading and possible gender-related differences in glucose catabolism in exercise before and after endurance training.
- Discussion of the synergy between enhanced glycogen storage and creatine supplementation.
- Manipulation of nutritional variables to impact responsiveness to resistance training via mechanisms that alter nutrient availability, circulating metabolites and hormonal secretions and interactions with receptors on target tissues, and gene translation and transcription.
- Expanded information on characteristic features and warning signs of anorexia nervosa and bulimia nervosa to help coaches and trainers identify athletes with eating disorders.
- Expanded discussion of Atkins-type low-carbohydrate ketogenic diets, including the South Beach Diet, on health-related variables and body-weight loss.
- Regional body fat distribution and associated health risks.
- Historical view of the BMI of Miss America contestants compared to the World Health Organization cut-off for undernutrition and the BMI for Behnke's standard for the reference woman.
- Discussion of the change in the way many men view the ideal male physique as reflected by the increasing prevalence of muscle dysmorphia or the "Adonis complex," the pathologic preoccupation with muscle size and overall muscularity.
- Discussion of whether ribose possess the ergogenic potential as the next creatine on the supplement scene.
- Usefulness of ingesting large quantities of (—)-hydroxycitrate (HCA) as an anti-obesity agent or ergogenic aid.
- Current standards for overweight and obesity.
- Health risks of obesity and its economic impact.
- Trends in overweight and obesity by racial, ethnic, and gender characteristics worldwide.
- Section on homocysteine and coronary heart disease risk and nutrition's role in controlling levels of this potentially harmful amino acid.
- Discussion of muscular strength related to bone density.
- Discussion of the energy balance equation has been moved to an earlier portion of the text from its previous introduction in the discussion of weight loss in Chapter 14. This was done because of the importance of maintaining proper energy balance, not only for weight control but also for sustaining a physically active lifestyle.
- Added sections on ginseng and ephedrine, two herbal and botanical remedies promoted to improve health, boost energy, control body weight, and enhance exercise performance.

Pedagogic Features

Each chapter contains numerous pedagogic features to engage the student and promote comprehension.

Test Your Knowledge. Each chapter begins with ten True-False statements about relevant chapter material. Tackling these questions before reading the chapter allows students to assess changes in their comprehension after completing the chapter. This approach also provides students the opportunity to evaluate the completeness of their answers with the answer key provided at the end of the chapter. The key includes complete rationales for each answer.

Case Study/Personal Health and Exercise Nutrition. Each chapter also contains at least one case study or a topic related to personal health and exercise nutrition. This unique part of the text more actively involves the student in specific areas of nutritional assessment and health appraisal, application of dietary guidelines, weight control, body composition assessment, overuse syndrome, and physical activity recommendations.

Equations and Data. Important equations and data are highlighted throughout the text for easy reference.

Key Terms. Key terms are bolded throughout the text and defined within the chapter.

References. A complete and up-to-date reference list is included at the end of every chapter.

Web sites. Where applicable, web sites related to nutrition, exercise, and health are included.

Art Program

The full-color art program continues to be a stellar feature of the textbook. Over 200 figures are included to illustrate important concepts in the text. New figures have been added to enhance the new and updated content.

Student Resources

To enhance the student learning experience outside of the classroom, we have included two CD-ROMs in the second edition of *Sports and Exercise Nutrition.*

1. **Nutritionist Pro™ Nutritional Analysis Software** created by First DataBank. For over seven years, thousands of nutrition and exercise professionals have found they can count on First DataBank nutrition software to save time, cut costs and raise their level of client service—in hospitals, clinics, universities, health and fitness centers, private practices and a host of other settings. Nutritionist Pro combines powerful nutrition analysis functions (diet analysis, recipe analysis, menu analysis, and reporting) with the most comprehensive, accurate and up-to-date nutrition knowledge base in the world. This student version is active for 180 days from first launch of the CD-ROM.

   The CD-ROM is PC compatible only. The system requirements for the CD-ROM are:

   - Windows 98, NT, 2000, and XP
   - Pentium processor 166 MHz (300 or better recommended)
   - 64 MB RAM (128 MB RAM recommended)
   - 200 MB available hard drive space to install
   - CD-ROM drive
   - SVGA monitor and video card that supports at least 800×600 pixels and 256 colors
   - HP or compatible laser printer

2. **Student Study CD-ROM.** This CD-ROM includes a quiz tool with approximately 300 multiple choice and true/false quiz questions so students can test their knowledge or prepare for exams.

Instructor Resources. We understand the demand on instructor's time, so to help make your job easier, you will have access to Instructor Resources upon adoption of *Sports and Exercise Nutrition.* An Instructor's Resource CD-ROM (ISBN: 0-7817-9331-9) is available which includes a test generator from Brownstone with approximately 1,500 multiple choice, true/false, and fill-in-the-blank questions; PowerPoint slides for every chapter; and an image bank that contains all of the figures from the textbook. Additionally, the images from the book and the PowerPoint slides are available on a companion website at *http://connection.lww.com/go/mkksen.*

HOW TO USE THIS BOOK

With *Sports and Exercise Nutrition* you will gain a strong foundation in the science of exercise nutrition and bioenergetics, plus insight to how the principles work in the real world of human physical activity and sports medicine. This guide shows you how to put the book's features to work for you.

Introductory Section

Outlines the historical precedent for exercise nutrition, helping you strengthen and ground your knowledge of the field.

Vivid full-color illustrations and photographs

Enhance your learning of important topics and add visual impact.

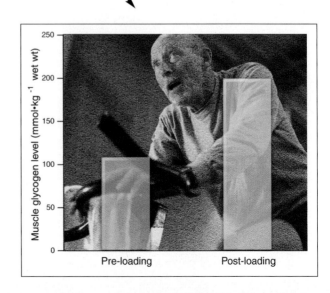

Test Your Knowledge Boxes

Offer true/false statements at the beginning of each chapter to quiz and challenge your current knowledge, allowing you to assess your comprehension after completing the chapter.

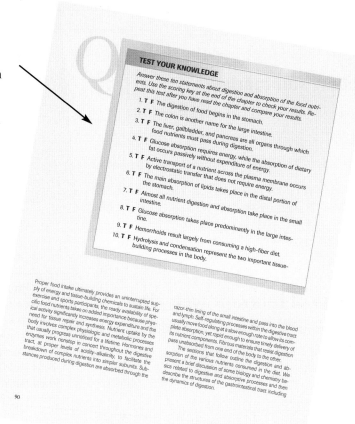

Case Studies and Personal Health and Exercise Nutrition Activities

Engage readers in specific areas of nutritional assessment and health appraisal, application of dietary guidelines, weight control, body composition, overuse syndrome, and physical activity recommendations.

Section summaries

Reinforce and review key concepts and material.

ADP concentrations function as a cellular feedback mechanism to maintain a relatively constant level (homeostasis) of energy currency available for biologic work. Other rate-limiting modulators include cellular levels of phosphate, cyclic AMP, calcium, NAD$^+$, and citrate and pH.

Summary

1. Food macronutrients provide the major sources of potential energy to rejoin ADP and phosphate ion to form ATP.

2. The complete breakdown of 1 mole of glucose liberates 689 kcal of energy. Of this, ATP bonds conserve about 263 kcal (38%), with the remainder dissipated as heat.

3. During glycolytic reactions in the cell's cytosol, a net of two ATP molecules forms during anaerobic substrate-level phosphorylation.

4. Pyruvate converts to acetyl-CoA during the second stage of carbohydrate breakdown within the mitochondrion. Acetyl-CoA then progresses through the citric acid cycle.

5. Hydrogen atoms released during glucose breakdown oxidize via the respiratory chain; the energy generated couples to ADP phosphorylation.

6. The complete oxidation of a glucose molecule in skeletal muscle theoretically yields a net total of 36 ATP molecules.

Figure 4.22 The "metabolic mill" shows important interconversions among carbohydrates, fats, and proteins. Note that all interconversions are possible except that fatty acids cannot contribute to glucose synthesis (note one-way red arrow).

Listings of relevant web sites

Direct you to reliable online exercise nutrition resources.

From the data in Table 6.1, the average net energy values can be rounded to simple whole numbers referred to as **Atwater general factors** (http://www.sportsci.org/news/-history/atwater/atwater.html).

These values, named for Wilbur Olin Atwater (1844–1907), the 19th century chemist who pioneered human nutrition and energy balance studies, represent the en-

References

At the end of each chapter list additional classic and up-to-date resources.

General References

Boyle M. Personal nutrition. 4th ed. Belmont, CA: Wadsworth Publishing, 2001.

Brody T. Nutritional biochemistry. 2nd ed. New York: Academic Press, 1999.

Brown J. Nutrition now. Belmont, CA: Wadsworth Publishing, 1999.

Campbell MK. Biochemistry. 3rd ed. Philadelphia: WB Saunders, 1999.

Emken EA. Metabolism of dietary stearic acid relative to other fatty acids in human subjects. Am J Clin Nutr 1994;60(suppl):1023S.

Fox SI. Human physiology. 7th ed. New York: McGraw-Hill, 2002.

Groff JL, Gropper SS. Advanced nutrition and human metabolism. 3rd ed. Belmont, CA: Wadsworth Publishing, 1999.

Guthrie HA, ed. Introductory nutrition. 7th ed. St. Louis: CV Mosby, 1988.

Guyton AC. Textbook of medical physiology. 10th ed. Philadelphia: WB Saunders, 2000.

Kraut J. How do enzymes work? Science 1988;242:533.

Mahan LK, Escott-Stump S. Krause's food, nutrition, & diet therapy. Philadelphia: WB Saunders, 2000.

Marieb EN. Essentials of human anatomy and physiology. 7th ed. Menlo Park, CA. Pearson Education: Benjamin Cummings, 2003.

Powers HJ Riboflavin (vitamin B-2) and health. Am J Clin Nutr 2003;77:1352.

Jennifer, Shils ME, et al. Modern nutrition in health and disease. 10th ed. Baltimore: Lippincott Williams & Wilkins, 2005.

Vander AJ, et al. Human physiology: the mechanisms of body function. 7th ed. New York: McGraw-Hill, 1997.

Whitney EN, Rolfes SR. Understanding nutrition (with InfoTrac). 9th ed. Stamford, CT: Thomson/Wadsworth, 2002.

Additional Readings

Albi E, Viola Magni MP. The role of intranuclear lipids. Biol Cell 2004;96:657.

Armas LA, et al. Vitamin D2 is much less effective than Vitamin D3 in humans. J Clin Endocrinol Metab 2004;89:5387.

Borsheim E, et al. Effect of carbohydrate intake on net muscle protein synthesis during recovery from resistance exercise. J Appl Physiol 2004;96:674.

Chan MA, et al. Influence of carbohydrate ingestion on cytokine responses following acute resistance exercise. Int J Sport Nutr Exerc Metab 2003;13:454.

Jeanes YM, et al. The absorption of Vitamin E is influenced by the amount of fat in a meal and the food matrix. Br J Nutr 2004;92:575.

Jeukendrup AE. Carbohydrate intake during exercise and performance. Nutrition 2004;20:669.

Korach-Andre M, et al. Glucose appearance in the peripheral circulation and liver glucose output in men after a large 13C starch meal. Am J Clin Nutr 2004;80:881.

Lancaster GI, et al. Effect of pre-exercise carbohydrate ingestion on plasma cytokine, stress hormone, and neutrophil degranulation responses to continuous, high-intensity exercise. Int J Sport Nutr Exerc Metab 2003;13:436.

Vuorilehto K, et al. Indirect electrochemical reduction of nicotinamide coenzymes. Bioelectrochemistry 2004;65:1.

Wasserman RH. Vitamin D and the dual processes of intestinal calcium absorption. J Nutr 2004;134:3137.

Student Resources

Nutritionist Pro™ Nutritional Analysis Software created by First DataBank. Nutritionist Pro combines powerful nutrition analysis functions (diet analysis, recipe analysis, menu analysis, and reporting) with the most comprehensive, accurate, and up-to-date nutrition knowledge base in the world. This student version is active for 180 days from first launch of the CD-ROM.

Student Study CD-ROM provides a quiz tool with approximately 300 multiple choice and true/false quiz questions so you can test your knowledge or prepare for exams.

ACKNOWLEDGMENTS

We gratefully acknowledge the following individuals at Lippincott Williams & Wilkins for their dedication and expertise with this project: Pete Darcy, executive editor; Paula Williams, Jennifer Glazer, and Sirkka Bertling, production editors, for helpful editing and quality suggestions; Jonathan Dimes for keen insights about art design, and for keeping a sharp eye on the art program; to illustrator Michael Kress-Russick who continues to turn our sketches into gorgeous art pieces using Macintosh magic; to Christen D. Murphy, marketing manager, for creatively promoting our text and interpreting its unique aspects to the appropriate markets: to Kate Staples, our editorial assistant; and a very special thanks to Rebecca Keifer, managing editor, for tolerating our unique idiosyncrasies, for gently keeping us focused and "on track," and for making what often becomes a difficult task a relatively enjoyable experience. We are also grateful to the numerous undergraduate and graduate students at our respective universities for keeping our "motors" going during our work on various projects related to this text.

WILLIAM MCARDLE • Sound Beach, NY
FRANK KATCH • Santa Barbara, CA
VICTOR KATCH • Ann Arbor, MI

Frank Katch, William McArdle (in chair), Victor Katch

CONTENTS

INTRODUCTION

Food provides the the source of essential elements and building blocks for preserving lean body mass, synthesizing new tissue, optimizing skeletal structure, repairing existing cells, maximizing oxygen transport and use, maintaining optimal fluid and electrolyte balance, and regulating all metabolic processes. "Good nutrition" encompasses more than preventing nutrient deficiencies related to disease, including overt endemic diseases ranging from beriberi (vitamin deficiency disease from inadequate thiamine [Vitamin B[1]]; damages heart and nervous system) to xerophthalmia (caused by vitamin A deficiency and general malnutrition leading to night blindness, corneal ulceration, and blindness). It also encompasses the recognition of individual differences in need for and tolerance of specific nutrients, and the role of genetic heritage on such factors. Borderline nutrient deficiencies (i.e., less than required to cause clinical manifestations of disease) negatively impact bodily structure and function and thus the capacity for exercise.

Proper nutrition also forms the foundation for physical performance; it provides the fuel for biologic work and the chemicals for extracting and using food's potential energy. Not surprisingly then, from the time of the ancient Olympics to the present, almost every conceivable dietary practice has been used to enhance exercise the performance. Writings from the first Olympic games in 776 BC to today's computerized era provide a glimpse at what athletes consume. Poets, philosophers, writers, and the physicians of ancient Greece and Rome tell of diverse strategies athletes undertook to prepare for competitions. They consumed various animal meats (oxen, goat, bull, deer), moist cheeses and wheat, dried figs, and special "concoctions" and liquors. For the next two thousand years, however, little reliable information existed about the food preferences of top athletes (except for rowers and pedestrian walkers during the nineteenth century). The 1936 Berlin Olympics offered a preliminary assessment of the food consumed by world-class athletes. From the paper by Schenk,[1]

> . . . the Olympic athletes competing at Berlin frequently focused upon meat, that athletes regularly dined on two steaks per meal, sometimes poultry, and averaged nearly half a kilogram of meat daily . . . pre-event meals regularly consisted of one to three steaks and eggs, supplemented with "meat-juice" extract. . . . Other athletes stressed the importance of carbohydrate. . . . Olympic athletes from England, Finland and Holland regularly consumed porridge, the Americans ate shredded wheat or corn flakes in milk, and the Chileans and Italians feasted on pasta . . . members of the Japanese team consumed a pound of rice daily.

During the 1996 Olympic Games, about 12,000 athletes from 197 countries consumed 5 million meals (about 1.1 million pounds of food, including 550,000 gallons of bottled water). Interestingly, five times as many black-eyed peas (3,333 lb) were eaten than anchovies (665 lb), while garlic (1,034 lb) equaled one-seventh the amount of spaghetti consumed (7,850 lb). Athletes ate more apples (270,000 lb) than any other staple; other foods consumed included beef (240,000 lb), poultry (150,000 lb), milk (70,000 lb), peaches (56,600 lb), pasta (52,000 lb), and rice and potatoes (34,000 lb). During this Olympiad, some countries applied specific dietary regimens, while athletes from less industrialized countries had free choice of what they ate, often combining ritual with novelty foods. The majority of athletes probably consumed dietary supplements including vitamins and minerals; a smaller percentage most likely ingested stimulants, narcotics, anabolic agents, diuretics, peptides, glycoprotein hormones and analogs, alcohol, marijuana, local anesthetics, corticosteroids, beta blockers, beta-2 agonists, and used blood doping, all prohibited by the International Olympic Committee.

Even today's technologically savvy world is inundated with trendy theories, misinformation, and outright quackery about links between nutrition and physical performance. Accomplishments during the last 100 years of Olympic competition have undeniably improved (**Fig. i.1**), but no one has yet established universal ties between food and these remarkable physical achievements. Athletes have every reason to desire any substance that might confer a competitive advantage because winning insures glory and multimillion dollar endorsement contracts. Their eagerness to shave milliseconds from a run or add centimeters to a jump convinces them to experiment with nutrition and polypharmacy supplementation, including illegal drugs.

The search for the Holy Grail to enhance physical performance has not been limited to the last few decades. Athletes and trainers in ancient civilization also sought to improve athletic prowess. Although lacking objective proof, they routinely experimented with nutritional substances and rituals, trusting that the natural and supernatural would provide an advantage. Over the past 25 centuries, the scientific method has gradually replaced dogma and ritual as the most effective approach healthful living and optimal physical performance. The emerging field of exercise nutrition uses the ideas of pioneers in medicine, anatomy, physics, chemistry, hygiene, nutrition, and physical culture to establish a robust body of knowledge.

A sound understanding of exercise nutrition enables one to appreciate the importance of adequate nutrition, and to critically evaluate the validity of claims concerning nutrient supplements and special dietary modifications to enhance physique, physical performance, and exercise training responses. Knowledge of the nutrition-metabolism interaction forms the basis for the preparation, performance, and recuperation phases of intense exercise and/or training. Not surprisingly, many physically active individuals, including some of the world's best athletes, obtain nutritional information in the locker room, and from magazine and newspaper articles, advertisements, video "infomercials," training partners, health-food shops, and testimonials from successful athletes, rather than from well-informed and well-educated coaches, trainers, physicians, and physical fitness and exercise nutrition professionals. Far too many devote considerable time and energy striving for optimum performance and training, only to fall short from inadequate, counterproductive, and sometimes harmful nutritional practices.

We hope the second edition of Sports and Exercise Nutrition continues to provide "cutting-edge" scientific information for all people involved in regular physical activity and exercise training, not just the competitive athlete. We agree with UC San Diego biology professor Paul Saltman who stated the following in a presentation to the American Medical Association in July 17, 1996 prior to the Atlanta Olympics:[2]

> Coaches, trainers and, above all, athletes, must have an understanding of the biochemical and physiological basis of foods and nutrients in order to translate this knowledge into "real world" training table regimens to provide the competitive edge. They need not be limited by these principles, but liberated by them.

Exercise Nutrition for the Future: A Fresh Look

And if we are ignorant of our past, if we are indifferent to our story and those people who did so much for us, we're not just being stupid, we're being rude. (From 146th Beloit College Commencement. May 12, 1996. Pulitzer Prize-winner David McCollough)

The accompanying timeline presents an historical overview of selected individuals from the Renaissance to the 21st century whose work and scientific experiments demonstrated the intimate interconnections among medicine, physiology, exercise, and nutrition. Their important accomplishments provide a powerful rationale for developing an integrated subject field of study that we call exercise nutrition.

Some consider an exercise nutrition curriculum (at a college or university) as a subset of nutrition, but we believe this designation requires updating. First we recommend a change in name from sports nutrition to

One hundred years of Olympic competition—Athens, 1896 to Atlanta, 1996. Records are plotted for the men in **blue** and women in red. The last point of each graph marks the world record (WR).

(World records as of November 9, 1997)

Figure i.1. One hundred years of Olympic competition—Athens, 1896 to Atlanta, 1996—in selected events for men in blue and women in red.

exercise nutrition. The term exercise encompasses more than the word sports, and more fully reflects the many active men and women who are not necessarily "sportsmen." An academic program would have as its core academic content applicable to the ever-increasing number of physically active individuals. Such a curriculum would neither be housed in a Department of Nutrition nor a Department of Exercise Science or Kinesiology. Rather, the curriculum deserves a unique identity. **Figure i.2** presents six core areas for research and study that constitute exercise nutrition, with specific topics listed within each area.

The focus of exercise nutrition becomes cross-disciplinary. It synthesizes knowledge from the separate but related fields of nutrition and exercise. A number of existing fields take a cross-disciplinary approach. Biochemists do not receive in-depth training as chemists or biologists. Instead, their training as biochemists makes them more competent biochemists than more narrowly focused chemists or biologists. The same inclusivity characterizes a biophysicist, a radio astronomer, a molecular biologist, and a geophysicist.

Historical precedents exist for linking two fields: those involving nutrition and those involving exercise. The chemist Lavoisier, for example, employed exercise to study respiration, probably not thinking that his discoveries would impact fields other than chemistry. A.V. Hill, a competent mathematician and physiologist, won a Nobel Prize in Physiology or Medicine, not for his studies of mathematics or physiology per se, but for his integrative work with muscle that helped to unravel secrets about the biochemistry of muscular contraction.

Nutritional Enhancement	**Health and Longevity**
• Optimal nutrition vs. optimal nutrition for exercise • Environmental stressors • Individual differences • Military • Spaceflight dynamics	• Eating patterns • Exercise patterns • Nutrition-exercise interactions • Reproduction • Mortality and morbidity • Epidemiology
Energy Balance and Body Composition • Metabolism • Exercise dynamics • Assessment • Weight control/obesity • Body size, shape, and proportion	**Peak Physiologic Function** • Protein, carbohydrate, and lipid requirement • Oxidative stress • Fatigue and staleness • Tissue repair and growth • Micronutrient needs • Gender related effects
Optimal Growth • Normal and abnormal • Bone, muscle, other tissues • Life span • Effects on cognitive behaviors • Effects of chronic exercise • Sport-specific interactions	**Safety** • Disordered eating • Ergogenic/ergolytic substances • Thermal stress and fluid replacement • Nutrient abuse • Exercise-stress-nutrient interactions • Food quality

Figure i.2. Six core areas for research and study in the field of Exercise Nutrition.

In the cross-discipline of exercise nutrition, students specialize neither in exercise nor nutrition. Instead, they are trained in aspects of *both* fields. Our concept of an academic discipline agrees with Professor Franklin Henry's ideas promoted in the late 1950s.[3] It is an organized body of information collectively embraced in a formal course of instruction worthy of pursuit on its own merits.

Exercise nutrition synthesizes data from physiology, chemistry, exercise physiology, biochemistry, medicine, and nutrition. Students of exercise nutrition may not be full-fledged chemists, exercise physiologists, or nutritionists; however, their cross-disciplinary training gives them a broader and more appropriate perspective to advance their discipline. The renal physiologist studies the kidney as an isolated organ to determine its functions, often utilizing exercise as the stressor. The exercise scientist measures the effects of exercise on kidney function. Here the researcher emphasizes exercise physiology more than renal physiology. By contrast, the exercise nutritionist might investigate how combining diet and exercise impact kidney function in general and in specific circumstances like physical activity under heat stress.

We urge the establishment of a separate discipline to unite previously disparate fields. We hope others share our vision.

References

1. Grivetti LE, Applegate EA. From Olympia to Atlanta: a cultural-historical perspective on diet and athletic training. J Nutr 869S, 1997.
2. Available at: http://www.newswisw.com//articles/Diet.AMA.html
3. Henry FM. Physical education: An academic discipline. Proceedings of the 67th Annual Meeting of the National College Physical Education Association for Men, AAHPERD, Washington DC, 1964.

Timeline: Exercise Nutrition through the ages

Leonardo da Vinci (1452–1519). Master anatomist produced exquisite drawings of the heart and circulation which showed that air reached pulmonary arteries via bronchi, not directly through the heart as taught by Galenic medicine.

Michelangelo Buonarroti (1475–1564). Realistic sculpture of "David" combined scientific anatomy with ideal body proportions.

"David"

Santorio (1561–1636). Accurately recorded changes in body weight over a 30-year period to understand metabolism. Published *De Medicina Statica Aphorismi* (Medical Aphorisms), 1614.

Santorio's scale used to assess his weight.

1450   1500   1600

Albrecht Dürer (1471–1528) "Quadrate Man" illustrated age-related differences in body segment ratios.

Andreas Vesalius (1514–1564). Incomparable *De Humani Corporis Fabrica* (On the Composition of the Human Body) and *De Fabrica* (1543) based on his own dissections demolished traditional Galenic pronouncements about human anatomy.

William Harvey (1578–1657). Proved the heart pumped blood one way through a closed circulatory system (see Chapter 1).

Giovanni Alfonso Borelli (1608–1679). Used mathematical models to explain locomotion (*De Motu Animaliu,* 1680, 1681). Showed that the lungs filled with air because the chest volume increased when diaphragm moved downward. Disproved the Galenic claim that air cooled the heart by showing how respiration, not circulation, required diffusion of air in the alveoli.

Robert Boyle (1627–1691) Proved that combustion and respiration required air. Boyle's Law of Gases states that at constant temperature, the pressure (P) of a given mass of gas varies inversely proportional to its volume (V): $P_1V_1 = P_2V_2$.

Boyle's "Pneumatical Engine" apparatus

René-Antoine Fercault de Réaumur (1683–1757). Proved by regurgitation experiments that gastric secretions digest foods (*Digestion in Birds*, 1752).

James Lind (1716–1794). Eradicated scurvy by adding citrus fruits to sailors' diets (see Chapter 2).

Joseph Priestley (1733-1804). Discovered oxygen by heating red oxide of mercury in a closed vessel (*Observations on Different Kinds of Air*, 1773).

Priestley's laboratory

1620   **1700**   **1735**

Stephen Hales (1677–1761). *Vegetable Statics* (1727) described how chemical changes occurred in solids and liquids upon calcination (oxidation during combustion), and how the nervous system governed muscular contraction.

Hale's combustion apparatus.

Joseph Black (1728–1799) Isolated carbon dioxide gas in air produced by fermentation (*Experiments Upon Magnesia Alba, Quicklime, And Some Other Alcaline Substances*, 1756).

Lazzaro Spallanzani (1729–1799). Proved that tissues of the heart, stomach, and liver consume oxygen and liberate carbon dioxide, even in creatures without lungs.

Henry Cavendish (1731–1810). Identified hydrogen produced when acids combined with metals (*On Factitious Air*, 1766). Proved that water formed when "inflammable air" (hydrogen) combined with "deflogisticated air" (oxygen) (*Experiments in Air*, 1784).

Antoine Laurent Lavoisier (1743–1794). Quantified effects of muscular work on metabolism by measuring increases in oxygen uptake, pulse rate, respiration rate. Proved that atmospheric air provides oxygen for animal respiration, and that the "caloric" (heat) liberated during respiration is itself the source of the combustion (see Chapter 3).

A.F. Fourcroy (1755–1809). Demonstrated that the same proportions of nitrogen occur in animals and plants.

Joseph Louis Proust (1755–1826). Formulated "Law of Definite Proportions" (chemical constancy of substances permits future analysis of major nutrients, including metabolic assessment by oxygen consumption).

1740   1755   1775

Carl Wilhelm Scheele (1742–1786). Described oxygen ("fire-air") independently of Priestley, and "foul air" (phlogisticated air-later called nitrogen) in a famous experiment with bees (*Chemical Treatise on Air and Fire*, 1777). Scheele's bees living in "fire air" in a closed vessel submerged in limewater.

Claude Louis Berthollet (1748–1822). Proved that animal tissues do not contain ammonia, but that hydrogen united with nitrogen during fermentation to produce ammonia. He disagreed with Lavoisier's concept of heat production: "the quantity of heat liberated in the incomplete oxidation of a substance is equal to the difference between the total caloric value of the substance and that of the products formed."

Humphrey Davey (1778–1829). Consolidated all of the contemporary chemical data related to nutrition, including 47 elements he isolated (*Elements of Agricultural Chemistry*, 1813). Tried to explain how heat and light affect the blood's ability to contain oxygen.

Davey's chemistry laboratory where he isolated 47 elements

Nineteenth Century Metabolism and Physiology

The untimely death of Lavoisier (1794) did not terminate fruitful research in nutrition and medicine. During the next half century, scientists discovered the chemical composition of carbohydrates, lipids, and proteins, and further clarified the energy balance equation.

Joseph-Louis Gay-Lussac (1778–1850). Proved that 20 animal and vegetable substances differed depending on the proportion of H to O atoms. Named one class of compounds ("saccharine") later identified as carbohydrates. Proved the equivalency of oxygen percentage in air at altitude and sea level.

François Magendie (1783–1855). Established experimental physiology as a science and founded its first journal (*Journal de Physiologie Expérimentale*). Proved that anterior spinal nerve roots control motor activities, while posterior roots control sensory functions. Categorized foods as nitrogenous or non-nitrogenous (*Précis élémentaire de Physiologie*, 1816), arguing that foods, not air, provided nitrogen to tissues.

Michel Eugène Chevreul (1786–1889). Explained that fats consists of fatty acids and glycerol (*Chemical Investigations of Fat*, 1823). Coined the term margarine, and showed that lard consists of two main fats he called "stearine and elaine." With Gay-Lussac, patented the manufacture of the stearic acid candle (still used today).

Gerardus Johannis Mulder (1802–1880). Established the field of physiological chemistry (*General Physiological Chemistry*, 1854). Researched albuminous substances he named "proteine." Strongly advocated society's role in promoting quality nutrition. Established minimum standards for protein consumption (laborers 120 g daily, others 60 g).

1778

1800

William Prout (1785–1850). First to separate foodstuffs into the modern classification of carbohydrates, fats, and proteins. Measured the carbon dioxide exhaled by men exercising to fatigue (*Annals of Philosophy*, 2: 328, 1813). Showed that walking raised carbon dioxide production to a plateau (ushering in the modern concept of steady-state gas exchange). Proved that free HCl appeared in the stomach's gastric juice. First prepared pure urea. Extolled milk as the perfect food in *Treatise on Chemistry, Meteorology, and the Function of Digestion* (1834).

William Beaumont (1785–1853). Explained in-vivo and in-vitro human digestion (see Chapter 4).

Jean Baptiste Boussingault (1802– 1884). Father of "scientific agriculture." Determined the effects of calcium, iron, and nutrient intake (particularly nitrogen) on energy balance in animals and humans.

Justus von Liebig (1803–1873). Dominant chemist of his time, yet asserted without evidence that vigorous exercise by humans and animals required a high protein intake (1850's experiments by others disproved his assertions) (see Chapter 5).

Claude Bernard (1813–1878). Perhaps the greatest experimental physiologist of all time. His discoveries in regulatory physiology helped future scientists understand how metabolism and nutrition affect exercise (see Chapter 6).

Edward Hitchcock, Jr. (1828–1911). Amherst College professor who pioneered anthropometric assessment of body build and scientific muscular strength training and testing.

Carl von Voit (1831–1908). Disproved Liebig's assertion about protein as a main energy fuel by demonstrating that protein breakdown does not increase in proportion to exercise intensity or duration.

1800   1820   1830

Henri Victor Regnault (1810–1878). Developed closed-circuit spirometry to determine respiratory quotient (VCO_2/VO_2). Established relationship between body size and metabolism (heat production).

Small animal respiration chamber.

Edward Smith (1819–1874). Used closed-circuit spirometry to assess energy metabolism during forced exercise. Disproved Liebig's claim that protein alone serves as the primary source of muscular power (see Chapter 7).

Eduard Pflüger (1829–1910). First demonstrated that minute changes in the partial pressure of gases in blood affects the rate of oxygen release and transport across capillary membranes, thus proving blood flow alone does not govern how tissues use oxygen.

Max Joseph von Pettenkofer (1818–1901).Perfected respiration calorimeter to study human and animal metabolism. Initiated studies of scientific hygiene (air quality, soil composition and ground water, moisture content of structures, building ventilation, functions of clothing, spread of disease, water quality). He discovered creatinine (amino acid in urine), and founded *Zeitschrift für Biologie* (1865 with Voit) and *Zeitschrift für Hygiene* (1885).

Pettenkofer's 1863 respiration chamber. Top image shows the entire apparatus.Image at left is cut-away view showing human experiment. Fresh air was pumped into the sealed chamber and exhausted air sampled for carbon dioxide

Nathan Zuntz (1847–1920). Devised first portable metabolic apparatus to assess respiratory exchange in animals and humans at different altitudes. Proved that carbohydrates are precursors of lipid synthesis, and that lipids and carbohydrates should not be consumed equally. Zuntz produced 430 articles concerning blood and blood gases, circulation, mechanics and chemistry of respiration, general metabolism and metabolism of specific foods, energy metabolism and heat production, and digestion.

Max Rubner (1854–1932). Discovered the Isodynamic Law and the calorific heat values of foods (4.1 kcal · g⁻¹ for protein and carbohydrates, 9.3 kcal · g⁻¹ for lipids). Rubner's Surface Area Law states that resting heat production is proportional to body surface area, and that consuming food increases heat production (SDA effect).

Frederick Gowland Hopkins (1861–1947). Isolated and identified the structure of the amino acid tryptophan (1929 Nobel Prize in Medicine or Physiology) (see Chapter 10).

1835   **1850**   **1860**

Austin Flint, Jr. (1836–1915). Prolific author and physiology researcher who chronicled topics of importance to the emerging science of exercise physiology and future science of exercise nutrition. His 987-page compendium of five prior textbooks (*The Physiology of Man; Designed to Represent the Existing State of Physiological Science as Applied to the Functions of the Human Body*, 1877) summarized knowledge about exercise, circulation, respiration, and nutrition from French, German, English, and American literature.

Wilbur Olin Atwater (1844–1907). Published the chemical composition of 2600 American foods (1896) still used in modern databases of food consumption; performed human calorimetric studies. Confirmed that the Law of Conservation of Energy governs transformation of matter in the human body and inanimate world (see Chapter 8).

Russel Henry Chittenden (1856–1943). Refocused scientific attention on man's minimal protein requirement while resting or exercising (no debilitation occurred from protein intake less than 1 g · kg⁻¹ body mass in either normal and athletic young men (*Physiological Economy In Nutrition, With Special Reference To The Minimal Proteid Requirement Of The Healthy Man. An Experimental Study*, 1897) (see Chapter 9).

Francis Gano Benedict (1870–1957). Conducted exhaustive studies of energy metabolism in newborn infants, growing children and adolescents, starving people, athletes and vegetarians. Devised "metabolic standard tables" on sex, age, height, and weight to compare energy metabolism in normals and patients (see Chapter 11).

Otto Fritz Meyerhof (1884–1951). 1923 Nobel Prize in Physiology or Medicine with A.V. Hill for elucidating the cyclic characteristics of intermediary cellular energy transformation (see Chapter 13).

1870   **1900**

August Krogh (1874–1949). 1920 Nobel Prize in Physiology or Medicine for discovering the mechanism that controls capillary blood flow in resting and active muscle (in frogs). Krogh's 300 published scientific articles link exercise physiology with nutrition and metabolism (see Chapter 12).

Archibald Vivian (A.V.) Hill (1886–1977). 1922 Nobel Prize in Physiology or Medicine with Meyerhof for discoveries about the chemical and mechanical events in muscle contraction (see Chapter 14).

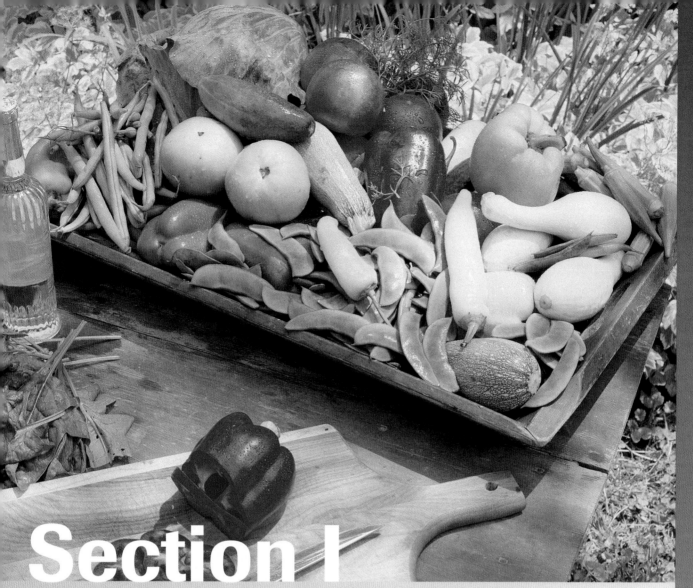

Section I

Food Nutrients: Structure, Function and Digestion, Absorption, and Assimilation

Outline

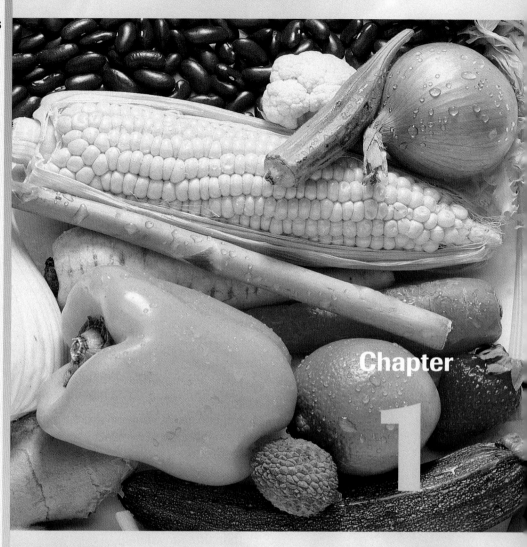

Chapter

1

The
Macronutrients

TEST YOUR KNOWLEDGE

Answer these ten statements about carbohydrates, fats, and proteins. Use the scoring key at the end of the chapter to check your results. Repeat this test after you have read the chapter and compare your results.

1. **T F** Carbohydrates consist of atoms of carbon, oxygen, nitrogen, and hydrogen.

2. **T F** Glucose can be synthesized from amino acids in the body.

3. **T F** Dietary fiber's main function is to provide energy for biologic work.

4. **T F** Carbohydrate intake for most physically active individuals should make up about 45% of the total caloric intake.

5. **T F** Individuals who consume simple carbohydrates run little risk of gaining weight.

6. **T F** A given quantity of sugar, lipid, and protein contains about the same amount of energy.

7. **T F** Although found predominantly in the animal kingdom, certain plant forms also contain cholesterol.

8. **T F** Vegans are at somewhat greater risk for nutrient and energy malnutrition than individuals who consume foods from plant and animal sources.

9. **T F** Consuming extra high-quality protein above recommended levels facilitates increases in muscle mass.

10. **T F** The protein requirement (per kg of body mass) for men is greater than that for women.

The carbohydrate, lipid, and protein nutrients ultimately provide energy to maintain body functions during rest and all forms of physical activity. In addition to their role as biologic fuels, these nutrients, called **macronutrients**, also maintain the organism's structural and functional integrity. This chapter focuses on each macronutrient's structure, function, and source in the diet.

ATOMS: NATURE'S BUILDING BLOCKS

Of the 103 different atoms or elements identified in nature, the mass of the human organism contains about 3% nitrogen, 10% hydrogen, 18% carbon, and 65% oxygen. These atoms play the major role in the chemical composition of nutrients and make up the structural units for the body's biologically active substances.

The union of two or more atoms forms a molecule whose particular properties depend on its specific atoms and their arrangement. Glucose is glucose because of the arrangement of three different kinds of 24 atoms within its molecule. Chemical bonding involves a common sharing of electrons between atoms, as occurs when hydrogen and oxygen atoms join to form a water molecule. The force of attraction between positive and negative charges serves as bonding, or "chemical cement," to keep the atoms within a molecule together. A larger aggregate of matter (a substance) forms when two or more molecules bind chemically. The substance can take the form of a gas, liquid, or solid, depending on the forces of interaction among molecules. Altering forces by removing, transferring, or exchanging electrons releases energy, some of which powers cellular functions.

CARBON: THE VERSATILE ELEMENT

All nutrients contain carbon except water and minerals. Almost all of the substances within the body consist of carbon-containing (**organic**) compounds. Carbon atoms share chemical bonds with other carbon atoms and with atoms of other elements to form large carbon-chain molecules. Specific linkages of carbon, hydrogen, and oxygen atoms form lipids and carbohydrates, while the addition of nitrogen and certain minerals creates a protein molecule. Carbon atoms linked with hydrogen, oxygen, and nitrogen also serve as atomic building blocks for the body's exquisitely formed structures.

 # Carbohydrates

THE NATURE OF CARBOHYDRATES

All living cells contain carbohydrates, a class of organic molecules that includes monosaccharides, disaccharides, and polysaccharides. Except for lactose and a small amount of glycogen from animals, plants provide the exclusive source of carbohydrate in the human diet. As the name suggests, carbohydrates contain carbon and water. Combining atoms of carbon, hydrogen, and oxygen forms a carbohydrate (sugar) molecule with the general formula $(CH_2O)n$, where n equals from 3 to 7 carbon atoms, with single bonds attaching to hydrogen and oxygen. Carbohydrates with 5 and 6 atoms interest nutritionists the most.

FIGURE 1.1 displays the chemical structure of **glucose**, the most typical sugar, along with other carbohydrates synthesized during photosynthesis. Glucose contains 6 carbon, 12 hydrogen, and 6 oxygen atoms having the chemical formula $C_6H_{12}O_6$. Each carbon atom has four bonding sites that link to other atoms, including carbons. Carbon bonds not linked to other carbon atoms remain "free" to accept hydrogen (with only one bond site), oxygen (with two bond sites), or an oxygen–hydrogen combination (OH), termed a hydroxyl. **Fructose** and **galactose**, two other simple sugars, have the same chemical formula as glucose, but with a slightly different carbon-to-hydrogen-to-oxygen linkage. This makes fructose, galactose, and glucose uniquely different in function, each with its own distinctive biochemical characteristics.

KINDS AND SOURCES OF CARBOHYDRATES

Four categories of carbohydrates exist: **monosaccharides**, **disaccharides**, **oligosaccharides**, and **polysaccharides**. The number of simple sugars linked within the molecule distinguishes each carbohydrate type. TABLE 1.1 classifies the different carbohydrates.

Monosaccharides

The monosaccharide molecule represents the basic unit of carbohydrates. More than 200 monosaccharides exist in nature. The number of carbon atoms in their ringed structure determines the category. The Greek word for this number, ending with "ose," indicates they represent sugars. For example, 3-carbon monosaccharides are trioses, 4-carbon sugars are tetroses, 5-carbon pentoses, 6-carbon hexoses, and 7-carbon sugars heptoses. The hexose sugars glucose, fructose, and galactose make up the nutritionally important monosaccharides. Glucose, also called dextrose or blood sugar, occurs naturally in food. The digestion of more complex carbohydrates also produces glucose. Furthermore, glucose can be produced by **gluconeogenesis**, synthesizing it (primarily in the liver) from carbon skeletons of specific amino acids and from glycerol, pyruvate, and lactate. The small intestine absorbs glucose, where it then can be *(a)* used directly by the cells for energy, *(b)* stored as glycogen in the muscles and liver for later use, or *(c)* converted to fat and stored for energy.

Fructose (also called levulose or fruit sugar), the sweetest of the simple sugars, occurs in large amounts in fruits and honey. It accounts for about 9% of the average energy intake in the United States. The small intestine absorbs some fructose directly into the blood, and the liver slowly converts it to glucose. Galactose does not occur freely in nature; rather, it forms milk sugar (lactose) in the mammary glands of lactating animals. In the body, galactose converts to glucose for energy metabolism.

Disaccharides and Oligosaccharides

Combining two monosaccharide molecules forms a disaccharide or double sugar. The monosaccharides and disaccharides are collectively called sugars or **simple sugars**.

Each disaccharide includes glucose as a principle component. The three disaccharides of nutritional significance are listed below.

- **Sucrose**, the most common dietary disaccharide, consists of glucose plus fructose; it constitutes up to 25% of the total caloric intake in the Unites States. Sucrose occurs naturally in most foods that contain

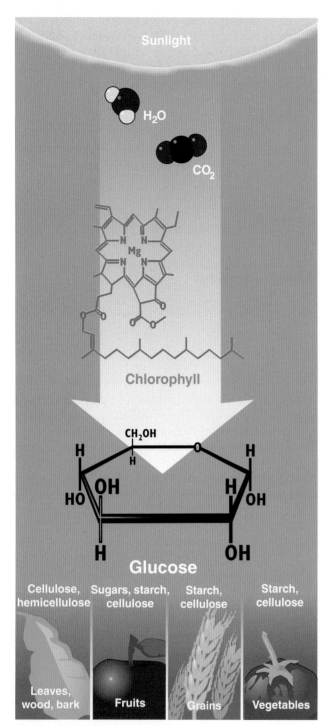

■ Figure 1.1. Three-dimensional ring structure of the simple sugar molecule glucose, formed during photosynthesis when the energy from sunlight interacts with water, carbon dioxide, and the green pigment chlorophyll. The molecule resembles a hexagonal plate to which H and O atoms attach. About 75% of the plant's dry matter consists of carbohydrate; photosynthesis forms approximately 100 billion tons of carbohydrates yearly.

carbohydrates, particularly in beet and cane sugar, brown sugar, sorghum, maple syrup, and honey. Honey, sweeter than table sugar because of its greater fructose content, offers no advantage nutritionally or as an energy source.

- **Lactose**, found in natural form only in milk (called milk sugar), consists of glucose plus galactose. The least sweet of the disaccharides, lactose can be artificially processed and is often present in carbohydrate-rich, high-calorie liquid meals. A substantial segment of the world's population is **lactose intolerant**; these individuals lack adequate quantities of the enzyme lactase that splits lactose to glucose and galactose during digestion.
- **Maltose**, composed of two glucose molecules, occurs in beer, cereals, and germinating seeds. Also called malt sugar, maltose makes only a small contribution to the carbohydrate content of a person's diet.
- **Oligosaccharides** (*oligo* in Greek, meaning a few) form from combining 3 to 9 monosaccharide residues. The main dietary sources for the oligosaccharides are vegetables, particularly seed legumes.

Sugar by Any Other Name

Many different terms refer to monosaccharides and disaccharides or to products containing these simple sugars. The box below gives names for sugars present either naturally in food products or added during their manufacture. Food labels (see Chapter 9) place all these simple carbohydrates into one category, "sugars."

TERMS THAT DENOTE SUGAR	
Sugar	Corn syrup
Sucrose	Natural sweeteners
Brown sugar	High-fructose corn syrup
Confectioner's sugar (powdered sugar)	Date sugar
Turbinado sugar	Molasses
Invert sugar	Maple sugar
Glucose	Dextrin
Sorbitol	Dextrose
Levulose	Fructose
Polydextrose	Maltose
Lactose	Caramel
Mannitol	Fruit sugar
Honey	

Table 1.1   GENERAL CLASSIFICATION OF CARBOHYDRATES

Monosaccharides[a,b]		Oligosaccharides		Polysaccharides		
Pentoses $C_5H_{10}O_5$	**Hexoses** $C_6H_{12}O_6$	**Disaccharides** $C_{12}H_{22}O_{11}$	**Pentosans** $(C_5H_6O_4)n^2$	**Hexosans** $(C_6H_{10}O_5)n^2$		**Mixed Polysaccharides**
Arabinose	Fructose	Lactose	Araban	Cellulose		Agar
Ribose	Galactose	Maltose	Xylan	Glycogen		Pectin
Xylose	Glucose	Sucrose		Inulin		Chitin
Deoxyribose	Mannose	Trehalose		Mannan		Hemicelluloses
				Starch (amylose and amylopectin)		Carrageenan
						Vegetable gums

[a] Also include trioses and tetroses
[b] **Derivatives of monosaccharides**
  Sugar alcohols: glycerol, inositol, mannitol, sorbitol
  Amino sugars: galactosamine (formed from galactose—present in cartilage, tendons, and aorta); glucosamine (formed from glucose—present in connective tissues)
  Sugar acids: ascorbic acid (vitamin C, not formed in the body); gluconic acid (formed from glucose); glucuronic acid (formed from glucose, aids in detoxification and excretion of other compounds, and is present in connective tissue)

Sugars Give Flavor and Sweetness to Foods

Receptors in the tip of the tongue recognize diverse sugars and even some noncarbohydrate substances. Sugars vary in sweetness on a per gram basis. For example, fructose is almost twice as sweet as sucrose under either acid or cold conditions; sucrose is 30% sweeter than glucose, and lactose is less than one-half as sweet as sucrose. Because of sweetness variations, some sugars improve the palatability of many foods and thus enhance the eating experience. TABLE 1.2 gives the sweetness of selected sugars and alternative sweeteners and their typical dietary sources.

Polysaccharides

The term *polysaccharide* refers to the linkage of from ten to thousands of monosaccharide residues by **glycosidic bonds**. Polysaccharides classify into plant and animal categories. Cells that store carbohydrate for energy link simple sugar into the more complex polysaccharide form. This reduces the osmotic effect within the cell that would result from storage of an equal energy value of a larger number of simple sugar molecules.

Plant Polysaccharides

Starch and **fiber** represent the two common forms of plant polysaccharides.

Starch. Starch serves as the storage form of carbohydrate in plants and represents the most familiar form of plant polysaccharide. Starch appears as large granules in the cell's cytoplasm and is plentiful in seeds, corn, and various grains that make bread, cereal, spaghetti, and pastries. Large amounts also exist in peas, beans, potatoes, and roots, where starch serves as an energy store for the plant's future use.

Plant starch remains an important source of carbohydrate in the American diet, accounting for approximately 50% of the total carbohydrate intake. Daily starch intake, however, has decreased about 30% since the turn of the 20th century, whereas simple sugar consumption correspondingly has increased from 30% to approximately 50% of total carbohydrate intake. The term **complex carbohydrate** commonly refers to dietary starch.

The Form Makes a Difference. Starch exists in two forms: **amylose**, a long straight chain of glucose units twisted into a helical coil, and **amylopectin**, a highly branched monosaccharide linkage (FIG. 1.2). The relative proportion of each starch form determines the specific characteristics of the starch in a particular plant species. For example, the predominance of one form or the other determines the "digestibility" of a food containing starch. The branching of the amylopectin polymer exposes greater surface area to digestive enzymes than starches whose glucose units link in a straight chain. *Starches with a relatively large amount of amylopectin digest and absorb rapidly, whereas starches with high amylose content have a slower rate of chemical breakdown* **(hydrolysis)**. Chapters 7 and 8 cover more about the importance of the different carbohydrate forms in feedings before, during, and after strenuous exercise.

Fiber: The Unheralded "Nutrient." Fiber, classified as a non-starch, structural polysaccharide, includes cellulose, the most abundant organic molecule on earth. Fibrous materials resist hydrolysis by human digestive enzymes, although a portion ferments by action of intestinal bacteria and ultimately participates in metabolic reactions following intestinal absorption. *Fibers exist exclusively in plants; they make up the structure of leaves, stems, roots, seeds, and fruit coverings.* Fibers differ widely in physical and chemical characteristics and in

Table 1.2. **RELATIVE SWEETNESS OF SIMPLE SUGARS AND ALTERNATIVE SWEETENERS**

Type of Sweetener	Relative Sweetness (sucrose = 1.0)	Dietary Sources
Sugars		
Lactose	0.2	Dairy products
Maltose	0.4	Sprouted seeds
Glucose	0.7	Corn syrup
Sucrose	1.0	Table sugar
Invert sugar	1.3	Candies, honey
Fructose	1.2–1.8	Fruit, honey, some soft drinks
Sugar alcohols		
Sorbitol	0.6	Dietetic candies
Mannitol	0.6	Dietetic candies
Xylitol	0.75	Sugarless gum
Alternative Sweeteners		
Cyclamate	30	Not currently in use in U.S.
Aspartame	200	Diet soft drinks, diet fruit
Acesulfame-K	200	drinks, sugarless gum,
Saccharin	500	powdered diet sweetener
Sucralose	600	diet drink mixes, puddings, gelatin desserts

physiologic action. They are located mostly within the cell wall as cellulose, gums (substances dissolved or dispersed in water that give a gelling or thickening effect), hemicellulose (sugar units containing 5 or 6 carbons; insoluble in water but soluble in alkali), pectin (forms gels with sugar and acid) imparts crispy texture to freshly picked apples), and the noncarbohydrate lignins that give rigidity to plant cell walls (increase in content with plant maturity).

Health Implications. Dietary fiber has received considerable attention by researchers and the lay press, largely from epidemiologic studies linking high fiber intake (particularly whole grains[71,82]) with lower occurrence of obesity, type 2 diabetes, hyperlipidemia, hypertension, intestinal disorders, and heart disease.[6,47,75,84,95] The Western diet, high in fiber-free animal foods and low in natural plant fiber lost through processing (refining), contributes to more intestinal disorders in industrialized countries than in countries that consume a more primitive-type diet high in unrefined, complex carbohydrates. For example, the typical American diet contains a daily fiber intake of about 12 to 15 g, far short of the most recent recommendations of the Food and Nutrition Board of the National Academy of Sciences of 38 g for men and 25 g for women up to age 50, and 30 g for men and 21 g for women over age 50.[34] In contrast, the fiber content of

diets from Africa and India range between 40 and 150 g per day.

Fiber retains considerable water and thus gives "bulk" to the food residues in the large intestine, often increasing stool weight and volume by 40 to 100%. Bulking action may aid gastrointestinal functions by *(a)* exerting a scraping action on the cells of the gut wall, *(b)* binding or diluting harmful chemicals or inhibiting their activity, and *(c)* shortening the transit time for food residues (and possibly carcinogenic materials) to pass through the digestive tract. The potential protective effect of fiber on rates and risks of colon cancer remains an inconclusive, hotly debated topic.[14,39] However, two recent studies—one by American scientists and one by a British team—showed that fibrous foods, particularly grains, cereals, and fruits, provide significant protection.[11,91]

Increased fiber intake modestly reduces serum cholesterol, particularly the **water-soluble** mucilaginous fibers such as pectin and guar gum in oats (rolled oats, oat bran, oat flour), legumes, barley, brown rice, peas, carrots, psyllium, and a variety of fruits (all rich in diverse phytochemicals and antioxidants).[5,32,54] In type 2 diabetic patients, a daily dietary fiber intake (50 g; 25 g soluble and 25 g insoluble) above that recommended by the American Diabetes Association (24 g; 8 g soluble and 16 g insoluble)

A. Straight chain linkage in amylose starch arranged in a helical coil

B. Branch point in amylopectin starch

Branch point

■ **Figure 1.2.** The two forms of plant starch. **A.** Straight-chain linkage with unbranched bonding of glucose residues (glycosidic linkages) in amylose starch. **B.** Branch point in the highly branched amylopectin starch molecule. Although the amylopectin structure appears linear, it exists as a helical coil.

improved glycemic control, decreased hyperinsulinemia, and lowered plasma lipid concentrations.[19] For men with elevated blood lipids, adding 100 g of oat bran to the daily diet reduced serum cholesterol by 13% and improved the ratio of the blood's lipoproteins.[56] A high-fiber oat cereal favorably altered low-density-lipoprotein cholesterol particle size and number in middle-aged and older men, without adversely changing blood triacylglycerol or high-density-lipoprotein cholesterol concentrations.[27] Increasing daily intake of quar gum fiber reduced cholesterol by lowering the harmful low-density-lipoprotein component of the cholesterol profile.[12,32] In contrast, the **water-insoluble** fibers of cellulose, hemicellulose, and lignin, and cellulose-rich wheat bran failed to lower cholesterol.[13] In January 1997, the Food and Drug Administration (FDA) ruled that manufacturers of oatmeal and other oat-based cereals could claim that their products may reduce heart disease risk, provided the health claim advises one to also eat "diet(s) low in saturated fat and cholesterol."

How dietary fibers favorably affect serum cholesterol remains unknown, although multiple mechanisms likely operate (FIG. 1.3A). Perhaps individuals who consume the most dietary fiber also lead more healthy overall lifestyles that include more physical activity, smoking fewer cigarettes, and eating a more nutritious diet.[122] Adding fiber to the diet also replaces cholesterol- and saturated fat-laden food choices. In addition, water-soluble fibers may hinder cholesterol absorption or reduce cholesterol metabolism in the gut. These actions would limit hepatic lipogenesis (less glucose as a substrate and less insulin as an activator) while facilitating

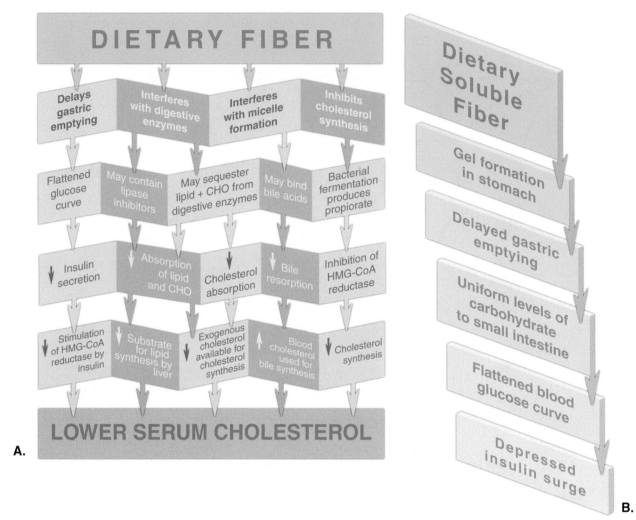

Figure 1.3. A. Possible mechanism by which dietary fiber lowers blood cholesterol. (CHO, carbohydrate; HMG-CoA reductase, hydroxy-3-methylglutaryl–coenzyme A reductase). **B.** Possible mechanisms by which dietary soluble fiber lowers blood glucose. (Modified from McIntosh M, Miller C. A diet containing food rich in soluble and insoluble fiber improves glycemic control and reduces hyperlipidemia among patients with type 2 diabetes. Nutr Revs 2001;59:52.)

excretion of existing cholesterol bound to fiber in the feces. Heart disease and obesity protection may relate to dietary fiber's regulatory role in favorably reducing insulin secretion by slowing nutrient absorption by the small intestine following a meal (Fig. 1.3B).[72] For nearly 69,000 middle-aged nurses, each 5-g daily increase in cereal fiber (1/2 cup of bran-flake cereal contains 4 g of fiber) translated into a 37% decrease in coronary risk.[121] Dietary fiber also contains micronutrients, particularly magnesium, which reduce risk for type 2 diabetes.[97] Magnesium possibly increases the body's sensitivity to insulin, thus reducing the required level of insulin production per unit rise in blood sugar.

The overall health benefits of a high-fiber diet may also come from other components in the food sources. Thus, one should obtain the diverse fibers from food in the daily diet, not from fiber supplements. Obtaining fiber in food rather than from over-the-counter supplements ensures intake of other important nutrients. *Present nutritional wisdom advocates a well-structured diet containing 20 to 40 g of fiber (depending on age) per day (ratio of 3:1 for water-insoluble to soluble fiber) by following the recommendations of the Food Guide Pyramid from the United States Department of Agriculture* (see Chapter 7). Chapter 9 points out that the nutrition labeling law requires packaged food to list fiber content. Examples of high-fiber common foods include 2/3 cup brown rice (3 g), 1/2 cup cooked carrots (3 g), 1 cup Wheaties (3 g), oatmeal (4 g), shredded wheat (5 g), 1 whole wheat pita (5 g), 1/2 grapefruit (6 g), Cracklin' Oat Bran (6 g), lentils (7 g), and Raisin Bran (7 g). One-half cup of the high-fiber bran cereals Fiber One and All-Bran With Extra Fiber contain 14 to 15 g.

TABLE 1.3 lists recommended daily fiber intake by age and gender and the total fiber content of common grains and grain products, nuts and seeds, vegetables and legumes,

Table 1.3 RECOMMENDED DAILY FIBER INTAKE BY AGE AND GENDER AND SOURCES OF TOTAL FIBER (G)^A IN COMMON GRAINS AND GRAIN PRODUCTS, NUTS AND SEEDS, VEGETABLES AND LEGUMES, FRUITS, AND BAKED GOODS

Food	Serving	Fiber/Serving	Food	Serving	Fiber/Serving
Grains			Broccoli, raw	1 cup	2.9
Oat bran	1 cup	16.4	Black beans	1 oz	2.5
Refined white flour, bleached	1 cup	3.4	Green beans, raw, cooked	1 cup	2.5
Spaghetti, whole wheat	1 cup	5.0	Artichoke, raw	1 oz	2.3
Penne, whole wheat	1 cup	10.0	Carrot	1	2.3
Bran muffin	1	4.0	Baked potato	1	2.3
Whole wheat flour	1 cup	15.1	Tomato, raw	1	1.8
Wheat germ, toasted	1 cup	15.6	Onions, sliced, raw	1 cup	1.8
Couscous	1 cup	8.7	Lentils, stir fry	1 oz	1.1
Popcorn, air-popped	1 cup	1.3	Chili w/beans	1 oz	0.9
Rice bran	1 oz	21.7	**Fruits**		
Millet	1 cup	17.0	Avocado	1	22.9
Corn grits	1 cup	4.5	Loganberries, fresh	1 cup	9.3
Barley, cooked, whole	1 cup	4.6	Pear, Bartlett	1	4.6
Bulgur wheat	1 cup	25.6	Figs	2	4.1
Rye flour-dark	1 cup	17.7	Blueberries	1 cup	3.9
Wild rice	1 cup	4.0	Strawberries, fresh	1 cup	3.9
All-Bran cereal	1/2 cup	8.5	Apple, raw	1	3.5
Barley	1 cup	31.8	Orange, navel	1	3.4
Oatmeal, cooked	1 cup	4.1	Grapefruit, sections, fresh	1	3.0
Grape Nuts	1 cup	10.0	Banana	1	2.3
Macaroni, cooked enriched	1 cup	2.2	Pineapple, chunks	1 cup	2.3
Rice, white	1 oz	1.5	Grapes, Thompson, seedless	1 cup	1.9
Almonds, dried	1 oz	3.5	Peach, fresh	1	1.5
Peanut butter	1 Tbsp	1.0	Plum, small	1	0.6
Macadamia nuts, dried	1 oz	1.5	**Baked goods**		
Low-fat granola	1 cup	4.5	Whole wheat toast	Slice	2.3
Cherrios	1 cup	5.0	Waffle, homemade	1	1.1
Nuts and seeds			Pumpkin pie	Slice	5.4
Pumpkin seeds, roasted, unsalted	1 oz	10.2	Oatmeal bread	Slice	1.0
Chestnuts, roasted	1 oz	3.7	French bread	Slice	0.7
Peanuts, dried, unsalted	1 oz	3.5	Danish pastry, plain	1	0.7
Sunflower seeds, dry	1 oz	2.0	Fig bar cookie	1	0.6
Walnuts, chopped, black	1 oz	1.6	Chocolate chip cookie, homemade	1	0.2
Vegetables and legumes			White bread	Slice	0.6
Pinto beans, dry, cooked	1 cup	19.5	Pumpernickel bread	Slice	1.7
Lima beans, fresh, cooked	1 cup	16.0	Rye bread	Slice	1.9
Black eyed peas, cooked from raw	1 cup	12.2	Seven-grain bread	Slice	1.7
Mixed vegetables (corn, carrots, beans)	1 cup	7.2			
Corn on cob	1	3.2			

Recommended Daily Fiber Intake (g)

Children 1–3 years	19
Children 4–8 years	25
Boys 9–13 years	31
Boys 14–18 years	38
Girls 9–18 years	26
Men 19–50 years	38
Men 51 years and older	30
Women 19–50 years	25
Women 51 years and older	21

Data from the United States Department of Agriculture.

^{a} The crude fiber content of foods reported in food composition tables (including the foods in the above table) refers to the organic portion of the dry, acid, and alkali-extracted residue from the ashing of the food after it is ground up, dried to a constant weight in a low-temperature oven, and had the fat removed with solvents. The fat-free food sample is then boiled in hot sulfuric acid, rinsed in hot water, and then boiled again in dilute sodium hydroxide to yield the food's crude fiber content.

fruits, and baked goods. Individuals who experience frequent constipation (infrequent or nonexistent bowel movements) should increase daily fiber intake. Seed coats of grains and legumes, and the skins and peels of fruits and vegetables, contain a relatively high fiber content. Adding the pulpy residues from the juices of fruits and vegetables significantly increases the fiber content of biscuits, breads, and other homemade dishes.

FIGURE 1.4 gives a sample daily 2200-kcal menu that includes 31 g of fiber (21 g of insoluble fiber). In this particular meal plan, lipid calories account for 30% (saturated fat, 10%), protein 16%, and carbohydrate 54% of total caloric

intake. Each 10-g increase in a subpar diet's fiber content reduces coronary risk by about 20%. Five daily servings of fruits and vegetables combined with 6 to 11 servings of grains (particularly whole grains) ensures dietary fiber intake at recommended levels. Whole grains provide a nutritional advantage over refined grains because they contain more fiber, vitamins, minerals, and diverse phytochemicals, all of which favorably affect health status.[76] Excessive fiber intake (particularly high-fiber foods with seed coats and thus large amounts of phytates) are ill advised for individuals with marginal levels of nutrition; these compounds generally blunt intestinal absorption of the major minerals calcium and phosphorus and some trace minerals including iron.

Animal Polysaccharides

Glycogen, the storage polysaccharide found in mammalian muscle and liver, consists of an irregularly shaped, branched polysaccharide polymer similar to amylopectin in plant starch. This macromolecule, synthesized from glucose during **glucogenesis**, ranges from a few hundred to thousands of glucose molecules linked together like a chain of sausages, with some branch points for additional glucose linkage. FIGURE 1.5 shows that glycogen synthesis occurs by adding individual glucose units to an already existing glycogen polymer.

FIGURE 1.6 illustrates that a well-nourished 80-kg person stores approximately 500 g of carbohydrate. Of this, the largest reserve (approximately 400 g) exists as muscle glycogen, 90 to 110 g as liver glycogen (highest concentration that represents between 3 to 7% of the liver's weight), and only about 2 to 3 g as blood glucose. Because each gram of either glycogen or glucose contains about 4 kcal of energy, the typical person stores between 1500 and 2000 kcal of carbohydrate energy—enough total energy to power a high-intensity 20-mile run.

Glycogen Dynamics. Several factors determine the rate and quantity of glycogen breakdown and subsequent synthesis. Muscle glycogen serves as the *major source* of carbohydrate energy for active muscles during exercise. In contrast to muscle glycogen, liver glycogen reconverts to glucose (controlled by a specific **phosphatase enzyme**) for transport in the blood to the working muscles. **Glycogenolysis** describes this reconversion process; it provides a rapid extramuscular glucose supply. Depleting liver and muscle glycogen through either *(a)* dietary restriction or *(b)* high-intensity exercise stimulates glucose synthesis from the structural components of other nutrients, principally amino acids, through gluconeogenic metabolic pathways.

Hormones control the level of circulating blood glucose and play an important role in regulating liver and muscle glycogen stores. Elevated blood glucose levels cause the beta cells of the pancreas to secrete additional **insulin**, forcing peripheral tissues to take up the excess glucose. This

Jazi's Diner

Breakfast

Whole grain cereal (0.75 cup)
Whole wheat toast (2 slices)
Margarine (2 tsp)
Jelly, strawberry (1 Tbsp)
Milk, 2% (1 cup)
Raisins (2 Tbsp)
Orange juice (0.5 cup)
Coffee (or tea)

Lunch

Bran muffin (1)
Milk, 2% (1 cup)
Hamburger on bun, lean beef patty (3 oz)
with 2 slices tomato and lettuce,
catsup (1 Tbsp) and mustard (1 Tbsp)
Whole wheat crackers (4 small)
Split-pea soup (1 cup)
Coffee (or tea)

Dinner

Green salad (3.5 oz)
Broccoli, steamed (0.5 cup)
Roll, whole wheat (1)
Margarine (2 tsp)
Brown rice (0.5 cup)
Chicken breast, skinless, broiled (3 oz)
Salad dressing, vinegar and oil (1 Tbsp)
Pear, medium (1)
Yogurt, vanilla, lowfat (0.5 cup)

Figure 1.4. Sample menu for breakfast, lunch, and dinner (2200 kcal) containing 31 g of dietary fiber. The diet's total cholesterol content is less than 200 mg, and total calcium equals 1242 mg.

Figure 1.5. Glycogen synthesis is a four-step process. *Stage 1.* ATP donates a phosphate to glucose to form glucose 6-phosphate. This reaction involves the enzyme hexokinase. *Stage 2.* Glucose 6-phosphate isomerizes to glucose 1-phosphate by the enzyme glucose 6-phosphate isomerase. *Stage 3.* The enzyme uridyl transferase reacts uridyl triphosphate (UTP) with glucose 1-phosphate to form UDP-glucose (a phosphate is released as UTP → UDP). *Stage 4.* UDP-glucose attaches to one end of an existing glycogen polymer chain. This forms a new bond (known as a glycoside bond) between the adjacent glucose units, with the concomitant release of UDP. For each glucose unit added, 2 moles of ATP converts to ADP and phosphate.

feedback mechanism inhibits further insulin secretion, which maintains blood glucose at an appropriate physiologic concentration. In contrast, when blood glucose falls below the normal range, the pancreas' alpha cells immediately secrete insulin's opposing hormone, **glucagon**, to normalize blood glucose levels. This "insulin antagonist" hormone stimulates liver glycogenolysis and gluconeogenesis to raise the blood glucose concentration.

The body stores comparatively little glycogen, so one's diet profoundly affects the amount available. For example, a 24-hour fast or a low-carbohydrate, normal-calorie (isocaloric) diet greatly reduces glycogen reserves. In contrast, maintaining a carbohydrate-rich isocaloric diet for several days enhances the body's carbohydrate stores to a level almost twice that of a normal, well-balanced diet. *The body's upper limit for glycogen storage averages about 15 g*

Figure 1.6. Distribution of carbohydrate energy in an average 80-kg man.

per kilogram (kg) of body mass, equivalent to 1050 g for an average-sized, 70-kg man and 840 g for a typical 56-kg woman.

RECOMMENDED DIETARY CARBOHYDRATE INTAKE

FIGURE 1.7 illustrates the carbohydrate content of selected foods. Rich carbohydrate sources include cereals, cookies, candies, breads, and cakes. Fruits and vegetables appear to be less valuable sources because carbohydrate percentage derives from the food's total weight, including water content. The dried portions of these foods, however, exist as almost pure carbohydrate. This makes them an ideal lightweight, "dehydrated" food source during hiking or long treks when one must transport the food supply during the activity. The bottom of the figure lists the amount of carbohydrate in various food categories.

On a worldwide basis, carbohydrates represent the most prevalent source of calories. In Africa, for example, nearly 80% of total caloric intake comes from carbohydrates, while in Caribbean countries the value reaches 65%. *Carbohydrates account for between 40 and 50% of the total calories in the typical American diet.* For a sedentary 70-kg person, this translates to a daily carbohydrate intake of about 300 g. For individuals who engage in regular physical activity, carbohydrates should supply about 60% (400 to 600 g) of total daily calories, predominantly as unrefined, fiber-rich fruits, grains, and vegetables. This quantity replenishes the carbohydrate used to power the increased level of physical activity. During intense training, carbohydrate intake should increase to 70% of total calories consumed when in energy balance.

Nutritious dietary carbohydrate sources consist of fruits, grains, and vegetables, but most persons do not consume these foods. In fact, the average American consumes about 50% of carbohydrates as simple sugars, predominantly as sucrose and high-fructose corn syrup (formed commercially by enzyme action on cornstarch that emphasizes fructose formation). Simple sugar intake represents more than the yearly equivalent of 70 pounds of table sugar (18 teaspoons of sucrose a day) and 50 pounds of corn syrup. About 100 years ago, the yearly intake of simple sugars averaged only 4 pounds per person!

Consuming excessive fermentable carbohydrate (principally sucrose) *causes* tooth decay, but dietary sugar's contributing role to diabetes, obesity, and coronary heart disease still remains an area of controversy (see next section). Substituting fructose for sucrose, a monosaccharide nearly 80% sweeter than table sugar, provides equal sweetness with fewer calories. In addition, fructose does not stimulate pancreatic insulin secretion. Consuming fructose thus helps to stabilize blood glucose and insulin levels. More is said in Chapter 8 concerning preexercise fructose feedings.

Some Confusion Concerning Dietary Carbohydrates

Concern exists about the negative effects of the high **glycemic load**—an index that incorporates both carbohydrate quantity and glycemic index (see Chapter 8)—of typical portions of food on risk for obesity, type 2 diabetes, abnormal blood lipids, and coronary heart disease, particularly among sedentary individuals.[25,69,70,81,90,104,111,113,120] Frequent and excessive consumption of more rapidly absorbed forms of carbohydrate (i.e., those with high glycemic index) may alter the metabolic profile and increase disease risk, particularly for individuals with excess body fat. For example, eating a high-carbohydrate, low-fat meal reduces fat breakdown and increases fat synthesis more in overweight men than in lean men.[73] Dietary patterns of women followed over 6 years showed that those who consumed a starchy diet (potatoes and low-fiber, processed white rice, pasta, and white bread, along with nondiet soft drinks) suffered

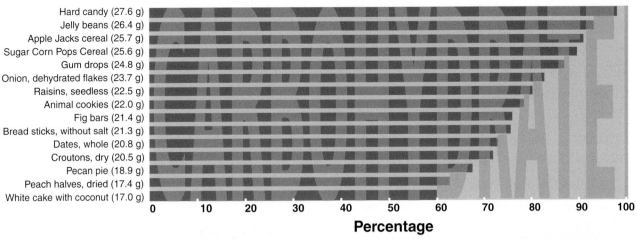

Hard candy (27.6 g)
Jelly beans (26.4 g)
Apple Jacks cereal (25.7 g)
Sugar Corn Pops Cereal (25.6 g)
Gum drops (24.8 g)
Onion, dehydrated flakes (23.7 g)
Raisins, seedless (22.5 g)
Animal cookies (22.0 g)
Fig bars (21.4 g)
Bread sticks, without salt (21.3 g)
Dates, whole (20.8 g)
Croutons, dry (20.5 g)
Pecan pie (18.9 g)
Peach halves, dried (17.4 g)
White cake with coconut (17.0 g)

Percentage

Good food sources of carbohydrates

Food	Amount	CHO (g)	Food	Amount	CHO (g)
Fruits			**Breakfast cereals**		
Prunes	10	53	Oatmeal, instant	1 packet	25
Banana	1 medium	26	Corn Flakes	0.5 cup	24
Pear	1 medium	25	Cream of Wheat	1 serving	22
Apple	1 medium	20	Raisin Bran	0.5 cup	21
Orange	1 medium	18			
Grapes	1 cup	16			
Fruit Roll-ups	1 roll	12			
			Beverages		
			Grape juice	8 oz	42
			Cola	12 oz	38
Vegetables			Orange juice	8 oz	27
			Milk, chocolate	8 oz	26
Potato	1 large	42	Milk, skim	8 oz	14
Lima beans	1 cup	39			
Winter squash	0.5 cup	15			
Peas	0.5 cup	12	**Grains, pastas, starches**		
Carrot	1 medium	10			50
			Rice, cooked	1 cup	45
			Spaghetti	2 oz dry	43
			Stuffing	1 cup	41
			Lentils	1 cup	40
Bread-type foods			**Sweets, snacks, desserts**		
Submarine roll	8-inch long	60			
Bran muffin	1 large	47	Fruit yogurt	1 cup	50
Pancakes	3, (4 in. dia)	45	Soft ice cream	1 medium	35
Bagel	1 whole	31	Fig newtons	3	33
Matzo	1 sheet	28	Honey	2 Tbsp	30
Whole wheat bread	1 slice	17	Maple syrup	2 Tbsp	25

■ **Figure 1.7.** Percentage of carbohydrate in common foods arranged by food type. The insert graph displays the number of grams of carbohydrate per ounce (28.3 g) of the food, expressed as a percentage.

2.5 times the rate of diabetes of women who consumed less of those foods and more fiber-containing whole-grain cereals, fruits, and vegetables.[97] Participants who became diabetic developed type 2 diabetes, the most common form of the disease that afflicts more than 16 million people in the United States. High blood glucose levels in type 2 diabetes can result from *(a)* decreased effect of insulin on peripheral tissue **(insulin resistance)**, *(b)* inadequate insulin production by the pancreas to control blood sugar **(relative insulin deficiency)**, or *(c)* the combined effect of both factors.

Diet-induced insulin resistance/hyperinsulinemia often precedes manifestations of the **metabolic syndrome**—defined as having three or more of the criteria indicated in TABLE 1.4.[10,85,101] In essence, the syndrome reflects a concurrence of four factors:

1. Disturbed glucose and insulin metabolism
2. Overweight and abdominal fat distribution
3. Mild dyslipidemia
4. Hypertension

These individuals exhibit a high risk of cardiovascular disease, diabetes, and all- cause mortality.[61] Estimates place the age-adjusted prevalence of the metabolic syndrome in the United States at 25% or about 47 million men and women.[36] The percentage increases from 6.7% among individuals aged 20 through 29 years to 43.5% for those aged 60 through 69 years. A particularly high prevalence occurs among Mexican Americans and African Americans.

Table 1.4.	**CLINICAL IDENTIFICATION OF THE METABOLIC SYNDROME**

Risk Factor	Defining Level
• Abdominal obesity[a] (waist circumference)[b]	
Men	>102 cm (>40 in)
Women	>88 cm (>35 in)
• Triacylglycerols	≥150 mg/dL
• High-density lipoprotein cholesterol	
Men	<40 mg/dL
Women	<50 mg/dL
• Blood pressure	≥130/≥85 mm Hg
• Fasting glucose	≥110 mg/dL

[a] Overweight and obesity are associated with insulin resistance and the metabolic syndrome. However, the presence of abdominal obesity is more highly correlated with the metabolic risk factors than is an elevated body mass index (BMI). Therefore, the simple measure of waist circumference is recommended to identify the body weight component of the metabolic syndrome.
[b] Some male patients can develop multiple metabolic risk factors when the waist circumference is only marginally increased, e.g., 94–102 cm (37–40 in). Such patients may have strong genetic contribution to insulin resistance and they should benefit from changes in life habits, similarly to men with categorical increases in waist circumference.

Not All Carbohydrates Are Physiologically Equal

Digestion rates of different carbohydrate sources possibly explain the carbohydrate intake–diabetes link. Low-fiber processed starches (and simple sugars) digest quickly and enter the blood at a relatively rapid rate (high glycemic index), whereas slow-release forms of high-fiber, unrefined complex carbohydrates minimize surges in blood glucose. The rapid rise in blood glucose with refined, processed starch intake increases insulin demand, stimulates overproduction of insulin by the pancreas to accentuate hyperinsulinemia, increases plasma triacylglycerol concentrations, and stimulates fat synthesis. Consuming such foods for prolonged periods may eventually reduce the body's sensitivity to insulin (more insulin resistant), thus requiring progressively greater insulin output to control blood sugar levels. *Type 2 diabetes results when the pancreas cannot produce sufficient insulin to regulate blood glucose.* In contrast, diets with fiber-rich, low-glycemic carbohydrates tend to lower blood glucose and insulin response after eating, improve the blood lipid profile, and increase insulin sensitivity.[40,79,83,92,114]

Regularly consuming high glycemic foods can increase cardiovascular risk because elevated blood glucose precipitates oxidative damage and inflammation that elevates blood pressure, stimulates clot formation, and reduces blood flow. For type 1 diabetic patients who require exogenous insulin, consumption of low glycemic index foods causes more favorable physiologic adaptations for glycemic control, high-density-lipoprotein cholesterol concentrations, serum leptin levels, resting energy expenditure, voluntary food intake, and nitrogen balance.[2,15]

A Role in Obesity?

About 25% of the population produce excessive insulin from consuming rapidly absorbed carbohydrates. These insulin-resistant individuals increase their risk for obesity if they consistently consume such a diet. Weight gain occurs because abnormal quantities of insulin *(a)* promote glucose entry into cells and *(b)* facilitate the liver's conversion of glucose to triacylglycerol, which then becomes stored as body fat in adipose tissue.[38]

The insulin surge in response to a sharp rise in blood glucose following ingestion of high-glycemic carbohydrates often abnormally decreases blood glucose. This **rebound hypoglycemia** sets off hunger signals that cause the person to overeat. This repetitive scenario of high blood sugar followed by low blood sugar exerts the most profound effect on the sedentary obese individual who shows the greatest insulin resistance and consequently the greatest insulin surge to a blood glucose challenge. For physically active people, regular low-to-moderate physical activity produces the following three beneficial effects:

1. Exerts a potent influence for weight control
2. Stimulates plasma-derived fatty acid oxidation, which decreases fatty acid availability to the liver

and blunts any increase in plasma very low density lipoprotein cholesterol–triacylglycerol concentrations

3. Improves insulin sensitivity, thus reducing the insulin requirement for a given glucose uptake

To reduce the risks for type 2 diabetes and obesity, consuming more slowly absorbed, unrefined complex carbohydrate foods provides a form of "slow-release" carbohydrate without producing rapid fluctuations in blood sugar. If rice, pasta, and bread remain the carbohydrate sources of choice, they should be consumed in unrefined form as brown rice and whole-grain pastas and breads. The same dietary modification would benefit individuals involved in heavy physical training and endurance competition. Their daily dietary carbohydrate intake should approach 800 g (8 to 10 g per kg of body mass; see Chapter 7).

ROLE OF CARBOHYDRATE IN THE BODY

Carbohydrates serve four important functions related to energy metabolism and exercise performance.

Energy Source

Carbohydrates primarily serve as an energy fuel, particularly during high-intensity exercise. Energy derived from blood-borne glucose and liver and muscle glycogen breakdown ultimately powers the contractile elements of muscle and other forms of more "silent" biologic work.

Carbohydrates exhibit the most dramatic use and depletion in intense exercise and heavy training, compared with fat and protein. For physically active people, adequate daily carbohydrate intake maintains the body's relatively limited glycogen stores. In contrast, exceeding the cells' capacity to store glycogen triggers conversion and storage of excess dietary carbohydrate calories as fat.

Affects Metabolic Mixture and Spares Protein

Carbohydrate availability affects the metabolic mixture catabolized for energy. TABLE 1.5 shows the effect of reduced energy intake during a 40-hour fast and 7 days of total food deprivation on plasma glucose and fat breakdown components. After almost 2 days of fasting, blood glucose decreases 35% but does not decrease to a lower level during further prolonged food abstinence. Concurrently, circulating fatty acid and ketone levels (acetoacetate and β-hydroxybutyrate byproducts of incomplete fat breakdown) increase rapidly, with plasma ketones rising dramatically after 7 days of starvation.

Adequate carbohydrate intake preserves tissue proteins. Normally, protein serves a vital role in tissue maintenance,

Table 1.5 CHANGES IN THE PLASMA CONCENTRATIONS OF GLUCOSE, FATTY ACIDS, AND KETONES FOLLOWING 40 HOURS OF FASTING AND SUBSEQUENT 7 DAYS OF STARVATION

Nutrient $(mmol \cdot L^{-1})$	Normal	40 Hours Fasting	7 Days Starvation
Glucose	5.5	3.6	3.5
Fatty acids	0.3	1.15	1.19
Ketones	0.01	2.9	4.5

Adapted from Bender DA. Introduction to nutrition and metabolism. London: UCL Press, 1993.

repair, and growth and, to a lesser degree, as a nutrient energy source. Glycogen reserves readily deplete during (a) starvation, (b) reduced energy intake and/or low-carbohydrate diets, and (c) strenuous exercise. Reduced glycogen reserves and plasma glucose levels trigger glucose synthesis from both protein (amino acids) and the glycerol portion of the fat (triacylglycerol) molecule. This gluconeogenic conversion provides a metabolic option to augment carbohydrate availability (and to maintain plasma glucose levels) with depleted glycogen stores. The price paid, however, strains the body's protein components, particularly muscle protein. In the extreme, gluconeogenesis reduces lean tissue mass and produces an accompanying solute load on the kidneys, which must excrete the nitrogen-containing byproducts of protein breakdown.

Metabolic Primer/Prevents Ketosis

Components of carbohydrate catabolism serve as "primer" substrate for fat catabolism. Insufficient carbohydrate metabolism—either through limitations in glucose transport into the cell (as in diabetes from too little insulin production or insulin insensitivity) or glycogen depletion through inadequate diet, particularly very low carbohydrate diets, or prolonged exercise—causes more fat mobilization than oxidation. This produces incomplete fat breakdown and the accumulation of acetone-like byproducts (chiefly acetoacetate and hydroxybutyrate) called **ketone bodies**. Excessive ketone formation increases body fluid acidity, a harmful condition called acidosis or with regard to fat breakdown, **ketosis**. Chapter 5 continues the discussion of carbohydrate as a primer for fat catabolism.

Fuel for the Central Nervous System

The central nervous system requires carbohydrate to function properly. Under normal conditions and with several days of total food deprivation, the brain relies on blood glucose almost exclusively as its fuel. In poorly regulated diabetes, during starvation, or with a low carbohydrate intake,

Diabetes 2003 Facts

Each year, at least one million people in the United States will be added to the number of people diagnosed with diabetes, predominantly of the type 2 variety. This segment on Personal Health and Exercise Nutrition is of a general nature in that it applies to the population rather than a single individual. It reflects the latest statistics about how diabetes—the body's inability to produce sufficient insulin (insulin insufficiency) or use it effectively (insulin resistance) to metabolize sugar—affects this country's 18.2 million adults and children. A chronic elevation in blood glucose level can lead to the following medical complications:

1. *Heart disease.* This is the leading cause of diabetes-related deaths. Adults with diabetes have heart disease death rates two to four times higher than adults without diabetes.
2. *Stroke.* Diabetics exhibit a two to four times higher stroke risk than nondiabetics.
3. *High blood pressure.* About 73% of adults with diabetes have elevated blood pressure of 140/90 mm Hg or higher or use prescription medications to control their hypertension.
4. *Blindness.* Diabetes is the leading cause of new cases of blindness among adults 20–74 years old. Diabetic retinopathy causes from 12,000 to 24,000 new cases of blindness yearly.
5. *Kidney disease.* Diabetes is the leading cause of treated, end-stage renal disease, accounting for 43% of new cases. In 2000, 41,046 people with diabetes began treatment for end-stage renal disease, and 129,183 diabetics underwent dialysis or kidney transplantation.
6. *Nervous system disease.* About 60 to 70% of persons with diabetes have mild-to-severe nervous system damage. This impairs sensation or pain in the feet or hands, slows digestion of food, and produces carpal tunnel syndrome and other nerve pathologies. Severe forms of diabetic nerve disease play a major role in lower-extremity amputations.
7. *Amputations.* More than 60% of nontraumatic lower-limb amputations in the United States occur among diabetics. From 1997 to 1999, about 82,000 of these amputations were performed.
8. *Dental disease.* Periodontal or gum diseases are more common among diabetics than nondiabetics. Young adults with diabetes experience twice the risk for these disorders. Almost one-third of diabetics have severe periodontal diseases with loss of attachment of the gums to the teeth measuring 5 mm or more.
9. *Complications of pregnancy.* Poorly controlled diabetes before conception and during the first trimester causes major birth defects in 5 to 10% of pregnancies and spontaneous abortions in 15 to 20% of pregnancies. Poorly controlled diabetes

during the second and third trimesters often results in excessively large babies, posing a risk to the mother and child.
10. *Other complications.* Uncontrolled diabetes often leads to biochemical imbalances and acute life-threatening diabetic ketoacidosis and hyperosmolar (nonketotic) coma. Diabetics are more susceptible to many other illnesses (e.g., pneumonia and influenza); once acquired, they often have a worse prognosis than persons without diabetes.

STATISTICS ABOUT DIABETES

- Diabetes is the sixth leading cause of death in the United States.
- An estimated 13 million Americans have been diagnosed with diabetes, and about 5.2 million additional Americans have the disease but remain undiagnosed.
- Diabetes is the leading cause of blindness among adults between 20 and 74 years of age.
- 14.9% of American Indians and Alaska Natives who are at least 20 years old and receive care from the Indian Health Service have diabetes. On average, American Indians and Alaska Natives are 2.3 times as likely to have diabetes than non-Hispanic whites of similar age.
- 1.4% of non-Hispanic blacks aged 20 years or older have diabetes. On average, non- Hispanic blacks are 1.6 times as likely to have diabetes than non-Hispanic whites of a similar age.
- 8.4% of non-Hispanic whites aged 20 years or older have diabetes.
- 8.2% of Hispanics aged 20 years or older have diabetes. On average, Hispanic Americans are 1.5 times more likely to have diabetes than non-Hispanic whites of similar age.
- Native Hawaiians and Japanese and Filipino residents of Hawaii aged 20 years or older are twice as likely to have diabetes as white residents of Hawaii.
- Direct medical and indirect expenditures attributable to diabetes in 2002 were estimated at $132 billion. Direct medical expenditures alone totaled $91.8 billion and comprised $23.2 billion for diabetes care, $24.6 billion for chronic complications attributable to diabetes, and $44.1 billion for excess prevalence of general medical conditions.
- Individuals can reduce the risk of diabetes by 50 to 70% by reducing their body weight by 5 to 7% and exercising at a moderate intensity for about 150 minutes weekly.
- Per capita yearly medical expenditures totaled $13,243 for persons with diabetes and $2,560 for persons without the disease. When adjusting for differences in age, sex, and race/ethnicity between the population with and without diabetes, diabetics' medical expenditures were 2.4 times higher than expenditures for nondiabetics.

the brain adapts after about 8 days by metabolizing relatively large amounts of fat (in the form of ketones) for alternative fuel. Adaptations also occur in skeletal muscle to chronic low-carbohydrate, high-fat diets that increase fat use during exercise, which spares muscle glycogen.[63,80]

Liver glycogenolysis primarily maintains normal blood glucose levels at rest and during exercise, usually at $100 \text{ mg} \cdot \text{dL}^{-1}$ (5.5 mM). In prolonged, intense exercise, blood glucose eventually falls below normal levels because liver glycogen depletes and active muscles continue to use the available blood glucose. Symptoms of reduced blood glucose or **hypoglycemia** include weakness, hunger, and dizziness. Reduced blood glucose ultimately impairs exercise performance and partially explains "central" fatigue associated with prolonged exercise. Sustained and profound hypoglycemia (e.g., induced by an overdose of exogenous insulin) can trigger loss of consciousness and produce irreversible brain damage. Blood sugar usually remains regulated within narrow limits for two main reasons: the important role of glucose (a) in nerve tissue metabolism and (b) as the energy fuel for red blood cells.

Summary

1. Atoms provide the basic building blocks of all matter and play the major role in the composition of food nutrients and biologically active substances.

2. Carbon, hydrogen, oxygen, and nitrogen serve as the primary structural units for most of the body's biologically active substances. Specific combinations of carbon with oxygen and hydrogen form carbohydrates and lipids. Proteins consist of combinations of carbon, oxygen, and hydrogen, with nitrogen and minerals.

3. Simple sugars consist of chains of three to seven carbon atoms with hydrogen and oxygen in the ratio of 2 to 1. Glucose, the most common simple sugar, contains a six-carbon chain: $C_6H_{12}O_6$.

4. There are three kinds of carbohydrates: monosaccharides (sugars like glucose and fructose), disaccharides (combinations of two monosaccharides as in sucrose, lactose, and maltose), and oligosaccharides (3 to 9 glucose residues). Polysaccharides that contain 10 or more simple sugars form starch and fiber in plants and glycogen, the large glucose polymer in animals.

5. Glycogenolysis reconverts glycogen to glucose, whereas gluconeogenesis synthesizes glucose predominantly from the carbon skeletons of amino acids.

6. The two basic starch configurations are (a) amylose, consisting of a long straight chain of glucose units and (b) amylopectin, constructed from a highly branched monosaccharide linkage. The "digestibility" of a starch-containing food depends upon the predominance of one starch form or the other.

7. Fiber, a nonstarch structural plant polysaccharide, resists human digestive enzymes. Although technically not a nutrient, water-soluble and water-insoluble dietary fibers confer health benefits for gastrointestinal functioning and reduce cardiovascular disease risks.

8. Heart disease and obesity protection may relate to dietary fiber's regulatory role in favorably reducing insulin secretion by slowing nutrient absorption in the small intestine following a meal.

9. Americans typically consume 40 to 50% of total calories as carbohydrates. Greater sugar intake in the form of sweets (simple sugars) occurs commonly in the population with possibly harmful effects for glucose-insulin regulation, cardiovascular disease, and obesity.

10. Physically active men and women should consume about 60% of daily calories as carbohydrates (400 to 600 g), predominantly in unrefined complex form. During intense training and prolonged physical activities, carbohydrate intake should increase to 70% of total calories or 8 to 10 g per kg of body weight.

11. Frequent and excessive consumption of carbohydrates with high glycemic index may alter the metabolic profile and increase risk for the metabolic syndrome of obesity, insulin resistance, glucose intolerance, dyslipidemia, and hypertension.

12. Carbohydrates stored in limited quantity in liver and muscles (a) serve as a major source of energy, (b) spare protein breakdown for energy, (c) function as a metabolic primer for fat metabolism, and (d) provide fuel for the central nervous system.

13. A carbohydrate-deficient diet rapidly depletes muscle and liver glycogen This profoundly affects high-intensity anaerobic and long-duration aerobic exercise capacity.

Lipids

THE NATURE OF LIPIDS

Lipid (from the Greek *lipos,* meaning fat), the general term for a heterogeneous group of compounds, includes oils, fats, and waxes and related compounds. Oils become liquid at room temperature, while fats remain solid. A lipid molecule contains the same structural elements as carbohydrate except that it differs markedly in its linkage of atoms. Specifically, the lipid's ratio of hydrogen to oxygen considerably exceeds that of carbohydrate. For example, the formula $C_{57}H_{110}O_6$ describes the common lipid stearin, with an H-to-0 ratio of 18.3:1; for carbohydrate, the ratio is 2:1. Approximately 98% of dietary lipids exist as triacylglycerols (see below), while about 90% of the body's total fat resides in the adipose tissue depots of the subcutaneous tissues.

KINDS AND SOURCES OF LIPIDS

Plants and animals contain lipids in long hydrocarbon chains. Lipids are generally greasy to the touch and remain insoluble in water but soluble in organic solvents such as ether, chloroform, and benzene. According to common classification, lipids belong to one of three main groups: **simple lipids**, **compound lipids**, and **derived lipids**. TABLE 1.6 lists the general classification for lipids, with specific examples of each form.

Simple Lipids

The simple lipids, or "neutral fats," consist primarily of **triacylglycerols**, the most plentiful fats in the body. They constitute the major storage form of fat in adipose (fat) cells. This molecule consists of two different clusters of atoms. One cluster, **glycerol**, consists of a 3-carbon alcohol molecule that by itself does not qualify as a lipid because of its high solubility in water. Three clusters of carbon-chained atoms, usually in even number, termed **fatty acids**, attach to the glycerol molecule. Fatty acids consist of straight hydrocarbon chains with as few as 4 carbon atoms or more than 20 in their chain, although chain lengths of 16 and 18 carbons prevail.

Three molecules of water form when glycerol and fatty acids join in the synthesis (**condensation**) of the triacylglycerol molecule. Conversely, during hydrolysis, when the fat molecule cleaves into its constituents by the action of **lipase enzymes**, three molecules of water attach at the point where the molecule splits. FIGURE 1.8 illustrates the basic structure of **saturated fatty acid** and **unsaturated fatty acid** molecules. All lipid-containing foods consist of a mixture of different proportions of saturated and unsaturated fatty acids. Fatty acids get their name because the organic acid (COOH) molecule forms part of their chemical structure.

Figure 1.8. The presence or absence of double bonds between the carbon atoms constitutes the major structural difference between saturated and unsaturated fatty acids. R represents the glycerol portion of the triacylglycerol molecule.

Type of Lipid	Example
Table 1.6 GENERAL CLASSIFICATION OF LIPIDS	
I. Simple lipids	
Neutral fats	Triglycerides (triacylglycerols)
Waxes	Beeswax
II. Compound lipids	
Phospholipids	Lecithins, cephalins, lipositols
Glycolipids	Cerebrosides, gangliosides
Lipoproteins	Chylomicrons, very low density lipoproteins (VLDLs), low density lipoproteins (LDLs), high density lipoproteins (HDLs)
III. Derived lipids	
Fatty acids	Palmitic acid, oleic acid, stearic acid, linoleic acid
Steroids	Cholesterol, ergosterol, cortisol, bile acids, vitamin D, estrogens, progesterone, androgens
Hydrocarbons	Terpenes

Saturated Fatty Acids

A saturated fatty acid contains only single covalent bonds between carbon atoms; all of the remaining bonds attach to hydrogen. The fatty acid molecule is referred to as saturated because it holds as many hydrogen atoms as chemically possible.

Saturated fatty acids occur primarily in animal products such as beef (52% saturated fatty acids), lamb, pork, chicken, and egg yolk, and in dairy fats of cream, milk, butter (62% saturated fatty acids), and cheese. Saturated fatty acids from the plant kingdom include coconut and palm oil (liquid at room temperature because they have short fatty acid chains), vegetable shortening, and hydrogenated margarine; commercially prepared cakes, pies, and cookies also contain plentiful amounts of these fatty acids.

Unsaturated Fatty Acids

Unsaturated fatty acids contain one or more double bonds along the main carbon chain. Each double bond reduces the number of potential hydrogen-binding sites; therefore, the molecule remains unsaturated relative to hydrogen. A **monounsaturated fatty acid** contains one double bond along the main carbon chain. Examples include canola oil, olive oil (77% monounsaturated fatty acids), peanut oil, and the oil in almonds, pecans, and avocados. A **polyunsaturated fatty acid** contains two or more double bonds along the main carbon chain; safflower, sunflower, soybean, and corn oil serve as examples.

Fatty acids from plant sources are generally unsaturated and tend to liquefy at room temperature. Lipids with longer (more carbons in the chain) and more saturated fatty acids remain solid at room temperature, while those with shorter and more unsaturated fatty acids stay soft. Oils exist as liquid and contain unsaturated fatty acids. **Hydrogenation** changes oils to semisolid compounds. This chemical process bubbles liquid hydrogen into vegetable oil, which reduces double bonds in the unsaturated fatty acid to single bonds to capture more hydrogen atoms along the carbon chain. This creates firmer fat because adding hydrogen to the carbons increases the lipid's melting temperature. Hydrogenated oil thus behaves as a saturated fat. The most common hydrogenated fats include lard substitutes and margarine.

Butter versus Margarine: A Health Risk in Trans Fatty Acids

One cannot distinguish butter and margarine by caloric content, but rather by their fatty acid composition. Butter contains about 62% saturated fatty acids (which dramatically raise low-density-lipoprotein cholesterol) compared with 20% in margarine. During manufacturing, margarine and other vegetable shortenings like unsaturated corn, soybean, or sunflower oil become partially hydrogenated. This process rearranges the chemical structure of the original polyunsaturated oil. The lipid remains hardened (saturated), but not as hard as butter. A **trans unsaturated fatty acid** forms in margarine when one of the hydrogen atoms along the restructured carbon chain moves from its naturally occurring *cis* position to the opposite side of the double bond that separates two carbon atoms (*trans* position). Although *trans* fatty acids are close in structure to most unsaturated fatty acids, the opposing hydrogens on its carbon chain make the physical properties similar to saturated fatty acids. Seventeen to 25% of margarine's fatty acids exist as *trans* unsaturated fatty acids, compared with only 7% in butterfat. A serving of French fries can contain up to 3.6 g of *trans* fat, and doughnuts and pound cake can have 4.3 g. (Liquid vegetable oils normally have no *trans* fatty acids, but they are sometimes added to extend the oil's shelf life.) Because margarine consists of vegetable oil, it contains no cholesterol; butter, on the other hand, originates from a dairy source and contains between 11 and 15 mg of cholesterol per teaspoon. *Trans* fatty acids represent about 5 to 10% of the fat in the typical American diet. Food packages need not label *trans* fatty acids, although labels may contain "hydrogenated fat" or "partially hydrogenated fat," which indicates the presence of these fats.

Current controversy over margarine versus butter centers on the detrimental health effects of *trans* fatty acids through their adverse effects on serum lipids and lipoproteins.[8,9,49,77] A diet high in margarine and commercial baked goods and deep-fried foods prepared with hydrogenated (hardened) vegetable oils increases low-density-lipoprotein cholesterol concentration by about the same amount as a diet high in saturated fatty acids. Unlike saturated fats, hydrogenated oils decrease the beneficial high-density-lipoprotein cholesterol concentration. *Trans* fatty acids also elevate plasma levels of triacylglycerols and may impair arterial wall flexibility.

Dietary *trans* fatty acids account for 30,000 deaths annually from heart disease.[117] In addition, a prospective study of more than 84,204 healthy middle-aged women demonstrated that diets high in *trans* fatty acids promote resistance to insulin, increasing the risk for type 2 diabetes.[98] Women with high tissue levels of *trans* fatty acids are also 40% more likely than those with the lowest levels to develop breast cancer.

In September 2002, to great fanfare, McDonald's corporation and their chain of thousands of eateries worldwide announced plans to reformulate a healthier cooking oil for its French fries, cutting by half the *trans* fatty acid content and reducing the saturated fat by 16%, but leaving overall fat and calorie levels unchanged. The company termed its decision (which it has yet to implement) "a major step" toward its goal of eliminating *trans* fatty acid from its cooking oil. After more than a decade of debate, the Food and Drug Administration (FDA) announced on July 9, 2003 that it would require food processors to include the amount of *trans* fatty acids in a serving, listed on a separate line under saturated fat on the nutrition panel label. This requirement does not go into effect until 2006. The FDA estimates that this change in regulations "will save between $900 million and $1.8 billion a year in medical costs, lost productivity, and pain and suffering."

Lipids in the Diet

FIGURE 1.9 shows the approximate percentage contribution of some common food groups to the total lipid content of the typical American diet. Vegetables generally contribute about 34% to the daily lipid intake; the remaining 66% comes from animal sources.

The average person in the United States consumes about 15% of total calories (over 50 lb) as saturated fats. The United States diet contrasts to that of the Tarahumara Indians of Mexico whose diet high in complex, unrefined carbohydrate contains only 2% of total calories as saturated fat.[23] The relationship between saturated fatty acid intake and coronary heart disease risk has prompted nutritionists and medical personnel to recommend replacing at least a portion of the saturated fatty acids and nearly all *trans* fatty acids in the diet with nonhydrogenated monounsaturated and polyunsaturated fatty acids.[16,88] Consuming both forms of unsaturated fatty acids lowers coronary risk even below normal levels. From a public health perspective, individuals are advised to consume no more than 10% of total energy intake as saturated fatty acids (about 250 kcal or 25 to 30 g per day for the average young adult male) and all lipid intake to less than 30% of total calories.

Fish Oils (and Fish) Are Healthful. Studies of the health profiles of Greenland Eskimos who consume large quantities of lipid from fish, seal, and whale, yet have a low incidence of coronary heart disease, indicated the potential for two essential long-chain polyunsaturated fatty acids to confer diverse health benefits. These oils, eicosapentaenoic acid (EPA) and docosahexaenoic acid (DHA), belong to an **omega-3** family of fatty acids (also termed n-3, characterized by the presence of a double bond three carbons from the n end of the molecule) found primarily in the oils of shellfish and cold-water herring, salmon, sardines, bluefish, and mackerel and sea mammals. Plant sources for alpha linolenic acid, another omega-3 oil and precursor of EPA and DHA, include dark green leafy vegetables and flax, hemp, canola, soy, and walnut oils.

Regular fish intake (two meals a week) and fish oil may benefit one's lipid profile (particularly plasma triacylglycerol),[60,99,105] overall heart disease risk (particularly risk of ventricular fibrillation and sudden death),[3,28,50,52,65] inflammatory disease risk,[22] and (for smokers) risk of contracting chronic obstructive pulmonary disease.[100] A long-term study of employees of the Western Electric Company in Chicago noted a reduction of 42% in heart attacks among men who ate 7 ounces or more of fish a week compared with men who rarely ate fish.[26] This benefit from regular yet moderate fish intake remained even when considering numerous other factors known to affect heart disease risk. Omega-3 fish oils, particularly DHA, may also prove beneficial in treating diverse psychological disorders and Alzheimer's disease. The relation between intake of fish and marine fatty acids and risk of hormone-related cancers (e.g., breast and prostate) remains unclear.[110]

Several mechanisms explain how eating fish with—its additional cardioprotective nutrients of selenium, various natural antioxidants, and protein not present in fish oil—protects against death from heart disease. Fish oil may act as an antithrombogenic agent to prevent blood clot formation on arterial walls. It also may inhibit the growth of atherosclerotic plaques, reduce pulse pressure and total vascular resistance (increase arterial compliance), and stimulate endothelial-derived nitric oxide to facilitate myocardial perfusion.[22,86] The oil's lowering effect on triacylglycerol also confers protection because plasma triacylglycerol level strongly predicts coronary heart disease risk.[31] On the negative side, elevation in atherogenic low-density-lipoprotein cholesterol may accompany the triacylglycerol-lowering effect of fish oil supplements.[1,42] For men with moderate hypercholesterolemia, daily supplements of 12 g of fish oil in capsule form for 12 weeks decreased triacylglycerols by 37.3%, reduced total cholesterol by 11.5%, but increased harmful low-density-lipoprotein cholesterol by 8.5%. Combining fish oil supple-

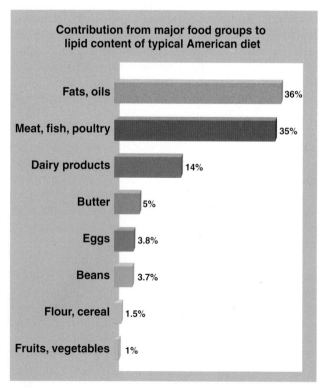

Contribution from major food groups to lipid content of typical American diet

Food group	Percentage
Fats, oils	36%
Meat, fish, poultry	35%
Dairy products	14%
Butter	5%
Eggs	3.8%
Beans	3.7%
Flour, cereal	1.5%
Fruits, vegetables	1%

■ **Figure 1.9.** Lipid content of the typical American diet as contributed from the major food sources.

ments with 900 mg of garlic eliminated fish oil's negative effect on low-density-lipoprotein cholesterol.[1] The possible health implications of these findings await further research.

Perhaps the most powerful cardioprotective benefit of fish oils relates to their antiarrhythmic effect on myocardial tissue.[4,21] This protection against ventricular arrhythmias occurs from the unique effects of dietary n-3 fatty acids on the respective n-3 fatty acid content of the myocardial cell membranes. In the event of severe physiologic stress (e.g., ischemic attack from reduced myocardial blood flow), the n-3 fatty acids in the cell membrane are released and locally protect the myocardium from the development and propagation of a rapid heart rate (tachycardia), which often causes cardiac arrest and sudden death.

All Lipid Intake in Moderation. In the quest for good health and optimal exercise performance, prudent practice entails cooking with and consuming lipids derived primarily from vegetable sources. This approach may be too simplistic, however, because total saturated *and* unsaturated fatty acid intake may constitute a risk for diabetes and heart disease. If so, then one should reduce the intake of all lipids, particularly lipids high in saturated fatty acids and *trans* fatty acids. Concerns also exist over the association of high-fat diets with ovarian, colon, endometrial, and other cancers. Another beneficial effect of reducing the diet's lipid content relates to weight control. The energy requirements of various metabolic pathways make the body particularly efficient in converting excess calories from dietary lipid to stored fat.[102] Consequently, greater increases in body fat may occur with a high-fat diet than with an equivalent caloric excess of carbohydrate.

FIGURE 1.10 lists the saturated, monounsaturated, and polyunsaturated fatty acid content of various sources of dietary lipid. All fats contain a mix of each fatty acid type, although different fatty acids predominate in certain lipid sources. In foods, α-linolenic acid is the major omega-3 fatty acid; linoleic acid is the major omega-6 fatty acid; and oleic acid is the major omega-9 fatty acid. These fatty acids provide components for vital body structures, perform important roles in immune function and vision, help form and maintain the integrity of plasma membranes, and produce hormonelike compounds called eicosanoids.

One can only obtain omega-3 and omega-6 polyunsaturated fatty acids (abundant in most vegetable oils except tropical ones) through the diet. Because of their role as precursors of other fatty acids that the body cannot synthesize they have been termed **essential fatty acids**. About 1 to 2% of the total energy intake should come from linoleic acid. For a 2500-kcal intake, this corresponds to about 1 tablespoon of plant oil per day. Mayonnaise, cooking oils and salad dressings, whole grains, vegetables, and other foods readily provide this amount. Fatty fish (salmon, tuna, or sardines) or canola, soybean, safflower, sunflower, sesame, and flax oils provide the best sources for α-linolenic acid or its related omega-3 fatty acids, EPA and DHA.

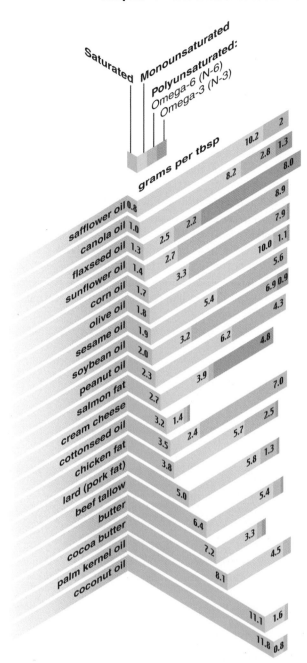

Figure 1.10. Saturated, monounsaturated, and polyunsaturated fatty acid content of various sources of dietary lipid.

Compound Lipids

Compound lipids consist of a triacylglycerol molecule combined with other chemicals and represent about 10% of the body's total fat. One group of modified triacylglycerols, the **phospholipids**, contains one or more fatty acid molecules combined with a phosphorus-containing group and a nitrogenous base. These lipids form in all cells, although the liver synthesizes most of them. The phosphorus part of the phospholipids within the plasma membrane bilayer attracts water (hydrophilic), while the lipid portion repels water (hydrophobic). Thus phospholipids interact with water and lipid to modulate fluid movement across cell membranes. Phospholipids also maintain the structural integrity of the cell, play an important role in blood clotting, and provide structural integrity to the insulating sheath around nerve fibers. **Lecithin**, the most widely distributed phospholipid in food sources (liver, egg yolk, wheat germ, nuts, soybeans), functions in fatty acid and cholesterol transport and use. Lecithin does not qualify as an essential nutrient because the body manufactures the required amount.

Other compound lipids include **glycolipids** (fatty acids bound with carbohydrate and nitrogen) and water-soluble **lipoproteins** (formed primarily in the liver when protein joins with either triacylglycerols or phospholipids). *Lipoproteins provide the major avenue for lipid transport in the blood.* If blood lipids did not bind to protein, they literally would float to the top like cream in nonhomogenized fresh milk.

High- and Low-Density-Lipoprotein Cholesterol

FIGURE 1.11 illustrates the general dynamics of dietary cholesterol and the lipoproteins, including their transport among the small intestine, liver, and peripheral tissues. Four types of lipoproteins exist according to gravitational density. **Chylomicrons** form when emulsified lipid droplets (including long-chain triacylglycerols, phospholipids, and free fatty acids) leave the intestine and enter the lymphatic vasculature. Under normal conditions, the liver metabolizes chylomicrons and sends them for storage in adipose tissue. Chylomicrons also transport the fat-soluble vitamins A, D, E, and K.

The liver and small intestine produce **high-density lipoprotein (HDL)**. HDL contains the greatest percentage of protein (about 50%) and the least total lipid (about 20%) and cholesterol (about 20%) compared with the other lipoproteins. Degradation of a **very-low-density lipoprotein (VLDL)** produces a **low-density lipoprotein (LDL)**. VLDL, formed in the liver from fats, carbohydrates, alcohol, and

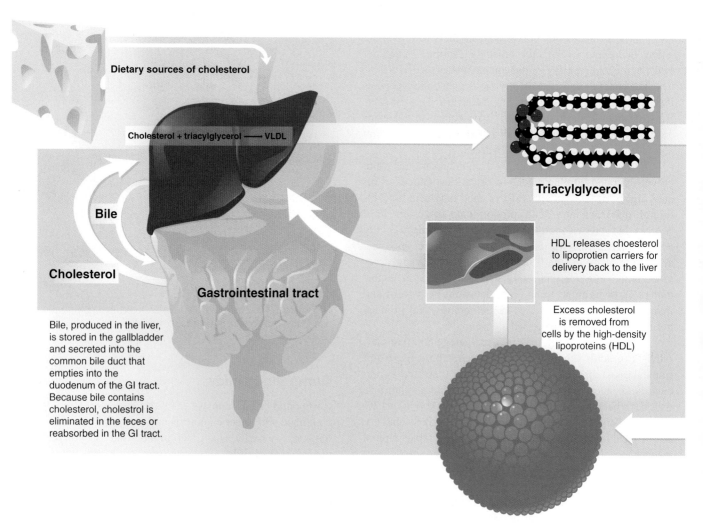

Dietary sources of cholesterol

Cholesterol + triacylglycerol —— VLDL

Bile

Cholesterol

Gastrointestinal tract

Triacylglycerol

HDL releases choesterol to lipoprotein carriers for delivery back to the liver

Excess cholesterol is removed from cells by the high-density lipoproteins (HDL)

Bile, produced in the liver, is stored in the gallbladder and secreted into the common bile duct that empties into the duodenum of the GI tract. Because bile contains cholesterol, cholestrol is eliminated in the feces or reabsorbed in the GI tract.

■ **Figure 1.11.** General interaction between dietary cholesterol and the lipoproteins and their transport among the small intestine, liver, and peripheral tissues.

cholesterol, contains the greatest percentage of lipid (95%), of which about 60% consists of triacylglycerol. VLDL transports triacylglycerols to muscle and adipose tissue. Action of the enzyme **lipoprotein lipase** produces a denser LDL molecule because now it contains more lipid. LDL and VLDL have the most lipid and least protein components.

"Bad" Cholesterol. Among the lipoproteins, LDL, which normally carries between 60 and 80% of the total serum cholesterol, has the greatest affinity for cells of the arterial wall. LDL delivers cholesterol to arterial tissue, where LDL oxidizes and participates in the proliferation of smooth muscle cells and other unfavorable changes that damage and narrow arteries. Regular aerobic exercise, visceral fat accumulation, and the diet's macronutrient composition all affect serum LDL concentrations.

"Good" Cholesterol. Unlike LDL, HDL protects against heart disease. HDL acts as a scavenger in the **reverse transport of cholesterol** by removing cholesterol from the arterial wall. It then delivers it to the liver for incorporation into bile and subsequent excretion via the intestinal tract.

The amount of LDL and HDL cholesterol and their specific ratios (e.g., HDL ÷ total cholesterol) and subfractions provide more-meaningful indicators of coronary artery disease risk than total cholesterol alone.[55,87] Regular aerobic exercise and abstinence from cigarette smoking significantly increase HDL, lower LDL, and favorably alter the LDL ÷ HDL ratio.[59,66,106,119]

Derived Lipids

Derived lipids form from simple and compound lipids. Unlike the neutral fats and phospholipids with hydrocarbon chains, derived lipids contain hydrocarbon rings. *Cholesterol, the most widely known derived lipid, exists only in animal tissue.* The chemical structure of cholesterol provides the backbone for synthesizing all of the body's steroid compounds (e.g., bile salts, vitamin D, sex hormones, and adrenocortical hormones). Cholesterol does not contain fatty acids,

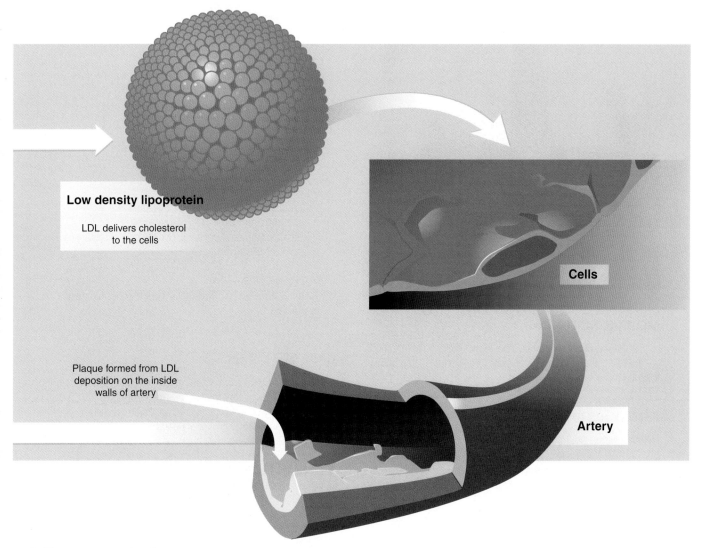

Low density lipoprotein

LDL delivers cholesterol to the cells

Cells

Plaque formed from LDL deposition on the inside walls of artery

Artery

■ **Figure 1.11** continued

CASE STUDY/PERSONAL HEALTH AND EXERCISE NUTRITION 1–2

Adult Hyperlipidemia

The following data were obtained on J.M., a 58-year-old executive, who has not had an annual physical examination in 5 years. He has gained weight and is now concerned about his health status.

MEDICAL HISTORY

J.M. has no history of chronic diseases or major hospitalization. He does not take medications or dietary supplements, and has no known food allergies.

FAMILY HISTORY

J.M.'s father died from a heart attack at age 61; his younger brother has had triple bypass surgery, and his uncle has type 2 diabetes. His mother, physically inactive for most of her adult life, classifies as obese with high serum cholesterol and triacylglycerol levels.

SOCIAL HISTORY

J.M. has been overweight since high school. He has gained 15 pounds during the last year, which he attributes to his job and changes in eating habits (eats out more frequently). J.M. wants to improve his diet but does not know what to do. He typically eats only two meals daily, with at least one meal consumed at a restaurant and several snacks interspersed. He drinks three to five cups of coffee throughout the day and two to three alcoholic drinks every evening. He also smokes one pack of cigarettes daily and reports high stress in his job and at home (two teenage children). J.M. states that he has little opportunity for exercise or leisure time activities given his present schedule.

PHYSICAL EXAMINATION/ANTHROPOMETRIC/ LABORATORY DATA

- Blood pressure: 135/90
- Height: 6 feet (182.9 cm)
- Body weight: 215 lb (97.1 kg)
- BMI: 29.0
- Abdominal girth: 40.9 inches (104 cm)
- Laboratory data
  - Nonfasting total cholesterol: 267 mg·dL^{-1}
  - HDL-C: 34 mg·dL^{-1}
  - LDL-C: 141 mg·dL^{-1}
  - Blood glucose: 124 mg·dL^{-1}
- Dietary intake from 24-hour food recall
  - Calories: 3001 kcal
  - Protein: 110 g (14.7% of total kcal)
  - Lipid: 121 g (36.3% of total kcal)
  - Carbohydrate: 368 g (49% of total kcal)
  - Saturated fatty acids: 18% of total kcal
  - Monounsaturated fatty acids (MUFA): 7% of total kcal
  - Cholesterol: 390 mg
  - Fiber: 10 g
  - Folic acid: 200 μg
- General impressions: overly fat male with possible metabolic syndrome

CASE QUESTIONS

1. Provide an overall assessment of J.M.'s health status.
2. What other laboratory tests could be performed?
3. Interpret J.M.'s blood lipid profile based on his history, physical examination, and laboratory data.
4. Give recommendations for improving the adequacy of J.M.'s diet.
5. Create the best dietary approach for J.M.
6. What course of action should J.M. consider to improve his blood lipid profile?

CASE STUDY/PERSONAL HEALTH AND EXERCISE NUTRITION 1–2

ANSWERS

1. Based on available data it appears that J.M. is hypercholesterolemic (elevated cholesterol, low HDL-C, elevated LDL-C) and perhaps prediabetic (elevated blood glucose) with a high risk for coronary heart disease (elevated cholesterol; elevated glucose; elevated diastolic blood pressure; high BMI; family history of chronic disease and larger than normal abdominal girth). According to the National Cholesterol Education Program (NCEP; <http://www.nhlbi.nih.gov/guidelines/cholesterol/index.htm>) all adults age 20 and older should have cholesterol and HDL-cholesterol measured at least every 5 years. Perform a fasting blood lipid profile when cholesterol exceeds 240 mg·dL^{-1}.

2. A fasting lipid profile is warranted on the basis of his cholesterol level and number of risk factors. The fasting blood sample should include total triacylglycerol level. Additionally, plasma homocysteine and lipoprotein (a) levels should be measured based on J.M.'s family history of heart disease. Perform a fasting blood glucose determination to rule out glucose intolerance or type 2 diabetes.

    The following 12-hour fasting blood profile indicates
    a. Total cholesterol: 266 mg·dL^{-1} (desirable <200 mg·dL^{-1})
    b. HDL-C: 31 mg·dL^{-1} (desirable >40 mg·dL^{-1})
    c. LDL-C: 150 mg·dL^{-1} (desirable <130 mg·dL^{-1})
    d. Triacylglycerol: 341 mg·dL^{-1} (desirable <150 mg·dL^{-1})
    e. Glucose: 110 mg·dL^{-1} (desirable <100 mg·dL^{-1})
    f. Homocysteine: 8 μmol·L^{-1} (desirable <12 μmol·L^{-1})
    g. Lipoprotein(a): 11 mg·dL^{-1} (desirable <20 mg·dL^{-1})

3. J.M. has "combined" hyperlipidemia, because both total triacylglycerol and LDL-C levels are higher than normal values for his age. This is sometimes referred to as "familial hyperlipidemia." In such a familial disorder, the diagnosis is based on (a) the combined hyperlipidemia in first-degree family members and (b) the elevated triacylglycerol and LDL-C concentrations. Familial hyperlipidemia represents the most common form of lipid disorder; it exists in 1 out of 100 Americans.

4. J.M.'s diet does not fall within recommended guidelines, with the following variables exceeding recommended levels: total fat intake (as % of total kcal) versus recommended 30% level; saturated fat versus recommended <10% of total kcal; cholesterol versus recommended <300 mg·dL^{-1}; fiber versus recommended > 30 g·dL^{-1}. Daily caloric intake of 3100 kcal is high relative to energy expenditure and promotes excess weight (fat) gain. J.M. must reduce daily caloric intake by at least

500 kcal and increase caloric expenditure to a similar extent through moderate physical activity to promote consistent weight loss while preserving fat-free body mass.

5. Recommendations for J.M. include lowering total cholesterol, LDL-C, and triacylglycerol levels, raising HDL-C levels, and reducing body weight (fat). To achieve these goals J.M. should follow the National Heart, Lung and Blood Institute guidelines for optimizing the blood lipid profile shown in the accompanying table. Translating these guidelines into specific recommendations includes the following: Eat (a) sufficient MUFA (up to 15% of total calories) from olive oil, peanuts, avocados, safflower and sunflower oils, cashew nuts; (b) 3 to 5 servings per day of fruits and vegetables; (c) 7 to 8 daily servings of whole grains, beans, and legumes; (d) only nonfat or low-fat dairy products, and chicken (without skin), fish, or lean meats limited to 6 oz per day. Fiber intake also needs to increase to 30 g per day, which should be accomplished by increasing fruit, whole grain, and vegetable intake.

National Cholesterol Education Program Diet Recommendations

Total fat	<30% total kcal
Saturated fat	8–10% total kcal
Polyunsaturated fat	Up to 10% total kcal
Monounsaturated fat	Up to 15% total kcal
Cholesterol	<300 mg/day
Carbohydrates	50–60% total kcal
Protein	10–20% total kcal
Calories	To achieve and maintain desired weight

6. Only after sufficient attempts at lifestyle changes that include dietary modification (see above) and initiating a regular exercise program (aerobic exercise such as daily walking, cycling, or swimming for 45–60 minutes at light-to-moderate intensity) should drug therapy be considered and only as an adjunct and not as a substitute for lifestyle modifications. J.M. also requires medical clearance including an exercise stress test prior to starting an exercise program.

    J.M.'s modifiable risk factors include obesity, high-fat diet, sedentary lifestyle, smoking, and excessive alcohol intake. Along with an improved diet and a regular exercise program, he should enroll in a smoking cessation program and limit his alcohol intake. Meeting with a lifestyle management consultant should be encouraged.

but shares some of the physical and chemical characteristics of lipids. Thus from a dietary viewpoint, cholesterol is considered a lipid.

Cholesterol, widespread in the plasma membrane of all cells, is obtained either through the diet (**exogenous cholesterol**) or through cellular synthesis (**endogenous cholesterol**). Even if an individual maintains a "cholesterol-free" diet, endogenous cholesterol synthesis varies between 0.5 and 2.0 g per day. More endogenous cholesterol forms with a diet high in saturated fatty acids, which facilitate cholesterol synthesis by the liver.[29,30,41] While the liver synthesizes about 70% of the body's cholesterol, other tissues—including the walls of the arteries and intestines—also synthesize it. The rate of endogenous synthesis usually meets the body's needs; hence, severely reducing cholesterol intake, except in pregnant women and infants, probably causes little harm.

Functions of Cholesterol

Cholesterol participates in many complex bodily functions, including building plasma membranes and as a precursor in synthesizing vitamin D and adrenal gland hormones as well as the sex hormones estrogen, androgen, and progesterone. Cholesterol provides a crucial component for the synthesis of bile, which emulsifies lipids during digestion, and plays an important role in forming tissues, organs, and body structures during fetal development.

TABLE 1.7 presents the cholesterol content per serving of common foods from meat and dairy sources. Egg yolk contributes a rich source of cholesterol, as do red meats and organ meats (liver, kidney, and brains). Shellfish, particularly shrimp, and dairy products (ice cream, cream cheese, butter, and whole milk) contain relatively large amounts of cholesterol. Foods of plant origin contain *no* cholesterol.

Cholesterol and Heart Disease

Powerful predictors of coronary artery disease include high levels of total serum cholesterol and the cholesterol-rich LDL molecule. The risk becomes particularly apparent when combined with other risk factors such as cigarette smoking, physical inactivity, obesity, and untreated hypertension. A continuous and graded relationship exists between serum cholesterol and death from coronary artery disease; thus, lowering cholesterol appears to offer prudent heart disease protection.[51,57,103] For heart disease patients, coronary blood flow improves (thus reducing myocardial ischemia during daily life) in 6 months or less when drug and diet therapy aggressively lower both total blood cholesterol and LDL-cholesterol.[7] (For example, drugs called statins reduce cholesterol by up to 60 $mg \cdot dL^{-1}$.) Studies with animals show that a diet high in cholesterol and saturated fatty acids raises serum cholesterol in "susceptible" animals. This diet

Table 1.7	**CHOLESTEROL CONTENT OF SOME COMMON FOODS**				
Food	*Quantity*	*Cholesterol (mg)*	*Food*	*Quantity*	*Cholesterol (mg)*
Meat			**Dairy**		
Brains, pan fried	3 oz	1696	Egg salad	1 cup	629
Liver, chicken	3 oz	537	Custard, baked	1 cup	213
Caviar	3 oz	497	Egg, yolk	1 large	211
Liver, beef, fried	3 oz	410	Ice cream, soft serve, vanilla	1 cup	153
Spare ribs, cooked	6 oz	198	Eggnog	1 cup	149
Shrimp, boiled	3 oz	166	Ice cream, rich	1 cup	88
Tuna, light, water pack	1 can	93	Pizza, cheese	1 slice	47
Chicken breast, fried, no skin	3 oz	91	Milk, whole	1 cup	34
Halibut, smoked	3 oz	86	Cottage cheese, large curd	1 cup	34
Lamb chop, broiled	1	84	Cheese, cheddar	1 oz	30
Abalone, fried	3 oz	80	Milk, low fat, 2%	1 cup	18
Hamburger patty	3 oz	75	Chocolate milk shake	1 cup	13
Corned beef	3 oz	73	Butter	1 pat	11
Chicken or turkey, light meat	3 oz	70	Cottage cheese, low-fat 1%	1 cup	10
Lobster, cooked	3 oz	61	Yogurt, low-fat with fruit	1 cup	10
Clams	3 oz	57	Buttermilk (>1% fat)	1 cup	9
Taco, beef	1	57	Milk, skim	1 cup	5
Swordfish, broiled	3 oz	50	Mayonnaise	1 Tbsp	5
Bacon strips	3 pieces	36			
Hot dog	1	29			
Hot dog, beef	1	27			
French fries, McDonald's	Regular	13			

combination eventually produces **atherosclerosis**, a degenerative process that forms cholesterol-rich deposits (**plaque**) on the inner lining of the medium and larger arteries, which narrow and eventually close. In humans, dietary cholesterol raises the ratio of total cholesterol to HDL-cholesterol to adversely affect the cholesterol risk profile.[116] In addition, reducing saturated fatty acid and cholesterol intake generally lowers serum cholesterol, although for most people the effect remains modest. Similarly, increasing dietary intake of mono- and polyunsaturated fatty acids lowers blood cholesterol.[96]

A controlled 7- to 10-year investigation of nearly 4000 healthy middle-aged men with elevated cholesterol showed a cause-and-effect relationship between serum cholesterol and heart disease.[67,68] Lowering cholesterol reduced heart attack risk and improved survival if a heart attack occurred. Coronary heart disease risk improvement is closely linked to the cholesterol decrease by the factor of 1:2. A 1% reduction in cholesterol reduced risk by 2%! These findings, corroborated in other clinical trials,[32,116] show the wisdom of reducing serum lipids through modifications that curtail intake of cholesterol-rich foods, increase physical activity, and control body weight. TABLE 1.8 recommends levels for total cholesterol and the LDL and HDL subfractions.

RECOMMENDED DIETARY LIPID INTAKE

Recommendations for dietary lipid intake for physically active individuals follow prudent recommendations for the general population. In the United States, dietary lipids represent about 36% of total caloric intake. Standards for optimal lipid intake have not been firmly established for the general population or for physically active groups, but most health professionals (American Heart Association [AHA]; www.americanheart.org) recommend that lipid intake should not exceed 30% of the diet's total energy content, and consuming less (American Cancer Society recommends 20%; www.aci.org) may confer even greater health benefits.[64,94] Unsaturated fatty acids should account for at least 70% and preferably 80% of the total lipid intake, equally distributed between polyunsaturates and monounsaturates. Compliance with current dietary recommendations ($\leq$30% of energy from lipid, <10% from saturated fat, and <300 mg of cholesterol per day) lowers total plasma cholesterol and LDL-cholesterol levels by about 5% compared with lipid intake in the typical American diet.[48] For coronary heart disease patients, a more drastic lowering of total dietary fat intake toward the 10% level produces more pronounced cholesterol-lowering effects accompanied by clinical improvements.[89]

TABLE 1.9 presents three daily menus, each consisting of 2000 kcal but with different percentages of total lipid. *Meal Plan A*, typical of the North American diet, consists of 38% of total calories from lipid. *Meal Plan B* contains 29% lipid, a value recommended by most health professionals. *Meal Plan C*, with 10% lipid, may be desirable from a health perspective but is difficult to maintain, particularly for physically active individuals with high daily energy expenditures.

Ratio of Polyunsaturated to Saturated Fatty Acids

TABLE 1.10 lists examples of foods high and low in saturated fatty acids, foods high in monounsaturated and polyunsaturated fatty acids, and the ratio of polyunsaturated to saturated fatty acids (**P/S ratio**). One should attempt to maintain the P/S ratio at least at 1:1 and preferably 2:1. Based on dietary surveys, the P/S ratio in the United States only ranges between 0.43 and 1.0. The P/S ratio has some limitations and should not be used exclusively to guide lipid intake. For example, the ratio does not consider the potential cholesterol-lowering role of monounsaturated fatty acids if they replace the diet's saturated fatty acids. Nevertheless, the P/S ratio provides the consumer with useful information about the fatty acid content of food, provided the food source lists the fatty acid types.

Ratio of Saturated to Monounsaturated to Polyunsaturated Fatty Acids

The AHA takes a slightly different approach to healthful eating. Previous guidelines recommended a lipid intake less

Table 1.8.	CLASSIFICATION LEVELS OF LDL, HDL, AND TOTAL CHOLESTEROL (MG PER DL)

LDL Cholesterol	Classification
<100	Optimal
100–129	Near or above optimal
130–159	Borderline high
160–189	High
≥190	Very high

Total Cholesterol	Classification
<200	Desirable
200–239	Borderline high
≥240	High

HDL Cholesterol	Classification
<40	Low
≥60	High

From Expert on Panel Detection, Evaluation, and Treatment of High Blood Cholesterol in Adults. Executive summary of the third report of the National Cholesterol Education Program (NCEP) Expert Panel on Detection. Evaluation, And Treatment of High Blood Cholesterol in Adults (Adult Treatment Panel III). JAMA 2001;285:2486.

LDL, low-density lipoprotein cholesterol; HDL, high-density lipoprotein cholesterol.

Table 1.9   THREE DIFFERENT DAILY MEAL PLANS, EACH CONSISTING OF 2000 CALORIES, BUT WITH DIFFERENT PERCENTAGES OF TOTAL FAT

Plan A. 38% Fat Diet

Breakfast
1 apple Danish pastry
1/2 cup orange juice
1 cup whole milk

Lunch
2 slices of wheat bread
2 oz turkey breast
1 oz Swiss cheese
1 teaspoon mayonnaise
1 small banana
1 small bag potato chips (15 chips)

Snack
1/2 cup vanilla ice cream

Dinner
4 oz T-bone steak
1 large baked potato
1 1/2 cup steamed broccoli
1 dinner roll
1 teaspoon margarine
2 tablespoons sour cream
1 1/4 cup fresh strawberries

Snack
15 grapes
2 chocolate chip cookies
Total calories: 1990
Total fat: 84 g; 38% of calories from fat
Saturated fat: less than 10%

Plan B. 29% Fat Diet

Breakfast
1 bagel
1 tablespoon cream cheese
1/2 cup orange juice
1 cup 1% milk

Lunch
2 slices of wheat bread
2 oz of turkey breast
1 teaspoon of mayonnaise
1 small banana
Lettuce salad with 2 cups of fresh vegetables—broccoli, cauliflower, carrots, cucumbers, cherry tomatoes
3 tablespoons reduced calorie salad dressing

Snack
1 cup low-fat yogurt
1 fresh peach
6 cups of air-popped popcorn

Dinner
4 oz sirloin (grilled or broiled)
1 large baked potato
1 1/2 cup steamed broccoli
1 dinner roll
1 tablespoon reduced-calorie margarine
2 tablespoons sour cream
1 1/4 cup strawberries

Snack
30 grapes
Total calories: 1971
Total fat: 63 g; 29% of calories from fat
Saturated fat: 7% of calories

Plan C. 10% Fat Diet

Breakfast
1/2 cup bran cereal with raisins
1 bagel
1 tablespoon cream cheese
1/2 cup orange juice
1 cup skimmed milk
1/2 grapefruit

Lunch
2 slices of wheat bread
2 oz turkey breast
1 teaspoon mayonnaise
1 small banana
Lettuce salad with 3 cups of fresh vegetables—broccoli, cauliflower, carrots, cucumbers, cherry tomatoes
3 tablespoons fat-free salad dressing

Snack
1 cup nonfat yogurt
1 fresh peach
6 cups of air-popped popcorn

Dinner
1 large baked potato
1 1/2 cup steamed broccoli
2 dinner rolls
1 teaspoon margarine
1 1/4 cup fresh strawberries
1 cup skimmed milk

Snack
30 grapes
1 cup skimmed milk
Total calories: 1990
Total fat: 21 g; 10% of calories from fat
Saturated fat: less than 3%

than 30% of total calories, with the percentage of lipid calories distributed in a ratio of 10:10:10 for saturated to monounsaturated to polyunsaturated fatty acids. Owing to difficulty determining the particular fat source percentage of a meal, the AHA now encourages Americans to focus more on replacing high-fat foods with fruits, vegetables, grains, fat-free and low-fat dairy products, fish, poultry, and lean meat.[58] Other new components of the AHA guidelines include a focus on weight control and the addition of two weekly servings of fish high in omega-3 fatty acids.

The AHA has also recommended that people consume no more than 300 mg (0.01 oz) of cholesterol daily—almost the amount of cholesterol in an egg yolk and about one-half the cholesterol ingested daily by the average American male—limiting intake to 100 mg per 1000 kcal of food ingested. More desirable benefits occur by reducing daily

Table 1.10   **EXAMPLES OF FOODS HIGH AND LOW IN SATURATED FATTY ACIDS, FOODS HIGH IN MONOUNSATURATED AND POLYUNSATURATED FATTY ACIDS, AND THE POLYUNSATURATED TO SATURATED FATTY ACID (P/S) RATIO OF COMMON FATS AND OILS**

High saturated	**%**	Peanut oil	48
Coconut oil	91	Cashews, dry roasted	42
Palm kernel oil	82	Peanut butter	39
Butter	68	Bologna	39
Cream cheese	57	Beef, cooked	33
Coconut	56	Lamb, roasted	32
Hollandaise sauce	54	Veal, roasted	26
Palm oil	51	**High polyunsaturated**	**%**
Half & half	45	Safflower oil	77
Cheese, Velveeta	43	Sunflower oil	72
Cheese, mozzarella	41	Corn oil	58
Ice cream, vanilla	38	Walnuts, dry	51
Cheesecake	32	Sunflower seeds	47
Chocolate almond bar	29	Margarine, corn oil	45
Low saturated	**%**	Canola oil	32
Popcorn	0	Sesame seeds	31
Hard candy	0	Pumpkin seeds	31
Yogurt, nonfat	2	Tofu	27
Crackerjacks	3	Lard	11
Milk, skim	4	Butter	6
Cookies, fig bars	4	Coconut oil	2
Graham crackers	5	**P/S Ratio, Fats & Oils**	
Chicken breast, roasted	6	Coconut oil	0.2/1.0
Pancakes	8	Palm oil	0.2/1.0
Cottage cheese, 1%	8	Butter	0.1/1.0
Milk, chocolate, 1%	9	Olive oil	0.6/1.0
Beef, dried	9	Lard	0.3/1.0
Chocolate, mints	10	Canola oil	5.3/1.0
High monounsaturated	**%**	Peanut oil	1.9/1.0
Olives, black	80	Soybean oil	2.5/1.0
Olive oil	75	Sesame oil	3.0/1.0
Almond oil	70	Margarine, 100% corn oil	2.5/1.0
Canola oil	61	Cottonseed oil	2.0/1.0
Almonds, dry	52	Mayonnaise	3.7/1.0
Avocados	51	Safflower oil	13.3/1.0

Data from the Science and Education Administration, Home and Garden Bulletin 72, Nutritive value of foods. Washington, DC: US Government Printing Office, 1985, 1986; Agricultural Research Service, United States Department of Agriculture, Nutritive value of American foods in common units. Agricultural Handbook no. 456. Washington, DC, US Government Printing Office, 1975.

cholesterol intake toward 150 to 200 mg. The main sources of dietary cholesterol include the same animal food sources rich in saturated fatty acids. Reducing the intake of these foods not only reduces intake of preformed cholesterol but, more importantly, reduces the intake of saturated fatty acids that stimulate endogenous cholesterol synthesis.

ROLE OF LIPID IN THE BODY

Four important functions of lipids in the body include:

1. Energy reserve
2. Protection of vital organs
3. Thermal insulation
4. Transport medium for fat-soluble vitamins and hunger suppressor.

Energy Source and Reserve

Fat constitutes the ideal cellular fuel because each molecule carries large quantities of energy per unit weight, transports and stores easily, and provides a ready source of energy. In well-nourished individuals at rest, fat provides as much as 80 to 90% of the energy requirement. One gram of pure lipid contains about 9 kcal (38 kJ) of energy, more than *twice* the energy available to the body in an equal quantity of carbohydrate or protein. This occurs from the greater quantity of hydrogen in the lipid molecule. Chapter 4 points out that the oxidation of hydrogen atoms provides the energy for bodily functions at rest and during exercise. Recall that the synthesis of a triacylglycerol molecule from glycerol and three fatty acid molecules creates three water molecules. In contrast, when glucose forms glycogen, 2.7 g of water stores with each gram. *Whereas fat exists as a relatively water-free, concentrated fuel, glycogen becomes hydrated and heavy relative to its energy content.*

FIGURE 1.12 illustrates the total mass (and energy content) from fat and various body fat depots in an 80-kg man. Approximately 15% of the body mass for males and 25% for females consists of fat. The potential energy stored in the fat molecules of a typical 80-kg young adult male translates to about 110,700 kcal (12,300 g body fat $\times$ 9.0 kcal·g^{-1}). Most of this energy—present as adipose tissue and intramuscular triacylglycerols and a small amount of plasma free fatty acids—is available for exercise. This amount of energy would fuel a run from New York City to Madison, Wisconsin (assuming an energy expenditure of about 100 kcal per mile). Contrast this fact to the limited 2000-kcal reserve of stored carbohydrate that could only fuel a 20-mile run. Viewed from a different perspective, the body's energy reserves from carbohydrate could power high-intensity running for about 1.6 hours, while fat reserves would allow the person to continue for about 120 hours! As was the case for carbohydrate, fat used as a fuel "spares" protein to carry out its important functions of tissue synthesis and repair.

Protection and Insulation

Up to 4% of the body's fat protects against trauma to the heart, liver, kidneys, spleen, brain, and spinal cord. Fats stored just below the skin (subcutaneous fat) provide insulation, determining ability to tolerate extremes of cold exposure.[74] Swimmers who excelled in swimming the English Channel showed only a slight fall in body temperature while resting in cold water and essentially no lowering effect while swimming.[93] In contrast, body temperature of leaner, non-Channel swimmers decreased markedly under rest and exercise conditions. The insulatory layer of fat probably affords little protection except in cold-related activities like deep-sea diving or ocean or channel swimming or among Arctic inhabitants. Excess body fat hinders temperature regulation during heat stress, most notably during sustained exercise in air when the body's heat production can increase 20 times above the resting level. The insulation shield from subcutaneous fat retards the flow of heat from the body.

For large-sized football linemen, excess fat storage provides additional cushioning to protect from the sport's normal hazards. Any possible protective benefit, however, must be evaluated against the liability imposed by the "dead weight" of excess fat and its effect on energy expenditure, thermal regulation, and exercise performance.

Vitamin Carrier and Hunger Depressor

Consuming about 20 g of dietary lipid daily provides a sufficient source and transport medium for the fat-soluble vitamins A, D, E, and K. Significantly reducing lipid intake depresses the body's level of these vitamins, which ultimately may lead to vitamin deficiency. Dietary lipid also facilitates absorption of vitamin A precursors from nonlipid plant sources like carrots and apricots. It takes about 3.5 hours after ingesting lipids to empty them from the stomach. Thus, some lipid in the diet can delay the onset of "hunger pangs" and contribute to satiety following the meal. This helps to explain why reducing diets containing a small amount of lipid sometimes prove initially more successful in blunting the immediate urge to eat than more extreme fat-free diets.

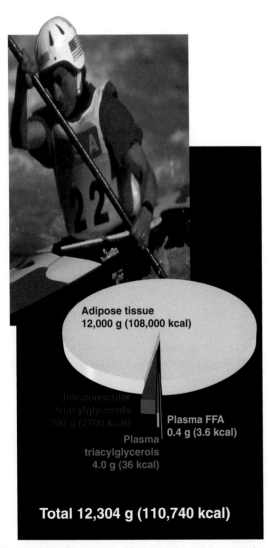

Adipose tissue
12,000 g (108,000 kcal)

Intramuscular triacylglycerols
300 g (2700 kcal)

Plasma FFA
0.4 g (3.6 kcal)

Plasma triacylglycerols
4.0 g (36 kcal)

Total 12,304 g (110,740 kcal)

■ **Figure 1.12.** Distribution of fat energy in an average 80-kg man.

Summary

1. Lipids, like carbohydrates, contain carbon, hydrogen, and oxygen atoms, but with a higher ratio of hydrogen to oxygen. For example, the lipid stearin has the formula $C_{57}H_{110}O_6$. Lipid molecules consist of one glycerol molecule and three fatty acid molecules.

2. Lipids, synthesized by plants and animals, are grouped into one of three categories: *(a)* simple lipids (glycerol plus three fatty acids), *(b)* compound lipids (phospholipids, glycolipids, and lipoproteins) composed of simple lipids combined with other chemicals, and *(c)* derived lipids like cholesterol, synthesized from simple and compound lipids.

3. Saturated fatty acids contain as many hydrogen atoms as chemically possible; thus, "saturated" describes this molecule with respect to hydrogen. Saturated fatty acids exist primarily in animal meat, egg yolk, dairy fats, and cheese. Dietary intakes high in saturated fatty acids elevate blood cholesterol and promote coronary heart disease.

4. Unsaturated fatty acids contain fewer hydrogen atoms attached to the carbon chain. Instead, double bonds connect carbon atoms and the fatty acid exists as either monounsaturated or polyunsaturated with respect to hydrogen. Heart disease protection occurs from increasing the diet's proportion of unsaturated fatty acids.

5. Dietary *trans* fatty acids may account for 30,000 deaths annually from heart disease. High intake of this fatty acid also increases risk for contracting type 2 diabetes.

6. Perhaps the most powerful cardioprotective benefit of fish oils relates to their antiarrhythmic effect on myocardial tissue. This protection against ventricular arrhythmias and sudden death is likely provided by the unique effects of these dietary fatty acids on the fatty acid content of the myocardial cell membranes.

7. Lowering blood cholesterol, especially that carried by LDL, significantly reduces coronary heart disease risk.

8. Dietary lipid currently provides about 36% of total energy intake. Prudent advice recommends a 30% level or lower for dietary lipid, of which 70 to 80% should consist of unsaturated fatty acids.

9. Lipids provide the largest nutrient store of potential energy for biologic work. They also protect vital organs, provide insulation from the cold, and transport the fat-soluble vitamins A, D, E, and K.

► Proteins

THE NATURE OF PROTEINS

The body of an average-sized adult contains between 10 and 12 kg of protein, primarily located within the skeletal muscle mass. Structurally, proteins (from the Greek word meaning "of prime importance") resemble carbohydrates and lipids because they too contain atoms of carbon, oxygen, and hydrogen. Protein molecules also contain about 16% nitrogen, along with sulfur and occasionally phosphorus, cobalt, and iron. Just as glycogen forms from many simple glucose subunits linked together, the protein molecule polymerizes from its **amino acid** "building-block" constituents in endlessly complex arrays. **Peptide bonds** link amino acids in chains that take on diverse forms and chemical combinations. The hydrogen from the amino acid side chain of one amino acid combines with the hydroxyl group of the carboxylic (organic) acid end of another amino acid. Two joined amino acids produce a **dipeptide**, and linking three amino acids produces a **tripeptide**, and so on. A linear configuration of up to 100 amino acids produces a **polypeptide**, while combining more than 100 amino acids forms a **protein**. Three amino acids make up thyrotropin-releasing hormone, whereas the muscle protein myosin forms from the linkage of 4500 amino acid units. Single cells contain thousands of different protein molecules. In total, approximately 50,000 different protein-containing compounds exist in the body. The biochemical functions and properties of each protein depend on the sequence of specific amino acids.

Each of the 20 different amino acids required by the body has a positively charged amine group at one end and a negatively charged organic acid group at the other end. The amine group consists of two hydrogen atoms attached to nitrogen (NH$_2$), whereas the organic acid group (technically termed a carboxylic acid group) contains one carbon atom, two oxygen atoms, and one hydrogen atom (COOH). The remainder of the amino acid molecule may take several different forms, referred to as the amino acid's functional group, or **side chain**. *The side chain's unique structure dictates the amino acid's particular characteristics.* FIGURE 1.13 *top* shows the structure for the amino acid alanine.

The potential for combining the 20 amino acids creates an almost infinite number of possible proteins. For example, proteins formed from linking just three different amino acids could generate 20^3 or 8000 different proteins, and just 6 different amino acids yields 64 million proteins (20^6)!

KINDS OF PROTEINS

The body cannot synthesize eight amino acids (nine in children and some older adults) so they must be ingested preformed in foods. Isoleucine, leucine, lysine, methionine,

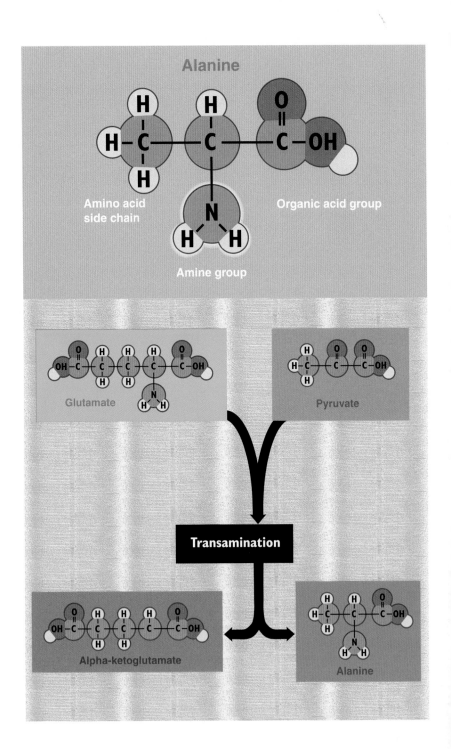

■ **Figure 1.13.** *Top,* Chemical structure of the amino acid alanine. *Bottom,* Transamination occurs when an amine group from a donor amino acid transfers to an acceptor acid to form a new amino acid.

phenylalanine, threonine, tryptophan, and valine make up these **essential amino acids**. The body also synthesizes cystine from methionine and tyrosine from phenylalanine. Infants cannot synthesize histidine, and children have reduced capability for synthesizing arginine. The body manufactures the remaining nine **nonessential** amino acids. The term *nonessential* does not mean they are unimportant; rather, they must be synthesized from other compounds already in the body at a rate to meet demands for normal growth and tissue repair.

Fortunately, animals and plants manufacture proteins that contain essential amino acids. No health or physiologic advantage exists from an amino acid derived from an animal compared with the same amino acid from vegetable origin. Plants synthesize amino acids by incorporating nitrogen in the soil along with carbon, oxygen, and hydrogen from air and water. In contrast, animals do not possess broad capability for protein synthesis; they ingest most of their protein.

Synthesizing a specific protein requires the availability of appropriate amino acids. **Complete proteins**, or higher-quality proteins, come from foods with all of the essential amino acids in the quantity and the correct ratio to maintain nitrogen balance and allow tissue growth and repair. An **incomplete protein**, or lower-quality protein, lacks one or more essential amino acid. Incomplete protein diets eventually lead to protein malnutrition. This occurs whether or not the food sources contain adequate energy or protein quantity.

Protein Sources

Sources of complete protein include eggs, milk, meat, fish, and poultry. Among all food sources, eggs provide the optimal mixture of essential amino acids; hence, eggs receive the highest quality rating of 100 for comparison with other foods. TABLE 1.11 rates common sources of dietary protein.

Table 1.11 **RATING OF PROTEIN QUALITY OF DIETARY SOURCES FOR PROTEIN**

Food	Protein Rating
Eggs	100
Fish	70
Lean beef	69
Cow's milk	60
Brown rice	57
White rice	56
Soybeans	47
Brewer's hash	45
Whole-grain wheat	44
Peanuts	43
Dry beans	34
White potato	34

Table 1.12 **GOOD FOOD SOURCES FOR PROTEIN**

Food	Serving	Protein (g)
Animal		
Tuna	3 oz	22
Turkey, light meat	4 oz	9
Fish	3 oz	17
Hamburger	4 oz	30
Egg, whole	1 large	6
Egg, white	1 large	4
Beef, lean	4 oz	24
Dairy		
Cottage cheese	0.5 cup	15
Yogurt, low fat	8 oz	11
Cheese	1 oz	8
Milk, skim	8 oz	8
Plant		
Peanuts	1 oz	7
Peanut butter	1 Tbsp	4
Pasta, dry	2 oz	7
Whole-wheat bread	2 slices	6
Baked beans	1 cup	14
Tofu	3.5 oz	11
Almonds, dried	12	3
Chick peas	0.5 cup	20
Lentils	0.5 cup	9

Presently, animal sources provide almost two-thirds of the dietary protein, whereas 85 years ago protein consumption occurred equally from plant and animal origins. Reliance on animal sources for dietary protein largely accounts for the relatively high intake of cholesterol and saturated fatty acids in the world's major industrialized nations.

The **biologic value** of a food refers to its completeness for supplying essential amino acids. Higher-quality protein foods come from animal sources, whereas vegetables (lentils, dried beans and peas, nuts, and cereals) remain incomplete in one or more essential amino acid; thus, these have a relatively lower biologic value. The animal protein collagen remains an exception because it lacks the essential amino acid tryptophan. This protein forms part of the connective tissue of animals. Unfortunately, some manufacturers add collagen to predigested powdered protein supplements. TABLE 1.12 lists examples of good food sources of protein.

The Vegetarian Approach

Eating a variety of plant foods (grains, fruits, and vegetables) supplies all of the essential amino acids, each providing a different quality and quantity of amino acids. Grains and legumes supply excellent protein content, but neither offers the full complement of essential amino acids. An exception may be well-processed, isolated soybean protein, termed *soy-protein isolates*, whose protein quality matches that of some animal proteins. Grains lack the essential amino acid lysine, while legumes contain lysine but lack the sulfur-containing essential amino acid methionine (found abundantly in grains). Tortillas and beans, rice and beans, rice and lentils, rice and peas, and peanuts and wheat (bread) serve as staples in many cultures because they provide **complementary protein** sources of all essential amino acids from the plant kingdom.

True vegetarians, or **vegans**, consume nutrients from only two sources—the plant kingdom and dietary supplements. Many physically active vegetarians are at somewhat greater risk for inadequate energy and nutrient intake because they eliminate meat and dairy products from the diet and increasingly rely on foods relatively low in energy, quality protein, and micronutrients. Vegans make up less than 1% of the United States population, although between 5 and 7% of Americans consider themselves "almost" vegetarians. Nutritional diversity remains the key for these men and women. For example, a vegan diet provides all the essential amino acids if the recommended dietary allowance for protein contains 60% of protein from grain products, 35% from legumes, and 5% from green leafy vegetables. A 70-kg person obtains all essential amino acids by consuming about 56 g of protein from approximately 1 1/4 cups of beans, 1/4 cup of seeds or nuts, 4 slices of whole-grain bread, 2 cups of vegetables (1 cup leafy green), and 2 1/2 cups from grain sources (brown rice, oatmeal, and cracked wheat).

An Increasing Number of Near-Vegetarian Athletes

An increasing number of competitive and champion athletes consume diets composed predominately of nutrients from varied plant sources, including some dairy and meat products. Considering how much time it requires to train and prepare for competition, vegetarian athletes often encounter difficulty in planning, selecting, and preparing nutritious meals from predominantly plant sources without relying on supplementation. The fact remains, however, that two-thirds of the world's population subsist on largely vegetarian diets, with little reliance on animal protein. Well-balanced vegetarian and vegetarian-type diets provide abundant carbohydrate, crucial in heavy, prolonged training. Such diets contain little or no cholesterol, are high in fiber, and rich in fruit and vegetable sources of antioxidant vitamins and diverse phytochemicals.

Controlled clinical trials generally conclude that substituting soy protein for animal protein decreases blood pressure, plasma homocysteine levels, triacylglycerols, total cholesterol, and harmful oxidized LDL-cholesterol, without reducing beneficial HDL-cholesterol.[5,53,115] For example, daily consumption of as little as 20 g of soy protein instead of animal protein for 6 weeks favorably modified blood lipid profiles.[109] Genistein, a component of soy also may offer protection against breast cancer.[62]

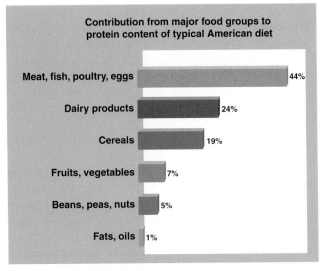

Figure 1.14. Typical American diet's contribution of protein from the major food sources.

Obtaining ample higher-quality protein becomes the strict vegetarian's main nutritional concern. Children on vegan diets should be monitored to ensure adequate vitamin D and calcium intake, which most Americans obtain from milk products. A **lactovegetarian diet** provides milk and related products like ice cream, cheese, and yogurt. The lactovegetarian approach minimizes the problem of consuming sufficient higher-quality protein and increases the intake of calcium, phosphorus, and vitamin B_{12} (produced by bacteria in the digestive tract of animals). Good meatless sources of iron include fortified ready-to-eat cereals, soybeans, and cooked farina, while cereals, wheat germ, and oysters contain high zinc levels. Adding an egg to the diet **(ovolactovegetarian diet)** ensures intake of higher-quality protein.

FIGURE 1.14 displays the contribution of various food groups to the protein content of the American diet. By far, the greatest protein intake comes from animal sources, with only about 30% derived from plant sources.

RECOMMENDED DIETARY PROTEIN INTAKE

Despite the beliefs of many coaches, trainers, and athletes, no benefit accrues from eating excessive protein. An intake exceeding three times the recommended level does *not* enhance work capacity during intensive training.[24] *For athletes, muscle mass does not increase simply by eating high-protein foods or special amino acid mixtures.* If lean tissue synthesis resulted from the extra protein consumed by the typical athlete, then muscle mass would increase tremendously. For example, consuming an extra 100 g (400 kcal) of protein daily translates into a daily 500-g (1.1-lb) increase in muscle mass. This obviously does not happen. Excessive dietary protein ultimately is used directly for energy (following deamination) or recycled as components of other molecules including stored fat in subcutaneous adipose tissue depots. Harmful side effects can occur when dietary protein intake significantly exceeds recommended values. A high protein catabolism strains liver and kidney function owing to the elimination of urea and other compounds.

Many cultures consume more than twice the protein requirement. On a population basis, protein intake relative to total energy consumed equals 11% (Germany), 12% (United States), 12% (Sweden), 12.6% (Italy), and 14.4% (Japan). The diets of endurance- and resistance-trained athletes often exceed by two to three times the recommended intake.[43–45] This occurs because the athletes' diet encourages meat consumption. Furthermore, an athlete's caloric intake (and output) surpasses that of a sedentary counterpart.

The RDA: A Liberal Standard

The **Recommended Dietary Allowance (RDA)** for protein, vitamins, and minerals represents a standard for nutrient intake expressed as a daily average. These guidelines were initially developed in May 1942 by the Food and Nutrition Board of the National Research Council/National Academy of Science (www2.nas.edu/iom) to evaluate and plan for the nutritional adequacy of groups rather than individuals. They have been revised 11 times.[35] RDA levels represent a liberal yet safe excess to prevent nutritional deficiencies in practically all healthy people. In the 11th edition (1999), RDA recommendations included 19 nutrients, energy intake, and the **Estimated Safe and Adequate Daily Dietary Intakes (ESADDI)** for seven additional vitamins and minerals and three electrolytes. The ESADDI should be viewed as more tentative and evolutionary than the RDA. ESADDI recommendations for certain essential micronutrients (e.g., vitamins biotin and pantothenic acid and trace elements copper, manganese, fluoride, selenium, chromium, and molybdenum) required sufficient scientific data to formulate an intake range considered adequate and safe, yet insufficient for a precise single RDA. Any intake within this range is considered acceptable for maintaining adequate physiologic function, and sufficient to prevent under- or overexposure. No RDA or ESADDI exists for sodium, potassium, and chlorine; instead, recommendations refer to a minimum requirement for health.

We emphasize that the RDA reflects an ongoing evaluation based on available data for the nutritional needs of a *population* over a prolonged period. Specific individual requirements only can be determined by laboratory measurements. Malnutrition occurs from cumulative weeks, months, and even years of inadequate nutrient intake. Also, someone who regularly consumes a diet containing nutrients below the RDA standards may not become malnourished. Rather, the RDA represents a probability statement for adequate nutrition; as nutrient intake falls below the RDA, the statistical probability for malnourishment increases for that person; the chance increases progressively with lower nutrient intake. In Chapter 2, we discuss the **Dietary Reference Intakes**, which represent the current set of standards for recommended intake of nutrients and other food components.[33,112]

TABLE 1.13 lists the protein RDAs for adolescent and adult men and women. On average, 0.83 g of protein per kg body mass represents the recommended daily intake. To determine protein requirement for men and women ages 18 to 65, multiply body mass in kg by 0.83. Thus, for a 90-kg man, total protein requirement equals 75 g (90 × 0.83). The protein RDA holds even for overweight persons; it includes a reserve of about 25% to account for individual differences in protein requirement for about 98% of the population. Generally, the protein RDA (and the quantity of the required essential amino acids) decreases with age. In contrast, the protein RDA for infants and growing children of 2.0 to 4.0 g per kg body mass facilitates growth and development. Pregnancy requires that daily protein intake increase by 20 g, and nursing mothers should increase intake by 10 g. *A 10% increase in the calculated protein requirement, particularly for a vegetarian-type diet, accounts for dietary fiber's effect in reducing the digestibility of many plant-based protein sources.* Stress, disease, and injury usually increase the protein requirement.

Protein Requirement for Physically Active Persons

Current debate focuses on the necessity of a larger than normal protein requirement for still growing adolescent athletes, individuals involved in strength development programs that enhance muscle growth and endurance training regimens that increase protein breakdown, and athletes subjected to recurring tissue microtrauma, like wrestlers and football players.[17,46,78,107,108] Inadequate protein and energy intake can induce a loss of body protein, particularly from skeletal muscle, with concomitant performance deterioration. If physically active individuals require additional protein, then more than likely, they meet their needs by additional food intake that compensates for the increased energy expenditure in training. However, this may not pertain to men and women with poor nutritional habits or those who reduce energy intake to achieve a desired aesthetic "look" or to compete at a lower weight-class category in the hopes of gaining a competitive advantage. Chapter 7 presents a more complete discussion of protein balance and requirements in exercise and training.

TABLE 1.13. **AVERAGE DAILY ENERGY ALLOWANCE AND RECOMMENDED PROTEIN INTAKES**

Category	Age (years) or Condition	Weight[a] (kg)	Weight[a] (lb)	Height[a] (cm)	Height[a] (in.)	Average Energy Allowance (kcal)[b] Per kg	Average Energy Allowance (kcal)[b] Per day[c]	RDA for Protein (g/day)
Infants	0.0–0.5	6	13	60	24	108	650	13
	0.5–1.0	9	20	71	28	89	850	14
Children	1–3	13	29	90	35	102	1300	16
	4–6	20	44	112	44	90	1800	24
	7–10	28	62	132	52	70	2000	28
Males	11–14	45	99	157	62	55	2500	45
	15–18	66	145	176	69	45	3000	59
	19–24	72	160	177	70	40	2900	58
	25–50	79	174	176	70	37	2900	63
	51+	77	170	173	68	30	2300	63
Females	11–14	46	101	157	62	47	2200	46
	15–18	55	120	163	64	40	2200	44
	19–24	58	128	164	65	38	2200	46
	25–50	63	138	163	64	36	2200	50
	51+	65	143	160	63	30	1900	50
Pregnant	1st trimester						0	60
	2nd trimester						+300	60
	3rd trimester						+500	60
Lactating	1st 6 months						+500	65
	2nd 6 months						+500	62

Source: National Research Council, Food and Nutrition Board.
[a]Weights and heights represent median values.
[b]In the range of light-to-moderate activity the coefficient of variation equals ±20%.
[c]Figure is rounded.

ROLE OF PROTEIN IN THE BODY

Blood plasma, visceral tissue, and muscle represent the three major sources of body protein. No body "reservoirs" of this macronutrient exist. All protein contributes to tissue structures or exists as important constituents of metabolic, transport, and hormonal systems. Protein constitutes between 12 and 15% of the body mass, but the protein content of different cells varies considerably. A brain cell, for example, consists of only about 10% protein, while red blood cells and muscle cells include up to 20% of their total weight as protein. The protein content of skeletal muscle represents about 65% of the body's total protein. This quantity can increase somewhat with exercise training, depending on the nature of the training regimen, training duration, type of workout, and many other interrelated factors.

Amino acids provide the major building blocks for synthesizing the body's various tissues. They also incorporate nitrogen into RNA and DNA compounds, into the coenzyme electron carriers NAD^+ and FAD (see Chapter 5), into the heme components of the oxygen-binding hemoglobin and myoglobin compounds, into the catecholamine hormones epinephrine and norepinephrine, and into the neurotransmitter serotonin. Amino acids activate vitamins that play a key role in metabolic and physiologic regulation. **Anabolism**

refers to tissue building processes; the amino acid requirement for anabolism can vary considerably. For example, tissue anabolism accounts for about one-third of the protein intake during rapid growth in infancy and childhood. As growth rate declines, so does the percentage of protein retained for anabolic processes. Once a person attains optimal body size and growth stabilizes, a continual turnover still occurs for the tissue's existing protein component.

Proteins serve as primary constituents for plasma membranes and internal cellular material. Proteins in the cell nuclei (nucleoproteins) "supervise" cellular protein synthesis and transmission of hereditary characteristics. Collagenous **structural proteins** compose the hair, skin, nails, bones, tendons, and ligaments. Another classification, **globular proteins**, makes up the nearly 2000 different enzymes that modulate the rate of chemical reactions and regulate catabolism of fats, carbohydrates, and proteins for energy release. Blood plasma also contains the specialized proteins thrombin, fibrin, and fibrinogen required for blood clotting. Within red blood cells, the oxygen-carrying compound hemoglobin contains the large globin protein molecule.

Proteins play a role in regulating the acid–base quality of the body fluids. Buffering neutralizes excess acid metabolites formed during relatively intense exercise. The structural proteins actin and myosin play an essential role in muscle action; these proteins slide past each other as muscles shorten and lengthen during movement. Even in older adults, the body's protein-containing structures "turn over" on a regular basis; normal protein dynamics require adequate protein intake simply to replace the amino acids continually degraded in the turnover process.

DYNAMICS OF PROTEIN METABOLISM

Dietary protein primarily supplies amino acids for the various anabolic processes. In addition, some catabolism of protein for energy takes place. In well-nourished individuals at rest, protein breakdown contributes between 2 and 5% of the body's total energy requirement. During **catabolism**, protein first degrades into its amino acid components. The amino acid molecule then loses its nitrogen (amine group) in the liver by the process of **deamination**. This "freed" nitrogen forms **urea** (H_2NCONH_2), which the body then excretes. The remaining deaminated carbon compound can take one of three routes: it can be *(a)* synthesized to a new amino acid, *(b)* converted to carbohydrate or fat, or *(c)* catabolized directly for energy. Urea formed in deamination (including some ammonia) leaves the body in solution as urine. Excessive protein catabolism promotes fluid loss because urea must be dissolved in water for excretion.

In muscle, enzymes facilitate nitrogen removal from certain amino acids and subsequently pass this nitrogen to other compounds in the biochemical reactions of **transamination** (see Fig. 1.13 *bottom*). An amino group shifts from a donor amino acid to an acceptor acid (keto acid), the acceptor thus becoming a new amino acid. A specific transferase enzyme accelerates the transamination reaction. This allows amino acid formation from non-nitrogen-carrying organic compounds formed in metabolism (e.g., pyruvate). In both deamination and transamination, the resulting carbon skeleton of the nonnitrogenous amino acid residue further degrades during energy metabolism.

Nitrogen Balance

Nitrogen balance exists when nitrogen intake (protein) equals nitrogen excretion. In **positive nitrogen balance**, nitrogen intake exceeds nitrogen excretion, with the additional protein used to synthesize new tissues. Positive nitrogen balance occurs in growing children, during pregnancy, in recovery from illness, and during resistance exercise training, in which overloading muscle cells promotes protein synthesis. The body does not develop a protein reserve as it does with fat storage in adipose tissue or as carbohydrate stored as liver and muscle glycogen. Individuals who consume adequate protein have a higher content of muscle and liver protein than individuals fed a subpar, low-protein diet. Also, labeling of protein (injecting protein with one or several of its carbon atoms "tagged") shows that some proteins become

recruited for energy metabolism. Other proteins in neural and connective tissues remain relatively "fixed" as cellular constituents; they cannot be mobilized without harming tissue functions.

Greater nitrogen output than nitrogen intake (**negative nitrogen balance**) indicates protein use for energy and possible encroachment on amino acids, primarily from skeletal muscle. Interestingly, a negative nitrogen balance occurs even when protein intake exceeds the recommended standard if the body catabolizes protein because it lacks other energy nutrients in the diet. For example, an individual engaged in arduous training may consume adequate or excess protein yet be deficient in energy as carbohydrate or lipid. In this scenario, protein becomes a primary energy fuel. This creates a negative protein (nitrogen) balance that reduces the body's lean tissue mass. The protein-sparing role of dietary lipid and carbohydrate discussed previously becomes important during tissue growth periods and the high-energy output requirements of intensive exercise training. Also, starvation produces the greatest negative nitrogen balance. *Starvation diets, or diets with reduced carbohydrate and/or energy, deplete glycogen reserves, which might trigger a protein deficiency with accompanying lean tissue loss.*

The Alanine–Glucose Cycle

Some body proteins do not readily metabolize for energy, but muscle proteins are more labile. Amino acids participate in energy metabolism when the exercise energy demand increases.[18,20,118] FIGURE 1.15 shows that alanine release (and possibly glutamine) from active leg muscles increases in proportion to exercise intensity.

A model indicates that alanine *indirectly* serves the energy requirements of exercise. Active skeletal muscle synthesizes alanine during transamination. This occurs from the glucose intermediate pyruvate (with nitrogen derived in part from the amino acid leucine). Alanine deaminates after it leaves the muscle and enters the liver. Gluconeogenesis then converts the remaining carbon skeleton of alanine to glucose, which then enters the blood for use by active muscle. The residual carbon fragment from the amino acid that formed alanine oxidizes for energy within the muscle cell. FIGURE 1.16 summarizes the sequence of the **alanine-glucose cycle**. After 4 hours of continuous light exercise, the liver's output of alanine-derived glucose accounts for about 45% of the liver's total glucose release. *During prolonged exercise, the alanine–glucose cycle generates from 10 to 15% of the total exercise energy requirement.* Regular exercise training enhances the liver's synthesis of glucose using the carbon skeletons of noncarbohydrate compounds. This facilitates blood glucose homeostasis during prolonged exercise. Chapters 5 and 7 discuss protein's role as a potential energy fuel in exercise and the protein requirements of physically active people.

Figure 1.15. Dynamics of alanine release from leg muscle during 40 minutes of exercise. Alanine release nearly doubles during mild exercise compared with resting conditions. During the most intense aerobic exercise the alanine flow from the active legs exceeds the resting value by more than sixfold. (From Felig P, Wahren J. Amino acid metabolism in exercising man. J Clin Invest 1971;50:2073.)

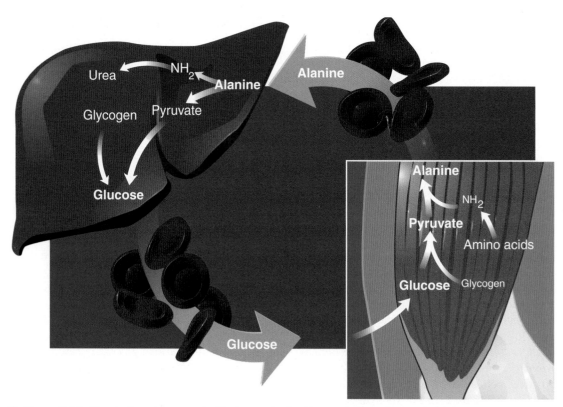

Figure 1.16. The alanine–glucose cycle. Alanine, synthesized in muscle from glucose-derived pyruvate via transamination, is released into the blood and converts to glucose and urea in the liver. Glucose release into the blood coincides with its subsequent delivery to the muscle for energy. During exercise, increased production and output of alanine from muscle helps to maintain blood glucose for nervous system and active muscle needs. Exercise training augments processes of hepatic gluconeogenesis. (From Felig P, Wahren J. Amino acid metabolism in exercising man. J Clin Invest 1971;50: 2703.)

Summary

1. Proteins differ chemically from lipids and carbohydrates because they contain nitrogen in addition to sulfur, phosphorus, and iron.

2. Proteins form from subunits called amino acids. The body requires 20 different amino acids, each containing an amino radical (NH_2) and an organic acid radical called a carboxyl group (COOH). Amino acids contain a side-chain that defines the amino acid's particular chemical characteristics.

3. An almost infinite number of possible protein structures can form because of the diverse combinations possible for the 20 different amino acids.

4. The body cannot synthesize 8 of the 20 amino acids. These are the essential amino acids that must be consumed in the diet.

5. Animal and plant cells contain protein. Proteins with all the essential amino acids are called complete (higher-quality) proteins; the others are called incomplete (lower-quality) proteins. Examples of higher-quality, complete proteins include animal proteins in eggs, milk, cheese, meat, fish, and poultry.

6. The diets of many physically active persons and competitive athletes consists predominantly of nutrients from plant sources. Consuming a variety of plant foods provides all of the essential amino acids because each food source contains a different quality and quantity of them.

7. Proteins provide the building blocks for synthesizing cellular material during anabolic processes. Amino acids also contribute their "carbon skeletons" for energy metabolism.

8. The RDA, the recommended quantity for nutrient intake, represents a liberal yet safe level of excess to meet the nutritional needs of practically all healthy persons. For adults, the protein RDA equals 0.83 g per kg of body mass.

9. Proteins in nervous and connective tissue generally do not participate in energy metabolism. The amino acid alanine, however, plays a key role in providing carbohydrate fuel via gluconeogenesis during prolonged exercise. During strenuous exercise of long duration, the alanine–glucose cycle accounts for up to 40 to 50% of the liver's glucose release.

10. Protein catabolism accelerates during exercise because carbohydrate reserves deplete. Thus, individuals who train vigorously on a regular basis must maintain optimal levels of muscle and liver glycogen to minimize lean tissue loss and deterioration in performance.

11. Regular exercise training enhances the liver's capacity to synthesize glucose from the carbon skeletons of noncarbohydrate compounds.

TEST YOUR KNOWLEDGE **ANSWERS**

1. False—Carbohydrates do not contain nitrogen, only carbon, oxygen, and hydrogen atoms. Protein is the only macronutrient to contain nitrogen.

2. True—Glucose can be formed by gluconeogenesis, a process that synthesizes glucose (primarily in the liver) from carbon skeletons of specific amino acids as well as from nonprotein sources like glycerol, pyruvate, and lactate.

3. False—Fibers exist exclusively in plants; they make up the structure of leaves, stems, roots, seeds, and fruit coverings. Because of its resistance to digestive enzymes, fiber cannot be absorbed by the body and used for energy. However, fiber does retain considerable water as it passes through the digestive tract and thus gives "bulk" to the food residues in the large intestine, often increasing stool weight and volume by 40 to 100%. This aids gastrointestinal function.

4. False—For regular exercisers, carbohydrates should supply about 60% of total daily calories (400–600 g), predominantly as unrefined, fiber-rich fruits, grains, and vegetables.

5. False—About 25% of the population produces excessive insulin in response to an intake of rapidly absorbed carbohydrates (high glycemic rating). These insulin-resistant individuals increase their risk for obesity if they consistently eat such a diet. Weight gain occurs because abnormal quantities of insulin *(a)* promote glucose entry into cells and *(b)* facilitate the liver's conversion of glucose to triacylglycerol, which then becomes stored as body fat in adipose tissue. Also, excess calories, regardless of dietary source, contribute to obesity.

6. False—Carbohydrate and protein each contains 4.0 kcal per gram. In contrast, each gram of lipid contains more than twice the amount at 9.0 kcal.

7. False—Cholesterol, the most widely known derived lipid, exists only in animal tissue; it is never found in plants of any origin.

8. True—True vegetarians or vegans consume nutrients from only two sources, the plant kingdom and dietary supplements. This places vegans at a somewhat greater risk for inadequate energy and nutrient intake because they eliminate meat and dairy products from the diet and increasingly rely on foods relatively low in energy, quality protein, and certain micronutrients. Nutritional diversity remains the key for these men and women. For example, a vegan diet provides all the essential amino acids if 60% of protein intake comes from grain products, 35% from legumes, and 5% from green, leafy vegetables. Vitamin B$_{12}$, found only in the animal kingdom, must be obtained in supplement form.

9. False—For athletes, muscle mass does not increase simply by eating high-protein foods or special amino acid mixtures. If lean tissue synthesis resulted from extra protein, then muscle mass would increase tremendously for individuals on the typical Western diet. For example, consuming an extra 100 g (400 kcal) of protein daily theoretically translates into a daily 500-g (1.1-lb) increase in muscle mass. This obviously does not happen. A proper resistance training program combined with a well-balanced diet increases muscle mass. Excessive dietary protein is used directly for energy or recycled as components of other molecules including fat stored in the subcutaneous adipose tissue depots.

10. False—On average, 0.83 g of protein per kg body mass represents the recommended daily intake for both women and men. For a 90-kg man, the total daily protein requirement equals 75 g (90 × 0.83) while a 50-kg woman requires 41.5 g (50 × 0.83). The protein RDA even holds for overweight persons; it includes a reserve of about 25% to account for individual differences in protein requirement for about 98% of the population.

References

1. Adler AJ, Holub BJ. Effect of garlic and fish-oil supplementation on serum lipid and lipoprotein concentrations in hypercholesterolemic men. Am J Clin Nutr 1997;67:445.
2. Agus MS, et al. Dietary composition and physiologic adaptations to energy restriction. Am J Clin Nutr 2000;71:901.
3. Albert CM, et al. Fish consumption and risk of sudden cardiac death. JAMA 1998;279:23.
4. Albert CM, et al. Blood levels of long-chain n-3 fatty acids and risk of sudden death. N Engl J Med 2002;346:1113.
5. Anderson JW, et al. Meta-analysis of the effects of soy protein intake on serum lipids. N Engl J Med 1995;333:276.
6. Anderson JW, et al. Cholesterol-lowering effects of psyllium intake adjunctive to diet therapy in men and women with hypercholesterolemia: meta-analysis of 8 controlled trials. Am J Clin Nutr 2000;71:472.
7. Andrews TC, et al. Effect of cholesterol reduction on myocardial ischemia in patients with coronary disease. Circulation 1997;95:324.
8. Aro A, et al. Stearic acid, *trans* fatty acids, and dairy fat: effects on serum and lipoprotein lipids, apolipoproteins, lipoprotein (a), and lipid transfer proteins in healthy subjects. Am J Clin Nutr 1997;65:1419.
9. ASCN/AIN Task Force on Trans Fatty Acids: position paper on trans fatty acids. Am J Clin Nutr 1996;63:663.
10. Barnard RJ, et al. Diet-induced insulin resistance precedes other aspects of the metabolic syndrome. J Appl Physiol 1998;84:1311.
11. Bingham SA, et al. Dietary fibre in food and protection against colorectal cancer in the European Prospective Investigation into Cancer and Nutrition (EPIC): an observational study. Lancet. 2003;361:1496.
12. Braaten JT, et al. Oat B-glucan reduces blood cholesterol concentration in hypercholesterolemic subjects. Eur J Clin Nutr 1994;48:465.
13. Brown I, et al. Cholesterol-lowering effects of dietary fiber: a meta-analysis. Am J Clin Nutr 1999;69:30.
14. Burkitt D. Dietary Fiber. In: Medical applications of clinical nutrition. New Canaan, CT: Keats, 1983.
15. Buyken AE, et al. Glycemic index in the diet of European outpatients with type 1 diabetes: relations to glycated hemoglobin and serum lipids. Am J Clin Nutr 2001;73:574.
16. Caggiula AW, Mustak VA. Effects of dietary fat and fatty acids on coronary artery disease risk and total and lipoprotein cholesterol concentrations: epidemiologic studies. Am J Clin Nutr 1997;65(suppl):1597S.
17. Carraro F, et al. Effect of exercise and recovery on muscle protein synthesis in human subjects. Am J Physiol 1990;259:E470.
18. Carraro F, et al. Alanine kinetics in humans during low-intensity exercise. Med Sci Sports Exerc 1994;26:48.
19. Chandalia M, et al. Beneficial effects of high dietary fiber intake in patients with type 2 diabetes mellitus. N Engl J Med 2000;342:1392.
20. Christensen HN. Role of amino acid transport and counter transport in nutrition and metabolism. Physiol Rev 1990;70:43.
21. Connor WE. Do the n-3 fatty acids from fish prevent deaths from cardiovascular disease? Am J Clin Nutr 1997;66:188.
22. Connor WE. Importance of n-3 fatty acids in health and disease. Am J Clin Nutr 2000;71 (suppl):171S.
23. Conner WE, et al. The plasma lipids, lipoproteins, and diet of the Tarahumara Indians of Mexico. Am J Clin Nutr 1978;31:1131.
24. Consolazio CF, et al. Protein metabolism during intensive physical training in the young adult. Am J Clin Nutr 1975;28:29.
25. Daly ME, et al. Dietary carbohydrates and insulin sensitivity: a review of the evidence and clinical implications. Am J Clin Nutr 1997;66:1072.
26. Daviglus ML, et al. Fish consumption and the 30-year risk of fatal myocardial infarction. N Engl J Med 1997;336:1046.
27. Davy BM, et al. High-fiber oat cereal compared with wheat cereal consumption favorably alters LDL-cholesterol subclass and particle numbers in middle-aged and older men. Am J Clin Nutr 2002;76:351.
28. Dewailly E, et al. N-3 Fatty acids and cardiovascular disease risk factors among the Inuit of Nunavik. Am J Clin Nutr 2001;74:474.
29. Dietschy JM. Theoretical considerations of what regulates low-density-lipoprotein and high-density-lipoprotein cholesterol. Am J Clin Nutr 1997;65(suppl):1581S.
30. Dreon DM, et al. Change in dietary saturated fat intake is correlated with change in mass of large low-density-lipoprotein particles in men. Am J Clin Nutr 1998;67:828.
31. Drexel H, et al. Plasma triglycerides and three lipoprotein cholesterol fractions are independent predictors of the extent of coronary arteriosclerosis. Circulation 1994;90:2230.
32. Fernandez ML, et al. Guar gum effects on plasma low-density lipoprotein and hepatic cholesterol metabolism in guinea pigs fed low-and high-cholesterol diets: a dose-response study. Am J Clin Nutr 1995;61:127.
33. Food and Nutrition Board, Institute of Medicine. Dietary reference intakes: a risk assessment model for establishing upper intake levels for nutrients. Washington, DC: National Academy Press, 1998.
34. Food and Nutrition Board, Institute of Medicine. Dietary reference intakes for energy, carbohydrates, fiber, fat, protein and amino acids. Washington, DC: National Academy Press, 2002.
35. Food and Nutrition Board. Recommended Dietary Allowances. 11th ed. Washington, DC: National Academy of Sciences, 1999.
36. Ford ES, et al. Prevalence of the metabolic syndrome among US adults. Findings from the Third National Health and Nutrition Examination Survey. JAMA 2002;287:356.
37. Frick MH, et al. Helsinki Heart Study: primary-prevention trial with gemfibrozil in middle-aged men with dyslipidemia. Safety of treatment, changes in risk factors, and incidence of coronary heart disease. N Engl J Med 1987;317:3217.
38. Friedman, MI. Fuel partitioning and food intake. Am J Clin Nutr 1998;67(suppl):513S.

39. Fuchs CF, et al. Dietary fiber and risk of colorectal cancer and adenoma in women N Engl J Med 1999;440:169.

40. Fung TT, et al. Whole-grain intake and risk of type-2 diabetes: a prospective study in men. Am J Clin Nutr 2002;76:535.

41. Grundy SM, Denke MA. Dietary influences of serum lipids and lipoproteins. Am J Clin Nutr 1994;60 (suppl):986S.

42. Harris WS. Fish oils and plasma lipid and lipoprotein metabolism: a critical review. J Lipid Res 1989;30:785.

43. Heyward VH, et al. Anthropometric, body composition and nutritional profiles of bodybuilders during training. J Appl Sports Sci Rev 1989;3:22.

44. Hickson JF, Wolinsky I. Research directions in protein nutrition for athletes. In: Wolinsky I, Hickson JF Jr, eds. Nutrition in exercise and sport. Boca Raton, FL: CRC Press, 1994.

45. Hickson JF, et al. Nutritional profile of football athletes eating from a training table. Nutr Res 1987;7:27.

46. Hickson JF, et al. Repeated days of body building exercise do not enhance urinary nitrogen excretions from untrained young males. Nutr Res 1990;10:723.

47. Howarth NC, et al. Dietary fiber and weight regulation. Nutr Res 2001;59:129.

48. Howell WM, et al. Plasma lipid and lipoprotein responses to dietary fat and cholesterol: a meta-analysis. Am J Clin Nutr 1997;65:1747.

49. Hu FB, et al. Dietary fat intake and the risk of coronary heart disease in women. N Engl J Med 1997;337:1491.

50. Hu FB, et al. Fish and omega-3 fatty acid intake on risk of coronary heart disease in women. 2002;287:1815.

51. Iribarren C, et al. Serum total cholesterol and mortality: compound factors and risk modification in Japanese-American men. JAMA 1995;273:1926.

52. Iso H, et al. Intake of fish and omega-3 fatty acids and risk of stroke in women. JAMA 2001;285:304.

53. Jenkins DJ, et al. Effects of high- and low-isoflavone soyfoods on blood lipids, oxidized LDL, homocysteine, and blood pressure in hyperlipidemic men and women. Am J Clin Nutr 2002;76:365.

54. Jenkins DJ, et al. Soluble fiber intake at a dose approved by the US Food and Drug Administration for a claim of health benefits: serum lipid risk factors for cardiovascular disease assessed in a randomized controlled crossover trial. Am J Clin Nutr 2002;75:834.

55. Kinosian B, et al. Cholesterol and coronary heart disease: predicting risk by levels and ratios. Ann Intern Med 1994;121:641.

56. Kirby RW, et al. Oat-bran intake selectively lowers serum low-density lipoprotein cholesterol concentrations of hypercholesterolemic men. Am J Clin Nutr 1981;34:824.

57. Klag MJ, et al. Serum cholesterol in young men and subsequent cardiovascular disease. N Engl J Med 1993;328:313.

58. Krauss RM, et al. AHA dietary guidelines revision 2000: a statement for health care professionals from the Nutrition Committee of the American Heart Association. Circulation 2000;102:2284.

59. Krauss WE, et al. Effect of the amount and intensity of exercise on plasma lipoproteins. N Engl J Med 2002;347:1483.

60. Laidlaw M, Holub BJ. Effects of supplementation with fish-oil derived n-3 fatty acids and γ-linoleic acid on circulating plasma lipids and fatty acid profiles in women. Am J Clin Nutr 2003;77:37.

61. Lakka HM, et al. The metabolic syndrome and total and cardiovascular disease mortality in middle-aged men. JAMA 2002;288:2709.

62. Lamartiniere CA. Protection against breast cancer with genistein: a component of soy. Am J Clin Nutr 2000;73:172.

63. Lambert EV, et al. Enhanced endurance in trained cyclists during moderate intensity exercise following 2 weeks adaptation to a high fat diet. Eur J Appl Physiol 1994;69:287.

64. Lauber RP, Sheard NF. The American Heart Association dietary guidelines for 2000: a summary report. Nutr Rev 2001;59:298.

65. Lemaitre RN, et al. n-3 Poly unsaturated fatty acids, fatal ischemic heart disease, and nonfatal myocardial infarction in obese adults. Am J Clin Nutr 2003;77:319.

66. LeMura LM, et al. Lipid and lipoprotein profiles, cardiovascular fitness, body composition, and diet during and after resistance, aerobic and combination training in young women. Eur J Appl Physiol 2000;82:451.

67. Lipid Research Clinics Program: The Lipid Research Clinics Coronary Primary Prevention Trial results. I. Reduction in incidence of coronary heart disease. JAMA 1984;251:351.

68. Lipid Research Clinics Program: The Lipid Research Clinics Coronary Primary Prevention Trial results. II. The relationship of reduction in incidence of coronary heart disease to cholesterol lowering. JAMA 1984;251:365.

69. Liu S, et al. A prospective study of dietary glycemic load, carbohydrate intake, and risk of coronary heart disease in US women. Am J Clin Nutr 2000;71:1455.

70. Liu S, et al. Dietary glycemic load assessed by food-frequency questionnaire in relation to plasma high-density-lipoprotein cholesterol and fasting triacylglycerols in postmenopausal women. Am J Clin Nutr 2001;73:560.

71. Liu S, et al. Is intake of breakfast cereals related to total and cause-specific mortality in men? Am J Clin Nutr 2003;77:594.

72. Ludwig DS, et al. Dietary fiber, weight gain, and cardiovascular disease risk factors in young adults. JAMA 1999;275:486.

73. Marques-Lopes I, et al. Postprandial de novo lipogenesis and metabolic changes induced by a high-carbohydrate, low-fat meal in lean and overweight men. Am J Clin Nutr 2001;73:253.

74. McArdle WD, et al. Thermal adjustment to cold-water exposure in resting men and women. J Appl Physiol 1984;56:1565.

75. McIntosh M, Miller C. A diet containing food rich in soluble and insoluble fiber improves glycemic control and reduces hyperlipidemia among patients with type 2 diabetes. Nutr Revs 2001;59:52.

76. McKeown NM, et al. Whole-grain intake is favorably associated with metabolic risk factors for type 2 diabetes and cardiovascular disease in the Framingham Offspring Study. Am J Clin Nutr 2002;76:390.

77. Mensink RP, et al. Effects of dietary fatty acids and carbohydrates on the ratio of serum total to HDL cholesterol and on serum lipids and apolipoproteins: a meta-analysis of 60 controlled trials. Am J Clin Nutr 2003;77:1146.

78. Meridith CN, et al. Dietary protein requirements and body protein metabolism in endurance-trained men. J Appl Physiol 1989;66: 2850.

79. Meyer KA, et al. Carbohydrates, dietary fiber, and incident type 2 diabetes in older women. Am J Clin Nutr 2000;71:921.

80. Miller VC, et al. Adaptations to high-fat diet that increase exercise endurance in male rats. J Appl Physiol 1984;56:78.

81. Mittendorfer B, Sidossis L. Mechanism for the increase in plasma triacylglycerol concentration after consumption of short-term, high-carbohydrate diets. Am J Clin Nutr 2001;73:892.

82. Montonen J, et al. Whole-grain and fiber intake and the incidence of type 2 diabetes. Am J Clin Nutr 2003;77:622.

83. Morris KL, Zemel MB. Glycemic index, cardiovascular disease, and obesity. Nutr Revs 1999;55:273.

84. Mozaffarian D, et al. Cereal, fruit, and vegetable fiber intake and risk of cardiovascular disease in elderly individuals. JAMA 2003;289:1659.

85. National Institutes of Health. Third report of the National Cholesterol Education Program Expert Panel on Detection, Evaluation, and Treatment of High Blood Cholesterol in Adults (Adult Treatment Panel III). Bethesda, MD: National Institutes of Health; 2001. NIH publication 01-3670.

86. Nestle P, et al. The n-3 fatty acids eicosapentaenoic and docosahaenoic acid increase systemic arterial compliance in humans. Am J Clin Nutr 2002;76:326.

87. NIH Consensus Conference. Triglyceride, high-density lipoprotein, and coronary heart disease. JAMA 1993;269:505.

88. Noakes M, Clifton PM. Changes in plasma lipids and other cardiovascular risk factors during 3 energy-restricted diets differing in total fat and fatty acid composition. Am J Clin Nutr 2000;71:706.

89. Ornish D, et al. Intensive lifestyle changes for reversal of coronary heart disease. JAMA 1998;280:2001.

90. Parks EJ, Hellerstein MK. Carbohydrate induced hypertriacylglycerolemia: historical perspective and review of biological mechanisms. Am J Clin Nutr 2000;71:412.

91. Peters U, et al. Dietary fibre and colorectal adenoma in a colorectal cancer early detection programme. Lancet. 2003;361:1491.

92. Poppitt SD, et al. Long-term effects of ad libitum low-fat, high-carbohydrate diets on body weight and serum lipids in overweight subjects with metabolic syndrome. Am J Clin Nutr 2002;75:11.

93. Pugh LGCE, Edholm OG. The physiology of channel swimmers. Lancet 1955;2:761.

94. Raeini-Sarjaz M, et al. Comparison of the effect of dietary fat restriction with that of energy restriction on human lipid metabolism Am J Clin Nutr 2001;73:262.

95. Rimm EB, et al. Vegetable, fruit, and cereal fiber intake and risk of coronary heart disease among men. JAMA 1996;275:447.

96. Roche HM, et al. Effect of long-term olive oil dietary intervention on postprandial triacylglycerol and factor VII metabolism. Am J Clin Nutr 1998;68:552.

97. Salmerón JE, et al. Dietary fiber, glycemic load, and risk of non-insulin-dependent diabetes mellitus in women. JAMA 1997;277:472.

98. Salmerón J.E, et al. Dietary fat intake and risk of type 2 diabetes in women. Am J Clin Nutr 2001;73:1019.

99. Schaefer EJ. Lipoproteins, nutrition, and heart disease. Am J Clin Nutr 2002;75:191.

100. Shahar E, et al. Dietary n-3 polyunsaturated fatty acids and smoking-related chronic obstructive pulmonary disease. N Engl J Med 1994;331:228.

101. Simonen P, et al. Introducing a new component of the metabolic syndrome; low cholesterol absorption. Am J Clin Nutr 2000;72:82.

102. Sims EAH, Danforth E Jr. Expenditure and storage of energy in man (perspective). J Clin Invest 1987;79:1019.

103. Stamler J, et al. Is the relationship between serum cholesterol and risk of premature death from coronary heart disease continuous or graded? Findings in 356,222 primary screenees of the Multiple Risk Factor Intervention Trial (Mr. Fit). JAMA 1986;256:2823.

104. Starc TJ, et al. Greater dietary intake of simple carbohydrate is associated with lower concentrations of high-density-lipoprotein cholesterol in hypercholesterolemic children. Am J Clin Nutr 1998;67:1147.

105. Stark KD, et al. Effect of fish-oil concentrate on serum lipids in postmenopausal women receiving and not receiving hormone replacement therapy in a placebo-controlled, double-blind trial. Am J Clin Nutr 2000;72:389.

106. Stefanick ML, et al. Effects of diet and exercise in men and postmenopausal women with low levels of HDL cholesterol and high levels of LDL cholesterol. N Engl J Med 1998;339:12.

107. Tarnopolsky MA, et al. Influence of protein intake and training status on nitrogen balance and lean body mass. J Appl Physiol 1988;64:187.

108. Tarnopolsky MA, et al. Effect of bodybuilding exercise on protein requirements. Can J Sport Sci 1990;15:225.

109. Teixeira SR, et al. Effects of feeding 4 levels of soy protein for 3 and 6 wk on blood lipids and apolipoproteins in moderately hypercholesterolemic men. Am J Clin Nutr 2000;71:1077.

110. Terry PD, et al. Intakes of fish and marine fatty acids and the risk of cancers of the breast and prostate and of other hormone-related cancers: a review of the epidemiologic evidence. Am J Clin Nutr 2003;77:532.

111. Tiollotson JL, et al. Relation of dietary carbohydrates to blood lipids in the special intervention and usual care groups in the Multiple Risk Factor Intervention Trial. Am J Clin Nutr 1997;65(suppl):3214S.

112. Trumbo P, et al. Dietary reference intakes: vitamin A, vitamin K, arsenic, boron, chromium, iodine, manganese, molybdenum, nickel, silicon, vanadium, and zinc. J Am Diet Assoc 2001;101:294.

113. Van Wijk JPH, et al. Effects of different nutrient intakes on daytime triacylglycerolemia in healthy, normolipemic, free-living men. Am J Clin Nutr 2001;74:171.

114. Vidon C, et al. Effects of isoenergetic high-carbohydrate compared with high-fat diets on human cholesterol synthesis and expression of key regulatory genes of cholesterol metabolism. Am J Clin Nutr 2001;73:878.

115. Wangen KE, et al. Soy isoflavones improve plasma lipids in normocholesterolemic and mildly hypercholesterolemic post menopausal women. Am J Clin Nutr 2001;73:225.

116. Weggemans RM, et al. Dietary cholesterol from eggs increases the ratio of total cholesterol to high-density lipoprotein cholesterol in humans: a meta-analysis. Am J Clin Nutr 2001;73:885.

117. Willett WC, Ascherio A. Trans fatty acids: are the effects only marginal? Am J Public Health 1994;84:722.

118. Williams BD, et al. Alanine and glutamine kinetics at rest and during exercise. Med Sci Sports Exerc 1998;30:1053.

119. Williams PT. High-density lipoprotein cholesterol and other risk factors for coronary heart disease in female runners. N Engl J Med 1996;334:1298.

120. Wolfe RR. Metabolic interactions between glucose and fatty acids in humans. Am J Clin Nutr 1998;67(suppl):519S.

121. Wolk A, et al. Long-term intake of dietary fiber and decreased risk of coronary heart disease among women. JAMA 1999;281:1998.

122. Wynder EL, et al. High fiber intake: indicator of a healthy lifestyle. JAMA 1996;275:486.

Additional Readings

Ardern CI, et al. Race and sex similarities in exercise-induced changes in blood lipids and fatness. Med Sci Sports Exerc 2004;36:161.

Barr SI, Rideout CA. Nutritional considerations for vegetarian athletes. Nutrition 2004;20:696.

Boisseau N, et al. Protein intake and nitrogen balance in male non-active adolescents and soccer players. Eur J Appl Physiol 2002;88:288.

Burke DG, et al. Effect of creatine and weight training on muscle creatine and performance in vegetarians. Med Sci Sports Exerc 2003;35:1946.

Collaku A, et al. A genome-wide linkage scan for dietary energy and nutrient intakes: The Health, Risk Factors, Exercise Training, and Genetics (HERITAGE) Family Study. Am J Clin Nutr 2004;79:881.

Hinton PS, et al. Nutrient intakes and dietary behaviors of male and female collegiate athletes. Int J Sport Nutr Exerc Metab 2004;14:389.

Luca-Moretti M, et al. Master amino acid pattern as substitute for dietary proteins during a weight-loss diet to achieve the body's nitrogen balance equilibrium with essentially no calories. Adv Ther 2003;20:282.

Nawrocki A, Gorski J. Effect of plasma free fatty acid concentration on the content and composition of the free fatty acid fraction in rat skeletal muscles. Horm Metab Res 2004;36:601.

Phillips SM. Protein requirements and supplementation in strength sports. Nutrition 2004;20:689.

Wang JS, Chow SE. Effects of exercise training and detraining on oxidized low-density lipoprotein-potentiated platelet function in men. Arch Phys Med Rehabil 2004;85:1531.

Wells AM, et al. Comparisons of vegetarian and beef-containing diets on hematological indexes and iron stores during a period of resistive training in older men. J Am Diet Assoc 2003;103:594.

Chapter

2

The Micronutrients and Water

TEST YOUR KNOWLEDGE

Answer these ten statements about vitamins, minerals, and water. Use the scoring key at the end of the chapter to check your results. Repeat this test after you have read the chapter and compare your results.

1. **T F** Vitamin supplementation above the Recommended Dietary Allowance (RDA) level does not improve exercise performance.

2. **T F** From a survival perspective, food is of greater importance than water.

3. **T F** Achieving the recommended intake of "major" minerals is more crucial to good health than achieving the recommended intake of "trace" minerals.

4. **T F** Plants provide a better source of minerals than do animal sources.

5. **T F** Sedentary adults require about 3.785 L (1 gal) of water each day to maintain optimal body functions.

6. **T F** Decreasing sodium in the diet represents the only important lifestyle approach to lowering high blood pressure.

7. **T F** None of the 13 vitamins required by the body is toxic if consumed in excess.

8. **T F** A telltale symptom of iron deficiency anemia is soft and brittle bones.

9. **T F** Stationary cycling is an excellent exercise to promote bone health.

10. **T F** Pharmacologic approaches to treating borderline hypertension are more effective than dietary approaches.

Effective regulation of all metabolic processes requires a delicate blending of food nutrients in the watery medium of the cell. Of special significance in this regard are the **micronutrients**—the small quantities of vitamins and minerals that facilitate energy transfer and tissue synthesis. For example, the body requires each year only about 350 g (12 oz) of vitamins from the 862 kg (1896 lb) of food consumed by the average adult who generally consumes fairly well balanced meals. With proper nutrition from a variety of food sources, the physically active person or competitive athlete need not consume vitamin and mineral supplements; such practices usually prove physiologically and economically wasteful. Furthermore, some micronutrients consumed in excess can adversely affect health and safety.

 # Vitamins

THE NATURE OF VITAMINS

Vitamins achieved importance centuries before scientists isolated and classified them. The Greek physician Hippocrates advocated ingesting liver to cure night blindness. While he did not know the reason for the cure, we now know that vitamin A, which helps to prevent night blindness, occurs plentifully in this organ meat. In 1897, Dutch physician

Christiaan Eijkman (1858–1930; shared the 1929 Nobel Prize in Physiology or Medicine for his discovery of the antineuritic vitamin) observed that a regular diet of polished rice caused beriberi in fowl, while adding thiamine-rich rice polishings to table scraps cured the disease. In the early 19th century, adding oranges and lemons to the diet of British sailors paved the way for eradicating the dreaded disease scurvy because of the protective effects of the vitamin C contained in the fruits. In 1932, scientific experiments demonstrated that ascorbic acid (technically a liver metabolite) was essentially identical in function to vitamin C. Interestingly, most animal species synthesize ascorbic acid except for man, guinea pigs, and certain monkeys; thus, these species must consume vitamin C in their diet.

The formal discovery of vitamins, initially called "vital amines," revealed they were organic substances needed by the body in minute amounts. Vitamins, their amine role having been discredited, have no particular chemical structure in common and often are considered accessory nutrients because they neither supply energy nor contribute substantially to body mass. Except for vitamin D, the body cannot manufacture vitamins; hence, the diet or supplementation must supply them.

Some foods contain an abundant quantity of vitamins. For example, the green leaves and roots of plants manufacture vitamins during photosynthesis. Animals obtain vitamins from the plants, seeds, grains, and fruits they eat or from the meat of other animals that previously consumed these foods. Several vitamins, notably vitamins A and D, niacin, and folate, become activated from their inactive precursor or **provitamin** form. **Carotenes**, the best known of the provitamins, comprise the yellow and yellow–orange pigment-precursors of vitamin A that give color to vegetables (carrots, squash, corn, pumpkins) and fruits (apricots, and peaches).

KINDS OF VITAMINS

Thirteen different vitamins have been isolated, analyzed, classified, and synthesized and had recommended dietary allowance (RDA) levels established. Vitamins are classified as either **fat soluble** or **water soluble**. The fat-soluble vitamins include vitamins A, D, E, and K. The water-soluble vitamins are vitamin C and the B-complex vitamins (based on their common source distribution and common functional relationships): thiamine (B_1), riboflavin (B_2), pyridoxine (B_6), niacin (nicotinic acid), pantothenic acid, biotin, folic acid (folacin or folate, its active form in the body), and cobalamin (B_{12}).

Fat-Soluble Vitamins

Fat-soluble vitamins dissolve and are stored in the body's fatty tissues, without a need to consume them daily. In fact, years may elapse before symptoms surface of a fat-soluble vitamin insufficiency. The liver stores vitamins A and D, whereas vitamin E distributes throughout the body's fatty tissues. Vitamin K is stored only in small amounts, mainly in the liver. Dietary lipid provides the source of fat-soluble vitamins; these vitamins, transported as part of lipoproteins in the lymph, travel to the liver for dispersion to various tissues. Consuming a true "fat-free" diet could certainly accelerate development of a fat-soluble vitamin insufficiency.

Fat-soluble vitamins should not be consumed in excess without medical supervision. Toxic reactions from excessive fat-soluble vitamin intake generally occur at a lower multiple of recommended intakes than those from water-soluble vitamins. For example, a daily moderate-to-large excess of vitamin A (as retinol but not in carotene form) and vitamin D produce serious toxic effects. Children are particularly susceptible; excess vitamin D, for example, can cause excessive calcium deposits and mental retardation. Consuming vitamin A in amounts not much greater than recommended values (RDA of 700 $\mu g \cdot d^{-1}$ for females and 900 $\mu g \cdot d^{-1}$ for males) precipitates bone fractures later in life. Also, high doses consumed early in pregnancy have been linked to a greater risk of birth defects. In young children, a large vitamin A accumulation (called hypervitaminosis A) causes irritability, swelling of the bones, weight loss, and dry itchy skin. In adults, symptoms can include nausea, headache, drowsiness, hair loss, diarrhea, and loss of calcium from bones, causing osteoporosis and increased risk of fractures.[103] An excess of vitamin A inhibits cells that produce new bone, stimulates cells that break down existing bone, and negatively affects the action of Vitamin D, which helps the body maintain normal calcium levels. Discontinuing high vitamin A intakes reverses its adverse effects. Kidney damage can result from a regular excess of vitamin D. Although "overdoses" from vitamins E and K are rare, intakes above the recommended levels yield no health benefits.

Water-Soluble Vitamins

The water-soluble vitamins act largely as **coenzymes**— small molecules combined with a larger protein compound (apoenzyme) to form an active enzyme that accelerates the interconversion of chemical compounds. Coenzymes participate directly in chemical reactions; when the reaction runs its course, coenzymes remain intact and participate in further reactions. Water-soluble vitamins, like their fat-soluble counterparts, consist of carbon, hydrogen, and oxygen atoms. They also contain nitrogen and metal ions including iron, molybdenum, copper, sulfur, and cobalt.

Water-soluble vitamins disperse readily in body fluids without the need to store them in the tissues to any appreciable extent. If the diet regularly contains less than 50% of the recommended values for these vitamins, then marginal deficiencies could develop within about 4 weeks. Generally, even an excess intake of water-soluble vitamins becomes voided in the urine. Water-soluble vitamins exert their influence for 8 to 14 hours after ingestion; thereafter, their potency decreases. For maximum benefit, for example, one should consume vitamin C (recommended daily intake at 75 mg for women and 90 mg for men) in food or supplement form at least every 12 hours. Some researchers recommend that the RDA for vitamin C for healthy people be increased to 200 mg (2–4 daily servings of fruits and 3–5 servings of vegetables) to ensure optimal cellular saturation.[85] TABLE 2.1 lists excellent dietary sources of vitamin C. Sweating, even during extreme physical activity, probably produces only a negligible loss of water-soluble vitamins.[11,56]

Table 2.1 GOOD DIETARY SOURCES OF VITAMIN C		
Food	Serving	Vitamin C (mg)
Vegetables		
Broccoli	1/2 cup, chopped, cooked	49
Brussels sprouts	1/2 cup, cooked	48
Cauliflower	1/2 cup, cooked	34
Kale	1/2 cup, chopped, cooked	27
Kohlrabi	1/2 cup, cooked slices	44
Peas with edible pods	1/2 cup, cooked	38
Sweet pepper	1 raw pepper	95
Potato, flesh and skin	7 oz, baked	26
Potato, flesh and skin	7 oz, microwaved	31
Rutabaga	1/2 cup cooked, mashed	26
Sweet potato	1/2 cup, baked, mashed	25
	4 oz, baked	28
Tomato	4 1/2 oz, raw	22
	1/2 cup, cooked	25
Tomato juice	1/2 cup	22
Vegetable juice	1/2 cup	34
Fruits		
Cantaloupe	1/2 cup cubes	34
Cranberry juice cocktail	8 oz (1 cup)	90
Grapefruit	half a fruit	41
	1 cup, sections with juice	79
	1/2 cup fresh juice	47
	1/2 cup canned juice	36
Grape juice	1/2 cup (from frozen concentrate)	30
Guava	3 oz, whole fruit	165
Honeydew	1/2 cup cubes	21
Kiwi	1 medium fruit	75
Lemon juice	3 oz, fresh	42
Mango	1/2 cup, sliced	23
Orange	One 5-oz navel	80
	1/2 cup fresh juice	62
	1/2 cup canned juice	43
	1/2 cup juice (from concentrate)	48
Papaya	1/2 cup cubes	43
Pineapple	1/2 cup canned in heavy syrup	60
Raspberries	1/2 cup, fresh	31
Strawberries	1/2 cup, fresh	43
	1/2 cup (frozen, sweetened)	53
Tangerine	2 1/2 oz, whole fruit	26

Vitamin Storage in the Body

The body does not readily excrete an excess of fat-soluble vitamins. In contrast, water-soluble vitamins continually leave the body because cellular water dissolves these compounds, which then leave via the kidneys. An exception is vitamin B_{12}, which stores more readily than the other water-soluble vitamins, and fat-soluble vitamin K. Because of their limited storage, water-soluble vitamins must be consumed regularly to prevent possible deficiency. A wide latitude exists, however, as an average person would require 10 days without consuming thiamine before deficiency symptoms emerge; it takes about 30 to 40 days of lack of vitamin C before symptoms of deficiency appear. Since a broad array of vitamins is readily available in the foods consumed in a well-balanced diet, little chance occurs for long-term vitamin deficiency. Exceptions include conditions of starvation, alcoholism (which compromises nutrient intake), or significant deviations from prudent dietary recommendations.

ROLE OF VITAMINS IN THE BODY

FIGURE 2.1 summarizes many of the biologic functions of vitamins. These important nutrients contain no useful energy for the body, but instead serve as essential links and regulators in numerous metabolic reactions that *release* energy from food. Vitamins also control processes of tissue synthesis and help to protect the integrity of the cells' unique plasma membrane. The water-soluble vitamins play important roles in energy metabolism (TABLE 2.2). *Vitamins participate repeatedly in metabolic reactions; thus, the vitamin needs of physically active people probably do not exceed those of sedentary counterparts.*

DEFINING NUTRIENT NEEDS

Controversy surrounding the RDAs caused the Food and Nutrition Board and scientific nutrition community to reexamine the usefulness of a single standard. This process, begun in 1997, led the National Academy's Institute of Medicine (in cooperation with Canadian scientists) to develop the **Dietary Reference Intakes.**

Dietary Reference Intakes

Dietary Reference Intakes (DRIs) represent a radically new and more comprehensive approach to nutritional recommendations for individuals.[181] Think of the DRIs as the umbrella term that encompasses the array of new standards—RDAs, Estimated Average Requirements, Adequate Intakes, and the Tolerable Upper Intake Levels—for nutrient recommendations in planning and assessing diets for healthy persons.

Similarities of dietary patterns caused the inclusion of both Canada and the United States in the target population.

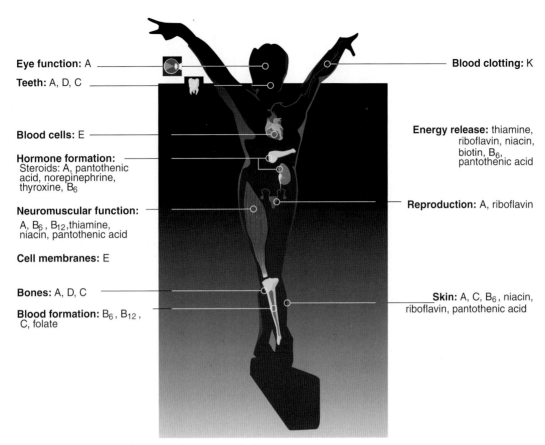

Eye function: A

Teeth: A, D, C

Blood cells: E

Hormone formation:
Steroids: A, pantothenic
acid, norepinephrine,
thyroxine, B_6

Neuromuscular function:
A, B_6, B_{12}, thiamine,
niacin, pantothenic acid

Cell membranes: E

Bones: A, D, C

Blood formation: B_6, B_{12},
C, folate

Blood clotting: K

Energy release: thiamine,
riboflavin, niacin,
biotin, B_6,
pantothenic acid

Reproduction: A, riboflavin

Skin: A, C, B_6, niacin,
riboflavin, pantothenic acid

Figure 2.1 Biologic functions of vitamins in the body.

Recommendations encompass not only daily intakes intended for health maintenance but also upper-intake levels that reduce the likelihood of harm from excess nutrient intake. The DRIs differ from their predecessor RDAs by focusing more on promoting health maintenance and risk reduction for nutrient-dependent diseases (e.g., heart disease, diabetes, hypertension, osteoporosis, various cancers, and age-related macular degeneration), rather than the traditional criterion of preventing deficiency diseases such as scurvy or beriberi. In addition to including values for energy, protein, and the micronutrients, DRIs also provide values for macronutrients and food components of nutritional importance, such as phytochemicals. Whenever possible, nutrient intakes are recommended in four categories instead of one. This concept of range places the DRIs more in line with the Estimated Safe and Adequate Daily Dietary Intakes (ESADDIs).

Unlike its RDA predecessor, the DRI value also includes recommendations that apply to gender and life stages of growth and development based on age and, when appropriate, pregnancy and lactation. The goal of a complete revision every 5 years as with the RDAs was abandoned, with the new modification of making immediate changes in the DRI as new scientific data become available. The National Academy Press presents the reports to date on the DRIs (www.nap.edu/; search for Dietary Reference Intakes).

The following definitions apply to the four different sets of values for the intake of nutrients and food components in the DRIs:

- **Estimated Average Requirement (EAR):**
  Average level of daily nutrient intake to meet the requirement of one-half of the healthy individuals in a particular life-stage and gender group. In addition to assessing nutritional adequacy of intakes of population groups, the EAR provides a useful value for determining the prevalence of inadequate nutrient intake by the proportion of the population with intakes below this value.
- **Recommended Dietary Allowance (RDA):** The average daily nutrient intake level sufficient to meet the requirement of nearly 97 to 98% of healthy individuals in a particular life-stage and gender group (FIG. 2.2). For most nutrients, this value represents the EAR plus two standard deviations of the requirement.
- **Adequate Intake (AI):** The AI provides an assumed adequate nutritional goal when no RDA exists. It represents a recommended average daily nutrient intake level based on observed or experimentally determined approximations or estimates of nutrient intake by a group (or groups) of apparently healthy persons and is used when an RDA cannot

be determined. Low risk exists with intakes at or above the AI level.

- **Tolerable Upper Intake Level (UL):** The highest average daily nutrient intake level likely to pose no risk of adverse health effects to almost all individuals in the specified gender and life-stage group of the general population. As intake increases above the UL, the potential risk of adverse effects increases.

The DRI report indicates that fruits and vegetables yield about one-half as much vitamin A than previously believed. Thus, individuals who do not eat vitamin-A rich, animal-derived foods should upgrade their intake of carotene-rich fruits and vegetables. The report also sets a daily maximum

Figure 2.2 Theoretical distribution of the number of persons adequately nourished by a given nutrient intake. The RDA (recommended dietary allowance) is set at an intake level than would meet the nutrient needs of 97 to 98% of the population (2 standard deviations [sd] above mean). EAR is the Estimated Average Requirement, which represents a nutrient intake value estimated to meet the requirement of one-half of the healthy individuals in a gender and life-stage group.

Table 2.2   WATER-SOLUBLE VITAMINS AND ENERGY TRANSFER

Vitamin B₁ (thiamine): Provides oxidizable substrate in citric acid cycle via oxidative decarboxylation of pyruvate to acetyl-CoA during carbohydrate breakdown; requirement related to total energy expenditure and total carbohydrate breakdown; needs may be somewhat higher in physically active people with large carbohydrate catabolism; membrane and nerve conduction; pentose synthesis; oxidative decarboxylation of α-keto acids in amino acid breakdown

Vitamin B₂ (riboflavin): Hydrogen (electron) transfer during mitochondrial metabolism in respiratory chain; combines with phosphoric acid to form flavin adenine dinucleotide (FAD) and flavin adenine mononucleotide (FMN)

Vitamin B₆ (pyridoxine): Important coenzyme in protein synthesis and glycogen metabolism; coenzyme in transamination reactions; formation of precursor compounds for heme in hemoglobin; coenzyme for phosphorylase, which facilitates glycogen release from liver

Vitamin B₁₂ (cyanocobalamin): Important coenzyme in the transfer of single-carbon units in nucleic acid metabolism; influences protein synthesis; role in gastrointestinal, bone, and nervous tissue function

Niacin (nicotinamide and nicotinic acid): Hydrogen (electron) transfer during glycolysis and mitochondrial metabolism; component of nicotine and nicotine adenine dinucleotide phosphate (NADP); role in fat and glycogen synthesis; amino acid tryptophan converted to niacin; excess niacin may depress fatty acid mobilization, which would facilitate carbohydrate depletion

Pantothenic acid: Component of the citric acid cycle intermediate acetyl-CoA; involved in synthesis of cholesterol, phospholipids, hemoglobin, and steroid hormones

Folate (folic acid, folacin): Coenzyme in amino acid metabolism and nucleic acid synthesis; essential for normal formation of red and white blood cells; protects against neural tube defects in fetus

Biotin: Essential role in carbohydrate, fat, and amino acid metabolism; involved in carboxyl unit transport and CO_2 fixing in tissues; role in gluconeogenesis and fatty acid synthesis and oxidation

Vitamin C (ascorbic acid): Antioxidant; may relate to exercise through its role in the synthesis of collagen and carnitine; enhances iron absorption and possibly heat acclimatization; facilitates iron availability; cofactor in some hydroxylation reactions (e.g., dopamine to noradrenaline)

---

intake level for vitamin A, in addition to boron, copper, iodine, iron, manganese, molybdenum, nickel, vanadium, and zinc. Specific recommended intakes are provided for vitamins A and K, chromium, copper, iodine, manganese, molybdenum, and zinc. The report concludes that one can meet the daily requirement for the nutrients examined without supplementation. The exception is the mineral iron, for which most pregnant women need supplements to obtain their increased daily requirement.

TABLE 2.3 lists the major bodily functions, dietary sources, and symptoms of a deficiency or excess of the water-soluble and fat-soluble vitamins. TABLES 2.4 AND 2.5 present the RDA, AI, and UL values for these vitamins. Well-balanced meals provide an adequate quantity of all vitamins, regardless of age and physical activity level. Indeed, individuals who expend considerable energy exercising generally need not consume special foods or supplements that increase vitamin intake above recommended levels. Also, at high levels of daily physical activity, food intake generally increases to sustain the added exercise energy requirements. Additional food through a variety of nutritious meals proportionately increases vitamin and mineral intakes. Chapter 7 summarizes recommendations from the DRI report on ranges for macronutrient and fiber intake and daily physical activity to optimize health and reduce risk of chronic illness.

Several possible exceptions exist to the general rule that discounts a need for supplementation if one consumes a well-balanced diet. First, vitamin C and folate exist in foods that usually make up only a small part of most American's total

Table 2.3 FOOD SOURCES, MAJOR BODILY FUNCTIONS, AND SYMPTOMS OF DEFICIENCY OR EXCESS OF THE FAT-SOLUBLE AND WATER-SOLUBLE VITAMINS FOR HEALTHY ADULTS (19–50 YEARS OF AGE)

Vitamin	Dietary Sources	Major Bodily Functions	Deficiency	Excess
Fat soluble				
Vitamin A (retinol)	Provitamin A (β-carotene) widely distributed in green vegetables. Retinol present in milk, butter, cheese, fortified margarine	Constituent of rhodopsin (visual pigment). Maintenance of epithelial tissues. Role in mucopolysaccharide synthesis	Xerophthalmia (keratinization of ocular tissue), night blindness, permanent blindness	Headache, vomiting, peeling of skin, anorexia, swelling of long bones
Vitamin D	Cod-liver oil, eggs, dairy products, fortified milk, and margarine	Promotes growth and mineralization of bones. Increases absorption of calcium	Rickets (bone deformities) in children; osteomalacia in adults	Vomiting, diarrhea, loss of weight, kidney damage
Vitamin E (tocopherol)	Seeds, green leafy vegetables, margarines, shortenings	Functions as an antioxidant to prevent cell damage	Possible anemia	Relatively nontoxic
Vitamin K (phylloquinone)	Green leafy vegetables, small amounts in cereals, fruits, and meats	Important in blood clotting (involved in formation of prothombin)	Conditioned deficiencies associated with severe bleeding; internal hemorrhages	Relatively nontoxic; synthetic forms at high doses may cause jaundice
Water soluble				
Vitamin B$_1$ (thiamin)	Pork, organ meats, whole grains, nuts, legumes, milk, fruits, and vegetables	Coenzyme (thiamin pyrophosphate) in reactions involving the removal of carbon dioxide	Beriberi (peripheral nerve changes, edema, heart failure)	None reported
Vitamin B$_2$	Widely distributed in foods: meats, eggs, milk products, whole grain and enriched cereal products, wheat germ, green leafy vegetables	Constituent of two flavin nucleotide coenzymes involved in energy metabolism (FAD and FMN)	Reddened lips, cracks at mouth corner (cheilosis), eye lesions	None reported
Niacin	Liver, lean meats, poultry, grains, legumes, peanuts (can be formed from tryptophan)	Constituent of two coenzymes in oxidation-reduction reactions (NAD and NADP)	Pellagra (skin and gastrointestinal lesions, nervous mental disorders)	Flushing, burning and tingling around neck, face, and hands
Vitamin B$_6$	Meats, fish, poultry, vegetables, whole-grain, cereals, seeds	Coenzyme (pyridoxal phosphate) involved in amino acid and glycogen metabolism	Irritability, convulsions, muscular twitching, dermatitis, kidney stones	None reported
Pantothenic acid	Widely distributed in foods: meat, fish, poultry, milk products, legumes, whole grains	Constituent of coenzyme A, which plays a central role in energy metabolism	Fatigue, sleep disturbances, impaired coordination, nausea	None reported
Folate	Legumes, green vegetables, whole wheat products, meats, eggs, milk products, liver	Coenzyme (reduced form) involved in transfer of single-carbon units in nucleic acid and amino acid metabolism	Anemia, gastrointestinal disturbances, diarrhea, red tongue	None reported
Vitamin B$_{12}$	Muscle meats, fish, eggs, dairy products, (absent in plant foods)	Coenzyme involved in transfer of single-carbon units in nucleic acid metabolism	Pernicious anemia, neurologic disorders	None reported
Biotin	Legumes, vegetables, meats, liver, egg yolk, nuts	Coenzymes required for fat synthesis, amino acid metabolism, and glycogen (animal starch) formation	Fatigue, depression, nausea, dermatitis, muscular pains	None reported
Vitamin C (ascorbic acid)	Citrus fruits, tomatoes, green peppers, salad greens	Maintains intercellular matrix of cartilage, bone, and dentine; important in collagen synthesis	Scurvy (degeneration of skin, teeth, blood vessels, epithelial hemorrhages)	Relatively nontoxic; possibility of kidney stones

Table 2.4 DIETARY REFERENCE INTAKES (DRIs): RECOMMENDED INTAKES FOR INDIVIDUALS: VITAMINS

Life Stage Group	Vitamin A (μg/d)[a]	Vitamin C (mg/d)	Vitamin D (μg/d)[b,c]	Vitamin E (mg/d)[d]	Vitamin K (μg/d)	Thiamin (mg/d)	Riboflavin (mg/d)	Niacin (mg/d)[e]	Vitamin B6 (mg/d)	Folate (μg/d)[f]	Vitamin B12 (μg/d)	Pantothenic Acid (mg/d)	Biotin (μg/d)	Choline (mg/d)[g]
Infants														
0–6 mo	400*	40*	5*	4*	2.0*	0.2*	0.3*	2*	0.1*	65*	0.4*	1.7*	5*	125*
7–12 mo	500*	50*	5*	5*	2.5*	0.3*	0.4*	4*	0.3*	80*	0.5*	1.8*	6*	150*
Children														
1–3 y	**300**	**15**	5*	**6**	30*	**0.5**	**0.5**	**6**	**0.5**	**150**	**0.9**	2*	8*	200*
4–8 y	**400**	**25**	5*	**7**	55*	**0.6**	**0.6**	**8**	**0.6**	**200**	**1.2**	3*	12*	250*
Males														
9–13 y	**600**	**45**	5*	**11**	60*	**0.9**	**0.9**	**12**	**1.0**	**300**	**1.8**	4*	20*	375*
14–18 y	**900**	**75**	5*	**15**	75*	**1.2**	**1.3**	**16**	**1.3**	**400**	**2.4**	5*	25*	550*
19–30 y	**900**	**90**	5*	**15**	120*	**1.2**	**1.3**	**16**	**1.3**	**400**	**2.4**	5*	30*	550*
31–50 y	**900**	**90**	5*	**15**	120*	**1.2**	**1.3**	**16**	**1.3**	**400**	**2.4**	5*	30*	550*
51–70 y	**900**	**90**	10*	**15**	120*	**1.2**	**1.3**	**16**	**1.3**	**400**	**2.4**[h]	5*	30*	550*
>70 y	**900**	**90**	15*	**15**	120*	**1.2**	**1.3**	**16**	**1.3**	**400**	**2.4**[h]	5*	30*	550*
Females														
9–13 y	**600**	**45**	5*	**11**	60*	**0.9**	**0.9**	**12**	**1.0**	**300**	**1.8**	4*	20*	375*
14–18 y	**700**	**65**	5*	**15**	75*	**1.0**	**1.0**	**14**	**1.2**	**400**[f]	**2.4**	5*	25*	400*
19–30 y	**700**	**75**	5*	**15**	90*	**1.1**	**1.1**	**14**	**1.3**	**400**[f]	**2.4**	5*	30*	425*
31–50 y	**700**	**75**	5*	**15**	90*	**1.1**	**1.1**	**14**	**1.3**	**400**[f]	**2.4**	5*	30*	425*
51–70 y	**700**	**75**	10*	**15**	90*	**1.1**	**1.1**	**14**	**1.5**	**400**	**2.4**[h]	5*	30*	425*
>70 y	**700**	**75**	15*	**15**	90*	**1.1**	**1.1**	**14**	**1.5**	**400**	**2.4**[h]	5*	30*	425*
Pregnancy														
≤18 y	**750**	**80**	5*	**15**	75*	**1.4**	**1.4**	**18**	**1.9**	**600**[f]	**2.6**	6*	30*	450*
19–30 y	**770**	**85**	5*	**15**	90*	**1.4**	**1.4**	**18**	**1.9**	**600**[f]	**2.6**	6*	30*	450*
31–50 y	**770**	**85**	5*	**15**	90*	**1.4**	**1.4**	**18**	**1.9**	**600**[f]	**2.6**	6*	30*	450*
Lactation														
≤18 y	**1200**	**115**	5*	**19**	75*	**1.4**	**1.6**	**17**	**2.0**	**500**	**2.8**	7*	35*	550*
19–30 y	**1300**	**120**	5*	**19**	90*	**1.4**	**1.6**	**17**	**2.0**	**500**	**2.8**	7*	35*	550*
31–50 y	**1300**	**120**	5*	**19**	90*	**1.4**	**1.6**	**17**	**2.0**	**500**	**2.8**	7*	35*	550*

Sources: Dietary Reference Intakes for Calcium, Phosphorous, Magnesium, Vitamin D, and Fluoride (1997); Dietary Reference Intakes for Thiamin, Riboflavin, Niacin, Vitamin B6, Folate, Vitamin B12, Pantothenic Acid, Biotin, and Choline (1998); Dietary Reference Intakes for Vitamin C, Vitamin E, Selenium, and Carotenoids (2000); and Dietary Reference Intakes for Vitamin A, Vitamin K, Arsenic, Boron, Chromium, Copper, Iodine, Iron, Manganese, Molybdenum, Nickel, Silicon, Vanadium, and Zinc (2001). These reports may be accessed via www.nap.edu. Copyright 2001 by the National Academy of Sciences. All rights reserved.

Note: This table (taken from the DRI reports, see www.nap.edu) presents Recommended Dietary Allowances (RDAs) in **bold type** and Adequate Intakes (AIs) in ordinary type followed by an asterisk **(*)**. RDAs and AIs may both be used as goals for individual intake. RDAs are set to meet the needs of almost all (97 to 98 percent) individuals in a group. For healthy breastfed infants, the AI is the mean intake. The AI for other life stage and gender groups is believed to cover needs of all individuals in the group, but lack of data or uncertainty in the data prevent being able to specify with confidence the percentage of individuals covered by this intake.

[a] As retinol activity equivalents (RAEs). 1 RAE = 1 μg retinol, 12 μg β-carotene, 24 μg α-carotene, or 24 μg β-cryptoxanthin. To calculate RAEs from REs of provitamin A carotenoids in foods, divide the REs by 2. For preformed vitamin A in foods or supplements and for provitamin A carotenoids in supplements, 1 RE = 1 RAE.

[b] Calciferol. 1 μg calciferol = 40 IU vitamin D.

[c] In the absence of adequate exposure to sunlight.

[d] As α-tocopherol. α-Tocopherol includes *RRR*-α-tocopherol, the only form of α-tocopherol that occurs naturally in foods, and the *2R*-stereoisometric forms of α-tocopherol (*RRR-, RSR-, RRS-,* and *RSS*-α-tocopherol) that occur in fortified foods and supplements. It does not include the *2S*-stereoisomeric forms of α-tocopherol (*SRR-, SSR-, SR-,* and *SSS*-α-tocopherol), also found in fortified foods and supplements.

[e] As niacin equivalents (NE). 1 mg of niacin = 60 mg of tryptophan; 0–6 months = preformed niacin (not NE).

[f] As dietary folate equivalents (DFE). 1 DFE = 1 μg food folate = 0.6 μg of folic acid from fortified food or as a supplement consumed with food = 0.5 μg of a supplement taken on an empty stomach.

[g] Although AIs have been set for choline, there are few data to asses whether a dietary supply of choline is needed at all stages of the life cycle and it may be that the choline requirement can be met by endogenous synthesis at some of these stages.

[h] Because 10 to 30 percent of older people may malabsorb food-bound B12, it is advisable for those older than 50 years to meet their RDA mainly by consuming foods fortified with B12 or a supplement containing B12.

[i] In view of evidence linking folate intake with neural tube defects in the fetus, it is recommended that all women capable of becoming pregnant consume 400 μg from supplements or fortified foods in addition to intake of food folate from a varied diet.

[j] It is assumed that women will continue consuming 400 μg from supplements or fortified food until their pregnancy is confirmed and they enter prenatal care, which ordinarily occurs after the end of the periconceptional period—the critical time for formation of the neural tube.

Table 2.5 DIETARY REFERENCE INTAKES (DRIs): TOLERABLE UPPER INTAKE LEVELS (UL[a]): VITAMINS

Life Stage Group	Vitamin A (µg/d)[b]	Vitamin C (mg/d)	Vitamin D (µg/d)	Vitamin E (mg/d)[c,d]	Vitamin K	Thiamin	Riboflavin	Niacin (mg/d)[d]	Vitamin B6 (mg/d)[d]	Folate (µg/d)[d]	Vitamin B12	Pantothenic Acid	Biotin	Choline (g/d)	Carotenoids[e]
Infants															
0–6 mo	600	ND[f]	25	ND	ND	ND	ND	ND	ND	ND	ND	ND	ND	ND	ND
7–12 mo	600	ND	25	ND	ND	ND	ND	ND	ND	ND	ND	ND	ND	ND	ND
Children															
1–3 y	600	400	50	200	ND	ND	ND	10	30	300	ND	ND	ND	1.0	ND
4–8 y	900	650	50	300	ND	ND	ND	15	40	400	ND	ND	ND	1.0	ND
Males, Females															
9–13 y	1700	1200	50	600	ND	ND	ND	20	60	600	ND	ND	ND	2.0	ND
14–18 y	2800	1800	50	800	ND	ND	ND	30	80	800	ND	ND	ND	3.0	ND
19–70 y	3000	2000	50	1000	ND	ND	ND	35	100	1000	ND	ND	ND	3.5	ND
>70 y	3000	2000	50	1000	ND	ND	ND	35	100	1000	ND	ND	ND	3.5	ND
Pregnancy															
≤18 y	2800	1800	50	800	ND	ND	ND	30	80	800	ND	ND	ND	3.0	ND
19–50 y	3000	2000	50	1000	ND	ND	ND	35	100	1000	ND	ND	ND	3.5	ND
Lactation															
≤18 y	2800	1800	50	800	ND	ND	ND	30	80	800	ND	ND	ND	3.0	ND
19–50 y	3000	2000	50	1000	ND	ND	ND	35	100	1000	ND	ND	ND	3.5	ND

Sources: Dietary Reference Intakes for Calcium, Phosphorous, Magnesium, Vitamin D, and Fluoride (1997); Dietary Reference Intakes for Thiamin, Riboflavin, Niacin, Vitamin B6, Folate, Vitamin B12, Pantothenic Acid, Biotin, and Choline (1998); Dietary Reference Intakes for Vitamin C, Vitamin E, Selenium, and Carotenoids (2000); and Dietary Reference Intakes for Vitamin A, Vitamin K, Arsenic, Boron, Chromium, Copper, Iodine, Iron, Manganese, Molybdenum, Nickel, Silicon, Vanadium, and Zinc (2001). These reports may be accessed via www.nap.edu. Copyright 2001 by the National Academy of Sciences. All rights reserved.

[a]UL = The maximum level of daily nutrient intake that is likely to pose no risk of adverse effects. Unless otherwise specified, the UL represents total intake from food, water, and supplements. Due to lack of suitable data, ULs could not be established for vitamin K, thiamin, riboflavin, vitamin B12, pantothenic acid, biotin, or carotenoids. In the absence of ULs, extra caution may be warranted in consuming levels above recommended intakes.

[b]As preformed vitamin A only.

[c]As α-tocopherol; applies to any form of supplemental α-tocopherol.

[d]The ULs for vitamin E, niacin, and folate apply to synthetic forms obtained from supplements, fortified foods, or a combination of the two.

[e]β-Carotene supplements are advised only to serve as a provitamin A source for individuals at risk of vitamin A deficiency.

[f]ND = Not determinable due to lack of data of adverse effects in this age group and concern with regard to lack of ability to handle excess amounts. Source of intake should be from food only to prevent high levels of intake.

caloric intake. The availability of these foods also varies by season. Second, different athletic groups have relatively low intakes of vitamins B1 and B6.[42,146] Their adequate intake occurs if the daily diet contains fresh fruit, grains, and uncooked or steamed vegetables. Individuals on meatless diets should consume a small amount of milk, milk products, or eggs because vitamin B12 exists only in foods of animal origin. Consuming recommended quantities of folate is crucial to fetal nervous system development in the early stage of pregnancy; as of January 1, 1998, the Food and Drug Administration (www.fda.gov) required that folate fortify all enriched foods. This constituted the first new fortification of foods since 1943, when vitamins and iron were added to enrich flour.

Antioxidant and Disease Protection Role of Specific Vitamins

Most of the oxygen consumed during mitochondrial energy metabolism combines with hydrogen to produce water. Normally, electron "leakage" along the electron transport chain allows about 2 to 5% of oxygen to form oxygen-containing **free radicals** such as superoxide (O_2^-), hydrogen peroxide (H_2O_2), and hydroxyl (OH^-) radicals. *A free radical represents a highly chemically reactive atom, molecule, or molecular fragment that contains at least one unpaired electron in its outer orbital or valence shell.* (Paired electrons, by way of contrast, represent a far more stable state.) These are the same free radicals produced by external factors such as heat and ionizing radiation and carried in cigarette smoke, environmental pollutants, and even some medications. Once formed, free radicals search out other compounds to create new free radical molecules.

When superoxide forms, it dismutates to hydrogen peroxide. Normally, superoxide rapidly converts to O_2 and H_2O by the action of **superoxide dismutase**, an enzyme in the body's first line of antioxidant defense. An accumulation of free radicals increases the potential for cellular damage (**oxidative stress**) to many biologically important substances in processes that add oxygen to cellular components. These substances include the genetic material of DNA and RNA, proteins, and lipid-containing structures, particularly the polyunsaturated fatty acid-rich bilayer membrane that isolates the cell against noxious toxins and carcinogens. Oxygen radicals have strong affinity for the polyunsaturated fatty acids that make up the lipid bilayer of the cell membrane.

During unrestrained oxidative stress, the plasma membrane's fatty acids deteriorate. Membrane damage occurs through a chain-reaction series of events termed **lipid peroxidation**. These reactions, which incorporate oxygen into lipids, increase the vulnerability of the cell and its constituents. Free radicals also facilitate LDL-cholesterol oxidation, thus leading to cytotoxicity and enhanced plaque formation in the coronary arteries.[167] Oxidative stress ultimately increases the likelihood of cellular deterioration associated with advanced aging, cancer, diabetes, coronary artery disease, exercise-related oxidative damage, and a general decline in central nervous system and immune functions.

No way exists to stop oxygen reduction and subsequent free radical production, but an elaborate natural defense against their damaging effects exists within the mitochondria and surrounding extracellular spaces. This defense includes the antioxidant scavenger enzymes catalase, glutathione peroxidase, superoxide dismutase, and metal-binding proteins. In addition, the non-enzymatic nutritive reducing agents vitamins A, C, and E and the vitamin A-precursor β-carotene (one of the "carotenoids" in dark green and orange vegetables) serve important protective functions.[64,80,129,168] These antioxidant vitamins protect the plasma membrane by reacting with and removing free radicals. This quenches the harmful chain reaction. Many of these vitamins also blunt the damaging effects to cellular constituents of high serum homocysteine levels (see page 55).[115]

Examples of Health Benefits

Dietary habits have frequently been linked to the occurrence of cardiovascular disease, diabetes, osteoporosis, cataracts, premature aging, and diverse cancers including postmenopausal breast, distal colon, prostate, pancreas, ovary, and endometrium.[190] Maintaining a diet with recommended levels of the antioxidant vitamins (particularly vitamin C) reduces risk for several types of cancer.[140] Significant protection against heart disease occurs with relatively high daily intakes from either foods or supplements of the B vitamins folate (400 μg) and vitamin B_6 (3 mg).[139] These two vitamins reduce blood levels of homocysteine, an amino acid that increases risk for heart attack and stroke. Good sources of folate include enriched whole-grain cereals, nuts and seeds, dark green, leafy vegetables, beans and peas, and orange juice.

A normal to above normal intake of vitamin E (in both α-tocopherol and γ-tocopherol forms[69]) and β-carotene and/or high serum levels of carotenoids also blunts the progression of coronary artery narrowing and reduces heart attack risk in men and women.[63,108] Unfortunately, this effect is not always observed for high-risk patients and those with congestive heart failure.[73,101,175,198] Postmenopausal women whose diets contained the most vitamin E had 62% less chance of dying from coronary heart disease (CHD) than women who consumed the least vitamin E.[81] In elderly men, a high plasma concentration of vitamins C and E and β-carotene associates with a reduced development and progression of early atherosclerotic lesions.[50] One model for heart disease protection proposes that the antioxidant vitamins, particularly vitamin E (recommended intake of 15 mg·d^{-1}), inhibit oxidation of LDL-cholesterol and its subsequent uptake into foam cells embedded in the arterial wall. The **oxidative modification hypothesis** maintains that the oxidation of LDL-cholesterol—a process similar to butter turning rancid—contributes to the plaque-forming, artery-clogging atherosclerotic process.[33,86] Additional benefits of vitamin E in the diet include protection against prostate cancer (risk reduced by one-third and death rate by 40%) and heart disease and stroke, perhaps by preventing blood clot formation from the anticoagulant properties of vitamin E quinone, a natural byproduct of vitamin E metabolism. All evidence does not support a reduced colorectal cancer risk from increased intake of vitamin-rich fruits and vegetables.[102,174]

Eat a Variety of Healthful Foods. Several randomized trials of supplements of β-carotene and vitamin A per se did not show a reduced incidence of cancer and cardiovascular disease.[61,125] Such findings have caused current nutritional guidelines to refocus more on the consumption of a broad array of foods rather than on isolated chemicals within these foods.[182] The current recommendation is to increase the consumption of fruits, vegetables, and whole grains and include lean meat or meat substitutes and low-fat dairy foods to gain substantial health benefits and reduce risk of early mortality.

Disease protection from diet can be linked to the myriad of accessory nutrients and substances within the vitamin-containing fruits, grains, and vegetables. Such nonvitamin substances (as yet unavailable in supplement form) include various plant phytochemicals such as isothiocyanates, the potent stimulators of natural detoxifying enzymes in the body, present in broccoli, cabbage, cauliflower, and other cruciferous vegetables. Researchers at the National Eye Institute (www.nei.nih.gov) observed that persons with higher intakes of two specific antioxidants, lutein and zeaxanthin (found primarily in green leafy vegetables such as spinach, kale, and collard greens), experienced 70% less age-related macular degeneration than individuals with lower intakes. This disease results from deterioration of the macular cells in the center of the retina, the light-sensitive layer in the back of the eye that enables us to see. Lycopene, a potent antioxidant substance in carotene-rich foods (and what makes tomatoes red, released largely by cooking) has been linked to reduced heart disease risk and reduced risk of developing several deadly forms of cancer (prostate, colon, and rectal).[6] Vitamin E pills contain the vitamin predominantly in its α-tocopherol form. However, the γ-tocopherol form of vitamin E (present in soybeans, nuts, and grains) may provide a complementary benefit in neutralizing harmful compounds within the body.[69]

Chapter 7 explores the possible interaction of exercise, free radical formation, and antioxidant vitamin requirements. Undoubtedly, the next decade will witness considerable research in the fascinating area of functional foods and **nutraceuticals**—the foods or parts of food that provide medical or health benefits including prevention and/or treatment of diseases.

BEYOND CHOLESTEROL: HOMOCYSTEINE AND CORONARY HEART DISEASE

In 1969, an 8-year old boy died of a stroke. Autopsy reveled that his arteries had the sclerotic look of the blood vessels of an elderly man, and his blood contained excess levels of the amino acid **homocysteine.** His rare genetic disorder, homocystinuria, causes premature hardening of the arteries and early death from heart attack or stroke. In the years following this observation, an impressive number of studies have shown an almost lockstep association between high homocysteine levels and both heart attack and all-cause mortality.[14,40,138,184,188] In the presence of other conventional CHD risks (e.g., smoking and hypertension), synergistic effects magnify the negative impact of homocysteine.[195] Elevated homocysteine levels also associate with increased risk of cognitive impairment, Alzheimer disease, and adverse outcomes and complications of pregnancy.[109,134,135,156]

All individuals produce homocysteine, but it normally converts to other nondamaging amino acids. Three B vitamins—folate, B_6, and B_{12}—facilitate the conversion. If the conversion slows from a genetic defect or vitamin deficiency, homocysteine levels increase and promote cholesterol's damaging effects on the arterial lumen. FIGURE 2.3A proposes a mechanism for homocysteine damage.[114,191] The homocysteine model points up the fact that CHD can be mediated through multiple biologic pathways and helps to explain why some people contract heart disease despite low-to-normal LDL-cholesterol levels.

Excessive homocysteine causes blood platelets to clump, thus fostering blood clots and deterioration of smooth muscle cells that line the arterial wall. Chronic homocysteine exposure can scar and thicken arteries and provides a fertile medium for circulating LDL-cholesterol to initiate damage and encourage plaque formation. Persons with elevated homocysteine levels run a 3 to 4.5 times greater risk of death from heart disease than individuals with normal levels.

Some Question as to the Strength of the Association

A recent report analyzed the data from 30 studies that encompassed almost 17,000 people who collectively suffered 5073 heart attacks and 1113 strokes.[176] After controlling for high blood pressure and stroke, a person who lowered homocysteine level by 25% reduced heart-attack risk by a modest 11% and stroke risk by 19%. More definitive assessments of homocysteine and cardiovascular disease risk will emerge from prospective, randomized clinical trials currently under way that involve administering vitamins B_6 and B_{12} and folate to healthy persons and evaluating disease outcome over at least 5 years.

Figure 2.3 A. Proposed mechanism for how the amino acid homocysteine damages the lining of arteries and sets the stage for cholesterol infiltration into a blood vessel. **B.** Proposed defense against the possible harmful effects of elevated homocysteine levels.

It remains uncertain what causes some persons to accumulate homocysteine, but evidence points to deficiency of B vitamins and lifestyle factors such as cigarette smoking, alcohol and coffee consumption, and high meat intake.[51,67,95,100,123,152,170] No clear standard for normal or desirable homocysteine levels currently exists. Research must show that normalizing homocysteine actually reduces risk of heart attack and stroke. In this regard, recent data indicate that homocysteine-lowering therapy with the combination of folate and vitamins B_{12} and B_6 improved the outcome for heart disease patients undergoing coronary angioplasty.[154] Sufficient evidence supports consuming adequate B vitamins, particularly folate. Even small amounts of this vitamin (plentiful in enriched whole-grain cereals, nuts and seeds, dark green, leafy vegetables, beans and peas, and orange juice) provides a cost-efficient means to lower homocysteine levels (Fig. 2.3B).[178] As of 1999, folate fortifies all white flour, breads, pasta, grits, white rice, and cornmeal. Between 300 and 400 μg represents the current recommended daily folate intake.

Summary

1. Vitamins are organic substances that neither supply energy nor contribute to body mass. Vitamins serve crucial functions in almost all bodily processes; they must be obtained from food or dietary supplementation.

2. Plants manufacture vitamins during photosynthesis. Animals obtain vitamins from the plants they eat or from the meat of other animals that previously consumed these foods. Animals also produce some vitamins from precursor substances known as provitamins.

3. Thirteen known vitamins are classified as either water soluble or fat soluble. The fat-soluble vitamins are vitamins A, D, E, and K; vitamin C and the B-complex vitamins compose the water-soluble vitamins.

4. Excess fat-soluble vitamins accumulate in body tissues and can increase to toxic concentrations. Except in relatively rare instances, excess water-soluble vitamins generally remain nontoxic and eventually are excreted in the urine. Their maximum potency for the body occurs within 8 to 14 hours following ingestion.

5. The Dietary Reference Intakes (DRIs) differ from their predecessor RDAs by focusing more on promoting health maintenance and risk reduction for nutrient-dependent diseases rather than the traditional criterion of preventing deficiency diseases.

6. Think of the DRIs as the umbrella term that encompasses the new standards—the RDAs, Estimated Average Requirements, Adequate Intakes, and the Tolerable Upper Intake Levels—for nutrient recommendations for use in planning and assessing diets for healthy people. DRI values include recommendations that apply to gender and life stages of growth and development based on age and, when appropriate, pregnancy and lactation.

7. Vitamins regulate metabolism, facilitate energy release, and serve important functions in bone and tissue synthesis.

8. Consuming vitamin supplements above the RDA does not improve exercise performance or the potential for sustaining intense physical training. In fact, serious illness occurs from regularly consuming an excess of fat-soluble and, in some instances, water-soluble vitamins.

9. Vitamins A, C, E, and β-carotene serve important protective functions as antioxidants. A diet with appropriate levels of these micronutrients can reduce the potential for free radical damage (oxidative stress) and may protect against heart disease and cancer.

10. All individuals produce homocysteine, but it normally converts to other nondamaging amino acids. Three B-vitamins—folate, B_6, and B_{12}—facilitate the conversion. If the conversion slows due to a genetic defect or vitamin deficiency, homocysteine levels increase and promote cholesterol's damaging effects on the arterial lumen.

➤ Minerals

THE NATURE OF MINERALS

In addition to the elements of carbon, oxygen, hydrogen, and nitrogen, approximately 4% of the body's mass (about 2 kg for a 50-kg woman) consists of a group of 22 mostly metallic elements collectively called **minerals.** Minerals serve as constituents of enzymes, hormones, and vitamins; they

THE ABCs OF SOUND NUTRITION AND GOOD HEALTH

AIM FOR FITNESS…
- Aim for a healthy weight.
- Be physically active each day.

BUILD A HEALTHY BASE…
- Let the Pyramid guide food choices.
- Choose a variety of grains daily, especially whole grains.
- Choose a variety of fruits and vegetables daily.
- Keep food safe to eat.

CHOOSE SENSIBLY…
- Choose a diet low in saturated fat and cholesterol and moderate in total fat.
- Choose beverages and foods to moderate intake of sugars.
- Choose and prepare foods with less salt.
- If you drink alcoholic beverages, do so in moderation.

combine with other chemicals (e.g., calcium phosphate in bone, iron in the heme of hemoglobin) or exist singularly (free calcium in body fluids).

The minerals essential to life include seven **major minerals** (required in amounts >100 mg daily) and 14 minor or **trace minerals** (required in amounts <100 mg daily). Trace minerals account for less than 15 g (approximately 0.5 oz) or 0.02% of the total body mass. Like excess vitamins, excess minerals serve no useful physiologic purpose and can produce toxic effects. RDAs and recommended ranges of intakes have been established for many minerals; if the diet supplies these recommended levels, this ensures an adequate intake of the remaining minerals.

Most major or trace minerals occur freely in nature, mainly in the waters of rivers, lakes, and oceans, in topsoil, and beneath the earth's surface. Minerals exist in the root systems of plants and in the body structure of animals that consume plants and water containing minerals.

KINDS AND SOURCES OF MINERALS

TABLE 2.6 lists the major bodily functions, dietary sources, and symptoms of deficiency or excess of the minerals. TABLES 2.7 AND 2.8 present the RDA, UL, and AI values for these minerals. Mineral supplements, like vitamin supplements, generally confer little benefit because the required minerals occur readily in food and water. Some supplementation may be necessary in geographic regions where the soil or water supply lacks a particular mineral. Relatively poor concentrations of the mineral iodine occur in certain areas of the United States, particularly the basin of the Great Lakes and Pacific Northwest, and in central Brazil and the Himalayan mountains. Iodine is required by the thyroid gland to synthesize the thyroxine and triiodothyronine, hormones

that accelerate resting metabolism. Adding iodine to the water supply or to table salt (iodized salt) easily prevents iodine deficiency. A common mineral deficiency in the United States results from a lack of iron in the diet. Between 30 and 50% of American women of childbearing age suffer some form of dietary iron insufficiency. As discussed on page 74, upgrading one's diet with iron-rich foods or prudent use of iron supplements alleviates this problem.

ROLE OF MINERALS IN THE BODY

Whereas vitamins activate chemical processes without becoming part of the byproducts of the reactions they catalyze, minerals often become incorporated within the structures and existing chemicals of the body. Minerals serve three broad roles in the body:

- Minerals provide *structure* in forming bones and teeth.
- In terms of *function*, minerals help to maintain normal heart rhythm, muscle contractility, neural conductivity, and acid–base balance.
- Minerals *regulate* metabolism by becoming constituents of enzymes and hormones that modulate cellular activity.

FIGURE 2.4 lists minerals that participate in catabolic and anabolic cellular processes. Minerals activate reactions that release energy during carbohydrate, fat, and protein breakdown. In addition, minerals are essential for synthesizing biologic nutrients: glycogen from glucose, triacylglycerol from fatty acids and glycerol, and protein from amino acids. A lack of the essential minerals disrupts the fine balance between catabolism and anabolism. Minerals also form important components of hormones. Inadequate thyroxine production from iodine deficiency, for example, significantly slows the body's resting metabolism. In extreme cases, this predisposes a person to develop obesity. The synthesis of insulin, the hormone that facilitates glucose uptake by cells, requires zinc (as do approximately 100 other enzymes), whereas the digestive acid hydrochloric acid forms from the mineral chlorine.

Mineral Bioavailability

The body varies considerably in its capacity to absorb and use the minerals in food. For example, spinach contains considerable calcium, but only about 5% of this calcium becomes absorbed. The same holds true for dietary iron, which the small intestine absorbs with efficiency averaging 5 to 10%. Factors that affect the **bioavailability** of minerals in food include

- *Type of food:* the small intestine readily absorbs minerals in animal products because plant binders and dietary fibers are unavailable to hinder digestion

Table 2.6	**THE IMPORTANT MAJOR AND MINOR (TRACE) MINERALS FOR HEALTHY ADULTS (19–50 YEARS OF AGE) AND THEIR DIETARY REQUIREMENTS, FOOD SOURCES, FUNCTIONS AND THE EFFECTS OF DEFICIENCIES AND EXCESSES**			
Mineral	*Dietary Sources*	*Major Bodily Functions*	*Deficiency*	*Excess*
Major				
Calcium	Milk, cheese, dark green vegetables, dried legumes	Bone and tooth formation, blood clotting, nerve transmission	Stunted growth, rickets, osteoporosis, convulsions	Not reported in humans
Phosphorus	Milk, cheese, yogurt, meat, poultry, grains, fish	Bone and tooth formation, acid–base balance, helps prevent loss of calcium from bone	Weakness, demineralization	Erosion of jaw (phossy jaw)
Potassium	Leafy vegetables, cantaloupe, lima beans, potatoes, bananas, milk, meats, coffee, tea	Fluid balance, nerve transmission, acid–base balance	Muscle cramps, irregular cardiac rhythm, mental confusion, loss of appetite can be life-threatening	None if kidneys function normally; poor kidney function causes potassium buildup and cardiac arrhythmias
Sulfur	Obtained as part of dietary protein and is present in food preservatives	Acid–base balance, liver function	Unlikely to occur if dietary intake is adequate	Unknown
Sodium	Common salt	Acid–base balance, body water balance, nerve function	Muscle cramps, mental apathy, reduced appetite	High blood pressure.
Chlorine (chloride)	Chloride is part of salt containing food; some vegetables and fruits	Important part of extracellular fluids	Unlikely to occur if dietary intake is adequate	Along with sodium contributes to high blood pressure
Magnesium	Whole grains, green leafy vegetables	Activates enzymes involved in protein synthesis	Growth failure, behavioral disturbances	Diarrhea
Minor				
Iron	Eggs, lean meats, legumes whole grains, green leafy vegetables	Constituent of hemoglobin and enzymes involved in energy metabolism	Iron deficiency anemia (weakness, reduced resistance to infection)	Siderosis; cirrhosis of the liver
Fluorine	Drinking water, tea, seafood	May be important in maintenance of bone structure	Higher frequency of tooth decay	Mottling of teeth, increased bone density
Zinc	Widely distributed in foods	Constituent of enzymes involved in digestion	Growth failure, small sex glands	Fever, nausea, vomiting, diarrhea
Copper	Meats, drinking water	Constituent of enzymes associated with iron metabolism	Anemia, bone changes (rare)	Rare metabolic condition (Wilson's disease)
Selenium	Seafood, meats, grains	Functions in close association with vitamin E	Anemia (rare)	Gastrointestinal disorders, lung irritations
Iodine (iodide)	Marine fish and shellfish, dairy products, vegetables, iodized salt	Constituent of thyroid hormones	Goiter (enlarged thyroid)	Very high intakes depress thyroid activity
Chromium	Legumes, cereals, organ meats, fats, vegetable oils, meats, whole grains	Constituent of some enzymes; involved in glucose and energy metabolism	Rarely reported in humans; impaired ability to metabolize glucose	Inhibition of enzymes Occupational exposures: skin and kidney damage

Food and Nutrition Board, National Academy of Sciences-National Research Council, Washington, DC. Recommended dietary allowances, revised 1989.

Table 2.7	DIETARY REFERENCE INTAKES (DRIs): RECOMMENDED INTAKES FOR INDIVIDUALS: MINERALS											
Life Stage Group	Calcium (mg/d)	Chromium (μg/d)	Copper (μg/d)	Fluoride (mg/d)	Iodine (μg/d)	Iron (mg/d)	Magnesium (mg/d)	Manganese (mg/d)	Molybdenum (μg/d)	Phosphorus (mg/d)	Selenium (μg/d)	Zinc (mg/d)
Infants												
0–6 mo	210*	0.2*	200*	0.01*	110*	0.27*	30*	0.003*	2*	100*	15*	2*
7–12 mo	270*	5.5*	220*	0.5*	130*	11*	75*	0.6*	3*	275*	20*	3
Children												
1–3 y	500*	11*	340	0.7*	90	7	80	1.2*	17	460	20	3
4–8 y	800*	15*	440	1*	90	10	130	1.5*	22	500	30	5
Males												
9–13 y	1,300*	25*	700	2*	120	8	240	1.9*	34	1,250	40	8
14–18 y	1,300*	35*	890	3*	150	11	410	2.2*	43	1,250	55	11
19–30 y	1,000*	35*	900	4*	150	8	400	2.3*	45	700	55	11
31–50 y	1,000*	35*	900	4*	150	8	420	2.3*	45	700	55	11
51–70 y	1,200*	30*	900	4*	150	8	420	2.3*	45	700	55	11
>70 y	1,200*	30*	900	4*	150	8	420	2.3*	45	700	55	11
Females												
9–13 y	1,300*	21*	700	2*	120	8	240	1.6*	34	1,250	40	8
14–18 y	1,300*	24*	890	3*	150	15	360	1.6*	43	1,250	55	9
19–30 y	1,000*	25*	900	3*	150	18	310	1.8*	45	700	55	8
31–50 y	1,000*	25*	900	3*	150	18	320	1.8*	45	700	55	8
51–70 y	1,200*	20*	900	3*	150	8	320	1.8*	45	700	55	8
>70 y	1,200*	20*	900	3*	150	8	320	1.8*	45	700	55	8
Pregnancy												
≤18 y	1,300*	29*	1,000	3*	220	27	400	2.0*	50	1,250	60	13
19–30 y	1,000*	30*	1,000	3*	220	27	350	2.0*	50	700	60	11
31–50 y	1,000*	30*	1,000	3*	220	27	360	2.0*	50	700	60	11
Lactation												
≤18 y	1,300*	44*	1,300	3*	290	10	360	2.6*	50	1,250	70	14
19–30 y	1,000*	45*	1,300	3*	290	9	310	2.6*	50	700	70	12
31–50 y	1,000*	45*	1,300	3*	290	9	320	2.6*	50	700	70	12

Sources: Dietary Reference Intakes for Calcium, Phosphorous, Magnesium, Vitamin D and Fluoride (1997); Dietary Reference Intakes for Thiamin, Riboflavin, Niacin, Vitamin B$_6$, Folate, Vitamin B$_{12}$, Pantothenic Acid, Biotin, and Choline (1998); Dietary Reference Intakes for Vitamin C, Vitamin E, Selenium, and Carotenoids (2000); and Dietary Reference Intakes for Vitamin A, Vitamin K, Arsenic, Boron, Chromium, Copper, Iodine, Iron, Manganese, Molybdenum, Nickel, Silicon, Vanadium, and Zinc (2001). These reports may be accessed via www.nap.edu.
Copyright 2001 by the National Academy of Sciences. Reprinted with permission.

Note: This table presents Recommended Dietary Allowances (RDAs) in **bold type** and Adequate Intakes (AIs) in ordinary type followed by an asterisk (*). RDAs and AIs may both be used as goals for individual intake. RDAs are set to meet the needs of almost all (97 to 98 percent) individuals in a group. For healthy breastfed infants, the AI is the mean intake. The AI for other life stage and gender groups is believed to cover needs of all individuals in the group, but lack of data or uncertainty in the data prevent being able to specify with confidence the percentage of individuals covered by this intake.

Table 2.8 DIETARY REFERENCE INTAKES (DRIs): TOLERABLE UPPER INTAKE LEVELS (ULᵃ): MINERALS

Life Stage Group	Arsenic[b]	Boron (mg/d)	Calcium (g/d)	Chromium	Copper (μg/d)	Fluoride (mg/d)	Iodine (μg/d)	Iron (mg/d)	Magnesium (mg/d)[c]	Manganese (mg/d)	Molybdenum (μg/d)	Nickel (mg/d)	Phosphorus (g/d)	Selenium (μg/d)	Silicon[d]	Vanadium (mg/d)[e]	Zinc (mg/d)
Infants																	
0–6 mo	ND	ND	ND	ND	ND	0.7	ND	40	ND	ND	ND	ND	ND	45	ND	ND	4
7–12 mo	ND	ND	ND	ND	ND	0.9	ND	40	ND	ND	ND	ND	ND	60	ND	ND	5
Children																	
1–3 y	ND	3	2.5	ND	1,000	1.3	200	40	65	2	300	0.2	3	90	ND	ND	7
4–8 y	ND	6	2.5	ND	3,000	2.2	300	40	110	3	600	0.3	3	150	ND	ND	12
Males, females																	
9–13 y	ND	11	2.5	ND	5,000	10	600	40	350	6	1,100	0.6	4	280	ND	ND	23
14–18 y	ND	17	2.5	ND	8,000	10	900	45	350	9	1,700	1.0	4	400	ND	ND	34
19–70 y	ND	20	2.5	ND	10,000	10	1,100	45	350	11	2,000	1.0	4	400	ND	1.8	40
>70 y	ND	20	2.5	ND	10,000	10	1,100	45	350	11	2,000	1.0	3	400	ND	1.8	40
Pregnancy																	
≤18 y	ND	17	2.5	ND	8,000	10	900	45	350	9	1,700	1.0	3.5	400	ND	ND	34
19–50 y	ND	20	2.5	ND	10,000	10	1,100	45	350	11	2,000	1.0	3.5	400	ND	ND	40
Lactation																	
≤18 y	ND	17	2.5	ND	8,000	10	900	45	350	9	1,700	1.0	4	400	ND	ND	34
19–50 y	ND	20	2.5	ND	10,000	10	1,100	45	350	11	2,000	1.0	4	400	ND	ND	40

Sources: Dietary Reference Intakes for Calcium, Phosphorous, Magnesium, Vitamin D and Fluoride (1997); Dietary Reference Intakes for Thiamin, Riboflavin, Niacin, Vitamin B₆, Folate, Vitamin B₁₂, Pantothenic Acid, Biotin, and Choline (1998); Dietary Reference Intakes for Vitamin C, Vitamin E, Selenium, and Carotenoids (2000); and Dietary Reference Intakes for Vitamin A, Vitamin K, Arsenic, Boron, Chromium, Copper, Iodine, Iron, Manganese, Molybdenum, Nickel, Silicon, Vanadium, and Zinc (2001). These reports may be accessed via www.nap.edu.

Copyright 2001 by the National Academy of Sciences. Reprinted with permission.

ᵃUL = The maximum level of daily nutrient intake that is likely to pose no risk of adverse effects. Unless otherwise specified, the UL represents total intake from food, water, and supplements. Due to lack of suitable data, ULs could not be established for arsenic, chromium, and silicon. In the absence of ULs, extra caution may be warranted in consuming levels above recommended intakes.

[b]Although the UL was not determined for arsenic, there is no justification for adding arsenic to food or supplements.

[c]The ULs for magnesium represent intake from a pharmacologic agent only and do not include intake from food and water.

[d]Although silicon has not been shown to cause adverse effects in humans, there is no justification for adding silicon to supplements.

[e]Although vanadium in food has not been shown to cause adverse effects in humans, there is no justification for adding vanadium to food and vanadium supplements should be used with caution. The UL is based on adverse effects in laboratory animals and this data could be used to set a UL for adults but not children and adolescents.

[f]ND = not determinable due to lack of data of adverse effects in this age group and concern with regard to lack of ability to handle excess amounts. Source of intake should be from food only to prevent high levels of intake.

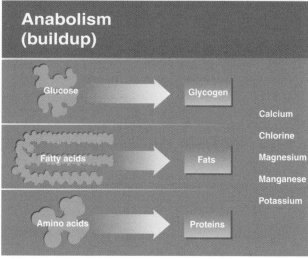

Figure 2.4 Minerals function in the catabolism and anabolism of macronutrients.

and absorption. Also, foods from the animal kingdom generally contain high mineral concentration (except for magnesium, which has a higher concentration in plants).

- *Mineral-mineral interaction:* many minerals have the same molecular weight and thus compete for intestinal absorption. This makes it unwise to consume an excess of any one mineral because it can retard another mineral's absorption.
- *Vitamin-mineral interaction:* various vitamins interact with minerals in a manner that affects mineral bioavailability. From a positive perspective, vitamin D facilitates calcium absorption, while vitamin C improves iron absorption.
- *Fiber-mineral interaction:* high fiber intake blunts the absorption of some minerals (e.g., calcium, iron, magnesium, phosphorus) by binding to them, causing them to pass unabsorbed through the digestive tract.

In the subsequent sections, we describe specific functions of the more important minerals related to physical activity.

CALCIUM

Calcium, the most abundant mineral in the body, combines with phosphorus to form bones and teeth. These two minerals represent about 75% of the body's total mineral content of about 2.5% of body mass. In its ionized form (about 1% of the body's 1200 mg), calcium plays an important role in muscle action, blood clotting, nerve transmission, activation of several enzymes, synthesis of calcitriol (active form of vitamin D), and transport of fluids across cell membranes. Calcium also may contribute to easing premenstrual syndrome and polycystic ovary syndrome, preventing colon cancer, and optimizing blood pressure regulation,[38,96] although its role in reducing heart disease risk remains unclear.[1]

Osteoporosis: Calcium, Estrogen, and Exercise

Bone is a dynamic tissue matrix of collagen, minerals, and about 50% water. **Bone modeling** promotes continual increases in skeletal size and shape during youth. Bone also exists in a continual state of flux, or **bone remodeling**, in which bone-destroying cells (osteoclasts) cause the breakdown (resorption) of bone while bone-forming osteoblast cells synthesize bone, governed by an array of growth factors, gonadal hormones, and pituitary hormones. Calcium availability combined with regular physical activity significantly affects the dynamics of bone remodeling. The plasma calcium level, regulated by hormonal action, is maintained either by calcium from food or calcium derived from the resorption of the bone mass. The two broad categories of bone are

- **Cortical bone:** dense, hard outer layer of bone such as the shafts of the long bones of the arms and legs
- **Trabecular bone:** spongy, less dense, and relatively weaker bone most prevalent in the vertebrae and ball of the femur

A Mineral Whose Requirement Is Often Not Met

Growing children require more calcium per unit body mass than do adults, yet many adults remain deficient in calcium intake. As a general guideline, adolescents and young adults require 1300 mg of calcium daily (1000 mg for adults ages 19 to 50 and 1200 mg for those older than 50) or about as much calcium as in five 8-oz glasses of milk. Unfortunately, calcium remains one of the most frequent nutrients lacking in the diet of both sedentary and physically active individuals, particularly adolescent girls. For an average adult, daily calcium intake ranges between 500 and 700 mg. *Female dancers, gymnasts, and endurance competitors are the athletes most prone to calcium dietary insufficiency.*[12,32,107]

NATIONAL ACADEMY OF SCIENCES RECOMMENDED DAILY CALCIUM INTAKE

Age	Amount (mg)
1–3 years	500
4–8 years	800
9–18 years	1300
19–50 years	1000
51 years and older	1200

Inadequate dietary calcium affects about 50% of American children under age 5, 65% of teenage boys, and 85% of teenage girls. Part of this calcium lack occurs because Americans now drink far less milk than soft drinks, or about 23 gallons of milk per year versus 49 gallons of soft drinks. Over 75% of adults consume less than the RDA, and about 25% of females in the United States consume less than 300 mg of calcium daily. Inadequate calcium intake forces the body to draw upon its bone calcium "reserves" to restore the deficit. Prolonging this restorative imbalance, either from inadequate calcium intake or low levels of calcium-regulating hormones, promotes one of two conditions:

1. **Osteoporosis**, literally meaning "porous bones," with bone density more than 2.5 standard deviations below normal for age and gender
2. **Osteopenia**—from the Greek words *osteo*, meaning bone and *penia*, meaning poverty—a midway condition in which bones weaken, with increased fracture risk

Osteoporosis develops progressively as bone loses its calcium mass (bone mineral content) and calcium concentration (bone mineral density) and progressively becomes porous and brittle (FIG. 2.5). The stresses of normal living often cause bone to break.

Currently, osteoporosis afflicts more than 28 million Americans, of whom 80 to 90% are women, with another 18 million individuals with low bone mass. Fifty percent of all women eventually develop osteoporosis. Men are not immune from osteoporosis, with about two million men in the Unites States currently suffering from this affliction. Among older individuals, particularly women above age 60, this disease has reached near-epidemic proportions. Osteoporosis accounts for more than 1.5 million fractures (the clinical manifestation of the disease) yearly, including about 700,000 spinal fractures, 300,000 hip fractures, 200,000 wrist fractures, and 300,000 fractures of other body parts. Nearly 15% of postmenopausal women will fracture a hip, and about 33% will suffer spine-shortening and often painful vertebral fractures. Of the women who suffer a bone fracture

■ **Figure 2.5** Micrograph of normal bone (left) and osteoporotic bone (right). Osteoporotic bone shows these characteristics: loss of mineral matter, brittleness, cortex thinning (concomitant medullary diameter increase), increased porosity, imbalance between bone formation and resorption, disrupted bone architecture and cross-sectional geometry, microfracture accumulation, loss of mechanical integrity, and less tolerance to bending stress and thus more susceptibility to fracture.

after age 85, 25% die within 1 year. Estimates from the largest study to date indicate that nearly one-half of postmenopausal women aged 50 and older with no previous osteoporosis diagnosis have low bone mineral density, including 7% with osteoporosis.[161] This indicates that one out

BONE HEALTH DIAGNOSTIC CRITERIA BASED ON VARIATION (STANDARD DEVIATION) OF OBSERVED BONE DENSITY VALUES COMPARED WITH VALUES FOR SEX-MATCHED YOUNG ADULT POPULATION

Normal	<1.0 SD below mean
Osteopenia	1.0–2.5 SD below mean
Osteoporosis	>2.5 SD below mean
Severe osteoporosis	>2.5 SD below mean plus one or more fragility fractures

of two women (lower risk among African American and Hispanic women) and one out of eight men over age 50 will experience an osteoporosis-related fracture in their lifetime. The annual medical cost of hip fractures in the United States equals about $10 billion and may exceed $240 billion by the mid-21st century.[131]

Increased susceptibility to osteoporosis among older women coincides with the marked decrease in estrogen secretion that accompanies menopause.[28] Whether estrogen exerts its protective effects on bone by inhibiting bone resorption or decreasing bone turnover remains unknown (see page 70 for estrogen's possible actions). Men normally produce some estrogen, which largely explains their relatively low prevalence of osteoporosis. In addition, a portion of circulating testosterone converts to estradiol (a form of estrogen), which also promotes positive calcium balance. Most men maintain adequate testosterone levels throughout life. Risk factors for men include low testosterone levels, cigarette smoking, and use of medications such as steroids.

A Progressive Disease

Between 60 and 80% of an individual's susceptibility to osteoporosis links to genetic factors, while 20 to 40% remains lifestyle related. Women normally show gains in bone mass throughout the third decade of life with proper nutrition (adequate calcium and vitamin D, which increases efficiency of calcium absorption) and regular moderate physical activity.[83,177] However, adolescence serves as the prime bone building years to maximize bone mass; fully 90% of bone mass accumulates by about age 17.[3,106] In reality, osteoporosis for many women begins early in life because the average teenager consumes suboptimal calcium to support growing bones. This imbalance worsens into adulthood, particularly among women with genetic predisposition that limits their ability to compensate for low calcium intake by increasing calcium absorption.[47,52,89] By middle age, adult women generally consume only one-third of the calcium required for optimal bone maintenance.

Beginning around age 50, the average man experiences a bone loss of about 0.4% each year, whereas the female begins to lose twice this amount at age 35. For men, the normal rate of bone mineral loss does not usually pose a problem until the eighth decade of life. Menopause makes women highly susceptible to osteoporosis because there is little or no release of estrogen from the ovaries. Muscle, adipose tissue, and connective tissue continue to produce estrogen, but only in limited quantities. The dramatic fall in estrogen production at menopause coincides with reduced intestinal calcium absorption, less calcitonin production (a hormone that inhibits bone resorption), and increased bone resorption as bone loss accelerates to 3 to 6% per year in the 5 years following menopause. The rate then drops to approximately 1% yearly. At this rate, the typical woman loses 15 to 20% of her bone mass in the first decade after menopause, and some

women lose as much as 30% by age 70. Women can augment their genetically determined bone mass through purposeful increases in weight-bearing exercise and calcium intake throughout life and through estrogen replacement therapy in postmenopausal years.

Prevention Through Diet

FIGURE 2.6A illustrates that the variation in bone mass within a population results from a complex interaction among the various factors that affect bone mass rather than the distinct effect of each factor.[93,122,164] Because of this lack of independence among factors that influence bone mass, the portion of bone mass variation attributable to diet within a group may actually reflect how diet interacts with genetic factors, physical activity patterns, body weight, and drug or medication use (e.g., estrogen therapy). *Despite these interactive effects, adequate calcium intake throughout life remains a prime defense against bone loss with aging.* In fact, milk intake during childhood and adolescence associates with increased bone mass and bone density in adulthood and reduced fracture risk, independent of current milk or calcium intake.[71] Increasing the calcium intake of adolescent girls from their typical 80% of RDA level to the 110% level through supplementation

---

IMPORTANT RISK FACTORS FOR OSTEOPOROSIS

- Advanced age
- White or Asian female
- Slight build or tendency to be underweight
- Anorexia nervosa or bulimia nervosa
- Sedentary lifestyle
- Postmenopause including early or surgically induced menopause
- Low testosterone levels in men
- High protein intake
- Excess sodium intake
- Cigarette smoking
- Excessive alcohol use
- Abnormal absence of menstrual periods (amenorrhea)
- Calcium-deficient diet in years before and after menopause
- Family history (genetic predisposition) of osteoporosis
- High caffeine intake (possible)
- Vitamin D deficiency, either through inadequate exposure to sunlight or dietary insufficiency (prevalent in about 40% of adults); aging skin loses much of its ability to synthesize vitamin D, even when exposed to sunlight

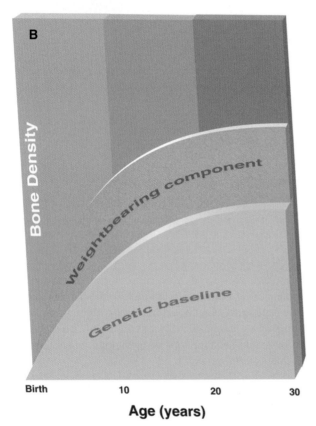

■ **Figure 2.6 A.** The variation in bone mass within the population is likely a function of how the different factors that affect bone mass interact with each other. (Modified from Specker BL. Should there be dietary guidelines for calcium intake. Am J Clin Nutr 2000;71:663.) **B.** Weightbearing exercise augments skeletal mass during growth above the genetic baseline. The degree of augmentation depends largely on the amount of mechanical loading to which a particular bone is subjected. (Modified from Turner CH. Site-specific effects of exercise: importance of interstitial fluid pressure. Bone 1999;24:161.)

significantly increased total body calcium and spinal bone mineral density. A National Institutes of Health consensus panel in 2000 recommended that adolescent girls consume 1500 mg of calcium daily, an intake level that does not adversely affect zinc balance.[98] Furthermore, increasing daily calcium intake for middle-aged women, particularly for es-

trogen-deprived women after menopause, to between 1200 and 1500 mg improves the body's calcium balance. The additional calcium slows the rate of bone loss, even with inadequate estrogen.[136] Additionally, a positive link exists between consuming diverse fruits and vegetables and bone health.[118] The association between carbonated beverage intake and increased bone fracture risk most likely results from the beverage displacing milk consumption rather than the effects on urinary calcium excretion of one or more of the beverage's constituents.[58] Conversely, drinking tea may protect against osteoporosis. Although tea contains caffeine (about one-half to one-third less than the same volume of coffee), it also contains other nutrients such as flavonoids that positively influence bone accretion.[59]

TABLE 2.9 *(top)* indicates that good dietary calcium sources include milk and milk products, calcium-fortified orange juice, canned sardines and canned salmon with bones, almonds, and dark green leafy vegetables.

Calcium supplements can correct dietary deficiencies regardless of whether extra calcium comes from fortified foods or commercial supplements (calcium citrate [less likely to cause stomach upset than other forms and also enhances iron absorption], calcium gluconate, calcium carbonate [can be constipating, especially for older people with low levels of stomach acid] or commercial products such as Tums).[110] Check the label for the amount of calcium, not the combined chemical, per dose. Calcium carbonate contains about 40% per dose, down to 21% in calcium citrate, and 9% in calcium gluconate. Because many calcium supplements, including those from refined sources, contain measurable lead, one should seek out brands that have been labeled as "tested for lead."[147] Adequate vitamin D facilitates calcium uptake, whereas excessive meat, salt, coffee, and alcohol consumption inhibit its absorption. For individuals who live and train in northern latitudes, primarily those who train indoors such as gymnasts and figure skaters, a vitamin D supplement of 200 IU is recommended.[3] The bottom of Table 2.9 indicates the calcium and vitamin D content of selected dietary supplements.

In postmenopausal women, estrogen supplements or low-dose, slow-release fluoride-plus-calcium supplements can treat severe osteoporosis. Estrogen therapy increases bone density of the spine and hip during the first several years of hormone treatment in both middle-aged and frail elderly women.[21,87,186] However, this treatment is not without risk as discussed in Case Study: Personal Health and Exercise Nutrition.

More Is Not Necessarily Better. The National Academy of Sciences has established an upper level intake of 2500 mg calcium per day—the equivalent of about 8 glasses of milk—for all age groups. Indiscriminate use of calcium supplements, particularly calcium carbonate antacids, in excess of twice the recommended amount places an individual at risk for developing kidney stones. Another possible downside from excessively high calcium intakes concerns reduced

Table 2.9 *(TOP)* CALCIUM CONTENT IN COMMON FOODS *(BOTTOM)* CALCIUM CONTENT AND VITAMIN D CONTENT IN SELECTED SUPPLEMENTS

Food	Amount	Calcium Content (mg)
Yogurt, plain, nonfat	8 oz	450
Yogurt, plain, low fat	8 oz	350–415
Yogurt, low fat with fruit	8 oz	250–350
Milk, skim	1 cup	302–316
Milk, 2%	1 cup	313
Cheddar cheese	1 oz	204
Provolone	1 oz	214
Mozzarella cheese, part skim	1 oz	207
Ricotta cheese, part skim	1 cup	337
Swiss cheese	1 oz	272
Almonds	1/2 cup	173
Figs, dried	10 figs	269
Orange juice, calcium fortified	1 cup	250
Orange	1 medium	56
Rhubarb, cooked with sugar	1/2 cup	174
Collards, turnip greens, spinach, cooked	1 cup	200–270
Broccoli, cooked	1 cup	178
Oatmeal with milk	1 cup	313
Salmon, canned with bones	3 1/2 oz	230
Sardines, canned with bones	3 1/2 oz	350
Halibut	Half fillet	95

Supplement	Elemental Calcium per Tablet (mg)	Vitamin D per Tablet (IU)
Calcium carbonate (generic)	600	200
Tums	200	0
Tums 500	500	0
Viactiv Soft Calcium chews	500	100
Citracal Caplets + D	315	200

zinc absorption and balance.[196] If this theory proves correct, individuals with high calcium intake should monitor the adequacy of dietary zinc intake (most readily available form of zinc occurs in red meats and poultry).

Exercise Is Helpful

Regular dynamic exercise helps to build bone mass and bone strength and slow the rate of skeletal aging. Children and adults, regardless of age, who maintain an active lifestyle show greater bone mass and bone density, with substantial improvements in mechanical strength of bone, than their sedentary counterparts.[13,43,74,78,120,127,165,185] Benefits of regular exercise and everyday physical activity on bone mass accretion (and perhaps bone shape and size) are greatest during childhood and adolescent years when peak bone mass can increase to the greatest extent (Fig. 2.6B).[2,68,70,79,88,116,183] For example, long-term soccer participation, starting at prepubertal age, relates to markedly increased bone mineral content and bone density at the femoral neck and lumber spine region.[19] Collegiate female gymnasts demonstrate significantly greater whole-body, spine, femur, and upper-limb bone mineral density and bone mineral content than controls.[130] These differences appear to reflect gymnastics activity rather than self-selection, because the athletes showed similar values between dominant and nondominant arms in contrast to controls. For these athletes, bone mineral density increases during the competitive season and decreases in the off season.[162]

The benefits of regular exercise often accrue into the seventh and even eighth decade of life.[171,187] The decline in vigorous physical activity typically observed in advancing age closely parallels the age-related bone mass loss. In this regard, moderate levels of physical activity, including walking, associate with substantially lower risk of hip fracture in postmenopausal women.[45] Even prior exercise and sports experience provides a residual effect on an adult's bone mineral density. For example, former female gymnasts had greater bone mass as adults than females with no previous athletic experience.[76] Consciously restricting food intake blunts the bone-building benefits of regular physical activity.[99]

The osteogenic effect of exercise becomes particularly effective during the growth periods of childhood and adolescence (Fig. 2.7) and may reduce fracture risk later in life.[72] FIGURE 2.8 illustrates the beneficial effects of weight-bearing exercise. *Short intense bouts of mechanical loading of bone through dynamic exercise performed three to five times a week provides a potent stimulus to maintain or increase bone mass.* This form of exercise includes walking, running, dancing, rope skipping, high-impact jumping, basketball, and gymnastics; high-intensity resistance exercises and circuit-resistance training also exert a positive effect. These exercises generate significant impact load and/or intermittent force against the long bones of the body.[20,37,88,173,187] Activities providing relatively high impact on the skeletal mass (e.g., volleyball, basketball, gymnastics, judo, and karate) induce the greatest increases in bone mass, particularly at weight-bearing sites.[4,26,34,44,160] Even walking 1 mile daily benefits bone mass during and after menopause.

Mechanism of Action. Intermittent muscle forces acting on bones during physical activity modify bone metabolism at the point of stress.[9,75,82,84] For example, the lower-limb bones of older cross-country runners have greater bone mineral content than the bones of less active counterparts. Likewise, the playing arm of tennis players and the throwing arm of baseball players show greater bone thickness than their less-used, nondominant arm.

Bone Health: Nutrition and Pharmacologic Therapy

Michelle became a near-vegan (consumes some fish) at age 12 years when she stopped eating meat and dairy products on urging from her mother, who had been a vegan her adult life. Now in her 20s and running regularly, Michelle remains a strict vegetarian. She plans to start a family in a year or so but is concerned that her diet may be inadequate in vitamins and minerals, particularly calcium, to ensure her and her baby's health. She also expresses concern she may be at high risk for osteoporosis because both her mother and grandmother have this disease. Michelle takes prednisone (a glucocorticoid drug) for psoriasis; she has normal estrogen levels.

CASE QUESTIONS

1. What bone assessment tests should Michelle undergo?
2. Review possible treatments options for Michelle.
3. Give the long-term outlook for Michelle's bone health status.

ANSWERS

1. Michelle should undergo a bone density test using dual-energy x-ray absorptiometry (DXA). If a DXA machine is unavailable, dual photon absorptiometry (measuring the spine, hip, and total body) and quantitative computed tomography (measuring the spine) can also evaluate bone density. If such devices are unavailable in her area, Michelle should contact a teaching hospital affiliated with a university.

> Michelle's bone mass is minus 2.1 Z-score values below the average for her age and classifies her as osteoporotic and a prime candidate for immediate treatment (see below).

DXA scans involve low-dose x-rays to capture images of the spine, hip, or entire body. A computer program compares the bone strength and risk of fracture with that of other people of the same age in the United States and with young people at peak bone density.

Scoring bone mineral density (BMD) uses Z-scores that represent standard deviation units above or below the average for the group. A BMD score below average by 2.0 Z-score standard deviations scores indicates osteoporosis. The box on page 62 presents the scoring system for diagnosing bone health.

2. Michelle is a prime candidate for aggressive dietary and pharmacologic interventions based on her BMD test results.

Dietary Approach:

Michelle needs to ensure adequate calcium intake. The 1000-mg per day Adequate Intake (AI) level for calcium (see Table 2.7 in text) for a person of Michelle's age is based on an estimated 40% total for calcium absorption. However, calcium absorption efficiency varies among persons; individuals who absorb calcium with poor efficiency should consume more. In all likelihood, Michelle falls into the category of a "poor absorber" because her diet contains adequate calcium from such foods as cooked spinach (1 cup = 280 mg calcium); canned sardines (2 oz = 220 mg calcium); cooked turnip greens (1 cup = 200 mg calcium); and canned salmon (3 oz = 180 mg calcium).

Michelle should increase her calcium intake to at least 1500 mg per day (food and/or supplements) along with the pharmacologic intervention listed below as recommended by her physician. For some persons, calcium intake in excess of 2000 mg per day causes inordinately high blood and urinary calcium concentrations, irritability, headache, kidney failure, soft tissue calcification, kidney stones, and decreased absorption of other minerals (2500 mg·d^{-1} represents the Tolerable Upper Intake value).

Pharmacologic Approach: Antiresorptive Medications

Currently, the US Food and Drug Administration (FDA) approves bisphosphonates (alendronate and risedronate), calcitonin, estrogens, parathyroid hormone, and raloxifene for the prevention and/or treatment of osteoporosis. These substances affect the bone remodeling cycle; they classify as antiresorptive medications. Bone remodeling progresses in two distinct stages: bone resorption and bone formation. During resorption, special osteoclast cells on the bone's surface dissolve bone tissue to create small cavities. During the formation stage, osteoblast cells fill the cavities with new bone tissue. Usually, bone resorption and bone formation occur in close sequence and remain balanced. A chronic negative balance in the bone-remodeling cycle causes bone loss that eventually leads to osteoporosis. Antiresorptive medications slow or stop the bone-resorbing portion of the remodeling cycle but do not slow the bone-forming stage. As such, new bone formation occurs at a greater rate than resorption, and bone density may increase over time. Teriparatide, a form of parathyroid hormone, is a newly approved osteoporosis medication. It is the first osteoporosis medication to increase the rate of bone formation in the bone-remodeling cycle.

Possible medications for Michelle include:

a. Bisphosphonates. These compounds incorporate into the bone matrix to inhibit cells that break down bone. Only these medications have been shown to reduce hip fracture risk.
- Alendronate sodium (brand name Fosamax)
- Risedronate sodium (brand name Actonel)

Both drugs are approved for prevention (5 mg·d^{-1} or 35 mg once weekly) and treatment (10 mg·d^{-1} or 70 mg once weekly) of postmenopausal osteoporosis in women and for treatment in men. It is taken on an empty stomach, first thing in the morning, with 8 oz of water (no other liquid) at least 30 minutes before eating or drinking. The patient must remain upright during this 30-minute period. Alendronate sodium is also approved for treatment of glucocorticoid-induced osteoporosis, as occurs with the long-term use of such drugs as prednisone and cortisone, which Michelle had been taking for her psoriasis. Major side effects include nausea, heartburn, or irritation of the esophagus.

b. Selective estrogen receptor modulators (SERMs)

• Calcitonin (brand names Miacalcin, Calcimar). Calcitonin, a naturally occurring hormone, is involved in calcium regulation and bone metabolism. In postmenopausal women calcitonin inhibits bone resorption, particularly in the presence of high levels of blood calcium, and increases spinal bone density. Injectable calcitonin may cause an allergic reaction and flushing of the face and hands, increase urinary frequency, promote nausea, and produce a rash. Side effects for nasal administration of this drug are uncommon but may include nasal irritation, backache, nosebleed, and headaches.

• Raloxifene (brand name Evista). Used for prevention and treatment in women, it has been shown to increase bone density at spine, hip, and neck and re-

duces spinal fractures. Common side effects include hot flashes and leg cramps. Blood clots are a rare side effect.

c. Estrogen replacement therapy (ERT) and hormone replacement therapy (HRT) (multiple brand names.) *In postmenopausal women, (ERT)/(HRT) is approved to prevent osteoporosis. Its use is not approved for premenopausal women with normal estrogen levels. Side effects may include vaginal bleeding, breast tenderness, mood disturbances, and gallbladder disease.*

A Word of Caution. A recent 8.5-year study of 16,808 healthy women ages 50 to 79 years showed that while combined estrogen and progestin therapy significantly reduced incidence of bone fractures and colorectal cancer, dramatic increases occurred in blood clots, strokes, heart attacks, and breast cancer.[197] These findings caused researchers to halt the study 3 years early. Consequently, hormone treatment for osteoporosis should be viewed as a more dramatic approach requiring medical consultation and supervision.

3. The long-term outlook for bone health remains positive. Michelle can increase her bone mineral content over the next several years with both nutritional and pharmacologic intervention. She should undergo bone density tests on a yearly basis to confirm treatment results.

Figure 2.7 Generalized curve for the association between age and the effects of regular bouts of intermittent, dynamic exercise on bone mass accretion.

Prevailing theory considers that dynamic loading creates hydrostatic pressure gradients within a bone's fluid-filled network. Fluid movement within this network in response to pressure changes from dynamic exercise generates fluid shear stress on bone cells that initiates a cascade of cellular events to ultimately stimulate the production of bone matrix protein.[183] The mechanosensitivity of bone and its subsequent buildup of calcium depends on two main factors: *(a)* the magnitude of the applied force (strain magnitude) and *(b)* its frequency or number of cycles of application. Owing to the transient sensitivity of bone cells to mechanical stimuli, shorter, more frequent periods of mechanical strain facilitate bone mass accretion.[144,145] As the applied force and strain increase, the number of cycles required to initiate bone formation decreases.[27] Chemicals produced in bone itself also may contribute to bone formation. Alterations in bone's geometric configuration to long-term exercise enhance its mechanical properties.[8] FIGURE 2.9 illustrates the anatomic structure and cross-sectional view of a typical long bone and depicts the dynamics of bone growth and remodeling.

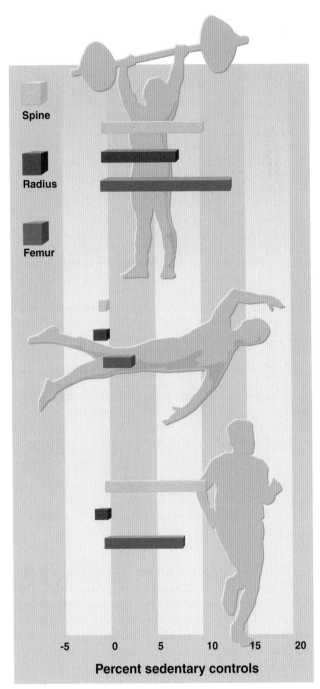

Percent sedentary controls

■ **Figure 2.8** Bone mineral density expressed as a percentage of sedentary control values at three skeletal sites for weightlifters, swimmers, and runners. (From Drinkwater BL. Physical activity, fitness, and osteoporosis. In: Bouchard C, et al., eds. Physical activity, fitness, and health. Champaign, IL: Human Kinetics, 1994.)

The Female Triad: An Unexpected Problem for Women Who Train Intensely

A paradox exists between exercise and bone dynamics for highly active premenopausal women, particularly young athletes who have yet to attain peak bone mass. Women who train intensely and emphasize weight loss often engage in disordered eating behaviors—a serious ailment that in the extreme causes diverse and life-threatening complications (see Chapter 15).[23] This further decreases energy availability, reducing body mass and body fat to a point at which significant alterations occur in secretion of the pituitary gonadotropic hormones. This, in turn, changes ovarian secretions, triggering irregular cycles (**oligomenorrhea**; six to nine menstrual cycles per year; 35 to 90 days between cycles) or cessation, a condition termed **secondary amenorrhea**. Clinicians define secondary amenorrhea as the cessation of monthly menstrual cycles for at least three consecutive months after regular cycles have been established. Chapter 13 more fully discusses the interactions between leanness, exercise, and menstrual irregularity.

The interacting, tightly bound continuum that generally begins with disordered eating (and a resultant energy drain) and leads to amenorrhea and then osteoporosis reflects the clinical entity labeled the **female athlete triad** (FIG. 2.10). Some researchers and physicians prefer the term **female triad** because this syndrome of disorders also afflicts physically active women in the general population who do not fit the typical competitive athlete profile.

Limited data exist as to the prevalence of the triad, mainly from a disagreement about how to define the disorder. Many young women who play sports likely suffer from at least one of the triad's irregularities, particularly disordered eating behaviors, which occur in 15 to 60% of female athletes based on informal surveys. FIGURE 2.11 illustrates the contributing factors associated with exercise-related amenorrhea, considered the "red flag" or most recognizable symptom for the triad's presence. Female athletes of the 1970s and 80s believed that the loss of normal menstruation reflected appropriately hard training and was an inevitable consequence of athletic success. The prevalence of amenor-

---

SIX PRINCIPLES FOR PROMOTING BONE HEALTH THROUGH EXERCISE

- **Specificity:** Exercise provides a local osteogenic effect.

- **Overload:** Progressively increasing exercise intensity promotes continued improvement.

- **Initial values:** Individuals with the smallest total bone mass have the greatest potential for improvement.

- **Diminishing returns:** As one approaches the biologic ceiling for bone density, further gains require greater effort.

- **More not necessarily better:** Bone cells become desensitized in response to prolonged mechanical-loading sessions.

- **Reversibility:** Discontinuing exercise overload reverses the positive osteogenic effects of exercise.

■ **Figure 2.9 A.** Anatomic structure and longitudinal view of a typical long bone. **B.** Bone dynamics during growth and continual remodeling.

rhea among female athletes in weight-related sports (distance running, gymnastics, ballet, cheerleading, figure skating, body building) probably ranges between 25 and 65%; while no more than 5% of the nonathletic women of menstruating age experience this condition.

In general, bone density relates closely to *(a)* menstrual regularity and *(b)* total number of menstrual cycles. Cessation of menstruation removes estrogen's protective effect on bone, making calcium loss more prevalent, with a concomitant decrease in bone mass. The most severe menstrual disorders exert the greatest negative effect on bone mass.[179,194] Lowered bone density from extended amenorrhea often occurs at multiple sites, including the lumbar spine and bone areas subjected to increased force and impact loading during exercise.[137] Concurrently, the problem worsens in individuals undergoing an energy deficit and accompanying low protein, lipid, and energy intakes.[199] In such cases, a poor diet also provides inadequate calcium intake. Persistent amenorrhea that begins at an early age diminishes the benefits of exercise on bone mass and increases risk for musculoskeletal injuries (particularly re-

Female Athlete Triad

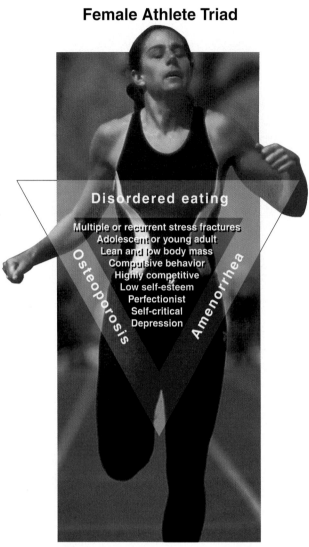

Disordered eating

Multiple or recurrent stress fractures
Adolescent or young adult
Lean and low body mass
Compulsive behavior
Highly competitive
Low self-esteem
Perfectionist
Self-critical
Depression

Osteoporosis Amenorrhea

▓ **Figure 2.10** The female athlete triad: disordered eating, amenorrhea, and osteoporosis.

peated stress fractures) during exercise.[55,111] For example, a 5% bone mass loss increases stress fracture risk by nearly 40%. Reestablishing normal menses causes some regain in bone mass, but it does *not* reach levels achieved with normal menstruation. Bone mass may *permanently* remain at suboptimal levels throughout adult life, leaving women at increased risk for osteoporosis and stress fractures even years after competitive athletic participation.[35,104]

ESTROGEN'S ROLE IN BONE HEALTH

• Increases intestinal calcium absorption

• Reduces urinary calcium excretion

• Facilitates calcium retention by bone

Professional organizations recommend that intervention begin within 3 months of the onset of amenorrhea. Successful treatment of athletic amenorrhea requires a nonpharmacologic, behavioral approach including[36]

• Reduce training level by 10 to 20%
• Gradually increase total energy intake
• Increase body weight by 2 to 3%
• Maintain daily calcium intake at 1500 mg

As with most medical ailments, prevention offers the most effective treatment for the female triad. Ideally, screening for the triad should begin in junior-high school and high school at the preparticipation medical examination and in subsequent evaluations. Such screenings provide insight about behaviors and symptoms related to disordered eating and menstrual irregularity. In addition, coaches and athletic trainers should routinely monitor athletes for changes in menstrual patterns and eating behaviors. *The identification of any one ailment in the triad requires prompt screening for the other two disorders.* Chapter 15 more fully discusses various eating disorders with emphasis on athletes and other physically active individuals.

Does Muscle Strength Relate to Bone Density?

Men and women who participate in strength and power activities have as much or more bone mass than endurance athletes.[143] Such findings have caused speculation about the possible relationship between muscular strength and bone mass. Laboratory experiments have documented greater maximum flexion and extension dynamic strength in postmenopausal women without osteoporosis than in their osteoporotic counterparts.[68,169] FIGURE 2.12 displays chest flexion and extension strength in normal and osteoporotic women. Unequivocal results emerged. The women with normal bone mineral density in the lumbar spine and femur neck exhibited 20% greater strength in 11 of 12 test comparisons for flexion; 4 of 12 comparisons for extension showed 13% higher values for women with normal bone density. Quite possibly, differences in maximum dynamic strength among postmenopausal women can serve a clinically useful role in screening for osteoporosis. Other data complement these findings; they indicate that regional lean tissue mass (often an indication of muscular strength) accurately predicts bone mineral density.[119] The lumbar spine and proximal femur bone mass of elite teenage weightlifters exceeds representative values for fully mature bone of reference adults.[25] In addition, a linear relation exists between increases in bone mineral density and total and exercise-specific weight lifted during a 1-year strength-training program.[29]

For female gymnasts, bone mineral density correlated moderately with maximal muscle strength and serum progesterone.[60] Despite oligomenorrhea and amenorrhea in many of these athletes, it is possible that they maintain bone

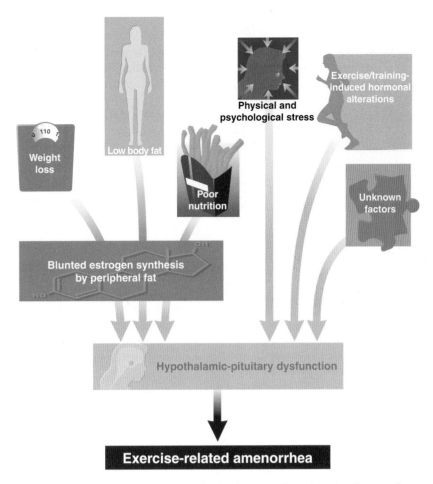

Figure 2.11 Factors contributing to the development of exercise-related amenorrhea.

mineral density levels that significantly correlate to muscular strength in the axial (L2-L4) and appendicular skeleton. For adolescent female athletes, absolute knee extension strength was moderately associated with total body, lumbar spine, femoral neck, and leg bone mineral density.[37]

Women at high risk for osteoporosis and those with osteoporosis reduce their *factor of risk* for fracture (defined as the ratio of load on the spine to the bone's failure load) by *(a)* strengthening bones by maintaining or increasing their density and *(b)* reducing the magnitude of spinal forces by avoiding higher-risk activities that increase spinal compression (e.g., heavy lifting activities).[112]

PHOSPHORUS

Phosphorus combines with calcium to form hydroxyapatite and calcium phosphate—compounds that give rigidity to bones and teeth. Phosphorus also serves as an essential component of the intracellular mediator, cyclic adenosine monophosphate (AMP), and the intramuscular high-energy compounds phosphocreatine (PCr) and adenosine triphosphate (ATP). ATP supplies the energy for all forms of

biologic work. Phosphorus combines with lipids to form phospholipid compounds, integral components of the cells' bilayer plasma membrane. The phosphorus-containing phosphatase enzymes help to regulate cellular metabolism. Phosphorus also participates in buffering acid end products of energy metabolism. For this reason, some coaches and trainers recommend consuming special "phosphate drinks" to reduce the effects of acid production in heavy exercise. "Phosphate loading" also has been proposed to facilitate oxygen release from hemoglobin at the cellular level. In Chapter 11, we discuss the usefulness of specific buffering drinks to augment exercise performance. Most studies confirm that the phosphorus intake of athletes generally attains recommended levels, with the possible exception of female dancers and gymnasts.[12,107] Rich dietary sources of phosphorus include meat, fish, poultry, milk products, and cereals.

MAGNESIUM

About 400 enzymes that regulate metabolism contain magnesium. Magnesium plays a vital role in glucose metabolism by helping to form muscle and liver glycogen from blood-

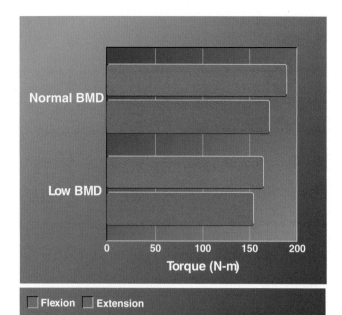

Figure 2.12 Comparison of chest press extension and flexion strength in age- and weight-matched postmenopausal women with normal and low bone mineral density (BMD). Women with low BMD scored significantly lower on each measure of muscular strength than the reference group. (From Stock JL, et al. Dynamic muscle strength is decreased in postmenopausal women with low bone density. J Bone Miner Res 1987;2:338; Janey C, et al. Maximum muscular strength differs in postmenopausal women with and without osteoporosis. Med Sci Sports Exerc 1987;19:S61.)

borne glucose. The 20 to 30 g of magnesium in the body also participates as a cofactor to break down glucose, fatty acids, and amino acids during energy metabolism. Furthermore, magnesium affects lipid and protein synthesis and contributes to proper functioning of the neuromuscular system. Magnesium also acts as an electrolyte, which, along with potassium and sodium, helps to maintain blood pressure. Sweating generally produces only small losses of magnesium. By regulating DNA and RNA synthesis and structure, magnesium regulates cell growth, reproduction, and the structure of plasma membranes. Because of its role as a Ca^{+2} channel blocker, inadequate magnesium could lead to hypertension and cardiac arrhythmias.

Conflicting data exist concerning the possible effects of magnesium supplements on exercise performance and the training response. In one study, magnesium supplementation did not affect quadriceps muscle strength or measures of fatigue in the 6-week period following a marathon.[180] Subsequent research showed that 4 weeks of a 212 mg per day magnesium oxide supplement increased resting magnesium levels but did not affect anaerobic or aerobic exercise performance, compared with a placebo.[46] In contrast, untrained men and women who supplemented with magnesium increased quadriceps power compared with a placebo treatment during 7 weeks of resistance training.[15]

The magnesium intake of athletes generally attains recommended levels, although female dancers and gymnasts have low intakes.[12,107] Green leafy vegetables, legumes, nuts, bananas, mushrooms, and whole grains provide a rich source of magnesium. We do not recommend taking magnesium supplements because these often are mixed with dolomite $(CaMg[CO_3]_2)$, an extract from dolomitic limestone and marble, which often contains the toxic elements mercury and lead.

IRON

The body normally contains between 3 to 5 g (about 1/6 oz) of the trace mineral iron. Approximately 80% of this amount exists in functionally active compounds, predominantly combined with **hemoglobin** in red blood cells. This iron–protein compound increases the oxygen-carrying capacity of blood approximately 65 times. FIGURE 2.13 displays the percentage composition of centrifuged whole blood for plasma and concentration of red blood cells (called the **hematocrit**), including average hemoglobin values for men and women.

Iron serves other important exercise-related functions besides its role in oxygen transport in blood. It is a structural component of **myoglobin** (about 5% of total iron), a compound with some similarities to hemoglobin, that aids in oxygen storage and transport within the muscle cell. Small

Figure 2.13 Percentage composition of centrifuged whole blood for plasma and red blood cell concentration (hematocrit). Also included are average values for hemoglobin for men and women per 100 mL of blood.

amounts of iron also exist in **cytochromes**, the specialized substances that facilitate energy transfer within the cell. About 20% of the body's iron does not combine in functionally active compounds and exists as **hemosiderin** and **ferritin** stored in the liver, spleen, and bone marrow. These stores replenish iron lost from the functional compounds and provide the iron reserve during periods of insufficient dietary iron intake. Another plasma protein, **transferrin**, transports iron from ingested food and damaged red blood cells for delivery to tissues in need. *Plasma levels of transferrin generally reflect the adequacy of current iron intake.*

Physically active individuals should include normal amounts of iron-rich foods in their daily diet. Persons with inadequate iron intake or with limited rates of iron absorption or high rates of iron loss often develop a reduced concentration of hemoglobin in red blood cells. This extreme condition of iron insufficiency, called **iron deficiency anemia**, produces general sluggishness, loss of appetite, and reduced capacity to sustain even mild exercise. "Iron therapy" with this condition normalizes the hemoglobin content of the blood and improves exercise capacity. TABLE 2.10 lists recommendations for iron intake for children and adults.

Females: A Population at Risk

Insufficient iron intake represents the most common micronutrient insufficiency, affecting between 20 and 50% of the world's population.[10] In the United States, estimates place between 10 and 13% of premenopausal women as deficient in iron intake and between 3 and 5% are anemic by conventional diagnostic criteria.[39,90] Inadequate iron intake frequently occurs among young children, teenagers, and females of childbearing age, including many physically active women.[22,132] In addition, pregnancy can trigger a moderate iron-deficiency anemia from the increased iron demand for both mother and fetus.

Table 2.10	RECOMMENDED DIETARY ALLOWANCES FOR IRON	
	Age (years)	*Iron (mg)*
Children	1–10	10
Males	11–18	12
	19+	10
Females	11–50	15
	51+	10
	Pregnant	30[a]
	Lactating	15[a]

Food and Nutrition Board, National Academy of Sciences-National Research Council, Washington, DC. Recommended dietary allowances, revised 1989.
[a] Generally, this increased requirement cannot be met by ordinary diets; therefore, the use of 30 to 60 mg of supplemental iron is recommended.

Iron loss from the 30 to 60 mL of blood lost during a menstrual cycle ranges between 15 and 30 mg. This loss requires an additional 5-mg dietary iron daily for premenopausal females, which increases the average monthly iron requirement by about 150 mg. Thus, an additional 20 to 25 mg of iron becomes available to females each month (assuming typical iron absorption) for synthesizing red blood cells lost during menstruation. Dietary iron insufficiencies of the large number of American premenopausal women relate to a limited supply of iron in the typical diet, which averages about 6 mg of iron per 1000 kcal of food ingested.

Iron Source Is Important

Intestinal absorption of iron varies closely with iron need, yet considerable variation in bioavailability occurs because of diet composition. For example, the intestine usually absorbs between 2 and 10% of iron from plants (trivalent ferric or **nonheme** elemental **iron**), whereas iron absorption from animal sources (divalent ferrous or **heme iron**) increases to between 10 and 35%. The body absorbs about 15% of ingested iron, depending on one's iron status, form of iron ingested, and composition of the meal. For example, intestinal absorption of nonheme (but not heme) iron significantly increases when consuming diets with low iron bioavailability.[65] Conversely, iron supplementation reduces nonheme iron but not heme iron absorption from food.[148] Despite this partial adaptation in iron absorption, iron stores remain greater after supplementation than after placebo treatment. The presence of heme iron in food also increases iron absorption from nonheme sources. Consuming more meat maintains iron status more effectively in exercising women than supplementing with commercial iron preparations.[92]

Of Concern to Vegetarians

The relatively low bioavailability of nonheme iron places women on vegetarian-type diets at increased risk for developing iron insufficiency. Female vegetarian runners have a poorer iron status than counterparts who consume the same quantity of iron from predominantly animal sources.[163] Including foods rich in vitamin C in the diet (see Table 2.1) upgrades the bioavailability of dietary iron. This occurs because ascorbic acid increases the solubility of nonheme iron, making it available for absorption at the alkaline pH of the small intestine. The ascorbic acid in a glass of orange juice, for example, significantly increases nonheme iron absorption from a breakfast meal.

The top panel of FIGURE 2.14 clearly illustrates the effect of exogenous vitamin C on nonheme iron absorption. Eight healthy men without iron deficiency were studied at rest after taking either 100 mg of ferric sodium citrate complex, 100 mg of ferric sodium citrate complex with 200 mg ascorbic acid, or no exogenous iron. The iron supplement alone caused an 18.4% increase in serum iron concentration compared with the control, no iron condition. Combining iron and vitamin C, however, induced a peak 72% increase in serum iron. Furthermore, taking the iron-only supplement followed by 1 hour of moderate exercise produced a 48.2% increase in serum iron concentration compared with only an 8.3% increase at rest (Fig. 2.14, *bottom*). Combining exercise and iron supplementation plus vitamin C did not significantly augment physical activity's effect on iron absorption. These data convincingly indicate that moderate exercise

does not impair the body's absorption of supplemental iron; instead, it facilitates iron uptake to the same amount as vitamin C supplementation without exercise. These findings also provide a nutrition-based justification for moderate exercise following eating.

Heme iron sources include tuna (3 oz = 1.6 mg), chicken (4.0 oz breast = 1.8 mg), clams (3 oz = 2.6 mg), beef (3 oz = 2.7 mg), oysters (3 oz = 5.9 mg), and beef liver (3 oz = 6.6 mg); **nonheme iron sources** include oatmeal (1 cup nonfortified = 1.6 mg; fortified with nutrient added = 6.3 mg), spinach (1/2 cup cooked = 2.0 mg), soy protein (tofu, piece 2 1/2 × 2 3/4 × 1 inch = 2.3 mg), dried figs (4 figs = 2.3 mg), beans (1/2 cup refried = 2.3 mg), raisins (1/2 cup = 2.5 mg), lima beans (1/2 cup = 2.5 mg), prune juice (1 cup = 3.0 mg), peaches (1/2 cup dried = 3.3 mg), and apricots (1 cup dried = 6.1 mg). Fiber-rich foods, coffee, and tea contain compounds that interfere with the intestinal absorption of iron (and zinc).

Are the Physically Active at Greater Risk for Iron Insufficiency?

Interest in endurance sports, combined with increased participation of women in these activities, has focused research on the influence of strenuous training on the body's iron status. The term **"sports anemia"** frequently describes reduced hemoglobin levels approaching clinical anemia (12 g·dL^{-1} of blood for women and 14 g·dL^{-1} for men) attributable to intense training.

Some maintain that exercise training creates an added demand for iron that often exceeds its intake. This would tax iron reserves and eventually depress hemoglobin synthesis and/or reduce iron-containing compounds within the cell's energy transfer system. Individuals susceptible to an "iron drain" could experience reduced exercise capacity because of iron's crucial role in oxygen transport and use.

Heavy training theoretically increases iron demand from iron loss in sweat and from the loss of hemoglobin in urine from red blood cell destruction with increased temperature, spleen activity, circulation rates, and mechanical trauma from runners' feet pounding on the running surface (foot-strike hemolysis).[126,155] Gastrointestinal bleeding unrelated to age, sex, or performance time can also occur with long-distance running.[97,113] Such iron loss would stress the body's iron reserves required to synthesize 260 billion new red blood cells daily in the bone marrow of the skull, upper arm, sternum, ribs, spine, pelvis, and upper leg. Iron loss poses an additional burden to premenopausal women who have a greater iron requirement yet lower iron intake than men.

Real or Pseudoanemia?

Apparent suboptimal hemoglobin concentrations and hematocrits occur more frequently among endurance athletes, supporting the possibility of an exercise-induced anemia. On

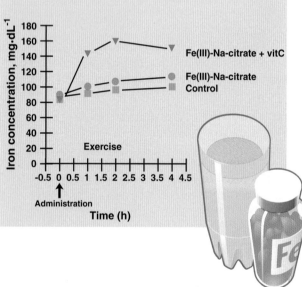

■ **Figure 2.14** *Top,* Serum iron concentrations following administration of a single dose of 100 mg ferric sodium citrate complex (Fe [III]-Na-citrate) or 100 mg of sodium citrate complex with 200 mg ascorbic acid (Fe [III]-Na-citrate + vit C) compared with controls at rest. *Bottom,* Serum iron concentrations following administration of a single dose of 100 mg of ferric sodium citrate complex (Fe [III]-Na-citrate) or 100 mg of sodium citrate complex with 200 mg ascorbic acid (Fe [III]-Na-citrate + vit C) compared with controls during moderate (60% V̇O$_2$ max) exercise. (From Schmid A, et al. Effect of physical exercise and vitamin C on absorption of ferric sodium citrate. Med Sci Sports Exerc 1996;28:1470.)

closer scrutiny, reductions in hemoglobin concentration appear transient, occurring in the early phase of training and then returning toward pretraining values. FIGURE 2.15 illustrates the general response for hematologic variables for high-school female cross-country runners during a competitive season. *The decrease in hemoglobin concentration generally parallels the disproportionately large expansion in plasma volume early in exercise training.*[53,155,159] For example, just several days of training increases plasma volume by 20%, while the total volume of red blood cells remains unchanged.[54] Consequently, **total hemoglobin** (an important factor in endurance performance) remains the same or increases somewhat with training, yet hemoglobin *concentration* decreases in the expanding plasma volume.

Despite hemoglobin's apparent dilution, aerobic capacity and exercise performance normally improve with training. Some mechanical destruction of red blood cells may occur with vigorous exercise (including minimal iron loss in sweat[17]), but no evidence shows that these factors strain an athlete's iron reserves sufficiently to precipitate clinical anemia as long as iron intake remains at recommended levels. Applying stringent criteria for both anemia and insufficient iron reserves makes sports anemia much less prevalent among highly trained athletes than generally believed.[189] For male collegiate runners and swimmers, no indications of the early stages of anemia were noted despite large changes in training volume and intensity during different phases of the competitive season.[128] Data from female athletes indicate the prevalence of iron deficiency anemia did *not* differ in comparisons among specific athletic groups or with a nonathletic control group.[141]

Should the Physically Active Supplement With Iron?

Losing any iron with exercise training (coupled with poor dietary habits) in adolescent and premenopausal females, particularly among those in the low-weight or body-appearance sports, could strain an already limited iron reserve. This does not mean that all physically active individuals should take supplementary iron or that all indications of sports anemia result from dietary iron deficiency or iron loss caused by exercise. It does suggest, however, the importance of monitoring an athlete's iron status by periodic evaluation of hematologic characteristics and iron reserves, particularly athletes who choose to supplement with iron.[31] This is important because reversal of full-blown iron deficiency anemia can require up to 6 months of iron therapy. Measuring **serum ferritin** concentration provides useful information about iron reserves. Values below 20 $\mu g \cdot L^{-1}$ for females and 30 $\mu g \cdot L^{-1}$ for males indicate depleted iron reserves.

Hemoglobin concentration of 12 g per dL represents the cutoff for the clinical classification of anemia for women. Low values within the "normal" range could reflect **functional anemia** or **marginal iron deficiency**, a condition characterized by depleted iron stores, reduced iron-dependent protein production (e.g., oxidative enzymes) but relatively *normal* hemoglobin concentrations. The ergogenic effects of iron supplementation on aerobic exercise performance and training responsiveness have been noted for such groups of iron-deficient athletes.[16,49] For example, physically active but untrained women classified as iron depleted (serum ferritin $< 16\ \mu g \cdot L^{-1}$) but not anemic (Hb >12 $g \cdot dL^{-1}$) received either iron therapy (50 mg ferrous sulfate) or a placebo twice daily for 2 weeks.[62] All subjects then

■ **Figure 2.15** Hemoglobin, red blood cell count, and hematocrit in female high school cross-country runners and a comparison group during the competitive season. (Adapted from Puhl JL, et al. Erythrocyte changes during training in high school women cross-country runners. Res Q Exerc Sport 1981;52:484.)

completed 4 weeks of aerobic training. The iron-supplemented group significantly increased serum ferritin levels with only a small (nonsignificant) increase in hemoglobin concentration. The supplemented group also had twice the improvement in 15-km endurance cycling time (3.4 vs 1.6 min faster) than the women who consumed the placebo. The researchers concluded that women with low serum ferritin levels but hemoglobin concentrations above 12 g·dL^{-1}, although not clinically anemic, might still be functionally anemic and thus benefit from iron supplementation to help exercise performance. Similarly, iron-depleted but nonanemic women received either a placebo or 20 mg of elemental iron as ferrous sulfate twice daily for 6 weeks.[18] FIGURE 2.16 shows that the iron supplement significantly attenuated the rate of decrease in maximal force measured sequentially during approximately 8 minutes of dynamic knee extension exercise.

These findings support current recommendations to use an iron supplement for physically active women with low serum ferritin levles.[121] Iron supplementation exerts little effect on hemoglobin concentration and red blood cell volume in iron-deficient but nonanemic groups. Any improved exercise capacity most likely comes from increased muscle oxidative capacity, not oxygen transport capacity by the blood.

Steer Clear of Iron Supplements Unless an Insufficiency Exists

For healthy individuals whose diets contain the recommended iron intake, iron supplementation does not increase hemoglobin, hematocrit, or other measures of iron status.[7,57] If dietary iron insufficiency causes subnormal hemoglobin levels, a physician may recommend supplementation with 325 mg ferrous sulfate two or three times weekly.

Potential harm exists from the overconsumption or overabsorption of iron, particularly with an excessive consumption of red meat and ready availability of iron and vitamin C supplements.[48] Supplements should not be used indiscriminately because excessive iron can accumulate to toxic levels and contribute to diabetes, liver disease, and heart and joint damage. Excess iron intake may even augment the growth of latent cancers (e.g., colorectal cancer) and infectious organisms.[117] Controversy exists as to whether individuals with high levels of body iron stores have a higher CHD risk than individuals with iron levels in the

■ **Figure 2.16** Maximal voluntary static contractions (MVCs) over the first 6 minutes of a progressive fatigue test of dynamic knee extensions before (●) and after (●) supplementation with either a placebo or iron. MVC$_{end}$ represents the last MVC of the protocol and occurred at different times (average ≈ 8 min) for each subject.

low-to-normal range.[30,77,133,151,157] If risk exists, one explanation postulates that high serum iron catalyzes free radical formation, which augments the oxidation of LDL-cholesterol, thus promoting atherosclerosis. Currently, the evidence supporting this hypothesis remains inconsistent and inconclusive.[158]

Approximately 1.5 million Americans have a genetic abnormality, **hereditary hemochromatosis**, that predisposes them to iron accumulation in the various body tissues. If undetected, this genetic abnormality produces excessive iron absorption and accumulation with early symptoms of chronic fatigue, abdominal pain, and menstrual dysfunction in females. In the extreme, hemochromatosis leads to cirrhosis or cancer of the liver, heart and thyroid disease, diabetes, arthritis, and infertility. Early diagnosis and treatment can prevent the serious complications of hemochromatosis.

SODIUM, POTASSIUM, AND CHLORINE

Sodium, potassium, and chlorine, collectively termed **electrolytes**, remain dissolved in the body as electrically charged particles called ions. Sodium and chlorine represent the chief minerals contained in blood plasma and extracellular fluid. Electrolytes modulate fluid exchange within the body's fluid compartments, allowing a well-regulated exchange of nutrients and waste products between the cell and its external fluid environment. Potassium is the chief intracellular mineral.

The most important function of sodium and potassium ions concerns their role in establishing the proper electrical gradient across cell membranes. This difference in electrical balance between the cell's interior and exterior allows the transmission of nerve impulses, the stimulation and action of muscle, and proper gland functioning. Electrolytes also maintain plasma membrane permeability and regulate the acid and base qualities of body fluids, particularly the blood. TABLE 2.11 lists values considered normal for electrolyte concentrations in serum and sweat, and the electrolyte and carbohydrate concentrations of common oral rehydration beverages.

How Much Sodium Is Enough?

With low-to-moderate sodium intake, the hormone **aldosterone** acts on the kidneys to conserve sodium. Conversely, high dietary sodium inhibits aldosterone release. Any excess sodium becomes excreted in the urine. Consequently, salt balance generally remains normal throughout a wide range of intakes. This does not occur in individuals who cannot adequately regulate excessive sodium intake. Abnormal sodium accumulation in body fluids increases fluid volume and elevates blood pressure to levels that pose a health risk. Such **sodium-induced hypertension** occurs in about one-third of individuals with hypertension.

Sodium is widely distributed naturally in foods, so one can readily obtain the daily requirement without adding "extra" salt to foods. Sodium intake in the United States regularly exceeds the daily level recommended for adults of 2400 mg, or the amount of sodium in one heaping teaspoon of table salt (sodium makes up about 40% of salt). The typical Western diet contains about 4500 mg of sodium (8–12 g of salt) each day with three-quarters coming from processed food and restaurant meals. This represents 10 times the 500 mg of sodium the body actually needs. Heavy reliance on table salt in processing, curing, cooking, seasoning, and preserving common foods accounts for the large sodium intake. Aside from table salt, common sodium-rich dietary sources include monosodium glutamate (MSG), soy sauce, condiments, canned foods, baking soda, and baking powder.

For decades, one low-risk, first-line of defense in treating high blood pressure eliminated excess sodium from the

Table 2.11	**ELECTROLYTE CONCENTRATIONS IN BLOOD SERUM AND SWEAT, AND CARBOHYDRATE AND ELECTROLYTE CONCENTRATIONS OF SOME COMMON BEVERAGES**						
	Na^+ $(mEq \cdot L^{-1})$	K^+ $(mEq \cdot L^{-1})$	Ca^{2+} $(mEq \cdot L^{-1})$	Mg^{2+} $(mEq \cdot L^{-1})$	Cl^- $(mEq \cdot L^{-1})$	Osmolality $(mOsm \cdot L^{-1})$	CHO $(g \cdot L^{-1})$
Blood serum	140	4.5	2.5	1.5–2.1	110	300	—
Sweat	60–80	4.5	1.5	3.3	40–90	170–220	—
Coca Cola	3.0	—	—	—	1.0	650	107
Gatorade	23.0	3.0	—	—	14.0	280	62
Fruit juice	0.5	58.0	—	—	—	690	118
Pepsi Cola	1.7	trace	—	—	trace	568	81
Water	trace	trace	—	—	trace	10–20	—

diet. Reducing sodium intake possibly lowers sodium and body fluid, thereby lowering blood pressure. This effect is particularly apparent for **"salt sensitive"** individuals; reducing dietary sodium decreases their blood pressure.[66,166] Debate concerns the magnitude of this reduction for most hypertensives.[5,41,91,105] If dietary constraints prove ineffective in lowering blood pressure, drugs that induce a water loss **(diuretics)** become the next line of defense. Unfortunately, diuretics also produce losses in other minerals, particularly potassium. A potassium-rich diet (potatoes, bananas, oranges, tomatoes, and meat) becomes a necessity for a patient using diuretics.

The DASH Dietary Intervention to Lower High Blood Pressure

Nearly 50 million Americans have hypertension, a condition if left untreated increases the risk of stroke, heart attack, and kidney failure. Fifty percent of hypertensives actually seek treatment and only about one-half of these individuals achieve long-term success. One reason for the lack of compliance concerns possible side effects of readily available antihypertensive medications. For example, fatigue and impotence often discourage patients from maintaining a chronic medication schedule required by pharmacologic treatment of hypertension.

Table 2.12	DIETARY APPROACHES TO STOP HYPERTENSION (DASH)	
Food Group	**Example of 1 Serving**	**Servings**
Vegetables	1/2 cup of cooked or raw chopped vegetables; 1 cup of raw leafy vegetables; or 6 oz of juice	8–12 daily
Fruit	1 medium apple, pear, orange, or banana; 1/2 grapefruit; 1/3 cantaloupe; 1/2 cup of fresh frozen or canned fruit; 1/4 cup of dried fruit; or 6 oz of juice	8–12 daily
Grains	1 slice of bread; 1/2 cup of cold, dry cereal; cooked rice or pasta	6–12 daily
Dairy	1 cup of no-fat or low-fat milk or 1 1/2 oz of low-fat or part-skim cheese	2–4 daily
Nuts, seeds, and beans	1/3 cup (1 1/2 oz) of nuts; 2 tablespoons of seeds; or 1/2 cup of cooked beans	4–7 weekly
Meat, poultry, or fish	3 oz chunk (roughly the size of a deck of cards)	1–2 daily
Oil or other fats	1 tsp. vegetable oil; butter; salad dressings; soft margarine	2–4 daily

THE DASH APPROACH

Research using **Dietary Approaches to Stop Hypertension (DASH)** to treat hypertension shows that this diet lowers blood pressure in the general population and in persons with stage 1 hypertension to the same extent as pharmacologic therapy and often more than other lifestyle changes.[24,149] Two months of the diet reduced systolic pressure by an average of 11.4 mm Hg; diastolic pressure decreased by 5.5 mm Hg. Every 2 mm Hg reduction in systolic pressure lowers heart disease risk by 5% and stroke risk by 8%.

TABLE 2.12 shows the specifics of the DASH diet with its high content of fruits, vegetables, and dairy products and low-fat composition. Further good news emerges from the latest research from the DASH group indicating that the standard DASH diet combined with a daily salt intake of 1150 mg—called the DASH-Sodium diet—produced greater blood pressure reductions than were achieved with the DASH diet only.[150,172] Blood pressure declined significantly for both normotensive and hypertensive subjects, with the greatest benefits for subjects with high blood pressure. The DASH diet alone and sodium restriction alone both lowered blood pressure, but the greatest reductions emerged with the DASH-low sodium combination. The best available scientific information currently available recommends the following lifestyle approaches to prevent

hypertension:[192,193]

- Regularly engage in moderate physical activity
- Maintain normal body weight
- Limit alcohol consumption
- Reduce sodium intake and maintain an adequate intake of potassium
- Consume a diet rich in fruits, vegetables, and low-fat dairy products and reduced in saturated fatty acids and total fat

TABLE 2.13 shows a sample DASH diet consisting of approximately 2100 kcal. This level of energy intake provides a stable body weight for a typical 70-kg person. More physically active and heavier individuals should boost portion size or the number of individual items to maintain weight. Individuals desiring to lose weight or who are lighter and/or sedentary should eat less, but not less than the minimum number of servings for each food group listed in Table 2.12.

Can Sodium Intake Be Too Low?

A low-sodium diet in conjunction with excessive perspiration, persistent vomiting, or diarrhea creates the potential to deplete the body's sodium content to critical levels, a condition termed **hyponatremia.** This condition causes a broad array of symptoms ranging from muscle cramps, nausea, vomiting, dizziness and, in the extreme, to shock, coma, and death. A minimal likelihood of hyponatremia exists for most persons because responses by the kidneys to low sodium status trigger sodium conservation. In addition, the availability of sodium in so many foods makes it improbable that sodium levels would fall to critically low levels.

Even when body weight loss from perspiration reaches 2 to 3% of body weight (about 5 to 7 lb), adding a bit of extra table salt to food usually restores sodium for most persons. Endurance athletes, basketball, baseball, soccer, and football players who routinely lose more than 4% of body weight following competition should consume salt-containing drinks prior to and after heavy sweating to ensure adequate sodium concentrations in the body. Chapter 10 discusses exercise, fluid intake, and risks of hyponatremia in greater detail.

Table 2.13 SAMPLE 2100-kcal DASH DIET

Food	Amount
Breakfast	
Orange juice	6 oz
1% low-fat milk	8 oz (used with corn flakes)
Corn flakes (1 tsp. sugar)	1 cup (dry) [equals 2 servings of grains]
Banana	1 medium
Whole-wheat bread	1 slice
Soft margarine	1 tsp.
Lunch	
Low-fat chicken salad	3/4 cup
Pita bread	1/2 large
Raw-vegetable medley	
Carrot and celery sticks	3–4 sticks each
Radishes	2
Lettuce	2 leaves
Part-skim mozzarella	1 1/2 slices (1.5 oz)
1% low-fat milk	8 oz
Fruit cocktail	1/2 cup
Dinner	
Herbed baked cod	3 oz
Scallion rice	1 cup [equals 2 servings of grain]
Steamed broccoli	1/2 cup
Stewed tomatoes	1/2 cup
Spinach salad (raw spinach)	1/2 cup
Cherry tomatoes	2
Cucumber	2 slices
Light Italian salad dressing	1 tbsp. (equals 1/2 fat serving)
Whole wheat dinner roll	1
Soft margarine	1 tsp.
Melon balls	1/2 cup
Snack	
Dried apricots	1 oz (1/4 cup)
Mixed nuts, unsalted	1.5 oz (1/3 cup)
Mini-pretzels, unsalted	1 oz (3/4 cup)
Diet ginger ale	12 oz (does not count as a serving of any food)

Summary

1. Approximately 4% of the body mass consists of 22 elements called minerals. Minerals become distributed in all body tissues and fluids.

2. Minerals occur freely in nature, in the waters of rivers, lakes, and oceans, and in soil. The root system of plants absorbs minerals; they eventually become incorporated into the tissues of animals that consume plants.

3. Minerals function primarily in metabolism as constituents of enzymes. Minerals provide structure in the formation of bones and teeth and synthesize the biologic macronutrients glycogen, fat, and protein.

4. A balanced diet generally provides adequate mineral intake, except in some geographic locations lacking specific minerals (e.g., iodine).

5. Osteoporosis has reached almost epidemic proportions among older individuals, particularly women. Adequate calcium intake and regular weight-bearing exercise and/or resistance training provide an effective defense against bone loss at any age.

6. Paradoxically, women who train intensely but cannot match energy intake to energy output reduce body weight and body fat to the point that may adversely affect menstruation. These women often show advanced bone loss at an early age. Restoration of normal menstruation does not totally restore bone mass.

7. The significant association between muscular strength and bone density raises the likelihood of using strength testing of postmenopausal women as a clinically useful tool to screen for osteoporosis.

8. About 40% of American women of childbearing age suffer from dietary iron insufficiency that could lead to iron-deficiency anemia. This condition negatively affects aerobic exercise performance and the ability to perform intense training.

9. For women on vegetarian-type diets, the relatively low bioavailability of nonheme iron increases the risk for developing iron insufficiency. Both vitamin C (in food or supplement form) and moderate physical activity increase intestinal absorption of nonheme iron.

10. Regular physical activity generally does not create a significant drain on the body's iron reserves. If it does, females, with the greatest iron

requirement and lowest iron intake, could increase their risk for anemia. Assessment of the body's iron status should evaluate hematologic characteristics and iron reserves.

11. The Dietary Approaches to Stop Hypertension (DASH) diet lowers blood pressure in some individuals to the same extent as pharmacologic therapy and often more than other lifestyle changes.

➤ Water

WATER IN THE BODY

Water makes up from 40 to 70% of an individual's body mass, depending on age, sex, and body composition; it constitutes 65 to 75% of the weight of muscle and about 50% of the weight of body fat (adipose tissue). Consequently, differences in the relative percentage of total body water among individuals result largely from variations in body composition (i.e., differences in lean vs fat tissue).

FIGURE 2.17 depicts the fluid compartments of the body, the normal daily body water variation, and specific terminology to describe the various states of human hydration. The body contains two fluid "compartments;" The first compartment, **intracellular**, refers to inside the cells; the second,

Daily euhydration variability of total body water
Temperature climate: 0.165 L (0.2% body mass)
Heat exercise conditions: 0.382 L (0.5% body mass)

Daily plasma volume variability
All conditions: 0.027 L (0.6% blood volume)

Hydration terminology
Euhydration: normal daily water variation
Hyperhydration: new steady-state condition of increased water content
Hypohydration: new steady-state condition of decreased water content
Dehydration: process of losing water either from the hyperhydrated state to euhydration, or from euhydration downward to hypohydration
Rehydration: process of gaining water from a hypohydrated state toward euhydration

■ **Figure 2.17** Fluid compartments, average volumes and variability, and hydration terminology. Volumes represent those for an 80-kg man. Approximately 60% of the body mass consists of water in striated muscle (80% water), skeleton (32% water), and adipose tissue (50% water). For a man and woman of similar body mass, the woman contains less total water because of her larger ratio of adipose tissue to lean body mass (striated muscle + skeleton).(Adapted from Greenleaf JE. Problem: thirst, drinking behavior, and involuntary dehydration. Med Sci Sports Exerc 1992;24:645.)

extracellular, indicates fluids surrounding the cells. Extracellular fluid includes the blood plasma and the interstitial fluids, which primarily compose the fluid that flows in the microscopic spaces among the cells. Also included as interstitial fluid are lymph, saliva, and fluid in the eyes, fluids secreted by glands and the digestive tract, fluids that bathe the nerves of the spinal cord, and fluids excreted from the skin and kidneys. Blood plasma accounts for 20% of the extracellular fluid (3 to 4 L). *Much of the fluid lost through sweating is extracellular fluid, predominantly from the blood plasma.* Of the total body water, an average of 62% (26 L of the body's 42 L of water for an average-sized man) represents intracellular water and 38% comes from extracellular sources. These volumes do not remain static but represent averages from a dynamic exchange of fluid between compartments, particularly in physically active individuals.[153] Exercise training often increases the percentage of water distributed within the intracellular compartment from increases in muscle mass and its accompanying large water content. In contrast, an acute bout of exercise temporarily shifts fluid from the plasma to the interstitial and intracellular spaces from the increased hydrostatic (fluid) pressure within the active circulatory system.

FUNCTIONS OF BODY WATER

Water is a ubiquitous, remarkable nutrient. Without water, death occurs within days. It serves as the body's transport and reactive medium; diffusion of gases always takes place across surfaces moistened by water. Nutrients and gases travel in aqueous solution; waste products leave the body through the water in urine and feces. Water, in conjunction with various proteins, lubricates joints and protects a variety of "moving" organs like the heart, lungs, intestines, and eyes. Because it is noncompressible, water gives structure and form to the body through the turgor provided for body tissues. Water has tremendous heat-stabilizing qualities because it absorbs considerable heat with only minor changes in temperature. This quality, combined with water's high heat of vaporization (energy required to change 1 g of a liquid into the gaseous state at the boiling point), facilitates maintenance of a relatively constant body temperature during *(a)* environmental heat stress and *(b)* the large increase in internal heat generated by exercise. Chapter 10 says more about the dynamics of thermoregulation during heat stress, particularly water's important role.

WATER BALANCE: INTAKE VERSUS OUTPUT

The body's water content remains relatively stable over time. Although considerable water output occurs in physically active individuals, appropriate fluid intake usually

■ **Figure 2.18** Water balance in the body. *Top,* Little or no exercise in normal ambient temperature and humidity. *Bottom,* Moderate to heavy exercise in a hot, humid environment.

restores any imbalance in the body's fluid level. FIGURE 2.18 displays the sources of water intake and output.

Water Intake

A sedentary adult in a thermoneutral environment requires about 2.5 L of water each day. For an active person in a hot environment the water requirement often increases to between 5 and 10 L daily. Three sources provide this water: *(a)* liquids, *(b)* foods, and *(c)* metabolic processes.

Water from Liquids

The average individual normally consumes 1200 mL or 41 oz of water each day. Exercise and thermal stress can increase fluid intake five or six times above normal. At the extreme, an individual lost 13.6 kg (30 lb) of water weight during a 2-day, 17-hour, 55-mile run across Death Valley, California (lowest point in the Western Hemisphere at almost 300 feet below sea level; recognized as one of the hottest places on earth with highest recorded temperature of 134°F). However, with proper fluid ingestion, including salt supplements, body weight loss amounted to only 1.4 kg. In this example, fluid loss and replenishment represented between 3.5 and 4 gallons of liquid!

Water in Foods

Fruits and vegetables contain considerable water (e.g., lettuce, watermelon and cantaloupe, pickles, green beans, and broccoli); in contrast, butter, oils, dried meats, and chocolate, cookies, and cakes have a relatively low water content.

Metabolic Water

Carbon dioxide and water form when food molecules catabolize for energy. Termed **metabolic water**, this fluid provides about 14% of a sedentary person's daily water requirement. The complete breakdown of 100 g of carbohydrate, protein, and fat yields 55, 100, and 107 g of metabolic water, respectively. Additionally, each gram of glycogen joins with 2.7 g of water as its glucose units link together; subsequently, glycogen liberates this bound water during its catabolism for energy.

Water Output

Water loss from the body occurs in one of four ways: *(a)* in urine, *(b)* through the skin, *(c)* as water vapor in expired air, and *(d)* in feces.

Water Loss in Urine

Under normal conditions the kidneys reabsorb about 99% of the 140 to 160 L of filtrate formed each day; consequently, the volume of urine excreted daily by the kidneys ranges from 1000 to 1500 mL or about 1.5 quarts.

Elimination of 1 g of solute by the kidneys requires about 15 mL of water. Thus, a portion of water in urine becomes "obligated" to rid the body of metabolic byproducts like urea, an end product of protein breakdown. Catabolizing large quantities of protein for energy (as occurs with a high-protein diet) actually accelerates the body's dehydration during exercise.

Water Loss through the Skin

A small quantity of water, perhaps 350 mL, termed **insensible perspiration**, continually seeps from the deeper tissues through the skin to the body's surface. Water loss through the skin also occurs as sweat produced by specialized sweat glands beneath the skin's surface. Evaporation of sweat's water component provides the refrigeration mechanism to cool the body. Daily sweat rate under normal conditions amounts to between 500 and 700 mL. This by no means reflects sweating capacity; the well-acclimatized person can produce up to 12 L of sweat (equivalent of 12 kg) at a rate of 1 L per hour during prolonged exercise in a hot environment.

Water Loss As Water Vapor

Insensible water loss through small water droplets in exhaled air amounts to 250 to 350 mL per day. The complete moistening of all inspired air as it passes down the pulmonary airways accounts for this avenue of water loss. Exercise affects this source of water loss because inspired air requires humidification. For physically active persons, the respiratory passages release 2 to 5 mL of water each minute during strenuous exercise, depending on climatic conditions. Ventilatory water loss is least in hot, humid weather and greatest in cold temperatures (inspired cold air contains little moisture) or at altitude, because inspired air volumes are significantly larger than at sea-level conditions.

Water Loss in Feces

Intestinal elimination produces between 100 and 200 mL of water loss because water constitutes approximately 70% of fecal matter. The remainder comprises nondigestible material including bacteria from the digestive process and the residues of digestive juices from the intestine, stomach, and pancreas. With diarrhea or vomiting, water loss increases to between 1500 and 5000 mL.

PHYSICAL ACTIVITY AND ENVIRONMENTAL FACTORS PLAY AN IMPORTANT ROLE

The loss of body water represents the most serious consequence of profuse sweating. The severity of physical activity, environmental temperature, and humidity determine the amount of water lost through sweating. Relative humidity (water content of the ambient air) significantly affects the efficiency of the sweating mechanism for temperature regulation. Ambient air becomes completely saturated with water vapor at 100% relative humidity. This blocks evaporation of fluid from the skin surface to the air, thus negating this important avenue for body cooling. Under such conditions, sweat beads on the skin and eventually rolls off, without providing an evaporative cooling effect. On a dry day, air can hold considerable moisture, and fluid rapidly evaporates from the skin. Thus, the sweat mechanism functions at optimal efficiency and body temperature remains regulated within a narrow range. Importantly, plasma volume begins to decrease when sweating causes a fluid loss equal to 2 or 3% of body mass. Fluid loss from the vascular compartment strains circulatory function, which ultimately impairs exercise capacity and thermoregulation. *Monitoring changes in body weight provides a convenient method for assessing fluid loss during exercise and/or heat stress. Each 0.45 kg (1 lb) of body weight loss corresponds to 450 mL of dehydration.*

Summary

1. Water constitutes 40 to 70% of the total body mass; muscle contains 72% water by weight, whereas water represents only about 50% of the weight of body fat (adipose tissue).

2. Of the total body water, roughly 62% exists intracellularly (inside the cells) and 38% occurs extracellularly in the plasma, lymph, and other fluids outside the cell.

3. The normal average daily water intake of 2.5 L comes from liquid (1.2 L) and food (1.0 L) intake and metabolic water produced during energy-yielding reactions (0.3 L).

4. Daily water loss occurs in urine (1–1.5 L), through the skin as insensible perspiration (0.50–0.70 L), as water vapor in expired air (0.25–0.30 L), and in feces (0.10 L).

5. Food and oxygen exist in the body in aqueous solution, while nongaseous waste products always leave in a watery medium. Water also provides structure and form to the body and plays a crucial role in temperature regulation.

6. Exercise in hot weather greatly increases the body's water requirement. In extreme conditions, fluid needs increase five or six times above normal.

TEST YOUR KNOWLEDGE ANSWERS

1. True Vitamin intake above the RDA does not improve exercise performance or the potential to sustain physical training. In fact, serious illness occurs from regularly consuming excess fat-soluble vitamins and, in some instances, water-soluble vitamins.

2. False While the body can conserve water, there is some loss every day. After only a few days, severe dehydration can result in death. In contrast, death from starvation takes much longer, perhaps 60 days or more.

3. False The terms *major* and *trace* do not reflect nutritional importance; rather, they are classifications referring to the amount needed for (daily) functioning. In essence, each of the micronutrients, major or trace, is critical to the maintenance of optimal physiologic functioning and good health.

4. False Most major and trace minerals occur freely in nature, mainly in the waters of rivers, lakes, and oceans, in topsoil, and beneath the earth's surface. Minerals exist in the root systems of plants and in the body structure of animals that consume plants and water containing minerals. Neither plant nor animal kingdom provides a "better" source for these micronutrients.

5. False Adults need about 1 mL of water per kcal of energy expended each day. If the average woman expends 2400 kcal per day she then requires about 2400 mL (2.4 L) of water on a daily basis. This volume transposes to about 0.63 gallons (2.4 L ÷ 3.785).

6. False While sodium is an important contributor to increased blood pressure in some hypertensive individuals, weight (fat) loss, regular exercise, and a well-balanced diet are also important changes a person can make to lower blood pressure.

7. False Fat-soluble vitamins should not be consumed in excess without medical supervision. Toxic reactions from excessive fat-soluble vitamin intake generally occur at a lower multiple of recommended intakes than water-soluble vitamins. An excess intake of certain water-soluble vitamins also causes untoward effects in certain individuals.

8. False Iron deficiency anemia impairs the body's ability to transport oxygen and process it in energy transfer reactions. This condition produces general sluggishness, loss of appetite, and reduced capacity to sustain even mild exercise.

9. False Short intense bouts of mechanical loading of bone through weightbearing exercise performed three to five times a week provides a potent stimulus to maintain or increase bone mass. This form of exercise includes walking, running, dancing, rope skipping; high-intensity resistance exercises, and circuit-resistance training also exert a positive effect. Sport activities providing relatively high impact on the skeletal mass (e.g., volleyball, basketball, gymnastics, judo, and karate) also induce increases in bone mass, particularly at weight-bearing sites.

10. False Research using Dietary Approaches to Stop Hypertension (DASH) to treat hypertension shows that this type of diet lowers blood pressure in the general population and in people with stage 1 hypertension to the same extent as pharmacologic therapy, and often more than other lifestyle changes.

References

1. Al-Delaimy WK, et al. A prospective study of calcium intake from diet and supplements and risk of ischemic heart disease among men. Am J Clin Nutr 2003;72:814.

2. American College of Sports Medicine. Position stand on physical activity and bone health. Med Sci Sports Exerc 2004;36:1985.

3. American College of Sports Medicine, American Dietetic Association and Dietitians of Canada. Joint position statement. Nutrition and athletic performance. Med Sci Sports Exerc 2000;32:2130.

4. Andreoli A, et al. Effects of different sports on bone density and muscle mass in highly trained athletes. Med Sci Sports Exerc 2001;33:507.

5. Apple LJ, et al, A clinical trial of the effects of dietary patterns on blood pressure: DASH Collaborative Research Group. N Engl J Med 1997;336:1117.

6. Arab L, Steck S. Lycopene and cardiovascular disease. Am J Clin Nutr 2000;71:1691S.

7. Asheden MJ, et al. The haematological response to an iron injection amongst female athletes. Int J Sports Med 1998;19:474.

8. Ashizawa N, et al. Tomographical description of tennis-loaded radius: reciprocal relation between bone size and volumetric BMD. J Appl Physiol 1999;86:1347.

9. Bailey DA, et al. Growth, physical activity, and bone mineral acquisition. Exerc Sport Sci Rev 1996;24:233.

10. Beard J, Stoltzfus R. Forward. J Nutr 2001;131(suppl):563S.

11. Beek EJ van der. Vitamin supplementation and physical exercise performance. Sports Sci 1991;9:77.

12. Benson J, et al. Inadequate nutrition and chronic calorie restriction in adolescent ballerinas. Phys Sportsmed 1985;13:79.

13. Boot AM, et al. Bone mineral density in children and adolescents: relation to puberty, calcium intake and physical activity. J Clin Endocrinol Metab 1997;82:57.

14. Bostom AG, et al. Nonfasting plasma total homocysteine levels and all-cause and cardiovascular disease mortality in the elderly Framingham men and women. Arch Intern Med 1999;159:1077.

15. Brilla L, Haley T. Effect of magnesium supplementation on strength training in humans. J Am Coll Nutr 1992;11:326.

16. Brownlie T IV, et al. Marginal iron deficiency without anemia impairs aerobic adaptation among previously untrained women. Am J Clin Nutr 2002;75:734.

17. Brune M, et al. Iron loss in sweat. Am J Clin Nutr 1986;43:438.

18. Brutsaert TD, et al. Iron supplementation improves progressive fatigue resistance during dynamic knee extensor exercise in iron-depleted, nonanemic women. Am J Clin Nutr 2003;77:441.

19. Cabet J, et al. High femoral bone mineral content and density in male football (soccer) players. Med Sci Sports Exerc 2001;33:1682.

20. Cassell C, et al. Bone mineral density in elite 7-9-yr-old female gymnasts and swimmers. Med Sci Sports Exerc 1996;28:1243.

21. Cauley JA, et al. Effects of estrogen plus progestin on risk of fracture and bone mineral density. JAMA 2003;290:1729.

22. Clarkson P M, Haymes EM. Exercise and mineral status of athletes: calcium, magnesium, phosphorus, and iron. Med Sci Sports Exerc 1995;27:831.

23. Cobb KL, et al. Disordered eating, menstrual irregularity, and bone mineral density in female runners. Med Sci Sports Exerc 2003;35:711.

24. Conlin PR, et al. The effect of dietary patterns on blood pressure control in hypertensive patients: results from the Dietary Approaches to Stop Hypertension (DASH) Trial. Am J Hypertens 2000;13:949.

25. Conroy BP, et al. Bone mineral density in elite junior Olympic weight lifters. Med Sci Sports Exerc 1993;25:1103.

26. Creighton DL, et al. Weight-bearing exercise and markers of bone turnover in female athletes. J Appl Physiol 2001;90:565.

27. Cullen DM, et al. Bone-loading response varies with strain magnitude and cycle number. J Appl Physiol 2001;91:1971.

28. Cummings SR, et al. Endogenous hormones and the risk of hip and vertebral fractures among older women. N Engl J Med 1998;339:733.

29. Cussler EC, et al. Weight lifted in strength training predicts bone change in postmenopausal women. Med Sci Sports Exerc 2003;35:10.

30. Derstine JL, et al. Iron status in association with cardiovascular disease risk in 3 controlled feeding studies. Am J Clin Nutr 2003;77:56.

31. Deugnier Y, et al. Increased body iron stores in elite road cyclists. Med Sci Sports Exerc 2002;34:876.

32. Deuster PA, et al. Nutritional survey of highly trained women runners. Am J Clin Nutr 1986;45:954.

33. Diaz MN, et al. Antioxidants and atherosclerotic heart disease. N Engl J Med 1997;337:408.

34. Dook JE, et al. Exercise and bone mineral density in mature female athletes. Med Sci Sports Exerc 1997;29:291.

35. Drinkwater BL, et al. Menstrual history as a determinant of current bone density in young athletes. JAMA 1990;263:545.

36. Dueck CA, et al. A diet and training intervention program for the treatment of athletic amenorrhea. Int J Sports Nutr 1996;6:134.

37. Duncan CS, et al. Bone mineral density in adolescent female athletes: relationship to exercise type and muscle strength. Med Sci Sports Exerc 2002;34:286.

38. Dwyer JH, et al. Dietary calcium, calcium supplementation, and blood pressure in African American adolescents. Am J Clin Nutr 1998;68: 648.

39. Eichner ER. Fatigue of anemia. Nutr Revs 2001;59:S17.

40. Eikelboom JW, et al. Homocyst(e)ine and cardiovascular disease: a critical review of epidemiologic evidence. Ann Intern Med 1999; 131:362.

41. Ely DL. Overview of dietary sodium effects on and interactions with cardiovascular and neuroendocrine functions. Am J Clin Nutr 1997; 65(suppl):594S.

42. Erp-Bart van AMJ, et al. Nationwide survey on nutritional habits in elite athletes. Part 1. Energy, carbohydrate, protein and fat intake. Int J Sports Med 1989;10(suppl 1):S3.

43. Faulkner RA, et al. Strength indices of the proximal femur and shaft in prepubertal female gymnasts. Med Sci Sports Exerc 2003;35:513.

44. Fehling PC, et al. A comparison of bone mineral densities among female athletes in impact loading and active loading sports. Bone 1995;17:205.

45. Feskanich D, et al. Walking and leisure-time activity and risk of hip fracture in postmenopausal women. JAMA 2002;288:2300.

46. Finstad EW, et al. The effects of magnesium supplementation on exercise performance. Med Sci Sports Exerc 2001;33:493.

47. Fleet J. How well you absorb calcium is important for limiting hip fracture risk. Nutr Revs 2001;59:338.

48. Flemming DJ, et al. Dietary factors associated with the risk of high iron stores in the elderly Framingham Heart Study cohort. Am J Clin Nutr 2002;76:1375.

49. Friedmann B, et al. Effects of iron repletion on blood volume and performance capacity in young athletes. Med Sci Sports Exerc 2001;33:741.

50. Gale CR. Antioxidant vitamin status and carotid atherosclerosis in the elderly. Am J Clin Nutr 2001;74:402.

51. Ganji V, Kafi MR. Demographic, health, lifestyle, and blood vitamin determinants of serum total homocysteine concentrations in the third National Health and Nutrition Examination Survey. Am J Clin Nutr 2003;77:826.

52. Giguere Y, Rousseau F. The genetics of osteoporosis: "complexities and difficulties." Clin Genet 2000;57:161.

53. Gledhill N, et al. Haemoglobin, blood volume, cardiac function, and aerobic power. Can J Appl Physiol 1999;24:54.

54. Green HJ, et al. Training induced hypervolemia: lack of an effect on oxygen utilization during exercise. Med Sci Sports Exerc 1987;19:202.

55. Gremion G, et al. Oligo-amenorrheic long-distance runners may lose more bone in spine than in femur. Med Sci Sports Exerc 2001;33:15.

56. Haymes EM. Vitamin and mineral supplementation to athletes. Int J Sports Nutr 1991;1:146.

57. Haymes EM, et al. Training for cross-country skiing and iron status. Med Sci Sports Exerc 1986;18:162.

58. Heaney R, Rafferty K. Carbonated beverages and urinary calcium excretion. Am J Clin Nutr 2001;74:343.

59. Hegarty VM, et al. Tea drinking and bone mineral density in older women. Am J Clin Nutr 2000;71:1003.

60. Helge EW, Kanstrup I-L. Bone density in female elite gymnasts: impact of muscle strength and sex hormones. Med Sci Sports Exerc 2002;34:174.

61. Hennekens CH, et al. Lack of effect of long-term supplementation with beta carotene on the incidence of malignant neoplasm and cardiovascular disease. N Engl J Med 1996;334:1145.

62. Hinton PS, et al. Iron supplementation improves endurance after training in iron-depleted, nonanemic women. J Appl Physiol 2000;88:1103.

63. Hodis HN, et al. Serial coronary angiographic evidence that antioxidant vitamin intake reduces progression of coronary artery disease. JAMA 1995;273:1849.

64. Huang H-Y, et al. Effects of vitamin C and vitamin E on in vivo lipid peroxidation: results of a randomized controlled trial. Am J Clin Nutr 2002;76:549.

65. Hunt JR, Roughead ZK. Adaptation of iron absorption in men consuming diets with high or low iron bioavailability. Am J Clin Nutr 2000;71:95.

66. Hunt SC, et al. Angiotensinogen genotype, sodium reduction, weight loss, and prevention of hypertension. Trials of Hypertension Prevention, Phase II. Hypertension 1998;32:393.

67. Jacques PF, et al. Determinants of plasma total homocysteine concentration in the Framingham Offspring cohort. Am J Clin Nutr 2001;73:613.

68. Janz KF, et al. Everyday activity predicts bone geometry in children: The Iowa Bone Development Study. Med Sci Sports Exerc 2004; 36:1124.

69. Jiang Q, et al. γ-Tocopherol, the major form of vitamin E in the US diet, deserves more attention. Am J Clin Nutr 2001;74:714.

70. Kahn K, et al. Does childhood and adolescence provide a unique opportunity for exercise to strengthen the skeleton? J Sci Med Sport 2000;3:150.

71. Kalkwarf HJ, et al. Milk intake during childhood and adolescence, adult bone density, and osteoporotic fractures in US women. Am J Clin Nutr 2003;77:257.

72. Karlsson MK, et al. Exercise during growth and young adulthood is associated with reduced fracture risk in old ages. J Bone Miner Res 2002;17(suppl 1):S297.

73. Keith ME, et al. A controlled clinical trial of vitamin E supplementation in patients with congestive heart failure. Am J Clin Nutr 2001; 73:219.

74. Kemmler W, et al. Exercise effects on fitness and bone mineral density in early postmenopausal women: 1-year EFOPS results. Med Sci Sports Exerc 2002;34:2115.

75. Kerr D, et al. Exercise effects on bone mass in postmenopausal women are site-specific and load-dependent. J Bone Min Res 1996; 11:218.

76. Kirchner EM, et al. Effect of past gymnastics participation on adult bone mass. J Appl Physiol 1996;80:226.

77. Klipstein-Grobusch K, et al. Dietary antioxidants and risk of myocardial infarction in the elderly: the Rotterdam Study. Am J Clin Nutr 1999;69:261.

78. Kohrt WM, et al. HRT preserves increases in bone mineral density and reductions in body fat after a supervised exercise program. J Appl Physiol 1998;84:1506.

79. Konyulsinrn D, et al. Good maintenance of exercise-induced bone gain with decreased training of female tennis and squash players: a prospective 5-year follow-up study of young and old starters and controls. J Bone Miner Res 2001;16:195.

80. Kritchevsky SB, et al. Provitamin A carotenoid intake and carotid artery plaques: the Atherosclerosis Risk in Communities Study. Am J Clin Nutr 1998;68:726.

81. Kushi LH, et al. Dietary antioxidant vitamins and death from coronary heart disease in postmenopausal women. N Engl J Med 1996;334:1156.

82. Layne JE, Nelson ME. The effects of progressive resistance training on bone density: a review. Med Sci Sports Exerc 1999;31:25.

83. LeBoff MS, et al. Occult vitamin D deficiency in postmenopausal US women with acute hip fracture. JAMA 1999;281:1505.

84. Lee EJ, et al. Variations in bone status of contralateral and regional sites in young athletic women. Med Sci Sports Exerc 1995;27:1354.

85. Levine M, et al. Criteria and recommendations for vitamin C intake. JAMA 1999;281:1485.

86. Lin Y, et al. Estimating the concentration of β-carotene required for maximal protection of low-density lipoproteins in women. Am J Clin Nutr 1998;67:837.

87. Lindsay R, et al. Effect of lower doses of conjugated equine estrogens with and without dedroxyprogesterone acetate on bone in early postmenopausal women. JAMA 2002;287:2668.

88. Lima F, et al. Effect of impact load and active load on bone metabolism and body composition of adolescent athletes. Med Sci Sports Exerc 2001;33:1318.

89. Livshits G, et al. Genes play an important role in bone aging. Hum Biol 1998;10:421.

90. Looker A, et al. Prevalence of iron deficiency in the United States. JAMA 1997;277:973.

91. Luft GS, Weinberger MH. Heterogeneous responses to changes in dietary salt intake: the salt-sensitivity paradigm. Am J Clin Nutr 1997;65(suppl):626S.

92. Lyle RM, et al. Iron status in exercising women: the effect of oral iron therapy vs increased consumption of muscle foods. Am J Clin Nutr 1992;56:1099.

93. Mackelvie KJ, et al. Lifestyle risk factors for osteoporosis in Asian and Caucasian girls. Med Sci Sports Exerc 2001;33:1818.

94. Malinow MR, et al. Plasma homocysteine levels and graded risk for myocardial infarction: findings in two populations at contrasting risk for coronary heart disease. Atherosclerosis 1996;126:27.

95. Malinow MR, et al. Reduction of plasma homocysteine levels by breakfast cereals fortified with folic acid in patients with coronary heart disease. N Engl J Med 1998;15:1009.

96. Martinez ME, et al. Physical activity, body mass index, and prostaglandin E_2 levels in rectal mucosa. J Natl Cancer Inst 1999; 91:950.

97. McCabe ME, et al. Gastrointestinal blood loss associated with running a marathon. Dig Dis Sci 1986;31:1229.

98. McKenna AA, et al. Zinc balance in adolescent females consuming a low- or high-calcium diet. Am J Clin Nutr 1997;65:1460.

99. McLean JA, et al. Dietary restraint, exercise, and bone density in young women: are they related? Med Sci Sports Exerc 2001;33:1292.

100. Mennen LI, et al. Homocysteine, cardiovascular disease risk factors, and habitual diet in the French Supplementation with Antioxidant Vitamins and Minerals Study. Am J Clin Nutr 2002;76:1279.

101. Meydani M. Vitamin E and prevention of heart disease in high-risk patients. Nutr Revs. 2000;58:278.

102. Michaels KB, et al. Prospective study of fruit and vegetable consumption and incidence of colon and rectal cancers. J Natl Cancer Inst 2000;92:1740.

103. Michaëlsson K, et al. Serum retinol levels and the risk of fracture. N Engl J Med 2003;348:287.

104. Micklesfield LK, et al. Bone mineral density in mature, premenopausal ultramarathon runners. Med Sci Sports Exerc 1995;27:688.

105. Midgley JP, et al. Effect of reduced dietary sodium on blood pressure: a meta-analysis of randomized controlled trials. JAMA 1996; 275:1590.

106. Modlesky CM, Lewis RD. Does exercise during growth have a long-term effect on bone health? Exerc Sport Sci Rev 2002;30:171.

107. Moffatt RJ. Dietary status of elite female high school gymnasts: inadequacy of vitamin and mineral intake. J Am Diet Assoc 1984;84:1361.

108. Morris D, et al. Serum carotenoids and coronary heart disease: the Lipid Research Clinics Coronary Prevention Trial and Follow-up Study. JAMA 1994;272:439.

109. Morris MS, et al. Hyperhomocysteinemia associated with poor recall in the third National Health and Sport Science Review Nutrition Examination Survey. Am J Clin Nutr 2001;73:927.

110. Mortensen L, Charles P. Bioavailability of calcium supplements and the effect of vitamin D: comparisons between milk, calcium carbonate, and calcium carbonate plus vitamin D. Am J Clin Nutr 1996;63:354.

111. Myburgh KH, et al. Low bone mineral density at axial and appendicular sites in amenorrheic athletes. Med Sci Sports Exerc 1993;25:1197.

112. Myers ER, Wilson SE. Biomechanics of osteoporosis and vertebral fracture. Spine 1997;22:25S.

113. Nachtigall D, et al. Iron deficiency in distance runners. A reinvestigation using ^{59}Fe-labeling and non-invasive liver iron quantification. Int J Sports Med 1996;17:473.

114. Nakayama MM, et al. T^{-786} mutation in the 5′-flanking of the region of the endothelial nitric oxide synthase gene is associated with coronary spasm. Circulation 1999;99:2855.

115. Nappo F, et al. Impairment of endothelial functions by acute hyperhomocystinemia and reversal by antioxidant vitamins. JAMA 1999; 281:2113.

116. Nelson DA, Bouxsein ML. Exercise maintains bone mass, but do people maintain exercise? J Bone Miner Res 2001;16:202.

117. Nelson RL. Iron and colorectal cancer risk: human studies. Nutr Res 2001;59:140.

118. New SA, et al. Dietary influences on bone mass and bone metabolism: further evidence of a positive link between fruit and vegetable consumption and bone health. Am J Clin Nutr 2000;71:142.

119. Nichols DL, et al. Relationship of regional body composition to bone mineral density in college females. Med Sci Sports Exerc 1995;27:178.

120. Nickols-Richardson SM, et al. Premenarcheal gymnasts possess higher bone mineral density than controls. Med Sci Sports Exerc 2000;32:62.

121. Nielsen P, Nachtigall D. Iron supplementation in athletes: current recommendations. Sports Med 1998;26:207.

122. Nieves JN, et al. Calcium potentiates the effect of estrogen and calcitonin on bone mass: review and analysis. Am J Clin Nutr 1998;67:18.

123. Nygård O, et al. Major lifestyle determinants of plasma total homocysteine distribution: The Horland Homocysteine Study. Am J Clin Nutr 1998;67:263.

124. Obarzanek E, et al. Effects on blood lipids of a blood pressure-lowering diet: the Dietary Approaches to Stop Hypertension (DASH) Trial. Am J Clin Nutr 2001;74:80.

125. Omenn GS, et al. Effects of a combination of beta carotene and vitamin A on lung cancer and cardiovascular disease. N Engl J Med 1996;334:1150.

126. O'Toole ML, et al. Hemolysis during triathlon races: its relation to race distance. Med Sci Sports Exerc 1988;20:172.

127. Pescatello LS, et al. Daily physical movement and bone mineral density among a mixed racial cohort of women. Med Sci Sports Exerc 2002;34:1966.

128. Pizza FX, et al. Serum haptoglobin and ferritin during a competitive running and swimming season. Int J Sports Med 1997;18:233.

129. Praticò D, et al. Vitamin E suppresses isoprostane generation in vivo and reduces atherosclerosis in apoE-deficient mice. Nature Med 1998;4:1189.

130. Proctor KL, et al. Upper-limb bone mineral density of female collegiate gymnasts versus controls. Med Sci Sports Exerc 2002;34:1830.

131. Raiz LG. The osteoporosis revolution. Ann Intern Med 1997;126:458.

132. Rajaram S, et al. Effects of long-term moderate exercise on iron status in young women. Med Sci Sports Exerc 1995;27:1105.

133. Ramakrishnan V, et al. Iron stores and cardiovascular disease risk factors in women of reproductive age in the United States. Am J Clin Nutr 2002;76:1256.

134. Ravaglia G, et al. Homocysteine and cognitive function in healthy elderly community dwellers in Italy. Am J Clin Nutr 2003;77:668.

135. Ray JG, Laskin CA. Folic acid and homocyst(e)ine metabolic defects and the risk of placental abruption, pre-eclampsia and spontaneous pregnancy loss: a review. Placenta 1999;20:519.

136. Reid IR. Effect of calcium supplementation on bone loss in postmenopausal women. N Engl J Med 1993;328:460.

137. Rencken ML, et al. Bone density at multiple skeletal sites in amenorrheic athletes. JAMA 1996;276:238.

138. Ridker PM, et al. Homocysteine and risk of cardiovascular disease among postmenopausal women. JAMA 1999;281:1817.

139. Rimm EB, et al. Folate and vitamin B_6 from diet and supplements in relation to risk of coronary heart disease among women. JAMA 1998;279:359.

140. Ripple MO, et al. Effect of antioxidants on androgen-induced AP-1 and NF-kB DNA-binding activity in prostate carcinoma cells. J Natl Cancer Inst 1999;91:1227.

141. Risser WL, et al. Iron deficiency in female athletes: its prevalence and impact on performance. Med Sci Sports Exerc 1988;20:116.

142. Robertson JO, et al. Fecal blood loss in response to exercise. Br Med J 1987;295:303.

143. Robinson TL, et al. Gymnasts exhibit higher bone mass than runners despite similar prevalence of amenorrhea and oligomenorrhea. J Bone Miner Res 1995;10:26.

144. Robling AG, et al. Recovery periods restore mechanosensitivity to dynamically loaded bone. J Exp Biol 2001;204:3389.

145. Robling AG, et al. Shorter, more frequent mechanical loading sessions enhance bone mass. Med Sci Sports Med 2002;34:196.

146. Rokitzk L, et al. Assessment of vitamin B_6 status of strength and speed power athletes. J Am Coll Nutr 1994;13:87.

147. Ross EA, et al. Lead content of calcium supplements. JAMA 2000;284:1425.

148. Roughead ZK, Hunt JR. Adaptation in iron absorption: iron supplementation reduces nonheme-iron but not heme-iron absorption from food. Am J Clin Nutr 2000;72:946.

149. Sacks FM, et al. Rationale and design of the dietary approaches to stop hypertension trial (DASH): a multicenter controlled feeding study of dietary patterns to lower blood pressure. Ann Epidemiol 1995;108:118.

150. Sacks FM, et al. Effects on blood pressure of reduced dietary sodium and the Dietary Approaches to Stop Hypertension (DASH) diet. DASH-Sodium Collaborative Research Group. N Engl J Med 2001;344:3.

151. Salonen JT, et al. High stored iron levels are associated with excess risk of myocardial infarction in eastern Finnish men. Circulation 1992;86:803.

152. Saw S-M, et al. Genetic, dietary, and other lifestyle determinants of plasma homocysteine concentrations in middle-aged and older Chinese men and women in Singapore. Am J Clin Nutr 2001;73:232.

153. Sawka MN, Coyle EF. Influence of body water and blood volume on thermoregulation and exercise performance in the heat. Exerc Sport Sci Rev 1999;27:167.

154. Schnyder G, et al. Effect of homocysteine lowering therapy with folic acid, vitamin B_{12} and vitamin B_6 on clinical outcome after percutaneous coronary intervention. JAMA 2002;288:973.

155. Schumacher YO, et al. Hematological indices and iron status in athletes of various sports and performances. Med Sci Sports Exerc 2002;34:869.

156. Selhub J, et al. B vitamins, homocysteine and neurocognitive function in the elderly. Am J Clin Nutr 2000;71(suppl):614S.

157. Sempos CT, et al. Body iron stores and risk of coronary heart disease. N Engl J Med 1994;330:1119.

158. Sempos CT, et al. Do body iron stores increase the risk of developing coronary heart disease? Am J Clin Nutr 2002;76:501.

159. Shoemaker JD, et al. Relationships between fluid and electrolyte hormones and plasma volume during exercise with training and detraining. Med Sci Sports Exerc 1998;30:497.

160. Singh R, et al. Maintenance of bone mass and mechanical properties after short-term cessation of high impact exercise in rats. Int J Sports Med 2002;23:77.

161. Siris E, et al. Identification and fracture outcomes of undiagnosed low bone mineral density in postmenopausal women: results from the National Osteoporosis Risk Assessment. JAMA 2001;286:2815.

162. Snow CM, et al. Bone gains and losses follow seasonal training and detraining in gymnasts. Calcif Tissue Int 2001;69:7.

163. Snyder AC, et al. Importance of dietary iron source on measures of iron status among female runners. Med Sci Sports Exerc 1989;21:7.

164. Specker BL. Should there be dietary guidelines for calcium intake? North Am J Clin Nutr 2000;71:663.

165. Stear SJ, et al. Effect of calcium and exercise intervention on the bone mineral status of 16–18-y-old adolescent girls. Am J Clin Nutr 2003;77:985.

166. Stamler J. The INTERSALT study: background, methods, findings, and implications. Am J Clin Nutr 1997;65(suppl):626S.

167. Steinberg D. Low density lipoprotein oxidation and its pathobiological significance. J Biol Chem 1997;272:20963.

168. Steinberg FM, Chait A. Antioxidant vitamin supplementation and lipid peroxidation in smokers. Am J Clin Nutr 1998;68:319.

169. Stock JL, et al. Dynamic muscle strength is decreased in postmenopausal women with low bone density. J Bone Miner Res 1987;2:338.

170. Stolzenberg-Solomon RZ, et al. Association of dietary protein intake and coffee consumption on serum homocysteine concentrations in an older population. Am J Clin Nutr 1999;69:467.

171. Suominen H, Rahkila P. Bone mineral density of the calcaneus in 70- to 81-yr-old male athletes and a population sample. Med Sci Sports Exerc 1991;23:1227.

172. Svetkey LP, et al. Effects of dietary patterns on blood pressure: subgroup analysis of the dietary approaches to Stop Hypertension (DASH) Randomized Clinical Trial. Arch Intern Med 1999;159:285.

173. Taaffle DR, et al. Differential effects of swimming versus weight bearing activity on bone mineral status of eumenorrheic athletes. J Bone Miner Res 1995;10:586.

174. Terry P, et al. Fruit, vegetables, dietary fiber, and risk of colorectal cancer. J Natl Cancer Inst 2001;93:525.

175. The Heart Outcomes Prevention Evaluation Study Investigators. Vitamin E supplementation and cardiovascular events in high-risk patients. N Engl J Med 2000;342:154.

176. The Homocysteine Studies Collaboration. Homocysteine and risk of ischemic heart disease. JAMA 2002;288:2015.
177. Thomas MK, et al. Hypovitaminosis D in medical inpatients. N Engl J Med 1998;338:784.
178. Tice JA, et al. Cost-effectiveness of vitamin therapy to lower plasma homocysteine levels for the prevention of coronary heart disease. Effect of grain fortification and beyond. JAMA 2001;286:936.
179. Tomten SE, et al. Bone mineral density and menstrual irregularities. A comparative study of cortical and trabecular bone structures in runners with alleged normal eating behavior. Int J Sports Med 1998;19:87.
180. Treblance S, et al. Failure of magnesium supplementation to influence marathon running performance or recovery in magnesium-replete subjects. Int J Sports Nutr 1992;2:154.
181. Trumbo B, et al. Dietary reference intakes: vitamin K, arsenic, boron, chromium, copper, iodine, manganese, molybdenum, nickel, silicon, vanadium, and zinc. Am Diet Assoc 2001;101:294.
182. Tucker KL. Eat a variety of healthful foods: old advice with new support. Nutr Rev 2001;59:156.
183. Turner CH, Robling AG. Designing exercise regimens to increase bone strength. Exerc Sport Sci Rev 2003;31:45.
184. Ueland PM, et al. The controversy over homocysteine and cardiovascular risk. Am J Clin Nutr 2000;72:324.
185. Ulrich CM, et al. Bone mineral density in mother-daughter pairs: relations to lifetime exercise, lifetime milk consumption, and calcium supplements. Am J Clin Nutr 1996;63:72.
186. Villareal DT, et al. Bone mineral density response to estrogen replacement in frail elderly women. A randomized controlled trial. JAMA 2001;286:815.
187. Vincent KR, Braith RW. Resistance exercise and bone turnover in elderly men and women. Med Sci Sports Exerc 2002;34:17.
188. Vollset SE, et al. Plasma total homocysteine and cardiovascular and noncardiovascular mortality: the Hordaland Homocysteine Study. Am J Clin Nutr 2001;74:130.
189. Weight LM, et al. Sports anemia: a real or apparent phenomenon in endurance-trained athletes. Int J Sports Med 1992;13:344.
190. Weisburger JH. Approaches for chronic disease prevention based on current understanding of underlying mechanisms. Am J Clin Nutr 2000;71(suppl):1710S.
191. Welch GN, Loscalzo J. Homocysteine and atherothrombosis. N Engl J Med 1999;338:1042.
192. Whelton PK, et al. Sodium reduction and weight loss in the treatment of hypertension in older persons: a randomized controlled trial of nonpharmacologic interventions in the elderly (TONE). JAMA 1998;279:839.
193. Whelton PK, et al. Primary prevention of hypertension: clinical and public health advisory from the National High Blood Pressure Prevention Program. JAMA 2002;288:1882.
194. Winters K, et al. Bone density and cyclic ovarian function in trained runners and active controls. Med Sci Sports Exerc 1996;28:776.
195. Wood D. Established and emerging cardiovascular risk factors. Am Heart J 2001;141(2 Pt 2).
196. Wood RJ, Zheng JJ. High dietary calcium intakes reduce zinc absorption and balance in humans. Am J Clin Nutr 1997;65:1803.
197. Writing Group for the Women's Health Initiative Investigators. Risk and benefits of estrogen plus progestin in healthy postmenopausal women: principal results from the women's Health Initiative Randomized Controlled Trial. JAMA 2002;288:321.
198. Yusuf S, et al. Vitamin E supplementation and cardiovascular events in high-risk patients. The Heart Outcomes Prevention Evaluation Study investigators. N Engl J Med 2000;342;154.
199. Zanker CL, Cooke CB. Energy balance, bone turnover, and skeletal health in physically active individuals. Med Sci Sports Exerc 2004;36:1372.

Additional Readings

Aguilo A, et al. Antioxidant diet supplementation influences blood iron status in endurance athletes. Int J Sport Nutr Exerc Metab 2004;14:147.
Barr SI, Rideout CA. Nutritional considerations for vegetarian athletes. Nutrition 2004;20:696.
Christ M, et al. Effects of a weight reduction program with and without aerobic exercise in the metabolic syndrome. Int J Cardiol 2004;97:115.
Deruisseau KC, et al. Iron status of young males and females performing weight-training exercise. Med Sci Sports Exerc 2004;36:241.
Gropper SS, et al. Copper status of collegiate female athletes involved in different sports. Int J Sport Nutr Exerc Metab 2003;13:343.
Lean ME, Hankey CR. Aspartame and its effects on health. BMJ 2004;329:755.
Leiper JB, Maughan RJ. Comparison of water turnover rates in young swimmers in training and age-matched non-training individuals. Int J Sport Nutr Exerc Metab 2004;14:347–357.
Peake JM. Vitamin C: Effects of exercise and requirements with training. Int J Sport Nutr Exerc Metab 2003;13:125–151.
Ramel A, et al. Plasma antioxidants and lipid oxidation after submaximal resistance exercise in men. Eur J Nutr 2004;43:2.
Reid SA, et al. Study of hematological and biochemical parameters in runners completing a standard marathon. Clin J Sport Med 2004;14:344.
Shirreffs SM, et al. Fluid and electrolyte needs for preparation and recovery from training and competition. J Sports Sci 2004;22:57.
Tsalis G, et al. Effects of iron intake through food or supplement on iron status and performance of healthy adolescent swimmers during a training season. Int J Sports Med 2004;25:306.
Von Duvillard SP, et al. Fluids and hydration in prolonged endurance performance. Nutrition 2004;20:651.
Wang JS, Chow SE. Effects of exercise training and detraining on oxidized low-density lipoprotein-potentiated platelet function in men. Arch Phys Med Rehabil 2004;85:1531.

Chapter

3

Digestion and Absorption of the Food Nutrients

TEST YOUR KNOWLEDGE

Answer these ten statements about digestion and absorption of the food nutrients. Use the scoring key at the end of the chapter to check your results. Repeat this test after you have read the chapter and compare your results.

1. **T F** The digestion of food begins in the stomach.

2. **T F** The colon is another name for the large intestine.

3. **T F** The liver, gallbladder, and pancreas are all organs through which food nutrients must pass during digestion.

4. **T F** Glucose absorption requires energy, while the absorption of dietary fat occurs passively without expenditure of energy.

5. **T F** Active transport of a nutrient across the plasma membrane occurs by electrostatic transfer that does not require energy.

6. **T F** The main absorption of lipids takes place in the distal portion of the stomach.

7. **T F** Almost all nutrient digestion and absorption take place in the small intestine.

8. **T F** Glucose absorption takes place predominantly in the large intestine.

9. **T F** Hemorrhoids result largely from consuming a high-fiber diet.

10. **T F** Hydrolysis and condensation represent the two important tissue-building processes in the body.

Proper food intake ultimately provides an uninterrupted supply of energy and tissue-building chemicals to sustain life. For exercise and sports participants, the ready availability of specific food nutrients takes on added importance because physical activity significantly increases energy expenditure and the need for tissue repair and synthesis. Nutrient uptake by the body involves complex physiologic and metabolic processes that usually progress unnoticed for a lifetime. Hormones and enzymes work nonstop in concert throughout the digestive tract, at proper levels of acidity–alkalinity, to facilitate the breakdown of complex nutrients into simpler subunits. Substances produced during digestion are absorbed through the razor-thin lining of the small intestine and pass into the blood and lymph. Self-regulating processes within the digestive tract usually move food along at a slow enough rate to allow its complete absorption, yet rapid enough to ensure timely delivery of its nutrient components. Fibrous materials that resist digestion pass unabsorbed from one end of the body to the other.

The sections that follow outline the digestion and absorption of the various nutrients consumed in the diet. We present a brief discussion of some biology and chemistry basics related to digestive and absorptive processes and then describe the structures of the gastrointestinal tract including the dynamics of digestion.

➤ Biology and Chemistry Basics Related to the Digestion, Absorption, and Assimilation of the Food Nutrients

HYDROLYSIS AND CONDENSATION: THE BASIS FOR DIGESTION AND SYNTHESIS

In general, hydrolysis reactions digest or break down complex molecules into simpler subunits, and condensation reactions build larger molecules by bonding their subunits together.

Hydrolysis Reactions

Hydrolysis catabolizes complex organic molecules carbohydrates, lipids, and proteins into simpler forms that the body absorbs and assimilates. During this basic decomposition process, chemical bonds split by the addition of hydrogen ions (H^+) and hydroxyl ions (OH^-), the constituents of water, to the reaction byproducts. Examples of hydrolytic reactions include the digestion of starches and disaccharides to monosaccharides, proteins to amino acids, and lipids to glycerol and fatty acids. A specific enzyme catalyzes each step in the breakdown process. For disaccharides, the enzymes are lactase (lactose), sucrase (sucrose), and maltase (maltose). The lipid enzymes (lipases) degrade the triacylglycerol molecule by adding water, cleaving the fatty acids from their glycerol backbone. During protein digestion, protease enzymes accelerate amino acid release when the addition of water splits the peptide linkages. The following equation represents the general form for all hydrolysis reactions:

$$AB + HOH \rightarrow A\text{-}H + B\text{-}OH$$

Water (HOH) added to substance AB decomposes the chemical bond that joins AB to produce the breakdown products A-H (H refers to hydrogen atom from water) and B-OH (OH refers to the remaining hydroxyl group from water). FIGURE 3.1A illustrates the hydrolysis reaction for the disaccharide sucrose to its end product molecules of glucose and fructose. Also shown is the hydrolysis of a dipeptide (protein) into its two constituent amino acid units. Intestinal absorption occurs rapidly following hydrolysis of the carbohydrate, lipid, and protein macronutrients.

Condensation Reactions

The reactions illustrated for hydrolysis also occur in the opposite direction. In this reversible reaction, governed by specific enzymes, the compound AB synthesizes from A-H and B-OH during **condensation** (also termed *dehydration synthesis*). A hydrogen atom is cleaved from one molecule and a hydroxyl group is removed from another. A water molecule forms in this building, or **anabolic**, process. The structural components of the nutrients bind together in condensation reactions to form more complex molecules and compounds. Figure 3.1B shows the condensation reactions for the synthesis of *(a)* maltose from two glucose units and *(b)* a more complex protein from two amino acid units. During protein synthesis, a hydroxyl removed from one amino acid and hydrogen from the other amino acid create a water molecule. The new bond for the protein is called a **peptide bond**. Water formation also occurs in synthesizing more complex carbohydrates from simple sugars. For lipids, water forms when glycerol and fatty acid components combine to form the triacylglycerol molecule.

ENZYMES: THE BIOLOGIC CATALYSTS

*An **enzyme**, a highly specific protein catalyst, accelerates the forward and reverse rates of chemical reactions without being consumed or changed in the reaction.* The great diversity of protein structures enables enzymes to perform highly specific functions. Enzymes only affect reactions that would normally take place but at a much slower rate. In a way, enzymes reduce the required **activation energy**, or energy input, to change the rate of the reaction. This occurs even though the equilibrium constants and total energy released (free energy change) per reaction remain unaltered. FIGURE 3.2 shows the effectiveness of a catalyst for initiating a chemical reaction compared with the uncatalyzed state. The horizontal axis represents the progress of the reaction; the vertical axis compares the energy required to initiate the reactions. Clearly, initiation (activation) of an uncatalyzed reaction requires considerably more energy than a catalyzed one. Without enzymes, digesting a simple meal would theoretically take 50 years!

Enzymes possess the unique property of not being readily altered by the reactions they affect. Consequently, the turnover of enzymes in the body remains relatively slow, and the specific enzymes are continually reused. A typical mitochondrion may contain up to 10 billion enzyme molecules, each carrying out millions of operations within a brief time. During strenuous exercise, enzyme activity rate

A. Hydrolysis

B. Condensation

■ **Figure 3.1** **A.** Hydrolysis chemical reaction of the disaccharide sucrose to the end-product molecules glucose and fructose and a hydrolysis reaction of a dipeptide (protein) into two amino acid constituents. **B.** Condensation chemical reaction to synthesize maltose from two glucose units and creation of a protein dipeptide from two amino acid units. Note that the reactions in **B** illustrate the reverse of the hydrolysis reaction for the dipeptide. The symbol *R* represents the remainder of the molecule.

increases tremendously within the cell, as energy demands increase some 100 times above the resting level. The rate of a catalyzed reaction can be 10^6 to 10^{20} times faster than an uncatalyzed reaction under similar conditions. A single cell's fluids contain as many as 4000 different enzymes, each with a specific function that catalyzes a specific chemical reaction. For example, glucose breakdown to carbon dioxide and water requires 19 different chemical reactions, each catalyzed by its own enzyme. Enzymes make contact at precise locations on the surfaces of cell structures; they also operate within the structure itself. Many enzymes function outside the cell—in the bloodstream, digestive mixture, or fluids of the small intestine.

Except for older enzyme names such as renin, trypsin, and pepsin, the suffix -*ase* appends to the enzyme based on its mode of operation or substance with which it interacts. For example, hydro*lase* adds water during hydrolysis reactions, prote*ase* interacts with protein, oxid*ase* adds oxygen to a substance, isomer*ase* rearranges atoms within a substrate to form structural isomers such as glucose and fructose, and

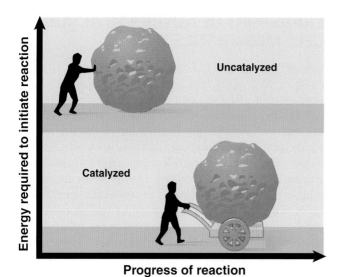

Figure 3.2 The presence of a catalyst greatly reduces the activation energy required to initiate a chemical reaction compared with the energy required for an uncatalyzed reaction. For the reaction to proceed, the reactant must have a higher free-energy level than the product.

Mode of Enzyme Action

A unique characteristic of an enzyme's three-dimensional globular protein structure is its interaction with its specific substrate. Interaction works similarly to a key fitting a lock. The enzyme turns on when its **active site**, usually a groove, cleft, or cavity on the protein's surface, joins in a "perfect fit" with the substrate's active site (FIGURE 3.3). By forming an **enzyme-substrate complex**, the splitting of chemical bonds produces a new product with new bonds. This frees the enzyme to act upon additional substrate. Figure 3.3 depicts the interaction sequence of the enzyme maltase as it disassembles maltose into its component glucose building blocks.

The **"lock and key mechanism"** describes the enzyme–substrate interaction. This interactive process ensures that the correct enzyme "mates" with its specific substrate to perform a particular function. Once the enzyme and substrate join, the enzyme changes shape as it molds to the substrate. Even if an enzyme links with a substrate, unless the specific conformational change occurs in the enzyme's shape, it will not interact chemically with the substrate.

ribonucle*ase* splits apart ribonucleic acid (RNA). Enzymes do not all operate at the same rate; some operate slowly, others more rapidly.

Enzymes often work cooperatively among their binding sites. While one substance "turns on" at a particular site, its neighbor "turns off" until the process completes. The operation then can reverse, with one enzyme becoming inactive and the other active. Enzymes also act along small regions of the **substrate** (any substance acted upon by an enzyme), each time working at a different rate than previously. Some enzymes delay beginning their work. The precursor digestive enzyme trypsinogen manufactured by the pancreas in inactive form serves as a good example. Trypsinogen enters the small intestine where, upon activation by intestinal enzyme action, it becomes the active enzyme trypsin that digests complex proteins into simple amino acids. **Proteolytic action** describes this process. Without the delay in activity, trypsinogen would literally digest the pancreatic tissue that produced it.

The temperature and hydrogen ion concentrations (acidity–alkalinity) of the reactive medium dramatically affect enzyme activity. Each enzyme performs its maximum activity at a specific pH. The optimum pH of an enzyme usually reflects the pH of the body fluids in which it bathes. For some enzymes, optimal activity requires a relatively high acidity level (e.g., the protein-digesting enzyme pepsin is optimally active in the hydrochloric acid of the gut); for others, the optimal pH occurs on the alkaline side of neutrality, as trypsin does in the pancreatic juice. Increases in temperature generally accelerate enzyme reactivity. As temperature rises above 40 to 50°C, the protein enzymes permanently denature and activity ceases.

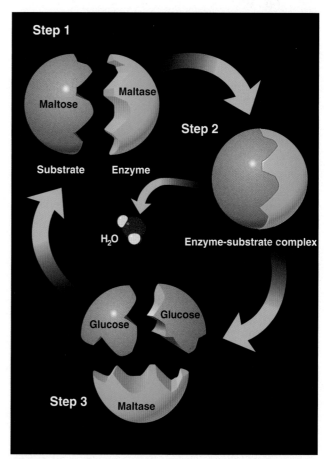

Figure 3.3 Sequence of steps in the "lock and key" mechanism of an enzyme with its substrate. The example shows how two monosaccharide molecules of glucose form when the enzyme maltase interacts with its disaccharide substrate maltose.

STEPS IN ENZYME ACTION

Step 1: The active site of the enzyme and substrate line up to achieve a perfect fit, forming an enzyme–substrate complex.

Step 2: The enzyme catalyzes (greatly speeds up) the chemical reaction with the substrate.

Step 3: An end product is formed.

The lock and key mechanism offers a protective function so only the correct enzyme activates the targeted substrate. Consider the enzyme hexokinase, which accelerates a chemical reaction by linking with a glucose molecule. When this linkage occurs, a phosphate molecule transfers from adenosine triphosphate (ATP) to a specific binding site on one of glucose's carbon atoms. Once the two binding sites join to form a glucose–hexokinase complex, the substrate begins its stepwise degradation (controlled by other specific enzymes) to form less complex molecules during energy metabolism.

Coenzymes

Some enzymes require activation by additional ions and smaller organic molecules termed **coenzymes**. These complex, nonprotein substances facilitate enzyme action by binding the substrate with its specific enzyme. Coenzymes then regenerate to assist in further similar reactions. The metallic ions iron and zinc play coenzyme roles, as do the B vitamins or their derivatives. Oxidation–reduction reactions use the B vitamins riboflavin and niacin, while other vitamins serve as transfer agents for groups of compounds in metabolic processes (see Table 2.2). Some advertisements imply that taking vitamin supplements provides immediate usable energy for exercise. Although vitamins "make the reactions go," they contain no chemical energy available for biologic work.

A coenzyme requires less specificity in its action than an enzyme because the coenzyme affects a number of different reactions. It acts as a "cobinder," or it can serve as a temporary carrier of intermediary products in the reaction. For example, the coenzyme **nicotinamide adenine dinucleotide (NAD$^+$)** forms NADH to transport the hydrogen atoms and electrons that split from food fragments during energy metabolism. The electrons then pass to special transporter molecules in another series of chemical reactions that ultimately deliver the electrons to molecular oxygen.

TRANSPORT OF NUTRIENTS ACROSS CELL MEMBRANES

Literally thousands of chemicals including ions, vitamins, minerals, acids, salts, water, gases, hormones, and carbohydrate, protein, and lipid components continually traverse the cell's bilayer plasma membrane during exchange between the cell and its surroundings. The plasma membrane remains highly permeable to some substances but not others. Such selective permeability allows cells to maintain reasonable consistency in chemical composition. Disrupting the equilibrium triggers immediate adjustments to restore constancy in the cell's "internal milieu." This occurs by two processes: *(a)* **passive transport** of substances through the plasma membrane (requires no energy) and *(b)* **active transport** through the plasma membrane, which requires metabolic energy to "power" the exchange of materials.

Passive Transport Processes

Simple diffusion, facilitated diffusion, osmosis, and filtration represent the four types of passive transport. FIGURE 3.4 shows an example of each.

Simple Diffusion

In the cellular environment, **simple diffusion** involves the free and continuous net movement of molecules in aqueous solution across the plasma membrane. In Figure 3.4, note that molecules of water, small lipids, and gases move unimpeded from outside the cell through the lipid bilayer into the intracellular fluid. *In simple diffusion, a substance moves from an area of higher concentration to lower concentration until it evenly disperses.* Only the kinetic energy of the molecules themselves, with no expenditure of stored cellular energy, powers this entirely passive process. When sugar and water mix, for example, the sugar molecules dissolve and evenly disperse by their continuous, random movement. Hot water speeds diffusion because higher temperature increases molecular movement and thus the diffusion rate. If the particles remain within a closed system, they eventually distribute evenly throughout, and the *net movement* of particles ceases.

Simple diffusion across the plasma membrane occurs for water molecules, dissolved gases (oxygen, carbon dioxide, and nitrogen), small uncharged polar molecules such as urea and alcohol, and various lipid-soluble molecules. These substances diffuse quickly because the plasma membrane consists of sheetlike, fluid structures composed mainly of lipids. This structure allows relatively small, uncomplicated molecules to easily traverse the membrane. For example, when a molecule of oxygen diffuses from its normal higher concentration outside the cell toward a lower concentration on the cell's inside, it moves down (or along) its concentration gradient. *The concentration gradient determines the direction and magnitude of molecular movement.* This explains

Figure 3.4 A. Simple diffusion. **B.** Facilitated diffusion, **C.** Osmosis. **D.** Filtration.

why oxygen molecules continuously diffuse into cells. In contrast, the higher concentration of carbon dioxide within the cell causes this gaseous end product of energy metabolism to move down its concentration gradient and continually diffuse from the cell into the blood.

Facilitated Diffusion

Facilitated diffusion involves the passive, highly selective binding of lipid-insoluble molecules (and other large molecules) to a lipid-soluble carrier molecule. This contrasts with simple diffusion by which molecules pass unaided through the semipermeable plasma membrane. The carrier molecule, a protein called a transporter, or **permease**, spans the plasma membrane. Its function facilitates the transfer of membrane-insoluble chemicals (hydrogen, sodium, calcium, and potassium ions, and glucose and amino acid molecules) down their concentration gradients across the cell's plasma membrane.

Glucose transport into the cell provides an excellent example of facilitated diffusion. Glucose, a large lipid-insoluble, uncharged molecule, would not pass readily into the cell without its specific permease. More specifically, if simple diffusion were the only means of glucose entrance

into a cell, its maximum rate of uptake would be nearly 500 times slower than glucose transport by facilitated diffusion. Facilitated diffusion allows glucose molecules to first attach to a binding site on a specific permease in the plasma membrane. A structural change then occurs in the permease that creates a "passageway" enabling the glucose molecule to penetrate the permease to enter the cytoplasm. Fortunately, facilitated diffusion of glucose keeps this important energy fuel readily available. Also, glucose transport does not require cellular energy. Consequently, facilitated diffusion serves as an energy-conserving mechanism that spares cellular energy for other vital functions.

Osmosis

Osmosis represents a special case of diffusion. Osmosis moves water (the solvent) through a selectively permeable membrane. This occurs because of a difference in the concentration of water molecules on both sides of the membrane, which is more permeable to water than to the solute. This passive process distributes water throughout the intracellular, extracellular, and plasma fluid body compartments.

In the example in Figure 3.4C, a semipermeable membrane separates compartments A and B. When an equal number of solute particles appear on sides A and B, the same water volume exists in both compartments. By adding a solute to an aqueous solution, the concentration of the solution increases by the amount of solute added. Adding more solute increases the concentration of particles while correspondingly decreasing the concentration of water molecules. In the example, adding nondiffusable solute to side B forces water from side A to move through the semipermeable membrane to side B. The volume of water then becomes greater on side B than side A. More water flows into an area containing more particles, leaving less water on the side with fewer solute particles. Eventually, by osmotic action, the concentration of solute particles equalizes on sides A and B.

Osmolality refers to the concentration of particles in solution, expressed as osmolal units of particles or ions formed when a solute dissociates. In living tissue, a difference always exists in the osmolality of the various fluid compartments. This occurs because the semipermeable membrane that separates different solutions retards the passage of many solute substances such as ions and intracellular proteins. Selective permeability maintains a difference in solute concentration on both sides of the membrane. Because water diffuses freely through the plasma membrane, a net movement of water occurs as the system attempts to equalize osmolality on both sides of the membrane. This can produce dramatic volume changes in the two fluid compartments. At some point, water no longer enters the cell because the hydrostatic pressure of water on one side of the cell balances the pressure tending to draw water through the membrane. **Osmotic pressure** of a solution refers to the physical pressure on one side of a membrane required to prevent the osmotic movement of water from the other side.

Altering the water volume inside a cell changes its shape or "tone," a characteristic referred to as *tonicity*. When a cell neither loses nor gains water when placed in a solution the solution becomes **isotonic** in relation to the cell. In isotonic solutions, the concentration of a nonpenetrating solute such as sodium chloride equalizes on the inside and outside of the cell, with no net movement of water. The body's extracellular fluid under normal conditions provides an example of an isotonic solution.

A **hypertonic** solution contains a higher concentration of nonpenetrating solutes outside the cell membrane than inside. When this occurs, water migrates out of the cell by osmosis, and the cell shrinks in size. Edema, an excess accumulation of water in body tissues, can be countered by infusing hypertonic solutions into the bloodstream. On the other hand, ingesting highly concentrated beverages containing salt or slowly absorbed fructose sugar creates an intestinal osmotic environment that actually causes water to move into the intestinal lumen. This sets the stage for intestinal cramping and impedes the rehydration process.

When the concentration of nondiffusible solutes outside the cell becomes diluted compared with the cell's interior, the extracellular solution becomes **hypotonic**. In such cases, the cell fills with water by osmosis and appears bloated. If the condition goes uncorrected, cells actually burst (lyse). Administering hypotonic solutions during dehydration returns the tissues to isotonic conditions.

For a membrane permeable to the solute and water (e.g., sugar in water), the solute and solvent molecules diffuse until the sugar molecules distribute equally. In contrast, for a membrane impermeable to the solute, osmotic pressure draws water in the direction that equalizes the solute concentration on both sides of the membrane. Water movement continues until solute concentration equalizes or until the hydrostatic pressure on one side of the membrane counteracts the force exerted by osmotic pressure. FIGURE 3.5 illustrates the osmotic effect on cells placed in isotonic, hypertonic, and hypotonic solutions.

Filtration

In **filtration**, water and its solutes flow passively from a region of higher hydrostatic pressure to one of lower pressure. The filtration mechanism allows plasma fluid and its solutes to move across the capillary membrane to literally bathe the tissues. Filtration moves the plasma filtrate (the fluid portion of the blood with no significant amount of proteins) through the kidney tubules during the production of urine.

Active Transport Processes

Energy-requiring **active transport** comes into play when a substance cannot move across the cell membrane by one of the four passive transport processes. Each active transport process requires the expenditure of cellular energy from ATP.

Sodium–Potassium Pump

FIGURE 3.6 illustrates the operation of the **sodium–potassium pump,** one of the active transport mechanisms for moving substances through semipermeable membranes. Energy from ATP "pumps" ions "uphill" against their electrochemical gradients through the membrane by a specialized carrier enzyme (sodium–potassium ATPase) that serves as the pumping mechanism. Recall that substances usually diffuse along their concentration gradients, from an area of higher to lower concentration. In the living cell, diffusion alone cannot provide optimal distribution of cellular chemicals. Instead, charged sodium and potassium ions and large amino acid molecules, insoluble in the lipid bilayer, must move against their concentration gradients to fulfill normal functions. Sodium ions, for example, exist in relatively low

Figure 3.6 The dynamics of the sodium–potassium pump. (ATP, adenosine triphosphate; ADP, adenosine diphosphate; P, phosphate.)

Figure 3.5 A. *Isotonic solution.* The cell retains its shape because of equal concentrations of solute inside and outside the cell. **B.** *Hypertonic solution.* The cell shrinks (crenates) because the outside of the cell has a higher concentration of nondiffusible solutes than the inside. **C.** *Hypotonic solution.* The concentration of nondiffusible solutes outside the cell is diluted compared to the concentration within the cell. The cell takes on water by osmosis, which can burst (lyse) the cell.

concentration inside the cell; thus, extracellular Na$^+$ tends to continually diffuse into the cell. In contrast, potassium ions exist in higher concentration inside the cell, and intracellular K$^+$ tends to diffuse toward the extracellular space. Consequently, to achieve proper Na$^+$ and K$^+$ concentrations about the plasma membrane for normal nerve and muscle functions, both ions continually move against their normal concentration gradients. This concentrates Na$^+$ extracellularly, whereas K$^+$ builds up within the cell. Countering the normal tendency of solutes to diffuse by means of the sodium–potassium pump provides the biologic way to establish normal electrochemical gradients for nerve and muscle stimulation.

Coupled Transport

Active transport absorbs nutrients through the epithelial cells of the digestive tract and reabsorbs important plasma

chemicals filtered by the kidneys. Absorption of intestinal glucose, for example, takes place by a form of active transport called **coupled transport**. FIGURE 3.7 shows molecules of glucose and Na$^+$ coupling together before they enter an intestinal villus; they then move in the same direction when "pumped" through the plasma membrane to the cell's inside and subsequently into the bloodstream. Amino acids also join with Na$^+$ for active absorption through the small intestine. A cotransporter, or **symport**, refers to the simultaneous transport of two chemicals in the same direction; each symport has its own specialized permease with a specific binding site for each substance. Coupled transport occurs in one direction only. When the glucose–sodium and amino acid–sodium symports move from the intestine to the blood, they cannot move back and reenter the intestine.

Bulk Transport

Bulk transport moves a large number of particles and macromolecules through cell membranes by an energy-

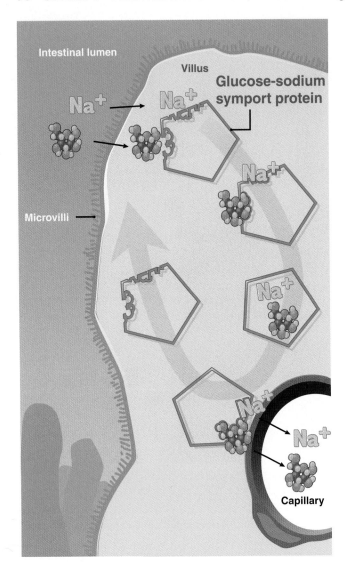

Figure 3.7 Coupled transport. A molecule of glucose and a sodium ion move together in the same direction through the plasma membrane in a symport protein.

requiring process. Bulk transport occurs in two ways: exocytosis and endocytosis.

Exocytosis. **Exocytosis** transfers hormones, neurotransmitters, and mucous secretions from intracellular to extracellular fluids. Exocytosis involves three distinct phases. First, the substance for transfer becomes enclosed within a membranous, saclike pouch. The pouch then migrates to the plasma membrane; once fused to the membrane, its contents eject into the extracellular fluids.

Endocytosis. In the transfer process of **endocytosis**, the cell's plasma membrane surrounds the substance, which then pinches away and moves into the cytoplasm.

ACID–BASE CONCENTRATION AND PH

Maintaining the acid–base balance of body fluids, a critical component of homeostasis, provides optimal functioning of digestion and overall physiologic regulation.

Acid

*An **acid** refers to any substance that dissociates (ionizes) in solution and releases hydrogen ions (H^+).* Acids taste sour, turn litmus indicators red, react with bases to form salts, and cause some metals to liberate hydrogen. Examples of acids in the body include hydrochloric, phosphoric, carbonic, citric, lactic, and carboxylic acids.

Base

*A **base** refers to any substance that picks up or accepts H^+ to form hydroxide ions (OH^-) in water solutions.* Basic or alkaline solutions taste bitter, are slippery to the touch, turn litmus indicators blue, and react with acids to form salts. Examples of bases in the body include sodium and calcium hydroxide and aqueous solutions of ammonia that form ammonium hydroxide.

pH

*The **pH** provides a quantitative measure of the acidity or alkalinity (basicity) of a liquid solution.* Specifically, pH refers to the concentration of protons or H^+; it computes as the logarithm of 1.0 divided by the H^+ concentration as follows:

$$pH = \log 1 \div [H^+]$$

where $[H^+]$ equals the molar concentration of H^+.

Solutions with relatively more OH^- than H^+ have a pH above 7.0 and are called basic, or alkaline. Conversely, solutions with more H^+ than OH^- have a pH below 7.0 and are termed acidic. Chemically pure (distilled) water has a neutral pH of 7.0 with equal amounts of H^+ and OH^-. The pH scale shown in FIGURE 3.8, devised in 1909 by the Danish chemist Sören Sörensen (1868–1939), ranges from 1.0 to 14.0. An inverse relation exists between pH and the concentration of H^+. Because of the logarithmic nature of the pH scale, a one-unit change in pH corresponds to a tenfold change in H^+ concentration. For example, lemon juice and gastric juice (pH = 2.0) have 1000 times greater H^+ concentration than black coffee (pH = 5.0), whereas hydrochloric acid (pH = 1.0) has approximately 1,000,000 times the H^+ concentration of blood (pH = 7.4).

The pH of body fluids ranges from a low of 1.0 for the digestive acid hydrochloric acid to a slightly basic pH between 7.35 and 7.45 for arterial and venous blood (and most other body fluids). The term **alkalosis** refers to an increase in pH above the normal average of 7.4; this results directly from a decrease in H^+ concentration (increase in pH). Con-

Concentration in moles per liter

Examples

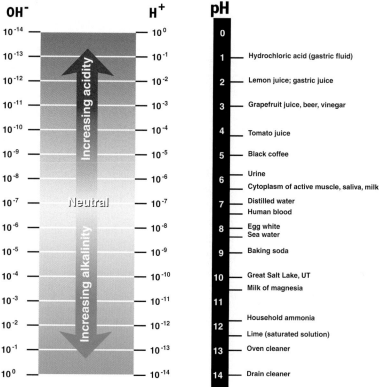

Figure 3.8 The pH scale quantifies the acidity or alkalinity (basicity) of a liquid solution. Blood pH remains regulated at the slightly alkaline pH of 7.4. Values for blood pH rarely fall below 6.9, even during the most vigorous exercise.

versely, **acidosis** refers to an increase in H^+ concentration (decrease in pH). The body regulates the diverse yet highly specific pH of various body fluids within narrow limits because metabolism remains highly sensitive to the H^+ concentration of the reacting medium.

Enzymes and pH

Many chemical processes in the body occur only at a specific pH. An enzyme that works at one pH becomes inactivated when the pH of its surroundings changes. For example, the lipid-digesting enzyme gastric lipase functions effectively in the stomach's highly acidic environment, but ceases to function within the slightly alkaline small intestine. The same occurs for salivary amylase, the enzyme that initiates starch breakdown in the mouth. The pH of the salivary fluids ranges between 6.4 and 7.0. When passed to the stomach (pH 1.0 to 2.0), salivary amylase ceases its digestive function because the stomach acids digest it as with any other protein. As a general rule, extreme changes in pH irreversibly damage enzymes. For this reason, the body maintains its acid–base balance within narrow limits.

Buffers

*The term **buffering** designates reactions that minimize changes in H^+ concentration.* The chemical and physiologic mechanisms that prevent H^+ changes are termed **buffers**. Inability of the buffer system to neutralize deviations in H^+ concentration disrupts effective body function, and coma or death ensues. Three mechanisms regulate the acid–base quality of the internal environment: *(a)* chemical buffers, *(b)* pulmonary ventilation, and *(c)* kidney function.

Chemical Buffers

The chemical buffering system consists of a weak acid and a base or salt of that acid. For example, the bicarbonate buffer consists of the weak carbonic acid and its salt sodium bicarbonate. Carbonic acid forms when the bicarbonate binds H^+. As long as H^+ concentration remains elevated, the reaction produces the weaker acid because the excess H^+ binds in accordance with the general reaction:

$$H^+ + Buffer \rightarrow H\text{–}Buffer$$

The strong stomach acid hydrochloric acid (HCl) combines with sodium bicarbonate to form the much weaker carbonic acid (H_2CO_3). This produces only a slight reduction in pH. When stomach acid remains elevated from inadequacy of the buffer response during digestion, many individuals seek "outside help" by ingesting neutralizing agents or antacids to provide buffering relief. If the concentration of H^+ decreases and body fluids become more alkaline, the buffering reaction moves in the opposite direction. This releases H^+ and acidity increases as follows:

$$H^+ + Buffer \leftarrow H\text{–}Buffer$$

The body continually produces other acids in addition to digestive juices. Much of the carbon dioxide generated in energy metabolism reacts with water to form the relatively weak carbonic acid ($CO_2 + H_2O \rightarrow H_2CO_3$), which then dissociates to H^+ and HCO_3^-. Sodium bicarbonate buffers lactic acid, a stronger acid produced during anaerobic metabolism, to form sodium lactate and carbonic acid; in turn, carbonic acid dissociates and increases the H^+ concentration of extracellular fluids. Other organic acids such as fatty acids dissociate and liberate H^+, as do sulfuric and phosphoric acids produced during protein breakdown. The buffering of hydrochloric acid by sodium bicarbonate occurs as follows:

$$HCl + NaHCO_3 \rightarrow NaCl + H_2CO_3 \rightarrow H^+ + HCO_3^-$$

Other available chemical buffers include the phosphate buffers phosphoric acid and sodium phosphate. These chemicals act similarly to the bicarbonate buffering system. The phosphate buffers regulate the acid–base quality of the kidney tubules and intracellular fluids that contain a relatively high concentration of phosphates. The protein-containing hemoglobin compound within red blood cells and other plasma proteins buffer carbonic acid.

Ventilatory Buffer

Any increase in H^+ concentration in body fluids stimulates the respiratory center in the brain to increase pulmonary ventilation. This adjustment causes greater than normal amounts of carbon dioxide to leave the blood. Carbon dioxide combines with water to form carbonic acid for transport dissolved in the blood. Thus, reducing the body's carbon dioxide content acts directly as a buffer by lowering carbonic acid concentration. This causes body fluids to become more alkaline. Conversely, ventilation below normal levels causes carbon dioxide (and carbonic acid) buildup, and the body fluids become more acidic.

Renal Buffer

The kidneys continually excrete H^+ to maintain long-term acid–base stability of body fluids. The renal buffer controls acidity by adjusting the concentration of bicarbonate ions, ammonia, and hydrogen ions secreted into the urine At the same time, it reabsorbs alkali, chloride, and bicarbonate.

Summary

1. Hydrolysis (catabolism) of complex organic molecules performs critical functions in digestion and energy metabolism. Condensation (anabolism) reactions synthesize complex biomolecules for tissue maintenance and growth.

2. Enzymes, highly specific protein catalysts, facilitate the interaction of substances to accelerate chemical reactions.

3. Coenzymes consist of nonprotein substances that assist enzyme action by binding a substrate to its specific enzyme.

4. Four passive processes transport nutrients throughout the body: simple diffusion, facilitated diffusion, osmosis, and filtration. Physical laws govern each of these processes, which do not require the input of chemical energy.

5. In active transport, substances move against their concentration gradients; metabolic energy "powers" the exchange of materials. Active transport absorbs nutrients from the digestive tract and reabsorbs plasma chemicals filtered by the kidneys.

6. Osmolality refers to the concentration of particles in a solution, expressed as osmolal units of particles or ions formed when a solute dissociates in solution.

7. Chemical and physiologic buffer systems normally regulate the acid–base quality of the body fluids within narrow limits.

8. The bicarbonate, phosphate, and protein chemical buffers serve as the rapid first line of defense to stabilize acid–base regulation. These buffers consist of a weak acid and the salt of that acid. Under acid conditions, buffering action converts a strong acid to a weaker acid and a neutral salt.

9. The lungs and kidneys help to regulate pH when a "stressor" affects the chemical buffer system. Changes in alveolar ventilation rapidly alter the free H^+ in extracellular fluids. With increased acidity, the renal tubules act as the body's final sentinels by secreting H^+ into the urine and reabsorbing bicarbonate.

➤ **Digestion and Absorption of Food Nutrients**

The physiology of human digestion had its origins when the Italian physiologist Spallanzani (1729–1799) first observed that gastric juice dissolved bread and animal tissues. However, pioneer American physician William Beaumont's classic experiments on Alexis St. Martin over an 8-year period (1825–1833) first detailed the human digestive processes. Beaumont discovered the function of the stomach's gastric juice and the time required for the digestion of different foods.

THE GASTROINTESTINAL TRACT

FIGURE 3.9A depicts the structures of the **gastrointestinal (GI) tract**; this includes the esophagus, gallbladder, liver, stomach, pancreas, small intestine, large intestine, rectum, and anus. The GI tract, also called the alimentary canal, essentially consists of a 7- to 9-m long tube that runs from the mouth to the anus. This serpentlike tube supplies the body with water and nutrients. Figure 3.9B shows the highly specialized connective tissue **mesentery** that weaves around and supports the approximately 2-kg mass of intestinal organs. This membrane contains a diffuse network of capillaries that transports absorbed nutrients. Figure 3.9C shows that the mesenteric blood vessels eventually converge to become the large **hepatic portal vein** that delivers nutrient-rich blood to the liver. The nutrients undergo processing in the liver and then return to the general circulation for transport throughout the body.

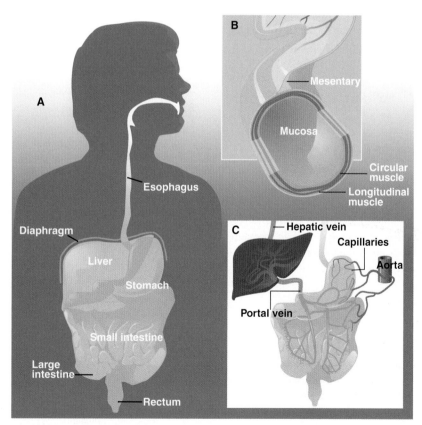

■ **Figure 3.9 A.** Structures of the gastrointestinal (GI) tract. **B.** Mesentery, which weaves around and gives support to the intestinal organs. **C.** The large portal vein collects blood from the mesenteric area and transports it to the liver for processing before the blood returns to the general circulation.

Mouth and Esophagus

The journey of a bite of food begins in the mouth. Crushing forces of up to 90 kg cut, grind, mash, and soften the food. **Mechanical digestion** increases the surface area of the food particles, making them easier to swallow and more accessible to enzymes and other digestive substances that start the degradation process. With swallowing, the bolus of food moves past the pharynx at the back of the mouth and enters the **esophagus**, the 25-cm portion of the GI tract that connects the pharynx to the stomach. Two layers of muscle tissue encircle the length of the esophagus; the inner layer consists of circular bands of muscle, while the outer tissue layer runs longitudinally. The esophagus constricts when the circular muscles reflexly contract and the longitudinal muscles relax; the reverse causes the esophagus to bulge. These powerful waves of rhythmic contraction and relaxation, called **peristalsis**, propel the small round food mass down the esophagus (see Fig. 3.12A).

Peristalsis involves progressive and recurring waves of smooth muscle contractions that compress the alimentary tube in a squeezing action, causing its contents to mix and move forward. This intrinsic means of food propulsion can occur in the microgravity of space flight and even when a person turns upside down. The end of the esophagus contains a one-way ring or valve of smooth muscle called the **esophageal sphincter**, which relaxes to allow the food mass entry into the **stomach**, the next section of the GI tract. This sphincter then constricts to help prevent the stomach contents from regurgitating back into the esophagus (gastric reflux). The stomach serves as a temporary holding tank for the partially digested food before moving it into the small intestine.

Sphincters That Control the Passage of Food

A sphincter is a circular muscle arrangement acting as a valve to regulate passage or flow of material through the GI tract. Several sphincters exist throughout the length of the GI tract; they respond to stimuli from nerves, hormones, and hormonelike substances and an increase in pressure around them. TABLE 3.1 lists all of the important sphincters, their location in the digestive tract, and the factors that control them.

Stomach

FIGURE 3.10 shows structural details of the approximately 25-cm long, J-shaped stomach, the most distensible portion of the GI tract; the inset details the stomach wall, showing the gastric glands. The **parietal cells** of the gastric glands secrete hydrochloric acid—stimulated by the hormones gastrin and acetylcholine released by the vagus nerve—and powerful enzyme-containing digestive juices that continually degrade the nutrients after they leave the esophagus and enter the stomach. Alkaline mucus, secreted from the mucous

neck cells, protects the mucosal lining of the gastric tissue. The buffering action of bicarbonate in alkaline pancreatic juice and alkaline secretions from glands in the submucosa of the duodenum (the first portion of the small intestine) normally protect the duodenum portion of the stomach from its highly acidic contents. The chief cells produce pepsinogen, the inactive form of the protein-digesting enzyme pepsin. Simple sugars are the easiest nutrients to digest, followed by proteins, and then lipids. *With the exception of alcohol and aspirin, little absorption takes place in the stomach.*

The stomach's volume averages about 1.5 L; however, it can hold a volume ranging from as little as 50 mL when nearly "empty" to about 6.0 L when fully distended after an excessively large meal. Regardless of its volume, the stomach contents mix with chemical substances to produce **chyme**, a slushy, acidic mixture of food and digestive juices.

After eating, the stomach usually takes 1 to 4 hours to empty, depending on the relative concentration of each nutrient and the volume of the meal. A large meal takes longer to clear the stomach than a smaller one. When eaten singularly, carbohydrates leave the stomach most rapidly, followed by proteins, and then lipids. The stomach may retain a high-fat meal for up to 6 hours before its chyme empties into the **small intestine**. Furthermore, food in liquefied form and fluids per

Table 3.1	**SPHINCTERS IN THE DIGESTIVE TRACT, THEIR LOCATION, AND FACTORS THAT INFLUENCE THEM**	
Sphincter	**Location**	**Comments**
Esophageal (upper and lower cardiac sphincter)	Junction between esophagus and stomach; prevents back flow (reflux) of stomach contents into esophagus	Opens only in response to muscle contractions in esophagus
Pyloric	Junction between stomach and first part of small intestine	Under hormonal and nervous system control; prevents back flow of intestinal contents into stomach
Oddi	End of the common bile duct	When hormone CCK stimulates gallbladder to contract during digestion, this sphincter relaxes to allow bile to flow down the common bile duct and enter the intestinal duodenum
Ileocecal	Terminus of small intestine	Opens in response to the presence of intestinal contents
Anal (two sphincters)	Terminus of large intestine	Under voluntary control

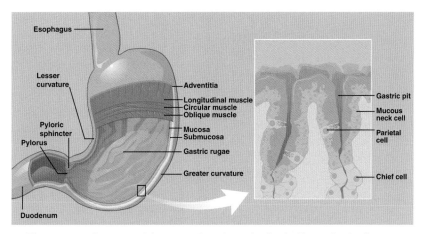

■ **Figure 3.10** Structure of the stomach and gastric glands. The parietal cells secrete hydrochloric acid, the neck cells secrete mucus, and chief cells produce pepsinogen.

se pass from the stomach most rapidly, whereas solids undergo a liquefaction phase. The nervous system, through hormonal regulation, largely controls the time and rate of stomach emptying via peristaltic waves that traverse the stomach toward the opening of the small intestine. A self-regulating feedback control also occurs between the stomach and small intestine. Excessive distension of the stomach from volume overload sends signals that cause the sphincter at the intestinal entrance to relax to allow more chyme to enter. Conversely, distention of the first portion of the intestine or the presence of excessive protein, lipid, or highly concentrated or acidic solutions, reflexly slows gastric emptying. A unique life-sustaining stomach function is its secretion of **intrinsic factor**, a polypeptide required for vitamin B_{12} absorption by the terminal portion of the small intestine.

Small Intestine

Approximately 90% of digestion (and essentially all lipid digestion) occurs in the first two sections of the 3-m long small intestine. This coiled structure consists of three sections: the **duodenum** (first 0.3 m), **jejunum** (next 1–2 m, where most of digestion occurs), and **ileum** (last 1.5 m). Absorption takes place through millions of specialized protruding structures of the intestinal mucosa. These fingerlike protrusions called **villi** move in wavelike fashion. *Most nutrient absorption through the villi occurs by active transport that uses a carrier molecule and expends ATP energy.* FIGURE 3.11 shows that the highly vascularized surfaces of villi contain small projections known as **microvilli**. These structures *(a)* contain the digestive enzymes embedded within its cell membranes and *(b)* absorb the smaller digested units of carbohydrates, proteins, and lipids, in addition to water, electrolytes (80% absorbed), alcohol, vitamins, and minerals.

Villi increase the absorptive surface of the intestine by up to 600-fold compared with a flat-surfaced tube of the same dimensions. If spread out, the 300-m^2 surface area of the small intestine would cover the area of a tennis court, or about 150 times the external surface of the body! This large surface greatly augments the speed and capacity for nutrient absorption. Each villus contains small lymphatic vessels called **lacteals** that absorb most digested lipids from the intestine. They transport via the lymphatic vessels that drain into the large veins near the heart.

■ **Figure 3.11** The microscopic structure of the small intestine. The tiny villi and microvilli projections (termed *brush border*) greatly increase the surface area of the mucosal cell's plasma membrane for nutrient absorption.

Intestinal Contractions

It usually takes 1 to 3 days after eating food before the GI tract eliminates it. The movement of chyme through the small intestine takes from 3 to 10 hours. Peristaltic contractions are much weaker in the small intestine than in the esophagus and stomach. The major contractile activity of the intestines occurs by segmentation contractions. These intermittent oscillating contractions and relaxations of the intestinal wall's circular smooth muscle augment mechanical mixing of intestinal chyme with bile, pancreatic juice, and intestinal juice. FIGURE 3.12B shows that segmentation contractions give the small intestine section of the GI tract a "sausage-link" look, because the alternating contraction and relaxation occur in nonadjacent segments of this structure. Thus, instead of propelling food directly forward as in peristalsis (Fig. 3.12A), the food actually moves slightly backward before advancing. This gives the digestive juices additional time to blend with the food mass before it reaches the large intestine. The propulsive movements of segmentation contractions continue to churn and mix the chyme before it passes the pyloric sphincter and enters the large intestine.

During digestion, **bile**, produced in the liver and stored and secreted by the **gallbladder**, increases the lipid droplets' solubility and digestibility through **emulsification**. The lipid content of the intestinal chyme stimulates the gallbladder's pulsatile release of bile into the duodenum. In a manner similar to the action of many household detergents, bile salts break apart fat into numerous smaller droplets that do not coalesce. This renders the fatty acid endproducts insoluble in water so the small intestine can absorb them. Some bile components are excreted in the feces, but the intestinal mucosa reabsorbs most of the bile salts; they return in the hepatic portal blood to the liver, where they become components in the resynthesis of new bile.

The **pancreas** secretes between 1.2 and 1.6 L of alkali-containing juice (digestive enzymes in an inactive form plus sodium bicarbonate) to help buffer the hydrochloric acid from the stomach that remains in the intestinal chyme. At a higher pH, pancreatic enzymes, released by neural and hormonal mechanisms, degrade the larger protein, carbohydrate, and lipid nutrients into smaller subunits for further digestion and absorption. The intestinal lining cannot withstand the highly acidic gastric juices from the stomach. Consequently, neutralizing this acid provides crucial protection against duodenal damage, which in extreme form triggers tissue ulceration or ulcers.

Large Intestine

FIGURE 3.13 depicts the components of the **large intestine**, which serves as the final digestive structure for absorbing water and electrolytes from the chyme it receives and storing digestive residues as fecal matter. This terminal 1.2-m (4-ft) portion of the GI tract, also known as the **colon** or bowel, contains no villi. Its major anatomic sections include the ascending colon, descending colon, transverse colon, sigmoid colon, rectum, and anal canal. Of the 8- to 12-L volume of food, fluid, and gastric secretions that enter the GI tract daily, only about 750 mL pass into the large

▓ **Figure 3.12** Propulsion of nutrients through the GI tract. **A.** Peristalsis involves the reflex-controlled alternate contraction and relaxation of adjacent segments of the GI tract, which causes one-directional flow of food (with some mixing). **B.** Segmentation contractions involve the alternate contraction and relaxation of nonadjacent segments of the intestine. This localized intestinal rhythmicity propels food forward and then backward causing food to mix with digestive juices.

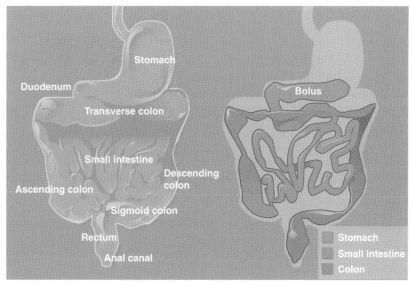

■ **Figure 3.13** Gross anatomic structures of the large intestine.

intestine. Here, bacteria ferment the remaining undigested food residue devoid of all but about 5% of useful nutrients. Intestinal bacteria (through their own metabolism) synthesize small amounts of vitamins K and biotin, which then become absorbed. Bacterial fermentation also produces about 500 mL of gas (flatus) each day. This gas consists of hydrogen, nitrogen, methane, hydrogen sulfide, and carbon dioxide. A small amount produces no outward effects, but excessive flatus can trigger severe abdominal distress as usually occurs from consuming large quantities of beans or dairy products. These foods leave partially digested sugars that contribute to larger than normal intestinal gas production. Mucus, the only significant secretion of the large intestine, protects the intestinal wall and helps to hold fecal matter together.

THE DIGESTIVE PROCESS

Digestion occurs almost entirely under involuntary control, in harmony with exquisite neural and hormonal regulation, to help maintain relative constancy in the internal environment. Polypeptides and polysaccharides degrade into simpler subunits to enter the epithelial cells of the intestinal villi for absorption into the blood. Fats, emulsified by bile, hydrolyze into their fatty acid and monoglyceride subunits for absorption by the intestinal villi. Within the epithelial cells of the villi, triacylglycerols resynthesize and combine with protein for secretion into the lymphatic fluid. The autonomic nervous system controls the entire GI tract: the parasympathetic system generally increases gut activity, while the sympathetic system exerts an inhibitory effect. Even without neural control, intrinsic autoregulatory mechanisms eventually return gut function to near-normal levels.

FIGURE 3.14 presents an overview of digestive processes throughout the GI tract. The diagram lists the major enzymes and hormones that act on proteins, lipids, and carbohydrates during their journey from the mouth through the GI tract. FIGURE 3.15 illustrates the sites and routes for nutrient absorption.

Hormones That Control Digestion

Four hormones that regulate digestion are gastrin, secretin, cholecystokinin (CCK), and gastric inhibitory peptide (TABLE 3.2). Hormonelike compounds, many of which occur in the small intestine and brain (e.g., vasoactive intestinal peptide, bombesin, substance P, and somatostatin), control other important aspects of GI function. These different compounds diffuse from cells or nerve endings throughout the GI tract to exert their influence on nearby cells.

Carbohydrate Digestion and Absorption

Starch hydrolysis begins once food enters the mouth. The **salivary glands**, located along the underside of the jaw, continually secrete lubricating mucous substances that combine with food particles during chewing. The enzyme **salivary α-amylase** (ptyalin) attacks starch and reduces it to smaller linked glucose molecules and the simpler disaccharide form maltose. When the food–saliva mixture enters the more acidic stomach, some additional starch breakdown occurs, but this quickly ceases because salivary amylase deactivates at the low pH of gastric juice.

Food entering the alkaline environment of the duodenum portion of the small intestine encounters **pancreatic amylase**, a powerful enzyme released from the pancreas. This enzyme, in conjunction with other enzymes, completes

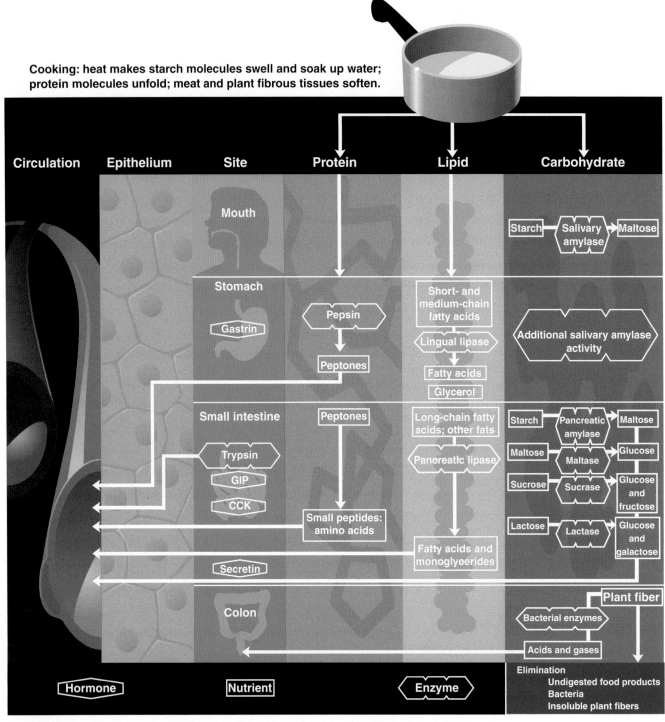

■ **Figure 3.14** Overview of human digestion. (GIP, gastric inhibitory peptide; CCK, cholecystokinin).

the hydrolysis of starch into smaller branched chains of glucose molecules (4–10 glucose linkages, called dextrins and oligosaccharides); the disaccharides cleave into simple monosaccharides. Enzyme action on the surface of the cells of the intestinal lumen's brush border completes the final stage of carbohydrate digestion to simple monosaccharide form. For example, **maltase** breaks down maltose to its glucose components, **sucrase** reduces sucrose to the simple sug-

ars glucose and fructose, and **lactase** degrades lactose to glucose and galactose. Active transport (common protein carriers) in the intestinal villi and microvilli (see Fig. 3.11) absorbs the monosaccharides. *Glucose and galactose absorption occurs by a sodium-dependent, carrier-mediated active transport process. The electrochemical gradient created with sodium transport (see Figs. 3.6 and 3.7) augments the absorption of these monosaccharides.*

The maximum rate of glucose absorption from the small intestine ranges between 50 and 80 g · h^{-1} for a person who weighs 70 kg. If we assume that high-intensity aerobic exercise (20 kcal · min^{-1}) derives 80% of its energy from carbohydrate breakdown, then roughly 4 g of carbohydrate (1 g carbohydrate = 4.0 kcal) are catabolized each minute (240 g · h^{-1}). Even under optimal conditions for intestinal absorption, carbohydrate intake during exercise cannot balance its utilization rate. Fructose is not absorbed via active transport, but in combination with a carrier protein by the much slower method of facilitated diffusion.

If disease affects intestinal enzymes or the villi themselves, the GI tract can indeed become "upset" and may take several weeks to resume normal functioning. For example, carbohydrates cannot completely break down when the digestive enzyme level is altered. A person recovering from

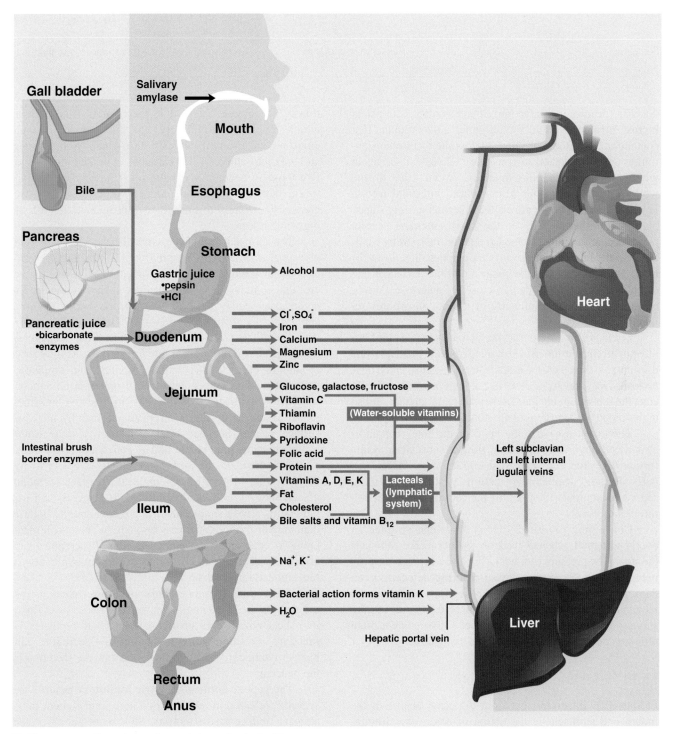

■ **Figure 3.15** Sites of secretion and absorption in the GI tract.

Table 3.2   **HORMONES THAT REGULATE DIGESTION**

Hormone	Origin	Secretion Stimulus	Action
Gastrin	Pyloric areas of stomach and upper duodenum	Food in stomach (protein, caffeine, spices, alcohol); nerve input	Stimulates flow of stomach enzymes and acid; stimulates action of lower esophageal sphincter; slows gastric emptying
Gastric inhibitory peptide (GIP)	Duodenum, jejunum	Lipids; proteins	Inhibits secretion of stomach acid and enzymes; slows gastric emptying
Cholecystokinin (CCK)	Duodenum, jejunum	Fat and protein in duodenum	Contraction of gallbladder and flow of bile to duodenum; causes secretion of enzyme-rich pancreatic juice and bicarbonate-rich pancreatic fluid; slows gastric emptying
Secretin	Duodenum, jejunum	Acid chyme; peptones	Secretion of bicarbonate-rich pancreatic fluid and slows gastric emptying

diarrhea (or intestinal infection) often experiences transient **lactose intolerance** and should avoid milk products that contain lactose. Reestablishing appropriate lactase concentration allows a person to consume this sugar once again without undesirable consequences. About 70% of the world's population suffer from reduced intestinal lactase levels to the point that it affects the digestion of milk sugar.

The epithelial cells of the small intestine secrete monosaccharides into the bloodstream for transport by capillaries to the hepatic portal vein that empties directly to the liver. The liver removes the greatest portion of glucose and essentially all of the absorbed fructose and galactose. Peripheral tissues, under the influence of insulin, absorb any remaining blood glucose.

Circulatory transport from the GI tract occurs via the **hepatic portal circulation**. Blood drained from the small intestine does not pass directly to the heart. Instead, intestinal blood travels to the liver, which processes its nutrients before they finally enter the general circulation. The hepatic portal circulation also drains blood from portions of the stomach and pancreas.

The colon provides the "end of the line" for undigested carbohydrates, including fibrous substances. Some further digestion and water reabsorption occur here; then peristaltic and segmentation actions push the remaining semisolid contents (stool) into the rectum for expulsion through the anus.

Consuming too much dietary fiber can produce an overly soft stool, whereas inadequate fiber intake compacts the stool. The pressure exerted during a bowel movement expels the stool. Excessive pressure during defecation can damage supporting tissues and expose blood vessels in the rectum **(hemorrhoids)**. Hemorrhoidal bleeding may require surgery. Gradually increasing the diet's fiber content often relieves constipation and hemorrhoid symptoms.

Lipid Digestion and Absorption

FIGURE 3.16 illustrates that lipid digestion begins in the mouth and stomach by the action of acid-stable **lingual lipase**, an enzyme secreted in the mouth. This enzyme, which operates effectively in the stomach's acid environment, primarily digests short-chain (4–6 carbons) and medium-chain (8–10 carbons) saturated fatty acids like those in coconut and palm oil. Chewing food mixes lipase with the food and reduces particle size; this increases the exposed surface to facilitate action of the digestive juices.

The stomach secretes **gastric lipase**, its own lipid-digesting enzyme. This enzyme works with lingual lipase to continue the hydrolysis of a small amount of triacylglycerol that contains short- and medium-chain fatty acids. *The major breakdown of lipids, particularly triacylglycerols containing long-chain (12–18 carbons) fatty acids, occurs in the small intestine.* When chyme enters the small intestine, mechanical mixing and bile act on the triacylglycerols (bound together as large lipid globules) and emulsifies them into a fine immersion of oil droplets in an aqueous suspension. Although bile contains no digestive enzymes, its action breaks up the fat droplets and thereby increases surface contact between lipid molecules and the water-soluble enzyme **pancreatic lipase**. Pancreatic lipase exerts a strong effect on the surface of the fat droplets to hydrolyze some triacylglycerol molecules further to monoglycerides (one fatty acid connected to glycerol) and free fatty acids. These simpler fats, which have greater polarity than unhydrolyzed lipids, pass through the microvilli membrane to enter intestinal epithelial cells. Pancreatic lipase effectively digests long-chain fatty acids common in animal fats and certain plant oils.

The peptide hormone **cholecystokinin**, released from the wall of the duodenum, controls the release of enzymes into the stomach and small intestine. CCK regulates GI functions including stomach motility and secretion, gallbladder contraction and bile flow, and enzyme secretion by the pancreas.

The peptide hormones **gastric inhibitory peptide** and **secretin**, released in response to a high lipid content in the stomach, reduce gastric motility. Slowing of gut movement

Fundamentals of Nutritional Assessment: Applying Analysis Skills

Nutritional assessment evaluates an individual's nutritional status and nutrient requirements on the basis of interpretation of clinical information from different sources Examples include diet history, medical history, review of symptoms, and physical examination, including anthropometric and laboratory data. Purposes of nutritional assessment include defining current nutritional status, determining levels of nutritional support, and monitoring changes in nutrient intake from a particular intervention program.

Nutritional deficiency usually develops over time, starting at a young age and then progressing in stages. An overt deficiency often remains unrecognized until the condition passes the individual's "clinical horizon" and moves into a disease state or becomes manifested by acute trauma (e.g., heart attack or type 2 diabetes complications). Nutritional assessment during any developmental stage of deficiency provides the basis for identifying a problem area and planning a prudent intervention.

ASSESSING DIETARY INTAKE

Several different methods commonly provide dietary information:

24–Hour Dietary Recall

This approach, usually a qualitative assessment by the individual or by another person, involves informal oral questioning about food and beverage intake during the previous 24 hours. The person recalls all foods and beverages consumed, starting from the last meal, and includes the approximate portion size and the specifics of food preparation. The method is relatively easy, particularly when administered by a registered dietitian. However, the information obtained may not be precise enough to yield conclusive information. Particular problems involve inaccuracy in quantity assessment and method of preparation. This frequently produces gross underestimation of hidden fats (and hence calories) in such foods as sauces and dressings. Repeat 24–hour recalls that span several days provide a more accurate and reliable estimate of a typical day.

Food Diary

With the food diary method, the individual records all foods and beverages at the time consumed (or as close to the time as possible). This approach also enables the recording of food by brand, weight, and portion size. Typically, the person maintains a food diary for 2 to 7 days. Assessment includes at least one weekend day because most people eat differently on the weekend than during a typical schoolday or workday. The method can become tedious;

individuals when confronted with having to record everything eaten often change what they eat or eat nothing to avoid the hassle.

Food Frequency Assessment

A food frequency questionnaire lists a variety of foods, and the individual estimates the frequency of consuming each item. This method does not itemize a specific day's intake; instead it provides a general picture of the typical food consumption pattern.

Diet History

A diet history yields general information about an individual's dietary patterns. Factors include eating habits (number of meals per day, who prepares meals, and patterns of food preparation), food preferences, eating locations, and typical food choices in different situations.

ANALYZING DIETARY INTAKE

A combination of methods proves more valid than a single method in developing a comprehensive dietary assessment. For a general picture of the adequacy of a person's dietary intake, compare the food record with an established guide for diet planning such as the Food Guide Pyramid (see Chapter 7). Evaluate the energy and macronutrient and micronutrient content of the diet through food labels and food composition tables. The most comprehensive food database is the USDA Nutrient Database for Standard Reference, available online at http://www.nal.usda.gov/fnic/foodcomp/Data/SR13/sr13.html. Other programs on the World Wide Web can be found at http://www.nat.uiuc.edu/main-nat.html. With most computer programs for diet analysis, one enters each food and the exact size of the portion consumed. Based on the input data, the program calculates the nutrients consumed for each day or provides an average over several days. In essence, a dietary analysis program compares nutrient intake to recommended values.

MEDICAL HISTORY

Personal Medical History

Medical history includes immunizations, hospitalizations, surgeries, and acute and chronic injuries and illness—each of these has nutritional implications. History of prescriptions and the use of vitamin and mineral supplements, laxatives, topical medications, and herbal remedies (herbs and other supplements not typically identified as medications) also provide valuable information.

Family Medical and Social History

Medical histories that include information about health/nutrition/exercise status of parents, siblings, children, and spouse reveal risk for chronic diseases that may have a genetic or social connection. Moreover, sociocultural relationships regarding food choices help in understanding individual eating patterns and

CASE STUDY/PERSONAL HEALTH AND EXERCISE NUTRITION 3–1 (*continued*)

practices. Information about duration and frequency of use of alcohol, tobacco, illicit drugs, and caffeine help to formulate a more effective treatment plan and assess risk for chronic diseases.

PHYSICAL EXAMINATION

Nutrition-oriented aspects of the physical examination focus on the mouth, skin, head, hair, eyes, mouth, fingernails, extremities, abdomen, skeletal musculature, and fat stores. Dry skin, cracked lips, or lethargy may indicate nutritional deficiencies. The accompanying table lists specific signs of vitamin or mineral deficiencies. Malnutrition often results from low calorie intake and protein deficiency. This produces a condition known as marasmus, which is characterized by severe tissue wasting, loss of subcutaneous fat, and usually dehydration. Marasmus typically occurs in individuals with anorexia nervosa (see Chapter 15).

Anthropometric Data

Use of anthropometric data permits nutritional classification of individuals by categories ranging from undernourished to obese.

Interpreting nutritional status involves comparing an individual with reference data from large numbers of healthy people of similar age and gender.

A typical nutritional assessment collects the following anthropometric data:

1. Height
2. Body weight
3. BMI—Normal BMI ranges between 19 and 25; individuals with a BMI of 25.1 to 29.9 are considered overweight, and BMIs of 30 and above classify as obese. While BMI may not accurately reflect actual body fat content, it has become a clinically acceptable "first approximation" measure of excess body weight.
4. Waist girth—Excess fat located in the abdominal area coincides with greater health risk. It most often occurs in individuals with type 2 diabetes, dyslipidemia, hypertension, and cardiovascular disease. The easily measured waist girth provides an independent predictor of disease risk and correlates reasonably well with the more difficult assessment of total abdominal fat. For individuals whose BMI exceeds 35, waist girth provides

CLINICAL SIGNS AND SYMPTOMS OF NUTRITIONAL INADEQUACY

Organ	Sign/Symptom	Probable Cause
Skin	Pallor (paleness)	Iron, folate, vit B12 def.
	Ecchymosis (purplish patch)	Vit K def.
	Pressure ulcers/delayed healing	Protein malnutrition
	Hair hyperkeratosis (excess eruption)	Vit A def.
	Petechiae (minute hemorrhagic spots)	Vit A, C, or K def.
	Purpura (hemorrhage into skin)	Vit C or K def.
	Rash/eczema/scaling	Zinc def.
Hair	Dyspigmentation, easy pluckability	Protein malnutrition
Head	Temporal muscle wasting	Protein–energy malnutrition
Eyes	Night blindness, xerosis (pathologic dryness)	Vit A def.
Mouth	Bleeding gum	Vit C, Riboflavin def.
	Tongue fissuring (splitting), raw tongue, tongue atrophy (wasting)	Niacin, riboflavin, niacin def.
Heart	Tachycardia	Thiamin def.
Genital/urinary	Delayed puberty	Protein–energy malnutrition
Extremities	Bone softening	Vit D, calcium, phosphorus def.
	Bone/joint aches	Vit C def.
	Edema	Protein def.
	Muscle wasting	Protein–energy malnutrition
	Ataxia (loss of coordination)	Vit B12 def.
Neurological	Tetany (muscle twitches, cramps)	Calcium, magnesium def.
	Paresthesia (abnormal sensation)	Thiamin, vit B12 def.
	Loss of reflexes, wrist/foot drop	Thiamin def.
	Dementia (loss of cognitive function)	Niacin def.

def., deficiency; vit, vitamin.

little additional risk information because a BMI this large already indicates severe risk. Waist girth becomes particularly useful for individuals with a family history of diabetes and who exhibit borderline excess weight. Waist girths above 102 cm (40 inches) in men and 88 cm (35 inches) in women indicate increased disease risk.

5. Percentage weight change—If personal history information reveals a body weight change, compute percentage weight change as follows:

Percentage weight change = (usual weight
— current weight ÷ usual weight) × 100

6. Triceps skinfold (TSF)—TSF in nutritional assessment indicates excess energy stored as subcutaneous fat. A TSF above the 95th percentile for age and gender indicates obesity.

Laboratory Data

Measures of nutrients or their byproducts in body cells or fluids (blood or urine) often detect nutrient deficiencies or excesses. Typical laboratory measures include serum albumin to indicate total body protein status and liver and renal disease; serum transferrin to assess protein balance and iron status; serum prealbumin to show protein status and liver disease; and concentrations of sodium, potassium, chloride, phosphorus, and magnesium to reflect overall mineral status. Other valuable laboratory tests that diagnose selected clinical conditions related to nutrition include iron and hemoglobin, zinc, cholesterol, triacylglycerol, the different lipid subfractions (HDL, LDL, and VLDL), and glucose.

APPLYING CRITICAL ANALYSES SKILLS

1. Keep a food diary of everything you eat for three days including one weekend day. Prepare a form that contains the following headings:

Food or Beverage	Kind/How Prepared	Amount
_____	_____	_____
_____	_____	_____
_____	_____	_____
_____	_____	_____

2. Record your food as you eat so as not to rely on memory at a later time. Increase accuracy with the following guidelines:
   a. Be specific when recording food intake; pay attention to size, type (chicken breast vs. thigh), and amount (i.e., number of chips or weight of food eaten).
   b. Record the method of preparation (i.e., baked vs. fried; peeled vs. not peeled; skinless vs. with skin).
   c. Include items like butter, ketchup, and salad dressing.
   d. Include all deserts and toppings.
   e. If you eat out, indicate where.
   f. If you eat mixed dishes, break them down into component ingredients. For example, a chicken sandwich might be listed as 2 slices of white bread, 1 tablespoon of mayonnaise, and 3 ounces of skinless chicken breast.

3. After completing the 3-day food diary, analyze your diet using a commercially available program or one from the World Wide Web. *HINT:* Use the Google search engine [www.google.com] using *free dietary analysis programs* as the key term.

4. Construct the following form to assess the adequacy of your diet versus the Food Guide Pyramid:

Food	Quantity	Pyramid Group	Number of Servings
_____	_____	_____	_____
_____	_____	_____	_____
_____	_____	_____	_____
_____	_____	_____	_____

5. Answer the following questions:
   a. How many servings from each Pyramid food group did you consume?
   b. Does your diet meet the Food Guide Pyramid guidelines (see Chapter 7). If not, what changes must you make to bring your diet more in line with these guidelines?
   c. Compare and contrast your nutrient intake with the DRIs for your age and gender on pages 52 and 59.
   d. Suppose you consumed two Krispy Kreme plain doughnuts extra each day (above your current energy balance). How much extra weight would you gain in 6 months? How much in 12 months? 36 months? What specific additional energy expenditure (with specific exercise examples) would you need to offset this weight gain?
   e. List and discuss specific changes you need to make in your energy and nutrient intake to improve your health profile.

Evans-Stoner N. Nutritional assessment. A practical approach. *Nurs Clin North Am* 1997;32:637.
Johansson L, et al. Under- and over-reporting of energy intake related to weight status and lifestyle in a nationwide sample. *Am J Clin Nutr* 1998; 68:266.
Mascarenas MR, et al. Nutritional assessment in pediatrics. *Nutrition* 1998;14:105.
Schaefer EJ, et al. Lack of efficacy of food frequency questionnaire in assessing dietary macronutrient intakes in subjects consuming diets of known composition. *Am J Clin Nutr* 2000;71:746.

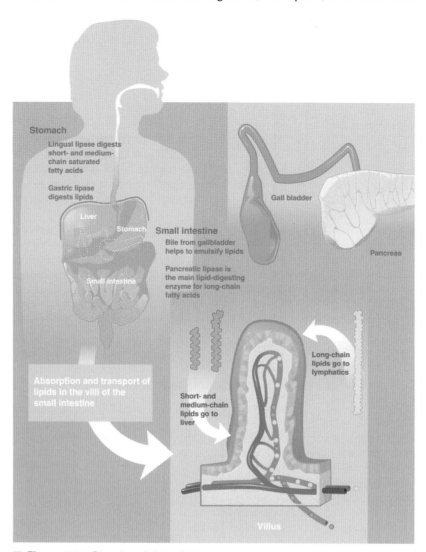

Stomach

Lingual lipase digests
short- and medium-
chain saturated
fatty acids

Gastric lipase
digests lipids

Gall bladder

Liver

Stomach

Small intestine

Bile from gallbladder
helps to emulsify lipids

Pancreas

Pancreatic lipase is
the main lipid-digesting
enzyme for long-chain
fatty acids

Small intestine

Long-chain
lipids go to
lymphatics

Absorption and transport of
lipids in the villi of the
small intestine

Short- and
medium-chain
lipids go to
liver

Villus

■ **Figure 3.16** Digestion of dietary lipids.

retains chyme in the stomach and explains why a high-fat meal prolongs digestion and gives a feeling of fullness compared with a meal of lower lipid content.

Micelles (fat–bile salt clusters) form when the water-insoluble monoglyceride and free fatty acid end products from lipid hydrolysis bind with bile salts. The outer brush border of the intestinal villi absorbs the micelles by diffusion. The micelles then split, bile returns to the liver, and triacylglycerol synthesis occurs within intestinal epithelial cells from fatty acids and monoglycerides.

Fatty Acid Carbon Chain Length Affects Digestive and Metabolic Processes

Triacylglycerols synthesized within the intestinal epithelium take one of two routes (hepatic portal system or lymphatic system), depending on their chain length. Most **medium-chain triacylglycerol** becomes absorbed directly into the portal vein (hepatic portal system) bound to albumin as glycerol and medium-chain free fatty acids. *Because medium-chain triacylglycerols bypass the lymphatic system, they enter the bloodstream rapidly for transport to the liver for subsequent use by various tissues in energy metabolism.* Medium-chain triacylglycerol supplementation has clinical application for patients with tissue-wasting disease or with intestinal malabsorption difficulties. Chapter 12 discusses the proposed use of medium-chain triacylglycerols as an energy aid in endurance exercise.

Once absorbed inside the epithelial cells, long-chain fatty acids (more than 12 carbons in the fatty acid chain) reform into triacylglycerols. These then combine with a small amount of phospholipid, protein, and cholesterol to form small fatty droplets called **chylomicrons**. The chylomicrons move slowly upward via the second route, the lymphatic system. They eventually empty into the venous blood of the systemic circulation in the neck region by way of the thoracic duct. Through the action of the enzyme **lipoprotein lipase** that lines capillary walls, the chylomicrons in the bloodstream readily hydrolyze to provide free fatty acids and glycerol for use by peripheral tissues. The liver then takes up the remaining cholesterol-containing remnant particles of the chylomicron. It generally takes 3 to 4 hours before ingested long-chain triacylglycerols enter the blood.

Protein Digestion and Absorption

The digestive efficiency for protein, particularly animal protein normally remains high, with less than 3% of this ingested macronutrient appearing in the feces. Indigestible components of this macronutrient include fibrous connective tissue of meat, some coverings of grains, and particles of nuts that remain unaffected by digestive enzymes. *In essence, protein digestion liberates the building blocks of ingested proteins to produce the final end products— simple amino acids and dipeptides and tripeptides—for absorption across the intestinal mucosa.* Specific enzymes within the stomach and small intestine promote protein hydrolysis.

The powerful enzyme **pepsin** initiates protein digestion chiefly to short-chain polypeptides in the stomach (see Fig. 3.14). Pepsin (actually a group of protein-digesting enzymes) represents the active form of its precursor pepsinogen. Pepsin's release from the cells of the stomach wall is controlled by the peptide hormone **gastrin**, secreted in response to external environmental cues (sight and smell of food) or internal cues (thought of food or stomach distention by food contents). Gastrin also stimulates secretion of gastric hydrochloric acid, a harsh acid that lowers the pH of gastric contents to about 2.0. The acidification of ingested food achieves the following: *(a)* activates pepsin, *(b)* kills pathogenic organisms, *(c)* improves absorption of iron and calcium, *(d)* inactivates hormones of plant and animal origin, and *(e)* denatures food proteins, making them more vulnerable to enzyme action. Pepsin, particularly effective in the stomach's acidic medium, easily degrades meat's collagenous connective tissue fibers. Once these fibers dismantle, other enzymes digest the remaining animal protein.

Stomach enzymes and acids attack the long, complex protein strands to hydrolyze about 15% of the ingested proteins. Uncoiling the three-dimensional shape of protein breaks it into smaller polypeptide and peptide units. Pepsin inactivates at the relatively high pH of the duodenum as the chyme passes into the small intestine.

The final steps in protein digestion occur in the small intestine. Here the peptide fragments dismantle further by alkaline enzyme action from the pancreas—most notably **trypsin** from its inactive precursor **trypsinogen**—into tripeptides, dipeptides, and single (free) amino acids. Free amino acid absorption occurs by active transport (coupled to the transport of sodium) and delivery to the liver via the hepatic portal vein. In contrast, dipeptides and tripeptides move into the intestinal epithelial cells by a single membrane carrier that uses an H^+ gradient for active transport. Once inside the cytoplasm, the dipeptides and tripeptides hydrolyze into their amino acid constituents and flow into the bloodstream.

One important function of the small intestine is to absorb amino acids and protein in more complex form. This argues against the widespread practice advocated in body building and strength magazines of ingesting a "predigested," hydrolyzed simple amino acid supplement to facilitate amino acid availability. The advertising hype does not justify the purchase of these products. When amino acids reach the liver, one of three events occurs:

- Conversion to glucose (glucogenic amino acids)
- Conversion to fat (ketogenic amino acids)
- Direct release into the bloodstream as plasma proteins such as albumin or as free amino acids

Free amino acids are synthesized into biologically important proteins, peptides (e.g., hormones), and amino acid derivatives such as phosphocreatine and choline, the essential component of the neurotransmitter acetylcholine.

Vitamin Absorption

Vitamin absorption occurs mainly by the passive process of diffusion in the jejunum and ileum portions of the small intestine (see Fig. 3.15). Absorption and storage by the body constitutes a basic difference between the fat-soluble and water-soluble vitamins.

Fat-Soluble Vitamins

Up to 90% of fat-soluble vitamins are absorbed with dietary lipids (as part of dietary fat containing micelles) throughout various sections of the small intestine. Once absorbed, chylomicrons and lipoproteins transport these vitamins to the liver and fatty tissues.

Water-Soluble Vitamins

The diffusion process absorbs water-soluble vitamins except for vitamin B_{12}. This vitamin combines with intrinsic factor produced by the stomach, which the intestine absorbs by endocytosis. Water-soluble vitamins do not remain in the tissues to any great extent. Instead, they pass into the urine when their concentration in plasma exceeds the renal capacity for reabsorption. Thus, food intake must regularly replenish water-soluble vitamins. The ingested B vitamins in food exist as part of coenzymes; digestion then releases the vitamins to their free vitamin form. This coenzyme breakdown occurs first in the stomach and then along sections of the small intestine where absorption proceeds. Ingestion of a variety of vitamin-laden nutrients, not their absorption, becomes the limiting factor in proper vitamin nutrition for healthy men and women.

ABSORPTION SITES FOR WATER-SOLUBLE VITAMINS

- **Vitamin C**: Approximately 90% of absorption takes place in the distal portion of the small intestine. Excess vitamin C intake above a threshold of approximately 1500 mg daily decreases the efficiency of kidney reabsorption, and large amounts void in the urine.

- **Thiamine**: Absorption occurs mainly in the jejunum of the small intestine. Alcoholics, individuals on extremely low-calorie diets, and the confined elderly often show symptoms of thiamine deficiency (beriberi, depression, mental confusion, loss of muscle coordination). Symptoms often become evident within 10 days because of the body's small thiamine reserve.

- **Riboflavin**: Absorption occurs mainly in the proximal portion of the small intestine.

- **Niacin**: Some absorption takes place in the stomach, but most occurs in the small intestine.

- **Pantothenic acid**: This vitamin exists as part of coenzyme A. Absorption occurs readily throughout the small intestine when the vitamin releases from its coenzyme.

- **Biotin**: Absorption occurs mainly in the upper one-third to one-half of the small intestine.

- **Folate**: Absorption occurs in the small intestine with the help of a specialized intestinal enzyme system (conjugase).

- **Vitamin B6 (pyridoxine)**: Absorption occurs mainly in the intestinal jejunum.

- **Vitamin B12**: A salivary enzyme initially acts on this vitamin in the stomach. The vitamin then combines with intrinsic factor, a glycoprotein secreted by the gastric glands, before it enters the small intestine. The pancreatic enzyme trypsin then liberates vitamin B12 from the intrinsic factor. The small intestine absorbs up to 70% in the ileum.

Mineral Absorption

Both extrinsic (dietary) and intrinsic (cellular) factors control the eventual fate of ingested minerals. Intestinal absorption increases to preserve the small micronutrient quantities when dietary intake of a particular mineral falls below the required level. The converse holds when mineral supplies exceed their limit, allowing little need for further increased absorption. Overall, the body does not absorb minerals very well. For most persons, this simply means that minerals exist in fairly generous amounts in a well-balanced normal diet. Thus, the body has little need to stockpile minerals. A possible exception exists for iron and calcium, two minerals that tend to be insufficient in the typical diet of American females.

Mineral availability in the body depends on its chemical form. For example, heme iron has an absorptive capacity of about 15% compared with nonheme iron absorption, which ranges between 2 and 10%. Variation in mineral absorption also exists between the sexes. Males absorb calcium better than females, yet total calcium absorption rarely exceeds 35% of the amount ingested, with the remaining two-thirds excreted in the feces. Of the calcium absorbed, one-half becomes voided in the urine. For phosphorus, about two-thirds is excreted daily in the urine. Poor absorption also occurs for magnesium (20–30%), and the trace minerals zinc (14–41%) and chromium (less than 2%). Determination of absorption rates for the other minerals requires further research. FIGURE 3.17 presents a generalized schema for major and trace mineral absorption, including the common pathways for their excretion.

Absorption of calcium, phosphorus, magnesium, and the trace minerals occurs mainly in the small intestine. The following six intrinsic factors affect mineral absorption: *(a)* bioavailability, *(b)* transit time from the source (diet) to the absorption site, *(c)* quantity of digestive juices, *(d)* pH of intestinal lumen contents, *(e)* presence of receptor sites in the intestine's mucosal lining and brush border, and *(f)* availability of substances that combine with the minerals during movement from the gut (via diffusion, facilitated diffusion, and/or active transport) and across cell membranes. Metallic minerals combine with a specific protein transporter (e.g., iron binds with transferrin) or a general protein carrier such as albumin, which binds with many minerals. Peptide and amino acid complexes also carry a small amount of each mineral in the blood. Although dietary fiber negatively affects absorption of certain minerals, consuming 20 to 30 g of fiber daily does not significantly impair absorption.

Water Absorption

The major absorption of ingested water and water contained in foods occurs by the passive process of osmosis in the small intestine. FIGURE 3.18 shows that in addition to the 2.0 L of water ingested daily by the typical sedentary adult, saliva, gastric secretions, bile, and pancreatic and intestinal secretions contribute an additional 7 L. This means that the intestinal tract absorbs about 9 L of water each day. Seventy-two percent of this water becomes absorbed in the proximal small intestine and 20% from its distal segment; the large intestine absorbs the remaining 8%.

The continuous secretion *and* absorption of water within the GI tract makes it difficult to quantify the body's net water uptake. The intestinal mucosa absorbs electrolytes and the components of macronutrient hydrolysis. This makes the intestinal medium progressively more hypotonic than the opposite side of the lumen membrane. This creates an osmotic gradient that forces water to move from the intestine to maintain isotonicity between the two fluid "compartments." In contrast, ingesting fluid hypertonic to plasma (greater than 280 $mOsm \cdot L^{-1}$) causes water secretion into the intestinal lumen. This retards net water absorption and increases the potential for GI distress. This can occur when consuming salt tablets, concentrated mixtures of simple amino acids, or a "sports drink" that contains a high percentage of simple sugars and minerals (see Chapter 10).

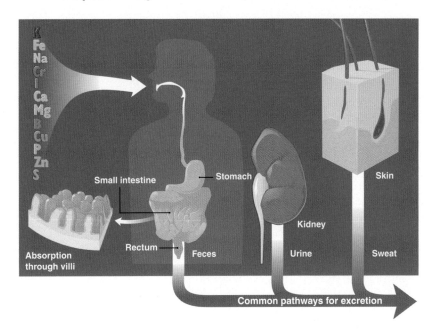

Figure 3.17 Absorption of minerals and their common excretion pathways.

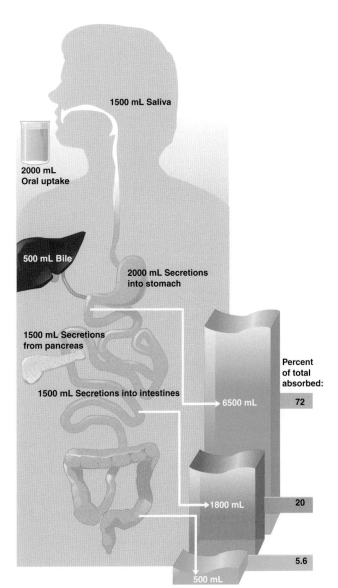

Figure 3.18 Estimated daily volumes of water that enter the small and large intestines of a sedentary adult and the volumes absorbed by each component of the intestinal tract. (From Gisolfi CV, Lamb DR, eds. Perspectives in exercise and sports medicine: fluid homeostasis during exercise. Indianapolis: Benchmark Press, 1990.)

Summary

1. Digestion hydrolyzes complex molecules into simpler substances for absorption. Self-regulating processes within the digestive tract largely control the liquidity, mixing, and transit time of the digestive mixture.

2. Physically altering food in the mouth makes it easier to swallow, while at the same time increasing its accessibility to enzymes and other digestive substances. Swallowing transfers the food mixture to the esophagus, where peristaltic action forces it into the stomach.

3. In the stomach, food contents mix as hydrochloric acid and enzymes continue the breakdown process. Little absorption occurs in the stomach except for some water and alcohol and aspirin.

4. The enzyme salivary α-amylase degrades starch to smaller linked glucose molecules and simpler disaccharides in the mouth. In the duodenum of the small intestine, pancreatic amylase continues carbohydrate hydrolysis into smaller chains of glucose molecules and simple monosaccharides.

5. Enzyme action on the surfaces of the intestinal lumen's brush border completes the final stage of carbohydrate digestion to simple monosaccharides.

6. Lipid digestion begins in the mouth and stomach by the action of lingual lipase and gastric lipase, respectively. The major lipid breakdown occurs in the small intestine by the emulsifying action of bile and the hydrolytic action of pancreatic lipase.

7. Medium-chain triacylglycerol rapidly absorbs into the portal vein bound to glycerol and medium-chain free fatty acids.

8. Once absorbed by the intestinal mucosa, long-chain fatty acids reform into triacylglycerols. They then form small fatty droplets called chylomicrons. These substances move slowly through the lymphatic system to eventually empty into the venous blood of the systemic circulation.

9. The enzyme pepsin initiates protein digestion in the stomach. The final steps in protein digestion occur in the small intestine, most notably under the action of the enzyme trypsin.

10. Vitamin absorption occurs mainly by the passive process of diffusion in the jejunum and ileum portions of the small intestine.

11. The large intestine serves as the final path for water and electrolyte absorption, including storage of undigested food residue (feces).

TEST YOUR KNOWLEDGE **ANSWERS**

1. False For many foods, digestion begins during cooking when protein structures break down, starch granules swell, and vegetables fibers soften. But for the most part, food breakdown begins in the mouth, where mechanical digestion increases the surface area of the food particles, making them easier to swallow and more accessible to enzymes and other digestive substances that start the breakdown process. For example, the enzyme salivary α-amylase (ptyalin) attacks starch and reduces it to smaller linked glucose molecules and the simpler disaccharide form maltose. Lipid digestion also begins in the mouth by the action of lingual lipase.

2. True The colon is the division of the large intestine extending from the cecum to the rectum. It comprises the ascending colon (portion between the ileocecal orifice and the right colic flexure), descending colon (portion that extends from the left colic flexure to the pelvic brim), transverse colon (portion between the right and left colic flexures), and sigmoid colon (S-shaped final portion of colon that is continuous with the rectum).

3. False While the liver, pancreas, and gallbladder play key roles in the process of digesting and assimilating food nutrients, they are not structures through which the nutrients pass directly during the digestive process.

4. True Glucose and galactose absorb from the small intestine into the blood against a concentration gradient, thus energy must be expended to power absorption of additional glucose across the intestinal mucosa. Absorption occurs by a sodium-dependent, carrier-mediated active transport process. The electrochemical gradient created with sodium transport augments absorption of these monosaccharides. In contrast, the low concentration of fat in intestinal cells allows for passive absorption of these molecules.

5. False Active transport of nutrients across cell membranes requires the expenditure of cellular energy from ATP. This process occurs when a substance cannot be transported by one of the four passive transport processes.

6. False With the exception of alcohol and aspirin, no nutrient absorption takes place in any portion of the stomach.

7. True Approximately 90% of digestion (and essentially all lipid digestion) and absorption occurs in the first two sections of the 3-m long small intestine. This coiled structure consists of three sections: the duodenum (first 0.3 m), jejunum (next 1–2 m, where most of digestion occurs), and ileum (last 1.5 m).

8. False Starch hydrolysis begins as food enters the mouth. The salivary glands continually secrete lubricating mucous substances that combine with food particles during chewing. The enzyme salivary α-amylase (ptyalin) attacks starch and reduces it to smaller linked glucose molecules and the disaccharide maltose. When the food–saliva mixture enters the more acidic stomach, some additional starch breakdown occurs, but this quickly ceases because salivary amylase deactivates under the low pH of stomach's gastric juices.

9. False Consuming excessive dietary fiber produces an overly soft stool, whereas inadequate fiber intake compacts the stool, making it more difficult to expel through the rectum. Extreme pressure during defecation can damage supporting tissues and expose blood vessels in the rectum (hemorrhoids). Gradually increasing the diet's fiber content often relieves constipation and hemorrhoid symptoms.

10. False In genzeral, hydrolysis reactions digest or break down complex molecules into simpler subunits, and condensation reactions build larger molecules by bonding their subunits together. Hydrolysis catabolizes complex organic molecules—carbohydrates, lipids, and proteins—to simpler forms that the body absorbs and assimilates. During this basic decomposition process, chemical bonds are split by addition of hydrogen ions (H^+) and hydroxyl ions (OH^-), the constituents of water, to the reaction byproducts. Examples of hydrolytic reactions include the digestion of starches and disaccharides to monosaccharides, proteins to amino acids, and lipids to glycerol and fatty acids. In contrast to hydrolysis reactions, reactions of condensation occur in the opposite direction and bind together the structural components of the nutrients to form more complex molecules and compounds.

General References

Boyle M. Personal nutrition. 4th ed. Belmont, CA: Wadsworth Publishing, 2001.

Brody T. Nutritional biochemistry. 2nd ed. New York: Academic Press, 1999.

Brown J. Nutrition now. Belmont, CA: Wadsworth Publishing, 1999.

Campbell MK. Biochemistry. 3rd ed. Philadelphia: WB Saunders, 1999.

Emken EA. Metabolism of dietary stearic acid relative to other fatty acids in human subjects. Am J Clin Nutr 1994;60(suppl):1023S.

Fox SI. Human physiology. 7th ed. New York: McGraw-Hill, 2002.

Groff JL, Gropper SS. Advanced nutrition and human metabolism. 3rd ed. Belmont, CA: Wadsworth Publishing, 1999.

Guthrie HA, ed. Introductory nutrition. 7th ed. St. Louis: CV Mosby, 1988.

Guyton AC. Textbook of medical physiology. 10th ed. Philadelphia: WB Saunders, 2000.

Kraut J. How do enzymes work? Science 1988;242:533.

Mahan LK, Escott-Stump S. Krause's food, nutrition, & diet therapy. Philadelphia: WB Saunders, 2000.

Marieb EN. Essentials of human anatomy and physiology. 7th ed. Menlo Park, CA. Pearson Education: Benjamin Cummings, 2003.

Powers HJ Riboflavin (vitamin B-2) and health. Am J Clin Nutr 2003;77:1352.

Jennifer, Shils ME, et al. Modern nutrition in health and disease. 10th ed. Baltimore: Lippincott Williams & Wilkins, 2005.

Vander AJ, et al. Human physiology: the mechanisms of body function. 7th ed. New York: McGraw-Hill, 1997.

Whitney EN, Rolfes SR. Understanding nutrition (with InfoTrac). 9th ed. Stamford, CT: Thomson/Wadsworth, 2002.

Additional Readings

Albi E, Viola Magni MP. The role of intranuclear lipids. Biol Cell 2004;96:657.

Armas LA, et al. Vitamin D2 is much less effective than Vitamin D3 in humans. J Clin Endocrinol Metab 2004;89:5387.

Borsheim E, et al. Effect of carbohydrate intake on net muscle protein synthesis during recovery from resistance exercise. J Appl Physiol 2004;96:674.

Chan MA, et al. Influence of carbohydrate ingestion on cytokine responses following acute resistance exercise. Int J Sport Nutr Exerc Metab 2003;13:454.

Jeanes YM, et al. The absorption of Vitamin E is influenced by the amount of fat in a meal and the food matrix. Br J Nutr 2004;92:575.

Jeukendrup AE. Carbohydrate intake during exercise and performance. Nutrition 2004;20:669.

Korach-Andre M, et al. Glucose appearance in the peripheral circulation and liver glucose output in men after a large 13C starch meal. Am J Clin Nutr 2004;80:881.

Lancaster GI, et al. Effect of pre-exercise carbohydrate ingestion on plasma cytokine, stress hormone, and neutrophil degranulation responses to continuous, high-intensity exercise. Int J Sport Nutr Exerc Metab 2003;13:436.

Vuorilehto K, et al. Indirect electrochemical reduction of nicotinamide coenzymes. Bioelectrochemistry 2004;65:1.

Wasserman RH. Vitamin D and the dual processes of intestinal calcium absorption. J Nutr 2004;134:3137.

Section II
Nutrient Bioenergetics in Exercise and Training

Outline

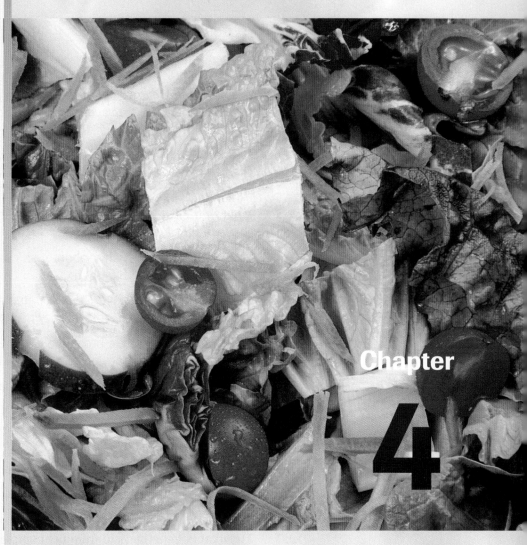

Chapter

4

Nutrient Role in Bioenergetics

TEST YOUR KNOWLEDGE

Answer these ten statements about nutrient bioenergetics. Use the scoring key at the end of the chapter to check your results. Repeat this test after you have read the chapter and compare your results.

1. **T F** Carbohydrates are used for energy and stored as glycogen in the liver and muscles. They also readily convert to fat for storage in adipose tissue.

2. **T F** Lipids are used for energy and stored as fat. Fatty acids also readily convert to carbohydrate.

3. **T F** An enzyme is an inorganic, nonprotein compound that catalyzes chemical reactions in the body.

4. **T F** Excessive protein intake does not contribute to body fat accumulation because of the lack of the enzymes to facilitate this conversion.

5. **T F** ATP forms only from the breakdown of the glycerol and fatty acid components of the triacylglycerol molecule.

6. **T F** The first law of thermodynamics refers specifically to the process of photosynthesis.

7. **T F** Oxidation and reduction refer to the conversion of oxygen into useful energy.

8. **T F** Energy is defined as the ability to perform work.

9. **T F** The main role for oxygen in the body is to combine with ADP in the synthesis of ATP.

10. **T F** The total net energy yield from the complete breakdown of a molecule of glucose is 36 ATPs.

Understanding each macronutrient's role in energy metabolism becomes crucial to optimizing the interaction between food intake and storage and exercise performance. No nutritional "magic bullets" exist per se, yet the quantity and blend of the daily diet's macronutrients profoundly affect exercise capacity, training response, and overall health.

A useful analogy shows how a car and the human body both obtain energy to make them "go." In an automobile engine, igniting the proper mixture of gasoline fuel with oxygen provides the energy required to drive the pistons. Gears and linkages harness the energy to turn the wheels; increasing or decreasing energy release either speeds up or slows down the engine. Similarly, the human body continuously extracts the energy from its fuel nutrients and harnesses it to perform its many complex biologic functions. Besides expending considerable energy for muscle action during physical activity, the body also expends energy for other "quieter" forms of biologic work including

- Digestion, absorption, and assimilation of food nutrients
- Glandular function that secretes hormones at rest and exercise
- Maintenance of electrochemical gradients along cell membranes for proper neuromuscular function
- Synthesis of new chemical compounds such as thick and thin protein structures in skeletal muscle tissue that enlarge with resistance training

NUTRITION–ENERGY INTERACTION

Bioenergetics refers to the flow of energy within a living system. The body's capacity to extract energy from food nutrients and transfer it to the contractile elements in skeletal muscle determines capacity to swim, run, bicycle, and ski long distances at high intensity. Energy transfer occurs through thousands of complex chemical reactions using a balanced mixture of macro- and micronutrients and a continual supply and use of oxygen. The term **aerobic** describes such oxygen-requiring energy reactions. In contrast, **anaerobic** chemical reactions generate energy rapidly for short durations without oxygen. Rapid anaerobic energy transfer maintains a high standard of performance in maximal short-term efforts like sprinting in track and swimming or repeated stop-and-go sports like soccer, basketball, lacrosse, water polo, volleyball, field hockey, and football, including the high power outputs generated during resistance training. The following point requires emphasis: *Anaerobic and aerobic breakdown of ingested food nutrients provides the energy source for synthesizing the chemical fuel that powers* all *forms of biologic work.*

➤ Introduction to Energy Transfer

ENERGY: THE CAPACITY FOR WORK

Extracting energy from the stored nutrients and ultimately transferring it to the contractile proteins of skeletal muscle greatly influences exercise performance. But unlike the physical properties of matter, energy cannot be defined in concrete terms of size, shape, or mass. Rather, motion plays a part in all forms of energy. This suggests a dynamic state related to change; thus the presence of energy emerges only when a change occurs. Within this context, energy relates to the performance of work—as work increases so does energy transfer.

The First Law of Thermodynamics

The **first law of thermodynamics** describes one of the most important principles related to work within biologic systems. The basic tenet states that energy is neither created nor destroyed, but instead, transforms from one state to another without being used up. In essence, this law describes the immutable principle of the **conservation of energy** that applies to both living and nonliving systems, first validated by chemists in the late 1890s. For example, the large amount of chemical energy "trapped" within the structure of fuel oil readily converts to heat energy in the home oil burner. In the body, chemical energy stored within the macronutrients' bonds does not immediately dissipate as heat. Rather, a large portion is conserved as chemical energy before changing into mechanical energy (and then ultimately to heat energy) by the musculoskeletal system. FIGURE 4.1 illustrates the interconversions for the six different forms of energy. *The first law of thermodynamics dictates that the body does not produce, consume, or use up energy; it merely transforms energy from one state to another as physiologic systems undergo continual change.*

Photosynthesis and Respiration

Photosynthesis and respiration provide the most fundamental examples of energy conversion in living cells.

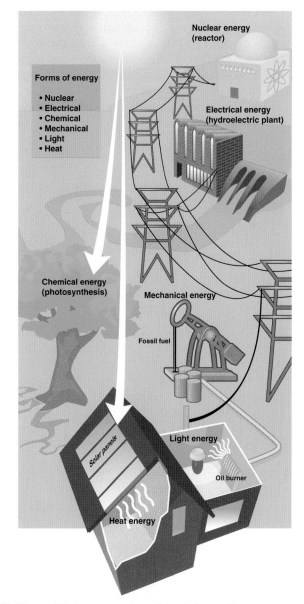

Forms of energy

- Nuclear
- Electrical
- Chemical
- Mechanical
- Light
- Heat

Nuclear energy (reactor)

Electrical energy (hydroelectric plant)

Chemical energy (photosynthesis)

Mechanical energy

Fossil fuel

Light energy

Oil burner

Solar panels

Heat energy

Figure 4.1 Interconversions of the six forms of energy.

Figure 4.2 Photosynthesis serves as the plant's mechanism for synthesizing carbohydrates, lipids, and proteins. In this example, a glucose molecule forms from the union of carbon dioxide and water.

Photosynthesis

In the sun, nuclear fusion releases part of the potential energy stored in the nucleus of the hydrogen atom. This energy, in the form of gamma radiation, converts to radiant energy.

FIGURE 4.2 depicts photosynthesis. The plant pigment chlorophyll (contained in chloroplasts, the large organelles located in the leaf's cells) absorbs radiant (solar) energy to synthesize glucose from carbon dioxide and water while oxygen flows to the environment. Animals subsequently use glucose and oxygen during respiration. Plants also convert carbohydrates to lipids and proteins. Animals then ingest plant nutrients to serve their own energy needs. *In essence, solar energy coupled with photosynthesis powers the animal world with food and oxygen.*

Cellular Respiration

FIGURE 4.3 shows that the reactions of respiration are the reverse of photosynthesis, as animals recover the plant's stored energy for use in biologic work. During respiration, the chemical energy stored in glucose, lipid, or protein molecules is extracted in the presence of oxygen. A portion of the energy remains in other chemical compounds that the body uses in diverse energy-requiring processes; the remaining energy flows as heat to the environment.

Biologic Work in Humans

Figure 4.3 also illustrates that biologic work takes one of three forms: *(a)* **mechanical work** of muscle contraction, *(b)* **chemical work** for synthesizing cellular molecules, and *(c)* **transport work** that concentrates diverse substances in the intracellular and extracellular fluids.

Figure 4.3 Respiration harvests the potential energy in food to form adenosine triphosphate (ATP). The energy in ATP powers all forms of biologic work.

Mechanical Work

Mechanical work generated by muscle contraction provides the most obvious example of energy transformation. A muscle fiber's protein filaments directly convert chemical energy into mechanical energy. However, this does not represent the only form of mechanical work. In the cell nucleus, for example, contractile elements literally tug at the chromosomes to facilitate cell division. Specialized structures such as cilia also perform mechanical work in many cells.

Chemical Work

All cells perform chemical work for maintenance and growth. Continuous synthesis of cellular components occurs as other components break down. The extreme of muscle tissue synthesis from chronic overload in resistance training vividly illustrates this form of biologic work.

Transport Work

The biologic work of concentrating substances in the body (transport work) progresses much less conspicuously than mechanical or chemical work. Cellular materials normally flow from an area of high concentration to one of lower concentration. This passive process of diffusion requires no energy. For proper physiologic functioning, certain chemicals require transport uphill, against their normal concentration gradients from an area of lower to one of higher concentration. Active transport describes this energy-requiring process (see Chapter 3). Secretion and reabsorption in the kidney tubules use active transport mechanisms, as does neural tissue in establishing the proper electrochemical gradients about its plasma membranes. These "quiet" forms of biologic work require continual expenditure of stored chemical energy.

Potential and Kinetic Energy

Potential energy and kinetic energy constitute the total energy of any system. FIGURE 4.4 shows potential energy as energy of position similar to water at the top of a hill before it flows downstream.

In this example, energy changes proportionally to the water's vertical drop—the greater the vertical drop, the greater the potential energy at the top. Other examples of potential energy include bound energy within the internal structure of a battery, a stick of dynamite, or a macronutrient before release of its stored energy through metabolism. *Releasing potential energy transforms it into kinetic energy of motion.* In some cases, bound energy in one substance directly transfers to other substances to increase their potential energy. Energy transfers of this type provide the necessary energy for the body's chemical work of biosynthesis. Specific building-block atoms of carbon, hydrogen, oxygen, and nitrogen join other atoms and molecules to synthesize important biologic compounds (e.g., cholesterol, enzymes,

Figure 4.4 Potential energy to perform work transforms into kinetic energy.

and hormones). Some newly created compounds serve structural needs of bone or the lipid-containing plasma membrane that encapsulates each cell. Other synthesized compounds such as adenosine triphosphate (ATP) and phosphocreatine (PCr) serve the cell's energy needs.

OXIDATION AND REDUCTION

Literally thousands of simultaneous chemical reactions occur in the body that involve the transfer of electrons from one substance to another. *Oxidation reactions transfer oxygen atoms, hydrogen atoms, or electrons.* A loss of electrons occurs in oxidation reactions, with a corresponding gain in valence. For example, removing hydrogen from a substance yields a net gain of valence electrons. *Reduction reactions involve any process in which the atoms in an element gain electrons with a corresponding decrease in valence.*

Oxidation and reduction reactions are always characteristically **coupled**, so that any energy released by one reaction incorporates into the products of another reaction. In essence, energy-liberating reactions couple to energy-requiring reactions. The term **reducing agent** describes the substance that donates or loses electrons as it oxidizes. The substance being reduced or gaining electrons is called the electron acceptor or **oxidizing agent**. The term **redox** reaction describes a coupled oxidation–reduction reaction.

An excellent example of an oxidation reaction involves electron transfer within the mitochondria. Here, special carrier molecules transfer oxidized hydrogen atoms and their removed electrons for delivery to oxygen, which becomes reduced. The carbohydrate, lipid, and protein nutrient substrates provide the source of hydrogen. Dehydrogenase (oxidase) enzymes tremendously speed up the redox reactions. Two hydrogen-accepting dehydrogenase coenzymes are the vitamin B-containing nicotinamide adenine dinucleotide (NAD^+), derived from the B vitamin niacin, and flavin adenine dinucleotide (FAD), derived from another B vitamin, riboflavin. Transferring electrons from NADH and $FADH_2$ harnesses energy in the form of ATP (see p. 127).

*The transport of electrons by specific carrier molecules constitutes the **respiratory chain**.* **Electron transport** represents the final common pathway in aerobic (oxidative) metabolism. For each pair of hydrogen atoms, two electrons flow down the chain and reduce one atom of oxygen. The process ends when oxygen accepts hydrogen and forms water. The coupled redox process constitutes hydrogen oxidation coupled to subsequent oxygen reduction. Chemical energy trapped or conserved in cellular oxidation–reduction reactions powers the various forms of biologic work.

FIGURE 4.5 illustrates a redox reaction during vigorous physical activity. As exercise intensifies, hydrogen atoms strip from the carbohydrate substrate at a greater rate than their oxidation in the respiratory chain. To continue energy metabolism, the nonoxidized excess hydrogens must be "accepted" by a substance other than oxygen. A molecule of pyruvate, an intermediate compound formed in the initial phase of carbohydrate catabolism, temporarily accepts a pair of hydrogens (electrons). A new compound called **lactic acid** (in the body as **lactate**) forms when reduced pyruvate accepts additional hydrogens. As illustrated in the figure, more intense exercise produces a greater flow of excess hydrogens to pyruvate, and lactate concentration rises rapidly within the active muscle. During recovery, the excess hydrogens in lactate now oxidize (electrons removed and passed to NAD^+) to re-form a pyruvate molecule. The enzyme lactate dehydrogenase (LDH) facilitates this reaction.

Summary

1. Energy, defined as the ability to perform work, appears only when a change occurs.

2. Energy exists in either potential or kinetic form. Potential energy refers to energy associated with a substance's structure or position; kinetic energy refers to energy of motion. Potential energy can be measured when it transforms to kinetic energy.

3. There are six forms of interchangeable energy states—chemical, mechanical, heat, light, electric, and nuclear—and each can convert or transform to another form.

4. In photosynthesis, plants transfer the energy of light into the potential energy of carbohydrates, lipids, and proteins. Respiration releases the stored energy in plants and couples it to other chemical compounds for biologic work.

5. Biologic work takes one of three forms: chemical (biosynthesis of cellular molecules), mechanical (muscle contraction), or transport (transfer of substances among cells).

6. Oxidation–reduction (redox) reactions couple so oxidation (a substance loses electrons) coincides with the reverse reaction of reduction (a substance gains electrons). Redox reactions power the body's energy-transfer processes.

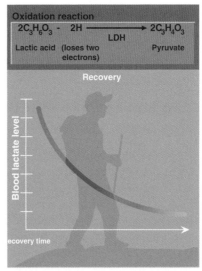

■ **Figure 4.5** Example of a redox (oxidation–reduction) reaction. During progressively strenuous exercise when the oxygen supply becomes inadequate, some pyruvate formed in energy metabolism gains two hydrogens (gains two electrons) and becomes *reduced* to a new compound, lactate. In recovery, when oxygen supply becomes adequate, lactate loses two hydrogens (two electrons) and *oxidizes* back to pyruvate. LDH, lactate dehydrogenase

Phosphate Bond Energy

The body demands a continual supply of chemical energy to perform its many complex functions. Energy transformations in the body largely depend upon *(a)* oxidation–reduction reactions and *(b)* chemical reactions that conserve and liberate the energy in ATP. Energy derived from the oxidation of food does not release suddenly at some kindling temperature because the body, unlike a mechanical engine, cannot use heat energy. If it did, the body fluids would actually boil, and tissues would burst into flames. Instead, extraction of chemical energy trapped within the bonds of the macronutrients releases in relatively small quantities during complex, enzymatically controlled reactions within the relatively cool, watery medium of cells. This temporarily conserves some energy that otherwise would dissipate as heat, to provide greater efficiency in energy transformations. In a sense, the cells receive energy as needed.

The story of how the body maintains its continuous energy supply begins with **adenosine triphosphate**, the body's special carrier for free energy.

ADENOSINE TRIPHOSPHATE: THE ENERGY CURRENCY

The energy in food does not transfer directly to the cells for biologic work. Instead, "nutrient energy" funnels through the energy-rich ATP compound. The potential energy within this molecule provides for *all* of the cell's energy-requiring processes. In essence, this energy receiver-energy donor role of ATP represents the cells' two major energy-transforming activities:

- Extract potential energy from food and conserve it within the bonds of ATP
- Extract and transfer the chemical energy in ATP to power biologic work

FIGURE 4.6 shows how ATP forms from a molecule of adenine and ribose (called adenosine) linked to three phosphate molecules. The bonds linking the two outermost phosphates are termed **high-energy bonds** because they represent a considerable quantity of potential energy within the ATP molecule.

During hydrolysis, adenosine triphosphatase catalyzes the reaction when ATP joins with water. In the degradation of one mole of ATP to **adenosine diphosphate** (**ADP**), the outermost phosphate bond splits and liberates approximately 7.3 kilocalories (kcal) of free energy (i.e., energy available for work).

$$ATP + H_2O \xrightarrow{ATPase} ADP + P - 7.3 \text{ kcal per mole}$$

The free energy liberated in ATP hydrolysis reflects the energy difference between the reactant and end products. Because this reaction generates considerable energy, we refer to ATP as a **high-energy phosphate** compound. Infrequently, additional energy releases when another phosphate splits from ADP. In some reactions of biosynthesis, ATP donates its two terminal phosphates simultaneously to synthesize cellular material. Adenosine monophosphate, or AMP, becomes the new molecule with a single phosphate group.

The energy liberated during ATP breakdown transfers directly to other energy-requiring molecules. In muscle, for example, this energy activates specific sites on the contractile elements causing the muscle fiber to shorten. *Because energy from ATP powers all forms of biologic work, ATP constitutes the cell's "energy currency."* FIGURE 4.7 illustrates the general role of ATP as energy currency.

The splitting of an ATP molecule takes place immediately and without oxygen. The cell's capability for ATP breakdown generates energy for rapid use; this would not occur if energy metabolism required oxygen at all times.

■ **Figure 4.6** Simplified illustration of ATP, the energy currency of the cell. The symbol ⊖ represents the high-energy bonds.

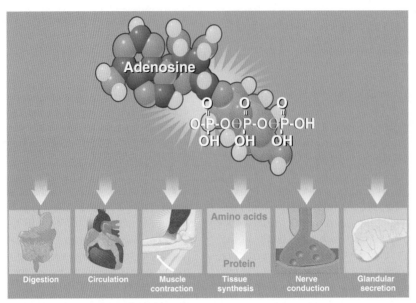

Figure 4.7 ATP, the energy currency, powers all forms of biologic work. The symbol ⊖ represents the high-energy bonds.

Anaerobic energy release can be thought of as a back-up power source called upon when the body requires energy in excess of what can be generated aerobically. For this reason, any form of physical activity can take place immediately without instantaneously consuming oxygen; examples include sprinting for a bus, lifting a weight, driving a golf ball, spiking a volleyball, doing a pushup, or jumping up in the air. The well-known practice of holding one's breath during a short sprint swim or run provides a clear example of ATP splitting without reliance on atmospheric oxygen. Withholding air (oxygen), although inadvisable can be done during a 60-yard sprint on the track, lifting a barbell, opening and closing your hand as fast as possible for 20 seconds, or dashing up multiple flights of stairs. In each case, energy metabolism proceeds uninterrupted because the energy for performing the activity comes almost exclusively from intramuscular anaerobic sources.

PHOSPHOCREATINE: THE ENERGY RESERVOIR

Cells store only a small quantity of ATP and must therefore continually resynthesize it at its rate of use. This provides a biologically useful mechanism for regulating energy metabolism. By maintaining only a small amount of ATP, its relative concentration (and corresponding concentration of ADP) changes rapidly, increasing a cell's energy demands. Any increase in energy requirement (i.e., disturbance in the cell's current state) immediately disrupts the balance between ATP and ADP. An imbalance immediately stimulates breakdown of other stored energy-containing compounds to

resynthesize ATP. This helps to explain why energy transfer increases rapidly when exercise begins. As one might expect, increases in energy transfer depend on exercise intensity. Energy transfer increases about fourfold in the transition from sitting in a chair to walking. However, changing from a walk to an all-out sprint almost immediately accelerates the rate of energy transfer about 120 times!

As pointed out above, a limited quantity of ATP serves as the energy currency for all cells. In fact, the body stores only 80 to 100 g (about 3.0 oz) of ATP at any one time. This provides enough intramuscular stored energy for several seconds of explosive, all-out exercise. To overcome this storage limitation, ATP resynthesis occurs continually to supply energy for biologic work. Fatty acids and glycogen represent the major energy sources for maintaining continual ATP resynthesis. Some energy for ATP resynthesis, however, comes directly from the anaerobic splitting of a phosphate from another intracellular high-energy phosphate compound **phosphocreatine (PCr)**, also known as creatine phosphate or CP. PCr is similar to ATP—it releases a large amount of energy when the bond splits between the creatine and phosphate molecules. FIGURE 4.8 schematically illustrates the release and use of phosphate-bond energy in ATP and PCr. The term **high-energy phosphates** describes these stored intramuscular compounds.

In each reaction, the arrow points in both directions, indicating a reversible reaction. In other words, phosphate (P) and creatine (Cr) join again to re-form PCr. This also applies to ATP, for ADP plus P re-forms ATP. Cells store approximately four to six times more PCr than ATP. *The onset of intense exercise triggers PCr hydrolysis for energy; it does not require oxygen and reaches a maximum in about*

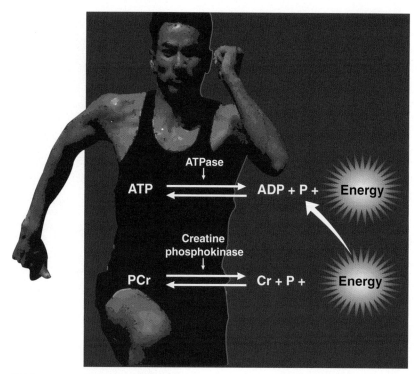

Figure 4.8 ATP and PCr provide anaerobic sources of phosphate-bond energy. The energy liberated from the hydrolysis (splitting) of PCr rebonds ADP and P to form ATP.

10 seconds.[26] Thus, PCr serves as a "reservoir" of high-energy phosphate bonds. PCr's speed for ADP phosphorylation considerably exceeds anaerobic energy transfer from stored muscle glycogen owing to the high activity rate of the creatine phosphokinase reaction.[10] If maximal effort continues beyond 10 seconds, the energy for continual ATP resynthesis must originate from the less rapid catabolism of the stored macronutrients.[8] Chapter 12 discusses the potential for exogenous creatine supplementation to increase intracellular levels of PCr and enhance short-term, all-out exercise performance.

Intramuscular High-Energy Phosphates

Energy release from the intramuscular energy-rich phosphates ATP and PCr sustains all-out exercise for approximately 5 to 8 seconds. Thus, in a 100-m sprint in world record time by 1996 Canadian Olympic champion Donovan Bailey (9.84 s, or 27.1 mph) the body cannot maintain maximum speed throughout this duration. During the last few seconds of the race, the runners actually slow down, with the winner often slowing down least! If all-out effort continues beyond 8 seconds or if moderate exercise continues for much longer periods, ATP resynthesis requires an additional energy source other than PCr. If resynthesis does not happen, the "fuel" supply diminishes and high-intensity movement ceases. As we discuss below, the foods we eat and store for ready access provide chemical energy to continually recharge cellular supplies of ATP and PCr.

Transfer of Energy by Chemical Bonds

Human energy dynamics involve transferring energy by means of chemical bonds. Potential energy releases by the splitting of bonds and is conserved by the formation of new bonds. Some energy lost by one molecule transfers to the chemical structure of other molecules without appearing as heat. In the body, biologic work occurs when compounds relatively low in potential energy become "juiced up" from the transfer of energy via high-energy phosphate bonds.

ATP serves as the ideal energy-transfer agent. In one respect, the phosphate bonds of ATP "trap" a relatively large portion of the original food molecule's potential energy. ATP also readily transfers this energy to other compounds to raise them to a higher activation level. **Phosphorylation** refers to energy transfer through phosphate bonds.

CELLULAR OXIDATION

Most of the energy for ATP phosphorylation comes from oxidation ("biologic burning") of the carbohydrate, lipid, and protein macronutrients consumed in the diet. Recall that a molecule reduces when it accepts electrons from an electron donor. In turn, the molecule that gives up electrons is oxidized. Oxidation reactions (donating electrons) and reduction reactions (accepting electrons) remain coupled because every oxidation coincides with a reduction. *In essence, cellular oxidation–reduction constitutes the mechanism for energy metabolism.* This process often involves the transfer of hydrogen atoms (contains one electron and one proton in its nucleus) rather than free electrons. Thus, a molecule that loses hydrogen oxidizes and one that gains hydrogen reduces. For example, the stored carbohydrate, fat, and protein molecules continually provide hydrogen atoms. The mitochondria, the cell's "energy factories," contain carrier molecules that remove electrons from hydrogen (oxidation) and eventually pass them to oxygen (reduction). Synthesis of the high-energy phosphate ATP occurs during oxidation–reduction reactions.

Electron Transport

FIGURE 4.9 illustrates the general scheme for hydrogen oxidation and accompanying electron transport to oxygen. During cellular oxidation, hydrogen atoms are not merely turned loose in the cell fluid. Rather, highly specific **dehydrogenase coenzymes** catalyze hydrogen's release from the nutrient substrate. The coenzyme part of the dehydrogenase (usually the niacin-containing coenzyme NAD^+) accepts pairs of electrons (energy) from hydrogen. While the substrate oxidizes and loses hydrogen (electrons), NAD^+ gains one hydrogen and two electrons and reduces to NADH; the other hydrogen appears as H^+ in the cell fluid.

The riboflavin-containing coenzyme **FAD** serves as the other important electron acceptor in oxidizing food fragments. FAD catalyzes dehydrogenations and accepts pairs of electrons. Unlike NAD^+, however, FAD becomes $FADH_2$ by accepting both hydrogens. *The NADH and $FADH_2$ formed in the breakdown of food are energy-rich molecules that carry electrons with a high energy transfer potential.* The coenzymes NAD^+ and FAD are derived from the water-soluble vitamins niacin and riboflavin, respectively; unfortunately, vitamin manufacturers often misleadingly link the consumption of these vitamins above recommended levels to increased energy capacity. To the contrary, once sufficient amounts of these coenzymes are available in the body, any excess vitamins are voided in the urine.

The **cytochromes**, a series of iron–protein electron carriers, then pass in "bucket brigade" fashion pairs of electrons carried by NADH and $FADH_2$ on the inner membranes of the mitochondria. The iron portion of each cytochrome exists in either its oxidized (ferric or Fe^{3+}) or reduced (ferrous or Fe^{2+}) ionic state. By accepting an electron, the ferric portion of a specific cytochrome reduces to its ferrous form. In turn, ferrous iron donates its electron to the next cytochrome, and so on down the line. By shuttling between these two iron forms, the cytochromes transfer electrons to their ultimate destination, where they reduce oxygen to form water. The NAD^+ and FAD then recycle for subsequent use in energy metabolism.

Electron transport by specific carrier molecules constitutes the respiratory chain; this serves as the final common

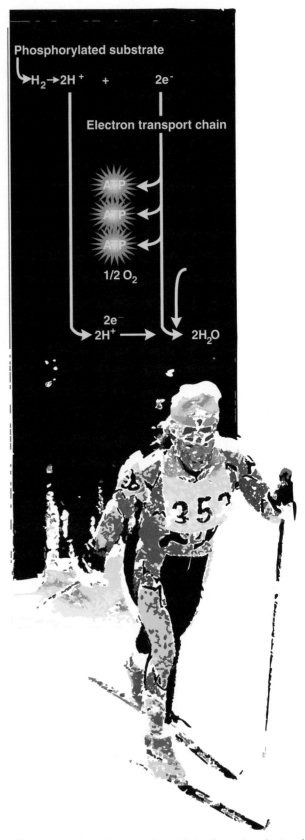

■ **Figure 4.9** General scheme for oxidation (removing electrons) of hydrogen and accompanying electron transport. In this process, oxygen becomes reduced (gain of electrons) and water forms. ATP, adenosine triphosphate.

pathway where the electrons extracted from hydrogen pass to oxygen. For each pair of hydrogen atoms, two electrons flow down the chain and reduce one atom of oxygen to form water. Of the five specific cytochromes, only the last one, cytochrome oxidase (cytochrome aa₃, with a strong affinity for oxygen) discharges its electron directly to oxygen. The right panel of FIGURE 4.10 shows the route for hydrogen oxidation, electron transport, and energy transfer in the respiratory chain. The respiratory chain releases free energy in relatively small amounts. In several of the electron transfers, energy conservation occurs by forming high-energy phosphate bonds.

Oxidative Phosphorylation

Oxidative phosphorylation synthesizes ATP by transferring electrons from NADH and FADH₂ to oxygen. This primary process represents the cell's way of extracting and trapping chemical energy in the high-energy phosphates. *More than 90% of ATP synthesis takes place in the respiratory chain by oxidative reactions coupled with phosphorylation.*

In a way, oxidative phosphorylation can be likened to a waterfall divided into several separate cascades by the intervention of water wheels at different heights. The left panel of Figure 4.10 depicts the water wheels harnessing the energy of the falling water. Similarly, electrochemical energy generated via electron transport in the respiratory chain is harnessed and transferred (or coupled) to ADP. Three distinct coupling sites during electron transport transfer the energy in NADH to ADP to re-form ATP (Fig. 4.10, *right panel*).

Oxidation of hydrogen and subsequent phosphorylation occur as follows:

$$NADH + H^+ + 3\ ADP + 3\ P + 1/2\ O_2 \rightarrow$$
$$NAD^+ + H_2O + 3\ ATP$$

Note in the above reaction that three ATPs form for each NADH plus H^+ oxidized. However, if FADH₂ originally donates hydrogen, then only two molecules of ATP form for each hydrogen pair oxidized. Two ATP molecules form because FADH₂ enters the respiratory chain at a lower energy level at a point beyond the site of the first ATP synthesis.

Efficiency of Electron Transport and Oxidative Phosphorylation

The formation of each mole of ATP from ADP conserves approximately 7 kcal of energy. Because 3 moles of ATP come from oxidizing 1 mole of NADH, about 21 kcal (7 kcal per mole × 3) are conserved as chemical energy. A relative efficiency of 40% occurs for harnessing chemical energy by electron transport-oxidative phosphorylation, since the oxidation of one mole of NADH liberates a total of 52 kcal (21 kcal ÷ 52 kcal × 100). The 60% remaining energy dissipates as heat. Considering that a steam engine transforms its fuel into useful energy at only about 30% efficiency, the value of 40% for the human body represents a remarkably high efficiency rate.

■ **Figure 4.10** Examples of harnessing potential energy. *Left: In industry,* energy from falling water becomes harnessed to turn the waterwheel, which in turn performs mechanical work. *Right: In the body,* the electron transfer chain removes electrons from hydrogens for ultimate delivery to oxygen. In oxidation–reduction, much of the chemical energy stored within the hydrogen atom does not dissipate to kinetic energy, but instead is conserved within ATP.

ROLE OF OXYGEN IN ENERGY METABOLISM

Three prerequisites exist for continual resynthesis of ATP during coupled oxidative phosphorylation from macronutrient catabolism. Satisfying the following three conditions causes hydrogen and electrons to shuttle uninterrupted down the respiratory chain to oxygen during energy metabolism:

1. Availability of the reducing agent NADH (or $FADH_2$) in the tissues
2. Presence of an oxidizing agent (oxygen) in the tissues
3. Sufficient concentration of enzymes and mitochondria in the tissues to ensure that energy transfer reactions proceed at their appropriate rate

In strenuous exercise, inadequate oxygen delivery (condition 2) or its rate of use (condition 3) creates a relative imbalance between hydrogen release and its final acceptance by oxygen. If either of these conditions occurs, electron flow down the respiratory chain "backs up," and hydrogens accumulate bound to NAD^+ and FAD. A subsequent section (see page 139) provides the details on how lactate forms when the compound pyruvate temporarily binds these excess hydrogens (electrons); lactate formation allows continuation of electron transport-oxidative phosphorylation.

Aerobic metabolism refers to energy-generating catabolic reactions. In this scenario, oxygen serves as the final electron acceptor in the respiratory chain and combines with hydrogen to form water. In one sense, the term *aerobic* is misleading because oxygen does not participate directly in ATP synthesis. On the other hand, oxygen's presence at the "end of the line" largely determines one's capacity for ATP production and, hence, ability for sustaining high-intensity, endurance exercises.

Summary

1. Energy within the chemical structure of carbohydrate, fat, and protein molecules does not suddenly release in the body at some kindling temperature. Rather, energy release occurs slowly in small amounts during complex enzymatically controlled reactions, thus enabling more efficient energy transfer and conservation.

2. About 40% of the potential energy in the food nutrients transfers to the high-energy compound adenosine triphosphate (ATP).

3. Splitting the terminal phosphate bond of ATP liberates free energy to power all forms of biologic work.

4. ATP serves as the body's energy currency, although its quantity amounts to only about 3.0 ounces.

5. Phosphocreatine (PCr) interacts with adenosine diphosphate (ADP) to form ATP. This nonaerobic, high-energy reservoir replenishes ATP rapidly.

6. Phosphorylation refers to energy transfer by phosphate bonds, in which ADP and creatine continually recycle into ATP and PCr.

7. Cellular oxidation occurs on the inner lining of the mitochondrial membranes; it involves transferring electrons from NADH and $FADH_2$ to oxygen. This process results in the release and coupled transfer of chemical energy to form ATP from ADP plus a phosphate ion.

8. During aerobic ATP resynthesis, oxygen serves as the final electron acceptor in the respiratory chain and combines with hydrogen to form water.

CASE STUDY/PERSONAL HEALTH AND EXERCISE NUTRITION 4-1

Overuse Injuries and Subsequent Pain

Bill, a former collegiate football athlete, has remained generally sedentary for the past 10 years. About once a month each weekend he participates in vigorous competitive sports like tennis, touch football, skiing, and roller hockey on consecutive days. He then complains of soreness and pain in his knees, back, shoulders, feet, and ankles. He stretches daily periodically to help "loosen" his back, but not on a regular basis. The stretching does not seem to help relieve the aches and pains of his skeletal maladies.

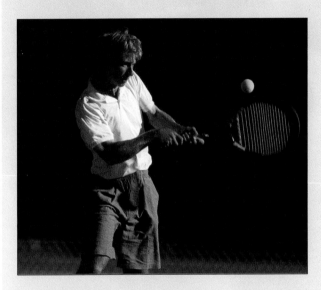

PAST MEDICAL HISTORY

Bill does not smoke, has no history of major disease, and maintains desirable body weight (although he weighs 10 pounds more than in college) and normal blood pressure. All laboratory data (blood work done yearly at a local hospital) fall within normal range. He is healthy, but more sedentary than he desires.

DIAGNOSIS

Weekend warrior with signs and symptoms of overuse injuries.

CASE QUESTIONS

1. Track the progression of an overuse injury.
2. Give the immediate first aid procedures for treating an overuse injury.
3. Describe different pain symptoms and possible treatments of an overuse injury.
4. How can Bill prevent recurring overuse injuries.

ANSWERS

1. Overuse injuries result from the repetitive use of muscles, tendons, and joints in the same way without sufficient rest. Such repeated muscle actions often occur in strenuous sports, but they also take place during any repeated motions such as cutting wood, digging in the ground, or raking leaves. Runners are particularly subject to overuse injuries of the knees and feet; likewise, tennis players frequently experience overuse injuries of the elbow and shoulder as do weight lifters and power athletes (discus and shot put athletes).

Pain that worsens with activity provides the main indication of an overuse injury. Symptoms often progress as follows:
- Initially, there exists a dull pain or discomfort and general fatigue (normally associated with strenuous exercise).
- Pain then becomes sharper and more localized (sensation can be pinpointed to a definite area such as the hip, knee, or elbow).
- Pain lingers from day to day, often accompanied by some swelling. In essence, tissue inflammation has occurred.
- Pain and/or swelling become severe enough to interfere with further activity.
- Pain and/or swelling interfere with normal daily activities such as standing, walking, and sleeping.

2. The five-letter acronym **P-R-I-C-E** (Protection, Rest, Ice, Compression, Elevation) describes the preferred immediate treatment sequence for soft tissue overuse injuries.

- **Protection:** Isolate the injured area to protect it from further damage.
- **Rest:** Restrict further activity and use of the injured area.
- **Ice:** Immediately surround the injured area with an ice pack secured with elastic wrap and continue application for 24 to 72 hours, depending on injury severity. Vasoconstriction from the ice helps to reduce bleeding, swelling (fluid seepage into surrounding tissues), and pain. The standard ice application interval lasts 15–20 minutes, with reapplication hourly or when pain persists. Ice or compression at bedtime is unnecessary unless the pain interferes with sleep. If the injury involves a contusion (bruise) to a muscle belly, place the muscle under mild stretch before applying ice; if possible, maintain that position for the duration of ice application.
- **Compression:** Compress the injured area firmly but not with excessive pressure. Begin the wrap distal to the injury and proceed toward and over the injured area.
- **Elevation:** If applicable, raise the injured area above heart level to minimize the hydrostatic effect of gravity on venous pooling and fluid efflux into injured tissues. Maintain limb elevation as long as practical. During sleep, elevate the injured limb with blankets or pillows.

CASE STUDY/PERSONAL HEALTH AND EXERCISE NUTRITION 4–1 *(continued)*

3. TABLES 1–4 list different pain symptoms for the shoulder, back, leg, and knee and possible causes.
4. Overuse injuries often take longer to heal than other injuries. Prevention thus becomes an important consideration. Bill can reduce the chance of incurring an overuse injury by doing the following:

   • Allow at least 48 hours between activities. Bill should consider interspersing a day of rest between sports days.
   • Decrease the intensity of activity (learn to ease up while playing). Bill needs to learn not to go "all-out" every time he plays.
   • Decrease the duration of activity (refrain from doing too

much at one time). Bill needs to limit the total time of exercise participation.
• Gradually increase the training level. Bill should consider joining a gym to upgrade his fitness for weekend sports participation.
• Make sure the exercise equipment is up-to-date and in good working order.
• Consider the participant's age. Bill needs to regard changes in his body as he ages and adjust his workouts accordingly. This includes devoting enough time for pre- and postexercise flexibility activities and for adequate warm-up prior to exercising and cool-down on completing the workout.

Table 1   SHOULDER PAIN: SYMPTOMS, CAUSES, AND TREATMENT

Symptoms	Possible Causes	Treatment
Severe pain and tenderness after exercising, especially when moving; numbness and tingling in arm; joint looks misshapen	Dislocation	Emergency treatment
Sudden joint pain along with flu or infection	Side effect of infection	Over-the-counter anti-inflammatory medication
Pain and swelling around shoulder; painful movements; sometimes fever	Bursitis	See physician
Pain and stiffness beginning in neck and moving to shoulder; numbness or tingling in arms, hands, and fingers; weakness in arms and legs	Cervical spondylosis—deterioration of joints in neck that put pressure on nerves and muscles	Call physician immediately; apply moist heat
Severe pain during movement; difficulty moving arm in any direction; aches when not being used	Frozen shoulder—inflammation of shoulder joint from lack of use (usually because of injury)	Apply P-R-I-C-E treatment; see physician
Pain or recurring dull ache in shoulder; difficulty raising or lowering arm; weakness in shoulder	Rotator cuff injury—inflammation of tendons that hold shoulder in place	See physician for advice
Pain in distinct spot that is worse with movement and follows injury, overexertion, or heavy lifting	Strained or torn tendon, ligament or muscle	Use P-R-I-C-E treatment; see physician
Pain and tenderness in shoulder, often worsens at night; muscle spasms	Tendonitis	Rest, use P-R-I-C-E treatment; antiinflammatory medication
Continual pain and stiffness in shoulder (and sometimes other joints)	Arthritis	See physician for advice and treatment

CASE STUDY/PERSONAL HEALTH AND EXERCISE NUTRITION 4–1 *(continued)*

Table 2   BACK PAIN: SYMPTOMS, CAUSES, AND TREATMENT

Symptoms	*Possible Causes*	*Treatment*
Severe lower back pain made worse by bending, twisting, coughing, or lifting (pain shoots down one leg); in severe cases, loss of bladder or bowel control	Protruded disk that irritates or presses on a nerve	With loss of bladder or bowel control, call physician for emergency advice; call doctor for advice and appointment; take pain relievers
Occasional or frequent lower back pain that may worsen at night; back or hip stiffness in morning that improves with activity; pain and stiffness in rib area; neck or chest pain; fatigue, weight loss, and poor appetite; fever; eye pain; blurred vision	Ankylosing spondylitis—a rare inflammatory form of arthritis that chiefly affects spinal column, usually in men under age 40	Call physician for advice; physical therapy, strength training, massage, and anti-inflammatory over-the-counter pain relievers
Numbness, weakness, and/or mild pain in back legs; worsens with walking, eases when sitting	Spinal stenosis—narrowing of spinal canal from arthritis, thickened spinal ligaments, or bulging disks	If overweight, weight loss and exercise to strengthen abdominal muscles
Pain and stiffness in back, buttocks, and thighs; difficulty moving or bending	Arthritis	Ask physician for treatment
Soreness and stiffness after exertion or injury, or soreness that develops gradually during the night; may spread to buttocks and thighs	Back sprain or strain	Rest; over-the-counter pain relievers
Aching, pain, and stiffness in back muscles; points on body feel sore when pressed; fatigue, headache, and insomnia	Fibromyalgia (can accompany chronic fatigue syndrome; affects women age 20–50; accompanied by sleep problems)	Treat with antidepressants, painkillers and muscle relaxants; exercise relieves discomfort
Backache, easily broken bones (especially in spine, wrists and hips), stooped or hunched posture	Osteoporosis	Over-the-counter pain relievers

Table 3   LEG PAIN: SYMPTOMS, CAUSES, AND TREATMENT

Symptoms	*Possible Causes*	*Treatment*
Severe leg pain, swelling, and tenderness after an injury; unable to move leg	Bone fracture	Go to emergency room immediately
Leg pain following injury, able to move leg	Strained, inflamed, or torn tendon, ligament, or muscle	Call physician for appointment
Pain and fatigue in muscles or thighs, calves, feet, or hips when walking or exercising; stops with rest; mostly in middle-aged and older adults	Peripheral vascular disease	Call physician for appointment
Pain and burning sensation with redness, tenderness, and itching; hard, cordlike swelling beneath skin along length of vein in leg (in phlebitis). Swelling, warmth, and redness throughout leg; bluish color in toes (in deep vein thrombosis)	Phlebitis (thrombophlebitis)—inflammation of vein near surface of skin, usually a result of infection or injury, which causes clotting; deep-vein thrombosis—blood clots in deep veins	Call physician for appointment; phlebitis is usually not harmful, but deep-vein thrombosis can cause clots that dislodge and travel to the lungs
Pain in front or side of lower leg that begins during or just after exercise	Shin splints—injury or inflammation of bone, tendon, or muscle in lower leg	Rest 2–3 weeks; use ice for inflammation and warm soaks for relief from discomfort
Leg muscles tighten suddenly and painfully for a few minutes, then return to normal	Leg cramps	Stretch; massage; immerse in warm water while stretching and massaging

Table 4   **KNEE PAIN: SYMPTOMS, CAUSES, AND TREATMENT**

Symptoms	Possible Causes	Treatment
Pain and possibly a "pop" at moment of injury; swelling, stiffness, instability, and difficulty walking	Ligament sprain or rupture and/or cartilage damage	Apply P-R-I-C-E treatment
Pain, swelling, and stiffness in joint	Arthritis	Call physician for advice
Tenderness, stiffness, and swelling above kneecap; pain when bending; possible fever or redness	Bursitis	Call physician for advice
Pain just below kneecap, especially when sitting or straightening leg; may be felt after running or jumping; knee pain and tightness that worsens with movement	Patellar tendonitis or "jumper's knee"	Apply P-R-I-C-E treatment for pain and swelling

Energy Release from Macronutrients

The energy released in macronutrient breakdown serves one crucial purpose—to phosphorylate ADP to re-form the energy-rich compound ATP (FIG. 4.11). Macronutrient catabolism favors the generation of phosphate-bond energy, yet the specific pathways of degradation differ depending on the nutrients metabolized. In the sections below, we show how ATP resynthesis occurs from the extraction of potential energy in the food macronutrients.

FIGURE 4.12 outlines the basic macronutrient fuel sources that supply substrate for oxidation and subsequent ATP formation. These sources consist primarily of the following:

- Glucose derived from liver glycogen
- Triacylglycerol and glycogen molecules stored within muscle cells
- Free fatty acids derived from triacylglycerol (in liver and adipocytes) that enter the bloodstream for delivery to active muscle
- Intramuscular and liver-derived carbon skeletons of amino acids

A small amount of ATP also forms from *(a)* anaerobic reactions in the cytosol in the initial phase of glucose or glycogen breakdown and *(b)* the phosphorylation of ADP by PCr under enzymatic control by creatine phosphokinase.

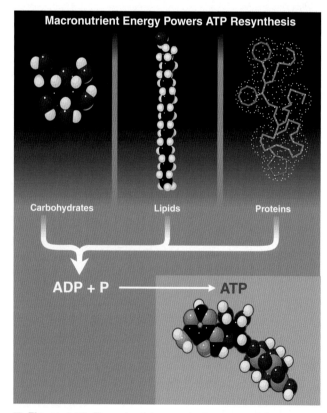

Macronutrient Energy Powers ATP Resynthesis

Carbohydrates   Lipids   Proteins

ADP + P → ATP

■ **Figure 4.11** The potential energy in the macronutrients powers ATP resynthesize. ADP, adenosine diphosphate; P, phosphate.

Figure 4.12 Basic macronutrient fuel sources that supply substrates for regenerating ATP. The liver provides a rich source of amino acid and glucose, while adipocytes generate large quantities of energy-rich fatty acid molecules. Once released, the bloodstream delivers these compounds to the muscle cell. Most of the cells' energy production takes place within the mitochondria. Mitochondrial proteins carry out oxidative phosphorylation in the inner membranous walls of this architecturally elegant complex. The intramuscular energy sources consist of the high-energy phosphates ATP and PCr and triacylglycerols, glycogen, and amino acids.

ENERGY RELEASE FROM CARBOHYDRATES

The *primary function of carbohydrates is to supply energy for cellular work.* The complete breakdown of one mole of glucose (180 g) to carbon dioxide and water yields a maximum of 686 kcal of chemical free energy available for work. In the body, however, complete glucose breakdown conserves only some of this energy in the form of ATP.

$$C_6H_{12}O_6 + 6O_2 \rightarrow 6CO_2 + 6H_2O + 686 \text{ kcal per mole}$$

Synthesizing one mole of ATP from ADP and phosphate ion requires 7.3 kcal of energy. Therefore, coupling all of the energy in glucose oxidation to phosphorylation could theoretically form 94 moles of ATP per mole of glucose (686 kcal ÷ 7.3 kcal·mole^{-1}). In muscle, however, the phosphate bonds only conserve 38% or 261 kcal of energy, with the remainder dissipated as heat. Consequently, glucose breakdown regenerates 36 moles of ATP (261 kcal ÷ 7.3 kcal·mole^{-1}) with an accompanying free energy gain of 261 kcal.

Anaerobic versus Aerobic

Glucose degradation occurs in two stages. In stage one, glucose breaks down relatively rapidly to two molecules of pyruvate. Energy transfers occur without oxygen (anaerobic). In stage two of glucose catabolism, pyruvate degrades further to carbon dioxide and water. Energy transfers from these reactions require electron transport and accompanying oxidative phosphorylation (aerobic).

IMPORTANCE OF CARBOHYDRATES IN ENERGY METABOLISM

- Carbohydrates are the only macronutrient whose stored energy generates ATP anaerobically. This becomes important in maximal exercise that requires rapid energy release above levels supplied by aerobic metabolic reactions. In this case, most of the energy for ATP resynthesis comes from stored intramuscular glycogen.

- During light and moderate aerobic exercise, carbohydrates supply about one-third of the body's energy requirements.

- Processing fat through the metabolic mill for energy requires some carbohydrate catabolism.

- Aerobic breakdown of carbohydrate for energy occurs more rapidly than energy generation from fatty acid breakdown. Thus, depleting glycogen reserves significantly reduces exercise power output. In prolonged high-intensity, aerobic exercise such as marathon running, athletes often experience nutrient-related fatigue—a state associated with muscle and liver glycogen depletion.

Glycolysis: Anaerobic Energy from Glucose Catabolism

The first stage of glucose degradation within cells involves a series of chemical reactions collectively termed **glycolysis** (also termed the Embden-Meyerhof pathway for its two biochemist discoverers). This series of reactions, summarized in FIGURE 4.13, occurs in the watery medium of the cell outside of the mitochondrion. In a sense, the reactions represent a more primitive form of energy transfer well developed in amphibians, reptiles, fish, and marine mammals. In humans, the cells' capacity for glycolysis becomes crucial during physical activities that require maximal effort for up to 90 seconds.

In the first reaction of Figure 4.13, ATP acts as a phosphate donor to phosphorylate glucose to glucose 6-phosphate. In most tissues of the body, phosphorylation "traps" the glucose molecule in the cell. (Liver and, to a small extent, kidney cells contain the enzyme **glucose 6-phosphatase** that splits the phosphate from glucose 6-phosphate, thus freeing glucose for transport across the cell membrane for delivery throughout the body.) In the presence of **glycogen synthase**, glucose joins (become polymerized) with other glucose

Figure 4.13 Glycolysis, a series of 10 enzymatically controlled chemical reactions creates two molecules of pyruvate from the anaerobic breakdown of glucose. Lactic acid (lactate) forms when NADH oxidation does not keep pace with its formation in glycolysis. ATP, adenosine triphosphate; ADP, adenosine triphosphate; NAD, nicotinamide adenine dinucleotide.

molecules to form glycogen. In energy metabolism, however, glucose 6-phosphate changes to fructose 6-phosphate. At this stage, no energy extraction occurs, yet energy incorporates into the original glucose molecule at the expense of one ATP molecule. In a sense, phosphorylation "primes the pump" for energy metabolism to proceed. The fructose 6-phosphate molecule gains an additional phosphate from ATP and changes to fructose 1,6-diphosphate under control of **phosphofructokinase (PFK)**. The activity level of PFK probably places a limit on the rate of glycolysis during maximum-effort exercise. Fructose 1,6-diphosphate then splits into two phosphorylated molecules, each with three carbon chains; these further decompose to pyruvate in five successive reactions. Fast-twitch muscle fibers contain relatively large quantities of PFK; this makes them ideally suited for generating rapid anaerobic energy from glycolysis.

Glycogen Catabolism

Glycogenolysis describes the cleavage of glucose from stored glycogen (glycogen → glucose). The **glycogen phosphorylase** enzyme in skeletal muscle regulates and limits glycogen's breakdown for energy. **Epinephrine**, a sympathetic nervous system hormone, influences the activity of this enzyme to cleave one glucose component at a time from the glycogen molecule.[4,6] The glucose residue then reacts with a phosphate ion to produce glucose 6-phosphate, bypassing step one of the glycolytic pathway. Thus, when glycogen provides a glucose molecule for glycolysis, a net gain of 3 ATPs occurs rather than the 2 ATPs that occur during this first phase of glucose breakdown (see next section).

Substrate-Level Phosphorylation in Glycolysis

Most of the energy generated in the reactions of glycolysis does not result in ATP resynthesis but instead dissipates as heat. In reactions 7 and 10, however, the energy released from the glucose intermediates stimulates the direct transfer of a phosphate group to ADP while generating four ATP molecules. *Because two molecules of ATP were lost in the initial phosphorylation of the glucose molecule, glycolysis generates a net gain of two ATP molecules.* These specific energy transfers from substrate to ADP by phosphorylation do not require oxygen. Rather, energy transfers directly via phosphate bonds in the anaerobic reactions called **substrate-level phosphorylation**. Energy conservation during glycolysis operates at an efficiency of about 30%.

Glycolysis generates only about 5% of the total ATP formed during the glucose molecule's complete breakdown. However, the high concentration of glycolytic enzymes and the speed of these reactions provide significant energy for muscle action during glycolysis. The following represent examples of activities that rely heavily on ATP generated by glycolysis: sprinting at the end of the mile run, performing all-out from start to finish in the 50- and 100-m swim, rou-

tines on gymnastics apparatus, and sprint running races up to 200 m. *Note that anaerobic energy transfer from the macronutrients occurs only from carbohydrate breakdown during glycolytic reactions.*

Hydrogen Release in Glycolysis

During glycolysis, two pairs of hydrogen atoms are stripped from the substrate (glucose) and their electrons passed to NAD^+ to form NADH (Fig. 4.13). Normally, if the respiratory chain processed these electrons directly, three molecules of ATP would generate for each molecule of NADH oxidized. However, the mitochondrion in skeletal muscle remains impermeable to NADH formed in the cytoplasm during glycolysis. Consequently, the electrons from extramitochondrial NADH shuttle indirectly into the mitochondria. In skeletal muscle, this route ends with electrons passing to FAD to form $FADH_2$ at a point below the first formation of ATP (see Fig. 4.10, *right panel*). *Thus, two rather than three ATP molecules form when the respiratory chain oxidizes cytoplasmic NADH. Because two molecules of NADH form in glycolysis, four molecules of ATP generate aerobically by subsequent electron transport-oxidative phosphorylation.*

Lactate Formation

Sufficient oxygen bathes the cells during light-to-moderate levels of energy metabolism. Consequently, the hydrogens (electrons) stripped from the substrate and carried by NADH oxidize within the mitochondria to form water when they join with oxygen. In a biochemical sense a "steady state," or more precisely a "steady rate," exists because hydrogen oxidizes at about the same *rate* that it becomes available. Biochemists frequently refer to this relatively steady dynamic condition as **aerobic glycolysis**, with pyruvate becoming the end product.

In strenuous exercise, when energy demands exceed either the oxygen supply or its rate of use, the respiratory chain cannot process all of the hydrogen joined to NADH. Continued release of anaerobic energy in glycolysis depends on NAD^+ availability for oxidizing 3-phosphoglyceraldehyde (see reaction 6 in Fig. 4.13), otherwise, the rapid rate of glycolysis "grinds to a halt." Under **anaerobic glycolysis**, NAD^+ re-forms as pairs of "excess" nonoxidized hydrogens combine temporarily with pyruvate to form lactate in an additional step, catalyzed by **lactate dehydrogenase**, in the reversible reaction shown in FIGURE 4.14.

The temporary storage of hydrogen with pyruvate represents a unique aspect of energy metabolism because it provides a ready "reservoir" to temporarily store the end products of anaerobic glycolysis. Also, once lactic acid forms in the muscle, it diffuses into the blood for buffering to sodium lactate and removal from the site of energy metabolism. In this way, glycolysis continues to supply ad-

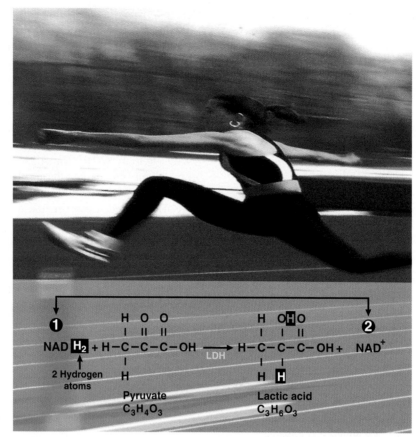

■ **Figure 4.14** *(1)* Lactic acid forms when excess hydrogens from NADH combine temporarily with pyruvate. *(2)* This frees up NAD$^+$ to accept additional hydrogens generated in glycolysis. LDH, lactate dehydrogenase; NAD, nicotinamide adenine dinucleotide.

ditional anaerobic energy for ATP resynthesis. This avenue for extra energy remains temporary; blood and muscle lactate levels increase, and ATP regeneration cannot keep pace with its utilization rate. Fatigue soon sets in, and exercise performance diminishes. Increased acidity from lactate accumulation (and perhaps the effect of the lactate anion itself) mediates fatigue by inactivating various enzymes involved in energy transfer and inhibiting some aspect of the muscle's contractile machinery.[3,9,13]

Even at rest, energy metabolism in red blood cells forms some lactate. This occurs because the red blood cells contain no mitochondria and thus must derive their energy from anaerobic glycolysis. Lactate should not be viewed as a metabolic "waste product." To the contrary, it provides a valuable source of chemical energy that accumulates in the body during heavy exercise. When sufficient oxygen once again becomes available during recovery, or when exercise pace slows, NAD$^+$ scavenges hydrogens attached to lactate; these hydrogens subsequently oxidize to synthesize ATP. Consequently, much circulating blood lactate becomes an energy source as it readily reconverts to pyruvate. In addi-

tion, the liver cells conserve the potential energy in the lactate and pyruvate molecules formed during exercise, as the carbon skeletons of these molecules become synthesized to glucose in the **Cori cycle** (FIG. 4.15). The Cori cycle not only removes lactate, but it also uses the lactate substrate to resynthesize blood glucose and muscle glycogen (gluconeogenesis in the liver) depleted in heavy exercise.[24]

Citric Acid Cycle: Aerobic Energy from Glucose Catabolism

Anaerobic glycolysis releases only about 10% of the energy within the original glucose molecule. Thus, extracting the remaining energy requires an additional metabolic pathway. This occurs when pyruvate *irreversibly* converts to acetyl-CoA, a form of acetic acid. Acetyl-CoA enters the second stage of carbohydrate breakdown, termed the **citric acid cycle**, also known as the Krebs cycle in honor of chemist Hans Krebs (1900–1981), who shared the 1953 Nobel Prize in Physiology or Medicine for his discovery of the citric acid cycle.

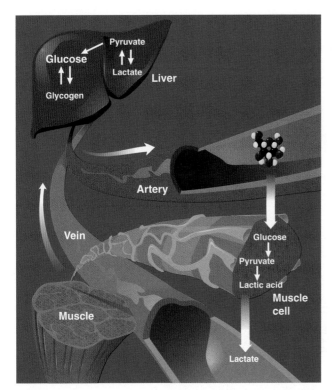

Figure 4.15 In the Cori cycle, lactic acid from muscle enters the venous system and converts to lactate. Lactate then enters the liver for conversion to pyruvate and synthesis to glucose for subsequent delivery to muscle. This gluconeogenic process helps to maintain carbohydrate reserves.

As shown schematically in FIGURE 4.16, the citric acid cycle degrades the acetyl-CoA substrate to carbon dioxide and hydrogen atoms within the mitochondria. Hydrogen atoms then oxidize during electron transport-oxidative phosphorylation with subsequent ATP regeneration. FIGURE 4.17 shows pyruvate preparing to enter the citric acid cycle by joining with the vitamin B (pantothenic acid)-derivative coenzyme A (A stands for acetic acid) to form the 2-carbon compound acetyl-CoA. This process releases two hydrogens and transfers their electrons to NAD^+, forming one molecule of carbon dioxide as follows:

$$Pyruvate + NAD^+ + CoA \rightarrow$$
$$Acetyl\text{-}CoA + CO_2 + NADH + H^+$$

The acetyl portion of acetyl-CoA joins with oxaloacetate to form citrate (citric acid), the same 6-carbon compound found in citrus fruits, which then proceeds through the citric acid cycle. The citric acid cycle continues its operations because it retains the original oxaloacetate molecule to join with a new acetyl fragment that then enters the cycle.

Each acetyl-CoA molecule entering the citric acid cycle releases two carbon dioxide molecules and four pairs of hydrogen atoms. One molecule of ATP also regenerates directly by substrate-level phosphorylation from citric acid cycle reactions (see reaction 7 in Fig. 4.17). As summarized at the bottom of Figure 4.17, four hydrogens release when acetyl-CoA forms from the two pyruvate molecules created in glycolysis, and 16 hydrogens are released in the citric acid cycle. *The most important function of the citric acid cycle generates electrons (H^+) for passage in the respiratory chain to NAD^+ and FAD.*

Oxygen does not participate directly in citric acid cycle reactions. The major portion of the chemical energy in pyruvate transfers to ADP through the aerobic process of electron transport-oxidative phosphorylation within the folding or cristae of the inner mitochondrial membrane. With adequate oxygen, including enzymes and substrate, NAD^+ and FAD regeneration takes place, and citric acid cycle metabolism proceeds unimpeded.

Net Energy Transfer from Glucose Catabolism

FIGURE 4.18 summarizes the pathways for energy transfer during glucose breakdown in skeletal muscle. Two ATPs (net gain) are formed from substrate-level phosphorylation in glycolysis. Similarly, 2 ATPs come from acetyl-CoA degradation in the citric acid cycle. Account for the 24 released hydrogen atoms as follows:

- Four extramitochondrial hydrogens (2 NADH) generated in glycolysis yield 4 ATPs during oxidative phosphorylation (6 ATPs in heart, kidneys, and liver).
- Four hydrogens (2 NADH) released in the mitochondrion as pyruvate degrades to acetyl-CoA yield 6 ATPs.
- Twelve of the 16 hydrogens (6 NADH) released in the citric acid cycle yield 18 ATPs.
- Four hydrogens joined to FAD (2 $FADH_2$) in the citric acid cycle yield 4 ATPs.

Thirty-eight ATPs represents the total ATP yield from the complete breakdown of glucose. *Because 2 ATPs initially phosphorylate glucose, 36 ATP molecules equal the net ATP yield from complete glucose breakdown in skeletal muscle. Four ATP molecules form directly from substrate-level phosphorylation (glycolysis and citric acid cycle), whereas 32 ATP molecules regenerate during oxidative phosphorylation.* One should temper these *theoretical* values for ATP generation in energy metabolism in light of biochemical information that suggests they may be overestimates because only 30 to 32 ATPs *actually* enter the cytoplasm of the cell. This differentiation between theoretical and actual ATP yield may result from the added energy cost required to transport ATP out of the mitochondria.[7] Chapter 5 explains the specifics of carbohydrate's role in energy release under anaerobic and aerobic exercise conditions.

Figure 4.16 Hydrogen formation and subsequent oxidation during aerobic energy metabolism. *Phase 1.* In the mitochondria, the citric acid cycle generates hydrogen atoms during acetyl-CoA breakdown. *Phase 2.* Significant quantities of ATP regenerate when these hydrogens oxidize via the aerobic process of electron transport-oxidative phosphorylation (electron transport chain). ADP, adenosine diphosphate; P, phosphate.

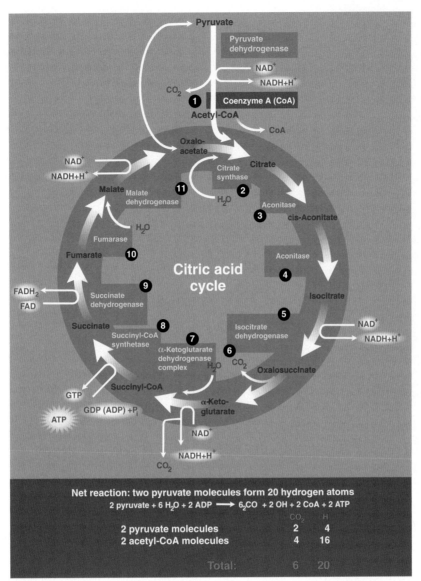

Figure 4.17 Schematic illustration and quantification for hydrogen (H) and carbon dioxide (CO_2) release in the mitochondrion during the breakdown of one pyruvate molecule. All values have been doubled when computing the net gain of H and CO_2 from pyruvate breakdown because glycolysis produces two molecules of pyruvate from one molecule of glucose. P_i, phosphate; ADP, adenosine diphosphate; ATP, adenosine triphosphate; NAD, nicotinamide adenine dinucleotide; FAD, flavin adenine dinucleotide; GDP, guanosine diphosphate; GTP, guanosine triphosphate.

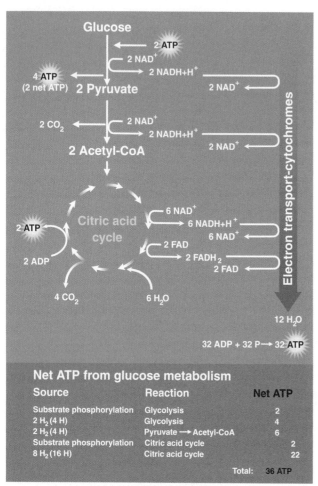

Net ATP from glucose metabolism

Source	Reaction	Net ATP
Substrate phosphorylation	Glycolysis	2
2 H_2 (4 H)	Glycolysis	4
2 H_2 (4 H)	Pyruvate → Acetyl-CoA	6
Substrate phosphorylation	Citric acid cycle	2
8 H_2 (16 H)	Citric acid cycle	22
	Total:	**36 ATP**

Figure 4.18 Net yield of 36 ATP molecules from energy transfer during the complete oxidation of one glucose molecule through glycolysis, the citric acid cycle, and electron transport.

ENERGY RELEASE FROM FAT

Stored fat represents the body's most plentiful source of potential energy. Relative to carbohydrate and protein, stored fat provides almost unlimited energy. The fuel reserves in a typical young adult male equal between 60,000 and 100,000 kcal from triacylglycerol in fat cells (**adipocytes**) and about 3000 kcal from intramuscular triacylglycerol (12 mmol·kg^{-1} muscle). In contrast, the carbohydrate energy reserve generally amounts to less than 2000 kcal. Energy sources for fat catabolism include:

- Triacylglycerol stored directly within the muscle fiber in close proximity to the mitochondria (more in slow-twitch than fast-twitch muscle fibers)
- Circulating triacylglycerol in lipoprotein complexes that hydrolyze on the surface of a tissue's capillary endothelium catalyzed by lipoprotein lipase
- Circulating free fatty acids mobilized from triacylglycerol in adipose tissue that serve as blood-borne energy carriers

Prior to energy release from fat, hydrolysis (**lipolysis** or fat breakdown) splits the triacylglycerol molecule into glycerol and three water-insoluble fatty acid molecules. The enzyme **hormone-sensitive lipase** catalyzes triacylglycerol breakdown as follows:

$$\text{Triacylglycerol} + 3\,H_2O \xrightarrow{\text{lipase}} \text{Glycerol} + 3 \text{ Fatty acids}$$

An intracellular mediator, **adenosine 3′,5′-cyclic monophosphate**, or **cyclic AMP**, activates hormone-sensitive lipase, and thus regulates fat breakdown.[21] Cyclic AMP in both adipocytes and muscle cells becomes activated by the various fat-mobilizing hormones—epinephrine, norepinephrine, glucagon, and growth hormone—which themselves cannot enter the cell.[20] Lactate, ketones, and insulin inhibit cyclic-AMP activation.[5]

Adipocytes: Site of Fat Storage and Mobilization

FIGURE 4.19 outlines the dynamics of fat storage and fat mobilization. Although all cells store some fat, adipose tissue serves as an active and major supplier of fatty acid molecules. Adipocytes specialize in synthesizing and storing triacylglycerol. Triacylglycerol fat droplets occupy up to 95% of the adipocyte cell's volume. Once hormone-sensitive lipase stimulates fatty acids to diffuse from the adipocyte into the circulation, nearly all bind to plasma albumin for transport as **free fatty acids (FFAs)** to active tissues.[19] Hence, FFAs are not truly "free" entities. At the muscle site, FFAs release from the albumin–FFA complex for transport across the plasma membrane (either by diffusion and/or a protein-mediated carrier system). Once inside the muscle cell, FFAs either reesterify to form intracellular triacylglycerols or they bind with intramuscular proteins and enter the mitochondria for energy metabolism (by action of **carnitine–acyl-CoA transferase**). Medium- and short-chain fatty acids do not depend on carnitine–acyl-CoA transferase transport, and most diffuse freely into the mitochondrion.

The water-soluble glycerol molecule formed during lipolysis readily diffuses from the adipocyte into the circulation. As a result, plasma glycerol levels often reflect the level of the body's triacylglycerol breakdown.[17] When delivered to the liver, glycerol serves as a gluconeogenic precursor for glucose synthesis. This relatively slow process explains why glycerol supplementation contributes little as an energy substrate during exercise.[14]

Breakdown of Glycerol and Fatty Acids

FIGURE 4.20 summarizes the pathways for the breakdown of the glycerol and fatty acid fragments of the triacylglycerol molecule.

potential energy in a fatty acid to ATP (a process termed *fatty acid oxidation*) cleaves 2-carbon acetyl fragments split from the long chain of the fatty acid. The process of converting an FFA to multiple acetyl-CoA molecules is called **beta (β)-oxidation**, because the second carbon on a fatty acid is termed the "beta carbon." ATP phosphorylates the reactions, water is added, hydrogens pass to NAD^+ and FAD, and the acetyl fragment joins with coenzyme A to form acetyl-CoA. β-*Oxidation provides the same two-carbon acetyl unit as acetyl generated from glucose breakdown.* β-Oxidation continues until the entire fatty acid molecule degrades to acetyl-CoA for direct entry into the citric acid cycle. The hydrogens released during fatty acid catabolism oxidize through the respiratory chain. *Note that fatty acid breakdown relates directly with oxygen uptake.* β-Oxidation proceeds only when oxygen joins with hydrogen. Under anaerobic conditions, hydrogen remains with NAD^+ and FAD, bringing a halt to fat catabolism.

Figure 4.19 Dynamics of fat mobilization and storage. Hormone-sensitive lipase stimulates triacylglycerol breakdown into glycerol and fatty acid components. After their release from adipocytes, the blood transports free fatty acids (FFAs) bound to plasma albumin. Fats stored within the muscle fiber also degrade to glycerol and fatty acids to provide energy. ATP, adenosine triphosphate.

Glycerol

The anaerobic reactions of glycolysis accept glycerol as 3-phosphoglyceraldehyde, which then degrades to pyruvate to form ATP by substrate-level phosphorylation. Hydrogen atoms pass to NAD^+, and the citric acid cycle oxidizes pyruvate. *The complete breakdown of the single glycerol molecule in a triacylglycerol molecule synthesizes a total of 19 ATP molecules.* Glycerol also provides carbon skeletons for glucose synthesis. This gluconeogenic role of glycerol becomes important when significant depletion of glycogen reserves occurs from dietary restriction of carbohydrates or in long-term exercise or heavy training.

Fatty Acids

Almost all fatty acids contain an even number of carbon atoms, ranging from 2 to 26. The first step in transferring the

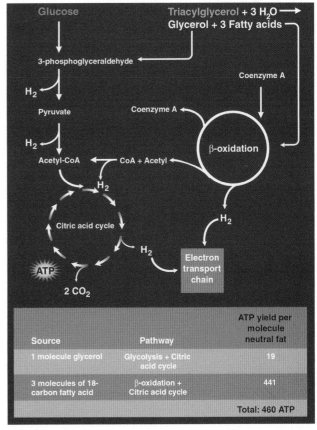

Source	Pathway	ATP yield per molecule neutral fat
1 molecule glycerol	Glycolysis + Citric acid cycle	19
3 molecules of 18-carbon fatty acid	β-oxidation + Citric acid cycle	441
		Total: 460 ATP

Figure 4.20 General scheme for the breakdown of the glycerol and fatty acid fragments of triacylglycerol. Glycerol enters the energy pathways during glycolysis. The fatty acid fragments prepare to enter the citric acid cycle through β-oxidation. The electron transport chain accepts hydrogens released during glycolysis, β-oxidation, and citric acid cycle metabolism. ATP, adenosine triphosphate.

Total Energy Transfer From Fat Catabolism

The breakdown of a fatty acid molecule progresses as follows:

- β-Oxidation produces NADH and $FADH_2$ by cleaving the fatty acid molecule into 2-carbon acetyl fragments.
- Citric acid cycle degrades acetyl Co-A into carbon dioxide and hydrogen atoms.
- Hydrogen atoms oxidize by electron transport-oxidative phosphorylation.

For each 18-carbon fatty acid molecule, 147 molecules of ADP phosphorylate to ATP during β-oxidation and citric acid cycle metabolism. Because each triacylglycerol molecule contains three fatty acid molecules, 441 ATP molecules form from the triacylglycerol's fatty acid components (3 × 147 ATP). Also, 19 molecules of ATP form during glycerol breakdown. This generates 460 ATP molecules for each typical triacylglycerol molecule catabolized. This number represents a considerable energy yield, because only 36 ATPs form during a glucose molecule's catabolism in skeletal muscle. The efficiency of energy conservation for fatty acid oxidation amounts to about 40%, a value similar to that for glucose oxidation.

Depending on a person's state of nutrition, level of training, and the intensity and duration of physical activity, intra- and extracellular lipid molecules usually supply between 30 and 80% of the energy for biologic work.[17,25] When high-intensity, long-duration exercise depletes glycogen reserves, fat serves as the *primary* fuel for exercise and recovery.[12]

FATS BURN IN A CARBOHYDRATE FLAME

Interestingly, fatty acid breakdown depends in part on a continual background level of carbohydrate breakdown. Recall that acetyl-CoA enters the citric acid cycle by combining with oxaloacetate to form citrate. This oxaloacetate is generated from pyruvate during carbohydrate breakdown (under the control of pyruvate carboxylase), which adds a carboxyl group to the pyruvate molecule. Carbohydrate depletion decreases pyruvate production during glycolysis. Diminished pyruvate reduces levels of citric acid cycle intermediates (oxaloacetate and malate), which slows citric acid cycle activity (see Fig. 4.21).[2,16,18,22,27] Citric acid cycle degradation of fatty acids depends on sufficient oxaloacetate availability to combine with the acetyl-CoA formed during β-oxidation. When the carbohydrate level decreases, the oxaloacetate level may become inadequate. In this sense, "fats burn in a carbohydrate flame."

A Slower Rate of Energy Release From Fat

A rate limit exists for fatty acid use by active muscle.[28] Aerobic training enhances this limit, but the power generated solely by fat breakdown still represents only about one-half that achieved with carbohydrate as the chief aerobic energy source. Thus, depleting muscle glycogen decreases a muscle's maximum aerobic power output. Just as the hypoglycemic condition coincides with a "central" or neural fatigue, muscle glycogen depletion probably causes "peripheral" or local muscle fatigue during exercise.[15]

While gluconeogenesis provides a metabolic option for synthesizing glucose from noncarbohydrate sources, it cannot replenish or even maintain glycogen stores unless one regularly consumes carbohydrates. Appreciably reducing carbohydrate availability seriously limits energy transfer capacity. Glycogen depletion could occur in prolonged exercise (marathon running), consecutive days of heavy training, inadequate energy intake, dietary elimination of carbohydrates (as advocated with high-fat, low-carbohydrate "ketogenic" diets), or diabetes. Diminished aerobic exercise intensity occurs even though large amounts of fatty acid substrate circulate to muscle. During extreme carbohydrate depletion, the acetate fragments produced in β-oxidation accumulate in the extracellular fluids because they cannot readily enter the citric acid cycle. The liver converts these compounds to ketone bodies (four-carbon long acidic derivatives, acetoacetic acid and β-hydroxybutyric acid together with acetone), some of which pass in the urine. If ketosis persists, the acid quality of the body fluids can increase to potentially toxic levels.

LIPOGENESIS

Lipogenesis describes the formation of fat, mostly in the cytoplasm of liver cells. It occurs as follows: ingested excess glucose or protein not used immediately to sustain metabolism converts into stored triacylglycerol. For example, when muscle and liver glycogen stores fill, as occurs after a large meal, any excess glucose (and amino acids) synthesizes to fatty acids. This lipogenic process requires ATP energy and the B vitamins biotin, niacin, and pantothenic acid.

Lipogenesis begins with carbons from glucose and the carbon skeletons from amino acid molecules that metabolize to acetyl-CoA (see section on protein metabolism). Liver cells bond together the acetate parts of the acetyl-CoA molecules in a series of steps to form the 16-carbon saturated fatty acid palmitic acid. Palmitic acid can then lengthen to an 18- or 20-carbon chain fatty acid in either the cytosol or the mitochondria. Ultimately, three fatty acid molecules join (esterify) with one glycerol molecule (produced during glycolysis) to yield one triacylglycerol molecule. Triacylglycerol releases into the circulation as a very-low-density lipoprotein (VLDL); cells may use VLDL for ATP production or store it in adipocytes along with other fats from dietary sources.

ENERGY RELEASE FROM PROTEIN

Chapter 1 emphasized that protein plays a role as an energy substrate during endurance-type activities and heavy training. The amino acids (primarily the branched-chain amino acids leucine, isoleucine, valine, glutamine, and aspartate) first convert to a form that readily enters pathways for energy release. This conversion requires nitrogen (amine) removal from the amino acid molecule. The liver serves as the main site for **deamination**, but skeletal muscle also contains enzymes that remove nitrogen from an amine group of an amino acid and pass it to other compounds during **transamination**. In this way, the "carbon skeleton" byproducts of donor amino acids participate directly in energy metabolism within muscle. Enzyme levels for transamination increase with exercise training to further facilitate protein's use as an energy substrate.

Once an amino acid loses its nitrogen-containing amine group, the remaining compound (usually a component of the citric acid cycle's reactive compounds) contributes to ATP formation. Some amino acids are **glucogenic** and when deaminated yield intermediate products for glucose synthesis via gluconeogenesis (FIG. 4.21). For example, pyruvate forms in the liver as alanine loses its amine group and gains a double-bond oxygen; pyruvate can then be synthesized to glucose. This gluconeogenic method serves as an important adjunct to the Cori cycle to provide glucose during prolonged exercise. Regular exercise training enhances the liver's capacity for gluconeogenesis from alanine.[23,24] Other amino acids such as glycine are **ketogenic** and when deaminated yield the intermediate acetyl-CoA or acetoacetate. These compounds cannot be synthesized to glucose, but instead are synthesized to fat or are catabolized for energy in the citric acid cycle.

Protein Breakdown Facilitates Water Loss

When protein provides energy, the body must eliminate the nitrogen-containing amine group and other solutes from protein breakdown. This requires excretion of "obligatory" water because the waste products of protein catabolism leave the body dissolved in fluid (urine). For this reason, excessive protein catabolism increases the body's water needs.

■ **Figure 4.21** Glucogenic and ketogenic amino acids. Carbon skeletons from amino acids that form pyruvate or directly enter the citric acid cycle are glucogenic because these carbon compounds can form glucose. Carbon skeletons that form acetyl-CoA are ketogenic because they cannot form glucose molecules but rather synthesize fat.

THE METABOLIC MILL

The citric acid cycle plays a much more important role than simply degrading pyruvate produced during glucose catabolism. Fragments from other organic compounds formed from fat and protein breakdown provide energy during citric acid cycle metabolism. FIGURE 4.22 illustrates that deaminated residues of excess amino acids enter the citric acid cycle at various intermediate stages, whereas the glycerol fragment of triacylglycerol catabolism gains entrance via the glycolytic pathway. Fatty acids become oxidized in β-oxidation to acetyl-CoA. This compound then enters the cycle directly.

The "metabolic mill" depicts the citric acid cycle as the vital link between food (macronutrient) energy and the chemical energy of ATP. The citric acid cycle also serves as a "metabolic hub" to provide intermediates that cross the mitochondrial membrane into the cytosol to synthesize bionutrients for maintenance and growth. For example, excess carbohydrates provide glycerol and acetyl fragments to synthesize triacylglycerol. Acetyl-CoA also functions as the branch point for synthesizing cholesterol, bile, and many hormones as well as ketone bodies and fatty acids. Fatty acids *cannot* contribute to glucose synthesis because the conversion of pyruvate to acetyl-CoA does not reverse (notice the one-way arrow in Fig. 4.22). Many of the carbon compounds generated in citric cycle reactions also provide the organic starting points for synthesizing nonessential amino acids.

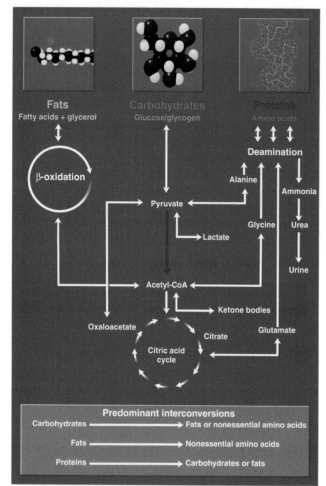

Figure 4.22 The "metabolic mill" shows important interconversions among carbohydrates, fats, and proteins. Note that all interconversions are possible except that fatty acids cannot contribute to glucose synthesis (note one-way RED arrow).

REGULATION OF ENERGY METABOLISM

Under normal conditions, electron transfer and subsequent energy release tightly couple to ADP phosphorylation. In general, without the availability of ADP for phosphorylation to ATP, electrons do not shuttle down the respiratory chain to oxygen. Compounds that either inhibit or activate enzymes at key control points in the oxidative pathways modulate regulatory control of glycolysis and the citric acid cycle.[1,11] Each pathway has at least one enzyme considered "rate-limiting" because it controls the speed of that pathway's reactions. By far, cellular ADP concentration exerts the greatest effect on the rate-limiting enzymes that control the energy metabolism of carbohydrates, fats, and proteins. This mechanism for respiratory control makes sense because any increase in ADP signals a need for energy to restore ATP levels. Conversely, high levels of cellular ATP indicate a relatively low energy requirement. From a broader perspective,

ADP concentrations function as a cellular feedback mechanism to maintain a relatively constant level (homeostasis) of energy currency available for biologic work. Other rate-limiting modulators include cellular levels of phosphate, cyclic AMP, calcium, NAD^+, and citrate and pH.

Summary

1. Food macronutrients provide the major sources of potential energy to rejoin ADP and phosphate ion to form ATP.

2. The complete breakdown of 1 mole of glucose liberates 689 kcal of energy. Of this, ATP bonds conserve about 263 kcal (38%), with the remainder dissipated as heat.

3. During glycolytic reactions in the cell's cytosol, a net of two ATP molecules forms during anaerobic substrate-level phosphorylation.

4. Pyruvate converts to acetyl-CoA during the second stage of carbohydrate breakdown within the mitochondrion. Acetyl-CoA then progresses through the citric acid cycle.

5. Hydrogen atoms released during glucose breakdown oxidize via the respiratory chain; the energy generated couples to ADP phosphorylation.

6. The complete oxidation of a glucose molecule in skeletal muscle theoretically yields a net total of 36 ATP molecules.

7. A biochemical "steady state" or "steady rate" exists when hydrogen atoms oxidize at their rate of formation.

8. During intense exercise, when hydrogen oxidation does not keep pace with its production, lactate forms as pyruvate temporarily binds hydrogen. This allows progression of anaerobic glycolysis for an additional time period.

9. The complete breakdown of a triacylglycerol molecule yields about 460 molecules of ATP. Fatty acid catabolism requires oxygen; the term *aerobic* describes such reactions.

10. Protein serves as a potentially important energy substrate. After nitrogen removal from the amino acid molecule during deamination, the remaining carbon skeletons enter various metabolic pathways to produce ATP aerobically.

11. Numerous interconversions take place among the food nutrients. Fatty acids represent a noteworthy exception, as they cannot be synthesized to glucose.

12. Fats require a certain level of carbohydrate breakdown for their continual catabolism for energy in the metabolic mill. To this extent, "fats burn in a carbohydrate flame."

13. Compounds that either inhibit or activate enzymes at key control points in the oxidative pathways modulate control of glycolysis and the citric acid cycle. Cellular ADP concentration exerts the greatest effect on the rate-limiting enzymes that control energy metabolism.

TEST YOUR KNOWLEDGE ANSWERS

1. True Carbohydrates provide energy (4 kcal per g) for the body to resynthesize ATP. They convert to glycogen in glycogenesis for storage in muscle and liver. Once the glycogen reserves become filled, any excess energy from carbohydrate readily converts to stored body fat, primarily in adipose tissue.

2. False Lipids provide energy (9 kcal per g) for ATP resynthesis. They store as fat in adipose tissue for future energy needs. Fatty acids cannot contribute to glucose formation because of the unavailability of the enzyme to convert acetyl-CoA (from fatty acid breakdown) to pyruvate for glucose synthesis.

3. False An enzyme is a highly specific and large organic protein catalyst that accelerates the rate of chemical reactions without being consumed or changed in the reactions.

4. False As in the case of carbohydrates and lipids, excess energy from dietary protein readily converts to fat for storage in adipose tissue. Thus, high-protein diets, if they constitute excess caloric intake, result in positive energy balance and a gain in body fat.

5. False The catabolism of all three macronutrients, carbohydrates, lipids, and proteins, results in ATP formation. On a relative basis, fat and carbohydrate provide their carbon skeletons for ATP synthesis more readily than protein, which primarily serves an anabolic role.

6. False The first law of thermodynamics states that energy is neither created nor destroyed but instead transforms from one form to another without being used up. In essence, the law dictates that the body does not produce, consume, or use up energy; it merely transforms energy from one form into another as physiologic systems undergo continual change.

7. False Oxidation reactions transfer oxygen atoms, hydrogen atoms, or electrons. A loss of electrons occurs in oxidation reactions with a corresponding gain in valence. Reduction reactions involve any process in which atoms gain electrons with a corresponding decrease in valence. Oxidation and reduction reactions always couple, so that the energy released by one reaction becomes incorporated into the products of the other reaction.

8. True The term *energy* suggests a dynamic state related to change; thus energy emerges only when a change occurs. Potential energy and kinetic energy constitute the total energy of a system. Potential energy refers to energy associated with a substance's structure or position, while kinetic energy refers to energy of motion. Potential energy can be measured when it transforms to kinetic energy. There are six forms of energy—chemical, mechanical, heat, light, electric, and nuclear—and each can convert or transform to another form.

9. False In essence, cellular oxidation–reduction constitutes the biochemical mechanism that underlies energy metabolism. The mitochondria, the cell's "energy factories," contain carrier molecules that remove electrons from hydrogen (oxidation) and eventually pass them to oxygen (reduction). ATP synthesis occurs during oxidation–reduction reactions. Aerobic metabolism refers to energy-generating catabolic reactions in which oxygen serves as the final electron acceptor in the respiratory chain and combines with hydrogen to form water. In one sense, the term *aerobic* seems misleading because oxygen does not participate directly in ATP synthesis. On the other hand, oxygen's presence at the end of the line largely determines the capacity for ATP production.

10. True Thirty-eight ATP molecules represents the total (gross) ATP yield from the complete breakdown of a glucose molecule. Because 2 ATPs initially phosphorylate glucose, 36 ATP molecules equal the net ATP yield from glucose breakdown in skeletal muscle. Four ATP molecules form directly from substrate-level phosphorylation (glycolysis and citric acid cycle), whereas 32 ATP molecules regenerate during oxidative phosphorylation.

References

1. Balban RS. Regulation of oxidative phosphorylation in the mammalian cell. Am J Physiol 1990;258:C377.
2. Campbell MK. Biochemistry. Philadelphia, WB Saunders, 1991.
3. Carins SP, et al. Role of extracellular $[Ca^{2+}]$ in fatigue of isolated mammalian skeletal muscle. J Appl Physiol 1998;84:1395.
4. Chasiotis D. Role of cyclic AMP and inorganic phosphate in the regulation of muscle glycogenolysis during exercise. Med Sci Sports Exerc 1988;20:545.
5. Coppack SW, et al. In vivo regulation of lipolysis in humans. J Lipid Res 1994;35:177.
6. Febbario MA, et al. Effect of epinephrine on muscle glycogenolysis during exercise in trained men. J Appl Physiol 1998;84:465.
7. Fox SI. Human physiology. 7th ed. New York: McGraw-Hill, 2002.
8. Greenhaff PL, Timmons JA. Interaction between aerobic and anaerobic metabolism during intense muscle contraction. Exerc Sport Sci Rev 1998;26:1.

9. Hogan MC, et al. Increased [lactate] in working dog muscle reduces tension development independent of pH. Med Sci Sports Exerc 1995; 27:371.

10. Hultman E, et al. Energy metabolism and fatigue. In: Taylor AW, et al., eds. Biochemistry of exercise VII. Champaign, IL: Human Kinetics, 1990

11. Jacobs I, et al. Effects of prior exercise or ammonium chloride ingestion on muscular strength and endurance. Med Sci Sports Exerc 1993; 25:809.

12. Kiens B, et al. Skeletal muscle substrate utilization during submaximal exercise in man: effect of endurance training. J Physiol 1993; 469:459.

13. Mainwood GW, Renaud JM. The effect of acid-base on fatigue of skeletal muscle. Can J Physiol Pharmacol 1985;63:403.

14. Murray R, et al. Physiological responses to glycerol ingestion during exercise. J Appl Physiol 1991;71:144.

15. Nybo L. CNS fatigue and prolonged exercise: effect of glucose supplementation. Med Sci Sports Exerc 2003;35:589.

16. Richter EA. Interaction of fuels in muscle metabolism during exercise. In: Intergration of Medical and Sports Sciences. Basal: Karger, 1992.

17. Romijn JA, et al. Regulations of endogenous fat and carbohydrate metabolism in relation to exercise intensity and duration. Am J Physiol 1993;265:E380.

18. Sahlin K, Broberg S. Tricarboxylic acid cycle intermediates in human muscle during prolonged exercise. Am J Physiol 1990;259:C834.

19. Seip RL, Semenkovich CF. Skeletal muscle lipoprotein lipase: molecular regulation and physiological effects in relation to exercise. Exerc Sport Sci Rev 1998;26:191.

20. Shepherd RE, Bah MD. Cyclic AMP regulation of fuel metabolism during exercise: regulation of adipose tissue lipolysis during exercise. Med Sci Sports Exerc 1988;20:531.

21. Stefanick ML, Wood PD. Physical activity, lipid and lipoprotein metabolism, and lipid transport. In: Bouchard C, et al., eds. Physical activity, fitness, and health. Champaign, IL: Human Kinetics, 1994.

22. Stryer L. Biochemistry. 4th ed San Francisco: WH Freeman, 1995.

23. Sumida KD, Donovan CM. Enhanced hepatic gluconeogenic capacity for selected precursors after endurance training. J Appl Physiol 1995; 79:1883.

24. Sumida KD, et al. Enhanced gluconeogenesis from lactate in perfused livers after endurance training. J Appl Physiol 1993;74:782.

25. Thompson DL, et al. Substrate use during and following moderate- and low-intensity exercise: implications for weight control. Eur J Appl Physiol 1998;78:43.

26. Trump ME, et al. Importance of muscle phosphocreatine during intermittent maximal cycling. J Appl Physiol 1996;80:1574.

27. Turcoatte LP, et al. Impaired plasma FFA oxidation imposed by extreme CHO deficiency in contracting rat skeletal muscle. J Appl Physiol 1994;77:517.

28. Vusse van der GJ, et al. Lipid metabolism in muscle. Handbook of physiology, section 12: Exercise: regulation and integration of multiple systems. New York: Oxford Press, 1996.

General References

Bodner GM. Metabolism: Part I. Glycolysis, or the Embden-Meyerhof pathway. J Chem Educ 1986;63:566.

Bodner GM. The tricarboxylic acid (TA), citric acid, Krebs cycle. J Chem Educ 1986;63:673.

Brooks GA, et al. Exercise physiology: human bioenergetics and its applications. 3rd ed. Mountain View, CA: Mayfield, 2000.

Cerretelli P. Energy sources for muscular exercise. Int J Sports Med 1992; 13(suppl 1):S106.

Hargreaves M. Interactions between muscle glycogen and blood glucose during exercise. Exerc Sport Sci Rev 1997;25:21.

Marieb EN. Human anatomy and physiology. 3rd ed. Redwood City, CA: Benjamin Cummings, 1999.

Nelson DL, Cox MM. Lehninger's principles of biochemistry. 3rd ed. New York: Worth Publishers, 2000.

Nicklas BJ. Effects of endurance exercise on adipose tissue metabolism. Exerc Sport Sci Rev 1997;25:77.

Shils ME, et al. Modern nutrition in health and disease. 9th ed. Baltimore: Lippincott Williams & Wilkins, 1999.

Stryer L. Biochemistry. 4th ed. San Francisco: WH Freeman, 1995.

Vander AJ, et al. Human physiology: the mechanisms of body function. 7th ed. New York: McGraw-Hill, 1997.

Additional Readings

Christ-Roberts CY, et al. Exercise training increases glycogen synthase activity and GLUT4 expression but not insulin signaling in overweight nondiabetic and type 2 diabetic subjects. Metabolism 2004;53:1233.

Cox KL, et al. Independent and additive effects of energy restriction and exercise on glucose and insulin concentrations in sedentary overweight men. Am J Clin Nutr 2004;80:308.

de Glisezinski I, et al. Aerobic training improves exercise-induced lipolysis in SCAT and lipid utilization in overweight men. Am J Physiol Endocrinol Metab 2003;285:E984

Holmes AG, et al. Suppressing lipolysis increases interleukin-6 at rest and during prolonged moderate-intensity exercise in humans. J Appl Physiol 2004;97:689.

Jeukendrup AE. Modulation of carbohydrate and fat utilization by diet, exercise and environment. Biochem Soc Trans 2003;31:1270

Mittendorfer B, et al. Excess body fat in men decreases plasma fatty acid availability and oxidation during endurance exercise. Am J Physiol Endocrinol Metab 2004;286:E354.

Richterova B, et al. Effect of endurance training on adrenergic control of lipolysis in adipose tissue of obese women. J Clin Endocrinol Metab 2004;89:1325.

Roepstorff C, et al. Regulation of plasma long-chain fatty acid oxidation in relation to uptake in human skeletal muscle during exercise. Am J Physiol Endocrinol Metab 2004;287:E696.

Schmitt B, et al. Transcriptional adaptations of lipid metabolism in tibialis anterior muscle of endurance-trained athletes. Physiol Genomics 2003;15:148.

Watt MJ, et al. Reduced plasma FFA availability increases net triacylglycerol degradation, but not GPAT or HSL activity, in human skeletal muscle. Am J Physiol Endocrinol Metab 2004;287:E120.

Zderic TW, et al. Manipulation of dietary carbohydrate and muscle glycogen affects glucose uptake during exercise when fat oxidation is impaired by β-adrenergic blockade. Am J Physiol Endocrinol Metab 2004;287:E1195.

Zderic TW, et al. High-fat diet elevates resting intramuscular triglyceride concentration and whole body lipolysis during exercise. Am J Physiol Endocrinol Metab 2004;286:E217.

Chapter

5

Macronutrient Metabolism in Exercise and Training

TEST YOUR KNOWLEDGE

Answer these ten statements about micronutrient metabolism in exercise and training. Use the scoring key at the end of the chapter to check your results. Repeat this test after you have read the chapter and compare your results.

1. **T F** Anaerobic sources supply the predominant energy for short-term, powerful movement activities.

2. **T F** Lipid provides the primary energy macronutrient for ATP resynthesis during high-intensity aerobic exercise.

3. **T F** As blood flow increases with light and moderate exercise, more free fatty acids leave adipose tissue depots for delivery to active muscle.

4. **T F** Carbohydrate provides the preferential energy fuel during high-intensity anaerobic exercise.

5. **T F** Severely lowered liver and muscle glycogen levels during prolonged exercise induce fatigue, despite sufficient oxygen availability to muscles and an almost unlimited potential energy from stored fat

6. **T F** A diet low in lipid content reduces fatty acid availability, which negatively affects endurance capacity in high-intensity aerobic exercise.

7. **T F** A decrease in blood sugar during prolonged exercise concomitantly increases fat catabolism for energy.

8. **T F** Exercise training enhances the ability to oxidize carbohydrate but not fat during exercise.

9. **T F** Because protein provides the building block molecules for tissue synthesis, its catabolism occurs only minimally (2% of total energy) during exercise.

10. **T F** Consuming a high-fat diet in the 7- to 10-day period before a bout of heavy exercise significantly improves exercise performance.

Gas exchange in the lungs along with biochemical and biopsy techniques, magnetic resonance imaging, and labeled nutrient tracers provide insight into contributions of the stored macronutrients and high-energy phosphates to exercise bioenergetics. The needle biopsy technique, for example, samples small quantities of active muscle to assess intramuscular nutrient kinetics throughout exercise. Such data provide an objective basis for recommending meal plans during exercise training, and specific nutritional modifications prior to, during, and in recovery from strenuous competition. *The fuel mixture that powers exercise generally depends on the intensity and duration of effort, and the exerciser's fitness and nutritional status.*

THE ENERGY SPECTRUM OF EXERCISE

FIGURE 5.1 depicts the relative contributions of anaerobic and aerobic energy sources during various durations of maximal exercise. In addition, TABLE 5.1 lists the approximate percentage of total energy for adenosine triphosphate (ATP) resynthesis from each energy transfer system for different competition running events. The data represent estimates from all-out running experiments in the laboratory, but they can relate to other activities by drawing the appropriate time relationships. For example, a 100-m sprint run equates to any all-out activity lasting about 10 seconds, while an 800-m run lasts approximately 2 minutes. All-out exercise for 1 minute includes the 400-m dash in track, the 100-m swim, and multiple full-court presses at the end of a basketball game.

The sources for energy transfer exist along a continuum. At one extreme, intramuscular high-energy phosphates ATP and phosphocreatine (PCr) supply most energy for exercise. The ATP–PCr and lactic acid systems provide about one-half of the energy required for intense exercise lasting 2 minutes; aerobic reactions provide the remainder. For top performance in all-out 2-minute exercise, a person must possess a well-developed capacity for *both* aerobic and anaerobic metabolism. Intense exercise of intermediate duration performed for 5 to 10 minutes, like middle-distance running and swimming or basketball, requires a greater demand for aerobic energy transfer. Performances of longer duration—marathon running, distance swimming and cycling, recreational jogging, and hiking and backpacking—require a fairly steady energy supply derived aerobically without reliance on lactate formation.

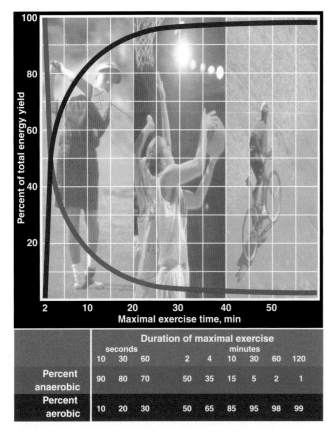

Duration of maximal exercise

	seconds			minutes					
	10	30	60	2	4	10	30	60	120
Percent anaerobic	90	80	70	50	35	15	5	2	1
Percent aerobic	10	20	30	50	65	85	95	98	99

▐ **Figure 5.1** Relative contributions of aerobic *(red)* and anaerobic *(blue)* energy metabolism during maximal physical effort of varying durations. Note that 2 minutes of maximal effort requires about 50% of the energy from both aerobic and anaerobic processes. At a world-class 4-minute per mile pace, approximately 65% of the energy comes from aerobic metabolism, with the remainder generated from anaerobic processes. For a marathon, on the other hand, the energy derived from aerobic processes almost totally powers the run.

Generally, anaerobic sources supply most of the energy for fast movements or during increased resistance to movement at a given speed. When movement begins at either fast or slow speed, the intramuscular high-energy phosphates provide immediate anaerobic energy for muscle action. After a few seconds, the glycolytic pathway (intramuscular glycogen breakdown in glycolysis) generates an increasingly greater proportion of energy for ATP resynthesis. Intense exercise continued beyond 30 seconds places a progressively greater demand on the relatively slower aerobic energy metabolism of the stored macronutrients. For example, power output during 30 seconds of maximal exercise (e.g., sprint cycling or running) is about twice the power output generated exercising all-out for 5 minutes at one's maximal oxygen uptake. Some activities rely predominantly on a single energy transfer system, whereas more than one energy system energizes most physical activities, depending on their intensity and duration. Higher-intensity and shorter-duration activities place greater demand on anaerobic energy transfer.

Two main macronutrient sources provide energy for ATP resynthesis during exercise: *(a)* liver and muscle glycogen and *(b)* triacylglycerols within adipose tissue and active muscle. To a lesser degree, amino acids within skeletal muscle donate carbon skeletons (minus nitrogen) to processes of energy metabolism. FIGURE 5.2 provides a generalized overview of the relative contribution to energy metabolism of carbohydrate, fat, and protein for adequately nourished individuals during rest and various exercise intensities. This illustration does not depict the significant alterations in metabolic mixture (increases in fat and protein breakdown) during prolonged, intense exercise with accompanying depletion of liver and muscle glycogen. The following sections discuss the specific energy contribution of each macronutrient during exercise and the adaptations in substrate use with training.

CARBOHYDRATE MOBILIZATION AND USE DURING EXERCISE

The liver markedly increases its release of glucose for use by active muscle as exercise progresses from low to high intensity.[11,53] Simultaneously, glycogen stored within muscle serves as the predominant carbohydrate energy source during the early stages of exercise and as exercise intensity increases.[22,41] Compared with fat and protein catabolism, carbohydrate remains the preferential fuel during high-intensity aerobic exercise because it rapidly supplies ATP during oxidative processes. In anaerobic effort (reactions of glycolysis), carbohydrate becomes the *sole* contributor of ATP.

Carbohydrate availability during exercise helps to regulate fat mobilization and its use for energy.[16,17] For example, increasing carbohydrate oxidation by ingesting rapidly

| Table 5.1 | AN ESTIMATE OF THE PERCENTAGE CONTRIBUTION OF DIFFERENT FUELS TO ATP GENERATION IN VARIOUS RUNNING EVENTS |

| | Percentage Contribution to ATP Generation | | | | |
| | | Glycogen | | | |
Event	Phosphocreatine	Anaerobic	Aerobic	Blood Glucose (Liver Glycogen)	Triacylglycerol (Fatty Acids)
100 m	50	50	—	—	—
200 m	25	65	10	—	—
400 m	12.5	62.5	25	—	—
800 m	6	50	44	—	—
1500 m	[a]	25	75	—	—
5000 m	[a]	12.5	87.5	—	—
10,000 m	[a]	3	97	—	—
Marathon	—	—	75	5	20
Ultramarathon (80 km)	—	—	35	5	60
24-h race	—	—	10	2	88

From Newsholme EA, et al. Physical and mental fatigue. Br Med Bull 1999;48:477.
[a]In such events, phosphocreatine will be used for the first few seconds and, if it has been resynthesized during the race, in the sprint to the finish.

absorbed (high-glycemic) carbohydrates prior to exercise (with associated hyperglycemia and hyperinsulinemia) significantly blunts long-chain fatty acid oxidation by skeletal muscle and free fatty acid liberation from adipose tissue during exercise. Perhaps increased carbohydrate availability (and resulting increased catabolism) inhibits long-chain fatty acid transport into the mitochondria, thus controlling the metabolic mixture in exercise. It also appears that the concentration of blood glucose provides feedback regulation of the liver's glucose output; an increase in blood glucose inhibits hepatic glucose release during exercise.[26]

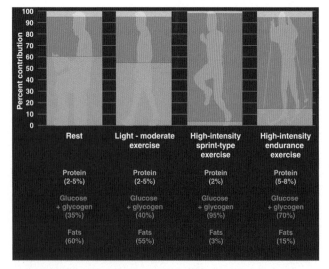

■ **Figure 5.2** Generalized illustration of the contribution of the carbohydrate (blue), fat (pink), and protein (yellow) macronutrients to energy metabolism or rest and during various intensities of exercise.

Intense Exercise

With strenuous exercise, neural–humoral factors increase hormonal output of epinephrine, norepinephrine, and glucagon and decrease insulin release. These actions stimulate **glycogen phosphorylase** to augment glycogen breakdown (glycogenolysis) in the liver and active muscles. In the early minutes of exercise when oxygen use fails to meet energy demands, stored muscle glycogen becomes the primary energy contributor because it provides energy without oxygen. As exercise duration progresses, blood-borne glucose from the liver increases its contribution as a metabolic fuel. Blood glucose, for example, can supply 30% of the total energy required by active muscle, with *most* of the remaining carbohydrate energy supplied by intramuscular glycogen.[18,44] *Carbohydrate availability in the metabolic mixture controls its use. In turn, carbohydrate intake dramatically affects its availability.*

One hour of high-intensity exercise decreases liver glycogen by about 55%, and a 2-hour strenuous workout just about depletes glycogen in the liver and specifically exercised muscles. FIGURE 5.3 illustrates that muscle uptake of circulating blood glucose increases sharply during the initial stage of exercise and continues to increase as exercise progresses. By the 40-minute mark, glucose uptake rises to between 7 and 20 times the resting uptake, depending on exercise intensity. Carbohydrate breakdown predominates when oxygen supply and/or use do not meet a muscle's needs, as in heavy anaerobic exercise. *During high-intensity aerobic exercise, the advantage of selective dependence on carbohydrate metabolism lies in its two times more rapid energy transfer compared with fat or protein.* Furthermore, compared with fat, carbohydrate generates about 6% more energy per unit of oxygen consumed.

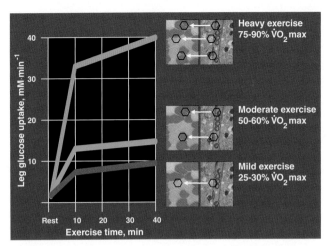

Figure 5.3 Exercise duration and intensity affect blood glucose uptake by the leg muscles. Exercise intensity is expressed as a percentage of an individual's VO₂max. (From Felig P, Wahren J. Fuel homeostasis in exercise. N Engl J Med 1975;293:1078.)

Moderate and Prolonged Exercise

Glycogen stored in active muscle supplies almost all of the energy in the transition from rest to moderate exercise, just as it does in intense exercise. During the next 20 minutes or so of exercise, liver and muscle glycogen supply between 40 and 50% of the energy requirement; the remainder is pro-

vided by fat breakdown (intramuscular triacylglycerols, including a small use of protein. (The nutrient energy mixture depends on the relative intensity of submaximal exercise. In light exercise fat remains the main energy substrate [see Fig. 5.9]). As exercise continues and muscle glycogen stores diminish, blood glucose from the liver becomes the major supplier of carbohydrate energy. Still, fat provides an increasingly larger percentage of the total energy metabolism. Eventually, plasma glucose concentration decreases because the liver's glucose output fails to keep pace with its use by muscles. During 90 minutes of strenuous exercise, blood glucose may actually decrease to **hypoglycemic levels** (less than 45 mg of glucose per 100 mL [dL] blood).[19]

FIGURE 5.4 depicts the metabolic profile during prolonged exercise in the glycogen-depleted and glycogen-loaded states. With glycogen depletion, blood glucose levels fall as submaximal exercise progresses. Concurrently, the level of fatty acids circulating in the blood increases dramatically compared with the same exercise with adequate glycogen reserves. Protein also provides an increased contribution to the energy pool. With carbohydrate depletion, exercise capacity (expressed as a percentage of maximum) progressively decreases after 2 hours to about 50% of the starting exercise intensity. The reduced power output level comes directly from the relatively slow rate of aerobic energy release from fat oxidation, which now becomes the primary energy source.[23,49]

Figure 5.4 Dynamics of nutrient metabolism in the glycogen-loaded and glycogen-depleted states. During exercise with limited carbohydrate (CHO) availability, blood glucose levels *(A)* progressively decrease, while fat metabolism *(B)* progressively increases compared with similar exercise when glycogen loaded. In addition, protein use for energy *(C)*, as indicated by plasma levels of 3-OH butyrate, remains considerably higher with glycogen depletion. After 2 hours, exercise capacity *(D)* decreases to about 50% of maximum in exercise begun in the glycogen-depleted state. (From Wagenmakers AJM, et al. Carbohydrate supplementation, glycogen depletion, and amino acid metabolism. Am J Physiol 1991;260:E883.)

Carbohydrate and fat breakdown use identical pathways for acetyl-CoA oxidation. Thus, metabolic processes that precede the citric acid cycle (e.g., β-oxidation, fatty acid activation, and intracellular and mitochondrial transport) most likely account for the relatively slow rate of fat versus carbohydrate oxidation. FIGURE 5.5 lists these possible rate-limiting factors.

Nutrient-Related Fatigue

Severely lowered levels of liver and muscle glycogen during exercise induce fatigue, despite sufficient oxygen availability to muscles and almost unlimited potential energy from stored fat. Endurance athletes commonly refer to this extreme sensation of fatigue as "bonking" or "hitting the wall." The image of hitting the wall suggests an inability to continue exercising, which in reality is not the case, although pain becomes apparent in the active muscles and exercise intensity decreases markedly. Because of the absence of the phosphatase enzyme in skeletal muscle (which releases glucose from liver cells), the relatively inactive muscles retain all of their glycogen. Controversy exists about why carbohydrate depletion during prolonged exercise coincides with reduced exercise capacity. Part of the answer relates to three factors:

1. Use of blood glucose as energy for the central nervous system
2. Muscle glycogen's role as a "primer" in fat metabolism
3. Slower rate of energy release from fat catabolism than from carbohydrate breakdown

Regular Exercise Improves Capacity for Carbohydrate Metabolism

Aerobically trained muscle exhibits a greater capacity to oxidize carbohydrate than untrained muscle. Consequently, considerable amounts of pyruvate move through the aerobic energy pathways during intense endurance exercise following training.[21] A trained muscle's augmented mitochondrial oxidative capacity and increased glycogen storage helps to explain its enhanced capacity for carbohydrate breakdown. During submaximal exercise, the endurance-trained muscle exhibits *decreased* reliance on muscle glycogen and blood glucose as fuel sources and greater fat use. This training adaptation represents a desirable response because it conserves the body's limited glycogen reserves.

Gender Differences in Substrate Use During Exercise

Available data support the notion of significant gender differences in carbohydrate metabolism in exercise. During submaximal exercise at equivalent percentages of $\dot{V}O_2$max (i.e., same relative workload), women derive a *smaller* proportion of total energy from carbohydrate oxidation than men.[27] This gender difference in substrate oxidation does not persist into recovery.[25]

Gender Differences in Training Effects on Substrate Use

With similar endurance-training protocols, both women and men show a significant decrease in glucose flux for a given submaximal power output.[12,20] But at the same relative work-

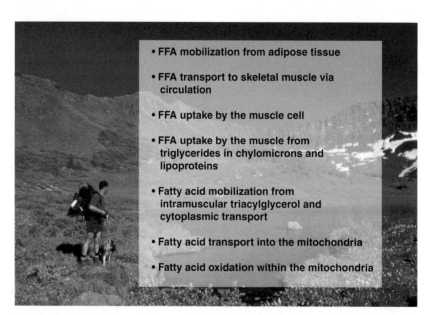

■ **Figure 5.5** Processes that potentially limit the magnitude of fat oxidation during aerobic exercise. FFA, free fatty acid.

load after training, women display an exaggerated shift toward fat catabolism, whereas men do not.[28] This suggests that endurance training induces greater glycogen-sparing at a given relative submaximal exercise intensity for women than for men. This gender difference in substrate metabolism's response to training may reflect differences in sympathetic nervous system adaptation to regular exercise (i.e., a more-blunted catecholamine response for women). The sex hormones estrogen and progesterone may affect metabolic mixture indirectly via interactions with the catecholamines or directly by augmenting lipolysis and/or constraining glycolysis.[5] Five potential sites for endocrine regulation of substrate use include

1. Substrate availability (via effects on nutrient storage)
2. Substrate mobilization from body tissue stores
3. Substrate uptake at tissue site of use
4. Substrate uptake within tissue itself
5. Substrate trafficking among storage, oxidation, and/or recycling

Any glycogen-sparing metabolic adaptations to training could benefit a woman's performance during high-intensity endurance competition.

CASE STUDY/PERSONAL HEALTH AND EXERCISE NUTRITION 5–1

Know What You Eat: Benefits of Phytochemicals

Background

Based on years of research in the field of nutrition, current consensus suggests that an optimum diet should

1. Supply an individual's needs for energy (calories) and macronutrients and micronutrients
2. Support health and promote successful aging
3. Provide pleasure, both individual and social, and reinforce personal and cultural identity

Within this framework, the following represent five major characteristics of an optimum diet that most scientists from diverse disciplines would agree with:

1. Contain foods of sufficient variety from all the major food groups
2. Contain as much fresh food as possible
3. Contain as few processed foods as possible
4. Contain an abundance of fruits and vegetables
5. Contain foods that provide health benefits (functional foods) beyond basic nutrition

Foods that provide health benefits beyond basic nutrition have been termed *functional foods* (see Case Study 6.1, p. 172). Beneficial substances in these foods include both *zoochemicals* (health- promoting compounds from the animal kingdom) and *phytochemicals* (health-promoting compounds from the plant kingdom). Much research has focused on phytochemicals because of their protective role in fighting chronic disease. Foods such as garlic, soybeans, cruciferous vegetables, legumes, onions, citrus fruits, tomatoes, whole grains, and diverse herbs and spices are excellent sources of chemoprotective phytochemicals. Specific phytochemicals with health benefits include allium compounds, isoflavones, saponins, indoles, isothiocyanates, dithiolthione, ellagic acid, polyacetylenes, flavonoids, carotenoids, phytates, lignins, glucarates, phthalides, and terpenoids.

Know Your Phytochemicals

Many different plants contain healthful phytochemicals. For example, carotenoids, polyphenols, and saponins exert strong antioxidant effects; sulfides and isothiocyanates stimulate enzymes that deactivate carcinogens; phytosterols and saponins alter the harmful effects of excess cholesterol; phytoestrogens possess a chemical structure similar to that of hormones and act by blocking deleterious effects of excessive hormone production. The accompanying table lists the more important phytochemicals, their biologic activity, and food sources.

KNOW YOUR PHYTOCHEMICALS

Phytochemical	*Activity and Effects*	*Food Sources*
Carotenoids (α-carotene, β-carotene, β-cryptoxanthin, luten, lycopene, zeaxanthin)	Vitamin-A precursors; antioxidants; increase cell-to-cell communication; decrease risk of macular degeneration	Yellow-orange fruits and vegetable (e.g., apricots, carrots, cantaloupe, broccoli, tomatoes, sweet potatoes); leafy greens such as spinach; dairy products, eggs, and margarine
Flavonoids (quercetin, kaempferol, myricetin), flavones (apigenin), flavonols (catechins)	Decrease capillary fragility and permeability; block carcinogens and slow growth of cancer cells	Fruits, vegetables, berries, citrus fruits, onions, purple grapes, tea, red wine
Phytoestrogens (isoflavones—genistein, biochanin A, daidzein, and lignins)	Metabolized to estrogen-like compounds in the GI tract; induce cancer cell death (apoptosis); slow cancer cell growth; reduce risk of breast, ovarian, colon, and prostate cancer; inhibit cholesterol synthesis; may reduce risk of osteoporosis	Isoflavones in soybeans and soy products; lignins in flax, rye, some berries, and some vegetables
Phytosterols (β-sitosterol, stigmasterol, campesterol)	Decrease cholesterol absorption; inhibit proliferation of colonic cells	Vegetable oils, nuts, seeds, cereals, legumes
Saponins (soyasaponins, soyasapogenols)	Bind bile acids and cholesterol in the GI tract to reduce absorption; toxic to tumor cells; antioxidant effects	Soybeans, modified margarines
Glucosinolates (glucobrassicin, isothiocyanates [sulphorophane], indoles [indole-3-carbinol])	Increase enzyme activity that deactivates carcinogens; favorably alter estrogen metabolism; affect regulation of gene expression	Cruciferous vegetables (broccoli, Brussels sprouts, cabbage), horseradish, mustard greens
Sulfides and **thiols** (dithiolthiones and allium compounds like diallyl sulfides, allyl methyl trisulfides)	Increase activity of enzymes that deactivate carcinogens; decrease conversion of nitrates to nitrites in intestines; may lower cholesterol, prevent blood clotting, and normalize blood pressure	Sulfides in onions, garlic, leeks, scallions; dithiolthiones in cruciferous vegetables
Inositol phosphates (phytate, inositol, pentaphosphate)	Bind metal ions and prevent them from generating free radicals; protect against cancer	Cereals, soybeans, soy-based foods, cereal grains, nuts, and seeds (especially abundant in sesame seeds and soybeans)
Phenolic acids (caffeic and ferulic acids, ellagic acid)	Anticancer properties; prevent formation of stomach carcinogens	Blueberries, cherries, apples, oranges, pears, potatoes
Protease inhibitors	Bind to trypsin and chymotrypsin; decrease cancer cell growth and inhibit malignant changes in cells; inhibit hormone binding; may aid DNA repair to slow cancer cell division; prevent tumors from releasing proteases that destroy neighboring cells	Soybeans; other legumes, cereals, vegetables
Tannins	Antioxidant effects; may inhibit activation of carcinogens and slow cancer promotion	Grapes, tea, lentils, red and white wine, black-eyed peas
Capsaicin	Modulates blood clotting	Hot peppers
Coumarin (phenolic)	Promotes enzyme function to protect against cancer	Citrus fruits
Curcumin (phenolic)	Inhibits enzymes that activate carcinogens; antiinflammatory and antioxidant properties	Turmeric, mustard
Monoterpene (limonene)	Triggers enzyme production to detoxify carcinogens; inhibits cancer promotion and cell proliferation; favorably affects blood clotting and cholesterol levels	Citrus fruit peels and oils, garlic

From Grosvenor MB, Smolin LA. Nutrition. From science to life. Philadelphia: Harcourt College Publishers, 2002.

Effect of Diet on Glycogen Stores and Endurance Capacity

We emphasized above that active muscle relies on ingested carbohydrate as a readily available energy nutrient. Diet composition profoundly affects glycogen reserves. FIGURE 5.6 shows the results from a classic experiment in which dietary manipulation varied muscle glycogen concentration. In one condition, caloric intake remained normal in six subjects for 3 days when lipid supplied most ingested calories (less than 5% as carbohydrate). In the second condition, the 3-day diet contained the recommended daily percentages of carbohydrate, lipid, and protein. With the third diet, carbohydrates supplied 82% of the calories. The needle biopsy technique determined glycogen content of the quadriceps femoris muscle; it averaged 0.63 g of glycogen per 100 g wet muscle with the high-fat diet, 1.75 g for the normal diet, and 3.75 g for the high-carbohydrate diet.

Endurance capacity during cycling exercise varied considerably depending upon each person's diet for the 3 days prior to the exercise test. With the normal diet, exercise lasted an average of 114 minutes, but only 57 minutes with the high-fat diet. Endurance capacity of subjects fed the high-carbohydrate diet averaged more than three times greater than that with the high-fat diet. In all instances, the point of fatigue coincided with the same low level of muscle glycogen. This clearly demonstrated the importance of muscle glycogen to maintain high-intensity exercise lasting more than 1 hour. These results emphasize the important role that diet plays in establishing appropriate energy reserves for long-term exercise and strenuous training.

A carbohydrate-deficient diet rapidly depletes muscle and liver glycogen; it subsequently affects performance in all-out short-term (anaerobic) exercise and in prolonged high-intensity endurance (aerobic) activities. These observations pertain to both athletes and physically active individuals who modify their diets by reducing carbohydrate intake below recommended levels (see Chapter 1). Reliance on starvation diets or potentially harmful low-carbohydrate, high-fat diets or low-carbohydrate, high-protein diets remains counterproductive for weight control, exercise performance, optimal nutrition, and good health. A low-carbohydrate diet makes it extremely difficult from the standpoint of energy supply to engage in vigorous physical activity.[2,15] Because of carbohydrate's important role in central nervous system function and neuromuscular coordination, training and competing under conditions of low glycogen reserves also increases the likelihood of injury. More is said in Chapter 8 concerning optimizing carbohydrate availability prior to, during, and in recovery from intense exercise training and competition.

■ **Figure 5.6** Effects of a low-carbohydrate (CHO) diet, mixed diet, and high-CHO diet on glycogen content of the quadriceps femoris muscle and duration of endurance exercise on a bicycle ergometer. With a high-CHO diet, endurance time increases 3 times more than with a low-CHO diet. (Adapted from Bergstrom J, et al. Diet, muscle glycogen and physical performance. Acta Physiol Scand 1967;71:140.)

FAT MOBILIZATION AND USE DURING EXERCISE

Depending on nutritional and fitness status of the individual and the exercise intensity and duration, fat supplies between 30 and 80% of the exercise energy requirement.[3,36,45,52] Three lipid sources supply the major energy for light-to-moderate exercise:

1. Fatty acids released from the triacylglycerol storage sites in adipocytes and delivered relatively slowly to muscles as free fatty acids (FFAs) bound to plasma albumin

2. Circulating plasma triacylglycerol bound to lipoproteins as very-low-density lipoproteins and chylomicrons
3. Triacylglycerol within the active muscle itself

Fat use for energy in light and moderate exercise varies closely with blood flow through adipose tissue (a threefold increase is not uncommon) and through active muscle. Adipose tissue releases more FFAs to active muscle as blood flow increases with exercise. Hence, somewhat greater quantities of fat from adipose tissue depots participate in energy metabolism. The energy contribution from intramuscular triacylglycerol ranges between 15 and 35%, with endurance-trained men and women using the highest percentage.[33,36]

Initiation of exercise produces a transient initial drop in plasma FFA concentration from the increased uptake by active muscles and the time lag in the release and delivery from adipocytes. Subsequently, increased FFA release from adipose tissue (and concomitant suppression of triacylglycerol formation) occurs through hormonal–enzymatic stimulation by sympathetic nervous system activation and decreased insulin levels. Subcutaneous abdominal adipocytes represent a particularly lively area for lipolysis compared with fat cells in the gluteal–femoral region. When exercise transitions to a high intensity, FFA release from adipose tissue fails to increase much above resting levels, which eventually produces a decrease in plasma FFAs. This, in turn, increases muscle glycogen usage, with a concurrent large increase in intramuscular triacylglycerol oxidation (see Fig. 5.9).[42]

On a relative basis, considerable fatty acid oxidation occurs during low-intensity exercise. For example, fat combustion almost totally powers light exercise at 25% of aerobic capacity. Carbohydrate and fat combustion contribute energy equally during moderate exercise. Fat oxidation gradually increases as exercise extends to an hour or more and glycogen depletes. Toward the end of prolonged exercise (with glycogen reserves low), circulating FFAs supply nearly 80% of the total energy required. FIGURE 5.7 shows this phenomenon for a subject who exercised continuously for 6 hours. A steady decline occurred in carbohydrate combustion (reflected by the respiratory quotient [RQ]; see Chapter 6) during exercise with an accompanying increase in fat combustion. Toward the end of exercise, 84% of the total energy for exercise came from fat breakdown! This experiment, conducted more than 70 years ago, illustrates fat oxidation's important contribution in prolonged exercise with glycogen depletion.

The hormones epinephrine, norepinephrine, glucagon, and growth hormone activate lipase. This causes lipolysis and mobilization of FFAs from adipose tissue. Exercise increases plasma levels of lipogenic hormones, so the active muscles receive a continual supply of energy-rich fatty acid substrate. Increased activity of skeletal muscle and adipose tissue lipases, including biochemical and vascular adaptations within the muscle, help to explain the training-induced enhanced use of fats for energy during moderate-intensity exercise.[13,14,30,46]

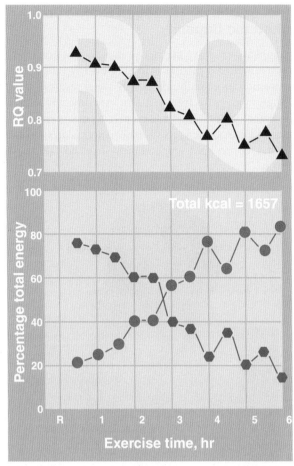

■ **Figure 5.7** *Top:* Reduction in respiratory quotient *(RQ)* at an oxygen uptake of 2.36 L · min⁻¹ during 6 hours of continuous exercise. *Bottom:* Percentage of energy derived from carbohydrate (CHO) *(purple)* and fat *(orange)* (1 kcal = 4.2 kJ). (Modified from Edwards HT, et al. Metabolic rate, blood sugar and utilization of carbohydrate. Am J Physiol 1934;108:203.)

Augmented fat metabolism in prolonged exercise probably results from a small drop in blood sugar, accompanied by a decrease in insulin (a potent inhibitor of lipolysis) and increased glucagon output by the pancreas as exercise progresses. These changes ultimately reduce glucose metabolism to further stimulate FFA liberation for energy. FIGURE 5.8 shows that FFA uptake by working muscle rises during 1 to 4 hours of moderate exercise. In the first hour fat supplies about 50% of the energy, while in the third hour, fat contributes up to 70% of the total energy requirement. *With carbohydrate depletion, exercise intensity decreases to a level governed by the body's ability to mobilize and oxidize fat.* Interestingly, prior exercise also partitions the trafficking of dietary fat fed in recovery toward a direction that favors its oxidation rather than storage.[48] This may partly explain the protection against weight gain offered by regular physical activity.[32,51]

Consuming a high-fat diet for a protracted period produces enzymatic adaptations that enhance capacity for fat

Figure 5.8 Uptake of oxygen and nutrients by the legs during prolonged exercise. *Green* and *yellow* areas represent the proportion of total oxygen uptake caused by oxidation of free fatty acids (FFAs) and blood glucose oxidation, respectively. *Orange* areas indicate the oxidation of non-blood-borne fuels (muscle glycogen and intramuscular fat and proteins). (From Ahlborg G, et al. Substrate turnover during prolonged exercise in man. J Clin Invest 1974;53:1080.)

oxidation during exercise.[34,38] We discuss the effectiveness of this dietary manipulation to improve endurance performance in Chapter 8.

Exercise Intensity Makes a Difference

The contribution of fat to the metabolic mixture in exercise differs depending on exercise intensity. For moderately trained subjects, the exercise intensity that maximizes fat burning ranges between 55 and 72% of $\dot{V}O_2max$.[1] FIGURE 5.9 illustrates the dynamics of fat use by trained men who cycled at 25 to 85% of their aerobic capacity. During light-to-mild exercise (40% of maximum or less), fat provided the main energy source, predominantly as plasma FFAs from

adipose tissue depots. Increasing exercise intensity produced an eventual *crossover* in the balance of fuel use. The total energy from fat breakdown (from all sources) remained essentially unchanged, while blood glucose and muscle glycogen supplied the added energy for more intense exercise. Total energy from fats during exercise at 85% of maximum and exercise at 25% of maximum did not differ. *Such data highlight the important role that carbohydrate, particularly muscle glycogen, plays as the major fuel source during high-intensity aerobic exercise.*

Nutritional Status Plays a Role

The dynamics of fat breakdown or its synthesis depend on availability of the "building block" fatty acid molecules. After a meal, when energy metabolism is low, digestive processes increase FFA and triacylglycerol delivery to cells. Increased fat delivery, in turn, promotes triacylglycerol synthesis through esterification. In contrast, with moderate exercise, increased use of fatty acids for energy reduces their concentration in the active cells, thus stimulating triacylglycerol breakdown into its glycerol and fatty acid components. Concurrently, hormonal release in exercise stimulates adipose tissue lipolysis, which further augments FFA delivery to

Figure 5.9 Steady-state substrate use calculated using three isotopes and indirect calorimetry in trained men performing cycle ergometer exercise at 25, 65, and 85% of $\dot{V}O_2max$. As exercise intensity increases, absolute use of glucose and muscle glycogen increases, while muscle triacylglycerol and plasma free fatty acid (FFA) use decreases. (From Romijn JA, et al. Regulation of endogenous fat and carbohydrate metabolism in relation to exercise intensity and duration. Am J Physiol 1993;265:E380.)

active muscle. Long-duration exercise in the fasted state places heavy demands on FFA use as an energy substrate.[35]

Exercise Training and Fat Metabolism

Regular aerobic exercise profoundly improves ability to oxidize long-chain fatty acids, particularly from triacylglycerol stored within active muscle, during mild- to moderate-intensity exercise.[29,31,37,39] FIGURE 5.10 shows the significant increase in fat catabolism during submaximal exercise following aerobic training, with a corresponding decrease in carbohydrate breakdown. *Adaptations in the responsiveness of adipocytes to lipolysis allow the trained person to exercise at a higher absolute level of submaximal exercise before experiencing the fatiguing effects of glycogen depletion.* However, even for endurance athletes, the improved capacity for fat oxidation cannot sustain the level of aerobic metabolism generated when oxidizing glycogen for energy. Consequently, well-nourished endurance athletes rely almost totally on oxidation of stored glycogen in near-maximal, sustained aerobic effort.

FIGURE 5.11 displays the contribution of various energy substrates to exercise metabolism of trained and untrained limb muscles. The important point concerns the greater uptake of FFAs (and concurrent conservation of limited glycogen reserves) by the trained limb during moderate exercise through six mechanisms shown in the shaded box below.

PROTEIN USE DURING EXERCISE

Nutritionists and exercise physiologists have long maintained that the protein RDA represents a liberal "margin of safety" to account for amino acids catabolized during exercise and amino acids required for protein synthesis following exercise. For the past 100 years, three reasons stand out as to why protein constitutes a limited fuel in exercise:

1. Protein's primary role provides amino-acid building blocks for tissue synthesis
2. Early studies show only minimal protein breakdown during endurance exercise as reflected by urinary nitrogen excretion
3. Theoretical computations and experimental evidence of protein requirements for muscle tissue synthesis with resistance training

More recent research on protein balance in exercise presents a compelling argument that protein serves as energy fuel to a much greater extent than previously believed, depending on energy expenditure and nutritional status.[4,10,40,47,50] *This applies primarily to the branched-chain amino acids (for the way the side chain branches from the molecule's amine core) leucine, valine, and isoleucine oxidized in skeletal muscle rather than in the liver.* As was shown in Figure 5.4, endurance exercise in a carbohydrate-

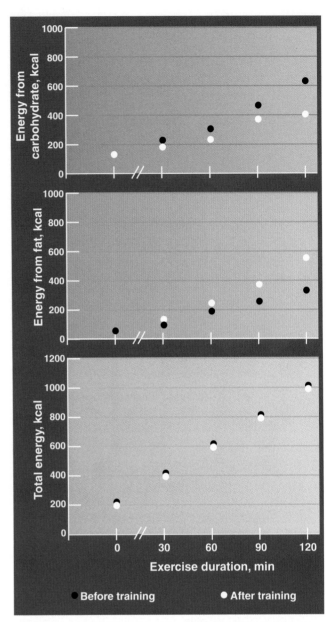

■ **Figure 5.10** Training enhances catabolism of fat. During constant-load prolonged exercise, energy from fat oxidation significantly increases following aerobic training, while corresponding decreases occur in carbohydrate breakdown. Carbohydrate-sparing adaptations can occur in two ways: *(a)* release of fatty acids from adipose tissue depots (augmented by a reduced level of blood lactate) and *(b)* greater intramuscular fat stores in the endurance-trained muscle. (From Hurley BF, et al. Muscle triglyceride utilization during exercise: effect of training. J Appl Physiol 1986;5:62.)

depleted state caused significantly more protein catabolism than protein breakdown with ample carbohydrate reserves. Also, if energy intake does not match energy expenditure in intense training even *twice* the protein RDA intake may not maintain nitrogen balance. Thus, dieting could negatively affect training regimens geared to increase muscle mass or maintain muscular strength and power.

FAT-BURNING ADAPTATIONS WITH AEROBIC TRAINING

- Facilitated rate of lipolysis and reesterfication within adipocytes
- Proliferation of capillaries in trained muscle to create a greater total number and density of these microvessels
- Improved transport of FFAs through the plasma membrane (sarcolemma) of the muscle fiber
- Augmented transport of fatty acids within the muscle cell by the action of carnitine and carnitine acyl transferase
- Increased size and number of muscle mitochondria
- Increased quantity of enzymes involved in β-oxidation, citric acid cycle metabolism, and the electron-transport chain within specifically trained muscle fibers

Figure 5.12 Protein synthesis stimulation during recovery from aerobic exercise. Values refer to differences between the exercise group and the control group who received the same diet for each time interval. (From Carraro F, et al. Whole body and plasma protein synthesis in exercise and recovery in human subjects. Am J Physiol 1990;258:E821.)

While protein breakdown generally increases only modestly with exercise, muscle protein synthesis rises markedly following both endurance and resistance-type exercise. FIGURE 5.12 shows that the rate of muscle protein synthesis (determined from labeled leucine incorporation into muscle) increased between 10 and 80% in the 4 hours following aerobic exercise. It then remained elevated for at least 24 hours.[9] Thus, two factors justify reexamining protein intake recommendations for those involved in exercise training: *(a)* increased protein breakdown during long-term exercise and heavy training and *(b)* increased protein synthesis in recovery from exercise. Chapter 7 further discusses the adequacy of the protein RDA for those who undertake heavy training.

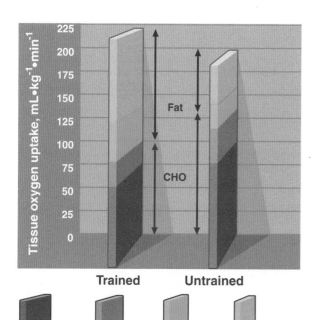

Figure 5.11 Estimated contribution of various substrates to energy metabolism in trained and untrained limb muscles. CHO, carbohydrate; FFA, free fatty acid. (From Saltin B, Åstrand P-O. Free fatty acids and exercise. Am J Clin Nutr 1993;57(suppl):752S.)

Summary

1. The major pathway for ATP production differs depending on exercise intensity and duration.

2. For all-out, short-duration efforts (100-m dash, lifting heavy weights), the intramuscular stores of ATP and PCr (immediate energy system) provide the required energy for exercise.

3. For intense exercise of longer duration (1–2 min), the anaerobic reactions of glycolysis (short-term energy system) provide the energy.

4. When exercise progresses beyond several minutes, the aerobic system predominates with oxygen uptake capacity becoming the important factor (long-term energy system).

5. Muscle glycogen and blood glucose serve as primary fuels during intense anaerobic exercise beyond 10-seconds duration. Glycogen stores also play an important energy metabolism role in sustained high levels of aerobic exercise such as marathon running, distance cycling, and endurance swimming.

6. Trained muscle exhibits an augmented capacity to catabolize carbohydrate aerobically for energy because of increased oxidative capacity of the mitochondria and increased glycogen storage.

7. Women derive a smaller proportion of the total energy from carbohydrate oxidation than do men during submaximal exercise at equivalent percentages of aerobic capacity. Following aerobic exercise training, women show a more exaggerated shift toward fat catabolism than men.

8. A carbohydrate-deficient diet rapidly depletes muscle and liver glycogen and profoundly affects both anaerobic capacity and prolonged, high-intensity aerobic physical effort.

9. Fat contributes about 50% of the energy requirement during light and moderate exercise. The role of stored fat (intramuscular and derived from adipocytes) becomes even more important at the latter stages of prolonged exercise. In this situation, the fatty acid molecules (mainly as circulating FFAs) provide more than 80% of the exercise energy requirements.

10. With carbohydrate depletion, exercise intensity decreases to a level determined by how well the body mobilizes and oxidizes fat.

11. Aerobic training increases long-chain fatty acid oxidation, particularly the fatty acids derived from triacylglycerols within active muscle during mild- to moderate-intensity exercise.

12. Enhanced fat oxidation spares glycogen, permitting trained individuals to exercise at a higher absolute level of submaximal exercise before experiencing the fatiguing effects of glycogen depletion.

13. A high-fat diet stimulates adaptations that augment fat use, yet reliable research has not yet demonstrated consistent exercise or training benefits from such dietary modifications.

14. Protein serves as an energy fuel to a much greater extent than previously thought, depending on nutritional status and the intensity of exercise training or competition. This applies particularly to branched-chain amino acids that oxidize within skeletal muscle rather than within the liver.

15. Reexamining the current protein RDA seems justified for those who engage in heavy exercise training. One must account for increased protein breakdown during exercise and the augmented protein synthesis in recovery.

TEST YOUR KNOWLEDGE **ANSWERS**

1. True Anaerobic sources supply most of the energy for fast, powerful movements, or during increased resistance to movement at a given speed. When movement begins at either fast or slow speed, the intramuscular high-energy phosphates (ATP and PCr) provide immediate anaerobic energy for muscle action. After a few seconds, the glycolytic pathway (intramuscular glycogen breakdown via glycolysis) generates an increasingly greater proportion of energy for ATP resynthesis.

2. False Liver and muscle glycogen provide the main macronutrient energy sources for ATP resynthesis during high-intensity aerobic exercise. The liver markedly increases its release of glucose as exercise progresses from low to high intensity. Concurrently, glycogen stored within the active muscles serves as the predominant energy source during the early stages of exercise and in high-intensity aerobic exercise. Compared with fat and protein catabolism, carbohydrate remains the preferential fuel during intense aerobic exercise because it more rapidly supplies ATP in oxidative processes. More specifically, dependence on carbohydrate during high-intensity aerobic exercise lies in its two-times more rapid rate of energy transfer than with fat and protein. Furthermore, carbohydrate generates about 6% more energy per unit oxygen consumed than fat.

3. True Depending on nutritional and fitness status of the individual and exercise intensity and duration, fat supplies between 30 and 80% of the exercise energy requirement. Fat use in light and moderate exercise varies closely with blood flow through adipose tissue and blood flow through active muscle. Adipose tissue releases more free fatty acids for delivery to active muscle as blood flow increases with exercise. Hence, somewhat greater quantities of fat from adipose tissue depots participate in energy metabolism.

4. True In predominantly anaerobic effort, carbohydrate becomes the sole macronutrient contributor of energy for ATP resynthesis. Carbohydrate breakdown in glycolysis provides the only available means for rapid anaerobic energy. This anaerobic energy is unavailable via the breakdown of fatty acids and amino acids, which provide energy only through aerobic metabolism.

5. True Controversy exists as to why carbohydrate depletion during prolonged exercise coincides with a reduced exercise capacity, commonly termed "bonking" or "hitting the wall." Part of the answer relates to the use of blood glucose as energy for the central nervous system, muscle glycogen's role as a "primer" in fat metabolism, and the slower rate of energy release from fat than from carbohydrate breakdown. In essence, with carbohydrate depletion, exercise intensity decreases to a level governed by the body's ability to mobilize and oxidize fat.

6. False A carbohydrate-deficient diet, not a diet deficient in fat, rapidly depletes muscle and liver glycogen This diet subsequently impairs performance in all-out short-term (anaerobic) exercise and in prolonged high-intensity endurance (aerobic) activities. These observations pertain to both athletes and physically active individuals who modify their diets by reducing carbohydrate intake below recommended levels.

7. True   Carbohydrate availability during exercise helps to regulate fat mobilization and its use for energy. Augmented fat metabolism in prolonged exercise probably results from a small drop in blood sugar, accompanied by a decrease in insulin (a potent inhibitor of lipolysis) and increased glucagon output by the pancreas as exercise progresses. These changes ultimately reduce glucose metabolism to further stimulate FFA liberation for energy. Toward the end of prolonged exercise (with glycogen reserves low), circulating FFAs supply nearly 80% of the total energy requirement.

8. False   Regular aerobic exercise profoundly improves the ability to oxidize long-chain fatty acids, particularly from triacylglycerol stored within active muscle, during mild- to moderate-intensity exercise. These adaptations allow the trained person to exercise at a higher absolute level of submaximal exercise before experiencing the fatiguing effects of glycogen depletion. Even for endurance athletes, however, improved capacity for fat oxidation cannot sustain the high level of aerobic metabolism generated when oxidizing glycogen for energy.

9. False   Protein serves as an energy fuel to a much greater extent than previously thought, depending on nutritional status and exercise intensity. This applies particularly to branched-chain amino acids that oxidize within skeletal muscle rather than within the liver. The use of protein for energy most frequently occurs in a glycogen-depleted state as amino acids donate their carbon skeletons for the synthesis of glucose by the liver.

10. False   Individuals consuming a high-carbohydrate diet perform significantly better after 7 weeks of training than individuals consuming a high-fat diet. While a high-fat diet stimulates adaptive responses that augment fat use, reliable research has yet to demonstrate consistent exercise or training benefits from such dietary modifications. Furthermore, one should carefully consider recommending a diet consisting of up to 60% total calories from lipid in terms of detrimental health risks, particularly those associated with cardiovascular disease.

References

1. Achten J, et al. Determination of the exercise intensity that elicits maximal fat oxidation. Med Sci Sports Exerc 2002;34:92.
2. Ball D, et al. The acute reversal of diet-induced metabolic acidosis does not restore endurance capacity during high-intensity exercise in man. Eur J Appl Physiol 1996;73:105.
3. Bergman BC, Brooks GA. Respiratory gas-exchange ratios during graded exercise in fed and fasted trained and untrained men. J Appl Physiol 1999;86:479.
4. Bowtell JL, et al. Modulation of whole body protein metabolism, during and after exercise, by variation of dietary protein. J Appl Physiol 1998;85:1744
5. Braun B, Horton T. Endocrine regulation of exercise substrate utilization in women compared to men. Exerc Sport Sci Rev 2001;29:149.
6. Deleted.
7. Deleted.
8. Deleted.
9. Carraro F, et al. Effect of exercise and recovery on muscle protein synthesis in human subjects. Am J Physiol 1990;259:E470.
10. Carraro F, et al. Alanine kinetics in humans during low-intensity exercise. Med Sci Sports Exerc 1994;26:48.
11. Coggan AR. Plasma glucose metabolism during exercise: effect of endurance training in humans. Med Sci Sports Exerc 1997;29:620,
12. Coggan AR, et al. Endurance training increases plasma glucose turnover and oxidation during moderate-intensity exercise in men. J Appl Physiol 1990;68:990.
13. Coggan AR, et al. Plasma glucose kinetics in subjects with high and low lactate thresholds. J Appl Physiol 1992;73:1873.
14. Coggan AR, et al. Isotopic estimation of CO_2 production before and after endurance training. J Appl Physiol 1993;75:70.
15. Costill DL, et al. Effects of repeated days of intensified training on muscle glycogen and swimming performance. Med Sci Sports Exerc 1988;20:249.
16. Coyle EF, et al. Fatty acid oxidation is directly regulated by carbohydrate metabolism during exercise. Am J Physiol 1997;273(Endocrinol Metab 36):E268.
17. De Glisezinski I, et al. Effects of carbohydrate ingestion of adipose tissue lipolysis during long-lasting exercise in trained men. J Appl Physiol 1998;84:1627.
18. Felig P, Wahren J. Fuel homeostasis in exercise. N Engl J Med 1975; 293:1078.
19. Felig P, et al. Hypoglycemia during prolonged exercise in normal men. N Engl J Med 1982;306:895.
20. Friellander AL, et al. Training induced alterations in carbohydrate metabolism in women: women respond differently than men. J Appl Physiol 1998;85:1175.
21. Fujimoto T, et al. Skeletal muscle glucose uptake response to exercise in trained and untrained men. Med Sci Sports Exerc 2003; 35:777.
22. Hargreaves M. Interactions between muscle glycogen and blood glucose during exercise. Exerc Sport Sci Rev 1997;25:21.
23. Hawley JA. Effect of increased fat availability on metabolism and exercise capacity. Med Sci Sports Exerc 2002;34:1485.
24. Deleted.
25. Horton TJ, et al. Fuel metabolism in men and women during and after long-duration exercise. J Appl Physiol 1998;85:1823.
26. Howlett K, et al. Effect of increased blood glucose availability on glucose kinetics during exercise. J Appl Physiol 1998;84:1423.
27. Jansson E. Sex differences in metabolic response to exercise. In: Saltin B, ed. Biochemistry of exercise, VI. Champaign, IL: Human Kinetics, 1986.
28. Jansson E, Kaijser L. Substrate utilization and enzymes in skeletal muscle of extremely endurance-trained men. J Appl Physiol 1987;62:999.
29. Jeukendrup AE, et al. Exogenous glucose oxidation during exercise in endurance-trained and untrained subjects. J Appl Physiol 1997;83:835.
30. Kiens B, et al. Skeletal muscle substrate utilization during submaximal exercise in man: effects of endurance training. J Physiol 1993; 469:459.
31. Kiens B. Effect of endurance training on fatty acid metabolism: local adaptations. Med Sci Sports Exerc 1997;29:640.
32. King G, et al. Relationship of leisure-time physical activity and occupational activity to the prevalence of obesity. Int J Obes 2001;25: 606.
33. Klein S, et al. Fat metabolism during low intensity exercise in endurance-trained and untrained men. Am J Physiol 1993;267:E708.
34. Lambert EV, et al. Enhanced endurance in trained cyclists during moderate intensity exercise following a 2 week adaptation to a high fat diet. Eur J Appl Physiol 1994;69:26.
35. Martin WH. Effect of acute and chronic exercise on fat metabolism. Exerc Sport Sci Rev 1996;24:203.
36. Martin WH III. Effect of endurance training on fatty acid metabolism during whole body exercise. Med Sci Spots Exerc 1997;29:635.
37. Martin WH III, et al. Effect of endurance training on plasma free fatty acid turnover and oxidation during exercise. Am J Physiol 1993;265: E708.
38. Mudio DM. Effect of dietary fat on metabolic adjustments to maximal VO_2 and endurance in runners. Med Sci Sports Exerc 1994;26:81.
39. Nicklas BJ. Effects of endurance exercise on adipose tissue metabolism. Exerc Sport Sci Revs 1997;25:77.
40. Rennie MJ, et al. Physical activity and protein metabolism. In: Bouchard C, et al., eds. Physical activity, fitness, and health. Champaign, IL: Human Kinetics, 1994.

41. Romijn JA, et al. Regulation of endogenous fat and carbohydrate metabolism in relation to exercise intensity and duration. Am J Physiol 1993;265:E380.
42. Romijn JA, et al. Relationship between fatty acid delivery and fatty acid oxidation during strenuous exercise. J Appl Physiol 1995;79: 1939.
43. Deleted.
44. Sherman WM. Metabolism of sugars and physical performance. Am J Clin Nutr 1995;62(suppl):228S.
45. Spirit LL. Regulation of skeletal muscle fat oxidation during exercise in humans. Med Sci Sports Exerc 2002;34:1477.
46. Stallknecht B, et al. Effect of training on epinephrine-stimulated lipolysis determined by microdialysis in human adipose tissue. Am J Physiol 1995;265:E1059.
47. Tarnopolosky MA, et al. Effect of bodybuilding exercise on protein requirements. Can J Sport Sci 1990;15:225.
48. Deleted.
49. Vusse, van der GJ, et al. Lipid metabolism in muscle. Handbook of physiology, section 12: Exercise: regulation and integration of multiple systems. New York: Oxford Press,1996.
50. Wagenmakers AJM. Muscle amino acid metabolism at rest and during exercise: role in human physiology and metabolism. Exerc Sport Sci Rev 1998;26:287.
51. Wier L, et al. Determining the amount of physical activity needed for long-term weight control. Int J Obes 2001;25:613.
52. Winder WW. Malonyl-CoA—Regulator of fatty acid oxidation in muscle during exercise. Exerc Sport Sci Rev 1998;26:117.
53. Wolfe R.R, et al. Role of changes in insulin and glucagon in glucose homeostasis in exercise. J Clin Invest 1986;77:900.

Additional Readings

Achten J, Jeukendrup AE. Optimizing fat oxidation through exercise and diet. Nutrition 2004;20:716.

Barnett C, et al. Muscle metabolism during sprint exercise in man: Influence of sprint training. J Sci Med Sport 2004;7:314.

Bishop D, et al. Induced metabolic alkalosis affects muscle metabolism and repeated-sprint ability. Med Sci Sports Exerc 2004;36:807.

De Feo P, et al. Metabolic response to exercise. J Endocrinol Invest 2003;26:851.

Dietrich Mde O, et al. Serum S100B protein: What does it mean during exercise? Clin J Sport Med 2004;14:368.

Duffield R, et al. Energy system contribution to 100-m and 200-m track running events. J Sci Med Sport 2004;7:302.

Fischer CP, et al. Endurance training reduces the contraction-induced interleukin-6 mRNA expression in human skeletal muscle. Am J Physiol Endocrinol Metab 2004;287:E1189.

LeBlanc PJ, et al. Effects of aerobic training on pyruvate dehydrogenase and pyruvate dehydrogenase kinase in human skeletal muscle. J Physiol 2004;1;559.

Peters SJ, Leblanc PJ. Metabolic aspects of low carbohydrate diets and exercise. Nutr Metab (Lond) 2004;1:7.

Pilegaard H, et al. Transcriptional regulation of pyruvate dehydrogenase kinase 4 in skeletal muscle during and after exercise. Proc Nutr Soc 2004;63:221.

Trappe TA, et al. Human soleus muscle protein synthesis following resistance exercise. Acta Physiol Scand 2004;182:189.

van Loon LJ. Use of intramuscular triacylglycerol as a substrate source during exercise in humans. J Appl Physiol 2004;97:1170.

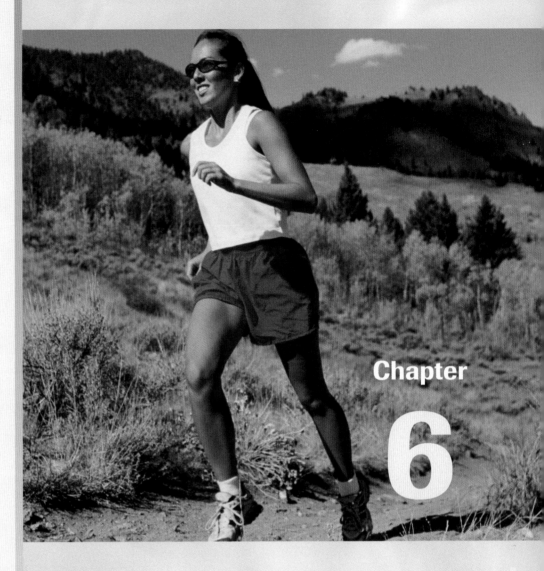

Chapter

6

Measurement of Energy in Food and During Physical Activity

All biologic functions require energy. Because the carbohydrate, lipid, and protein macronutrients contain the energy that ultimately powers biologic work, this makes energy the common denominator for classifying both food and physical activity.

➤ Measurement of Food Energy

THE CALORIE—A UNIT OF ENERGY MEASUREMENT

In nutritional terms, one calorie expresses the quantity of heat necessary to raise the temperature of 1 kg (1 L) of water 1°C (specifically, from 14.5 to 15.5°C). Thus, **kilogram calorie** or kilocalorie (**kcal**) more accurately defines calorie.

(Note the use of the letter k to designate a kilocalorie, as compared to a small calorie (c) that indicates the quantity of heat necessary to raise the temperature of 1 g of water 1°C.) For example, if a particular food contains 300 kcal, then releasing the potential energy trapped within this food's chemical structure increases the temperature of 300 L of water 1°C.

Different foods contain different amounts of potential energy. One-half cup of peanut butter with a caloric value of 759 kcal contains the equivalent heat energy to increase the temperature of 759 L of water 1°C. A corresponding unit of heat using Fahrenheit degrees is the British thermal unit or BTU. One BTU represents the quantity of heat necessary to raise the temperature of one pound (weight) of water 1°F from 63 to 64°F. A clear distinction exists between temperature and heat. Temperature reflects a quantitative measure of an object's hotness or coldness. Heat describes energy transfer (exchange) from one body or system to another. The following conversions apply:

1 cal = 4.186 J
1 kcal = 1000 cal = 4186 J = 4.184 kJ
1 BTU = 778 ft lb = 252 cal = 1055 J

The joule, or **kilojoule (kJ)**, reflects the standard international unit (SI unit) for expressing energy. To convert kilocalories to kilojoules, multiply the kilocalorie value by 4.184. The kilojoule value for 1/2 cup of peanut butter, for example, would equal 759 kcal × 4.184, or 3176 kJ. The **megajoule (MJ)** equals 1000 kJ; its use avoids unmanageably large numbers. The name joule honors British scientist Sir Prescott Joule (1818–1889) who studied how vigorous stirring of a paddle wheel warmed water. Joule determined that the movement of the paddle wheel added energy to the water, raising the water temperature in direct proportion to the work done.

GROSS ENERGY VALUE OF FOODS

Laboratories use **bomb calorimeters** similar to the one illustrated in FIGURE 6.1 to measure the total energy value of the various food macronutrients. Bomb calorimeters operate on the principle of **direct calorimetry**, measuring the heat liberated as the food burns completely.

Figure 6.1 shows food within a sealed chamber charged with oxygen at high pressure. An electrical current moving through the fuse at the tip ignites the food–oxygen mixture. As the food burns, a water jacket surrounding the bomb absorbs the heat (energy) liberated. Because the calorimeter is fully insulated from the outside environment, the increase in water temperature *directly* reflects the heat released during a food's oxidation (burning).

Heat of combustion refers to the heat liberated by oxidizing a specific food; it represents the food's total energy value. For example, a teaspoon of margarine releases 100 kcal of heat energy when burned completely in a bomb calorimeter. This equals the energy required to raise 1.0 kg (2.2 lb) ice water to its boiling point. The oxidation pathways of food in the intact organism and the bomb calorimeter differ, but the energy liberated in the complete breakdown of a food remains the same, regardless of the combustion pathways.

■ **Figure 6.1** A bomb calorimeter directly measures the energy value of food.

Carbohydrates

The heat of combustion for carbohydrate varies depending on the arrangement of atoms in the particular carbohydrate molecule. For glucose, heat of combustion equals 3.74 kcal per gram, about 12% less than for glycogen (4.19 kcal) and starch (4.20 kcal). *For 1 g of carbohydrate, a value of 4.2 kcal generally represents the average heat of combustion.*

Lipids

The heat of combustion for lipid varies with the structural composition of the triacylglycerol molecule's fatty acid components. For example, 1 g of either beef or pork fat yields 9.50 kcal, whereas oxidizing 1 g of butterfat liberates 9.27 kcal. The average energy value for 1 g of lipid in meat, fish, and eggs equals 9.50 kcal. In dairy products, the energy equivalent amounts to 9.25 kcal per gram, and 9.30 kcal in vegetables and fruits. *The average heat of combustion for lipid equals 9.4 kcal per gram.*

Proteins

Two factors affect energy release from protein combustion: *(a)* type of protein in the food and *(b)* relative nitrogen content of the protein. Common proteins in eggs, meat, corn (maize), and beans (jack, Lima, navy, soy) contain approximately 16% nitrogen, and have a corresponding heat of combustion that averages 5.75 kcal per gram. Proteins in other foods have a somewhat higher nitrogen content; most nuts and seeds contain 18.9% nitrogen, and whole-kernel wheat, rye, millets, and barley, 17.2%. Other foods contain a slightly lower nitrogen percentage, for example, whole milk has 15.7% and bran, 15.8%. *The heat of combustion for protein averages 5.65 kcal per gram.*

Comparing Macronutrient Energy Values

The average heats of combustion for the three macronutrients (carbohydrate, 4.2 kcal·g^{-1}; lipid, 9.4 kcal·g^{-1}; protein, 5.65 kcal·g^{-1}) demonstrates that the complete oxidation of lipid in the bomb calorimeter liberates about 65% more energy per gram than protein oxidation, and 120% more energy than carbohydrate oxidation. Recall from Chapter 1 that a lipid molecule contains more hydrogen atoms than either carbohydrate or protein molecules. The common fatty acid palmitic acid, for example, has the structural formula $C_{16}H_{32}O_2$. The ratio of hydrogen atoms to oxygen atoms in fatty acids always greatly exceeds the 2:1 ratio in carbohydrates. Simply stated, lipid molecules have more hydrogen atoms available for cleavage and subsequent oxidation for energy than carbohydrates and proteins.

One can conclude from the above discussion that lipid-rich foods have a higher energy content than foods relatively fat free. One cup of whole milk contains 160 kcal, whereas the same quantity of skimmed milk contains only 90 kcal. If a person who normally consumes 1 quart of whole milk each day switches to skimmed milk, the total calories ingested each year would decrease by the equivalent calories in 25 pounds of body fat. In 3 years, all other things remaining constant, body fat loss would approximate 75 pounds! Such a theoretical comparison merits serious consideration because of the almost identical nutritional composition between whole milk and skimmed milk except for fat content. Drinking an 8-oz glass of skimmed milk rather than whole milk also significantly reduces saturated fatty acid intake (0.4 vs. 5.1 g) and cholesterol (0.3 vs. 33 mg).

NET ENERGY VALUE OF FOODS

Differences exist in the energy value of foods when comparing the heat of combustion determined by direct calorimetry (**gross energy value**) to the **net energy value** actually available to the body. This pertains particularly to proteins, because the body cannot oxidize the nitrogen component of this nutrient. Rather, nitrogen atoms combine with hydrogen to form urea (NH_2CONH_2) for excretion in the urine. Elimination of hydrogen in this manner represents a loss of approximately 19% of the protein molecule's potential energy. This hydrogen loss reduces protein's heat of combustion in

the body to approximately 4.6 kcal per gram instead of 5.65 kcal per gram released during oxidation in the bomb calorimeter. In contrast, *identical* physiologic fuel values exist for carbohydrates and lipids (which contain no nitrogen) compared with their respective heats of combustion in the bomb calorimeter.

Coefficient of Digestibility

The efficiency of the digestive process influences the ultimate caloric yield from macronutrients. Numerically defined as the **coefficient of digestibility**, digestive efficiency represents the percentage of ingested food digested and absorbed to serve the body's metabolic needs. The food remaining unabsorbed in the intestinal tract becomes voided in the feces. Dietary fiber reduces the coefficient of digestibility: A high-fiber meal has less total energy absorbed than does a fiber-free meal of equivalent caloric content. This difference occurs because fiber moves food more rapidly through the intestine, reducing absorption time. Fiber also may cause mechanical erosion of the intestinal mucosa, which then becomes resynthesized through energy-requiring processes.

Table 6.1 shows different digestibility coefficients, heats of combustion, and net energy values for nutrients in the various food groups. *The relative percentage of macronutrients completely digested and absorbed averages 97% for carbohydrate, 95% for lipid, and 92% for protein.* Little difference exists in digestive efficiency between obese and lean individuals. However, considerable variability exists in efficiency percentages for any food within a particular category. Proteins in particular have variable digestive efficiencies, ranging from a low of about 78% for high-fiber legumes to a high of 97% for protein from animal sources. Some advocates promote the use of vegetables in weight loss diets because of plant protein's relatively low coefficient of digestibility. Those on a vegetarian-type diet should consume adequate and diverse protein food sources to obtain all essential amino acids (see Chapter 1).

From the data in Table 6.1, the average net energy values can be rounded to simple whole numbers referred to as **Atwater general factors** (http://www.sportsci.org/news/history/atwater/atwater.html).

These values, named for Wilbur Olin Atwater (1844–1907), the 19th century chemist who pioneered human nutrition and energy balance studies, represent the energy available to the body from ingested foods. Except when requiring exact energy values for experimental or therapeutic diets, the Atwater general factors accurately estimate the *net metabolizable energy* of typically consumed foods. For alcohol, 7 kcal (29.4 kJ) represents each g (mL) of pure (200-proof) alcohol ingested. In terms of metabolizable energy available to the body, alcohol's efficiency of use equals that of other carbohydrates.[15]

Table 6.1   **FACTORS FOR DIGESTIBILITY, HEATS OF COMBUSTION, AND NET PHYSIOLOGIC ENERGY VALUES[a] OF DIETARY PROTEIN, LIPID, AND CARBOHYDRATE**

Food Group	Digestibility (%)	Heat of Combustion (kcal·g^{-1})	Net Energy (kcal·g^{-1})
Protein			
Meats, fish	97	5.65	4.27
Eggs	97	5.75	4.37
Dairy products	97	5.65	4.27
Animal food (Average)	97	5.65	4.27
Cereals	85	5.80	3.87
Legumes	78	5.70	3.47
Vegetables	83	5.00	3.11
Fruits	85	5.20	3.36
Vegetable food (Average)	85	5.65	3.74
Total protein	**92**	**5.65**	**4.05**
Lipid			
Meat and eggs	95	9.50	9.03
Dairy products	95	9.25	8.79
Animal food	95	9.40	8.93
Vegetable food	90	9.30	8.37
Total lipid	**95**	**9.40**	**8.93**
Carbohydrate			
Animal food	98	3.90	3.82
Cereals	98	4.20	3.11
Legumes	97	4.20	4.07
Vegetables	95	4.20	3.99
Fruits	90	4.00	3.60
Sugars	98	3.95	3.87
Vegetable food	97	4.15	4.03
Total carbohydrate	**97**	**4.15**	**4.03**

From Merrill AL, Watt BK. Energy values of foods: basis and derivation. Agricultural handbook no. 74, Washington, DC: U.S. Department of Agriculture, 1973.
[a] Net physiologic energy values computed as the coefficient of digestibility times the heat of combustion adjusted for energy loss in urine.

ATWATER GENERAL FACTORS

- 4 kcal per gram for carbohydrate
- 9 kcal per gram for lipid
- 4 kcal per gram for protein

ENERGY VALUE OF A MEAL

The Atwater general factors can determine the caloric content of any portion of food (or an entire meal) from the food's composition and weight. TABLE 6.2 illustrates the method for calculating the kcal value of 100 g (3.5 oz) of chocolate-chip ice cream. Based on laboratory analysis, this ice cream contains approximately 3% protein, 18% lipid, and 23% carbohydrate, with the remaining 56% being essentially water. Thus, each gram of ice cream contains 0.03 g protein, 0.18 g lipid, and 0.23 g carbohydrate. Using these compositional values and the Atwater factors, the following represents the kcal value per gram of the chocolate-chip ice cream: Net kcal values show that 0.03 g of protein contains 0.12 kcal (0.03 × 4.0 kcal·g^{-1}), 0.18 g lipid contains 1.62 kcal (0.18 × 9 kcal·g^{-1}), and 0.23 g carbohydrate contains 0.92 kcal (0.23 × 4.0 kcal·g^{-1}). Combining the separate values for the nutrients yields a total energy value for each gram of chocolate-chip ice cream of 2.66 kcal (0.12 + 1.62 + 0.92). A 100-g serving yields a caloric value 100 times as large or 266 kcal. The percentage of total calories derived from lipid equals

CASE STUDY/PERSONAL HEALTH AND EXERCISE NUTRITION 6–1

How to Identify Functional Foods

Proper evaluation of foods no longer entails analysis of its macronutrient (carbohydrate, fat, protein) or micronutrient (vitamin, mineral) content. Other substances such as phytochemicals (plant chemicals) have been identified in a variety of fruits, vegetables, grains, legumes, nuts, seeds, herbs, spices, and teas. To date over 4000 phytochemicals have been identified, and about 150 have been studied in detail. These phytochemicals not only protect the plant itself from solar radiation or insect invasion, but consumption of these food chemicals by humans exerts beneficial effects. Such active food components are also found in animal sources (zoochemicals) like the omega-3 fatty acids in some cold-water fish, which reduce the risk of heart disease.

WHAT ARE FUNCTIONAL FOODS?

While there is no accepted definition of functional foods, and they remain undefined under current U.S. food regulations, they are generally viewed as any food or food ingredient that provides a potential health benefit beyond the traditional nutrients found in foods (e.g., protein, lipid, carbohydrate, vitamins, minerals, calories).

Unmodified whole food such as fruits and vegetables represent the simplest functional food. Foods fortified with nutrients or enhanced with phytochemicals or zoochemicals are referred to as "modified" functional foods.

U.S. REGULATION OF FUNCTIONAL FOODS

Regulation of functional foods remains confusing because they can be placed into a number of existing categories, including *conventional foods, food additives, dietary supplements, medical foods,* and foods for *special dietary use.* The category to define a specific functional food or component depends on how the manufacturer positions and markets the product. The most common approach to labeling and marketing uses the Food and Drug Administration (FDA)-approved health claims represented by law under the Nutrition Labeling and Education Act of 1990 (Table 1). The health claims authorized under this law describe a relationship between a food substance and a disease or other health-related condition (risk-reduction relationship). Some functional foods are classified as dietary supplements and therefore do not require FDA approval.

LEVELS OF INTAKE AND HEALTH BENEFITS

Only a few functional foods have established levels of intake. Table 2 presents a partial list of approximate intake levels for selected functional foods or food components that promote optimal health.

Table 1   FUNCTIONAL FOODS APPROVED BY THE FOOD AND DRUG ADMINISTRATION

Functional Food	Key Component	Functional Health Benefits	Scientific Evidence
Low-fat foods as part of a low-fat diet (e.g., cheese, snack foods, meats, fish dairy)	Low in total fat or saturated fat	Reduce cancer and CHD risk	Clinical trials
Foods containing sugar alcohols in place of sugar (gum, sugar candies, beverages, snack foods)	Sugar alcohols	Reduce tooth decay risk	Clinical trials
Oatmeal/oat bran/whole oat products	Beta glucan soluble fiber	Reduce cholesterol	Clinical trials
Milk, low fat	Calcium	Reduce osteoporosis risk	Clinical trials
Vegetables and fruits	Vitamins, phytochemicals, fiber	Reduce cancer and CHD risk	Epidemiologic studies/animal studies
Cereal with added folic acid	Folic acid	Reduce neural tube defect risk	Clinical trials
Juice, pasta, rice, snack bars, other high-calcium foods	Calcium	Reduce osteoporosis risk	Clinical trials
Modified margarine products	Plant sterols, plant stanol esters	Reduce CHD risk	Clinical trials
Soy	Soy protein	Support normal, healthy cholesterol levels	Clinical trials
Psyllium-containing foods (e.g., pasta, bread, snack foods)	Psyllium fiber	Reduce CHD risk	Clinical trials

From Position of the American Dietetic Association, functional foods. J Am Diet Assoc 1999;99:1278.

CASE STUDY/PERSONAL HEALTH AND EXERCISE NUTRITION 6–1 *(continued)*

Table 2   APPROXIMATE INTAKE LEVELS FOR SELECTED FUNCTIONAL FOODS AND THEIR EFFECTS

Food/Food Component	Level of Intake	Disease Association
Green or black tea	4–6 cups/day	Reduced risk for gastric and esophageal cancer
Soy protein	25 g (1 oz)/day	Reduced low-density-lipoprotein cholesterol, improved overall cholesterol profile
	60 g (2 oz)/day	Reduced menopausal symptoms
Garlic	600–900 mg/day (a fresh clove/day)	Reduced menopausal symptoms
Vegetables and fruits	5–9 servings/day	Reduced risk for cancer (colon, breast, prostate) reduced blood pressure
Fructo-oligosaccharides (FOS) (carbohydrate substitute used to add texture to foods, found in Jerusalem artichokes, shallots, onion powder)	3–10 g (1/10–1/3 oz)/day	Reduced blood pressure and serum cholesterol; beneficial effect on lipid metabolism; improved gastrointestinal health
Fish rich in n-3 fatty acids	>180 g (6 oz)/week	Reduced risk for heart disease
Grape juice	8–16 oz/day	Platelet aggregation reduction
Red wine	8 oz/day	Platelet aggregation reduction

From: Position of The American Dietetic Association, functional foods. J Am Diet Assoc 1999;99:1278.

60.9% (162-lipid kcal ÷ 266 total kcal). Similar computations estimate the caloric value for any food serving. Of course, increasing or decreasing portion sizes (or adding lipid-rich sauces or creams, or using fruits or calorie-free substitutes) affects caloric content accordingly.

Computing the caloric value of foods is time-consuming and laborious. Various governmental agencies in the Unites States and elsewhere have evaluated and compiled nutritive values for thousands of foods. The most comprehensive data bank resources include the U.S. Nutrient Data Bank (US-NDB) maintained by the U.S. Department of Agriculture's (USDA) Consumer Nutrition Center,[10] and a computerized data bank maintained by the Bureau of Nutritional Sciences of Health and Welfare Canada.[8] Many commercial software programs make use of the original USDA nutritional databases, which are available for download to the public for a nominal fee. (The USDA Nutrient Database for Standard Reference Release 11 can be viewed or downloaded from http://www.nal.usda.gov/fnic/foodcomp/Data/SR11/sr11.html; access the Nutrient Data Laboratory at http://

| Table 6.2 | **METHOD FOR CALCULATING THE CALORIC VALUE OF A FOOD FROM ITS COMPOSITION OF MACRONUTRIENTS** |

Food: *ice cream (chocolate with chocolate chips)*
Weight: *3/4 cup = 100 g*

	Composition		
	Protein	*Lipid*	*Carbohydrate*
Percentage	3%	18%	23%
Total grams	3	18	23
In 1 g	0.03	0.18	0.23
Calories per gram	0.12	1.62	0.92

$(0.04 \times 4.0 \text{ kcal}) + (0.18 \times 9.0 \text{ kcal}) + (0.23 \times 4.0 \text{ kcal})$

Total calories per gram: $0.12 + 1.62 + 0.92 = 2.66$ kcal

Total calories per 100 g: $2.66 \times 100 = 266$ kcal

Percentage of calories from lipid: $(18 \text{ g} \times 9.0 \text{ kcal} \cdot \text{g}^{-1})$ $\div 266 \text{ kcal} = 60.9\%$

www.nal.usda.gov/fnic/foodcomp/ ; and access the Food and Nutrition Information Center, National Agricultural Library, Agricultural Research Service of the USDA at http://www.nalusda.gov/fnic/)

Appendix A presents energy and nutritive values for common foods including specialty and fast-food items. Compute nutritive values for specialty dishes like chicken or beef tacos from standard recipes; actual values vary considerably depending on the method of preparation. Examination of Appendix A reveals large differences among the energy values of various foods. Consuming an equal number of calories from diverse foods often requires increasing or decreasing the quantity of a particular food. For example, to consume 100 kcal from each of six common foods—a carrots, celery, green peppers, grapefruit, medium-sized eggs, and mayonnaise—one must eat 5 carrots, 20 stalks of celery, 6.5 green peppers, 1 large grapefruit, 1 1/4 eggs, but only 1 tablespoon of mayonnaise. Consequently, an average sedentary adult female would need to consume either 420 celery stalks, 105 carrots, 136 green peppers, or 26 eggs, yet only 1 1/2 cup of mayonnaise or 8 oz of salad oil to meet her daily 2100-kcal energy needs. These examples dramatically illustrate that foods high in lipid content contain considerably more calories than foods low in lipid with correspondingly higher water content.

Note that a calorie reflects food energy *regardless* of the food source. Thus, from a standpoint of energy, 100 kcal from mayonnaise equals the same 100 kcal in 20 celery stalks. The more one eats of any food, the more calories one consumes. However, a small quantity of fatty foods represents a considerable quantity of calories; thus, the term "fattening" often describes these foods. An individual's caloric intake equals the sum of *all* energy consumed from either small or large food portions. Indeed, celery becomes a "fattening" food if consumed in excess! Chapter 7 considers variations in daily energy intake among sedentary and active individuals including diverse groups of athletes.

S u m m a r y

1. A kilocalorie (kcal) represents a measure of heat that expresses the energy value of food.

2. Burning food in the bomb calorimeter directly quantifies the food's energy content.

3. The heat of combustion represents the amount of heat liberated by the complete oxidation of a food in the bomb calorimeter. Average gross energy values equal 4.2 kcal per gram for carbohydrate, 9.4 kcal per gram for lipid, and 5.65 kcal per gram for protein.

4. The coefficient of digestibility indicates the proportion of food consumed that the body digests and absorbs.

5. Coefficients of digestibility average 97% for carbohydrates, 95% for lipids, and 92% for proteins. Thus, the net energy values (known as Atwater general factors) are 4 kcal per gram of carbohydrate, 9 kcal per gram of lipid, and 4 kcal per gram of protein.

6. The Atwater calorific values allow one to compute the caloric content of any meal from the food's carbohydrate, lipid, and protein content.

7. The calorie represents a unit of heat energy regardless of food source. From an energy standpoint, 500 kcal of chocolate ice cream topped with whipped cream and hazel nuts is no more fattening than 500 kcal of watermelon, 500 kcal of cheese and pepperoni pizza, or 500 kcal of a bagel with salmon, onions, and sour cream.

► Measurement of Human Energy Expenditure

ENERGY PRODUCED BY THE BODY

Direct calorimetry and **indirect calorimetry** and the **doubly labeled water technique** represent the most common approaches to accurately quantifying the energy generated by the body (energy expenditure) during rest and physical activity.

Direct Calorimetry

Heat represents the ultimate fate of all of the body's metabolic processes. The early experiments of French chemist Antoine Lavoisier (1743–1794) and his contemporaries (http://scienceworld.wolfram.com/biography/Lavoisier.html) in the 1770s provided the impetus to directly measure energy expenditure during rest and physical activity. The idea, similar to that used in the bomb calorimeter depicted in Figure 6.1, provides a convenient though elaborate way to directly measure heat production in humans.

The human calorimeter illustrated in FIGURE 6.2 consists of an airtight chamber with an oxygen supply where a person lives and works for an extended period.[1] A known water volume at a specified temperature circulates through a series of coils at the top of the chamber. This water absorbs

Figure 6.2 A human calorimeter directly measures energy metabolism (heat production). In the Atwater-Rosa calorimeter, a thin copper sheet lines the interior wall to which heat exchangers attach overhead and through which water passes. Water cooled to 2°C moves at a high flow rate, rapidly absorbing the heat radiated from the subject during exercise. As the subject rests, warmer water flows at a slower flow rate. In the original bicycle ergometer shown in the schematic, the rear wheel contacts the shaft of a generator that powers a light bulb. In a later version of the ergometer, copper made up part of the rear wheel. The wheel rotated through the field of an electromagnet producing an electric current for accurately determining power output.

the heat produced and radiated by the individual while in the calorimeter. Insulation protects the entire chamber so any change in water temperature relates directly to the individual's energy metabolism. For adequate ventilation, the person's exhaled air continually passes from the room through chemicals that remove moisture and absorb carbon dioxide. Oxygen added to the air recirculates through the chamber. Direct measurement of heat production in humans has considerable theoretical implications, yet its application is limited. Accurate measurements of heat production in the calorimeter require considerable time, expense, and formidable engineering expertise. Thus, use of the calorimeter remains inapplicable for energy determinations for most sport, occupational, and recreational activities.

Indirect Calorimetry

All energy-releasing reactions in the body ultimately depend on oxygen use. Measuring a person's oxygen uptake during aerobic exercise provides an indirect yet accurate estimate of energy expenditure. Indirect calorimetry remains relatively simple to operate and less expensive to maintain and staff than direct calorimetry.

Caloric Transformation for Oxygen

Studies with the bomb calorimeter show that approximately 4.82 kcal release when a blend of carbohydrate, lipid, and protein burns in 1 L of oxygen. Even with large variations in the metabolic mixture, this calorific value for oxygen varies only slightly (generally within 2 to 4%). Assuming the metabolism of a mixed diet, a rounded value of 5.0 kcal per liter of oxygen consumed designates the appropriate conversion factor for estimating energy expenditure under steady-rate conditions of aerobic metabolism. An energy-oxygen equivalent of 5.0 kcal per liter provides a convenient yardstick for transposing any aerobic physical activity to a caloric (energy) frame of reference. In fact, indirect calorimetry through oxygen-uptake measurement serves as the basis to quantify the energy (caloric) stress of most physical activities (refer to Appendix B).

Closed-circuit spirometry and open-circuit spirometry represent the two common methods of indirect calorimetry.

Closed-Circuit Spirometry

FIGURE 6.3 illustrates the technique of closed-circuit spirometry developed in the late 1800s and now used in hospitals and research laboratories to estimate resting energy expenditure. The subject breathes 100% oxygen from a prefilled container (spirometer). The equipment consists of a "closed

Figure 6.3 The closed-circuit method uses a spirometer prefilled with 100% oxygen. As the subject breathes from the spirometer, soda lime removes the expired air's carbon dioxide content.

system" because the person rebreathes only the gas in the spirometer. A canister of soda lime (potassium hydroxide) in the breathing circuit absorbs the carbon dioxide in exhaled air. A drum attached to the spirometer revolves at a known speed and records oxygen uptake from changes in the system's volume.

Oxygen uptake measurement using closed-circuit spirometry becomes problematic during exercise. The subject must remain close to the bulky equipment, the circuit's resistance to the large breathing volumes in exercise is considerable, and the speed of carbon dioxide removal becomes inadequate during heavy exercise. For these reasons, open-circuit spirometry, not the closed-circuit method, remains the most widely used procedure to measure exercise oxygen uptake.

Open-Circuit Spirometry

With open-circuit spirometry, a subject inhales ambient air with a constant composition of 20.93% oxygen, 0.03% carbon dioxide, and 79.04% nitrogen. The nitrogen fraction also includes a small quantity of inert gases. The changes in oxygen and carbon dioxide percentages in expired air compared with those in inspired ambient air indirectly reflect the ongoing process of energy metabolism. Thus, analysis of two factors—volume of air breathed during a specified time period and composition of exhaled air—provides a useful way to measure oxygen uptake and infer energy expenditure.

Four common indirect calorimetry procedures measure oxygen uptake during various physical activities:

1. Portable spirometry
2. Bag technique
3. Computerized instrumentation
4. Doubly labeled water technique

Portable Spirometry. German scientists in the early 1940s perfected a lightweight, portable system (first devised by German respiratory physiologist Nathan Zuntz [1847–1920] at the turn of the 20th century) to determine indirectly the energy expended during physical activity.[11] Activities included war-related operations such as traveling over different terrain with full battle gear, operating transportation vehicles including tanks and aircraft, and physical tasks that soldiers encounter during combat operations. The subject carried like a backpack the 3-kg box-shaped apparatus shown in FIGURE 6.4. Ambient inspired air passed through a two-way valve, and the expired air exited through a gas meter. The meter measured total expired air volume and collected a small gas sample for later analysis of oxygen and carbon dioxide content. Subsequent determination was made of oxygen uptake and energy expenditure for the measurement period.

Carrying the portable spirometer allows considerable freedom of movement for estimating energy expenditure in diverse activities such as mountain climbing, downhill skiing, sailing, golf, and common household activities

■ **Figure 6.4** Portable spirometer to measure oxygen uptake by the open-circuit method during **(A)** golf and **(B)** calisthenics exercise.

and size to evaluate the energy requirements of a specific occupational task. The technique also has recently determined energy expenditure during common household and garden tasks.[7]

Computerized Instrumentation. Advances in computer and microprocessor technology allow accurate and rapid measurement of metabolic and cardiovascular responses to exercise. A computer interfaces with at least three instruments: a system that continuously samples the subject's expired air, a flow-measuring device that records air volume breathed, and oxygen and carbon dioxide analyzers that measure the composition of the expired gas mixture. The computer performs metabolic calculations based on electronic signals it receives from the instruments. A printed or graphic display of the data appears throughout the measurement period. More advanced systems include automated blood pressure, heart rate, and temperature monitors and preset instructions to regulate speed, duration, and workload of a treadmill, bicycle ergometer, stepper, rower, swim flume, or other exercise

■ **Figure 6.5** Measurement of oxygen uptake during open-circuit spirometry (bag technique) during stationary cycle ergometer exercise **(A)** and box loading and unloading **(B)**.

(Appendix B). The equipment becomes cumbersome during vigorous activity. Also, the meter underrecords airflow volume during heavy exercise when breathing is rapid.[13]

Bag Technique. Figure 6.5A-B depicts the bag technique. The subject in Figure 6.5A rides a stationary bicycle ergometer, wearing headgear containing a two-way, high-velocity, low-resistance breathing valve. He breathes ambient air through one side of the valve and expels it out the other side. The air then passes into either large canvas or plastic Douglas bags (named for distinguished British respiratory physiologist Claude G. Douglas, 1882–1963) or rubber meteorologic balloons, or directly through a gas meter that continually measures expired air volume. The meter collects a small sample of expired air for analysis of oxygen and carbon dioxide composition. Assessment of oxygen uptake (as with all indirect calorimetric techniques) uses an appropriate calorific transformation for oxygen to compute energy expenditure. Figure 6.5B illustrates oxygen uptake measured by the bag technique while lifting boxes of different weight apparatus. FIGURE 6.6 depicts the computerized systems approach for collecting, analyzing, and displaying metabolic and physiologic responses during exercise.

The system illustrated in FIGURE 6.7 enables wireless telemetric transmission of data for metabolic measurement—pulmonary ventilation and oxygen and carbon dioxide analysis—during a broad range of exercise, sport, and occupational activities. The lightweight and miniaturized components include a voice-sensitive chip that provides feedback on pacing, duration of exercise, energy expenditure, heart rate, and pulmonary ventilation. The unit's microprocessor stores several hours of exercise data for later downloading to a computer. Telemetry provides "real time" data on a host computer.

With proper calibration, commercially available miniaturized equipment provides reasonable accuracy for quantifying the energy cost "in vivo" of diverse physical activities.[3] *Regardless of the apparent sophistication of a particular automated system, the output data still reflect the accuracy of the measuring device. Thus, accuracy and validity of the data require careful and frequent calibration of the measurement device using established reference standards.*

Doubly Labeled Water Technique. The doubly labeled water technique provides a useful way to estimate total daily energy expenditure of children and adults in free-living conditions without the normal constraints imposed by other indirect procedures.[5,18,21] The technique does not furnish sufficient refinement for accurate estimates of an individual's energy expenditure, but is more applicable for group estimates.[16] Because of the expense involved in using doubly labeled water, relatively few subjects participate in research studies. Its accuracy allows doubly labeled water to serve as a criterion for validating other methods (e.g., physical activity questionnaires and physical activity records) for estimating total daily energy expenditure of groups over prolonged time periods.[2,4,6,13]

The subject consumes a quantity of water containing a known concentration of the stable isotopes of hydrogen (^2H or deuterium) and oxygen (^{18}O or oxygen-18)—hence the

■ **Figure 6.6** Computer systems approach to the collection, analysis, and output of physiologic and metabolic data. (Photos courtesy of Fitco, a division of PhysioDyne Instrument Corporation, Farmingdale, NY; www.physiodyne.com)

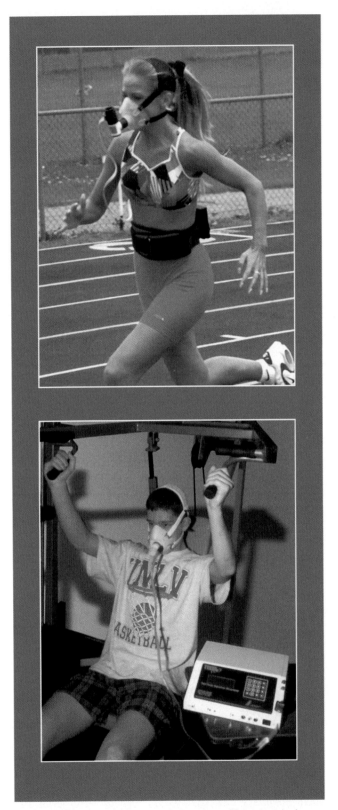

Figure 6.7 Miniaturized metabolic system. The 3 × 6-inch system fits in a chest-vest containing the electronic instrumentation, battery, oxygen and carbon dioxide sensors, and telemetry connections to a microcomputer that permits infrared transmission to a source computer. Easily transported during physical activity, the metabolic system weighs approximately 1.13 kg (2.5 lb). (Photo courtesy of V. Katch. Ann Arbor, MI.)

term *doubly labeled water*. The isotopes distribute throughout all body fluids. Labeled hydrogen leaves the body as water (^2H_2O) in sweat, urine, and pulmonary water vapor, while labeled oxygen leaves as water ($H_2{}^{18}O$) and carbon dioxide ($C^{18}O_2$) produced during macronutrient oxidation in energy metabolism. An isotope ratio mass spectrometer determines the differences between the two isotopes' elimination relative to the body's normal "background" levels. This procedure estimates total carbon dioxide production during the measurement period. Oxygen consumption (uptake) is easily estimated based on carbon dioxide production and an assumed (or measured) RQ value of 0.85 (see next section).

Under normal circumstances, a control baseline value for ^{18}O and ^2H is determined by analyzing the subject's urine or saliva before ingesting the doubly labeled water. The ingested isotopes require about 5 hours to distribute throughout the body water. The initial enriched urine or saliva sample is then measured and every day (or week) thereafter for the study's duration (usually up to 2 or 3 weeks). The progressive decrease in the sample concentrations of the two isotopes permits computation of carbon dioxide production rate.[17] Accuracy of the doubly labeled water technique versus energy expenditure with oxygen consumption in controlled settings averages between 3 and 5%. This magnitude of error probably increases in field studies, particularly among physically active individuals.[20]

The doubly labeled water technique provides an ideal way to assess total energy expenditure of groups over prolonged time periods including bed rest and during extreme activities like climbing Mt. Everest, cycling the Tour de France, rowing, and endurance running and swimming.[9,14,19] Major drawbacks of the method include the cost of enriched ^{18}O and the expense of spectrometric analysis of the two isotopes.

THE RESPIRATORY QUOTIENT

Research in the early part of the 19th century discovered a way to evaluate the metabolic mixture in exercise from measures of gas exchange in the lungs.[12] Because of inherent chemical differences in the composition of carbohydrates, lipids, and proteins, complete oxidation of a molecule's carbon and hydrogen atoms to the carbon dioxide and water end products requires different amounts of oxygen. Thus, the substrate metabolized determines the quantity of carbon dioxide produced relative to oxygen consumed. The **respiratory quotient (RQ)** refers to this ratio of metabolic gas exchange as follows:

$$RQ = CO_2 \text{ produced} \div O_2 \text{ consumed}$$

The RQ provides a convenient guide to approximate the nutrient mixture catabolized for energy during rest and aerobic exercise. Also, because the caloric equivalent for oxygen differs somewhat, depending on the macronutrients oxidized, precisely determining the body's heat production or energy expenditure requires knowledge of both the RQ and the oxygen uptake.

RQ for Carbohydrate

The complete oxidation of one glucose molecule requires six oxygen molecules and produces six molecules of carbon dioxide and water as follows:

$$C_6H_{12}O_6 + 6\ O_2 \rightarrow 6\ CO_2 + 6\ H_2O$$

Gas exchange during glucose oxidation produces a number of carbon dioxide molecules equal to the oxygen molecules consumed; therefore, the RQ for carbohydrate equals 1.00.

$$RQ = 6\ CO_2 \div 6O_2 = 1.00$$

RQ for Lipid

The chemical composition of lipids differs from that of carbohydrates in that lipids contain considerably fewer oxygen atoms in proportion to carbon and hydrogen atoms. (Note the 2:1 ratio of hydrogen to oxygen in carbohydrate matches the ratio in water, whereas fatty acids have a much larger ratio.) Consequently, catabolizing fat for energy requires considerably more oxygen consumed relative to carbon dioxide produced. Palmitic acid, a typical fatty acid, oxidizes to carbon dioxide and water, producing 16 carbon dioxide molecules for every 23 oxygen molecules consumed. The following equation summarizes this exchange to compute RQ:

$$C_{16}H_{32}O_2 + 23\ O_2 \rightarrow 16\ CO_2 + 16\ H_2O$$
$$RQ = 16\ CO_2 \div 23\ O_2 = 0.696$$

Generally, a value of 0.70 represents the RQ for lipid, with variation ranging between 0.69 and 0.73. The value depends on the oxidized fatty acid's carbon chain length.

RQ for Protein

Proteins do not simply oxidize to carbon dioxide and water during energy metabolism. Rather, the liver first deaminates the amino acid molecule. The body excretes the nitrogen and sulfur fragments in the urine, sweat, and feces. The remaining "keto acid" fragment then oxidizes to carbon dioxide and water to provide energy for biologic work. These short-chain keto acids, as with fat catabolism, require more oxygen consumed in relation to carbon dioxide produced to achieve complete combustion. The protein albumin oxidizes as follows:

$$C_{72}H_{112}N_2O_{22}S + 77\ O_2 \rightarrow 63\ CO_2 + 38\ H_2O$$
$$+ SO_3 + 9\ CO(NH_2)_2$$
$$RQ = 63\ CO_2 \div 77\ O_2 = 0.818$$

The general value 0.82 characterizes the RQ for protein.

Estimating Energy Expenditure by Use of the Weir Method

In 1949, J. B. Weir, a Scottish physician/physiologist from Glasgow University, Scotland, presented a simple method to estimate caloric expenditure from measures of pulmonary ventilation and the expired oxygen percentage, accurate to within ±1% of the traditional RQ method.

Basic Equation

Weir showed that the following formula calculated caloric expenditure ($kcal \cdot min^{-1}$) if energy production from protein breakdown averaged about 12.5% of total energy expenditure (a reasonable percentage for most persons under typical conditions):

$$kcal \cdot min^{-1} = \dot{V}_{E(STPD)} \times (1.044 - [0.0499 \times \%\ O_{2E}])$$

where $\dot{V}_{E(STPD)}$ represents expired ventilation (corrected to STPD conditions), and $\%O_{2E}$ represents expired oxygen percentage. The value in parenthesis ($1.044 - [0.0499 \times \% O_{2E}]$) represents the "Weir factor." TABLE 6.3 displays Weir factors for different $\%O_{2E}$ values.

To use the table, find the $\%O_{2E}$ and corresponding Weir factor. Compute energy expenditure in $kcal \cdot min^{-1}$ by multiplying the Weir factor by $\dot{V}_{E(STPD)}$.

Example

During a steady-rate jog on a treadmill, $\dot{V}_{E(STPD)} = 50$ $L \cdot min^{-1}$ and $O_{2E} = 16.0\%$. Energy expenditure by the Weir method computes as follows:

$$kcal \cdot min^{-1} = \dot{V}_{E(STPD)} \times (1.044 - [0.0499 \times \%O_{2E}])$$
$$= 50 \times (1.044 - [0.0499 \times 16.0]$$
$$= 50 \times 0.2456$$
$$= 12.3$$

RQ for a Mixed Diet

During activities ranging from complete bed rest to moderate aerobic exercise (walking or slow jogging), the RQ seldom reflects the oxidation of pure carbohydrate or pure fat. Instead, metabolism of a mixture of these two nutrients occurs, with an RQ intermediate between 0.70 and 1.00. *For most purposes, we assume an RQ of 0.82 from the metabolism of a mixture of 40% carbohydrate and 60% fat, applying the caloric equivalent of 4.825 kcal per liter of oxygen for the energy transformation.* Using 4.825, a value of 4% represents the maximum error possible when estimating energy metabolism from steady-rate oxygen uptake.

Table 6.3 **WEIR FACTORS FOR DIFFERENT EXPIRED OXYGEN PERCENTAGES ($\%O_{2E}$).**

$\%O_{2E}$	Weir Factor	$\%O_{2E}$	Weir Factor	$\%O_{2E}$	Weir Factor	$\%O_{2E}$	Weir Factor
14.50	.3205	15.80	.2556	17.10	.1907	18.30	.1308
14.60	.3155	15.90	.2506	17.20	.1807	18.40	.1268
14.70	.3105	16.00	.2456	17.30	.1857	18.50	.1208
14.80	.3055	16.10	.2406	17.40	.1757	18.60	.1168
14.90	.3005	16.20	.2366	17.50	.1658	18.70	.1109
15.00	.2955	16.30	.2306	17.60	.1707	18.80	.1068
15.10	.2905	16.40	.2256	17.70	.1608	18.90	.1009
15.20	.2855	16.50	.2206	17.80	.1558	19.00	.0969
15.30	.2805	16.60	.2157	17.90	.1508	19.10	.0909
15.40	.2755	16.70	.2107	18.00	.1468	19.20	.0868
15.50	.2705	16.80	.2057	18.10	.1308	19.30	.0809
15.60	.2556	16.90	.2007	18.20	.1368	19.40	.0769
15.70	.2606	17.00	.1957				

From Weir JB. J Physiol 1949;109:1. If $\%O_{2expired}$ does not appear in the table, compute individual Weir factors as $1.044 - 0.0499 \times \%O_{2E}$.

TABLE 6.4 presents the energy expenditure per liter of oxygen uptake for different nonprotein RQ values, including their corresponding percentages and grams of carbohydrate and fat used for energy. The nonprotein value assumes that the metabolic mixture comprises *only* carbohydrate and fat. Interpret the table as follows:

Suppose oxygen uptake during 30 minutes of aerobic exercise averages 3.22 $L \cdot min^{-1}$ with carbon dioxide production of 2.78 $L \cdot min^{-1}$. The RQ, computed as $V_{CO_2} \div V_{O_2}$ (2.78 ÷ 3.22), equals 0.86. From Table 6.4, this RQ value (left column) corresponds to an energy equivalent of 4.875 kcal per liter of oxygen uptake or an exercise energy output of 13.55 $kcal \cdot min^{-1}$ (2.78 L $O_2 \cdot min^{-1} \times 4.875$ kcal). Based on a nonprotein RQ, 54.1% of the calories come from the combustion of carbohydrate and 45.9% from fat. The total calories expended during the 30-minute exercise equals 406 kcal (13.55 $kcal \cdot min^{-1} \times 30$).

THE RESPIRATORY EXCHANGE RATIO

Application of the RQ assumes that oxygen and carbon dioxide exchange measured at the lungs reflects the actual gas exchange from macronutrient metabolism in the cell. This assumption remains reasonably valid for rest and during steady-rate (mild to moderate) aerobic exercise when no lactate accumulation takes place. However, factors can spuriously alter the exchange of oxygen and carbon dioxide in the lungs so the ratio of gas exchange no longer reflects only the substrate mixture in cellular energy metabolism. Respiratory physiologists term the ratio of carbon dioxide produced to oxygen consumed under such conditions the **respiratory exchange ratio (R or RER)**. This ratio computes in exactly the same manner as RQ.

For example, carbon dioxide elimination increases during hyperventilation because the breathing response increases to disproportionately high levels compared with actual metabolic demand. By overbreathing, normal carbon dioxide level in blood decreases as this gas "blows off" in expired air. A corresponding increase in oxygen uptake does not occur with this additional carbon dioxide elimination; thus, the rise in respiratory exchange ratio cannot be attributed to the oxidation of foodstuff. In such cases, R usually increases above 1.00.

Exhaustive exercise presents another situation that causes R to rise above 1.00. In such cases, sodium bicarbonate in the blood buffers or "neutralizes" the lactate generated during anaerobic metabolism to maintain proper acid-base balance in the following reaction:

$$HLa + NaHCO_3 \rightarrow NaLa + H_2CO_3 \rightarrow H_2O + CO_2 \rightarrow Lungs$$

Buffering of lactate produces carbonic acid, a weaker acid. In the pulmonary capillaries, carbonic acid degrades to carbon dioxide and water components, and carbon dioxide readily exits through the lungs. The R increases above 1.00 because buffering adds "extra" carbon dioxide to the expired air, in excess of the quantity normally released during energy metabolism.

Relatively low values for R occur following exhaustive exercise when carbon dioxide remains in cells and body fluids to replenish the bicarbonate that buffered the accumulating lactate. This action reduces the expired carbon dioxide without affecting oxygen uptake. This causes the R to dip below 0.70.

| Table 6.4 | THERMAL EQUIVALENTS OF OXYGEN FOR THE NONPROTEIN RESPIRATORY QUOTIENT (RQ), INCLUDING PERCENTAGE KILOCALORIES AND GRAMS DERIVED FROM CARBOHYDRATE AND LIPID |

Nonprotein RQ	kcal per LO_2	Percentage kcal derived from		Grams per LO_2	
		Carbohydrate	Lipid	Carbohydrate	Lipid
0.707	4.686	0.0	100.0	0.000	0.496
0.71	4.690	1.1	98.9	0.012	0.491
0.72	4.702	4.8	95.2	0.051	0.476
0.73	4.714	8.4	91.6	0.090	0.460
0.74	4.727	12.0	88.0	0.130	0.444
0.75	4.739	15.6	84.4	0.170	0.428
0.76	4.750	19.2	80.8	0.211	0.412
0.77	4.764	22.8	77.2	0.250	0.396
0.78	4.776	26.3	73.7	0.290	0.380
0.79	4.788	29.9	70.1	0.330	0.363
0.80	4.801	33.4	66.6	0.371	0.347
0.81	4.813	36.9	63.1	0.413	0.330
0.82	4.825	40.3	59.7	0.454	0.313
0.83	4.838	43.8	56.2	0.496	0.297
0.84	4.850	47.2	52.8	0.537	0.280
0.85	4.862	50.7	49.3	0.579	0.263
0.86	4.875	54.1	45.9	0.621	0.247
0.87	4.887	57.5	42.5	0.663	0.230
0.88	4.889	60.8	39.2	0.705	0.213
0.89	4.911	64.2	35.8	0.749	0.195
0.90	4.924	67.5	32.5	0.791	0.178
0.91	4.936	70.8	29.2	0.834	0.160
0.92	4.948	74.1	25.9	0.877	0.143
0.93	4.961	77.4	22.6	0.921	0.125
0.94	4.973	80.7	19.3	0.964	0.108
0.95	4.985	84.0	16.0	1.008	0.090
0.96	4.998	87.2	12.8	1.052	0.072
0.97	5.010	90.4	9.6	1.097	0.054
0.98	5.022	93.6	6.4	1.142	0.036
0.99	5.035	96.8	3.2	1.186	0.018
1.00	5.047	100.0	0	1.231	0.000

Summary

1. Direct calorimetry and indirect calorimetry are two methods for determining the body's rate of energy expenditure. Direct calorimetry measures actual heat production in an appropriately insulated calorimeter. Indirect calorimetry infers energy expenditure from measurements of oxygen uptake and carbon dioxide production, using closed-circuit spirometry, open-circuit spirometry, or the doubly labeled water technique.

2. The doubly labeled water technique estimates energy expenditure in free-living conditions without the normal constraints of laboratory procedures. Although serving as a "gold standard" for other long-term energy expenditure estimates, drawbacks include the cost of enriched ^{18}O and the expense of spectrometric analysis of the two isotopes.

3. The complete oxidation of each macronutrient requires a different quantity of oxygen uptake compared to carbon dioxide production. The ratio of carbon dioxide produced to oxygen consumed, termed the *respiratory quotient,* or *RQ,* provides key information about the nutrient mixture catabolized for energy. The RQ equals 1.00 for carbohydrate, 0.70 for fat, and 0.82 for protein.

4. For each RQ value, a corresponding caloric value exists for each liter of oxygen consumed. This RQ–kcal relationship provides an accurate estimate of exercise expenditure during steady-rate exercise.

5. The RQ does not indicate specific substrate use during non-steady rate exercise because of non-metabolic carbon dioxide production in the buffering of lactate.

6. The respiratory exchange ratio (R) reflects pulmonary exchange of carbon dioxide and oxygen under various physiologic and metabolic conditions; R does not fully mirror the macronutrient mixture catabolized.

TEST YOUR KNOWLEDGE ANSWERS

1. True In nutritional terms, one calorie expresses the quantity of heat needed to raise the temperature of 1 kg (1 L) of water 1°C (specifically, from 14.5 to 15.5°C). Thus, kilogram-calorie or kilocalorie (kcal) more accurately defines a calorie.

2. False Laboratories use the bomb calorimeter to measure the total energy value of the various food macronutrients. Bomb calorimeters operate on the principle of direct calorimetry, measuring the heat liberated as the food burns completely.

3. False Heat of combustion refers to the heat liberated by oxidizing a specific food; it represents the food's total energy value as measured by the bomb calorimeter. Although the oxidation pathways of food in the intact organism and bomb calorimeter differ, the energy liberated in the complete breakdown of food remains the same, regardless of the combustion pathways.

4. False The heat of combustion for carbohydrate varies depending upon the arrangement of atoms in the particular carbohydrate molecule. On average, for 1 g of carbohydrate, a value of 4.2 kcal generally represents the average heat of combustion.

5. False The heat of combustion for lipid varies with the structural composition of the triacylglycerol molecule's fatty acid components. The average heat of combustion for lipid equals 9.4 kcal per gram.

6. False The coefficient of digestibility represents the percentage of an ingested macronutrient actually digested and absorbed by the body. The quantity of food remaining unabsorbed in the intestinal tract becomes voided in the feces. The relative percentage digestibility coefficients average 97% for carbohydrate, 95% for lipid, and 92% for protein.

7. False The doubly labeled water technique provides a way to estimate total daily energy expenditure of children and adults in free-living conditions without the normal constraints imposed by other procedures of indirect calorimetry. It involves the ingestion of stable isotopes of hydrogen and oxygen, which distribute throughout all body fluids. Differences between elimination rates of the two isotopes relative to the body's normal "background" level estimates total carbon dioxide production from energy metabolism during the measurement period.

8. False The average net energy values can be rounded to simple whole numbers and are referred to as Atwater general factors, which are as follows: 4 kcal per gram for carbohydrate; 9 kcal per gram for lipid; 4 kcal per gram for protein.

9. True The more one eats of any food, the more calories one consumes. An individual's caloric intake equals the sum of all energy consumed from either small or large quantities of foods. Thus, celery becomes a "fattening" food if consumed in excess. However, achieving this excess involves consuming a considerable quantity of celery. For example, the typical sedentary woman needs to consume 420 celery stalks yet only 8 oz of salad oil to meet her daily 2100 kcal energy needs.

10. True Because of inherent chemical differences in the composition of carbohydrates, lipids, and proteins, complete oxidation of a molecule's carbon and hydrogen atoms to carbon dioxide and water end products requires different amounts of oxygen. Gas exchange during glucose oxidation produces six carbon dioxide molecules for six oxygen molecules consumed. Therefore, the RQ (CO_2 produced ÷ O_2 consumed) for carbohydrate equals 1.00. (RQ = 6 CO_2 ÷ 6 O_2 = 1.00)

References

1. Atwater WO, Rosa EB. Description of a new respiration calorimeter and experiments on the conservation of energy in the human body. US Department of Agriculture, Office of Experiment Stations, bulletin no. 63. Washington, DC: Government Printing Office, 1899.
2. Conway JM, et al. Comparison of energy expenditure estimates from doubly labeled water, a physical activity questionnaire, and physical activity records. Am J Clin Nutr 2002;75:519.
3. Crandall CG, et al. Evaluation of the Cosmed K2 portable telemetric oxygen uptake analyzer. Med Sci Sports Exerc 1994;26:108.
4. Ekelund U, et al. Energy expenditure assessed by heart rate and doubly labeled water in young athletes. Med Sci Sports Exerc 2002;34:1360.
5. Ekelund U, et al. Physical activity but not energy expenditure is reduced in obese adolescents: a case-controlled study. Am J Clin Nutr 2002;76:935.
6. Fogelholm M, et al. Assessment of energy expenditure in overweight women. Med Sci Sports Exerc 1998;30:1191.
7. Gunn SM, et al. Determining energy expenditure during some household and garden tasks. Med Sci Sports Exerc 2002;34:895.
8. Health and Welfare Canada. Nutrient value of some common foods. Ottawa, Canada: Health Services and Promotion Branch, Health and Welfare Canada, 1988.
9. Hill RJ, Davies PS. Energy intake and energy expenditure in elite lightweight female rowers. Med Sci Sports Exerc 2002;34:1823.
10. Katch FI. U.S. government raises serious questions about reliability of U.S. Department of Agriculture's food composition tables. Int J Sports Nutr 1995;5:62.
11. Koffranyi E, Michaelis HF. Ein tragbarer Apparat zur Bestimmung des Gasstoffwechsels. Arbeitsphysiologie 1940;11:148.
12. Krogh A, Lindhard J. The relative value of fat and carbohydrate as sources of muscular energy. Biochem J 1920;14:290.
13. Montoye HJ, et al. Measuring physical activity and energy expenditure. Boca Raton, FL: Human Kinetics, 1996.
14. Mudambo KS, et al. Adequacy of food rations in soldiers during exercise in hot, day-time conditions assessed by double labeled water and energy balance methods. Eur J Appl Physiol 1997;76:346.
15. Rumpler WW, et al. Energy value of moderate alcohol consumption by humans. Am J Clin Nutr 1996;64:108.
16. Speakman JR. The history and theory of the doubly labeled water technique. Am J Clin Nutr 1998;68(suppl):932S.
17. Speakman JR, et al. Revised equations for calculating CO_2 production from doubly labeled water in humans. Am J Physiol 1993;61:1200.
18. Starling RD, et al. Energy requirements and physical activity in free-living older women and men: a doubly labeled water study. J Appl Physiol 1998;85:1063.
19. Stroud MA, et al. Energy expenditure using isotope-labeled water ($^2H^{18}O$), exercise performance, skeletal muscle enzyme activities and plasma biochemical parameters in humans during 95 days of endurance exercise with inadequate energy intake. Eur J Appl Physiol 1997;76:243.
20. Westerterp KR, et al. Comparison of doubly labeled water with respirometry at low- and high-activity levels. J Appl Physiol 1988;65:53.
21. Withers RT, et al. Energy metabolism in sedentary and active 49- to 70-yr-old women. J Appl Physiol 1998;84:1333.

General References

Atwater WO, Woods CD. The chemical composition of American food materials. USDA bulletin no. 28. Washington, DC: USDA, 1896.

Boyle M. Personal nutrition. 4th ed. Belmont, CA: Wadsworth Publishing, 2001.
Brody T. Nutritional biochemistry. New York: Academic Press, 1998.
Brooks GA, et al. Exercise physiology: human bioenergetics and its applications. 2nd ed. Mountain View, CA: Mayfield, 2000.
Gibson RS. Principles of nutritional assessment. New York: Oxford University Press. 1990.
Guyton AC. Textbook of medical physiology. 10th ed. Philadelphia: WB Saunders, 2000.
Hamilton EM, et al. Nutrition: concepts and controversies. 5th ed. St. Paul, MN: West, 1991.
Health and Welfare Canada. Nutrient value of some common foods. Ottawa, Canada: Health Services and Promotion Branch, Health and Welfare, 1988.
Mahan IK, Escott-Stump S. Krause's food, nutrition, & diet therapy. Philadelphia: WB Saunders, 2000.
McCance A, Widdowson EM. The composition of foods. 5th ed. London: Royal Society of Chemistry. Ministry of Agriculture, Fisheries and Food, 1991.
Pennington JAT, Church HN. Bowes and Church's food values of portions commonly used. 15th ed. Philadelphia: JB Lippincott, 1989.
Shils ME, et al. Modern nutrition in health and disease. 9th ed. Baltimore: Lippincott Williams & Wilkins, 1999.
U.S. Department of Agriculture. *Composition of foods—raw, processed, and prepared.* no. 8. Washington, DC: U.S. Department of Agriculture, 1963–1987.

Additional Readings

Ainslie P. Estimating human energy expenditure: A review of techniques with particular reference to doubly labeled water. Sports Med 2003;33:683.
Bosy-Westphal A, et al. Effect of organ and tissue masses on resting energy expenditure in underweight, normal weight and obese adults. Int J Obes Relat Metab Disord 2004;28:72.
Donahoo WT, et al. Variability in energy expenditure and its components. Curr Opin Clin Nutr Metab Car 2004;7:599.
Ekelund U, et al. Body movement and physical activity energy expenditure in children and adolescents: How to adjust for differences in body size and age. Am J Clin Nutr 2004;79:851.
Gibney ER, et al. Measurement of total energy expenditure in grossly obese women: Comparison of the bicarbonate-urea method with whole-body calorimetry and free-living doubly labeled water. Int J Obes Relat Metab Disord 2003;27:641.
Hukshorn CJ, Saris WH. Leptin and energy expenditure. Curr Opin Clin Nutr Metab Care 2004;7:629.
Kien CL, Ugrasbul F. Prediction of daily energy expenditure during a feeding trial using measurements of resting energy expenditure, fat-free mass, or Harris-Benedict equations. Am J Clin Nutr 2004;80:876.
King GA, et al. Comparison of activity monitors to estimate energy cost of treadmill exercise. Med Sci Sports Exerc 2004;36:1244.
Levine JA. Nonexercise activity thermogenesis (NEAT): Environment and biology. Am J Physiol Endocrinol Metab 2004;286:E675.
Moran DS, et al. Metabolic rate monitoring and energy expenditure prediction using a novel actigraphy method. Med Sci Monit 2004;10:MT117.
Westerterp KR, Plasqui G. Physical activity and human energy expenditure. Curr Opin Clin Nutr Metab Care 2004;7:607.
Westerterp KR. Impacts of vigorous and non-vigorous activity on daily energy expenditure. Proc Nutr Soc 2003;62:645.

Section III

Optimal Nutrition for the Physically Active Person: Making Informed and Healthful Choices

Outline

Chapter

7

Nutritional Recommendations for the Physically Active Person

TEST YOUR KNOWLEDGE

Answer these ten statements about optimal nutrition for the physically active person. Use the scoring key at the end of the chapter to check your results. Repeat this test after you have read the chapter and compare your results.

1. **T F** Humans differ from machines in that they do not conform to the laws of thermodynamics, at least in terms of energy balance.

2. **T F** One pound of stored body fat contains approximately 3500 kcal of energy.

3. **T F** A major problem with the Food Guide Pyramid is that it lumps all foods within a food category together (e.g., bread, cereal, rice and pasta group) without distinguishing between healthful and not so healthful foods within that category.

4. **T F** Recent government guidelines for good nutrition emphasize specific numeric goals for different individual nutrients.

5. **T F** Physically active individuals require additional micronutrients above recommended values to support their increased level of energy expenditure.

6. **T F** Serious weight trainers benefit from taking high doses of amino acid supplements to increase muscle mass.

7. **T F** To promote good health, lipid intake should not exceed 10% of total caloric intake.

8. **T F** High-carbohydrate (60–70% total caloric intake), high-fiber (30–50 g per day) diets do not promote good health as they deprive an individual of needed quantities of lipid.

9. **T F** Athletes in heavy training require vitamin and mineral intake above recommended values for optimal physical performance and training responsiveness.

10. **T F** Saturated fatty acids provide an excellent source of antioxidant vitamins.

The past 25 years have witnessed considerable research interest in nutritional factors related to exercise and sports performance for physically active adults and competitive athletes. Less than optimal fluid, nutrient, and energy intakes profoundly affect thermoregulatory functions, substrate availability, exercise capacity, recovery from exercise, and training responsiveness. *An optimal diet supplies required nutrients in adequate amounts for tissue maintenance, repair, and growth without excess energy intake.* As the understanding of human nutrition evolves, a reasonable estimate of nutritional needs of men and women considers normal variation in nutrient digestion, absorption, and assimilation and daily energy expenditure. Dietary recommendations for physically active men and women must account for the energy requirements of a particular activity or sport and its training demands, including individual dietary preferences. Although no "one" food or diet exists for optimal health and exercise performance, careful planning and evaluation of food intake should follow sound nutritional guidelines. The physically active person must obtain sufficient energy and macronutrients to replenish liver and muscle glycogen, provide amino acid building blocks for tissue growth and repair, and maintain a desirable body weight. Lipid intake must also provide essential fatty acids and fat-soluble vitamins. Supplementing with vitamin and minerals is unnecessary provided a well-balanced diet provides for the body's energy needs. TABLE 7.1 outlines the recommendations of a joint position statement from the American College of Sports Medicine, American Dietetic Association, and Dietitians of Canada about how qualified health, exercise, and nutrition professionals can counsel individuals who engage regularly in physical activity.

THE ENERGY BALANCE EQUATION

The concept of energy balance most typically applies in discussions of body weight maintenance and weight loss as discussed in Chapter 14. Proper attainment of energy balance becomes an important goal for physically active people, particularly during heavy training or multiple daily workouts when maintaining energy balance with proper nutrient intake optimizes exercise performance and the training response.

The human body functions in accord with the laws of thermodynamics. If total food calories exceed daily energy expenditure, excess calories accumulate as fat in adipose tissue. One must consider the rationale underlying the **energy balance equation** when replenishing the body's macronutrient energy reserves in heavy training or in planning to favorably modify body weight and body composition. *In accord with the first law of thermodynamics, the energy balance equation dictates that body mass remains constant when caloric intake equals caloric expenditure.* FIGURE 7.1 depicts factors that contribute to daily energy balance and imbalance. The middle example shows what happens all too frequently when energy input exceeds energy output and the calories consumed in excess of daily requirements become stored as fat in adipose tissue. Obesity occurs with a long-term positive energy imbalance that often results from subtle regulatory alterations between energy intake and energy expenditure. *Thirty-five hundred "extra" kcal through either increased energy intake or decreased energy output approximates 1 lb (0.45 kg) of stored body fat.* The lower example illustrates what occurs when energy output exceeds energy input. In this case, the body obtains the required calories from its energy stores, resulting in reduced body mass and body fat. Little fluctuation occurs in body mass if an equilibrium exists in which energy input (calories in food) balances energy output (calories expended in daily activities) as shown in the top panel of the figure. This situation most typically applies to physically active individuals who must regularly replenish the energy to power exercise through nutrient-rich food sources as outlined in sections that follow.

PRINCIPLES OF GOOD EATING

Key principles of good eating include variety, balance, and moderation. This does not mean one must give up enjoyable

---

Table 7.1   WAYS THAT EXERCISE NUTRITIONISTS CAN HELP PHYSICALLY ACTIVE INDIVIDUALS, PARTICULARLY COMPETITIVE ATHLETES

- Educate athletes about energy requirements for their sport and the role of food in fueling the body. Discourage unrealistic weight and body composition goals and emphasize the importance of adequate energy intake for good health, prevention of injury, and exercise performance.
- Assess the body size and composition of an athlete for the determination of an appropriate weight and composition for the sports in which he or she participates. Provide the athlete with nutritionally sound techniques for maintaining an appropriate body weight and composition without the use of fad or severe diets. Undue pressure on athletes for weight loss or the maintenance of a lean body build can increase the risk of restrictive eating behaviors and, in extreme cases, lead to a clinical eating disorder.
- Assess the athlete's typical dietary and supplement intake during training, competition, and the off-season. Use this assessment to provide appropriate recommendations for energy and nutrient intakes for the maintenance of good health, appropriate body weight and composition, and optimal sport performance throughout the year. Give specific guidelines for making good food and fluid selections while traveling and eating away from home.
- Assess the fluid intake and weight loss of athletes during exercise and make appropriate recommendations regarding total fluid intake and fluid intake before, during, and after exercise. Help athletes to determine appropriate types and amounts of beverages to use during exercise, especially if the athlete is exercising in extreme environments.
- For athletes such as the vegetarian athlete with special nutrition concerns, provide appropriate nutritional guidelines to ensure adequate intakes of energy, protein, and micronutrients.
- Carefully evaluate any vitamin/mineral or herbal supplements, ergogenic aids, or performance-enhancing drugs an athlete wants to use. These products should be used with caution and only after careful review of their legality and the current literature pertaining to the ingredients listed on the product label; these products should not be recommended until after evaluating the athlete's health, diet, nutrition needs, current supplement and drug use, and energy requirements.

From American College of Sports Medicine, American Dietetic Association and Dietitians of Canada. Joint position statement. Nutrition and athletic performance. Med Sci Sports Exerc 2000;32:2130.

■ **Figure 7.1** The energy balance equation (*TEF* refers to the thermic effect of food).

foods to eat healthfully. To the contrary, a healthful diet requires some simple planning that does not demand a lifetime of deprivation and misery. In reality, eliminating enjoyable foods often proves detrimental in the long run and creates a diet program doomed to failure.

Variety

Choosing foods from a variety of sources creates a diet that contains sufficient amounts of all required nutrients. For example, each vegetable form contains a unique set of phytochemicals (see Case Study 6-1, p. 172), so consuming a variety of vegetables provides a broad array of these beneficial food constituents. A diverse diet also makes mealtime more interesting and something to look forward to.

Balance

Balance in one's diet indicates the intake of nutrients from the major food groups and thus enables the person to benefit from the variety of accessory chemicals unique to each food. Prolonged intake of a diet that inordinately focuses on one food group often creates nutritional deficiency, despite intake of sufficient energy. For example, if a person dislikes milk or milk products (yogurt, ice cream, and cheese), the likelihood of calcium deficiency increases because this food group constitutes the major source of calcium.

Moderation

Eating moderately requires appropriate planning to maintain a balanced nutrient intake throughout the day. For example,

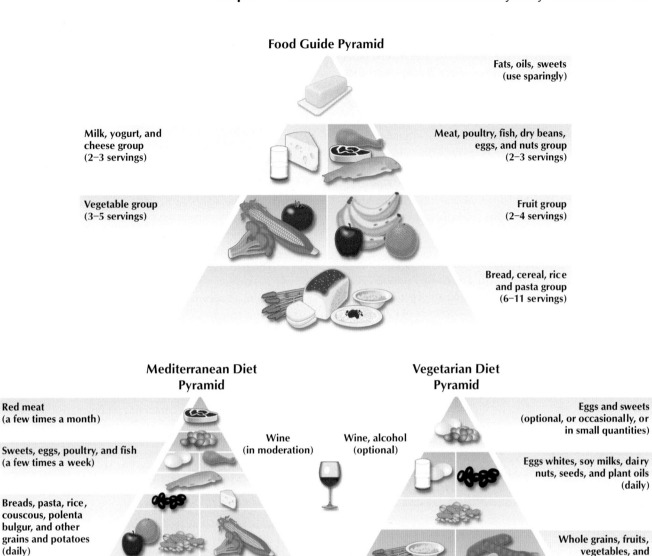

Figure 7.2 The Food Guide Pyramid emphasizes grains, vegetables, and fruits as important sources of nutrients.

if one meal contains high-fat foods, other meals during the day must contain less fat. A good action plan moderates rather than eliminates the intake of certain foods. In this way one can enjoy all types of foods during the day.

THE FOOD GUIDE PYRAMID

Lobbyists for the beef and dairy industries greatly influenced earlier approaches to recommending sound nutrition such as

the Four-Food-Group Plan. However, research in nutrition, cancer, and heart disease over the past 40 years uncovered the shortcomings of this plan, with its overemphasis on meat and milk products as a guide to healthful eating. In the typical American diet, energy-dense but nutrient-poor foods frequently substitute for more nutrient-rich foods. This pattern of food intake increases risk for obesity, marginal micronutrient intakes, low serum concentrations of vitamins, carotenoids, and HDL-cholesterol, and elevated levels of homocysteine.[69]

The **Food Guide Pyramid** (soon to be revamped as the Food Guidance System) represents a model of the *Dietary Guidelines for Americans* (see below) age 2 years and older (Fig. 7.2). The *Guidelines*, revised every 5 years with sixth edition evidence-based revisions due out in 2005, are formulated for the general population to help people without special nutrition training estimate whether the foods they choose meet nutritional needs. They provide a sound framework for meal planning for the physically active. They also serve as the basis for food labeling and provide a reference for meal planning at schools in the Federal lunch program. This practical approach to a healthful diet translates the RDAs and *Dietary Guidelines* by categorizing foods that make similar nutrient contributions; it also recommends the number of servings from each category. The Food Guide Pyramid recommendations also apply to individuals who consume a mostly vegetarian diet. Meat, fish, and poultry provide good sources of B-vitamins and iron and zinc, so vegetarians must emphasize these nutrients in the plant sources of their diet.

The current Food Guide Pyramid represents a total diet that provides sufficient protein, vitamins, and minerals. This plan goes beyond earlier nutrient-intake models to suggest a pattern of food choices for the entire day, rather than simply to provide a foundation diet. Major changes from the earlier food guide recommendations include an increase in total fruit and vegetable servings from 4 per day to 5 to 9 per day and an increase in bread and cereal servings from 4 per day to 6 to 11 per day. These changes provide the bulk of energy intake from carbohydrates while moderating fat intake.

A Closer Look

TABLE 7.2 presents the Pyramid's six food group categories, the major nutrients each food group supplies, and sample foods and servings sizes for each group. Although similarities exists among food groups, the daily recommended number of servings are as follows:

- Two servings from the milk, yogurt, and cheese group
- Two to three servings from the meat, poultry, fish, dry beans, eggs, and nuts group (5–7 oz total)
- Three to five servings from the vegetable group
- Two to four servings from the fruit group
- Six to 11 servings from the bread, cereals, rice, and pasta group

Planning Food Menus

TABLE 7.3 presents a sample diet prepared from recommendations of the Food Guide Pyramid. Use of the Pyramid creates nutritious daily diets containing as few as 1600 to 1800 kcal, an energy intake sufficient for a sedentary adult or an

Table 7.2 **THE FOOD GUIDE PYRAMID: SIX FOOD GROUP CATEGORIES, THE MAJOR NUTRIENTS EACH FOOD GROUP SUPPLIES, AND SAMPLE FOODS AND SERVING SIZES FOR EACH GROUP**

Food Category	*Major Nutrients*	*Foods and Serving Sizes*
Milk, yogurt, and cheese	Calcium, phosphorus, carbohydrate, protein, riboflavin, vitamin D, magnesium, zinc	1 cup milk 1.5 oz cheese 2 oz processed cheese 1 cup yogurt 2 cups cottage cheese
Meat, poultry, fish, dry beans, eggs, and nuts	Protein, thiamin, riboflavin, niacin, vitamin B_6, folate (plant protein), vitamin B_{12} (only in animals); phosphorus, magnesium (plant sources), iron, zinc	2–3 oz cooked meat, poultry, or fish 1–1.5 cups cooked dry beans 4 tbsp peanut butter 2 eggs 2/3–1 cup nuts
Fruits	Carbohydrate, vitamin C, folate, magnesium, potassium, dietary fiber	1/4 cup dried fruit 1/2 cup cooked or canned fruit 3/4 cup juice 1 melon wedge 1/2 cup berries
Vegetables	Carbohydrate, vitamin C, vitamin A, folate, magnesium, potassium, dietary fiber	1/2 cup raw or cooked vegetables 1 cup raw leafy vegetables 3/4 cup vegetable juice
Bread, cereal, rice, and pasta	Carbohydrate, thiamin, riboflavin (if enriched), niacin, folate (whole grains and enriched), magnesium (whole grains and enriched), iron (if enriched), zinc, dietary fiber	1 slice bread 1 oz (3/4 cup) ready-to-eat cereal 1/2 cup cooked cereal, rice, or pasta 1/2 hamburger roll, bagel, or English muffin 3–4 plain crackers 1 small roll, biscuit, or muffin one 6" tortilla
Fats, oils, and sweets	These foods should not replace any foods from the other groups; amounts consumed are determined by energy needs	

Table 7.3. **SAMPLE MENU GUIDED BY THE FOOD GUIDE PYRAMID**

Meal	Servings/Groups[a]
Breakfast	
1 peach	1 fruit
1.5 cups dry cereal	2 bread
1/2 cup low-fat milk	1/2 milk
1 slice bread	1 bread
1 tsp. butter	1 fat/sweet
Coffee (black)	
Lunch	
Chicken sandwich,	
2 slices bread	2 bread
2 oz chicken, 2 tsp mustard	1 meat
1 orange	1 fruit
2 small chocolate chip cookies	2 fat/sweet
1 diet soda	
Snack	
2 English muffin	2 bread
tsp. peanut butter	1/4 meat
1/2 cup yogurt	1/2 milk
Dinner	
Salad	
1 cup lettuce	1 vegetable
1/2 cup cucumber	1 vegetable
1 Tbs. salad dressing	1 fat/sweet
1/2 carrot	1/2 vegetable
3 oz fish (halibut)	1 meat
Small potato	1 bread
3/4 cup green beans	1 vegetable
1 tsp butter	1 fat/sweet
1 diet soda	
Snack	
2 cups cottage cheese	1 milk

[a] Milk: milk, yogurt and cheese group; Meat: Meat, poultry, fish, dry beans, eggs, and nuts group; Bread: bread, cereal, rice, and pasta group; Fat/sweet: fats, oils, and sweets group; fruit: fruit group
Nutrient summary:
1800 kcal
Carbohydrate: 55% of total kcal
Protein: 20% of total kcal
Fat: 25% of total kcal

older person. Weight gain on a 1600- to 1800-kcal diet suggests the necessity to gradually increase energy expenditure with regular physical activity.

When planning menus with the Food Guide Pyramid keep in the following points in mind:

- Each food in a group is deficient in at least one essential nutrient; thus no one food provides complete nutrition.
- Each food group is deficient in at least one essential nutrient, thus obtaining foods from the different groups becomes important.
- Choosing a variety of foods from all groups provides the essential nutrients for good health.
- Foods within a group differ with respect to nutrient and energy content. Thus, one must exercise care in both selection and quantity to ensure adequate nutrition without excess energy intake.
- The nutritional adequacy of the Pyramid depends on choosing a variety of foods from each of the food groups.
- Choose primarily low-fat and nonfat items from the milk, yogurt, and cheese group.
- Include protein-rich plant foods such as beans several times per week.
- Include a dark green vegetable each day as a rich source of vitamin A and vitamin C.
- Choose whole-grain varieties of breads, cereals, rice, and pasta often.

A Word About Serving Size

Much confusion exists about serving size and portion size. For example, the USDA defines a standard *serving* of pasta as one-half cup, while the Food and Drug Administration, which regulates food labels, claims a standard serving is one cup. Contrast these sizes with a typical restaurant pasta *portion* that averages about three cups—equal to six servings from the Food Guide Pyramid. To add further confusion, most people consider a serving to be the amount of food they typically consume (actually a portion) when, for the government's purpose, it represents a far smaller standard unit of measure. Within the perspective of "real world" standards and government standards, the USDA recommendation to consume 6 to 11 servings of grains or breads daily seems an unattainable goal. Keep in mind, however, that one serving by government standards represents a relatively small portion size: a 6-oz glass of fruit or vegetable juice; a medium-size orange, banana, or apple; one cup of salad greens, about the size of your fist; 1 egg; 1 cup of milk or yogurt; 1 slice of bread; two tablespoons of peanut butter, about the size of a ping-pong ball; one-half cup of chopped fruits and vegetables; three medium asparagus spears, eight carrot sticks, one ear of corn; one-fourth cup of dried fruit like raisins; 3 oz of meat, fish, or poultry, about the size of a deck of playing cards; a teaspoon of butter or mayonnaise, the size of a fingertip; or 2 oz of cheese, the size equivalent of two whole thumbs.

The 5th edition of *Dietary Guidelines for Americans 2000* recommends diet and lifestyle choices to promote health, support physically active lives, and reduce chronic disease risks. It also includes advice to exercise moderately for 30 minutes (e.g., walking, jogging, bicycling, and lawn, garden, and house work) "most, preferably all, days of the week." The *Guidelines* advise children to exercise moderately for 60 minutes daily. They acknowledge that good nutrition and regular exercise provide an important approach to ensure good health and combat the obesity epidemic in the United States. The *Guidelines* separate fruits and vegetables from grains and emphasize whole grain consumption.

TEN SUPER FOODS YOU SHOULD EAT

1. Cantaloupe
A quarter of a delicious melon supplies almost as much vitamin A and C as most people need in an entire day

2. Sweet potatoes
A nutritional All-Star - one of the best vegetables you can eat. They're loaded with carotenoids, vitamin C, potassium, and fiber. Mix in unsweetened applesauce or crushed pineapple for extra moisture and sweetness

3. Fat free (skim) or low-fat milk (1%, not 2%)
Excellent source of calcium, vitamins, and protein with little or no artery-clogging fat and cholesterol. (Soy milk can have just as many nutrients - if the company adds them.)

4. Salmon or other fatty fish
The omega-3 fats in fish, especially fatty fish like salmon, swordfish, and rainbow trout, can help reduce the risk of sudden-death heart attacks.

5. Oranges
Great-tasting and rich in vitamin C, folic acid and fiber

6. Broccoli
Lots of vitamin C, carotenoids, and folic acid.

7. Whole-grain bread
It's higher in fiber and about a dozen vitamins and minerals than enriched white bread or "wheat" bread"

8. 100% bran cereal
A half-cup serving provides about one-third of the fiber you need for an entire day -to reduce the risk of constipation, diverticulosis, and heart disease.

9. Beans
Inexpensive, low in fat, and rich in protein, iron, folic acid, and fiber. Choose garbanzo, pinto, black, navy, kidney or lentils. Eat them as a side dish or snack, in a tortilla with salsa, or in soup.

10 Spinach or kale
Loaded with vitamin C, carotenoids, calcium and fiber. Steam 'em and eat 'em.

LIMITATIONS OF THE FOOD GUIDE PYRAMID

- Grouping all fats and oils together (with sweets) fails to distinguish differences among good fats (olive oil and canola oil, high in monounsaturated fats and omega-3 fatty acids), which fend off heart disease by relaxing arteries and fighting inflammation, and harmful saturated fats and *trans*-unsaturated fatty acids in margarine, salad dressing, cookies, potato chips, French fries, and other fast or processed foods

- Vegetable category includes potatoes, which are mainly starch

- Fails to distinguish between high-fat and low-fat dairy products

- Grouping protein-containing meat, poultry, fish, dry beans, eggs, and nuts together does not recognize the various protein sources and their different effects on health

- Does not clarify differences between refined carbohydrates (white rice, white bread, refined cereal grains) and the more nutritious, fiber-rich healthful ones (whole grains, brown rice)

- Gives no emphasis to the role of daily exercise and weight control, which some argue should form the base of any pyramid designed to implement long-term health

USING THE DIETARY GUIDELINES

Proper use of the *Dietary Guidelines* produces nutritional practices that can reduce the incidence of obesity, hypertension, heart disease, and type 2 diabetes. Implementation involves making changes in typical food choices to adhere more closely to guideline recommendations. TABLE 7.4 lists examples of food substitutions that apply the *Dietary Guidelines*.

American Heart Association Recommendations

The most recent dietary guidelines from the American Heart Association (AHA; www.americanheart.org/) for the general public over the age of 2 years (formerly known as the "Step 1" diet) address the growing rates of obesity, hypertension, and type 2 diabetes in the United States.[77,83] Because of the strong association between excess body weight and cardiovascular disease, the recommendations also emphasize achieving and maintaining a healthful body weight. Lifestyle modifications include increasing the level of regular physical activity and eliminating all tobacco. These guidelines are essentially similar to guidelines from other agencies (including the USDA). They place great emphasis on the adoption of healthy eating patterns and lifestyle behaviors instead of targeting specific numeric goals as in the number of grams to consume for dietary fat. TABLE 7.5 outlines four major goals and associated guidelines for the general population; TABLE

Table 7.4. EXAMPLES OF APPROPRIATE SUBSTITUTIONS TO BRING EXISTING EATING BEHAVIORS MORE IN LINE WITH THE *DIETARY GUIDELINES*

If you eat this	Try this
White bread	Whole-wheat or whole grain bread
Breakfast cereal with sugar	Low-sugar cereal; shredded wheat
Cole slaw/potato salad	Bean salad with yogurt
Chips/salty snacks	Low salt, baked pretzels
Donuts	Bran muffin; corn bread
Vegetables, boiled	Vegetables steamed
Vegetables, canned	Vegetables frozen
Fried foods	Broiled or barbecued
Whole milk	Nonfat or low-fat milk
Ice cream	Sherbet or frozen yogurt
Mayonnaise-based salad dressing	Oil and vinegar or diet dressings
Cookies	Air-popped corn
Salted foods	Flavor foods with herbs and spices or lemons

7.6 presents specific dietary recommendations for the general population and for those men and women at higher disease risk (formerly known as the "Step 2" diet).

The principle message advises consuming a varied but balanced diet. To maintain a healthful body weight, attention must focus on portion size and number. Importance is placed on consuming a diet rich in fruits and vegetables, cereals and whole grains, nonfat and low-fat dairy products, legumes, nuts, fish, poultry, and lean meats.[7,35,59,85]

In July 2002, the AHA updated its guidelines (*Guide to the Primary Prevention of Cardiovascular Diseases*) for preventing heart attacks and strokes, listing secondhand smoke for the first time as a risk factor. They also recommend screening for risk factors beginning at age 20 and every 5 years thereafter to asses smoking habits, family medical history, and blood pressure. Men should maintain a waistline of 40 inches or less and women, 35 inches or less. Persons 40 years of age and older should be screened for additional risk factors such as cholesterol levels. Based on the latest research, the new guidelines drop passages recommending hormone supplements and antioxidant vitamins to reduce cardiovascular risk. Also, a daily dose of aspirin, previously recommended for individuals who have already suffered a heart attack or stroke, is now suggested for those whose risk assessment indicates at least a 10% risk of a heart attack in the next decade.

AN EXPANDING EMPHASIS ON HEALTHFUL EATING AND REGULAR PHYSICAL ACTIVITY

Scientists have responded to the rapidly rising number of adults and children who are overweight or obese and the

The ABCs of Good Nutrition: Applying the Dietary Guidelines for Americans

The current (2000) version of the *Dietary Guidelines for Americans* (http://www.usda.gov/cnpp), jointly developed by the U.S. Department of Agriculture and Department of Health and Human Services, represents medical and scientific consensus as a foundation for nutrition education for healthy Americans 2 years of age and older. When followed, the guidelines provide a prudent road map to reduce chronic disease risk and ensure nutritional adequacy.

One should learn the ABCs of the Dietary Guidelines and how to apply them to individual situations. After reviewing this information, you can evaluate your dietary habits, strengths, and shortcomings in comparison to the recommendations (Table 1).

DIETARY GUIDELINES FOR AMERICANS

The ABCs of the *D*ietary Guidelines consist of three components: (1) AIM FOR FITNESS, (2) BUILD A HEALTHY BASE, and (3) CHOOSE SENSIBLY. Refer to the following web site for more specific up-to-date information: http://www.pueblo.gsa.gov/cic_text/food/dietguide2000/toc.htm

AIM FOR FITNESS

1. *Aim for a healthy body weight as categorized by the body mass index (BMI).* Maintain or improve body weight. See Chapter 13 for a discussion about the BMI, and consult the following web site for easy means of computation: http://www.keepkidshealthy.com/welcome/bmicalculator.html
2. *Become more physically active each day.* Balance food intake with regular physical activity. The following web site provides handy calculators to estimate calorie expenditure during exercise, determine target heart rates, and even compute how much exercise "burns off" your favorite desert: http://my.webmd.com/content/tools/1/calc_dessert.htm?2-3628_81000_0000_07_04

BUILD A HEALTHY BASE

1. Let the Food Guide Pyramid (page 194) guide your food choices. http://www.nal.usda.gov/fnic/Fpyr/pymid.gif
2. Choose diverse grains on a daily basis, particularly unrefined, whole grains. http://www.cspinet.org/nah/wwheat.html

3. Choose a variety of fruits and vegetables daily.
4. Keep food safe to eat. http://www.fightbac.org/main.cfm

CHOOSE SENSIBLY

1. Choose a diet low in saturated fat and cholesterol and moderate in total fat. Eliminate *trans* fatty acids when possible.
2. Choose beverages and foods that lower intake of refined simple sugars. http://www.usda.gov/cnpp
3. Choose and prepare foods with less salt. http://www.pueblo.gsa.gov/cic_text/food/dietguide2000/lesssalt.htm
4. Drink alcoholic beverages in moderation. Some persons should not drink alcoholic beverages at all. http://www.pueblo.gsa.gov/cic_text/food/dietguide2000/alcohol.htm

APPLYING THE DIETARY GUIDELINES

Once you understand the *Dietary Guidelines* you can assess your diet and fitness goals in relation to them. Assessment also helps you make wise decisions about changing current diet and exercise habits.

CASE STUDY/PERSONAL HEALTH AND EXERCISE NUTRITION 7–1 *(continued)*

Table 1   THE ABCs OF YOUR DIETARY HABITS

Part I. Aim for Fitness

1. Determine your BMI.   _____

                                                                                                          Evaluation:

2. Choose a physical activity that you do (e.g., jogging). Calculate the calories (kcal) you burn do-   Activity: _____
   ing this activity for 10 and 45 minutes. How long would you have to do this activity to offset the   kcal in 10 minutes _____
   calories in one small bag of M&Ms?   kcal in 45 minutes _____

                                                                                                          Number of minutes _____

3. Determine your target heart rate (THR) for aerobic exercise training.   THR =

4. Determine how many calories you need to maintain your current level of body weight.   Calories =

5. Determine the number of calories in one pound of body fat.   Calories =

Part II. Build a Healthy Base

1. Draw and label the Food Guide Pyramid.

2. List five foods you eat often and the corresponding Pyramid category.   Food _____ Category

                                                                                                          Food _____ Category

                                                                                                          Food _____ Category

                                                                                                          Food _____ Category

                                                                                                          Food _____ Category

   Identify one whole-grain cereal that you eat.   Whole grain cereal _____

   Identify one whole-grain bread that you eat.   Whole grain bread _____

   Identify one whole-grain food that you eat.   Whole grain food _____

3. List the four principles of food safety and give an example of each from your experience   1.

                                                                                                          2.

                                                                                                          3.

                                                                                                          4.

4. List one food as a potential source of harmful microorganisms. Have you ever eaten this food?   Food _____
   Any consequences?   Consequences:

Part III. Choose Sensibly

Go to the Interactive Healthy Eating Index at the USDA site [http://147.208.9.133/]. Enter the food
you ate yesterday and compare your Healthy Eating Index score with the recommendations. View
your personal Food Guide Pyramid.

Table 7.5 NUTRITIONAL GUIDELINES FOR THE GENERAL POPULATION

Population Goals	Major Guidelines
Overall healthy eating pattern	• Consume a varied diet that includes foods from each of the major food groups with an emphasis on fruits, vegetables, whole grains, low-fat or nonfat dairy products, fish, legumes, poultry, and lean meats. • Monitor portion size and number to ensure adequate, not excess, intake.
Appropriate body weight BMI ≤25[a]	• Match energy intake to energy needs. • When weight loss is desirable, make appropriate changes to energy intake and expenditure (physical activity). • Limit foods with a high sugar content, and those with a high caloric density.
Desirable cholesterol profile	• Limit foods high in saturated fat, *trans* fat, and cholesterol. • Substitute unsaturated fat from vegetables, fish, legumes, and nuts.
Desirable blood pressure Systolic <140 mm Hg Diastolic <90 mm Hg	• Maintain a healthy body weight. • Consume a varied diet with an emphasis on vegetables, fruits, and low-fat or nonfat dairy products. • Limit sodium intake. • Limit alcohol intake.

Modified from Krauss RM, et al. AHA dietary guidelines revision 2000: a statement for healthcare professionals from the Nutrition Committee of the American Heart Association. Circulation 2000;102:2284.
[a] BMI, body mass index (kg/m²).

increasing incidence of comorbidities associated with the overweight condition. In September, 2002, the Institute of Medicine (www.iom.edu/), the medical division of the National Academies, issued guidelines as part of their *Dietary Reference Intakes* (see Chapter 2).[33] They recommend that Americans spend at least *one hour* (about 400–500 kcal) over the course of each day in moderately intense physical activity (brisk walking, swimming, or cycling) to maintain health and normal body weight. This amount of regular physical activity—based on an assessment of the amount of exercise healthy persons engage in each day—represents twice as much as previously recommended in 1996 in a report from the United States Surgeon General! The advice is in agreement with the 2003 recommendations by the World

Health Organization (WHO; www.who.int) and the Food and Agriculture Organization of the United Nations. It represents a bold increase in exercise duration considering that *(a)* 30 minutes of similar type exercise on most days significantly decreases disease risk and *(b)* more than 60% of the U.S. population fails to incorporate even a moderate level of exercise into their lives, and 25% do no exercise at all. Underlying the Institute's 60-minute exercise recommendation is the belief that 30 minutes of daily exercise burns insufficient calories to prevent weight gain; thus, a greater amount of regular exercise becomes necessary.

The team of 21 experts also recommended for the first time a range for macronutrient intake plus how much dietary fiber to consume in the daily diet (previous reports over the past

Table 7.6 SPECIFIC DIETARY RECOMMENDATIONS FOR THE GENERAL POPULATION AND FOR THOSE MEN AND WOMEN AT HIGHER DISEASE RISK

For the General Population	For Populations at Higher Risk[a]
• Restrict total fat to ≤30% of total calories. • Restrict saturated fat to <10% of total calories. • Limit the total intake of cholesterol-raising fatty acids (saturated and *trans*) to ≤10% of calories. • Limit cholesterol intake to <300 mg/day. • Replace cholesterol-raising fatty acids with whole grains and unsaturated fatty acids from fish, vegetables, legumes, and nuts. • Limit sodium intake to ≤2400 mg/day (≤6.0 g/day of salt). • If alcohol is consumed, limit intake to 2 drinks/day for men, 1 drink/day for women. • Eat at least 2 servings of fish per week. • Eat 5 or more servings of vegetables and fruits per day. • Eat 6 or more servings of grain products per day. • Emphasize daily intake of low-fat or nonfat dairy products.	*Elevated LDL-cholesterol or Preexisting cardiovascular disease* • Restrict saturated fat to <7% of total calories. • Limit cholesterol intake to <200 mg/day. • Weight loss when appropriate. • Include soy protein with isoflavones. *Dyslipidemia characterized by low HDL-cholesterol, elevated triglycerides, and small, dense LDL* • Replace saturated fat calories with unsaturated fat. • Limit carbohydrate intake, especially sugars and refined carbohydrates. • Weight loss when appropriate. • Increase physical activity. *Diabetes mellitus and insulin resistance* • Restrict saturated fat to <7% of total calories. • Limit cholesterol intake to <200 mg/day. • When selecting carbohydrates, choose those with high fiber content.

Modified from Krauss RM, et al. AHA dietary guidelines revision 2000: a statement for healthcare professionals from the Nutrition Committee of the American Heart Association. Circulation 2000;102:2284.
[a] Elevated LDL, low-density lipoprotein cholesterol; low HDL, high-density lipoprotein cholesterol.

60 years have dealt only with micronutrient recommendations). These recommendations are intended for professional nutritionists and the general public. To meet daily energy and nutrient needs while minimizing risk for chronic diseases such as heart disease and type 2 diabetes, adults should consume between 45 and 65% of their total calories from carbohydrates. This relatively wide range provides for flexibility, in recognition that both the high-carbohydrate, low-fat diet of Asian peoples and the higher-fat diet of peoples from the Mediterranean region, with its high monounsaturated fatty acid olive oil content, contribute to good health. The maximum intake of added sugars—the caloric sweeteners added to manufactured foods and beverages such as soda, candy, fruit drinks, cakes, cookies, and ice cream—is placed at 25% of total calories. The panel suggested that this relatively high 25% level represented the threshold above which a significant decline would occur for several important micronutrients such as vitamin A and calcium. This recommendation was considerably above WHO's 2003 recommendation of 10%. Acceptable lipid intake ranges between 20 and 35% of caloric intake, a range at the lower end of most recommendations and at the upper end of the 30% limit set by the AHA, American Cancer Society, and National Institutes of Health. The panel noted that very low fat intake combined with high intake of carbohydrate tends to lower HDL-cholesterol and raise triacylglycerol levels. Conversely, high intake of dietary fat (and accompanying increased caloric intake) contributes to obesity and its related medical complications. Moreover, high-fat diets usually link with an increased saturated fatty acid intake, raising plasma LDL-cholesterol concentrations, which further potentiates coronary heart disease risk. "As low as possible" saturated fat intake was recommended; the panel also recognized that no safe level existed for *trans* fatty acid intake.

Recommended protein intake ranges between 10 and 35% of calories, which remains consistent with prior recommendations. For the first time, age-based recommendations are provided for all of the essential amino acids contained in dietary protein. TABLE 7.7 presents an example of the macronutrient composition for a 2500-kcal diet based on these new guidelines.

The panel also recommended that adult men age 50 and younger should consume 38 g of fiber daily, and adult women, 21 g a day, values significantly above the 12 to 15 g currently consumed. For adults over the age of 50 who typically eat less food, the recommended intake equals 30 g of fiber for men and 21 g of fiber for women. Particularly important is the consumption of water-soluble fibers (pectin from fruits and oat and rice bran); these reduce plasma cholesterol levels and slow digestion to increase satiety and decrease the risk of overeating.

Clearly, no one food or meal provides optimal nutrition and associated health-related benefits. Perhaps the following statement best summarizes the metabolic, epidemiologic, and clinical trial evidence over the past several decades regarding diet and lifestyle behaviors and coronary heart disease:[58]

> Substantial evidence indicates that diets using nonhydrogenated unsaturated fats as the predominant form of dietary fat, whole grains as the main form of carbohydrates, an abundance of fruits and vegetables, and adequate omega-3 fatty acids can offer significant protection against coronary heart disease. Such diets, together with regular physical activity, avoidance of smoking, and maintenance of a healthy body weight, may prevent the majority of cardiovascular disease in Western populations.

MEDITERRANEAN AND VEGETARIAN DIET PYRAMIDS

The two bottom illustrations in Figure 7.2 present modifications of the basic pyramid for application to individuals whose diet consists largely of *(a)* foods from the plant kingdom (**Vegetarian Diet Pyramid**) or *(b)* fruits, nuts, vegetables, legumes, and all manner of unrefined grains, and protein derived from fish, beans, and chicken, with dietary fat composed mostly of monounsaturated fatty acids with mild ethanol consumption (**Mediterranean Diet Pyramid**). A Mediterranean-type diet—possibly mediated via several plant foods in the diet—substantially reduces the rate of recurrence after a first myocardial infarction.[26] Its high monounsaturated fatty acid content (generally olive oil with its associated phytochemicals[147]) also staves off age-related memory loss, heart disease, cancer, and overall mortality rate in healthy, elderly people.[82,146,155] Dietary focus of all three pyramids on fruits and vegetables, particularly cruciferous and green leafy vegetables and citrus fruit and juice, also reduces risk for ischemic stroke[67] and may enhance the beneficial effects of cholesterol-lowering drugs.[68]

PERSONAL ASSESSMENT

An objective assessment of energy and nutrient intake provides the frame of reference for judging the adequacy of one's diet in relation to recommended guidelines. Such

Table 7.7	**POSSIBLE MACRONUTRIENT COMPOSITION OF A 2500-KCAL DIET BASED ON RECOMMENDATIONS OF EXPERT PANEL OF THE INSTITUTE OF MEDICINE, NATIONAL ACADEMIES.**

	Composition of 2500-kcal Intake		
	Carbohydrate	*Lipid*	*Protein*
Percentage	60	15	25
kcal	1500	375	625
Grams	375	94	69
Ounces	13.2	3.3	2.4

determinations from careful daily food intake records provide a reasonably close estimate compared with more direct measurements. Appendix C outlines the *Three-Day Dietary Survey* procedure to assess a diet's adequacy.

Diet Quality

The **Diet Quality Index** appraises the "healthfulness" of one's diet; it gives a score based on a composite of the eight food-and-nutrient-based recommendations of the National Academy of Sciences.[101] This index, presented in FIGURE 7.3, offers a simple scoring schema based on the risk gradient associated with diet and the major diet-related chronic diseases. It evaluated the diets of participants in three national surveys conducted in the United States between 1965 and 1989–91.[123] Respondents who meet or exceed a given dietary goal receive a score of 0; a score of 1 applies to an intake that falls within 30% of a dietary goal; the score becomes 2 when intake fails to fall within 30% of the goal. The

scores for all eight categories are then totaled. The index ranges from 0 to 16, with the lower score representing a higher quality diet. A score of *4 or less* reflects a more healthful diet, while an index of *10 or higher* pinpoints a less healthful diet needing improvement.

The Healthy Eating Index

The USDA designed the **Healthy Eating Index (HEI)** presented in TABLE 7.8 for nutrition promotion activities and to monitor changes in diet quality over time. This 100-point analytic tool evaluates how well a person's diet conforms to such recommendations as the Food Guide Pyramid and *Dietary Guidelines for Americans* based on dietary balance, moderation, and variety.[45,158] Total scores can range from a "poor" diet (HEI score, 65) to a "good" diet (HEI score, >85), with 65 to 74 and 75 to 84 in between. HEI scores for each component of the index are defined as "poor" (score, <5), "needs improvement" (score between 5 and 8), and "good" (score, >8).

MACRONUTRIENT NEEDS FOR THE PHYSICALLY ACTIVE

Many physically active individuals receive either inadequate or incorrect information concerning prudent dietary practices. *Research in exercise nutrition, although far from complete, indicates that the large number of teenagers and adults, including competitive athletes, who exercise regularly to keep fit do not require additional nutrients beyond those obtained through the regular intake of a nutritionally well-balanced diet.*

What the Physically Active Actually Eat

Inconsistencies exist among studies that relate diet quality to physical activity level and/or physical fitness. Some studies have shown a positive association between healthier diets and higher physical activity levels, while others have not. Part of the inconsistency results from use of relatively crude and imprecise self-reported measures of physical activity, small sample size, or unreliable dietary assessments.[29,42,47,92] TABLE 7.9 contrasts the nutrient and energy intakes with national dietary recommendations of a large population-based cohort of nearly 8000 men and 2500 women classified as low, moderate, and high for cardiorespiratory fitness who participated in the Aerobics Center Longitudinal Study. The most significant findings of this study indicate:

- A progressively lower body mass index for both men and women with increasing levels of physical fitness
- Remarkably small differences in energy intake in relation to physical fitness classification for women (≤94 kcal per day) and men (≤82 kcal per day),

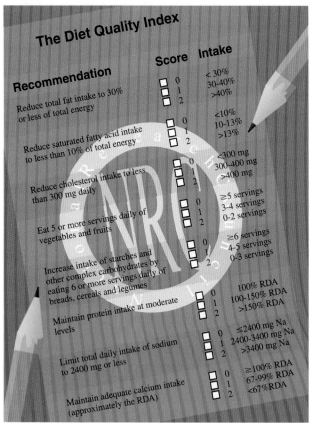

■ **Figure 7.3** The Diet Quality Index assesses risk for chronic diseases associated with overall dietary pattern. A score of 0 indicates that a respondent's diet meets the desired dietary goal for the item; a score of 1 means the intake falls within 30% of the goal; and an intake that fails to fall within 30% of the goal receives a score of 2. Scores are then added (range from 0 to 16), with the lower score indicating a better quality of diet. (From National Research Council, Committee on Diet and Health. Diet and health implications for reducing chronic disease risk. Washington, DC: National Academy Press, 1989.)

Table 7.8 **COMPONENTS OF THE HEALTHY EATING INDEX**[a]

Component	Scoring Range	Criteria for Maximum Score of 10	Criteria for Minimum Score of 0
Grain consumption	0–10	9[b,c] or 7.4[d] servings	0 servings
Vegetable consumption	0–10	4[b,c] or 3.5[d] servings	0 servings
Fruit consumption	0–10	3[b,c] or 2.5[d] servings	0 servings
Milk consumption	0–10	3[b] or 2[c,d] servings	0 servings
Meat consumption	0–10	2.4[b,c] or 2.2[d] servings	0 servings
Total fat intake	0–10	≤30% of energy from fat	≥45% of energy from fat
Saturated fat intake	0–10	<10% of energy from saturated fat	≥15% of energy from saturated fat
Cholesterol intake	0–10	≤300 mg	≥450 mg
Sodium intake	0–10	≤2400 mg	≥4800 mg
Dietary variety	0–10	≥24 different items over 3 days	≤9 different items over 3 days

Modified from Krauss RM, et al. AHA dietary guidelines revision 2000: a statement for healthcare professionals from the Nutrition Committee of the American Heart Association. Circulation 2000;102:2284.
[a] Intakes between the maximum and minimum cutoffs were assigned scores proportionally.
[b] For women aged 20–24 years
[c] For women aged 25–50 years
[d] For women aged ≥51 years

with the moderate fitness group consuming the fewest calories for both sexes
- A progressively higher dietary fiber intake and significantly lower cholesterol intake across fitness categories
- Men and women with higher fitness levels generally consumed diets that more closely approached dietary recommendations (with respect to dietary fiber, percentage of energy from total fat, percentage of energy from saturated fat, and dietary cholesterol) than peers of lower fitness

Endurance athletes and others who engage regularly in intense training must maintain adequate energy and protein intake and appropriate carbohydrate consumption to match this macronutrient's use for energy during exercise. Attention to proper diet does not mean that a physically active person must join the ranks of the more than 40% of Americans who take supplements (spending about $6 billion yearly) to micromanage nutrient intake.

FIGURE 7.4 lists the recommended intakes for protein, lipid, and carbohydrate and food sources for these macronutrients for active men and women. A daily energy requirement of 2000 kcal for women and 3000 kcal for men represents average values for typical young U.S. adults. *After meeting basic nutrient requirements (as recommended in Figure 7.4), a variety of food sources based on individual preference supply the extra energy needs for physical activity.*

Proteins

As discussed in Chapter 1, 0.8 g per kilogram of body mass (0.35 g·lb^{-1}) represents the RDA for protein intake. Thus, a person weighing 77 kg (170 lb) requires about 62 g or 2.2 oz of protein daily. Assuming that even during exercise rela-

tively little protein loss occurs through energy metabolism (an assumption not entirely correct), this protein recommendation remains adequate for most active individuals. Also, the protein intake for the typical American significantly exceeds the protein RDA; the competitive athlete's diet usually contains two to four times more protein than recommended values. One nutritional dilemma for the physically active vegetarian concerns obtaining an adequate balance of essential amino acids from a diet that obtains its protein from the plant kingdom. Chapter 1 discusses the use of complementary protein food sources to minimize this problem. It remains unclear if physically active children and adolescents require more protein for optimal growth and development than their sedentary counterparts.

Is the RDA Really Enough?

Studies of human protein needs in the mid-1800s postulated that muscular contraction destroyed a portion of the muscle's protein content to provide energy for biologic work. Based on this belief, prevailing wisdom recommended a high-protein diet for persons involved in heavy physical labor to provide for the structural content of skeletal muscle and its energy needs. In many ways, many modern-day athletes mimic these beliefs and practices. For men and women who devote considerable time and effort training with resistive equipment, dietary protein often represents their most important macronutrient. For one reason, many believe that resistance training in some way damages or "tears down" a muscle's inherent protein structure. This drain of muscle protein would require additional dietary protein above the RDA for subsequent tissue resynthesis to a new larger and more powerful state. In addition, many endurance athletes believe that training increases protein catabolism to sustain

Table 7.9　AVERAGE VALUES FOR NUTRIENT INTAKE BASED ON 3-DAY DIET RECORDS BY LEVELS OF CARDIORESPIRATORY FITNESS IN 7059 MEN AND 2453 WOMEN

Men

Variable	Low Fitness (N = 786)	Moderate Fitness (N = 2457)	High Fitness (N = 4716)
Demographic and health data			
Age (yr)	$47.3 \pm 11.1^{a,b}$	47.3 ± 10.3^{c}	48.1 ± 10.5
Apparently healthy (%)	$51.5^{a,b}$	69.1^{c}	77.0
Current smokers (%)	$23.4^{a,b}$	15.8^{c}	7.8
BMI (kg·m^{-2})	$30.7 \pm 5.5^{a,b}$	27.4 ± 3.7^{c}	25.1 ± 2.7
Nutrient data			
Energy (kcal)	2378.6 ± 718.6^{a}	2296.9 ± 661.9^{c}	2348.1 ± 664.3
Kcal·kg^{-1}·d^{-1}	25.0 ± 8.1^{a}	26.7 ± 8.4^{c}	29.7 ± 9.2
Carbohydrate (% kcal)	43.2 ± 9.4^{b}	44.6 ± 9.1^{c}	48.1 ± 9.7
Protein (% kcal)	18.6 ± 3.8	18.5 ± 3.8	18.1 ± 3.8
Total fat (% kcal)	36.7 ± 7.2^{b}	35.4 ± 7.1^{c}	32.6 ± 7.5
SFA (% kcal)	11.8 ± 3.2^{b}	11.3 ± 3.2^{c}	10.0 ± 3.2
MUFA (% kcal)	$14.5 \pm 3.2^{a,b}$	13.8 ± 3.1^{c}	12.6 ± 3.3
PUFA (% kcal)	$7.4 \pm 2.2^{a,b}$	7.5 ± 2.2	7.4 ± 2.3
Cholesterol (mg)	349.5 ± 173.2^{b}	314.5 ± 147.5^{c}	277.8 ± 138.5
Fiber (g)	21.0 ± 9.5^{b}	22.0 ± 9.7^{c}	26.2 ± 11.9
Calcium (mg)	$849.1 \pm 371.8^{a,b}$	860.2 ± 360.2^{c}	924.4 ± 386.8
Sodium (mg)	4317.4 ± 1365.7	4143.0 ± 1202.3	4133.2 ± 1189.4
Folate (μg)	336.4 ± 165.2^{b}	359.5 ± 197.0^{c}	428.0 ± 272.0
Vitamin B6 (mg)	2.4 ± 0.9^{b}	2.4 ± 0.9^{c}	2.8 ± 1.1
Vitamin B12 (μg)	6.6 ± 5.5^{a}	6.8 ± 6.0	6.6 ± 5.8
Vitamin A (RE)	$1372.7 \pm 1007.3^{a,b}$	1530.5 ± 1170.4^{c}	1766.3 ± 1476.0
Vitamin C (mg)	117.3 ± 80.4^{b}	129.2 ± 108.9^{c}	166.0 ± 173.2
Vitamin E (AE)	11.5 ± 9.1^{b}	12.1 ± 8.6^{c}	13.7 ± 11.4

Women

Variable	Low Fitness^{a,b} (N = 233)	Moderate Fitness^{c} (N = 730)	High Fitness (N = 1490)
Demographic and health data			
Age (yr)	47.5 ± 11.2^{b}	46.7 ± 11.6	46.5 ± 11.0
Apparently healthy (%)	$55.4^{a,b}$	71.1^{c}	79.3
Current smokers (%)	$12.0^{a,b}$	9.0^{c}	4.2
BMI (kg·m^{-2})	$27.3 \pm 6.7^{a,b}$	24.3 ± 4.9^{c}	22.1 ± 3.0
Nutrient data			
Energy (kcal)	1887.4 ± 607.5^{a}	1793.0 ± 508.2^{c}	1859.7 ± 514.7
Kcal·kg^{-1}·d^{-1}	27.1 ± 9.4^{a}	28.1 ± 8.8^{c}	31.7 ± 9.8
Carbohydrate (% kcal)	47.7 ± 9.6^{b}	48.2 ± 9.0^{c}	51.1 ± 9.4
Protein (% kcal)	17.6 ± 3.7^{a}	18.1 ± 3.9	17.7 ± 3.9
Total fat (% kcal)	34.8 ± 7.6^{b}	33.7 ± 6.8^{c}	31.3 ± 7.5
SFA (% kcal)	11.1 ± 3.3^{b}	10.6 ± 3.2^{c}	9.6 ± 3.1
MUFA (% kcal)	$13.4 \pm 3.4^{a,b}$	12.8 ± 3.0^{c}	11.9 ± 3.2
PUFA (% kcal)	7.5 ± 2.2	7.5 ± 2.2	7.4 ± 2.4
Cholesterol (mg)	244.7 ± 132.8^{b}	224.6 ± 115.6^{c}	204.1 ± 103.6
Fiber (g)	$18.9 \pm 8.2^{a,b}$	20.0 ± 8.3^{c}	23.2 ± 10.7
Calcium (mg)	$765.2 \pm 361.8^{a,b}$	774.6 ± 342.8^{c}	828.3 ± 372.1
Sodium (mg)	3350.8 ± 980.8	3256.7 ± 927.7	3314.4 ± 952.7
Folate (μg)	$301.8 \pm 157.6^{a,b}$	319.7 ± 196.2	356.2 ± 232.5
Vitamin B6 (mg)	2.0 ± 0.8^{b}	2.0 ± 0.8^{c}	2.2 ± 0.9
Vitamin B12 (μg)	4.7 ± 4.2	4.9 ± 4.2	5.0 ± 4.2
Vitamin A (RE)	1421.9 ± 1135.3^{b}	1475.1 ± 1132.9^{c}	1699.0 ± 1346.9
Vitamin C (mg)	116.7 ± 7.5^{b}	131.5 ± 140.0	153.5 ± 161.1
Vitamin E (AE)	10.8 ± 7.5	10.3 ± 6.5^{c}	11.5 ± 8.1

From Brodney S, et al. Nutrient intake of physically fit and unfit men and women. Med Sci Sports Exerc 2001;33:459.

BMI, body mass index; SFA, saturated fatty acid; PUFA, polyunsaturated fatty acid; MUFA, monounsaturated fatty acid; RE, retinol equivalents; AE, α-tocopherol units.

[a] Significant difference between low and moderate fitness. $P<.05$.

[b] Significant difference between low and high fitness. $P<.05$.

[c] Significant difference between moderate and high fitness. $P<.05$.

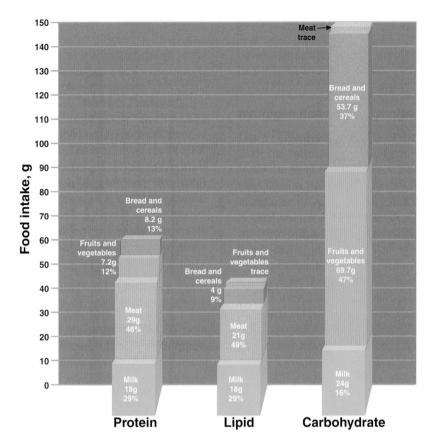

Figure 7.4 Basic recommendations for carbohydrate, lipid, and protein components and the general categories of food sources in a balanced diet.

the energy requirements of exercise, particularly when glycogen reserves are low. They thus believe that consuming added dietary protein offsets the protein–energy drain and provides building blocks to resynthesize depleted muscle mass. To some extent, the reasoning of both groups of athletes has merit. The relevant question, however, concerns whether the protein RDA provides a sufficient reserve should heavy training increase demands for protein synthesis and/or catabolism.

Some Modification Required for Recommended Protein Intake? Much of current understanding of protein dynamics in exercise derives from studies that expanded the classic method to determine protein breakdown by measuring urea excretion. For example, the output of "labeled" carbon dioxide from amino acids either injected or ingested increases during exercise in proportion to metabolic rate. As exercise progresses, the concentration of plasma urea also increases, coupled with a dramatic rise in nitrogen excretion in sweat. This often occurs without any change in urinary nitrogen excretion. These observations run counter to prior conclusions concerning minimal protein breakdown during endurance exercise, because the early studies only measured nitrogen in urine. FIGURE 7.5 illustrates that the sweat mechanism serves an important role in excreting the nitrogen from protein

breakdown during exercise. Furthermore, urea production does not reflect all aspects of protein breakdown because the oxidation of both plasma and intracellular leucine (a branched-chain essential amino acid) increases significantly during moderate exercise, independent of changes in urea production.[169]

Figure 7.5 also shows that protein use for energy reaches its highest level when subjects exercise in a glycogen-depleted state (indicated *low CHO*). This emphasizes the important role carbohydrate plays as a protein sparer. It further indicates that carbohydrate availability inhibits protein catabolism in exercise.[162] Protein breakdown for energy and its role in gluconeogenesis undoubtedly serve important needs in endurance exercise (or in frequent intense training) when glycogen reserves diminish.

Increased protein catabolism during endurance exercise and heavy training often mirrors the metabolic mixture during short-term starvation. With depleted glycogen reserves, gluconeogenesis from amino acid-derived carbon skeletons largely sustains the liver's glucose output. More than likely, augmented protein breakdown reflects the body's attempt to maintain blood glucose concentration for central nervous system functioning. *Eating a high-carbohydrate diet (with adequate energy intake) conserves muscle protein in individuals who engage in protracted hard training.* The poten-

Figure 7.5 Excretion of urea in sweat at rest, and during exercise after carbohydrate loading *(High CHO)* and carbohydrate depletion *(Low CHO)*. The largest use of protein (as reflected by sweat urea) occurs with low glycogen reserves. (From Lemon PWR, Nagel F. Effects of exercise on protein and amino acid metabolism. Med Sci Sports Exerc 1981;13:141.)

tial for increased protein use for energy (and the depression of protein synthesis) during strenuous exercise helps to explain why individuals who resistance-train to augment muscle size generally refrain from glycogen-depleting, endurance-type exercise.

The beginning phase of an exercise training regimen also places a transient but increased demand on body protein, perhaps resulting from both muscle injury and associated increased energy requirements. A continuing area of controversy concerns whether initial increased protein demand contributes to a true long-term increase in protein requirement above the RDA.[11,125] *Although a definitive answer remains elusive, protein breakdown above the resting level occurs during endurance exercise (and with resistance training) to a degree greater than previously believed.* Protein catabolism becomes most apparent when exercising with low carbohydrate reserves and/or low energy intake. Additionally, protein use may increase from a need to repair exercise-induced damaged tissue and from extra protein required for gains in lean tissue mass. Unfortunately, research has yet to pinpoint the protein requirements for individuals who train 4 to 6 hours daily by resistance-type exercise. These individuals' protein requirement may be only slightly greater than that of sedentary individuals, particularly if they consume normal amounts of carbohydrate.[150] Despite increased protein use for energy during heavy training, adaptations may augment the body's efficiency in dietary protein use and thus enhance amino acid balance.

One hopes that future research will target protein intake recommendations for individuals who typically use resis-

tance exercise to increase muscle size, strength, and power and individuals involved in prolonged endurance competitions and heavy training. *At this point, and without convincing evidence to the contrary, it seems safe to suggest that those in endurance training should consume between 1.2 and 1.4 g of high-quality protein per kg of body mass daily; those who resistance train may benefit from 1.6 g per kilogram of body mass.* This level of protein intake falls within the range typically consumed by physically active men and women, thus obviating the need to consume supplementary protein. Increase these values by 10% for vegetarians, to adjust for less-efficient digestion of plant protein. If protein intake remains adequate, consuming animal sources of protein does not facilitate muscle strength or size gains with resistance training compared with a similar protein intake from plant sources.[48]

Preparations of Simple Amino Acids

The usual reasons for using protein and amino supplements include stimulation of muscle growth and strength, enhanced energy capacity, and increased growth hormone output (see Chapter 12).[168] Supplement manufacturers often advertise that *only* simple amino acids are absorbed from the gut into the blood at a rate fast enough to stimulate muscle growth during resistance training. Male and female weightlifters, body builders, and other power athletes consume up to four times the RDA for protein.[73] This level of excess takes the form of liquids, powders, or pills of "purified" protein at a cost often in excess of $50 per pound of actual protein. Such preparations often contain proteins "predigested" to simple amino acids through chemical action in the laboratory. Advocates believe the body absorbs the simple amino acid molecule more readily (increased bioavailability) to optimize the expected muscle growth induced by training or to improve strength, power, and "vigor" in the short term for a heavy workout. This does not occur. The healthy intestine absorbs amino acids rapidly when they exist in more complex di- and tripeptide molecules, not just in simple amino acid form (see Chapter 3). The intestinal tract handles protein quite efficiently in its more complex form. A concentrated amino acid solution creates an osmotic effect that draws water into the intestine, often precipitating irritation, cramping, and diarrhea. In addition, carbohydrate remains the preferred energy source to power the anaerobic energy system primarily relied on in resistance training. Multiple sets of single exercises can reduce a muscle's glycogen content by 40%. *Simply stated, adequate research design and methodology has not shown that protein (amino acid) supplementation in any form above the RDA significantly increases muscle mass or improves muscular strength, power, or endurance.* Most individuals obtain adequate protein to sustain muscle growth with resistance training by consuming ordinary foods in a well-balanced diet. Provided caloric intake balances energy output by consuming a wide variety of foods, no need exists to consume supplements of protein or simple amino acids.

Lipids

Standards for optimal lipid intake are not firmly established. The amount of dietary lipid varies widely according to personal taste, money spent on food, and the availability of lipid-rich foods. For example, lipid furnishes only about 10% of the energy in the average diet of people living in Asia, whereas in many Western countries lipid accounts for 40 to 45% of the energy intake. *To promote good health, lipid intake should probably not exceed 30% of the diet's energy content. Of this, at least 70% should come from unsaturated fatty acids.* For those who consume a Mediterranean-type diet, rich in monounsaturated fatty acids, a somewhat higher total fat percentage (35–40%) becomes tolerable.

No exercise performance benefit occurs by reducing the percentage lipid intake below the 30% value. In fact, significant reductions in dietary lipid compromise exercise performance. A diet of 20% lipid produced poorer endurance performance scores than a diet of identical caloric value containing about 40% lipid.[117] Such findings further fuel the controversy concerning the importance of dietary lipid for individuals involved in heavy training and endurance competition (see "High-Fat versus Low-Fat Diets for Training and Endurance" in Chapter 8).[50,100] Consuming low-fat diets during strenuous training also creates difficulty in increasing carbohydrate and protein intake enough to furnish energy to maintain body weight and muscle mass. In addition, essential fatty acids and fat-soluble vitamins enter the body in dietary lipids; thus, sustaining a low-fat or "fat-free" diet could create a relative state of malnutrition. A low-fat diet (~20% total calories as lipid; see Chapter 12) also blunts the normal rise in plasma testosterone following a short-term bout of resistance exercise.[161] If additional research verifies these findings and if changes in hormonal milieu actually diminish training responsiveness and tissue synthesis, a low-fat intake may be contraindicated for heavy training.

Carbohydrates

The negative end of the nutrition continuum includes low-calorie "semistarvation" diets and other potentially harmful practices such as high-fat, low-carbohydrate diets, "liquid-protein" diets, or single-centered-food diets. These extremes counter good health, exercise performance, and optimum body composition. *A low-carbohydrate diet rapidly compromises energy reserves for vigorous physical activity or regular training.* Excluding sufficient carbohydrate energy from the diet causes an individual to train in a state of relative glycogen depletion; this may eventually produce "staleness" that hinders exercise performance.

The prominence of dietary carbohydrates varies widely throughout the world, depending on availability and relative cost of lipid-rich and protein-rich foods. Complex carbohydrate-rich foods (unrefined grains, starchy roots, and dried peas and beans) usually are cheapest compared with their energy value. In the Far East, carbohydrates (rice) contribute 80% of the total energy intake; in contrast, in the United States, carbohydrate supplies only about 40 to 50% of the energy intake. *No hazard to health exists when subsisting chiefly on a variety of fiber-rich complex unrefined carbohydrates, with adequate intake of essential amino acids, fatty acids, minerals, and vitamins.* The diet of the Tarahumara Indians of Mexico consists of high-fiber, complex carbohydrates (75% of calories) and correspondingly low intake of cholesterol (71 mg·day^{-1}), lipid (12% of calories), and saturated fat (2% of calories).[21] These nomads exhibit remarkable physical endurance. They reportedly run distances of up to 200 miles in a competitive soccer-type sports event that often lasts several days. This type of diet may also confer health benefits, because the Tarahumaras exhibit little or no hypertension, obesity, or death from cardiac and circulatory complications.

Stored muscle glycogen and blood-borne glucose become prime energy contributors in maximal exercise with inadequate oxygen supply to active muscles. Stored glycogen also provides substantial energy during intense levels of aerobic exercise. Consequently, dietary carbohydrate plays an important role for individuals who maintain a physically active lifestyle. *Their diet should contain at least 55 to 60% of calories as carbohydrates, predominantly starches from fiber-rich, unprocessed grains, fruits, and vegetables.* For competitive swimmers, rowers, and speed skaters, the importance of maintaining a relatively high daily carbohydrate intake relates more to the considerable and prolonged energy demands of their training than to the short-term demands of actual competition.

More Specific Carbohydrate Recommendations

Carbohydrate intake recommendations for physically active individuals assume that daily energy intake balances energy expenditure. Unless this condition exists, even consuming a relatively large *percentage* of carbohydrate calories will not adequately replenish this important energy macronutrient.

General recommendations for carbohydrate range between 6 and 10 g per kg of body mass per day. This amount will vary with an individual's daily energy expenditure and type of exercise performed. *Individuals undergoing heavy endurance training should consume on a daily basis 10 g of carbohydrate per kg of body mass.* Thus, the daily carbohydrate intake for a small 46-kg (100-lb) person who expends about 2800 kcal each day should be approximately 450 g, or 1800 kcal. In contrast, the person weighing 68 kg (150 lb) should consume 675 g of carbohydrate (2700 kcal) daily to sustain an energy requirement of 4200 kcal. In both examples, carbohydrates represent 65% of total energy intake. Chapter 12 presents specific diet–exercise techniques to facilitate glycogen storage in the days prior to endurance competition.

Carbohydrate and the "Overtraining Syndrome"

Endurance runners, swimmers, cross-country skiers, and cyclists frequently experience chronic fatigue in which successive days of hard training become progressively more difficult. Normal exercise performance usually deteriorates because the individual undergoes increasing difficulty recovering from exercise training. The overtrained condition, commonly termed the **overtraining syndrome**, represents more than just a short-term inability to train as hard as usual or a slight dip in competition-level performance. Rather, it reflects chronic fatigue experienced during workouts and in subsequent recovery periods. It also relates to increased incidence of infections, persistent muscle soreness, and general malaise and loss of interest in sustaining high-level training. Injuries occur more frequently in the overtrained state.[156] Specific symptoms of overtraining are highly individualized. The symptoms outlined in TABLE 7.10 generally represent the most common consequences of overtraining; they usually persist until the person rests. Complete recovery requires weeks or even months.

Depletion of carbohydrate reserves with repeated strenuous training probably contributes to the overtraining syndrome. FIGURE 7.6 illustrates that three successive days of running 16.1 km (10 miles) nearly depleted glycogen in the thigh muscle. This occurred even though the runners' diets contained 40 to 60% of total calories as carbohydrates. In addition, glycogen use on the third day of the run averaged about 72% less than use on day 1. Presumably, the body's fat reserves supplied the major energy for exercise.

It Takes Time to Replenish Glycogen

Even with a diet high in carbohydrates, muscle glycogen does not rapidly replenish to preexercise levels. It takes at least 24 hours to replenish muscle glycogen levels following prolonged exhaustive exercise; liver glycogen restores at a faster rate. *One to 2 days of rest (or lighter exercise) com-*

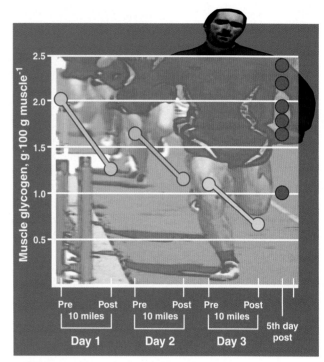

Figure 7.6 Average changes in muscle glycogen concentration for six male subjects before and after each 16.1-km run performed on three successive days. Muscle glycogen measured 5 days after the last run is referred to as "5th day post." (From Costill DL, et al. Muscle glycogen use during prolonged exercise on successive days. J Appl Physiol 1971;31:834.)

bined with a high-carbohydrate intake reestablishes preexercise muscle glycogen levels after exhaustive training or competition. Chapter 8 discusses in detail how to facilitate carbohydrate replenishment following exhaustive exercise.

Unmistakably, if a person performs unduly intense exercise on a regular basis, carbohydrate allowance must be adjusted to permit optimal glycogen resynthesis to maintain optimal training. This certainly provides a nutritional justification for the recommendation of many coaches and trainers to gradually reduce or *taper* the intensity of workouts several days before competition, while still maintaining a high-quality, carbohydrate-rich diet. TABLE 7.11 outlines practical nutritional guidelines to diminish the likelihood of chronic athletic fatigue or **staleness**. These guidelines were prepared for competitive swimmers, but the recommendations apply to all individuals in heavy training.

VITAMINS AND EXERCISE PERFORMANCE: THE ATHLETE'S DILEMMA

The money spent on dietary supplements in the United States continues to grow at a rate better than 10% per year. One report places the sale of dietary supplements at $17.1 billion in 2001. Worldwide sales of dietary supplements totaled

Table 7.10	THE OVERTRAINING SYNDROME: SYMPTOMS OF STALENESS

- Unexplained, persistently poor performance
- Disturbed mood states characterized by general fatigue, depression, and irritability
- Elevated resting pulse, painful muscles, and increased susceptibility to upper respiratory infections and gastrointestinal disturbances
- Insomnia
- Weight loss
- Overuse injuries

| Table 7.11 | **PRACTICAL NUTRITIONAL GUIDELINES FOR PREVENTION OF CHRONIC ATHLETIC FATIGUE AMONG ATHLETES**[a] |

- Consume easily digested high-carbohydrate drinks or solid foods 1–4 h before training and/or competition. Roughly 1 g of carbohydrate/kg body weight is the recommended intake 1 h before exercise, and up to 5 g of carbohydrate/kg body weight/h is suggested if the feeding occurs 4 h prior to exercise. For example, a 70-kg swimmer could drink 350 mL (12 oz) of a 20% carbohydrate beverage 1 h before exercise or eat 14 "energy bars," each containing 25 g carbohydrate, 4 h before exercise.
- Consume an easily digested, high-carbohydrate, liquid or solid food containing at least 0.35–1.5 g of carbohydrate/kg body weight/h immediately after exercise for the first 4 h after exercise. Thus, a 70-kg swimmer could drink 100–450 mL (3.6–16 oz) of a 25% carbohydrate beverage or 1–4.5 energy bars, each containing 25 g of carbohydrate, immediately after exercise and every hour thereafter for 4 h.
- Consume a 15–25% carbohydrate drink or a solid high-carbohydrate supplement with each meal. For example, reduce consumption of normal foods by 250 kcal and consume a high-carbohydrate beverage or solid food containing 250 kcal of carbohydrate with each meal.
- Maintain a stable body weight during all phases of training by matching energy consumption to the energy demands of training. This will also help maintain body carbohydrate reserves.

From Sherman WJ, Maglischo EW. Minimizing chronic athletic fatigue among swimmers: special emphasis on nutrition. Sports Sci Exchange, Gatorade Sports Sci Inst 1991;35(4).)

[a] In cooperation with a nutritionist or dietitian, athletes should maintain a record of foods consumed so that an accurate assessment can be made of total energy and total carbohydrate intake. Based on this assessment, dietary adjustments can be made to ensure that during intense training seasons, the athlete consumes roughly 10 g of carbohydrate/kg body weight daily.

nearly $32 billion in 1999, with an expected increase to $51 billion by 2010. Surveys show that over 158 million American consumers use dietary supplements. Vitamin–mineral pills represent the most common form of nutritional supplement used by the general public—they account for 70 to 90% of all supplements marketed. Estimates indicate that more than 40% of men and 50% of women age 60 and older use at least one vitamin or mineral supplement. Particularly susceptible marketing targets include the exercise enthusiast, the competitive athlete, and those who assist athletes to achieve peak performance. The following excerpts (including the letter writer's emphasis with underlining) come from a letter to a college athletic trainer from a physician extolling his concoction of micronutrients (with dosages as high as 15 to 25 times recommended levels) developed for the "unique" needs of the physically active individual. Such pseudoscientific promotional pitches from so-called experts continually bombard coaches, athletic trainers, and all individuals involved in regular exercise:

Dear _____:

I'm a physician with an interest in biochemistry and nutrition and the effects of both on athletes.

Today, good nutrition requires supplementation.

The product I developed is an "all-natural nutritional foundation for building strong, healthy bodies that perform at peak levels without harmful side effects. Using this formula, athletes notice increased energy and improved performance."

This product "is an alternative to steroids and other quick fixes."

This product "is the only complete supplement of its kind that combines 23 essential vitamins, miner-als and antioxidants in the proper amounts needed for powerful performance. (You may be startled to see how dramatically my formulation exceeds the RDAs.) The amounts shown on the back of this letter are based on the latest research in nutrition . . . NOT outdated government information."

While developing this product, "I consulted with world famous biochemists . . . collaborated with leading nutritionists (the same ones physicians have ignored for years) . . . walked miles of miles in health food stores . . . completed a comprehensive search of current medical literature."

The above letter applies the typical psychological "tools" of advertising: *respect for authority* (I'm a physician, of course I am correct), *safety* (try it, it can't hurt you and it might help); *disdain for the conventional wisdom of science and governmental agencies* (the new scientists have the answers but the "old club" will not publish them), *prestige by association* (I've checked with experts [unnamed biochemists and nutritionists] and gone to the library), and *if a little is good, more must be better* (you'll get a dose dramatically above recommended values). One of the few items missing is a testimonial from a renowned athlete, perhaps wearing a nostril-dilating adhesive strip!

More than 50% of athletes in certain sports consume vitamin–mineral supplements on a regular basis. They undertake such practices either to ensure adequate micronutrient intake or to achieve excess in hopes of enhancing exercise performance and training responsiveness.[17–19,72,103] If vitamin–mineral deficiencies become apparent in active people, they often occur among *(a)* vegetarians or groups with low energy intake (dancers, gymnasts, and weight-class sport athletes who continually strive to maintain or reduce body weight), *(b)* those who eliminate one or more food groups from their diet, or *(c)* individuals who consume large amounts of processed foods and simple sugars with low micronutrient density (endurance athletes). Under these adverse situations, a multivitamin–mineral supplement at recommended dosages can upgrade the micronutrient density of the daily diet. *Vitamins synthesized in the laboratory are no less effective for bodily functions than vitamins from natural sources.* Compared with the deficient state, vitamin supplements reverse the symptoms of vitamin deficiency and improve exercise performance. Once cured of a deficiency, supplements do not further improve normal nutritional status.

VITAMIN SUPPLEMENTS: THE COMPETITIVE EDGE?

Over 45 years of research fails to support the use of vitamin supplements to improve exercise performance or ability to train arduously in nutritionally adequate healthy peo-

ple.[124,151,153,164] When vitamin intake achieves recommended levels, supplements neither improve exercise performance nor increase the blood levels of these micronutrients. The facts, however, remain clouded by "testimonials" from coaches and elite athletes who attribute their success to a particular dietary modification or specific vitamin supplements.

As noted in Chapter 2, many vitamins serve as coenzyme components or precursors of coenzymes to help regulate energy metabolism. FIGURE 7.7 illustrates that B complex vitamins play a key role as coenzymes in important energy-yielding reactions during carbohydrate, fat, and protein catabolism. They also contribute to hemoglobin synthesis and red blood cell production. However, the belief that "if a little is good, more must be better" has led many coaches, athletes, fitness enthusiasts, and even some "expert" scientists to advocate supplementing with vitamins above recommended levels.

Supplementing with vitamin B_6 (pyridoxine), an essential cofactor in glycogen and amino acid metabolism, did not

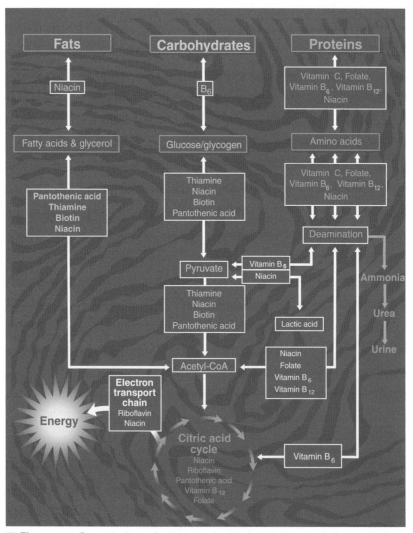

Figure 7.7 General schema for the role of water-soluble vitamins in the metabolism of carbohydrates, fats, and proteins.

benefit the metabolic mixture metabolized by women during high-intensity aerobic exercise.[91] In fact, the status of athletes for this vitamin normally equals reference standards for the population;[89] it does not decrease with strenuous exercise to levels warranting supplementation.[129] Supplementing for 4 days with a highly absorbable derivative of thiamin—a component of the five-enzyme complex pyruvate dehydrogenase that catalyzes movement of pyruvate into the citric acid cycle—offered no advantage over a placebo on measures of oxygen uptake, lactate accumulation, and cycling performance during exhaustive exercise.[164] The loss of water-soluble vitamins in sweat, even during extreme physical activity, is probably negligible.[49]

No exercise benefit exists for vitamins C and E with intakes above recommended values. Vitamin C, for example, serves as a factor to synthesize collagen and the adrenal hormone norepinephrine. Supplementing with vitamin C has negligible effects on endurance performance and does not alter the rate, severity, and duration of injuries, compared with placebo treatment. Vitamin C status, assessed by serum concentration and urinary ascorbate levels, in diverse groups of highly trained athletes does not differ from that of untrained subjects, despite large differences in daily physical activity level.[132] Other investigators report similar findings for this and other vitamins.[32,44,131] Furthermore, the energy intake of active persons usually increases to match the increased energy requirement of physical activity; thus a proportionate increase also occurs in micronutrient intake, often in amounts greatly exceeding recommended levels.

While vitamin E deficiencies may impair muscular function,[22] no scientific data have established that vitamin E consumed in excess of the RDA benefits stamina, circulatory function, or energy metabolism. Chronic high-potency multivitamin–mineral supplementation for well-nourished healthy, individuals does not benefit aerobic fitness, muscular strength, and athletic performance.[142]

A Unique Case for Vitamin C

Consuming vitamin C above recommended daily levels (75 mg for women and 90 mg for men) does not protect the general population against upper respiratory tract infection (URTI). However, daily supplements of 500 to 1500 mg of vitamin C per day may confer some benefit to individuals engaged in strenuous exercise who experience frequent viral infections.[52,118,120]

Moderate exercise heightens immune function, whereas a prolonged period of intense physical activity (marathon running or an exceedingly heavy training session) transiently suppresses and stresses the body's first line of defense against infectious agents. This increases risk of URTI within 1 or 2 weeks of exercise stress. For these individuals, additional vitamin C and E and perhaps carbohydrate ingestion before, during, and after a workout

may boost the normal immune mechanisms for combating infection.[62,102,109] Page 212 presents a more complete discussion of exercise, nutritional supplementation, and URTI.

Megavitamins

Most nutritionists believe little harm occurs in taking a multivitamin capsule containing the recommended quantity of each vitamin. For some people, the psychological effects of supplementation may even confer a benefit. Of concern are those individuals who take **megavitamins**, or doses at least *10* and up to 1000 times the RDA, hoping that "supercharging" with vitamins improves exercise performance and training responsiveness. Such practices can be harmful, except for serious medical illness that requires above-normal vitamin intake.

Vitamins Behave As Chemicals

Once the enzyme systems catalyzed by specific vitamins become saturated, any excess taken in megadose function as chemicals or drugs in the body. For example, a megadose of water-soluble vitamin C raises serum uric acid levels and precipitates gout in people predisposed to this disease. At intakes above 1000 mg daily, urinary excretion of oxalate (a breakdown product of vitamin C) increases, accelerating kidney stone formation in susceptible individuals. Also, some American blacks, Asians, and Sephardic Jews have a genetic metabolic deficiency that becomes activated to hemolytic anemia with excessive vitamin C intake. For iron-deficient individuals, megadoses of vitamin C may destroy significant amounts of vitamin B_{12}. In healthy persons, vitamin C supplements frequently irritate the bowel and cause diarrhea.

Excess vitamin B_6 can induce liver disease and nerve damage. Excessive riboflavin (B_2) can impair vision, whereas a megadose of nicotinic acid (niacin) acts as a potent vasodilator and inhibitor of fatty acid mobilization during exercise. A blunted fatty acid metabolism could cause a more rapid than normal depletion of muscle glycogen. Folate in concentrated supplement form can trigger an allergic response producing hives, light-headedness, and breathing difficulties. Possible side effects of a vitamin E megadose include headache, fatigue, blurred vision, gastrointestinal disturbances, muscular weakness, and low blood sugar. Because unsaturated fatty acids usually contain vitamin E, it is difficult to "construct" a vitamin E-deficient diet. The toxicity to the nervous system of megadoses of vitamin A and the damaging effects to the kidneys of excess vitamin D are well known.

If vitamin supplementation does offer benefits to physically active individuals, benefits only apply to those with marginal vitamin stores or who restrict energy intake or make poor dietary choices.[90] Well-controlled research must fully determine if and under what circumstances such supplementation confers benefits.

EXERCISE, FREE RADICALS, AND ANTIOXIDANTS: THE POTENTIALLY PROTECTIVE MICRONUTRIENTS FOR PHYSICALLY ACTIVE PEOPLE

The benefits of physical activity are well known, but the possibility for negative effects remain controversial. Potentially negative effects occur because elevated aerobic exercise metabolism increases the production of free radicals (see Chapter 2).[2,70,84,157] Free-radical production in humans and subsequent tissue damage are not directly measured, but rather inferred from markers of free radical byproducts. Increased free radicals could possibly overwhelm the body's natural defenses and pose a health risk from an elevated oxidative stress level.[63,133] Free radicals also play a role in muscle injury from exercise, particularly eccentric muscle actions and unaccustomed exercise. Muscle damage of this nature releases muscle enzymes and initiates inflammatory cell infiltration into the damaged tissue.

The opposing position maintains that while free radical production increases during exercise, the body's normal antioxidant defenses remain either adequate[160] or improve as natural enzymatic defenses become "upregulated" through exercise training adaptations.[37,51,60,138] Upregulation of antioxidant defenses accompanies a reduced exercise-induced lipid peroxidation in red blood cell membranes, which increases their resistance to subsequent oxidative stress.[97] *Convincing epidemiologic evidence also supports the beneficial effects of regular aerobic exercise on cancer and heart disease incidence, the occurrences of which link to oxidative stress.*[34]

Increased Metabolism and Free Radical Production

Exercise produces reactive oxygen (free radicals) in at least two ways. The first occurs via a mitochondrial electron leak, probably at the cytochrome level, that produces superoxide radicals. The second happens during alterations in blood flow and oxygen supply—underperfusion during intense exercise followed by reperfusion in recovery, which triggers excessive free radical generation. Some argue that the potential for free radical damage increases during trauma, stress, contraction-induced muscle damage from exercise, and from environmental pollutants including smog. With exercise, the risk depends on intensity and the participant's state of training, because exhaustive exercise by the untrained often produces oxidative damage in active muscles. FIGURE 7.8 illustrates how regular exercise affects oxidative response and potential for tissue damage, including protective adaptive responses.

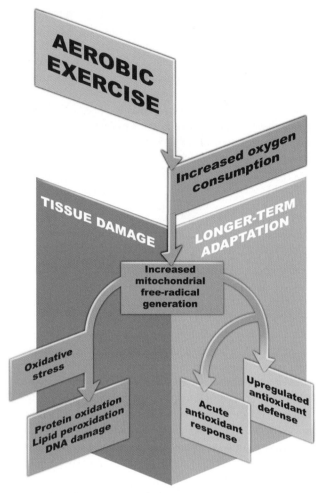

■ **Figure 7.8** Cascade of events and adaptations produced by regular aerobic exercise that lessen the likelihood of tissue damage.

Important Questions

Two questions arise concerning physical activity and free-radical production:

1. Are physically active individuals more prone to free-radical damage?
2. Are nutritional agents with antioxidant properties required in increased quantities by the physically active person?

In answer to the first question, research suggests that for well-nourished individuals, the body's natural defenses respond adequately to increased physical activity. A single bout of exercise increases oxidant formation, but the natural antioxidant defenses cope effectively in both healthy individuals and trained heart transplant recipients.[64] Even repeating multiple exercise bouts on consecutive days, various indices of oxidative stress indicated no depletion of antioxidant defenses. The second question requires an equivocal answer.[159] Some evidence indicates that exogenous antioxidant compounds either slow exercise-induced free-radical formation or augment the body's natural antioxidant defense system. This would limit the extent and progression of muscle damage following and acute exercise bout.

If supplementation proves beneficial, vitamin E may be the most important antioxidant related to exercise.[20,40,61,130,133] In one study, vitamin E-deficient animals began exercise with plasma membrane function compromised from oxidative damage. These animals reached exhaustion earlier than animals with normal vitamin E levels. For animals fed a normal diet, vitamin E supplements diminished exercise-induced oxidative damage to skeletal muscle fibers[39] and myocardial tissue.[41] FIGURE 7.9 shows the effects of 3 weeks of a daily 200-mg vitamin E supplement on pentane elimination (pentane serves as a primary marker of free radical production).[122] The vitamin E-supplemented trials dramatically reduced free radical production. Humans fed a daily antioxidant vitamin mixture of β-carotene, ascorbic acid, and vitamin E had lower serum and breath markers of lipid peroxidation at rest and following exercise than subjects not receiving supplements.[71] Five months of vitamin E supplementation in racing cyclists produced a protective effect on markers of oxidative stress induced by extreme endurance exercise. Two weeks of daily supplementation with 120 IU of vitamin E decreased free-radical interaction with cellular membranes and slowed muscle tissue disruption from heavy resistance training.[95] In contrast, 30 days of vitamin E supplementation (1200 IU·d^{-1}) produced a 2.8-fold increase in serum vitamin E concentration without affecting contraction-induced indices of muscle damage (including postexercise force decrement) or inflammation caused by eccentric muscle actions.[8] Similarly, a 4-week daily vitamin E supplement of 1000 IU produced no effect on biochemical or ultrastructural indices of muscle damage in experienced runners after a half marathon.[25] Differences in exercise severity and oxidative stress could account for discrepancies in research findings.

Selenium and some trace minerals such as copper, manganese, and zinc possess antioxidant properties owing to their incorporation within the structure of glutathione peroxidase and other enzymes that protect plasma membranes from free radical damage.[152] In a double-blind, placebo-controlled cancer prevention trial, individuals received a selenium supplement of 200 μg daily or about 3 to 4 times the recommended value.[16] Supplementation significantly reduced incidence of, and mortality from, prostate (71%), esophageal (67%), colorectal (62%), and lung (46%) cancers.

Proposed mechanisms for selenium's protection include its function as an essential component of antioxidant enzymes, how it alters carcinogen metabolism and inhibits tumor growth, its effects on the endocrine and immune systems, and its action through molecular mechanisms to regulate the programmed death *(apoptosis)* of damaged precancerous cells. The recommended daily selenium intake is 70 μg for adult men and 55 μg for women; intakes in excess of 1000 μg can produce toxicity—hair and fingernail loss and gastrointestinal dysfunction. Selenium-rich foods include cereals and other grains, Brazil nuts, seafood, meat, mushrooms, and asparagus.

Coenzyme Q$_{10}$ probably acts as an antioxidant either singularly within the respiratory chain or as a recycler of vitamin E. Little evidence exists that coenzyme Q$_{10}$ exerts the same direct antioxidant effect as vitamin E.

A Prudent Recommendation. Some evidence suggests that supplementing with various antioxidant compounds slows exercise-induced free radical formation and perhaps augments the body's natural defense system. Further research will contribute new insights in this important area. A prudent recommendation includes consuming a well balanced diet containing fruits, grains, and vegetables. Nutrient antioxidants are best obtained from diverse food sources, *not* from supplements. We endorse this position because of uncertainty whether health protection derives from the antioxidant per se or its interaction with the broad array of active compounds within the food source (e.g., the numerous "chemoprotectant" phytochemicals contained in plants). Three potential mechanisms for antioxidant health benefits include

1. Influencing molecular mechanisms and gene expression
2. Providing enzyme-inducing substances that detoxify carcinogens
3. Blocking uncontrolled growth of cells

According to the director of the division of cancer prevention and control at the National Cancer Institute (NCI; www.cancer.gov/), "More than 150 studies have clearly shown that groups of people who eat plenty of fruits and vegetables get less cancer at a number of cancer sites." The

■ **Figure 7.9** Pentane levels before and after 20 minutes of exercise at 100% V̇O$_2$max with and without vitamin E supplementation. (Adapted from Pincemail J, et al. Pentane measurement in man as an index of lipid peroxidation. Bioelectrochem Bioenerg 1987;18:117.)

RICH DIETARY SOURCES OF VITAMIN ANTIOXIDANTS

- β-Carotene: pigmented compounds or carotenoids that give color to yellow, orange, and green leafy vegetables and fruits; examples include carrots, dark-green leafy vegetables such as spinach, broccoli, turnips, beet and collard greens; sweet potatoes; winter squash; apricots, cantaloupe, mangos, and papaya

- Vitamin C: citrus fruits and juices; cabbage, broccoli, turnip greens; cantaloupe; green and red sweet peppers, and berries

- Vitamin E: poultry, seafood, vegetable oils, wheat germ, fish liver oils, whole-grain breads and fortified cereals, nuts and seeds, dried beans, green leafy vegetables, and eggs

Figure 7.10 Theoretical model of the interrelationships among stress, exercise, illness, and the immune system. (From MacKinnon LT. Current challenges and future expectations in exercise immunology: back to the future. Med Sci Sports Exerc 1994;26:191.)

NCI encourages consumption of five or more servings (nine recommended for men) of fruits and vegetables daily, while the USDA's *Dietary Guidelines* recommend two to four servings of fruits and three to five servings of vegetables daily.

EXERCISE, INFECTIOUS ILLNESS, CANCER, AND THE IMMUNE RESPONSE

"Don't exercise until you're fatigued or you'll get sick," is a common perception held by many parents, athletes, and coaches that too much strenuous exercise increases susceptibility to certain illnesses. In contrast, the belief also exists that regular, more moderate exercise improves health and reduces susceptibility to infectious illness such as the common cold.

Studies as early as 1918 reported that most cases of pneumonia among boys in boarding school occurred among athletes. Respiratory infections seemed to progress toward pneumonia after intense sports training. Anecdotal reports also related the severity of poliomyelitis to participation in heavy physical activity at a critical time of infection. Current epidemiologic and clinical findings from the flourishing field of **exercise immunology**—the study of the interactions of physical, environmental, and psychologic factors on immune function—support the contention that unusually strenuous physical activity affects immune function to increase susceptibility to illness, particularly URTI.

The immune system comprises a highly complex and self-regulating grouping of cells, hormones, and interactive modulators that defend the body from invasion from outside microbes (bacterial, viral, and fungal), foreign macromolecules, and abnormal cancerous cell growth. This system has two functional divisions: *(a)* **innate immunity** and *(b)* **acquired immunity**. The innate immune system includes

anatomic and physiologic components (skin, mucous membranes, body temperature, and specialized defenses such as natural killer cells, diverse phagocytes, and inflammatory barriers). The acquired immune system consists of specialized B- and T-lymphocyte cells. These cells when activated regulate a highly effective immune response to a specific infectious agent. If infection does occur, an optimal immune system blunts the severity of illness and speeds recovery.

FIGURE 7.10 proposes a model for interactions among exercise, stress, illness, and the immune system. Within this framework, exercise, stress, and illness interact, each with its own effect on immunity. For example, exercise affects susceptibility to illness, and certain illnesses clearly affect exercise capacity. Likewise, psychologic factors (via links between the hypothalamus and immune function) and other forms of stress, including nutritional deficiencies and acute alterations in normal sleep schedule, influence resistance to illness. Concurrently, exercise either positively or negatively moderates the body's response to stress. Each factor—stress, illness, and short- and long-term exercise—exerts an independent effect on immune status, immune function, and resistance to disease.

Upper Respiratory Tract Infections

FIGURE 7.11 displays the general J-shaped curve to describe the relationship between short-term exercise (and unusually intense training) and susceptibility to URTI. The figure also indicates that markers of immune function follow an inverted J-shaped curve.[112,170] While one may draw overly simplistic implications from these relationships, light-to-moderate physical activity does appear to offer more protection against URTI and possibly diverse cancers than a sedentary lifestyle.[66,88,94] In addition, moderate exercise does not exacerbate the severity and duration of illness if infection does occur.[165] In contrast, strenuous physical activity

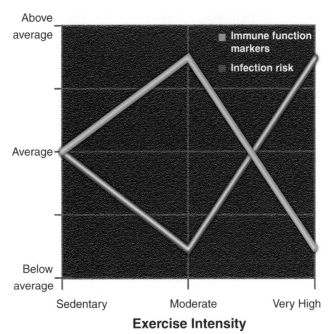

Figure 7.11 Exercise intensity affects immune function and risk of infection.

(marathon run or intense training session) provides an "open window" (3–72 hours) that decreases antiviral and antibacterial resistance and increases risk of UTRI (by two to six times) that manifests itself within 1 or 2 weeks.[24,57] For example, approximately 13% of the participants in a Los Angeles marathon reported an episode of URTI during the week following the race. For runners of comparable ability who did not compete for reasons other than illness, the infection rate approximated 2%.[104] Future research must establish a precise causal link and the degree of relationship between the magnitude of immunosuppression following a bout of heavy exertion and subsequent infection occurrence.

Acute Exercise Effects

- **Moderate exercise:** *A bout of moderate exercise boosts natural immune functions and host defenses for up to several hours.*[76,93] Noteworthy effects include the increase in natural killer (NK) cell activity. These phagocytic lymphocyte subpopulations enhance the disease-fighting capacity of the blood. They also provide the body's first line of defense against diverse pathogens. The NK cell does not require prior or specific sensitization to foreign bodies or neoplastic cells. Rather, these cells demonstrate spontaneous cytolytic activity that ultimately ruptures and/or inactivates viruses and the metastatic potential of tumor cells.[115,167]
- **Exhaustive exercise:** *A prolonged period of exhaustive exercise (and other forms of extreme stress or increased training) severely impairs the body's first line of defense against infection.*[74,75,80,114,140,166]

Repeated cycles of unusually intense exercise further compound the risk. For example, impaired immune function from strenuous exercise "carries over" to a second bout of exercise on the same day to produce even more pronounced changes in neutrophils, lymphocytes, and select CD cells.[134] Elevated temperature, cytokines, and various stress-related hormones (epinephrine, growth hormone [GH], cortisol, β-endorphins) with exhaustive exercise may mediate depression of the body's innate (NK cell and neutrophil activity) and adaptive (T- and B-cell function) immune defenses.[6,105,148] The transient but diminished immunity after strenuous exercise remains apparent in the mucosal immune system of the upper respiratory tract.[93,99] This negative effect of strenuous exercise on immune response clearly supports the wisdom of advising individuals with URTI symptoms to refrain from physical activity (or at least "go easy") to optimize normal immune mechanisms that combat infection.

Chronic Exercise Effects

Aerobic training positively affects natural immune functions and resistance to stress in young and older individuals and in the obese during periods of weight loss.[30,31,136] Areas of improvement include *(a)* enhanced functional capacity of natural cytotoxic immune mechanisms (e.g., antitumor actions of NK cell activity) and *(b)* slowing of the age-related decrease in T-cell function and associated cytokine production.[65,107] The cytotoxic T cells defend directly against viral and fungal infections and contribute to regulating other immune mechanisms.

If exercise training enhances immune function, one might question why trained individuals show increased susceptibility to URTI after intense competition. The **open window hypothesis** maintains that an inordinate increase in training or actual competition exposes even the highly conditioned person to "nonnormal" stress that transiently but severely depresses NK cell function. This period of immunodepression ("open window") decreases natural resistance to infection. The inhibitory effect of strenuous exercise on adrenocorticotropic hormone output and cortisol's maintenance of optimal blood glucose concentrations may negatively affect the immune process. For individuals who exercise regularly but only at moderate levels, the window of opportunity for infection remains "closed," thus preserving the protective benefits of regular exercise on immune function.

Resistance Training. Nine years of prior resistance exercise training did not affect resting NK cell number or activity level when compared with sedentary controls.[108] Comparisons also indicated that resistance training activated monocytes more than typically observed for regular aerobic exercise. Monocyte activation releases prostaglandins that downregulate NK cells following exercise; this inhibits the long-term positive effect of exercise on NK cells. These investigators had previously shown that NK cells increase a substantial 225% following an acute bout of resistance exercise,[113] a response similar to the immediate effect of moderate aerobic exercise.[36,46]

Perhaps a Role for Nutritional Supplements

Nutritional factors influence immune function (and possibly susceptibility to infection) in response to strenuous exercise and training.[14,38,53,137] For example, consuming a fat-rich diet (62% energy from lipids) negatively affected the immune system compared with a carbohydrate-rich diet (65% energy from carbohydrates).[116] Supplementing with a 6% carbohydrate beverage (0.7l L before; 0.25 L every 15 min during; 500 mL every hour throughout a 4.5-h recovery) beneficially lowered cytokine levels in the inflammatory cascade after 2.5 hours of endurance running.[102] Subsequent research by the same laboratory showed that ingesting carbohydrates (4 mL per kg body mass) every 15 minutes during 2.5 hours of high-intensity running or cycling maintained higher plasma glucose levels in 10 triathletes during exercise than a placebo.[110] Similar beneficial results with carbohydrate ingestion for cortisol and select antiinflammatory cytokines have been observed following competition, regardless of age or gender.[111] A blunted cortisol response and diminished pro- and antiinflammatory cytokine response accompanied the higher plasma glucose levels with carbohydrate supplementation in exercise. *This suggests a carbohydrate-induced reduction in overall physiologic stress in prolonged high-intensity exercise.*

Combined supplementation with the antioxidant vitamins C and E produces more prominent immunopotentiating effects (enhanced cytokine production) in young, healthy adults than supplementation with either vitamin alone.[62] Also, a 200-mg daily vitamin E supplement enhanced clinically relevant indices of T-cell–mediated function for healthy elderly subjects.[96] However, long-term daily supplementation with a physiologic dose of vitamins and minerals or with 200 mg of vitamin E did *not lower* the incidence and severity of acute respiratory tract infections in noninstitutionalized persons aged 60 and older. Among individuals experiencing an infection, those receiving vitamin E had *longer* total illness duration and restriction of activity.[43]

Additional research must determine whether intake of vitamins C and E (and other antioxidants such as β-carotene) above recommended levels upgrades immune function to protect the general population against URTI. Daily supplementation with vitamin C does appear to benefit individuals engaged in heavy exercise, particularly those predisposed to frequent viral URTI.[52,121] Runners who received a 600-mg daily vitamin C supplement before, and for 3 weeks after, a 90-km ultramarathon competition experienced significantly fewer symptoms of URTI—running nose, sneezing, sore throat, coughing, fever—than runners receiving a

placebo.[118] Interestingly, infection risk inversely related to race performance; those with the fastest times suffered more symptoms. URTI also appeared most frequently in runners with strenuous training regimens. For these individuals, additional vitamin C and E and perhaps carbohydrate ingestion before, during, and after prolonged stressful exercise may boost normal immune mechanisms to combat infection.[105,109] More than likely, the presence of other stressors—lack of sleep, mental stress, poor nutrition, or weight loss—magnify the stress on the immune system from a single bout (or repeated bouts) of exhaustive exercise.[14,105]

Glutamine and the Immune Response

The nonessential amino acid glutamine plays an important role in normal immune function. One protective aspect of glutamine concerns its use as an energy fuel for nucleotide synthesis by disease-fighting cells, particularly the lymphocytes and macrophages that defend against infection.[5,141] Sepsis, injury, burns, surgery, and endurance exercise lower glutamine levels in plasma and skeletal muscle. Lowered plasma glutamine most likely occurs because glutamine demand by the liver, kidneys, gut, and immune system exceeds its supply from the diet and skeletal muscle. A lowered plasma glutamine concentration contributes, at least in part, to the immunosuppression that accompanies extreme physical stress.[9,54,135,145] Thus, glutamine supplementation might reduce susceptibility to URTI following strenuous physical exertion.[139]

Marathoners who ingested a glutamine drink (5 g of L-glutamine in 330 mL of mineral water) at the end of a race and then 2-hours later reported fewer URTI than unsupplemented runners.[12] Subsequent studies by the same researchers to determine a possible mechanism for glutamine's protective effect on postexercise infection risk reported no effect of supplementation on changes in blood lymphocyte distribution.[13] Appearance of URTI in athletes during intense training does not fluctuate with changes in plasma glutamine concentration. Preexercise glutamine supplementation does not affect the immune response following a single bout of sustained high-intensity exercise or repeated bouts of intense exercise.[79,128,163] Glutamine supplements taken 0, 30, 60, and 90 minutes following a marathon race prevented the drop in glutamine concentrations following the race but did not influence three factors: *(a)* lymphokine-activated killer cell activity, *(b)* the proliferative responses, or *(c)* exercise-induced changes in leucocyte subpopulations.[127] Currently, insufficient data exist to recommend glutamine supplements to reliably blunt immunosuppression from exhaustive exercise.

A General Recommendation

A lifestyle that emphasizes regular physical activity, maintenance of a well-balanced diet, reducing stress to a minimum, and obtaining adequate sleep generally optimizes immune function. For prudent weight loss, use a gradual approach, because more rapid weight loss with accompanying severe caloric restriction suppresses immune function.[106] With prolonged, high-intensity exercise, carbohydrate ingestion (about $1 \, L \cdot h^{-1}$ of a typical sports drink) lessens the negative changes in immunity brought about by physiologic stress and carbohydrate depletion. In general, endurance athletes who ingest carbohydrate during a race experience much lower disruption in hormonal and immune measures than do athletes not consuming carbohydrate. These responses indicate a diminished level of physiologic stress.

MINERALS AND EXERCISE PERFORMANCE

The use of single-mineral supplements is ill advised unless prescribed by a physician or registered dietitian because of potential adverse consequences. For example, excess magnesium supplementation can cause gastrointestinal disturbances including diarrhea. Magnesium intake also can impair iron and zinc nutrition, while a 15-mg zinc excess per day inhibits copper absorption and adversely affects HDL-cholesterol concentrations. Concern also exists about the long-term effects of chromium supplementation on tissue chromium accumulation and toxic side effects. *Short- and long-term mineral supplementation above recommended levels does not benefit exercise performance or enhance training responsiveness.*

Mineral Loss in Sweat

Loss of water and accompanying mineral salts, primarily sodium chloride and some potassium chloride in sweat, poses an important challenge during prolonged exercise, especially in hot weather. Excessive water and electrolyte loss impairs heat tolerance and exercise performance and can cause severe dysfunction in the form of heat cramps, heat exhaustion, or heat stroke. The yearly number of heat-related deaths during spring and summer football practice tragically illustrates the importance of fluid and electrolyte replacement. During practice or a game, an athlete may lose up to 5 kg of water from sweating. This corresponds to about 8.0 g of salt depletion because each kg (1 L) of sweat contains about 1.5 g of salt (40% of NaCl represents sodium). *Replacement of water lost through sweating, however, becomes the crucial and immediate need.*

Defense Against Mineral Loss

Vigorous exercise triggers a rapid and coordinated release of the hormones **vasopressin** and **aldosterone** and the enzyme **renin** to minimize sodium and water loss through the kidneys.[27,98] Sodium conservation by the kidneys occurs even under extreme conditions such as running a marathon in warm, humid weather when sweat output often reaches 2 L per hour. Electrolytes lost in sweat are usually replenished by adding a slight amount of salt to fluid or food ingested. Runners in a 20-day road race in Hawaii maintained plasma minerals at normal levels by consuming an unrestricted diet without mineral supplements.[28] Ingesting "athletic drinks" offers no special benefit in replacing the minerals lost through sweating compared with consuming the same minerals in a well-balanced diet. Salt supplements may be necessary for prolonged exercise in the heat when fluid loss exceeds 4 or 5 kg. One can achieve proper supplementation by drinking a 0.1 to 0.2% salt solution (adding 0.3 tsp of table salt per L of water).[3] Chapter 10 presents more specific recommendations for electrolyte replacement via the rehydration beverage.

A mild potassium deficiency occurs with intense exercise during heat stress, but a diet with the recommended amount of potassium generally ensures adequate levels. Drinking an 8-oz glass of orange or tomato juice replaces the calcium, potassium, and magnesium lost in 3 L (7 lb) of sweat, a sweat loss not likely to occur with less than 60 minutes of vigorous exercise.

Trace Minerals and Exercise

Many athletes believe that supplementing with certain trace minerals enhances exercise performance and counteracts the demands of heavy training. Strenuous exercise may increase excretion of the following trace elements:

- Chromium: Necessary for carbohydrate and lipid catabolism and proper insulin function and protein synthesis
- Copper: Required for red blood cell formation; influences specific gene expression, and serves as a cofactor or prosthetic group for several enzymes
- Manganese: Component of superoxide dismutase in the antioxidant defense system
- Zinc: Component of lactate dehydrogenase, carbonic anhydrase, superoxide dismutase, and enzymes related to energy metabolism, cell growth and differentiation, and tissue repair

Urinary losses of zinc and chromium were 1.5- and 2.0-fold higher on the day of a 6-mile run than on a rest day.[4] A relatively large loss of copper and zinc occurs in sweat during exercise.[23,81] However, the normal plasma volume expansion with aerobic training combined with zinc redistribution from the plasma to other body tissues (e.g., liver and skeletal muscles) dilutes plasma zinc concentrations to indicate an *apparent* zinc inadequacy.

Trace mineral losses with exercise do not necessarily mean that physically active individuals should supplement with these micronutrients. For example, no benefit occurred from short-term 25 mg daily zinc supplementation on metabolic and endocrine responses and performance during strenuous exercise in eumenorrheic women.[143] Collegiate football players who supplemented with 200 μg of chromium (as chromium picolinate) daily for 9 weeks showed no beneficial changes in body composition or muscular strength during intense weightlifting compared with a control group that received a placebo.[15] Power and endurance athletes had significantly higher, not lower, plasma levels of copper and zinc than nontraining controls.[126] However, men and women who train strenuously (with large sweat production) and show marginal nutrition and low body weight (e.g., weight-class wrestlers, endurance runners, ballet dancers, female gymnasts) should carefully monitor trace mineral intake to prevent overt deficiency.[87] *For most physically active men and women only transient, trace mineral losses occur with exercise; these losses do not impair exercise performance, training responsiveness, and overall health.*

Iron, zinc, and copper interact and compete for the same carrier during intestinal absorption. Thus, excessive intake of one mineral often causes deficiency in the other.[86] For example, consuming excess iron reduces zinc absorption, while excess zinc blunts copper absorption. In addition, supplementing with zinc above recommended levels can lower HDL-cholesterol, diminishing the beneficial effect of aerobic exercise on this cardioprotective plasma lipoprotein. Chapter 12 discusses the possible ergogenic effects of chromium supplements and other trace minerals such as boron and vanadium. TABLE 7.12 outlines exercise-related functions and food sources of four minerals—zinc, copper, chromium, and selenium—associated with exercise and training.

Extremes of Physical Inactivity Present a Different Picture

Continuous periods of bed rest deplete stores of the trace minerals copper and zinc.[78] Because one-half of copper and zinc become constituents of muscle and bone mass, excessive bed rest (and perhaps physical inactivity) can drain these minerals. In this regard, delineating trace mineral balance in abnormal situations such as prolonged bed rest becomes important to clarify possible variations in require-

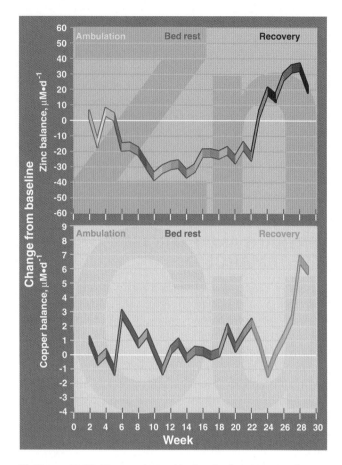

Figure 7.12 Changes in weekly zinc *(top)* and copper *(bottom)* balance during a 5-week control period, a 17-week period of bed rest, and a 7-week recovery period. (From Krebs JM, et al. Zinc and copper balances in healthy adult males during and after 17 wk of bed rest. Am J Clin Nutr 1993;58:897.)

ments for these elements. FIGURE 7.12 shows the time course for zinc and copper balance during a 30-week period; the study included a 5-week control period with ambulation, 17 weeks of continuous bed rest, and a 7-week recovery period with ambulation. Dietary intake remained constant at approximately 2688 kcal (11,115 kJ) throughout the observation period. Clear results emerged; bed rest markedly

Table 7.12	EXERCISE-RELATED FUNCTIONS AND FOOD SOURCES OF SELECTED TRACE MINERALS	
	Function	*Prominent Food Sources*
Zinc	Component of several enzymes involved in energy metabolism; cofactor to carbonic anhydrase	Oysters, wheat germ, beef, dark poultry meat, whole grains, liver
Copper	Required to synthesize cytochrome oxidase and for use of iron; constituent of ceruloplasmin; constituent of superoxide dismutase	Liver, kidney, shellfish, whole grains, legumes, nuts, eggs
Chromium	Enhances action of insulin	Mushrooms, prunes, nuts, whole grain bread and cereal, Brewer's yeast
Selenium	Functions as an antioxidant with glutathione peroxidase; complements vitamin E function	Seafood, kidney, liver

decreased cooper and zinc stores. During recovery with modest physical activity, trace mineral retention increased and remained greater than that with bed rest.

This study represents an extreme sedentary condition, yet it indicates that *physical inactivity* affects trace mineral dynamics. One hopes that future research will focus on the fascinating area of trace mineral metabolism in general, the effects of exercise and training (and detraining) on mineral requirements in particular, and relationships among indices of trace mineral status and peak exercise performance. At this time, it seems prudent to support the recommendations for trace mineral intake. Consuming a diet diverse in fruits, vegetables, grains, milk, and some meat supplies all the necessary trace minerals. If one chooses to supplement to enhance the diet's micronutrient density, intake should not exceed recommended levels.

EXERCISE AND FOOD INTAKE

Balancing energy intake with energy expenditure represents a primary goal for the physically active individual of normal body weight. Energy balance not only optimizes physical performance, it also helps to maintain lean body mass, training responsiveness, and immune and reproductive function. The most important factor affecting daily energy expenditure is level of physical activity (see Chapter 14). A person can estimate daily energy requirements from tabled energy cost values for diverse activities (considering frequency, intensity, and duration) such as those presented in Appendix B. However, the amount of energy that *maintains* an appropriate body weight and body composition represents the ultimate energy intake guideline.

FIGURE 7.13 illustrates age-related average daily energy intakes for males and females in the U.S. population. Energy intakes peak between ages 16 and 29 years and then decline for succeeding age groups. A similar pattern occurs for males and females, although males achieve higher energy intakes than females at all ages. Between ages 20 and 29 years, women consume on average 35% fewer kcal than men on a daily basis (3025 kcal [12,657 kJ] vs. 1957 kcal [8188 kJ]). Thereafter, the sex-related difference in energy intake becomes smaller; at age 70, women consume about 25% fewer kcal than their male counterparts.

Physical Activity Makes a Difference

Individuals who engage regularly in moderate-to-intense physical activity eventually increase daily energy intake to match their higher level of energy expenditure. Lumber workers, who expend approximately 4500 kcal each day, unconsciously adjust energy intake to balance energy output. Consequently, body mass remains stable despite a relatively large food intake. The body requires several days to attain energy equilibrium when balancing food intake to meet a

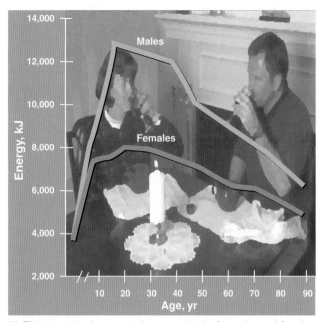

■ **Figure 7.13** Average daily energy intake for males and females by age in the U.S. population during the years 1988 to 1991. Multiply by 0.239 to convert kJ to kcal. (From Briefel RR, et al. Total energy intake of the US population: The third National Health and Nutrition Examination Survey, 1988–1991. Am J Clin Nutr 1995;62(suppl):1072S.)

new level of energy output. *Sedentary persons often do not maintain a fine energy balance, and energy intake exceeds daily energy expenditure.* The lack of precision in regulating food intake at the low end of the physical activity spectrum undoubtedly contributes to the "creeping obesity" in highly mechanized and technically advanced sedentary societies.

Daily food intake of athletes in the 1936 Olympics reportedly averaged more than 7000 kcal, or roughly three times the average intake.[1] These often-quoted energy values justify what many believe to be an enormous food requirement of athletes in training. However, these figures represent estimates, because objective dietary data did not appear in the original report. In all likelihood, they are inflated estimates of the energy expended (and required) by the athletes. For example, distance runners who train upward to 100 miles per week (6 min per mile pace at about 15 kcal per min) do not expend more than 800 to 1300 "extra" calories each day. For these endurance athletes, about 4000 kcal from daily food intake should balance the increased exercise energy expenditure.

Potential for Negative Energy Balance With High-Volume Training

Many athletes, particularly females, do not meet energy intake recommendations. Research with elite female swimmers, using the doubly labeled water technique, noted that total daily energy expenditure increased to 5593 kcal daily during high-volume training. This value represents the highest level of sustained daily energy expenditure reported for female athletes.[154] Daily energy intake did not increase enough to match training demands and averaged only 3136 kcal, implying a negative energy imbalance. The possibility of a negative energy balance in the transition from moderate to heavy training may ultimately compromise a person's full potential to train and compete.

FIGURE 7.14 presents energy intakes from a large sample of elite male and female endurance, strength, and team sport athletes in the Netherlands. For the males, daily energy intake ranged between 2900 and 5900 kcal, whereas the intakes of female competitors ranged between 1600 and 3200 kcal. With the exception of the large energy intakes of athletes at extremes of performance and training, daily energy intake generally did not exceed 4000 kcal for the men and 3000 kcal for the women. TABLE 7.13 lists additional energy and macronutrient intakes for elite male and female athletes. The data, presented as daily caloric intake, include the percentage of total energy as carbohydrate, protein, and lipid. For men, daily energy intake ranges from 3034 to 5222 kcal; for women, it ranges between 1931 and 3573 kcal. Averaging values across studies for percentage of total calories for each macronutrient results in values of 14.8% protein, 35.0% lipid, and 49.8% carbohydrate for the men and 14.4% protein, 31.8% lipid, and 54.0% carbohydrate for the women.

FIGURE 7.15 displays nutritional information for eight groups of male and female athletes, including four separate groups of male athletes. The data represent percentage of total calories consumed as carbohydrate, protein, and lipid,

■ **Figure 7.14** Daily energy intake (in kcal) of elite male and female endurance, strength, and team sport athletes. (Modified from van Erp-Baart AMJ, et al. Nationwide Survey on Nutritional Habits in Elite Athletes. Int J Sports Med 1989;10:53.)

Table 7.13 **EXAMPLES OF DAILY INTAKES OF ENERGY, PROTEIN, LIPID, AND CARBOHYDRATE (CHO) OF WELL-TRAINED MALE AND FEMALE ATHLETES**

Group	Energy Intake (kcal)	Protein (g)	Protein (%)	Lipid (g)	Lipid (%)	CHO (g)	CHO (%)	Research Study
Well-Trained Males								
Distance runners (n = 50)	3170	114	14	116	33	417	52	7
Distance runners (n = 10)	3034	128	17	115	34	396	49	4
Triathletes (n = 25)	4095	134	13	127	27	627	60	2
Marathon runners (n = 19)	3570	128	15	128	32	487	52	2
Football players (n = 56)	3395	126	15	141	38	373	44	2
Weight lifters (n = 19)	3640	156	18	155	39	399	43	2
Soccer players (n = 8)	4952	170	14	217	39	596	47	6
Swimmers (n = 22)	5222	166	12	248	43	596	45	1
Swimmers, male (n = 9)	3072	108	15	102	30	404	55	5
Well-Trained Females								
Distance runners (n = 44)	1931	70	19	60	28	290	53	7
Distance runners, eumenorrheic (n = 33)	2489	81	12	97	35	352	53	3
Distance runners, amenorrheic (n = 12)	2151	74	13	67	27	344	60	3
Swimmers (n = 21)	3573	107	12	164	41	428	48	1
Swimmers, females (n = 11)	2130	79	16	63	28	292	55	5

From Williams C. Carbohydrate needs of elite athletes. In: Simopoulos AP, Parlou KN, eds. Nutrition and fitness for athletes. Basel: Karger, 1993.
[1] Berning JR, et al. The nutritional habits of adolescent swimmers. Int J Sports Nutr 1991;1:240.
[2] Burke LM, et al. Dietary intakes and food use of groups of elite Australian male athletes. Int J Sports Nutr 1991;1:278.
[3] Deuster PA, et al. Nutritional intakes and status of highly trained amenorrheic and eumenorrheic women runners. Fertil Steril 1986;46:636.
[4] Grandjean AC. Macro-nutrient intake of US athletes compared with the general population and recommendations for athletes. Am J Clin Nutr 1989;49:1070.
[5] Hawley JA, Williams MM. Dietary intakes of age-group swimmers. Br J Sports Med 1991;25:154.
[6] Jacobs I, et al. Muscle glycogen concentration and elite soccer players. Eur J Appl Physiol 1982;48:297.
[7] (Unpublished)

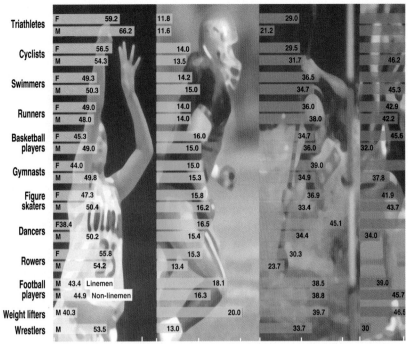

Figure 7.15 Percentage of total calories consumed as carbohydrates, proteins, and lipids, including total daily kcal per kilogram of body mass, for eight groups of male and female athletes and four additional groups of male athletes. The data represent averages for each group of athletes based on the world literature. (Data for lightweight rowers courtesy of Likomitrou M. Comparison of physical performance, nutritional and calorie intake, and body composition among heavyweight and lightweight oarsmen. Unpublished master's thesis. University of Massachusetts, Amherst, MA, 1995.)

including total kcal per kilogram of body mass. Not surprisingly, male triathletes and cyclists consume the most energy in relation to body mass, while female dancers and football lineman consume the least energy per unit size. Protein intake percentage ranged from 13.4% (male lightweight rowers) to 20% (male weight lifters); carbohydrate percentage ranged from 66.2% (male triathletes) to 38.4% (male dancers); and lipid percentage ranged from a surprisingly high 45.1% in male dancers to a low 23.7% in male lightweight rowers. In many instances, the percentage contribution of each macronutrient to total energy intake resembled that for the general population. Because of the athletes' generally larger energy intake, the absolute amount of each nutrient in grams exceeded values for the general population.

Tour de France

Some physical activities require extreme energy output (in excess of 1000 kcal per hour in elite marathoners and professional cyclists) and a correspondingly large energy intake during competition or periods of high-intensity training. For example, the daily energy requirements of elite cross-country skiers during 1 week of training averaged 3740 to 4860 kcal for women and 6120 to 8570 kcal for men.[144] These values for women agree with recent evaluations of daily energy expenditure of seven elite lightweight

female rowers, which averaged 3957 kcal over a 14-day training period.[56] FIGURE 7.16 outlines variation in daily energy expenditure for a male competitor during the most grueling event in sports, the Tour de France professional cycling race. Daily energy expenditure averaged 6500 kcal for nearly 3 weeks. Large variation occurred, depending on the level of activity for a particular day; energy expenditure decreased to 3000 kcal on a "rest" day and increased to 9000 kcal cycling over a mountain pass. By combining liquid nutrition with normal meals, this cyclist nearly matched daily energy expenditure with energy intake.

Ultraendurance Running Competition

Energy balance has been studied during a 1000-km (approximately 600-mile) race from Sidney to Melbourne, Australia. The Greek ultramarathon champion Kouros completed the race in 5 days, 5 hours, and 7 minutes, finishing 24 hours and 40 minutes ahead of the next competitor. Kouros did not sleep during the first 2 days of competition. He covered 463 km (287.8 miles) at an average speed of 11.4 km · h⁻¹ during day 1 and 8.3 km · h⁻¹ on day 2. During the remaining days, he took frequent rest periods, including periodic breaks for short "naps." Weather ranged from spring to winter conditions (30 to 8°C), and terrain varied. Table 7.14 lists the pertinent details of distance covered, energy expenditure, and food and water intake.

■ **Figure 7.16** Daily energy expenditure *(purple squares)* and energy intake *(yellow circles)* for a cyclist during the Tour de France competition. For 3 weeks in July, nearly 200 cyclists push themselves over and around the perimeter of France covering 2405 miles, more than 100 miles daily (only 1 day rest), at an average speed of 24.4 mph. Note the extremely high energy expenditure values and ability to achieve energy balance with liquid nutrition plus normal meals. *P,* stage; *R,* rest day. (Modified from Saris WHM, et al. Adequacy of vitamin supply under maximal sustained workloads; the Tour de France. In: Walter P, et al., eds. Elevated dosages of vitamins. Toronto: Huber Publishers, 1989.)

Table 7.14 FEATURES ABOUT DISTANCE COVERED AND DAILY AND TOTAL ENERGY BALANCE, NUTRIENT DISTRIBUTIONS IN FOOD, AND WATER INTAKE DURING AN ELITE ULTRA ENDURANCE PERFORMANCE

Day of the Race	Distance Covered (km)	Estimated Energy Expenditure (kcal)	Estimated Energy Intake (kcal)	Carbohydrates (g)	(%)	(kcal)	Lipids (g)	(%)	(kcal)	Proteins (g)	(%)	(kcal)	H₂O (L)
1	270	15,367	13,770	3375	98.0	13,502	20	1.3	180	22	0.7	88	22.0
2	193	10,741	8600	1981	92.2	7923	53	5.5	477	50	2.3	200	19.2
3	152	8919	12,700	3074	96.8	12,297	27	1.9	243	40	1.3	160	22.7
4	165	9780	7800	1758	90.1	7032	56	6.5	504	66	3.4	264	14.3
5	135	7736	12,500	3014	96.4	12,058	30	2.2	270	43	1.4	172	18.3
5 h	45	2536	550	138	100.0	550	—	—	—	—	—	—	3.2
Total	960	55,079	55,970	13,340		53,364	186		1674	221		734	99.7

Modified from Rontoyannis GP, et al. Energy balance in ultramarathon running. Am J Clin Nutr 1989;49:976.
The runner weighed 65 kg, was 171 cm tall, had a percentage body fat of 8%, and a $\dot{V}O_2$max of 62.5 mL·kg⁻¹·min⁻¹.

Table 7.15	HIGH-RISK SPORTS FOR MARGINAL NUTRITION

Criterion	Sports Discipline
Low weight—chronically low energy intakes to achieve low body fat	Gymnastics, jockeys, ballet, dancing, rhythmic gymnastics, ice dancing, aerobics
Competition weight—drastic weight loss regimens to achieve desired weight category	Weight class sports (e.g., judo, boxing, wrestling, rowing, ski jumping)
Low fat—drastic weight loss to achieve lowest possible fat	Body building
Vegetarian athletes	Endurance events

From Brouns F. Nutritional needs of athletes. New York: John Wiley & Sons, 1993.

The near equivalence between Kouros' estimated total energy intake (55,970 kcal) and energy expenditure (59,079 kcal) represents a remarkable aspect of energy homeostasis during extremes of physical exertion. Of the total energy intake from food, carbohydrates represented 95.3%, lipids 3%, with the remaining 1.7% proteins. Protein intake from food averaged considerably below the RDA level (although protein supplements were taken in tablet form). The unusually large daily energy intake (between 8600 and 13,770 kcal) came from Greek sweets (baklava, cookies, and donuts), some chocolate, dried fruit and nuts, various fruit juices, and fresh fruits. Every 30 minutes after the first 6 hours of running, Kouros replaced sweets and fruit with a small biscuit soaked in honey or jam. He consumed a small amount of roasted chicken on day 4, and drank coffee every morning. He took a 500-mg vitamin C supplement every 12 hours and a protein tablet twice daily.

The remarkable achievement by this champion exemplifies a highly conditioned athlete's exquisite regulatory control for energy balance during strenuous exercise. Kouros performed at a pace requiring a continuous energy supply averaging 49% of aerobic capacity during the first 2 days of competition (and 38% for days 3–5). He finished the competition without compromising overall health, with no muscular injuries or thermoregulatory problems, and his body mass remained unchanged. Reported difficulties included a severe bout of constipation during the competition and frequent urination that persisted for several days after the race.

Another case study of a 37-year-old male ultramarathoner further demonstrates the tremendous capacity for prolonged, high daily energy expenditure. The doubly labeled water technique evaluated energy expenditure during a 2-week period of a 14,500-km run around Australia in 6.5 months (average 70–90 km · d^{-1}) with no days for rest.[55] Daily energy expenditure over the measurement period averaged 6321 kcal; daily water turnover equaled 6.083 L. The subject ran about the same distance each day over the study

period as in the entire race period. As such, these data likely represent energy dynamics for the entire run.

High-Risk Sports for Marginal Nutrition

Gymnasts, ballet dancers, ice dancers, and weight-class athletes in boxing, wrestling, and judo engage in arduous training. Yet due to the nature of their sport, these men and women continually strive to maintain a lean, light body mass (TABLE 7.15).[10,149] As a result, energy intake often intentionally falls short of energy expenditure, and a relative state of malnutrition develops. The daily nutrient intake (% of RDA) of 97 competitive female gymnasts 11 to 14 years of age, indicate that nutritional supplementation could prove beneficial to these individuals (FIG. 7.17). Twenty-three percent of the girls consumed less than 1500 kcal daily, and more than 40% consumed less than two-thirds of the RDA for vitamin E, folate, iron, magnesium, calcium, and zinc. Clearly, a large number of these adolescent gymnasts needed to upgrade the nutritional quality of their diets or consider supplementation. For such athletes, carbohydrate intake fails to reach the level required by intense training. Consequently, they often train and perform in a carbohydrate-depleted state. Some protein supplementation to achieve a daily intake between 1.2 and 1.6 g per kg of body mass also may be warranted to maintain nitrogen balance and reduce the potential for impaired training status.

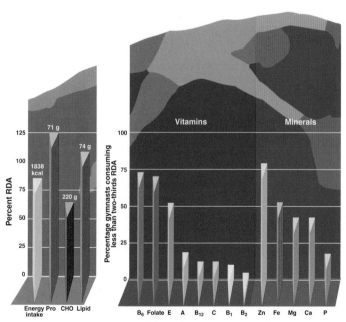

■ **Figure 7.17** Average daily nutrient intake for 97 adolescent female gymnasts (11–14 years) related to recommended values. The RDA on the *y* axis reflects only protein, while energy, CHO, and lipid reflect "recommended" values *(left)*. Percentage of gymnasts consuming less than two-thirds of the RDA *(right)*. Mean age, 13.1 years; mean stature, 152.4 cm (60 in.); mean body mass, 43.1 kg (94.8 lb). (Modified from Loosli AR, Benson J. Nutritional intake in adolescent athletes. Sports Med 1990;37:1143.)

Table 7.16	AN ACTIVE ATHLETE REQUIRES APPROXIMATELY 50 CALORIES OF FOOD PER KILOGRAM (23 CALORIES PER POUND) OF BODY MASS EACH DAY TO PROVIDE ENOUGH CALORIES FOR "OPTIMAL" ATHLETIC PERFORMANCE. A SAMPLE TRAINING DIET WOULD IDEALLY CONSIST OF APPROXIMATELY 60% CARBOHYDRATES, 15 TO 20% PROTEINS, AND LESS THAN 25% LIPIDS.

Body Weight	110 lb (50 kg)	132 lb (60 kg)	154 lb (70 kg)	176 lb (80 kg)
Total kcal	2500	3000	3500	4000
Recommended Number of Daily Servings				
Milk group (90 kcal) Skim milk, 1 cup Plain, low-fat yogurt, 1 cup	4[a]	4	4	4
Meat group (55–75 kcal) Cooked, lean meat (fish, poultry), 1 oz Egg, 1 Peanut butter, 1 tbsp Low-fat cheese, 1 oz Cottage cheese, 1/4 cup	5	5	6	6
Fruits	7	9	10	12
Vegetables	3	5	6	7
Grains	16	18	20	24
Lipids	5	6	8	10
Sample high-carbohydrate (350 g) 2500-kcal menu				

Breakfast	Lunch	Dinner	Snack #1	Snack #2
1 cup bran cereal 8 oz low-fat milk 1 English muffin 1 tsp margarine 4 oz orange juice	3 oz lean roast beef 1 hard roll 2 tsp mayonnaise or mustard, lettuce and tomato 1/2 cup cole slaw 2 fresh plums 2 oatmeal cookies 8 oz seltzer water with lemon	Chicken stir-fry: 3 oz chicken 1 cup diced vegetables 2 tsp oil 2 cup rice 1 cup orange and grapefruit sections 1 cup vanilla yogurt Iced tea with lemon	3 cups popcorn	8 oz apple cider

Modified from Carbohydrate and athletic performance. Sports Science Exchange, vol 7. Chicago: Gatorade Sports Science Institute, 1988.
[a] Bolded numbers below total kcal values represent recommended number of daily servings.

EAT MORE, WEIGH LESS

The energy intakes of 61 middle-aged men and women who ran 60 km per week ranged between 40 and 60% more calories per kg of body mass than intakes of sedentary controls. The extra energy required to run between 8 and 10 km daily accounted for the runners' larger caloric intake. Paradoxically, the most active runners who ate considerably more on a daily basis weighed considerably less than runners who exercised at a lower total caloric expenditure. These data agree with other studies of physically active people; they also support the argument that regular exercise provides an effective means for a person to actually "eat more yet weigh less" while maintaining a lower percentage of body fat. *Physically active people maintain a lighter, leaner body and a more healthful disease risk profile, despite increased intake of the typical American diet.* TABLE 7.16 presents a general model for food intake for physically active individuals, including an example of a 2500 kcal menu containing 350 g of carbo-hydrates. Chapter 14 more fully discusses the important role of regular exercise for weight control.

Summary

1. The Food Guide Pyramid provides broad recommendations for healthful nutrition for physically active men and women. It emphasizes fruits, grains, and vegetables and deemphasizes foods high in animal protein, lipids, and dairy products.

2. The Diet Quality Index, a composite score based on eight food-and-nutrient recommendations of the National Academy of Sciences, provides a general indication of the "healthfulness" of one's diet.

3. Within rather broad limits, a balanced diet provides the nutrient requirements of athletes and other individuals engaged in exercise training programs. Well-planned menus of about 1200 kcal a day offer the vitamin, mineral, and protein requirements. Consuming additional food (depending on physical activity level) then meets daily energy needs.

4. The protein RDA of 0.8 g per kilogram of body mass represents a liberal requirement believed adequate for all people, regardless of physical activity level.

5. A protein intake between 1.2 and 1.8 g per kg of body mass should adequately meet the possibility for added protein needs during strenuous training.

6. Physically active individuals readily achieve these values because they consume two to five times the protein RDA with their increased energy intake.

7. Precise recommendations do not exist for daily lipid and carbohydrate intake. A prudent recommendation suggests not exceeding 30 to 35% of daily calories from lipids; of this amount, most should be as unsaturated fatty acids.

8. For physically active people, carbohydrates should provide 60% or more of the daily calories (400–600 g), particularly as unrefined polysaccharides.

9. The American Heart Association (AHA) recommends lifestyle modifications that include increasing regular physical activity and eliminating use of all tobacco products.

10. Diet should emphasize fruits and vegetables, cereals and whole grains, nonfat and low-fat dairy products, legumes, nuts, fish, poultry, and lean meats.

11. To address the nation's obesity epidemic, the AHA urges men to maintain a waistline of 40 inches or less and for women, 35 inches or less.

12. Americans should devote at least an hour daily to moderately intense physical activity (brisk walking, swimming, or cycling) to maintain good health and a normal body weight.

13. To meet daily energy and nutrient needs and minimize chronic disease risk, adults should consume between 45 and 65% of total calories from carbohydrates, with maximum intake of added sugars placed at 25% of total calories.

14. Acceptable lipid intake ranges between 20 and 35% of caloric intake, with protein intake between 10 to 35%. Recommended fiber intake is 38 g daily for men and 21 g for women.

15. Successive days of hard training gradually deplete carbohydrate reserves, even when maintaining the recommended carbohydrate intake. This could lead to "staleness," making continued training more difficult.

16. Vitamin supplementation above amounts in a well-balanced diet does not improve exercise performance or the potential for training. Serious illness can result from consuming a regular excess of fat-soluble and, in some instances, water-soluble vitamins.

17. Elevated metabolism in physical activity increases the production of potentially harmful free radicals. To reduce the possibility for oxidative stress and cellular damage, the daily diet should contain foods rich in antioxidant vitamins and minerals.

18. A J-shaped curve generally describes the relationship between short-term exercise intensity and susceptibility to upper respiratory tract infection (URTI).

19. Light-to-moderate physical activity offers greater protection against URTI and diverse cancers than a sedentary lifestyle. A bout of intense physical activity provides an "open window" that decreases antiviral and antibacterial resistance and increases UTRI risk.

20. Glutamine supplements are not recommended to reliably blunt immunosuppression from exhaustive exercise.

21. Excessive sweating during exercise causes loss of body water and related minerals. Mineral loss should be replaced following exercise through well-balanced meals.

22. Intensity of daily physical activity largely determines energy intake requirements. The daily caloric needs of athletes in strenuous sports probably do not exceed 4000 kcal unless *(a)* body mass is large or *(b)* training level or competition is extreme.

TEST YOUR KNOWLEDGE **ANSWERS**

1. False The human body functions in accord with the laws of thermodynamics. This also includes the dynamics of energy balance. In accord with the first law of thermodynamics, the energy balance equation dictates that body mass remains constant when caloric intake equals caloric expenditure. If the total food calories exceed daily energy expenditure, excess calories accumulate as fat in adipose tissue. Conversely, weight loss occurs when daily energy expenditure exceeds daily energy intake.

2. True Thirty-five hundred "extra" kcal through either increased energy intake or decreased energy output approximates the energy contained in 1 pound (0.45 kg) of stored body fat.

3. True Grouping of all fats and oils together (with sweets) does not distinguish differences between good fats (olive oil and canola oil, high in monounsaturated fats and omega-3 fatty acids) that fend off heart disease and fight inflammation and harmful fats such as saturated fats and *trans*-unsaturated fatty acids. Also, such a grouping does not clarify differences between refined carbohydrates (white rice, white bread) and the more healthful ones (whole grains, brown rice).

4. False Guidelines from the U.S. government are essentially similar to those formulated by other agencies (including the USDA) and place great emphasis on the adoption of healthy eating patterns and lifestyle behaviors rather than focusing on specific numeric goals such as for dietary fat intake.

5. False Research in exercise nutrition, although far from complete, indicates that the large number of teenagers and adults who exercise regularly to keep fit, including competitive athletes, do not require additional nutrients beyond those obtained through the regular intake of a nutritionally well-balanced diet. Endurance athletes and others who engage regularly in heavy training must maintain adequate energy and protein intake and appropriate carbohydrate consumption to match this macronutrient's use for energy during exercise. However, attention to proper diet does not mean that a physically active person must join the ranks of the more than 40% of Americans who take supplements (spending about $6 billion yearly) to micromanage nutrient intake.

6. False Adequate research design and methodology has not shown that amino acid supplementation in any form above the RDA significantly increases muscle mass or improves muscular strength, power, or endurance. Most individuals obtain adequate protein to sustain muscle growth with resistance training by consuming ordinary foods in a well-balanced diet. Provided caloric intake balances energy output and one consumes a wide variety of foods, no need exists to consume supplements of protein or simple amino acids.

7. False Standards for optimal lipid intake are not firmly established, but to promote good health, lipid intake should probably not exceed 25 to 30% of the diet's energy content. Of this, at least 70% should come from unsaturated fatty acids.

8. False No hazard to health exists when subsisting chiefly on a variety of fiber-rich complex unrefined carbohydrates, with adequate intake of essential amino acids, fatty acids, minerals, and vitamins. The diet of the Tarahumara Indians of Mexico, for example, consists of high-fiber, complex carbohydrates (75% of calories) and correspondingly low intake of cholesterol (71 mg $\cdot$ day^{-1}), lipid (12% of calories), and saturated fat (2% of calories), and they exhibit excellent long-term health with low morbidity and mortality rates.

9. False Over 45 years of research fails to support the use of vitamin supplements by nutritionally adequate healthy people to improve exercise performance or the ability to train arduously. When vitamin intake achieves recommended levels via diet, supplements neither improve performance nor increase the blood levels of these micronutrients.

10. False The best sources of antioxidants are β-carotene found in pigmented compounds that give color to yellow and orange vegetables and fruits including carrots, dark-green leafy vegetables such as spinach, broccoli, turnips, beet and collard greens, and sweet potatoes, winter squash, apricots, cantaloupe, mangos, and papaya; vitamin C found in citrus fruits and juices, cabbage, broccoli, turnip greens, cantaloupe, green and red sweet peppers, and berries; vitamin E found in poultry, seafood, vegetable oils, wheat germ, fish liver oils, whole-grain breads and fortified cereals, nuts and seeds, dried beans, green leafy vegetables, and eggs.

References

1. Abrahams A. The nutrition of athletes. Br J Nutr 1948;2:266.
2. Aleisso HM, et al. Generation of reactive oxygen species after exhaustive aerobic and isometric exercise. Med Sci Sports Exerc 2000;32:1576.
3. American College of Sports Medicine: Position statement on prevention of heat injuries during distance running. Med Sci Sports Exerc 1984;16:ix.
4. Anderson RA, et al. Strenuous running: acute effects on chromium, copper, zinc, and selected variables in urine and serum of male runners. Biol Trace Element Res 1984;6:327.
5. Ardawi MN, Newsholme EA. Metabolism in lymphocytes and its importance in the immune response. Essays Biochem 1985;21:1.
6. Baum M, et al. Moderate and exhaustive endurance exercise influences the interferon-levels in whole-blood culture supernatants. Eur J Appl Physiol 1997;76:165.
7. Bazzano LA, et al. Fruit and vegetable intake and risk of cardiovascular disease in US adults: the first National Health and Nutrition Examination Survey Epidemiologic Follow-up Study. Am J Clin Nutr 2002;76:93.
8. Beaton LJ, et al. Contraction-induced muscle damage is unaffected by vitamin E supplementation. Med Sci Sports Exerc 2002;34:L798.
9. Blanchard MA, et al. The influence of diet and exercise on muscle and plasma glutamine concentrations. Med Sci Sports Exerc 2001;33:69.
10. Brouns F. Nutritional needs of athletes. New York: John Wiley & Sons, 1993.
11. Carraro F, et al. Urea kinetics in humans at two levels of exercise intensity. J Appl Physiol 1993;75:1180.
12. Castell LM, et al. Does glutamine have a role in reducing infections in athletes? Eur J Appl Physiol 1996;73:488.
13. Castell LM, et al. Some aspects of the acute phase response after a marathon race, and the effects of glutamine supplementation. Eur J Appl Physiol 1997;75:47.
14. Chandra .K. Nutrition and the immune system: an introduction. Am J Clin Nutr 1997;60(suppl):460S.

15. Clancy SP, et al. Effects of chromium picolinate supplementation on body composition, strength, and urinary chromium loss in football players. Int J Sport Nutr 1994;4:142.

16. Clark LC, et al. Effects of selenium supplementation for cancer prevention in patients with carcinoma of the skin: a randomized trial. JAMA 1996;276:1957.

17. Clarkson PM. Minerals: exercise performance and supplementation in athletes. J Sports Sci 1991;9:91.

18. Clarkson PM, Haymes EM. Trace mineral requirements for athletes. Int J Sports Nutr 1994;4:104.

19. Clarkson PM, Haymes EM. Exercise and mineral status of athletes: calcium, magnesium, phosphorus, and iron. Med Sci Sports Exerc 1995;27:831.

20. Clarkson PM, Thompson HS. Antioxidants: what role do they play in physical activity and health? Am J Clin Nutr 2000;72:637.

21. Connor WE, et al. The plasma lipids, lipoproteins, and diet of the Tarahumara Indians of Mexico. Am J Clin Nutr 1978;31:1131.

22. Coombes JS, et al. Effect of vitamin E deficiency on fatigue and muscle contractile properties. Eur J Appl Physiol 2002;87:272.

23. Couzy DL, et al. Zinc metabolism in the athlete: influence of training, nutrition and other factors. Int J Sports Med 1990;11:263.

24. Davis JM, et al. Exercise, alveolar macrophage function, and susceptibility to respiratory infection. J Appl Physiol 1997;83:1461.

25. Dawson B, et al. Effect of vitamin C and vitamin E supplementation on biochemical and ultrastructural indices of muscle damage after a 21 km run. Int J Sports Med 2002;23:10.

26. DeLorgeril M, et al. Mediterranean diet, traditional risk factors, and the rate of cardiovascular complications after myocardial infarction. Circulation 1999;99:779.

27. De Souza MJ, et al. Menstrual status and plasma vasopressin, renin activity, and aldosterone exercise responses. J Appl Physiol 1989;67:736.

28. Dressendorfer RH, et al. Plasma mineral levels in marathon runners during a 20-day road race. Phys Sportsmed 1982;10:113.

29. Eaton CB, et al. Cross-sectional relationship between diet and physical activity in two southeastern New England communities. Am J Prev Med 1995;11:238.

30. Fahlman M, et al.: Effects of endurance training on selected parameters of immune function in elderly women. Gerontology 46:97, 2000.

31. Fleshner M. Exercise and neuroendocrine regulation of antibody production: protective effect of physical activity of stress-induced suppression of the specific antibody response. Int J Sports Med 2000;21(suppl 1):S214.

32. Fogelholm GM, et al. Dietary and biochemical indices of nutritional status in male athletes and controls. J Am Coll Nutr 1992;11:181.

33. Food and Nutrition Board, Institute of Medicine. Dietary reference intakes for energy, carbohydrates, fiber, fat, protein and amino acids. Washington, DC: National Academy Press, 2002.

34. Friedenreic CM. Physical activity and cancer: lessons learned from nutritional epidemiology. Nutr Rev 2001;59:349.

35. Fung TT, et al. Whole-grain intake and risk of type-2 diabetes: a prospective study in men. Am J Clin Nutr 2002;76:535.

36. Gabriel HA, et al. Circulating leukocyte and lymphocyte subpopulations before and after intensive endurance exercise to exhaustion. J Appl Physiol 1991;63:449.

37. Ginsburg GS, et al. Effects of a single bout of ultraendurance exercise on lipid levels and susceptibility of lipids to peroxidation in triathletes. JAMA 1996;276:221.

38. Gleeson M, Bishop NC. Elite athlete immunology: importance of nutrition. Int J Sports Nutr 2000;21(suppl 1):S44.

39. Goldfarb AH, et al. Antioxidants: role of supplementation to prevent exercise-induced oxidative stress. Med Sci Sports Exerc 1993;25:232.

40. Goldfarb AH, et al. Vitamin E effects on indexes of lipid peroxidation in muscle from DHEA-treated and exercised rats. J Appl Physiol 1994;76:1630.

41. Goldfarb AH, et al. Vitamin E attenuates myocardial oxidative stress induced by DHEA in rested and exercised rats. J Appl Physiol 1996;80:486.

42. Grandjean AC. Macronutrient intakes of U.S. athletes compared with the general population and recommendations made for athletes. Am J Clin Nutr 1989;49:1070.

43. Gratt JM, et al. Effect of daily vitamin E and multivitamin-mineral supplementation on acute respiratory tract infections in elderly persons. JAMA 2002;288:715.

44. Guilland JC, et al. Vitamin status of young athletes including the effects of supplementation. Med Sci Sports Exerc 1989;4:441.

45. Hann CS, et al. Validation of the Healthy Eating Index with use of biomarkers in a clinical sample of healthy women. Am J Clin Nutr 2001;74:479.

46. Hansen JB, et al. Biphasic changes in leukocytes induced by strenuous exercise. Eur J Appl Physiol 1991;62:157.

47. Haraldsdottir J, Andersen LB. Dietary factors related to fitness in young men and women. Prev Med 1994;23:490.

48. Haub MD, et al. Effect of protein source on resistive-training-induced changes in body composition and muscle size in older men. Am J Clin Nutr 2002;76:511.

49. Haymes EM. Vitamin and mineral supplementation to athletes. Int J Sport Nutr 1991;1:146.

50. Helge JW, et al. Interaction of training and diet on metabolism and endurance during exercise in man. J Physiol 1996;492:1.

51. Hellsten Y, et al. Effect of sprint cycle training on activities of antioxidant enzymes in human skeletal muscle. J Appl Physiol 1996;81:1484.

52. Hemilüa H. Vitamin C and common cold incidence: a review of studies with subjects under heavy physical stress. Int J Sports Med 1996;17:379.

53. Henson DA, et al. Carbohydrate supplementation and lymphocyte proliferative response to long endurance running. Int J Sports Med 1998;19:574.

54. Hickson RC, et al. Glutamine prevents down-regulation of myosin heavy-chain synthesis and muscle atrophy from glucocorticoids. Am J Physiol 1995;31:E730.

55. Hill RJ, Davies PS. Energy expenditure during 2 wk of an ultra-endurance run around Australia. Med Sci Sport Exerc 2001;33:148.

56. Hill RJ, Davies PS. Energy intake and energy expenditure in elite lightweight female rowers. Med Sci Sports Exerc 2002;34:1823.

57. Hoffman-Goetz L, Pedersen BK. Exercise and the immune system: a model of the stress response? Immunol Today 1994;15:382.

58. Hu FB, Willett WC. Optimal diets for prevention of coronary heart disease. JAMA 2002;288:2569.

59. Hu FB, et al. Prospective study of major dietary patterns and risk of coronary heart disease in men. Am J Clin Nutr 2001;72:912.

60. Inal M, et al. Effect of aerobic and anaerobic metabolism on free radical generation in swimmers. Med Sci Sports Exerc 2001;33:564.

61. Itoh H, et al. Vitamin E supplementation attenuates leakage of enzymes following 6 successive days of running training. Int J Sports Med 2000;21:369.

62. Jeng KCG, et al. Supplementation with vitamins C and E enhances cytokine production by peripheral blood mononuclear cells in healthy adults. Am J Clin Nutr 1996;64:960.

63. Ji LL. Exercise and oxidative stress: role of the cellular antioxidant systems. Exerc Sport Sci Rev 1995;23:135.

64. Jimenez K, et al. Exercise does not induce oxidative stress in trained heart transplant recipients. Med Sci Sports Exerc 2001;32:2018.

65. Jonsdottir IH, et al. Voluntary chronic exercise augments in vivo natural immunity in rats. J Appl Physiol 1997;80:1799.

66. Jonsdottir IH, et al. Enhancement of natural immunity seen after voluntary exercise in rats. Role of central opioid receptors. Life Sci 2000;66:1231.

67. Joshipura KJ, et al. Fruit and vegetable intake in relation to risk of ischemic stroke. JAMA 1999;282:1233.

68. Jula A, et al. Effects of a diet and simvastatin on serum lipids, insulin and antioxidants in hypercholesterolemic men. A randomized controlled trial. JAMA 2002;287:598.

69. Kant AK. Consumption of energy-dense, nutrient-poor foods by adult Americans: the third National Health and Nutrition Examination Survey, 1988–1994. Am J Clin Nutr 2000;72:929.

70. Kanter MM. Free radicals and exercise: effects of nutritional antioxidant supplementation. Exerc Sport Sci Rev 1995;23:375.

71. Kanter MM, et al. Effects of an antioxidant vitamin mixture on lipid peroxidation at rest and postexercise. J Appl Physiol 1993;74:965.

72. Khoo C-S, et al. Nutrient intake and eating habits of triathletes. Ann Sports Med 1987;3:144.

73. Kleiner SM, et al. Metabolic profiles, diet and health practices of championship male and female body builders. J Am Diet Assoc 1990;90:962.

74. Kohut ML, et al. Prolonged exercise suppresses antigen-specific cytokine response to upper respiratory infection. J Appl Physiol 2001;90:678.

75. Koppel M, et al. Effects of elevated plasma noradrenaline concentration on the immune system in humans. Eur J Appl Physiol 1998;79:93.

76. Kosta T, et al. The symptomatology of upper respiratory tract infections and exercise in elderly. Med Sci Sports Exerc 2000;32:46.

77. Krauss RM, et al. AHA dietary guidelines revision 2000: a statement for health care professionals from the Nutrition Committee of the American Heart Association. Circulation 2000;102:2284.

78. Krebs JM, et al. Zinc and copper balances in healthy adult males during and after 17 wk of bed rest. Am J Clin Nutr 1993;58:897.

79. Krzywkowski K, et al. Effect of glutamine and protein supplementation on exercise-induced decreases in salivary IgA. J Appl Physiol 2001;91:832.

80. Lambert CP, et al. Influence of acute submaximal exercise on T-lymphocyte suppressor cell function in healthy young men. Eur J Appl Physiol 2000;82:151.

81. Lane HW. Some trace elements related to physical activity: zinc, copper, selenium, chromium and iodine. In: Hickson JE, Wolinski I, eds. Nutrition in exercise and sport. Boca Raton, FL: CRC Press, 1989.

82. Lasheras C, et al. Mediterranean diet and age with respect to overall survival in institutionalized, nonsmoking elderly people. Am J Clin Nutr 2000;71:987.

83. Lauber RP, Sheard NF. The American Heart Association dietary guidelines for 2000: a summary report. Nutr Rev 2001;59:298.

84. Leaf DA, et al. The effect of exercise intensity on lipid peroxidation. Med Sci Sports Exerc 1997;29:1036.

85. Liu S, et al. Fruit and vegetable intake and risk of cardiovascular disease: the Women's Health Study. Am J Clin Nutr 2000;72:922.

86. Lönnerdal B. Bioavailability of copper. Am J Clin Nutr 1996;63(suppl):821S.

87. Lukaski HC. Magnesium, zinc, and chromium nutriture and physical activity. Am J Clin Nutr 2000;72(suppl):585S.

88. Mackinnon LT. Future directions in exercise and immunology: regulation and integration. Int J Sports Med 1998;19:S205.

89. Manore MM. Vitamin B_6 and exercise. Int J Sports Nutr 1994;5:89.

90. Manore MM. Effects of physical activity on thiamine, riboflavin, and vitamin B_6 requirements. Am J Clin Nutr 2000;72(suppl):598S.

91. Manore MM, Leklem JE. Effect of carbohydrate and vitamin B_6 on fuel substrates during exercise in women. Med Sci Sports Exerc 1988;20:233.

92. Matthews CE, et al. Relationship between leisure-time physical activity and selected dietary variables in the Worcester Area Trial for Counseling in Hyperlipidemia. Med Sci Sports Exerc 1997;29:1199.

93. Matthews CE, et al. Physical activity and risk of upper-respiratory tract infection. Med Sci Sports Exerc 2000;32:S292.

94. Matthews CE, et al. Moderate to vigorous physical activity and risk of upper-respiratory tract infection. Med Sci Sports Exerc 2002;34:1242.

95. McBride JM, et al. Effect of resistance exercise on free radical production. Med Sci Sports Exerc 1998;30:67.

96. Meydani SN, et al. Vitamin E supplementation and in vivo immune response in healthy elderly subjects. JAMA 1997;277:1380.

97. Miyazaki H, et al. Strenuous endurance training in humans reduces oxidative stress following exhausting exercise. Eur J Appl Physiol 2001;84:1.

98. Montain SJ, et al. Aldosterone and vasopressin response in the heat: hydration level and exercise intensity effects. Med Sci Sports Exerc 1997;29:661.

99. Müuns G, et al. Impaired nasal mucociliary clearance in long-distance runners. Int J Sports Med 1995;16:209.

100. Mudio DM, et al. Effect of dietary fat on metabolic adjustments to maximal VO_2 and endurance in runners. Med Sci Sports Exerc 1994;26:81.

101. National Research Council, Committee on Diet and Health: Health implications for reducing chronic disease risk. Washington, DC: National Academy Press, 1989.

102. Nehlsen-Cannarella S, et al. Carbohydrate and cytokine response to 2.5 hr of running. J Appl Physiol 1997;82:1662.

103. Nieman B, et al. Supplementation patterns in marathon runners. J Am Diet Assoc 1989;89:1615.

104. Nieman DC. Physical activity, fitness, and infection. In: Bouchard C, et al, eds. Physical activity, fitness, and health. Champaign, IL: Human Kinetics, 1994.

105. Nieman DC. Immune response to heavy exertion. J Appl Physiol 1997;82:1385.

106. Nieman DC, Pedersen BK. Nutrition and exercise immunology. Boca Raton, FL: CRC Press, 2000.

107. Nieman DC, et al. Physical activity and immune function in elderly women. Med Sci Sports Exerc 1993;25:823.

108. Nieman D., et al. Natural killer cell cytotoxic activity in weight trainers and sedentary controls. J Strength Condit Res 1994;8:251.

109. Nieman DC, et al. Carbohydrate supplementation affects blood granulocyte and monocyte trafficking but not function following 2.5 hours of running. Am J Clin Nutr 1997;66: 153.

110. Nieman DC, et al. Influence of mode and carbohydrate on the cytokine response to heavy exertion. Med Sci Sports Exerc 1998;30:671.

111. Nieman DC, et al. Cytokine changes after a marathon race. J Appl Physiol 2001;91:109.

112. Novas A, et al. Total daily energy expenditure and incidence of upper respiratory tract infection symptoms in young females. Int J Sports Med 2002;23:465.

113. Pedersen BK. Influence of physical activity on the cellular immune system: mechanism of action. Int J Sports Med 1991;12:S23.

114. Pedersen BK, Hoffman-Goetz L. Exercise and the immune system: regulation, integration, and adaptation. Physiol Rev. 2000;80:1055.

115. Pedersen BK, et al. Exercise and the immune system—influence of nutrition and aging. J Sci Sports Med 1999;2:234.

116. Pedersen BK, et al. Training and natural immunity: effects of diets rich in fat or carbohydrate. Eur J Appl Physiol 2000;82:98.13.

117. Pendergast DR, et al.: The role of dietary fat on performance, metabolism and health. Am J Sports Med 1996;24:s53.

118. Peters EM, et al. Vitamin C supplementation reduces the incidence of postrace symptoms of upper-respiratory-tract infection in ultramarathon runners. Am J Clin Nutr 1993;57:170.

119. Peters EM, et al. Attenuation of the increase in circulating cortisol and enhancement of the acute phase response in vitamin C-supplemented ultramarathon runners. Int J Sports Med 2001;22:120.

120. Peters EM, et al. Vitamin C supplementation attenuates the increases in circulating cortisol, adrenaline and anti-inflammatory polypeptides following ultramarathon running. Int J Sports Med 2001;22:537.

121. Peters-Futre EM. Vitamin C, neutrophil function, and URTI risk in distance runners: the missing link. Exerc Immunol Rev 1997;3:32.

122. Pincemail J, et al.: Pentane measurement in man as an index of lipoperoxidation. Bioelectrochem Bioenerg 1987;18:117.

123. Popkin BM, et al. A comparison of dietary trends among racial and socioeconomic groups in the United States. N Engl J Med 1996;335:716.

124. Position of the American Dietetic Association. Nutrition for physical fitness and athletic performance for adults. ADA Reports 1987;87:933.

125. Rennie MJ, et al. Physical activity and protein metabolism. In: Bouchard C, et al., eds. Physical activity, fitness, and health. Champaign, IL: Human Kinetics, 1994.

126. Rodriguez Tuya I, et al. Evaluation of the influence of physical activity on plasma concentrations of several trace metals. Eur J Appl Physiol 1996;23:299.

127. Rohde T, et al. Competitive sustained exercise in humans, lymphokine activated killer cell activity, and glutamine—an intervention study. Eur J Appl Physiol 1998;78:448.

128. Rohde T, et al. Effect of glutamine supplementation on changes in the immune system induced by repeated exercise. Med Sci Sports Exerc 1998;30:856.

129. Rokitzke L, et al. Acute changes in vitamin B_6 status in endurance athletes before and after a marathon. Int J Sports Nutr 1994;4:154.

130. Rokitzki L, et al. α-Tocopherol supplementation in racing cyclists during extreme endurance training. Int J Sports Nutr 1994;4:255.

131. Rokitzki L, et al. Assessment of vitamin B_2 status in performance athletes of various types of sports. J Nutr Sci Vitaminol 1994;40:11.

132. Rokitzki L, et al. Dietary, serum and urine ascorbic acid status in male athletes. Int J Sports Med 1994;15:435.

133. Rokitzki L, et al. Lipid peroxidation and antioxidative vitamins under extreme endurance stress. Acta Physiol Scand 1994;151:149.

134. Rosen O, et al. Leukocyte counts and lymphocyte responsiveness associated with repeated bouts of strenuous endurance exercise. J Appl Physiol 2001;91:425.

135. Rowbottom DG, et al. The emerging role of glutamine as an indicator of exercise stress and overtraining. Sports Med 1996;21:80.

136. Scanga CB, et al. Effects of weight loss and exercise training on natural killer cell activity in obese women. Med Sci Sports Exerc 1998;30:1668.

137. Scharhag J, et al. Mobilization and oxidative burst of neutrophils are influenced by carbohydrate supplementation during prolonged cycling in humans. Eur J Appl Physiol 2002;87:584.

138. Senturk UK, et al. Exercise-induced oxidative stress affects erythrocytes in sedentary rats but not exercise-trained rats. J Appl Physiol 2001;91:1999.

139. Sharp NCC, Koutedakis Y. Sport and the overtraining syndrome: immunological aspects. Br Med Bull 1992;48:518.

140. Shephard RJ, et al. The impact of exercise on the immune system: NK cells, interleukins 1 and 2, and related responses. Exerc Sport Sci Rev 1995;23:215.

141. Shewchuk LD, et al. Dietary L-glutamine does not improve lymphocyte metabolism or function in exercise-trained rats. Med Sci Sports Exerc 1997;29:474.

142. Singh A, et al. Chronic multivitamin-mineral supplementation does not enhance physical performance. Med Sci Sports Exerc 1992;24:726.

143. Singh A, et al. Neuroendocrine response to running in women after zinc and vitamin E supplementation. Med Sci Sports Exerc 1999;31:536.

144. Sjödin AM, et al. Energy balance in cross-country skiers: a study using doubly labeled water. Med Sci Sports Exerc 1994;26:720.

145. Smith DJ, Norris SR. Changes in glutamine and glutamate concentrations for tracking training tolerance. Med Sci Sports Exerc 32:684, 2000.

146. Solfrizzi V, et al. High monounsaturated fatty acid intake protects against age-related cognitive decline. Neurology 1999;52:1563.

147. Stark AH, Madar Z. Olive oil as a functional food: epidemiology and nutritional approaches. Nutr Rev 2002;60:170.

148. Steensberg A, et al. Strenuous exercise decreases the percentage of type 1 T cells in the circulation. J Appl Physiol 2001;91:1708.

149. Sundgot-Borgen J. Prevalence of eating disorders in elite female athletes. Int J Sports Nutr 1993;3:30.

150. Tarnopolosky MA, et al. Influence of protein intake and training status on nitrogen balance and lean body mass. J Appl Physiol 1988;64:187.

151. Telford R, et al. The effect of 7 to 8 months of vitamin/mineral supplementation on athletic performance. Int J Sports Nutr 1992;2:135.

152. Tessier F, et al. Selenium and training effects on the glutathione system and aerobic performance. Med Sci Sports Exerc 1995;27:390.

153. Tiidus PM, Houston ME. Vitamin E status and response to exercise training. Sports Med 1995;26:12.

154. Trappe TA, et al. Energy expenditure of swimmers during high volume training. Med Sci Sports Exerc 1997;29:950.

155. Trichopoulou A, et al. Adherence to a Mediterranean diet and survival in a Greek population. N Engl J Med. 2003;348:2599.

156. Uusitalo AL, et al. Overtraining: making a difficult diagnosis and implementing targeted treatment. Phys Sportsmed 2001;29(5):35.

157. Van Remmen H, et al. Oxidative damage to DNA and aging. Exerc Sport Sci Rev 2003;31:149.

158. Variyam JN, et al. USDA's Healthy Eating Index and nutrition information. Washington, DC: USDA, 1998.

159. Vasankari TJ, et al. Increased serum and low-density-lipoprotein antioxidant potential after antioxidant supplementation in endurance athletes. Am J Clin Nutr 1997;65:1052.

160. Viquie CA, et al. Antioxidant status and indexes of oxidative stress during consecutive days of exercise. J Appl Physiol 1993;75:566.

161. Volek JS, et al. Testosterone and cortisol in relationship to dietary nutrients and resistance exercise. J Appl Physiol 1997;82:49.

162. Wagenmakers A.JM, et al. Carbohydrate supplementation, glycogen depletion, and amino acid metabolism. Am J Physiol 1991;260:E883.

163. Walsh NP, Blannin AK. Effect of oral glutamine supplementation on human neutrophil lipopolysaccharide-stimulated degranulation following prolonged exercise. Int J Sport. Nutr Exerc Metab 2000;1:39.

164. Webster MJ, et al. The effect of a thiamin derivative on exercise performance. Eur J Appl Physiol 1997;75:520.

165. Weidner TG, et al. The effect of exercise training on the severity and duration of viral upper respiratory illness. Med Sci Sports Exerc 1998;30:1578.

166. Weinstock C, et al. Effect of exhaustive exercise stress on the cytokine response. Med Sci Sports Exerc 1997;29:345.

167. Whiteside TL, Herberman RB. Short analytical review: the role of natural killer cells in human diseases. Clin Immunol Immunopathol 1989;53:1.

168. Wolfe RR. Protein supplements and exercise. Am J Clin Nutr 2000;72(suppl):551S.

169. Wolfe RR, et al. Isotopic analysis of leucine and urea metabolism in exercising humans. J Appl Physiol 1982;52:458.

170. Woods JA, et al. Exercise and cellular innate immune function. Med Sci Sports Exerc 1999;31:57.

Up-to-Date Complementary Readings

Akobundu UO, et al. Vitamins A and C, calcium, fruit, and dairy products are limited in food pantries. J Am Diet Assoc 2004;104:811.

Bloomer RJ, et al. Effects of antioxidant therapy in women exposed to eccentric exercise. Int J Sport Nutr Exerc Metab 2004;14:377.

Brooks GA, et al. Chronicle of the Institute of Medicine physical activity recommendation: How a physical activity recommendation came to be among dietary recommendations. Am J Clin Nutr 2004;79:921S.

Campbell WW, Geik RA. Nutritional considerations for the older athlete. Nutrition 2004;20:603.

Cavas L, Tarhan L. Effects of vitamin-mineral supplementation on cardiac marker and radical scavenging enzymes, and MDA levels in young swimmers. Int J Sport Nutr Exerc Metab 2004;14:133.

Cotton PA, et al. Dietary sources of nutrients among US adults, 1994 to 1996. J Am Diet Assoc 2004;104:921.

Feskanich D, et al. Modifying the Healthy Eating Index to assess diet quality in children and adolescents. J Am Diet Assoc 2004;104:1375.

Goldberg JP, et al. The obesity crisis: Don't blame it on the pyramid. J Am Diet Assoc 2004;104:1141.

Hinton PS, et al. Nutrient intakes and dietary behaviors of male and female collegiate athletes. Int J Sport Nutr Exerc Metab 2004;14:389.

Lukaski HC. Vitamin and mineral status: Effects on physical performance. Nutrition 2004;20:632.

Tande DL, et al. The associations between blood lipids and the Food Guide Pyramid: Findings from the Third National Health and Nutrition Examination Survey. Prev Med 2004;38:452.

Unnithan VB, Goulopoulou S. Nutrition for the pediatric athlete. Curr Sports Med Rep 2004;3:206.

Viitala PE, et al. The effects of antioxidant vitamin supplementation on resistance exercise induced lipid peroxidation in trained and untrained participants. Lipids Health Dis 2004;3:14.

Weinberg LG, et al. Nutrient contributions of dairy foods in the United States, Continuing Survey of Food Intakes by Individuals, 1994-1996, 1998. J Am Diet Assoc 2004;104:895.

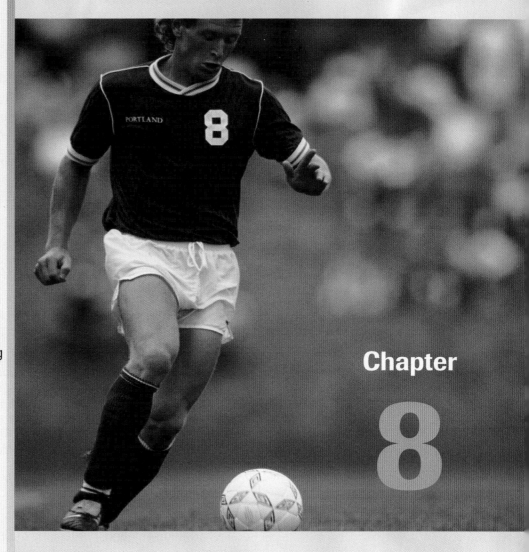

Chapter

8

Nutritional Considerations for Intense Training and Sports Competition

The need to maintain optimal nutrient intake to sustain energy and tissue-building requirements of regular physical activity also requires unique dietary modifications to facilitate intense training and competition.

THE PRECOMPETITION MEAL

Athletes often compete in the morning following the overnight fast. As pointed out in Chapter 1, significant depletion occurs in carbohydrate reserves over an 8- to 12-hour period without eating, even if the person normally follows appropriate dietary recommendations. Consequently, precompetition nutrition takes on considerable importance. *The precompetition meal should provide adequate carbohydrate energy and ensure optimal hydration.* Within this framework, fasting before competition or intense training makes no sense physiologically because it rapidly depletes liver and muscle glycogen, which subsequently impairs exercise performance. Thus, if a person trains or competes in the afternoon, breakfast becomes the important meal to optimize glycogen reserves. For late afternoon training or competition, lunch becomes the important source for topping off glycogen stores. Consider the following three factors when individualizing the precompetition meal plan:

1. Food preferences
2. "Psychological set" of the competitor
3. Digestibility of the foods

As a general rule, eliminate foods high in lipid and protein content on the day of competition because these foods digest slowly and remain in the digestive tract longer than carbohydrate foods of similar energy content. Timing of the precompetition meal also deserves consideration. The increased stress and tension that usually accompany competition decrease blood flow to the digestive tract, depressing intestinal absorption. *It takes 3 to 4 hours to digest, absorb, and store as muscle and liver glycogen a carbohydrate-rich, precompetition meal.*

Protein or Carbohydrate?

Many athletes become psychologically accustomed to, and even depend on, the classic "steak and eggs" precompetition meal. Such a meal may satisfy the athlete, coach, and restaurateur, but it provides no benefit to exercise performance. This type of meal, with its low carbohydrate content, can hinder optimal performance.

There are five reasons for modifying or even abolishing the high-protein precompetition meal in favor of one high in carbohydrates:

1. Dietary carbohydrates replenish the significant liver and muscle glycogen depletion from the overnight fast.
2. Carbohydrates digest and absorb more rapidly than either proteins or lipids. Thus, carbohydrates provide energy faster and reduce the feeling of fullness following a meal.
3. A high-protein meal elevates resting metabolism considerably more than a high-carbohydrate meal owing to greater energy requirements for digestion, absorption, and assimilation. This additional metabolic heat potentially strains the body's heat-dissipating mechanisms and impairs hot weather exercise performance.
4. Protein breakdown for energy facilitates dehydration during exercise because the byproducts of amino acid breakdown require water for urinary excretion. For example, approximately 50 mL of water "accompanies" excretion of each gram of urea in the urine.
5. Carbohydrate serves as the primary energy nutrient for short-term anaerobic activity and for prolonged, high-intensity aerobic exercise.

CASE STUDY/PERSONAL HEALTH AND EXERCISE NUTRITION 8–1

Applying the USDA Food Guide Pyramid to Children, Seniors, and Women During Pregnancy and Lactation

The Food Guide Pyramid provides a planning guide for diets that meet nutrient requirements and recommendations for health promotion and disease prevention. The following five food groups form the basis of the plan:
1. Bread, cereal, rice, and pasta
2. Vegetables
3. Fruits
4. Milk, yogurt, and cheese
5. Meat poultry, fish, dry beans, eggs, and nuts

The Pyramid also includes a recommendation to use fats, oils, and sweets sparingly. It meets a variety of energy needs and provides flexibility to suit preferences of persons from diverse cultures and lifestyles.

APPLICATION TO YOUNG CHILDREN (2–6 YEARS OF AGE)

Children have small stomachs and high nutrient needs relative to their body size. Consequently, they should consume nutritious meals and snacks throughout the day. Children require a varied diet based on whole grains, vegetables, and fruits combined with adequate milk and other high-protein foods. The USDA has designed a version of the Food Guide Pyramid for appeal to children 2 to 6 years of age (left-hand figure). Children ages 2 to 4 years should consume the low end of the range of number of servings recommended for adults. Recommended number of servings for children 4 to 6 years are the same as for adults, but the servings may need to be split between several meals or snacks consumed

throughout the day. Reduce serving size for children ages 2 and 3. For all children 2 to 6 years of age, 2 cups of milk should be consumed each day (or other choices from the dairy group).

Creativity ensures that a child's diet includes selections from each of the Pyramid's food groups. For example, serve fruits on cereals or as a juice; add milk to hot cereal, cream soup, pudding, and custard; use meats in spaghetti sauces, stews, casseroles, burritos, or pizza.

APPLICATION TO SENIORS (>70 YEARS OF AGE)

A modified Food Guide Pyramid emphasizes the nutrients and food selections of particular concern to older adults. This Pyramid, shown in the middle figure, builds from a base of water—eight 8-oz glasses per day. The Pyramid for seniors has a narrower base than the traditional Pyramid to emphasize the typically reduced energy needs of the elderly. Serving n umber equals or exceeds the minimum recommended by the regular Pyramid. Nutrient-dense choices from each food group are recommended. The "senior" pyramid also emphasizes the importance of dietary fiber and includes a flag at the top to indicate the possible need for dietary supplements.

APPLICATION DURING PREGNANCY AND LACTATION

During pregnancy, food (and supplements) must supply all the nutrients for fetal growth and development, while at the same time continuing to meet the mother's nutritional needs. Because energy needs for pregnant women increase proportionately less than the increased need for protein and micronutrients, a well-balanced, nutrient-dense diet becomes essential.

The energy and protein needs of pregnancy can easily be met by following the Food Guide Pyramid recommendations for pregnant women in right-hand figure. Additional servings recommended from the bread, cereal, rice, vegetable, and pasta group provide energy, protein, micronutrients, and fiber, particularly if one consumes whole grains.

Human Nutrition Information Service. The food guide pyramid. Home and Garden Bulletin no. 252. Hyattsville, MD: Human Nutrition Information Service. U.S. Department of Agriculture, 1992, rev 1996.

USDA's Food and Nutrition Information Center <www.nal.usda.gov/fnic/dga/index.html> National Center for Nutrition and Dietetics, the American Dietetic Association, ADAF, 1997.

Hadedad EH, et al. Vegetarian food guide pyramid: a conceptual framework. Am J Clin Nutr 1999;70(suppl);6152.

Russell RM, et al. Modified food guide pyramid for people over seventy years of age. J Nutr 1999;129:751.

Make It Carbohydrate Rich

The ideal precompetition meal maximizes muscle and liver glycogen storage and provides glucose for intestinal absorption during exercise. The meal should :

- Contain 150 to 300 g of carbohydrate (3–5 g per kg of body mass in either solid or liquid form)
- Be consumed 3 to 4 hours before exercising
- Contain relatively little fat and fiber to facilitate gastric emptying and minimize gastrointestinal distress.

The real significance of precompetition feeding occurs only if the person maintains a nutritionally sound diet throughout training. Preexercise feedings cannot correct existing nutritional deficiencies or inadequate nutrient intake in the weeks before competition. Chapter 11 discusses how endurance athletes can augment precompetition glycogen storage with the specific exercise/diet modifications of carbohydrate loading.

LIQUID AND PREPACKAGED BARS, POWDERS, AND MEALS

Commercially prepared nutrition bars, powders, and liquid meals offer an alternative approach to precompetition feeding or supplemental feedings during periods of competition.

These nutrient supplements also effectively enhance energy and nutrient intake in training, particularly if energy output exceeds energy intake from lack of interest or mismanagement of feedings.

Liquid Meals

Liquid meals provide a high-carbohydrate content but contain enough lipid and protein to contribute to satiety. They also supply the person with fluid because they exist in liquid form. The liquid meal digests rapidly, leaving essentially no residue in the intestinal tract. Liquid meals prove particularly effective during day-long swimming and track meets or during tennis, soccer, and basketball tournaments. In these situations, the person usually has little time for (or interest in) food. Liquid meals offer a practical approach to supplementing caloric intake during the high-energy output phase of training. Athletes can also use liquid nutrition if they have difficulty maintaining body weight and as a ready source of calories to gain weight.

Nutrition Bars

Nutrition bars (also called "energy bars," "protein bars," and "diet bars") contain a relatively high protein content that ranges between 10 and 30 g per bar. The typical 60-g bar contains 25 g (100 kcal) of carbohydrate (equal amounts of starch and sugar), 15 g (60 kcal) of protein, and 5 g (45 kcal) of lipid (3 g or 27 kcal of saturated fat), with the remaining weight as water. This represents about 49% of the bar's total 205 calories from carbohydrates, 29% from protein, and 22% from lipid. The bars often include vitamins and minerals (30–50% of recommended values), and some contain dietary supplements such as β-hydroxy-β-methylbutyrate (HMB). These bars must be labeled as dietary supplements, rather than foods.

Nutrient composition of nutrition bars generally varies with their purpose. For example, so-called energy bars contain a greater proportion of carbohydrates while "diet" or "weight loss" bars are lower in carbohydrate content and higher in protein. The "meal-replacement bars" have the largest energy content (240–310 kcal), with proportionately more of the three macronutrients. "Protein bars" simply contain a larger amount of protein. While nutrition bars provide a relatively easy way to obtain important nutrients, they should not totally substitute for normal food intake because they lack the broad array of plant fibers and phytochemicals found in food and contain a relatively high level of saturated fatty acids. As an added warning, because these bars are generally sold as dietary supplements, no independent assessment by the Food and Drug Administration (FDA) or other federal or state agency exists to validate the labeling claims for macronutrient content and composition.

Nutrition Powders and Drinks

A high protein content, between 10 and 50 g per serving, represents a unique aspect of nutrition powders and drinks. They also contain added vitamins, minerals, and other dietary supplement ingredients. The powders come in canisters or packets that readily mix with water (or other liquid), while the drinks come premixed in cans. These products often serve as an alternative to nutrition bars; they are marketed as meal replacements, dieting aids, energy boosters, or concentrated protein sources.

Nutrient composition of nutrition powders and drinks varies considerably from that of nutrition bars. For one thing, nutrition bars contain at least 15 g of carbohydrates to provide texture and taste, whereas powders and drinks do not. This accounts for the relatively high protein content of powders and drinks. Nutrition powders and drinks generally contain fewer calories per serving than do bars, but this can vary for a powder, depending on the liquid used for mixing.

The recommended serving of a powder averages about 45 g, the same amount as a nutrition bar (minus its water content), but wide variation exists in this recommendation. A typical serving of a high-protein powder mix contains about 10 g of carbohydrate (two-thirds as sugar), 30 g of protein, and 2 g of lipid. This amounts to a total of 178 kcal or 23% of calories from carbohydrate, 67% from protein, and 10% from lipid. Thus, when mixed in water, these powdered nutrient supplements far exceed the recommended protein intake percentage and fall below recommended lipid and carbohydrate percentages. A drink typically contains slightly more carbohydrate and less protein than does a powder.

Do not use powders and drinks to substitute for regular food intake because of their relatively high protein content and lack of the broad array of plant fibers and phytochemicals in a well-balanced diet. As with nutrition bars, the FDA or other federal or state agency makes no independent assessment of the validity of labeling claims for macronutrient content and composition.

TABLE 8.1 provides the macronutrient composition for commercially packaged liquid food supplements (rapid stomach emptying with low residue and gastrointestinal distress), high-carbohydrate drinks, and "high-energy" bars typically advocated for physically active individuals. Prudent use of some of these supplements can replenish glycogen reserves before and after high-intensity exercise and competition, especially because an athlete's appetite for "normal" food wanes.

CARBOHYDRATE FEEDINGS BEFORE, DURING, AND FOLLOWING INTENSE EXERCISE

The "vulnerability" of the body's glycogen stores during intense, prolonged exercise has focused considerable research on potential benefits of carbohydrate feedings immediately before and during exercise. This has also included ways to optimize carbohydrate replenishment in the postexercise recovery period.

Carbohydrate Feedings Before Exercise

Confusion exists about potential endurance benefits of preexercise ingestion of simple sugars. Some in exercise nutrition argue that consuming high-glycemic, rapidly absorbed carbohydrates (see Fig. 8.3) within 1 hour before exercising affects endurance performance negatively by:

- Inducing an overshoot in insulin from the rapid rise in blood sugar. Insulin excess causes a relative hypoglycemia (**rebound hypoglycemia**). Blood sugar reduction impairs central nervous system function during exercise to produce a fatiguing effect.
- Facilitating glucose influx into muscle (through large insulin release) to increase carbohydrate catabolism for energy in exercise. At the same time, high insulin levels inhibit lipolysis, which reduces free fatty acid mobilization from adipose tissue. Both augmented carbohydrate breakdown and depressed fat mobilization contribute to premature glycogen depletion and early fatigue.

Research in the late 1970s indicated that drinking a highly concentrated sugar solution 30 minutes before

Table 8.1 COMPOSITION OF COMMERCIAL CARBOHYDRATE SUPPLEMENTS IN LIQUID AND SOLID FORM

Sports Nutrition and "Metabolic Optimizer"

Beverage	No. of kcal per 8-oz Serving	Carbohydrate, g	Lipid, g	Protein, g
GatorPro Sports Nutrition	360	58 (65%)	7 (17%)	16 (18%)
Nutrament	240	34 (57%)	6.5 (25%)	11 (18%)
SportShake	310	45 (58%)	10 (29%)	11 (13%)
SegoVery	180	30 (67%)	2.5 (13%)	9 (20%)
Go	190	27 (56%)	3 (13%)	15 (31%)
Sustacal	240	33 (55%)	5.5 (21%)	14.5 (24%)
Ensure	254	35 (54%)	9 (32%)	9 (14%)
Endura Optimizer	279	57 (82%)	<1 (2%)	11 (16%)
Metabolol II	258	40 (62%)	2 (7%)	20 (31%)
ProOptibol	266	44 (66%)	2 (7%)	18 (27%)
Muscle Pep	261	45 (69%)	1 (3%)	18 (28%)
Protein Repair Formula	200	26 (52%)	1.5 (8%)	20 (40%)

High Carbohydrate Beverages

Beverage	Carbohydrate, type	Serving Size, oz	Carbohydrate, g per oz	% Carbohydrate
GatorLode	Maltodextrin & glucose	12	5.9	20
Carboplex	Maltodextrin		7.1	24
Exceed	Maltodextrin & sucrose	32	7.1	24
Carbo Fire	Glucose, polymers, fructose		7.1	24
Ultra Fuel	Maltodextrin	16	6.25	23
Carbo Power	Maltodextrin, high-fructose corn syrup		7.9	18

Sports Energy Bars

Bar	Size, oz	Total kcal	Carbohydrate, g	Protein, g	Lipid, g
Power Bar	2.25	225	42 (75%)	10 (17%)	2 (8%)
Exceed Sports Bar	2.9	280	53 (76%)	12 (17%)	2 (7%)
Edgebar	2.5	234	44 (75%)	10 (17%)	2 (8%)
K-Trainer	2.25	220	40 (73%)	10 (18%)	2 (9%)
Tiger Sport	2.3	230	40 (70%)	11 (19%)	3 (11%)
Thunder Bar	2.25	220	41 (74%)	10 (18%)	2 (8%)
Ultra Fuel	4.87	290	100 (82%)	15 (12%)	3 (6%)
Clif Bar	2.4	252	52 (80%)	5 (8%)	3 (12%)
Gator Bar	2.25	220	48 (87%)	3 (5%)	2 (8%)
Forza	2.5	231	45 (78%)	10 (18%)	1 (4%)
BTU Stoker	2.6	252	46 (73%)	10 (16%)	3 (11%)
PR Bar	1.6	190	19 (40%)	14 (30%)	6 (30%)

Carbohydrate content of common foods: 4 chocolate chip cookies = 28 g; 1 cup Wheaties (1 oz) = 23 g; 1 apple = 21 g; 1 cup apple juice = 29 g; 1 banana = 27 g

Protein content of common foods: 1 cup milk = 8 g; 3 oz baked salmon = 21 g; 1 cup cooked peas = 16 g; 3 oz steak = 22 g; 1 large egg = 6 g.

exercise precipitated early fatigue in endurance activities. For example, endurance on a bicycle ergometer declined 19% when subjects consumed a 300-mL solution containing 75 g of glucose 30 minutes before exercise compared with riding time preceded by the same volume of plain water or a liquid meal of protein, lipid, and carbohydrate.[25] Paradoxically, consuming the concentrated preevent sugar drink (in contrast to drinking plain water) prematurely depleted muscle glycogen reserves. This occurred because the dramatic rise in blood sugar within 5 to 10 minutes after ingestion produced an overshoot in insulin release from the pancreas (accentuated hyperinsulinemia) followed by a rapid decline in blood sugar (rebound hypoglycemia) as glucose moved rapidly into muscle.[33,95] At the same time, insulin inhibited fat mobilization for energy, an effect that can last for several hours after consuming a concentrated sugar solution. During exercise, therefore, intramuscular carbohydrate catabolized to a greater degree than under normal conditions. This increased the rate of glycogen depletion.

Although these negative research findings seem impressive and their explanation reasonable, subsequent investigations have *not* been replicated in healthy subjects[1,17,24,30] or patients with type-1 diabetes.[64] In fact, preexercise glucose ingestion *increased* muscle glucose uptake but *reduced* liver glucose output during exercise, to conserve liver glycogen.[50] The discrepancy among studies has no clear explanation. However, one way to eliminate any potential for negative effects of preexercise simple sugars is to consume them at least 60 minutes before exercising. This provides sufficient time to reestablished hormonal balance before exercise begins. In all likelihood, individual differences exist in the response to specific carbohydrate ingestion prior to exercise and the subsequent insulin release. The individual's preexercise glucose or glycogen status plays a role as well as the glycemic index of the food ingested (see page 238).

Preexercise Fructose: Not a Good Alternative

Fructose absorbs more slowly from the gut than either glucose or sucrose. This causes only minimal insulin response with essentially no decline in blood glucose. These observations have stimulated debate about the possible benefits of fructose as an immediate preexercise exogenous carbohydrate fuel source for prolonged exercise. The theoretical rationale for fructose use appears plausible, but its exercise benefits remain inconclusive. From a practical standpoint, consuming a high-fructose beverage often produces significant gastrointestinal distress (vomiting and diarrhea); this negatively affects exercise performance. Once absorbed by the small intestine, fructose must first enter the liver for conversion to glucose. This further limits how quickly fructose becomes available as an energy source.

Carbohydrate Feedings During Exercise

High-intensity aerobic exercise for 1 hour decreases liver glycogen by about 55%, whereas a 2-hour strenuous workout almost totally depletes the glycogen content of the liver and specifically exercised muscles (muscle fibers). Even maximal, repetitive 1- to 5-minute bouts of exercise interspersed with periods of lower-intensity exercise—as occurs in soccer, ice hockey, field hockey, European handball, and tennis— dramatically lower liver and muscle glycogen reserves.[35,74] Physical and mental performance improves with carbohydrate supplementation during exercise.[58,88,91] Carbohydrate feed-

ings during high-intensity prolonged exercise also allows individuals to exercise at greater intensity, although their perception of effort remained no different than for a placebo group.[82]

No Abnormal Insulin Response During Exercise

Consuming high-glycemic sugars during exercise does *not* augment the insulin response (and possible resulting hypoglycemia) that could occur with sugar consumption in the preexercise condition. This occurs because the release of sympathetic nervous system hormones in exercise inhibits insulin release. Concurrently, exercise augments glucose uptake by muscle so the exogenous glucose moves into these cells with a lower insulin requirement.

Consuming about 60 g of liquid or solid carbohydrates each hour benefits high-intensity, long-duration (≥ 1 h) aerobic exercise and repetitive short bouts of near-maximal effort.[2,20,41,55] As discussed in Chapter 5, sustained exercise at or below 50% of maximum intensity relies primarily on energy from fat oxidation, with relatively little demand on carbohydrate breakdown. This level of exercise does not tax glycogen reserves to a degree that would limit endurance. On the other hand, glucose feedings provide supplementary carbohydrate during high-intensity exercise when glycogen demand for energy increases greatly. In fact, mixtures of combinations of glucose, fructose, and sucrose ingested at a high rate (about 1.8 g·min^{-1}) result in a 20 to 55% higher exogenous carbohydrate oxidation rate (with reduced oxidation of endogenous carbohydrate) compared with ingestion of an isocaloric amount of glucose.[40,70] Exogenous carbohydrate intake during exercise provides the following benefits:

- Spares muscle glycogen, particularly in the type I, slow-twitch muscle fibers, because the ingested glucose powers exercise.[79–81]
- Maintains a more optimal level of blood glucose. This elevates plasma insulin levels and lowers cortisol and growth hormone levels, and prevents headache, lightheadedness, nausea, and other symptoms of central nervous system distress.[8,96] Blood glucose maintenance also supplies muscles with glucose when glycogen reserves deplete in the later stages of prolonged exercise.[16,32]

FIGURE 8.1 shows that training status does not alter the ability to oxidize glucose during exercise when the trained and untrained exercise are at the same relative intensity. Seven trained cyclists and seven untrained subjects exercised for 2 hours at 60% of aerobic capacity. At the onset of exercise, each subject consumed 8 mL · kg^{-1} of an 8% naturally labeled [^{13}C]-glucose solution with 2 mL · kg^{-1} of the fluid ingested every 20 minutes thereafter. Total exogenous [^{13}C]-glucose use (3.2 kcal · min^{-1}) was similar in both groups despite a 24% higher absolute oxygen uptake in the trained subjects (36 vs. 29 mL O$_2$ · kg^{-1} · min^{-1}; Fig. 8.1A) and higher total fat oxidation. (About 1 g [4.0 kcal] per

Oxygen consumption

Figure 8.1 A. Absolute (kJ per 60-min of exercise) and **B,** relative (%) contributions of substrates to energy expenditure in endurance trained and untrained men. (*) indicates statistically significant difference between trained and untrained. Multiply by 0.239 to convert kilojoules to kilocalories. (From Jeukendrup AE, et al. Exogenous glucose oxidation during exercise in endurance-trained and untrained subjects. J Appl Physiol 1997;83:835.)

minute represents the upper limit for oxidizing exogenous carbohydrate.[42,89]) Equivalence in exogenous glucose use between trained and untrained subjects occurred even with a relatively smaller contribution of exogenous and endogenous carbohydrate to the higher total energy expenditure of the trained subjects (Fig. 8.1 B). This suggests that carbohydrate absorption from the gastrointestinal tract into the circulation limits ingested carbohydrate's catabolism rate during exercise independent of training state.

Do not substitute exogenous fructose for glucose during prolonged exercise, because less fructose oxidizes when consuming equivalent amounts of both sugars.[51] Also, adding polylactate (a carbohydrate supplement of molecules of lactate ionically bound to amino acids) to a glucose polymer solution did not measurably affect physiologic or endurance performance variables compared with that with a glucose polymer only.[77]

A Distinct Ergogenic Advantage in Intense Aerobic Exercise

Carbohydrate feeding during exercise at 60 to 80% of aerobic capacity postpones fatigue by 15 to 30 minutes, with performance improvement generally ranging between 15 and 35%.[19] This effect, potentially significant in marathon running, occurs because fatigue in well-nourished individuals usually becomes noticeable within 2 hours of intense exercise. A person can ward off fatigue and extend endurance with a single concentrated carbohydrate feeding approximately 30 minutes before anticipated fatigue. FIGURE 8.2 shows that this feeding restores the level of blood glucose, which then sustains the energy needs of active muscles.

Endurance benefits from carbohydrate feedings become apparent at about 75% of aerobic capacity. When exercise initially exceeds this intensity, an individual must reduce intensity to the 75% level during the final stages to maintain the benefits from exogenous carbohydrate intake.[16] Repeated feedings of solid carbohydrate (43 g sucrose with 400 mL water) at the beginning and at 1, 2, and 3 hours during exercise maintain blood glucose and slow glycogen depletion during 4 hours of cycling. Maintaining blood glucose and glycogen reserves also enhances high-intensity exercise performance to exhaustion at the end of the activity.[2,4,67,75] The winner in a marathon run is usually the athlete who sustains high-intensity aerobic effort and sprints to the finish.

Figure 8.2 Average plasma glucose concentration during prolonged high-intensity aerobic exercise when subjects consumed either a placebo or glucose polymer (3 g per kg body mass in a 50% solution). (Modified from Coggan AR, Coyle EF. Metabolism and performance following carbohydrate ingestion late in exercise. Med Sci Sports Exerc 1989;21:59.)

REPLENISHING GLYCOGEN RESERVES: REFUELING FOR THE NEXT BOUT OF INTENSE TRAINING OR COMPETITION

All carbohydrates do not digest and absorb at the same rate. As mentioned in Chapter 1, plant starch composed primarily of amylose, represents a resistant carbohydrate because of its relatively slow hydrolysis rate. Conversely, starch with relatively high amylopectin content is digested and absorbed more rapidly.

The Glycemic Index

*The **glycemic index** serves as a relative (qualitative) indicator of how carbohydrate-containing food affects blood glucose levels.* The rise in blood sugar—termed the *glycemic response*—is determined after ingesting a food containing 50 g of a digestible carbohydrate (total carbohydrate minus fiber) and comparing it over a 2-hour period with a "standard" for carbohydrate (usually white bread or glucose) with an assigned value of 100.[5,94] The glycemic index expresses the percentage of total area under the blood glucose response curve for a specific food compared with that for glucose (FIG. 8.3). Thus, a food with a glycemic index of 45 indicates that ingesting 50 g of the food raises blood glucose concentrations to levels that reach 45% of that reached with 50 g of glucose. The glycemic index provides a more useful physiologic concept than simply classifying a carbohydrate on the basis of its chemical configuration as simple or complex, sugar or starch, or available or unavailable. The most updated international listing of glycemic index values contains nearly 1300 entries that represent values of more than 750 different food types.[26] Differences in values exist within the literature, depending on the laboratory and exact food type evaluated (e.g., slight variations in type of white bread, rice, and potatoes used as the standard of comparison). Do not view the glycemic index as an unwavering standard as considerable variability exists among individuals in response to consuming a specific carbohydrate-containing food. Also, a high glycemic index rating does not necessarily indicate poor nutritional quality. For example, carrots, brown rice, and corn, with their rich quantities of health-protective micronutrients, phytochemicals, and dietary fiber, have relatively high indices.

Individual differences in response to how food is digested and its preparation and ripeness affect the glycemic index. For example, a ripe banana has a higher glycemic index than a "greener" banana. Once foods are combined (i.e., a ripe banana eaten with three flavors of ice cream topped with nuts and chocolate fudge), the meal's glycemic index for that combination of foods differs from the glycemic index for each separate item. Also, eating foods based just on their published glycemic index may not deliver the expected nutritional benefits.[62,93]

The revised glycemic index listing also includes the **glycemic load** associated with the consumption of specified serving sizes of different foods. Whereas the glycemic index compares equal quantities of a carbohydrate-containing food, the glycemic load quantifies the overall glycemic effect of a typical *portion* of food. This represents the product of the amount of available carbohydrate in that serving and the glycemic index of the food. A high glycemic load reflects a greater expected elevation in blood glucose and a greater insulin release. An increased risk for type 2 diabetes and coronary heart disease coincides with the chronic consumption of a diet with a high glycemic load.[39,49]

Not All Carbohydrates Are Equal

FIGURE 8.4 lists the glycemic index for common items in various food groupings. For easy identification, we have placed foods into high, medium, and low categories for glycemic index. Interestingly, a food's index rating does not depend simply on its classification as a "simple" (mono- and disaccharides) or "complex" (starch and fiber) carbohydrate. This is because the plant starch in white rice and potatoes has a higher glycemic index than the simple sugars (particularly fructose) in apples and peaches. A food's fiber content slows digestion rate, thus many vegetables (e.g., peas, beans, and other legumes) have a low glycemic index. Ingesting lipids and proteins tends to slow the passage of food into the small intestine, thus reducing the glycemic index of the meal's accompanying carbohydrate content. *Clearly, the most rapid method of replenishing glycogen after exercise is to consume foods with moderate-to-high glycemic indices rather than foods rated low,[9,17,18,90] even if the replenishment meal*

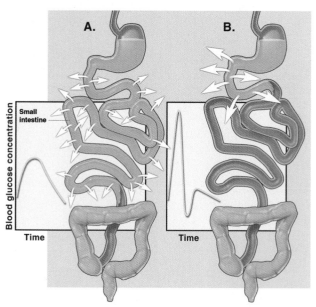

■ **Figure 8.3** General response of intestinal glucose absorption following feeding of foods with either (**A**) low glycemic index or (**B**) high glycemic index. Note that the low glycemic food absorbs at a slower rate throughout the full length of the small intestine to produce a more gradual rise in blood glucose.

High glycemic

Glucose	100
Carrots	92
Honey	87
Corn flakes	80
Whole meal bread	72
White rice	72
New potatoes	70
White bread	69
Shredded wheat	67
Brown rice	66
Beets	64
Raisins	64
Bananas	62

Corn	59
Sucrose	59
All-bran	51
Potato-chips	51
Peas	51
White pasta	50
Oatmeal	49
Sweet potatoes	48
Whole wheat pasta	42
Oranges	40

Apples	39
Fish sticks	38
Butter beans	36
Navy beans	31
Kidney beans	29
Lentils	29
Sausage	28
Fructose	20
Peanuts	13

Figure 8.4 Glycemic index categorization of common food sources of carbohydrates.

contains a small amount of lipid and protein.[10] During the first 2 hours of recovery when muscle glycogen content is at its lowest level, consuming a glucose polymer solution (low osmolality) restores glycogen more rapidly than an energy-equivalent solution of monomers with high osmolality.[61] This beneficial effect of low osmolality solutions on glycogen replenishment probably results from two factors: *(a)* more rapid gastric emptying and glucose delivery to the small intestine and *(b)* augmented postexercise-stimulated non-insulin-dependent glucose uptake by the muscles. The addition of L-arginine to a carbohydrate-containing beverage offers no additional benefit to carbohydrate replenishment.[68]

The need for glycogen in previously active muscle significantly affects glycogen resynthesis in the postexercise period. When food becomes available following exercise, the following factors facilitate cellular uptake of glucose:

- Hormonal milieu reflected by elevated insulin
- Increased tissue sensitivity to insulin and other transporter proteins (e.g., GLUT 1 and GLUT 4,

members of a family of facilitative monosaccharide transporters that mediate much of glucose transport activity)
- Low catecholamine levels
- Increased activity of a specific form of the glycogen-storing enzyme glycogen synthase

To speed glycogen replenishment after an intense bout of training or competition, one should consume high-glycemic carbohydrate-rich foods as soon as possible.

Follow this practical advice to rapidly restore depleted glycogen reserves: Within 15 minutes after stopping exercise, consume 50 to 75 g (2 to 3 oz, or 1.0 to 1.5 g per kg body mass) of high- to moderate-glycemic carbohydrates. Continue eating 50 to 75 g of carbohydrate every 2 hours until achieving 500 to 700 g (7 to 10 g per kg of body mass), or until eating a large high-carbohydrate meal. If immediately ingesting carbohydrate after exercise proves impractical, an alternative strategy involves eating meals containing 2.5 g of high-glycemic carbohydrate per kg body mass at 2, 4, 6, 8, and 22 hours postexercise. This replenishes glycogen to levels similar to those achieved with the same protocol begun immediately postexercise.[60]

Insulin–Stimulating Effect of Protein Ingestion in Recovery: Does It Augment Glycogen Replenishment?

Consuming an amino acid-protein mixture of wheat protein hydrolysate with free leucine and phenylalanine ($0.4 \ g \cdot kg^{-1} \cdot h^{-1}$) in a carbohydrate-containing beverage ($0.8 \ g \cdot kg^{-1} \cdot h^{-1}$) facilitates more muscle glycogen storage without gastrointestinal discomfort than ingesting a carbohydrate-only beverage of the same concentration.[84] This benefit appears to relate to the insulinotropic effect of a higher level of plasma amino acids.[83,97] This benefit of added protein and/or amino acids (and the associated increased insulin release) on glycogen replenishment, however, is no greater than that achieved by simply adding additional carbohydrate to the recovery supplement.[69] For example, trained athletes attained glycogen synthesis rates equivalent to those with a glucose plus protein supplement with a carbohydrate-only intake of $1.2 \ g \cdot kg^{-1} \cdot h^{-1}$.[84] Supplements were given at 30-minute intervals over a 5-hour recovery period. This carbohydrate replenishment protocol produced maximal glycogen resynthesis. Additional intake of protein or amino acids, while increasing the insulin response, does not increase the rate of glycogen synthesis.

What Is the Optimal Approach?

Research has addressed the following question: Is it better to consume large meals or more frequent snacks of high-glycemic carbohydrates to optimize glycogen replenishment? One study compared 24-hour carbohydrate replenishment with two patterns of consuming an energy-equivalent meal of high-glycemic carbohydrates: *(a)* "gorging" on a single large meal, with its greater incremental glucose and insulin response or *(b)* "nibbling" on frequent smaller snacks, which produces a more stable glucose and insulin response.[11] The two styles of eating produced *no difference* in final glycogen levels. These findings indicate that individuals should eat high-glycemic carbohydrates following heavy exercise; the frequency of the meals and snacks should dovetail with a person's appetite and the availability of food after exercising.

Glycogen Replenishment Takes Time

Avoid legumes, fructose, and milk products when rapidly replenishing glycogen reserves because of their slow rates of intestinal absorption. More-rapid glycogen resynthesis takes place if the person remains inactive during recovery.[15] *With optimal carbohydrate intake, glycogen stores replenish at about 5 to 7% per hour. Thus, even under the best of circumstances, it takes at least 20 hours to reestablish glycogen stores following a glycogen-depleting exercise bout.*

Optimal glycogen replenishment benefits individuals involved in *(a)* regular intense training, *(b)* tournament competition with qualifying rounds, or *(c)* competitive events scheduled with only 1 or 2 days for recuperation. Wrestlers who lose considerable glycogen (and water) using food and fluid restriction prior to the weigh-in to "make weight" also benefit from a proper glycogen replenishment strategy.[38] For collegiate wrestlers, short-term weight loss through energy restriction without dehydration significantly impaired anaerobic exercise capacity.[65] Anaerobic performance recovered to near-baseline values when these athletes then consumed meals containing 75% carbohydrate (21 kcal per kg body mass) over the next 5 hours. No improvement occurred if the refeeding diet contained only 45% carbohydrate. Even without full glycogen replenishment, some replenishment in recovery benefits endurance in the next exercise bout. For example, replenishing carbohydrate after only a 4-hour recovery period from glycogen-depleting exercise yields better endurance in subsequent exercise than a similar scenario with no carbohydrate eaten in recovery.

Choose the Right Form of Carbohydrate

To evaluate the influence of a carbohydrate's structure on glycogen replenishment, eight male cyclists decreased the glycogen content of the vastus lateralis muscle with 60-minutes of cycling at 75% $\dot{V}O_2max$ followed by six 1-minute sprints at 125% $\dot{V}O_2max$.[43] Twelve hours after the glycogen-depleting exercise, they consumed a 3000 kcal meal (ratio of 65%:20%:15% carbohydrate to lipid to protein). A solution of either glucose, maltodextrin (glucose polymer), waxy starch (100% amylopectin), or resistant starch (100% amylose) provided all of the recovery meal's carbohydrate. Muscle biopsies 24 hours into recovery (FIG. 8.5) revealed a significantly lower glycogen repletion level from the resistant starch meal (high amylose content, low glycemic index) than from meals with the other, more rapidly hydrolyzed carbohydrates. Keeping to the prescribed carbohydrate intake in the immediate recovery period produces more desirable glycogen replenishment than letting athletes eat the amount they wish.[44]

THE GLYCEMIC INDEX AND PREEXERCISE FEEDINGS

Use the glycemic index to formulate the immediate preexercise feeding. The ideal meal immediately before exercising should provide a source of glucose to maintain blood sugar and sustain muscle metabolism; it also should not trigger a spike in insulin release. A relatively normal plasma insulin level theoretically preserves blood glucose availability and optimizes fat mobilization and catabolism while sparing glycogen reserves. As mentioned previously, consuming

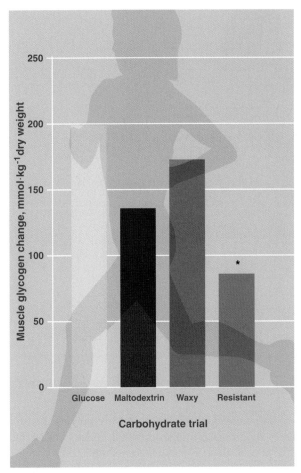

■ **Figure 8.5** Changes in muscle glycogen with various carbohydrate feedings of similar energy content in the 24-hour period following glycogen-depleting exercise. (*) Denotes significantly lower value than glucose, maltodextrin, and waxy starch. (From Jozsi AC, et al. The influence of starch structure on glycogen resynthesis and subsequent cycling performance. Int J Sports Med 1996;17:373.)

simple sugars (concentrated high-glycemic carbohydrates) immediately before exercising causes blood sugar to rise rapidly, often triggering excessive insulin release. The resulting rebound hypoglycemia, depressed fat catabolism, and the possible early depletion of glycogen reserves negatively affects exercise performance.

In contrast, consuming low-glycemic index foods (starch with high amylose content) immediately before exercise provides a relatively slow rate of glucose absorption into the blood. This eliminates the insulin surge, while a steady supply of "slow-release" glucose becomes available from the digestive tract as exercise progresses. This effect theoretically proves beneficial during long-term, high-intensity exercise, particularly in unusual events such as ocean swimming where the practicality of attempting to consume carbohydrate during exercise remains a challenge.

Several studies support the wisdom of consuming low-glycemic carbohydrates prior to exercise. In one study of

trained cyclists who performed high-intensity aerobic exercise, a preexercise low-glycemic meal of lentils significantly extended endurance over that with feedings of either glucose or a high-glycemic meal of potatoes of equivalent carbohydrate content.[9] Higher blood glucose levels near the end stages of exercise accompanied the low-glycemic, preexercise feeding.[22,31,78] Despite inducing potentially favorable alterations in blood glucose and fat catabolism, all research has not observed ergogenic benefits from low-glycemic preexercise carbohydrates.[24,30,78] Further study of the topic seems warranted.

GLUCOSE, ELECTROLYTES, AND WATER UPTAKE

As we discuss in Chapter 10, fluid ingestion before and during exercise minimizes the detrimental effects of dehydration on cardiovascular dynamics, temperature regulation, and exercise performance. Adding carbohydrate to the **oral rehydration solution** provides additional glucose energy for exercise as glycogen reserves deplete. Adding electrolytes to the rehydration beverage maintains the thirst mechanism and reduces the risk of hyponatremia. The coach and athletes should work together to determine the optimal fluid/carbohydrate mixture and volume to minimize fatigue and prevent dehydration. Concern focuses on the dual observations that a large fluid volume intake impairs carbohydrate uptake, while a concentrated sugar/electrolyte solution impairs fluid replacement.

Important Considerations

Stomach emptying rate greatly affects fluid and nutrient absorption by the small intestine. FIGURE 8.6 illustrates important factors that influence gastric emptying. Little negative effect of exercise on gastric emptying occurs until an intensity of about 75% of maximum, after which, emptying rate slows.[48] Gastric volume, however, greatly influences gastric emptying because emptying rate declines exponentially as fluid volume decreases. *A major factor to speed gastric emptying and compensate for any inhibitory effects of the beverage's carbohydrate content, involves maintaining a relatively large stomach fluid volume.*[3,23,]

Practical Recommendations

Consuming 400 to 600 mL of fluid 20 minutes before exercise optimizes the beneficial effect of increased stomach volume on fluid and nutrient passage into the small intestine. Regularly ingesting 150 to 250 mL of fluid (at 15-min intervals) throughout exercise continually replenishes fluid passed into the intestine; this maintains a relatively large and constant gastric volume.[23,46,59] This protocol delivers about 1 L of fluid per hour to the small intestine, a volume

Figure 8.6 Major factors that affect gastric emptying (stomach) and fluid absorption (small intestine).

that meets the needs of most endurance athletes. Prior research indicated that colder fluid emptied from the stomach more rapidly than fluid at room temperature, yet fluid temperature does *not* exert a major influence during exercise. Beverages containing alcohol or caffeine induce a diuretic effect (alcohol most pronounced), which facilitates water loss. Both beverages are contraindicated for fluid replacement.

Consider Fluid Concentration

Concern exists about the potential negative effect of sugar drinks on water absorption from the digestive tract. Gastric emptying slows when ingested fluids either contain increased concentrations of particles in solution (osmolality) or possess high caloric content.[6,66] Rehydration beverages hypertonic to plasma (>280 mOsm·kg^{-1}) retard net fluid uptake by the intestine. This negatively affects prolonged exercise in hot weather, when adequate fluid intake *and* absorption play prime roles in the participant's health and safety. The negative effect of concentrated sugar molecules on gastric emptying is diminished (and plasma volume maintained) if the drink contains a short-chain glucose polymer (**maltodextrin**) rather than simple sugars. Short-chain polymers (from 3 to 20 glucose units) derived from cornstarch breakdown reduce the number of particles in solution. Fewer particles facilitate water movement from the stomach for intestinal absorption.

Adding a small amount of glucose and sodium (glucose being the more important factor) to the oral rehydration so-

lution does not negatively affect gastric emptying. It also facilitates fluid uptake by the intestinal lumen because rapid cotransport of glucose–sodium across the intestinal mucosa stimulates water's passive uptake by osmotic action.[27,28,29] Water replenishes effectively, and the additional glucose uptake contributes to blood glucose maintenance. This glucose then spares muscle and liver glycogen, and/or provides blood glucose should glycogen reserves fall during the later stage of exercise.

Rehydration solutions that combine two different transportable carbohydrate substrates (glucose, fructose, sucrose, or maltodextrins) produce greater water uptake at a particular intestinal lumen osmolality than solutions containing only one substrate from enhanced solute flux (and thus water flux) from the intestine (Fig. 8.7).[73] The second substrate stimulates more intestinal transport mechanisms, thus facilitating net water absorption by osmosis. *To optimize water and carbohydrate absorption, consume a 6% carbohydrate–electrolyte solution that combines fructose and sucrose, each transported by separate noncompetitive pathways.*

Potential Benefit of Sodium. Adding moderate amounts of sodium (the most abundant ion in the extracellular space) to the ingested fluid minimally affects glucose absorption and does not alter the contribution of ingested glucose to the total energy yield in prolonged exercise.[29,34,52] The extra sodium (0.5–0.7 g per L) does, however, help to maintain plasma sodium concentrations. This effect benefits ultraendurance athletes at risk for hyponatremia. Hyponatremia occurs from a large sweat–sodium loss coupled with drinking copious

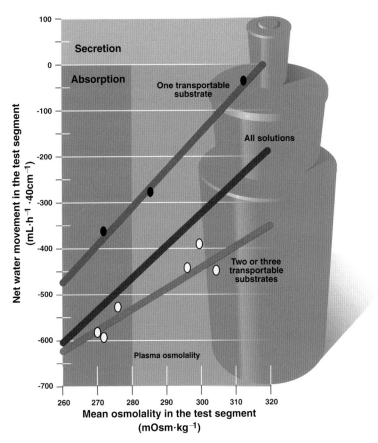

Figure 8.7 Net water movement related to mean osmolality in the intestinal test segment. Water absorption from the intestine shows as a negative value (high negative values indicate greater absorption) while secretion into the intestinal lumen would show as a positive value. The *purple line* shows the relationship among the three test solutions containing one transportable substrate, while the *orange line* refers to six solutions containing two or three transportable substrates. The middle line *(red)* represents the relationship among all test solutions. For each test solution, net water absorption increases as osmolality decreases. However, for any osmolality value, greater net water absorption occurs from the gut into the body with solutions containing more than one transportable substrate. (From Shi X, et al. Effects of carbohydrate type and concentration and solution osmolality on water absorption. Med Sci Sports Exerc 1996;27:1607.)

amounts of plain water (see Chapter 10). Maintaining plasma osmolality with added sodium in the rehydration beverage also reduces urine output and sustains the sodium-dependent osmotic drive to drink. These factors promote continued fluid intake *and* fluid retention during recovery.[53,54,92] Chapter 10 discusses the optimal characteristics of a rehydration beverage following exercise-induced dehydration.

RECOMMENDED ORAL REHYDRATION SOLUTION: EVALUATING THE SPORTS DRINKS

A 5 to 8% carbohydrate–electrolyte beverage consumed while exercising in the heat helps to regulate temperature and fluid balance as effectively as plain water. As an added bonus, this drink maintains glucose metabolism (provides an
intestinal delivery rate of 5.0 kcal · min^{-1}) and preserves glycogen during prolonged exercise.[13,23,56,72] Consuming this solution in recovery from prolonged exercise in a warm environment also improves endurance capacity for subsequent exercise.

THE IDEAL ORAL REHYDRATION BEVERAGE

- Tastes good
- Absorbs rapidly
- Causes little or no gastrointestinal distress
- Maintains extracellular fluid volume and osmolality
- Offers the potential to enhance exercise performance

Table 8.2 COMPARISON OF VARIOUS BEVERAGES USED BY ATHLETES TO REPLACE THE FLUID LOST IN EXERCISE

Beverages	Flavors	CHO Source	CHO conc (%)	Sodium (mg)	Potassium (mg)	Other Minerals and Vitamins	Osmolality (mOsm · L⁻¹)
GATORADE[a] Thirst Quencher Stokely-Van Camp, Inc., a subsidiary of the Quaker Oats Company	Lemon-lime, lemonade, fruit punch, orange, citrus cooler	Sucrose/glucose (powder) Sucrose/glucose syrup solids (liquid)	6	110	25	Chloride, phosphorus	280–360
Exceed[a] Ross Laboratories	Lemon-lime, orange	Glucose polymers/fructose	7.2	50	45		250
Quickick[a] Cramer Products, Inc.	Lemon-lime, fruit punch, orange, grape, lemonade	Fructose/sucrose	4.7	116	23	Chloride, calcium, magnesium, phosphorus	
Sqwincher, the Activity Drink Universal Products, Inc	Lemon-lime, fruit punch, lemonade, orange, grape, strawberry, grapefruit	Glucose/fructose	6.8	60	36	Calcium, chloride, phosphorus	305
10-K Beverage Products, Inc.	Lemon-lime, orange, fruit punch, lemonade, iced tea	Sucrose/glucose/fructose	6.3	52	26	Chloride, phosphorus, calcium, magnesium, vitamin C	470
USA Wet Texas Wet, Inc	Lemon-lime, orange, fruit punch	Sucrose	6.8	62	44	Vitamin C, chloride, phosphorus	350
Coca-Cola Coca-Cola, USA	Regular, Classic, Cherry	High-fructose corn syrup/sucrose	10.7–11.3	9.2	trace		
Sprite Coca-Cola, USA	Lemon-lime	High-fructose corn syrup/sucrose	10.2	28	trace	Chloride, phosphorus	450
Cranberry juice cocktail		High-fructose corn syrup/sucrose	15	10	61		
Orange juice		Fructose/sucrose/glucose	11.8	2.7	510	Phosphorus	600–715
Water				low[b]	low[b]		
PowerAde		High-fructose corn syrup/maltodextrin	8	73	33		695
All-Sport		High-fructose corn syrup	8–9	55	55	Phosphorus, vitamin C	890
10 K		Sucrose/glucose/fructose	6.3	54	25	Phosphorus, calcium, iron, vitamins C and A, niacin, riboflavin, thiamine	690
Cytomax		Fructose corn syrup/sucrose	7–11	10	150		
Breakthrough		Maltodextrin/fructose	8.5	60	45		
Everlast		Sucrose/fructose	6	100	20		
Hydra Charge		Maltodextrin/fructose	8	–	trace		
SportaLYTE		Maltodextrin/ fructose/glucose	7.5	100	60		

[a] Serving size, 8 fluid ounces.
[b] Depends on water source.

Figure 8.8 Fluid volume to ingest each hour to obtain the noted amount of carbohydrate (CHO). (Modified from Coyle EF, Montain SJ. Benefits of fluid replacement. Med Sci Sports Exerc 1992;24: S324.)

To determine the percentage carbohydrate in a drink, divide carbohydrate content (in grams) by fluid volume (in milliliters) and multiply by 100. For example, 80 g of carbohydrate in 1 L (1000 mL) of water provides an 8% solution. Environmental and exercise conditions interact to influence the optimal composition of the rehydration solution. Fluid replenishment becomes of utmost importance to health and safety when intense aerobic effort in hot, humid weather lasts between 30 and 60 minutes. Under these conditions, we recommend a more dilute carbohydrate–electrolyte solution containing less than 5% carbohydrate. In cooler weather, when dehydration is not a major factor, a more concentrated beverage of 15% carbohydrate suffices. Little difference exists among liquid glucose, sucrose, or starch as the preferred ingested carbohydrate fuel source during exercise.

Optimal carbohydrate replenishment ranges between 30 and 60 g (about 1–2 oz) per hour. TABLE 8.2 compares the carbohydrate and mineral content and osmolality of popular fluid replacement beverages. FIGURE 8.8 presents a general guideline for fluid intake each hour during exercise for a given amount of carbohydrate replenishment. Although a tradeoff exists between carbohydrate ingestion and gastric emptying, the stomach empties up to 1700 mL of water per hour, even when drinking an 8% carbohydrate solution. However, 1000 mL (about 1 quart) of fluid consumed per hour probably represents the optimal volume to offset dehydration, because larger fluid intakes can cause gastrointestinal discomfort.

HIGH-FAT VERSUS LOW-FAT DIETS FOR ENDURANCE TRAINING AND PERFORMANCE

Debate concerns the wisdom of maintaining a high-fat diet (or even fasting) during training or prior to endurance competition.[21,45,57,86] Adaptations to high-fat diets consistently show a shift in substrate use toward higher fat oxidation in exercise.[12,36,37,87] Proponents of high-fat diets argue that a long-term increase in dietary fat stimulates fat burning by augmenting the capacity to mobilize and catabolize this energy nutrient. Any fat-burning enhancement should conserve glycogen reserves and/or contribute to improved endurance capacity under low glycogen conditions. To investigate possible benefits, research compared endurance capacity in two groups of 10 young men matched for aerobic capacity who consumed either a high-carbohydrate diet (65% kcal from carbohydrate) or high-fat diet (62% kcal from lipid) for 7 weeks. Each group trained for 60 to 70 minutes at 50 to 85% of aerobic capacity, 3 days a week during weeks 1 to 3, and 4 days a week during weeks 4 to 7. Following 7 weeks of training, the group consuming the high-fat diet switched to the high-carbohydrate diet. FIGURE 8.9 displays the exercise performance for both groups. Endurance results were clear:

PRACTICAL RECOMMENDATIONS FOR FLUID AND CARBOHYDRATE REPLACEMENT DURING EXERCISE

- Monitor dehydration rate from changes in body weight. Require urination before postexercise body weight determination. Each pound of weight loss corresponds to 450 mL (15 fl oz) of dehydration.

- Drink fluids at the same rate as their estimated depletion (or at least at a rate close to 80% of the sweating rate) during prolonged exercise with accompanying cardiovascular stress, high metabolic heat, and dehydration.

- Endurance athletes can meet both carbohydrate (30–60 g per hour) and fluid requirements by drinking during each hour between 625 to 1250 mL (average about 250 mL every 15 min) of a beverage that contains 4 to 8% carbohydrate.

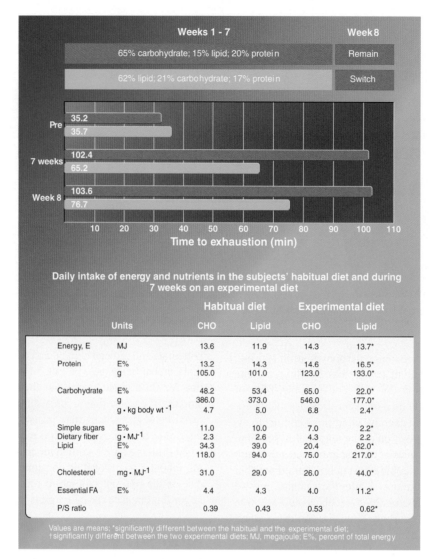

Figure 8.9 Effects of a high-carbohydrate (CHO) versus a high-fat diet on endurance performance. The group consuming the high-fat diet for 7 weeks switched to the high-CHO diet during week 8. The endurance test consisted of pedaling a bicycle ergometer at the desired rate. The inset table compares the average daily energy and nutrient intakes during the habitual and experimental diets. P/S ratio, polyunsaturated-to-saturated fatty acid ratio. (From Helge JW, et al. Interaction of training and diet on metabolism and endurance during exercise in man. J Physiol 1996;492:293.)

the group consuming the high-carbohydrate diet performed significantly better after 7 weeks of training than the group consuming the high-fat diet (102.4 vs. 65.2 minutes). When the high-fat diet group switched to the high-carbohydrate diet during week 8, only a small additional improvement in endurance of 11.5 minutes occurred. Consequently, total overall endurance improvement over the 8-week period reached 115% for the high-fat diet group, whereas endurance for the group on the high-carbohydrate diet improved by 194%. The inset table shows daily energy and nutrient intakes prior to the experimental treatment (habitual diet) and during the 7-week experimental diet. The high-fat diet produced suboptimal

adaptations in endurance performance, which were not fully remedied by switching to a high-carbohydrate diet.

Subsequent research from the same laboratory failed to demonstrate any endurance-enhancing effect of a high-fat diet containing only moderate carbohydrate (15% total calories) in rats, regardless of their training status. For sedentary humans, maintaining either a low or high dietary fat intake for 4 weeks did not affect maximal or submaximal aerobic exercise performance.[63] A 6-day exposure to a high-fat, low-carbohydrate diet, followed by 1 day of carbohydrate restoration with a high-carbohydrate diet increased fat oxidation during prolonged submaximal exercise. This carbohydrate-sparing effect did not enhance 1-hour time trial performance following 4 hours of continuous cycling.[14]

While a high-fat diet stimulates adaptive responses that augment fat catabolism, reliable research has yet to demonstrate consistent exercise or training benefits from this dietary modification. Compromised training capacity and symptoms of lethargy, increased fatigue, and higher ratings of perceived exertion usually accompany exercise when subsisting on a high-fat diet[12,36,76] One must carefully consider the potential detrimental health risks when recommending a diet with 60% of total calories from lipid. However, this concern may prove unwarranted for athletes with high levels of daily energy expenditure. For example, increasing the diet's percentage of lipid calories to 50% for physically active individuals who maintain a stable body weight does not adversely affect heart disease risk factors, including plasma lipoprotein profiles.[7,47] Overall, available research does not support the popular notion that reducing carbohydrate while increasing fat intake above a 30% level optimizes the metabolic "zone" for endurance performance.[71,85] Conversely, significant restriction of dietary fat intake below recommended levels also impairs endurance exercise performance.[36,84]

Summary

1. The precompetition meal should include readily digestible foods and contribute to the energy and fluid requirements of exercise. Meals high in carbohydrates and relatively low in lipids and proteins serve this purpose. Three hours should provide sufficient time to digest and absorb the precompetition meal.

2. Commercially prepared liquid meals offer a practical approach to precompetition nutrition and energy supplementation. These "meals" *(a)* provide balance in nutritive value, *(b)* contribute to fluid needs, and *(c)* absorb rapidly, leaving practically no residue in the digestive tract.

3. High-intensity aerobic exercise for 1 hour decreases liver glycogen by about 55%, whereas a 2-hour strenuous workout nearly depletes the glycogen content of the liver and specifically exercised muscles

4. Carbohydrate-containing rehydration solutions consumed during exercise enhance endurance performance by maintaining blood sugar concentration. Glucose supplied in the blood can *(a)* spare existing glycogen in active muscles or *(b)* serve as "reserve" blood glucose for later use should muscle glycogen become depleted.

5. All carbohydrates do not digest and absorb at the same rate. The glycemic index provides a relative measure of blood glucose increase after consuming a food containing 50 g of a digestible carbohydrate (total carbohydrate minus fiber) and compares it over a 2-hour period to a "standard" for carbohydrate (usually white bread or glucose) with an assigned value of 100. The glycemic load quantifies the overall glycemic effect of a typical portion of food.

6. For rapid carbohydrate replenishment after exercise, begin immediately to consume moderate-to-high glycemic index carbohydrate-containing foods (50–75 g of carbohydrate each hour). With optimal carbohydrate intake, glycogen stores replenish at a rate of about 5 to 7% per hour.

7. Use the glycemic index to formulate the immediate preexercise feeding. Foods with a low-glycemic index digest and absorb at a relatively slow rate. Ingesting these carbohydrates in the immediate preexercise period provides a steady supply of "slow- release" glucose from the intestinal tract during exercise.

8. Maintaining a relatively large stomach fluid volume throughout exercise enhances gastric emptying. Optimal gastric volume occurs by consuming 400 to 600 mL of fluid immediately before exercise, followed by regular fluid ingestion of 250 mL every 15 minutes thereafter.

9. Drinking concentrated sugar-containing beverages slows the gastric emptying rate. This could negatively upset fluid balance during exercise and heat stress.

10. The ideal oral rehydration solution contains between 5 and 8% carbohydrates. This formulation permits carbohydrate replenishment without adversely affecting fluid balance and thermoregulation.

11. Adding moderate amounts of sodium to the ingested fluid helps to maintain plasma sodium concentration. This benefits the ultraendurance athlete at risk for hyponatremia.

12. Maintaining plasma osmolality with added sodium in the rehydration beverage reduces urine output and sustains the sodium-dependent osmotic drive to drink.

13. A high-fat diet stimulates adaptive responses that augment fat use—but reliable research.has not yet demonstrated consistent exercise or training benefits from this dietary modification approach.

TEST YOUR KNOWLEDGE **ANSWERS**

1. False Significant depletion occurs in carbohydrate reserves over an 8- to 12-hour period without eating, even if the person normally follows appropriate dietary recommendations. Thus, fasting before competition or intense training makes no sense physiologically because it rapidly depletes liver and muscle glycogen, which subsequently impairs exercise performance. In individualizing the precompetition meal plan, consider the following factors *(a)* food preference, *(b)* "psychological set" of the competitor, and *(c)* digestibility of the foods.

2. False The ideal precompetition meal maximizes muscle and liver glycogen storage, and provides glucose for intestinal absorption during exercise. The meal should contain 150 to 300 g of carbohydrate (3–5 g per kg of body mass in either solid or liquid form), be consumed 3 to 4 hours before exercising, and contain relatively little fat and fiber to facilitate gastric emptying and minimize gastrointestinal distress.

3. False High-intensity aerobic exercise for 1 hour decreases liver glycogen by about 55%, whereas a 2-hour strenuous workout almost totally depletes the glycogen content of the liver and the exercised muscle fibers. Also, maximal, repetitive 1- to 5-minute bouts of exercise interspersed with periods of lower-intensity exercise—as occurs in soccer, ice hockey, field hockey, European handball, and tennis—dramatically lower liver and muscle glycogen reserves. Research shows that physical and mental performance under such conditions improves with carbohydrate supplementation during exercise. Carbohydrate feedings during high-intensity prolonged exercise also enables individuals to exercise at greater intensity of effort.

4. False The glycemic index serves as an indicator of a carbohydrate's ability to raise blood glucose levels. This index expresses the percentage of total area under the blood glucose response curve for a specific food, compared with glucose. Blood sugar increase—termed the *glycemic response*—is determined after ingesting a food containing 50 g of a carbohydrate and comparing it over a 2-hour period with a "standard" for carbohydrate (usually white bread or glucose) with an assigned value of 100.

5. True The most rapid method of replenishing carbohydrate after exercise requires consuming foods with moderate-to-high glycemic indices rather than foods rated low, even if the replenishment meal contains a small amount of lipid and protein. Furthermore, ingesting lipids and proteins slows the passage of food into the small intestine, reducing the glycemic index of the meal's accompanying carbohydrate content.

6. False More-rapid glycogen resynthesis takes place if the person remains inactive during recovery. With optimal carbohydrate intake (high glycemic foods), glycogen stores replenish at a rate of about 5 to 7% per hour. Thus, even under the best of circumstances, it takes at least 20 hours to reestablish glycogen stores following a glycogen-depleting exercise bout.

7. False Consuming 400 to 600 mL of fluid 20 minutes before exercise optimizes the beneficial effect of an increased stomach volume on fluid and nutrient passage into the small intestine. Then, regularly ingesting 150 to 250 mL of fluid (at 15-min intervals) throughout exercise continually replenishes fluid in the stomach; this maintains a relatively large and constant gastric volume. Such a protocol delivers about 1 L of fluid per hour to the small intestine, a volume that meets the needs of most endurance athletes.

8. False A 5 to 8% carbohydrate–electrolyte beverage consumed during exercise in the heat contributes to temperature regulation and fluid balance as effectively as plain water. As an added bonus, this drink aids in maintaining glucose metabolism (providing an intestinal delivery rate of 5.0 kcal · min^{-1}) and glycogen reserves in prolonged exercise.

9. True Adding moderate amounts of sodium to ingested fluids exerts a minimal effect on glucose absorption or the contribution of ingested glucose to the total energy yield in prolonged exercise. The extra sodium (0.5–0.7 g per L) does, however, contribute to maintaining plasma sodium concentrations and benefits the ultraendurance athlete at risk for hyponatremia. Hyponatremia occurs from large sweat–sodium loss coupled with drinking large amounts of plain water. Maintaining plasma osmolality with added sodium in the rehydration beverage also reduces urine output and sustains the sodium-dependent osmotic drive to drink.

10. False Drinking concentrated sugar-containing beverages slows gastric emptying rate, which could ultimately upset fluid balance during exercise and heat stress. The ideal oral rehydration solution contains between 5 and 8% carbohydrates. This beverage formulation permits carbohydrate replenishment without adversely affecting fluid balance and thermoregulation.

References

1. Anantaraman R, et al. Effects of carbohydrate supplementation on performance during 1 hour of high-intensity exercise. Int J Sports Med 1995;16:461.
2. Ball TC, et al. Periodic carbohydrate replacement during 50 min of high-intensity cycling improves subsequent sprint performance. Int J Sports Nutr 1995;5:151.
3. Beckers EJ, et al. Comparison of aspiration and scintigraphic techniques for the measurement of gastric emptying rates in man. Gut 1992;33:115.
4. Below PR, et al. Fluid and carbohydrate ingestion independently improve performance during 1 h of intense exercise. Med Sci Sports Exerc 1995;27:200.
5. Brand-Miller J, et al. The G.I. factor: the glycaemic index solution. Sydney, Australia: Hodder & Stoughton, 1996.
6. Brouns F, Beckers E. Is the gut an athletic organ? Sports Med 1993;15:242.
7. Brown R., Cox CM. Effects of high fat versus high carbohydrate diets on plasma lipids and lipoproteins in endurance athletes. Med Sci Sports Exerc 1998;30:1677.
8. Burelle Y, et al. Oxidation of an oral [^{13}C] glucose load at rest and prolonged exercise in trained and sedentary subjects. J Appl Physiol 1999;86:52.
9. Burke LM, et al. Muscle glycogen storage after prolonged exercise: effect of the glycemic index on carbohydrate feedings. J Appl Physiol 1993;74:1019.

10. Burke LM, et al. Effect of coingestion of fat and protein with carbohydrate feedings on muscle glycogen storage. J Appl Physiol 1995;78:2187.

11. Burke LM, et al. Muscle glycogen storage after prolonged exercise: effect of the frequency of carbohydrate feeding. Am J Clin Nutr 1996;64:115.

12. Burke LM, et al. Effect of fat adaptation and carbohydrate restoration on metabolism and performance during prolonged cycling. J Appl Physiol 2000;89:2413.

13. Burstein R, et al. Glucose polymer ingestion—effect on fluid balance and glycemic state during a 4-d march. Med Sci Sports Exerc 1994;26:360.

14. Carey AL, et al. Effects of fat adaptation and carbohydrate restoration on prolonged endurance exercise. J Appl Physiol 2001;91:225.

15. Choi D, et al. Effect of passive and active recovery on the resynthesis of muscle glycogen. Med Sci Sports Exerc 1994;26:992.

16. Coggan AR, Coyle EF. Metabolism and performance following carbohydrate ingestion late in exercise. Med Sci Sports Exerc 1989;21:59.

17. Coyle EF. Timing and method of increased carbohydrate intake to cope with heavy training, competition and recovery. J Sports Sci 1991;9:29.

18. Coyle EF. Substrate utilization during exercise in active people. Am J Clin Nutr 1995;61(suppl):968S.

19. Coyle EF, Coggan AC. Effectiveness of carbohydrate feeding in delaying fatigue during prolonged exercise. Sports Med 1984;1:446.

20. Coyle EF, et al. Muscle glycogen utilization during prolonged strenuous exercise when fed carbohydrate. J Appl Physiol 1986;61:165.

21. Cox CM, et al. The effects of high-carbohydrate versus high-fat dietary advice on plasma lipids, lipoproteins, apolipoproteins, and performance in endurance trained cyclists. Nutr Metab Cardiovasc Dis 1996;6:227.

22. DeMarco HD, et al. Pre-exercise carbohydrate meals: application of the glycemic index. Med Sci Sports Exerc 1999;31:164.

23. Duchman SM, et al. Upper limit for intestinal absorption of a dilute glucose solution in men at rest. Med Sci Sports Exerc 1997;29:482.

24. Febbraio MA, Stewart, KL. CHO feeding before prolonged exercise: effect of glycemic index on muscle glycogenolysis and exercise performance. J Appl Physiol 1996;81:1115.

25. Foster C, et al. Effects of pre-exercise feedings on endurance performance. Med Sci Sports 1979;11:1.

26. Foster-Powell K, et al. International table of glycemic index and glycemic load values: 2002. Am J Clin Nutr 2002;76:5.

27. Gisolfi CV, et al. Human intestinal water absorption: direct vs indirect measurements. Am J Physiol 1990;258:G216.

28. Gisolfi CV, et al. Intestinal water absorption from select carbohydrate solutions in humans. J Appl Physiol 1992;7:2142.

29. Gisolfi CV, et al. Effect of sodium concentration in a carbohydrate-electrolyte solution on intestinal absorption. Med Sci Sports Exerc 1995;27:1414.

30. Goodpaster BH, et al. The effects of pre-exercise starch ingestion on endurance performance. Int J Sports Med 1996;17:366.

31. Guezennec CY, et al. The role of type and structure of complex carbohydrates on response to physical exercise. Int J Sports Nutr 1993;14:224.

32. Hargreaves M, Briggs CA. Effect of carbohydrate ingestion on exercise metabolism. J Appl Physiol 1988;65:1553.

33. Hargreaves M, et al. Effect of fructose ingestion on muscle glycogen usage during exercise. Med Sci Sports Exerc 1985;17:360.

34. Hargreaves M, et al. Influence of sodium on glucose bioavailability during exercise. Med Sci Sports Exerc 1994;26:365.

35. Hawley JA, et al. Carbohydrate, fluid, and electrolyte requirements of the soccer player: a review. Int J Sports Med 1994;4:221.

36. Helge JW, et al. Interaction of training and diet on metabolism and endurance during exercise in man. J Physiol 1996;492:293.

37. Helge JW, et al. Impact of a fat-rich diet on endurance in man: role of the dietary period. Med Sci Sports Exerc 1998;30:456.

38. Horswill CA. Weight loss and weight cycling in amateur wrestlers: implications for performance and resting metabolic rate. Int J Sports Nutr 1993;3:245.

39. Jenkins DJ, et al. Glycemic index: an overview of implications in health and disease. Am J Clin Nutr 2002;76(suppl):266S.

40. Jentjens RL. Oxidation of combined ingestion of glucose and fructose during exercise. J Appl Physiol 2004;96:1277.

41. Jeukendrup AE, et al. Carbohydrate-electrolyte feedings improve 1 h time trial cycling performance. Int J Sports Med 1997;18:125.

42. Jeukendrup AE, et al. Exogenous glucose oxidation during exercise in endurance-trained and untrained subjects. J Appl Physiol 1997;83:835.

43. Jozsi AC, et al. The influence of starch structure on glycogen resynthesis and subsequent cycling performance. Int J Sports Med 1996;17:373.

44. Keizer HA, et al. Influence of liquid and solid meals on muscle glycogen resynthesis, plasma fuel hormone response, and maximal physical working capacity. Int J Sports Med 1987;8:99.

45. Lambert EV, et al. Enhanced endurance in trained cyclists during moderate intensity exercise following 2 weeks adaptation to a high fat diet. Eur J Appl Physiol 1994;69:287.

46. Lambert GP, et al. Simultaneous determination of gastric emptying and intestinal absorption during cycle exercise in humans. Int J Sports Med 1996;17:48.

47. Leddy J, et al. Effect of a high or a low fat diet on cardiovascular risk factors in male and female runners. Med Sci Sports Exerc 1997;29:17.

48. Leiper JB, et al. Effect of intermittent high-intensity exercise on gastric emptying in man. Med Sci Sports Exerc 2001;33:1270.

49. Liu S, et al. A prospective study of dietary glycemic load, carbohydrate intake, and risk of coronary heart disease in US women. Am J Clin Nutr 2000;71:1455.

50. Marmy-Conus N, et al. Preexercise glucose ingestion and glucose kinetics during exercise. J Appl. Physiol 1996;81:853.

51. Massicotte D, et al. Effect of metabolic rate on the oxidation of ingested glucose and fructose during exercise. Int J Sports Med 1994;15:177.

52. Massicotte D, et al. Lack of effect of NaCl and/or metoclopramide on exogenous (^{13}C)-glucose oxidation during exercise. Int J Sports Med 1996;17:165.

53. Maughan RJ, Lieper JB. Sodium intake and post-exercise rehydration in man. Eur J Appl Physiol 1995;71:311.

54. Maughan RJ, et al. Restoration of fluid balance after exercise-induced dehydration: effect of food and fluid intake. Int J Appl Physiol 1996;73:317.

55. McConell G, et al. Effect of timing of carbohydrate ingestion on endurance exercise performance. Med Sci Sports Exerc 1996;28:1300.

56. Millard-Stafford ML, et al. Carbohydrate-electrolyte replacement improves distance running performance in the heat. Med Sci Sports Exerc 1992;24:934.

57. Mudio DM. Effect of dietary fat on metabolic adjustments to maximal VO$_2$ and endurance in runners. Med Sci Sports Exerc 1994;26:81.

58. Nicholas CW, et al. Influence of ingesting a carbohydrate-electrolyte solution on endurance capacity during intermittent, high intensity shuttle running. J Sports Sci 1996;13:283.

59. Noakes TD, et al. The importance of volume in regulating gastric emptying. Med Sci Sports Exerc 1991;23:307.

60. Pabkin JAM, et al. Muscle glycogen storage following prolonged exercise: effect of timing of ingestion of high glycemic index food. Med Sci Sports Exerc 1997;29:220.

61. Piehl Aulin K, et al. Muscle glycogen resynthesis rate in humans after supplementation of drinks containing carbohydrates with low and high molecular masses. Eur J Appl Physiol 2000;81:347.

62. Pi-Sunyer X. Glycemic index and disease. Am J Clin Nutr 2002;76(suppl): 290S.

63. Pogliaghi S, Veicsteinas A. Influence of low and high dietary fat on physical performance in untrained males. Med Sci Sports Exerc 1999;31:149.

64. Ramires PR, et al. Oral glucose ingestion increases endurance capacity in normal and diabetic (type I) humans. J Appl Physiol 1997;83:608.

65. Rankin JW, et al. Effect of weight loss and refeeding diet composition on anaerobic performance in wrestlers. Med Sci Sports Exerc 1996;28:1292.

66. Rehrer NJ. The maintenance of fluid balance during exercise. Int J Sports Med 1994;15:122.

67. Riddell MC, et al. Substrate utilization during exercise with glucose and glucose plus fructose ingestion in boys ages 10-14 yr. J Appl Physiol 2001;90:903.

68. Robinson TM, et al. L-Arginine ingestion after rest and exercise: effects on glucose disposal. Med Sci Sports Exerc 2003:35:1309.

69. Roy LP, et al. Addition of protein and amino acids to carbohydrates does not enhance postexercise muscle glycogen synthesis. J Appl Physiol 2001;91:839.

70. Roy LP, et al. High oxidation rates from combined carbohydrates ingested during exercise. Med Sci Sports Exerc 2004;36:1551.

71. Sears B, Lawren W. The zone. New York: Harper Collins, 1995.

72. Shi X, Gisolfi CV. Fluid and carbohydrate replacement during intermittent exercise. Sports Med 1998;25:157.

73. Shi X, et al. Effects of carbohydrate type and concentration and solution osmolality on water absorption. Med Sci Sports Exerc 1995;27:1607.

74. Simard C, et al. Effect of carbohydrate intake before and during and ice hockey match on blood and muscle energy substrates. Res Q Exerc Sport 1988;59:144.

75. Spendiff O, Campbell IG. The effect of glucose ingestion on endurance upper-body exercise and performance. Int J Sports Med 2002;23:142.

76. Stepto NK, et al. Effect of short-term fat adaptation on high-intensity training. Med Sci Sports Exerc 2002;34:449.

77. Swensen T, et al. Adding polylactate to a glucose polymer solution does not improve endurance. Int J Sports Med 1994;15:430.

78. Thomas DE, et al. Plasma glucose levels after prolonged strenuous exercise correlate inversely with glycemic response to food consumed before exercise. Int J Sports Nutr 1994;4:361.

79. Tsintzas O-K, et al. Carbohydrate ingestion and glycogen utilization in different muscle fibre types in man. J Physiol (Lond) 1995;489:243.

80. Tsintzas O-K, et al. Carbohydrate ingestion and single muscle fiber glycogen metabolism during running in men. J Appl Physiol 1996;81:801.

81. Tsintzas O-K, et al. Influence of carbohydrate supplementation early in exercise on endurance running capacity. Med Sci Sports Exerc 1996;28:1373.

82. Utter AC, et al. Effect of carbohydrate ingestion on ratings of perceived exertion during a marathon. Med Sci Sports Exerc 2002;24:1779.

83. van Loon KJC. Plasma insulin responses after ingestion of different amino acid or protein mixtures with carbohydrate. Am J Clin Nutr 2000;72:2000.

84. van Loon KJC, et al. Maximizing postexercise muscle glycogen synthesis: carbohydrate supplementation and the application of amino acid or protein hydrolysate mixtures. Am J Clin Nutr 2000;72:106.

85. Venkatraman JT, Pendergast D. Effects of the level of dietary fat intake and endurance exercise on plasma cytokines in runners. Med Sci Sports Exerc 1998;30:1198.

86. Venkatraman JT, et al. Influence of the level of dietary lipid intake and maximal exercise on the immune status in runners. Med Sci Sports Exerc 1997;29:333.

87. Vogt M, et al. Effects of dietary fat on muscle substrates, metabolism, and performance in athletes. Med Sci Sports Exerc 2003;35:952.

88. Wagenmakers AJ. Carbohydrate feedings improve 1 h time trial cycling performance. Med Sci Sports Exerc 1996;28:S37.

89. Wagenmakers AJ, et al. Oxidation rates of orally ingested carbohydrates during prolonged exercise in men. J Appl Physiol 1993;75:2274.

90. Walton P, Rhodes EC. Glycaemic index and optimal performance. Sports Med 1997;33:164.

91. Welsh RS, et al. Carbohydrates and physical/mental performance during intermittent exercise to fatigue. Med Sci Sports Exerc 2002;34:723.

92. Wilk B, Bar-Or O. Effect of drink flavor and NaCl on voluntary drinking and hydration in boys exercising in the heat. J Appl Physiol 1996;80:1112.

93. Wolever T, et al. The glycemic index: methodology and clinical implications. Am J Clin Nutr 1991;54:846.

94. Wolever TMS, et al. Glycaemic index of 102 complex carbohydrate foods in patients with diabetes. Nutr Res 1994;14:651.

95. Yannick C, et al. Oxidation of corn starch, glucose, and fructose ingested before exercise. Med Sci Sports Exerc 1989;21:45.

96. Yaspelkis BB III, et al. Carbohydrate supplementation spares muscle glycogen during variable intensity exercise. J Appl Physiol 1993;75:1477.

97. Zawadzki KM, et al. Carbohydrate-protein complex increases the rate of muscle glycogen storage after exercise. J Appl Physiol 1992;72:1584.

Additional Readings

Billat V, et al. Training effect on performance, substrate balance and blood lactate concentration at maximal lactate steady state in master endurance-runners. Pflugers Arch 2004;447:875.

Campbell WW, Geik RA. Nutritional considerations for the older athlete. Nutrition 2004;20:603.

Chen KT, Yang RS. Effects of exercise on lipid metabolism and musculoskeletal fitness in female athletes. World J Gastroenterol 2004;10:122.

Clark SA, et al. Intensified exercise training does not alter AMPK signaling in human skeletal muscle. Am J Physiol Endocrinol Metab 2004;286:E737.

Gomez JE. ATHENA (Athletes Targeting Healthy Exercise and Nutrition Alternatives): A promising program up against stiff competition. Arch Pediatr Adolesc Med 2004;158:1084.

Kemmler W, et al. Benefits of 2 years of intense exercise on bone density, physical fitness, and blood lipids in early postmenopausal osteopenic women: Results of the Erlangen Fitness Osteoporosis Prevention Study (EFOPS). Arch Intern Med 2004;24;164:1084.

Koopman R, et al. Combined ingestion of protein and carbohydrate improves protein balance during ultra-endurance exercise. Am J Physiol Endocrinol Metab 2004;287:E712.

Lange KH. Fat metabolism in exercise—with special reference to training and growth hormone administration. Scand J Med Sci Sports 2004;14:74.

Leiper JB, Maughan RJ. Comparison of water turnover rates in young swimmers in training and age-matched non-training individuals. Int J Sport Nutr Exerc Metab 2004;14:347.

McCarty MF. An elevation of triglycerides reflecting decreased triglyceride clearance may not be pathogenic—relevance to high-carbohydrate diets. Med Hypotheses 2004;63;1065.

Viitala PE, et al. The effects of antioxidant vitamin supplementation on resistance exercise induced lipid peroxidation in trained and untrained participants. Lipids Health Dis 2004;22;3:14.

Watson TA, et al. Antioxidant restricted diet reduces plasma non-esterified fatty acids in trained athletes. Asia Pac J Clin Nutr 2004;13(Suppl):S81.

Yanai H, Morimoto M. Significant association between fluctuations in serum urate and high density lipoprotein cholesterol during exhaustive training. Br J Sports Med 2003;37:370.

Yanai H, Morimoto M. Effect of ascorbate on serum lipids and urate metabolism during exhaustive training. Clin Sci (Lond) 2004;106:107.

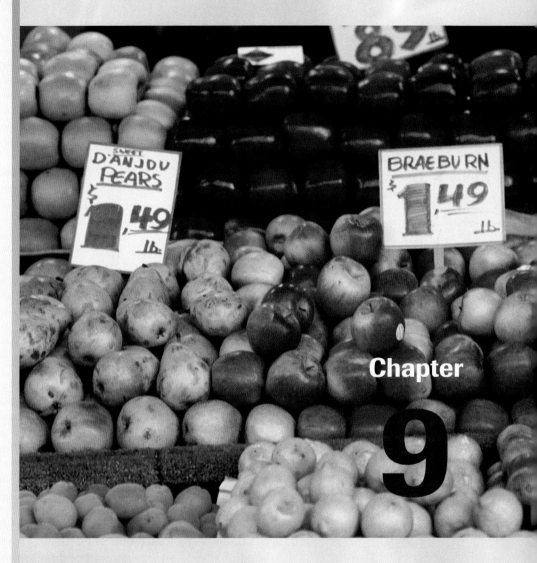

Chapter

9

Making Wise Choices in the Nutrition Marketplace

TEST YOUR KNOWLEDGE

Answer these ten statements about making wise choices in the nutrition marketplace. Use the scoring key at the end of the chapter to check your results. Repeat this test after you have read the chapter and compare your results.

1. **T F** The U.S. government oversees and guarantees that a nutritional supplement has been checked and rated safe to consume.

2. **T F** FTC stands for Federal Trade Commission; it regulates food-product advertising in different media.

3. **T F** FDA stands for the office of the Federal District Attorney; it prosecutes violators of food standards set by the Food and Drug Administration.

4. **T F** Federal law dictates that sellers of dietary supplements must guarantee their products as safe and effective.

5. **T F** Dietary supplements must provide precise information about their contents, clearly listed on the package.

6. **T F** The ATF stands for the Bureau of Alcohol, Tobacco and Firearms; it enforces laws related to alcohol, tobacco, and firearms.

7. **T F** The Daily Reference Values on food labels assume a 3000-kcal daily intake as representative of the average caloric intake for most adults.

8. **T F** The term "healthy" can be used on a food label without meeting any established criteria for making a claim for health benefits.

9. **T F** Computing a food's nutrient density provides a convenient way to compare the energy content of different foods.

10. **T F** Obesity continues to grow at an epidemic rate in the United States despite any significant change in eating patterns and behaviors.

Dramatic changes, both positive and negative, have affected the food and nutrition scene for the past 55 years. The most blatant example of negativism concerns how multinational companies focus on profit rather than consumer well-being. Companies allocate hundreds of millions of dollars annually to espouse supposed "health benefits" of micronutrient vitamins and minerals, specialty foods, and dietary supplements. Similarly, manufacturers of home exercise equipment use false and deceptive advertising to entice customers to purchase their products. Undoubtedly, big-budget advertising pays off. In 2000, approximately 158 million Americans consumed $17.1 billion worth of dietary supplements of dubious benefit, while exercising on $2.4 billion worth of equipment

ranging from abdominal "slimming" boards, stationary bicycles, beltless treadmills and "gliders," to face and neck "shapers."

The Food and Drug Administration (FDA) cannot provide adequate scientific data for many of these products to render an opinion about their safety, let alone their effectiveness. Nutrition supplements include ordinary vitamin and mineral capsules and exotically named potions, powders, creams, gels, lotions, liquids, gums, aerosols (e.g., bee pollen, royal jelly, germanium, coenzyme Q10, evening primrose oil, Cel-U-Lite, Maximum Memory Capsules, BioZonePlus Nutrition Enhancers, VitaManPlus, Chitosan, Cardio-Endurance Powder), and literally thousands of other "health-nutrition-fitness" products. About two-thirds of the U.S. population incorrectly believe that the government requires supplement labels to include warnings about side effects and dangers. Whereas pharmaceutical companies must test their drugs to verify that they do not cause cancer, interfere with reproduction, cause organ damage, or create other problems greater than those they can prevent, supplement companies have no obligation to test their products for safety or efficacy before they market them (see page 259). The FDA only intervenes when a supplement causes documented injury or illness, as occurred in 1990 when the agency banned the popular amino acid supplement L-tryptophan following 38 deaths and 1500 illnesses linked to its use.

Our point about this topic is straightforward: consumers must remain continually aware of advertising hype in the various media that promote the health and fitness benefits of products. Far too few "watchdog" organizations and adequately staffed and funded governmental agencies exist to patrol overzealous promoters whose products often pledge longer life, improved bodily functions, and instant cure for just about every possible ailment and misfortune.

FOOD ADVERTISING AND PACKAGING

In the late 1970s, renewed interest in nutrition and healthful eating sparked worldwide attention when the medical community linked cholesterol-rich diets to high blood cholesterol, a primary risk factor for heart disease. In addition, large-scale epidemiologic studies linked many forms of cancer to dietary practices. Coincidentally, the emerging physical fitness movement that swept North America became superimposed on the diet-heart disease and diet-cancer connections. Health clubs flourished, and articles in the lay press championed the latest tips on how to improve fitness and health by eating well and exercising regularly. However, the notion of a physically active and fit American culture seemed more illusory than real. While many people began to exercise, few actually stuck with it. At best, only 20% (and possibly less than 10%) of adults in the United States (and Australia, Canada, and England) obtain regular physical activity that translates to discernible health and fitness benefits.[2,7,11]

Advertising's Goal: To Shape Behavior

Advertising purposely attempts to create, shape, and alter perceptions about what we eat and how we exercise. The food industry, for example, spends more than $40 billion a year for advertising and promotion to sell its products and countless millions more for lobbying. In addition, food companies provide funds to academic departments and research institutes; they support conventions, meetings, and conferences and contribute to the production of "fact

---

EIGHT SUPPLEMENTS THAT CAN CAUSE SERIOUS PROBLEMS

- **Aristolochic acid.** The ingredient in some traditional Chinese medicines is toxic to the kidneys.

- **Chaparral.** In 1992, the FDA advised consumers to "stop taking chaparral immediately" because it can cause hepatitis.

- **Comfrey.** It can cause chronic liver disease.

- **Ephedra.** It has been linked to high blood pressure, strokes, and heart attacks and is 200 times more likely to cause an adverse reaction than all other herbs combined.

- **Kava.** It's a suspect in liver damage that has resulted in 11 liver transplants over the last several years.

- **PC SPES and SPES.** These supplements, which held promise as prostate-cancer fighters, turned out to be frauds. They worked like hormones only because they were spiked with hormones, a blood thinner, an antiinflammatory, and several other drugs.

- **Tiratricol.** In 2000, the FDA warned consumers not to use weight-loss supplements containing this thyroid hormone, which can cause strokes and heart attacks.

- **Usnic acid.** This "natural" compound (it's found in lichen), which is used in some herbal mixtures, appears to be toxic to the liver.

Sources: Food and Drug Administration (*www.dsan.fdo.gov/ %7Edms/ds-worn.html*) and CSPI.

---

sheets" such as those produced by the American Dietetic Association. Companies like Coca-Cola, Monsanto, Procter & Gamble, and Slim-Fast often sponsor nutrition journals. Food and drug companies underwrite the cost of publishing journal supplements of papers presented at conferences they frequently support. In some instances, corporate funding underwrites entire departments at universities.

McDonald's spends more than any other company in the world to advertise its products. McDonald's is the largest purchaser in the United States of pork, beef, and potatoes—and the second largest purchaser of chicken. Contrast this with the $750,000 the National Cancer Institute spends to promote fruits and vegetables. Soft drink

SAFETY OF THE TOP TEN HERBAL SUPPLEMENTS

Supplement	What Consumers Expect	Reported Reactions	Who Should Be Especially Careful	May Interact With
Black cohosh	To relieve symptoms of menopause	Mild gastrointestinal distress	Women who have had breast cancer (in an animal study, black cohosh caused cancer to spread)	No known drug interactions
Cranberry	To prevent or treat urinary tract infections	Regular use of cranberry concentrate tablets might increase the risk of kidney stones	Persons susceptible to kidney stones	Antidepressants and prescription painkillers
Echinacea	To prevent or treat colds or other infections	Minor gastrointestinal symptoms; increased urination; allergic reactions	Persons with autoimmune diseases (like multiple sclerosis, lupus, and rheumatoid arthritis); may also trigger episodes of erythema nodosum, an inflammation that produces tender nodules under the skin	No known drug interactions
Garlic	To lower cholesterol levels	Unpleasant breath odor; heartburn and flatulence	Persons who are about to have—or have just had—surgery (garlic thins the blood); women just before or after labor or delivery	Blood-thinning drugs like Coumadin (warfarin), heparin, or aspirin; blood-thinning supplements like ginkgo or high doses of vitamin E; chloroxazone, which is used to treat painful muscle conditions; HIV drugs
Ginkgo biloba	To improve memory	Mild headache; upset stomach; seizures (possibly caused by contamination with ginkgo seeds, which are toxic)	Persons with bleeding disorders like hemophilia; those who are about to have—or have just had—surgery; women just before or after labor or delivery; persons with diabetes	Blood-thinning drugs like Coumadin (warfarin), heparin, or aspirin; blood-thinning supplements like high doses of vitamin E; the antidepressant trazodone; antidiabetes drugs; thiazide diuretics
Ginseng	To increase energy and relieve stress	Insomnia; menstrual abnormalities and breast tenderness with long-term use	Women who have had breast cancer (ginseng stimulated the growth of breast cancer cells in test tubes); persons with high blood pressure who aren't taking medication to lower it	Any drug metabolized by the enzyme CYP 3A4 (ask your physician); MAO inhibitor drugs or digitalis; may increase the activity of insulin and oral hypoglycemics and decrease the activity of Coumadin (warfarin) and ticlopidine
Saw palmetto	To prevent or relieve the symptoms of an enlarged prostate	Mild gastrointestinal distress	Persons with bleeding disorders like hemophilia; those who are about to have—or have just had—surgery	Blood-thinning drugs like Coumadin (warfarin), heparin, or aspirin; blood-thinning supplements like ginkgo or high doses of vitamin E
Soy isoflavones	To relieve menopausal symptoms, prevent breast or prostate cancer, and strengthen bones	None reported	Women who have had—or are at high risk for—breast cancer (soy isoflavones may increase cell proliferation); pregnant women; persons with impaired thyroid function	No known drug interactions
St. John's wort	To alleviate depression	Mild gastrointestinal distress; rash; tiredness; restlessness	Persons with skin sensitive to sunlight; persons taking UV treatment; persons with bipolar disorder	Ritalin, ephedrine (found in ephedra), and caffeine; may increase the activity of protease inhibitors (for HIV), digitalis (for heart disease, statin drugs (for high cholesterol), warfarin (blood-thinner), chemotherapy drugs, oral contraceptives, tricyclic antidepressants, olanzapine and clozapine (for schizophrenia), and theophylline (for asthma); may increase sensitivity to sunlight if combined with sulfa drugs, Feldene (antiinflammatory), or Prilosec or Prevacid (for acid reflux)
Valerian	To induce sleep or relaxation	May impair attention for a few hours	Persons about to operate heavy machinery or drive	May increase the activity of central-nervous system depressants like barbiturates (such as Seconal) and benzodiazepines (such as Vallum or Halcion)

manufacturers commit about $500 million to $1 billion each year to advertise products, compared with $60 to $100 million by the dairy industry. Small wonder the average American drinks over 50 gallons of soft drinks yearly compared with about 21 gallons of milk!

The food industry does not stand alone when it comes to advertising hype and success. In 1996, American Consumers purchased $2.4 billion worth of exercise equipment (4% gain above 1995), with treadmill sales topping the list, and abdominal exercisers representing the fastest-growing product category. Television infomercials, newspapers, catalogs, direct phone marketing, magazines, and print-ads target specific groups for sales, often using misleading and deceptive advertising.

Product imagery definitely affects consumer purchases. Food manufacturers, for example, often pay a premium to supermarkets to locate and display products for easy identification. Obviously, such payments from a large manufacturer can cripple a less wealthy competitor's attempts to make inroads in a particular market segment. The practice, generally unknown to the consumer, makes good business sense (although morally questionable) because increased sales with fewer competitors trigger larger profits.

Governmental agencies try to police the food industry by legislating how manufacturers advertise their products. Unfortunately, no state or federal guidelines require that all the facts about a product need be made known to support a particular claim. Manufacturers of many dietary supplements, for example, retain the luxury of interpreting the "facts" about their product's effectiveness. Consequently, the consumer must decipher what the advertising actually means as well as interpret the information provided on food labels. According to the Federal Trade Commission (FTC) in a report made public in 2002 (http://www.ftc.gov/opa/2002/09/weightlossrpt.htm), nearly 40% of ads that appeared in mainstream, national publications made at least one representation that is "almost certainly false," and 55% of the ads made at least one representation that is "very likely to be false."

As we discuss below, the current food labeling law puts "teeth" into what manufacturers can and cannot state on food labels and what they can promote about their products' health benefits. TABLE 9.1 presents an almost 100-year chronology starting at 1906 of the U.S. government's role in regulating the quality and safety of food available to the American public.

GOVERNMENT "WATCHDOG" AGENCIES

Four governmental agencies create the rules, regulations, and legal requirements concerning advertising, packaging, and labeling of foods and alcoholic beverages.

Federal Trade Commission (FTC)[a]

The FTC regulates food product advertising in various media (TV, radio, newsprint) and pursues legal action against manufacturers who advertise unsubstantiated claims or deceptive ads. For example, if a TV ad states, "Consuming this supplement reduces your chances of colon cancer," the FTC can require the manufacturer to substantiate the claim. The FTC has authority to remove a product from the marketplace if the product's claims lack verification. Manufacturers often cooperate with the FTC and take affirmative corrective action of violations. In 1996, for example, this included a consent order against Mrs. Fields Cookies from misrepresenting the lipid, saturated fat, cholesterol, and caloric content of its baked food products (*Federal Register,* Jan 31, 1997, vol 62, no. 21,4769). In the same year, the FTC ordered a cease and desist order against Diet Workshop, Inc. from misrepresenting the results of any weight-loss program they offered, requiring them to provide scientific data substantiating any claims concerning weight-loss and weight maintenance (*Federal Register,* Jan 31, 1997, vol 62, no. 21,4767).

In September 1997, the FTC settled charges with Life Fitness, a manufacturer of exercise equipment, that it made unsubstantiated claims about the weight-loss benefits of its Lifecycle stationary exercise cycle. The order required Life Fitness to substantiate future claims about the weight-loss, calorie-burning, or fat-burning benefits of any exercise equipment it marketed. It also prohibits them from misrepresenting the result of any test, study, or research relating to such benefits (FTC; Sept 12, 1997, docket no. C-3766). The FTC also settled charges that Icon Health and Fitness, Inc., the world's largest manufacturer of home fitness equipment (treadmills, stair steppers, weight benches, "riders"), made unsubstantiated claims about the weight-loss benefits of the "Proform Cross Walk Treadmill." The order required the respondents to substantiate future claims about the weight-loss, calorie-burning, or fat-burning benefits of any exercise equipment. In addition, the order required that testimonials in the Icon Health and Fitness advertising either represent the typical experience of users or include disclosures of the generally expected results or some statement making clear that consumers should not

[a] FTC internet site: http://www.ftc.gov. The FTC describes its mission as follows: "To enforce a variety of federal antitrust and consumer protection laws. The Commission seeks to ensure that the nation's markets function competitively, and are vigorous, efficient, and free of undue restrictions." The Commission also works to enhance the smooth operation of the marketplace by eliminating acts or practices that are unfair or deceptive. In general, the Commission's efforts are directed toward stopping actions that threaten consumers' opportunities to exercise informed choice. Finally, the Commission undertakes economic analysis to support its law enforcement efforts and to contribute to the policy deliberations of the congress, the executive branch, other independent agencies, and state and local governments when requested. Additional consumer information from the FTC exists concerning tips for buying exercise equipment. (http://www.ftc.gov/ bcp/conline/edcams/exercise/index.html) as part of *Project Workout,* the FTC consumer education campaign (http://www.ftc.gov/opa/ 9706/workout.htm).

Table 9.1	CHRONOLOGY OF PROGRESS IN GOVERNMENTAL SUPPORT OF FOODS AND FOOD-RELATED PRACTICES

Year	Action	Description
1906	The Federal Food and Drugs Act and Federal Meat Inspection Act	Authorized the federal government through its Bureau of Chemistry to regulate the safety and quality of food. The responsibility eventually fell to the USDA, the agency that superseded the Bureau of Chemistry.
1913	GOULD Amendment	Food packages were required to state the quantity of its contents.
1924	US. vs. 96 Barrels Alleged Apple Cider Vinegar	Supreme Court ruled that the Food and Drug Act condemned every statement, design, or device that may mislead, misdirect, or deceive, even if technically true.
1938	Federal Food, Drug, and Cosmetic Act	This Act replaced the 1906 Food and Drug Act. Among other things, it requires the label of every processed packaged food to contain the name of the food, its net weight, and the name and address of the manufacturer or distributor. A list of ingredients also is required on certain products. The law also prohibits statements in food labeling that are false or misleading.
1950	The Oleomargarine Act	Requires prominent labeling of colored oleomargarine to distinguish it from butter.
1957	The Poultry Products Inspection Act	Authorized the USDA to regulate the labeling of poultry products along with other products.
1966	Fair Packaging and Labeling Act	Required all consumer products in interstate commerce to contain accurate information and to facilitate value comparisons.
1969	White House Conference on Food, Nutrition, and Health	Recommended that the federal government develop a system to identify the nutritional qualities of food.
1973	FDA Guidelines	FDA issues regulations requiring nutrition labeling on food containing one or more added nutrients or whose label or advertising includes claims about the food's nutritional properties or its usefulness in the daily diet. Nutrition labeling is voluntary for almost all other foods.
1975	FDA action	Voluntary nutrition labeling, postponed from its originally planned 1974 date, goes into effect.
1984	FDA action	FDA adds sodium to the list of required nutrients and potassium to the list of optional nutrients on the nutrition panel. Effective in 1985, the new regulation also defines terms, such as "low sodium," that may be used on labels to make sodium content claims.
1988	Surgeon General's Report on Nutrition and Health	The federal government's first formal recognition of the role of diet in certain chronic diseases.
1989	National Research Council of the National Academy of Sciences issues Diet and Health Implications for Reducing Chronic Disease Risk	This document presented additional evidence of the growing acceptance of diet as a factor in the development of chronic diseases such as coronary heart disease and cancer. Under contract with FDA and USDA's Food Safety and Inspection Service (FSIS), the Food and Nutrition Board of the National Academy of Sciences convenes a committee to consider how food labels could be improved to help consumers adopt or adhere to healthy diets. Its recommendations are presented in Nutrition Labeling: Issues and Directions. FDA publishes an advance notice of proposed rulemaking on food labeling and, with FSIS participating holds a series of four public hearings around the world.
1990	FDA action	FDA proposes extensive food labeling changes, which include mandatory nutrition labeling for most foods, standardized serving sizes, and uniform use of health claims. When Congress passed the Nutrition Labeling and Education Act of 1990 (NLEA), the Act reaffirmed the legal basis for FDA's labeling initiative and established an explicit timetable for implementation.

(continues)

Table 9.1 **CHRONOLOGY OF PROGRESS IN GOVERNMENTAL SUPPORT OF FOODS AND FOOD-RELATED PRACTICES (continued)**

Year	Action	Description
1991	FDA action	FDA issues more than 20 proposals to implement NLEA. In addition, the agency issues a final rule that sets up a voluntary point-of-purchase nutrition information program for raw produce and fish. FSIS unveils its proposals for mandatory nutrition labeling of processed meat and poultry and voluntary point-of-purchase nutrition information for raw meat and poultry.
1992	FDA action	FDA's voluntary point-of-purchase nutrition information program for fresh produce and raw fish became effective.
1993	FDA action	FDA issued final regulations implementing NLEA. Regulations covering health claims became effective May 8, 1993. Those pertaining to nutrition labeling and nutrient content claim became effective May 8, 1994. Food Safety and Inspection Services issues regulations for nutrition labeling of meat and poultry, effective July 6, 1994. In addition, the regulations established voluntary programs for nutrition information of many raw foods (the 20 most frequently eaten raw fruits, vegetables and fish), the 45 best-selling cuts of meat, supervised under the USDA program.
1994	FDA action	Implementation of nutrition labeling and nutrient content claim became effective May 8, 1994.
1995,1996	FDA action	Exemptions to the nutrition labeling act take effect between May 9, 1995, and May 8, 1996, and after May, 1997. These exemptions relate to foods produced by small businesses and to companies that meet requirements for number of employees and number of units of the food item within a product line produced yearly. Foods exempt from nutrition labeling include food served in hospital cafeterias and airplanes, food sold by food service vendors (mall cookie counters, sidewalk vendors, and vending machines), ready-to-eat foods not for immediate consumption (bakery, deli, and candy store items), foods shipped in bulk not for sale in that form to consumers, medical foods for patients with certain diseases, and plain coffee and tea, some spices, and other foods that contain no significant amounts of any nutrients.
1996	Federal Tea Tasters Repeal Act	Repeals the Tea Importation Act of 1897 to eliminate the Board of Tea Experts and user fees for FDA's testing of all imported tea. Tea itself is still regulated by the FDA.
	Saccharin Notice Repeal Act	Repeals the saccharin notice requirements
	Animal Drug Availability Act	Adds flexibility to animal drug approval process, providing for flexible labeling and more direct communication between drug sponsors and FDA
	Food Quality Protection Act	Amends the Food, Drug, and Cosmetic Act, eliminating application of the Delaney proviso to pesticides.
1997	Food and Drug Administration Modernization Act	Reauthorizes the Prescription Drug User Fee Act of 1992 and mandates the most wide-ranging reforms in agency practices since 1938. Provisions include measures to accelerate review of devices, regulating advertising of unapproved uses of approved drugs and devices, and regulating health claims on food.
1998	Mammography Quality Standards Reauthorization Act	Continues the 1992 Act until 2002. First phase to consolidate FDA laboratories nationwide from 19 facilities to 9 by 2014. Includes dedication of the first of five new regional laboratories.

expect to experience similar results (FTC; Sept 12, 1997, docket no. C-3765).

In October 2000, the FTC settled a claim that Weider Nutrition International, Inc., a leading manufacturer and marketer of nutritional supplements, vitamins, and sports nutrition products, did not have a reasonable basis to substantiate its claims that two of its products, PhenCal and

PhenCal 106, achieved the following:

- Caused significant weight loss
- Significantly increased ability to maintain a reduced-calorie diet and exercise regimen
- Significantly reduced food cravings and eating binges
- Prevented regain of lost weight

- Achieved the same effectiveness as the prescription weight loss treatment Phen-Fen

The complaint further alleged that Weider's claims that scientific studies that prove the safety and effectiveness of PhenCal are false.

The proposed consent agreement prohibited Weider from making the specific unsubstantiated claims. It also requires Weider, when advertising any food, drug, dietary supplement, or program, to have adequate scientific evidence before making claims relating to the safety of such product or program, the effect of such product or program on any disease, or the comparative or superior health benefit of such product or program (http://www.ftc.gov/os/2000/10/weider-agree.htm).

Food and Drug Administration (FDA)[b]

The FDA represents one of 13 agencies within the Department of Health and Human Services (DHHS). With the exception of poultry and meat products, the FDA regulates what manufacturers state on food labels; the safety of cosmetics, medicines, and medical devices; and feed and drugs for pets and farm animals. The FDA also decides what additives manufacturers can add to foods, including potential hazards with food additives (contaminants), food-borne infections, toxicants, artificially constituted foods, and pesticide residues.

One of six major FDA agencies, the **Center for Food Safety and Applied Nutrition (CFSAN)**[c] regulates $240 billion worth of domestic food, $15 billion of imported food, and $15 billion of cosmetic products sold across state lines. The CFSAN employs 800 people to carry out its mission that (a) the food supply remains safe, nutritious, and wholesome and (b) labels on foods and cosmetics maintain a high degree of accuracy. These two goals make sense when one considers that one-fifth of every consumer dollar in the United States goes for food and cosmetic products. In fiscal year 2000 (October 1, 1999 to September 30, 2000), the FDA spent more than $280 million on food and cosmetic safety activities. Interestingly, consumers spend 25 cents of every consumer dollar on products regulated by the FDA. Of this amount, approximately 75% is spent on food.

The CFSAN specialized support staff includes chemists, microbiologists, toxicologists, food technologists, pathologists, pharmacologists, nutritionists, epidemiologists, mathematicians, and sanitarians. Their areas of responsibility include

- Cosmetics and colors
- Food labeling
- Plant and diary foods and beverages
- Premarket approval
- Special nutritionals such as dietary supplements and infant formulas

The law defines a "dietary supplement" as a product taken by mouth that contains a "dietary ingredient" intended to supplement the diet. "Dietary ingredients" may include vitamins, minerals, herbs or other botanicals, amino acids, and substances (e.g., enzymes, organ tissues, glandular material, and metabolites). Dietary supplements may also be extracts or concentrates from plants or foods. Products sold as dietary supplements must be clearly labeled dietary supplements.

In 1994, Congress passed the Dietary Supplement Health and Education Act (DSHEA). This reduced the FDA's control over vitamin, mineral, enzyme, hormone, botanical, amino acid, and herb supplements, which it reclassified as foods not drugs. The law defines a dietary supplement (typically sold in the form of tablets, capsules, soft gels, liquids, powders, and bars) as a product taken by mouth that contains a dietary ingredient to supplement the diet. Under the DSHEA, FDA approval stringently requires proof of purity, safety, and effectiveness (via clinical trials) for public consumption of over-the-counter and prescription pharma-

---

[b] FDA Internet site: http://www.fda.gov. The FDA, a large public health agency, has the responsibility for protecting American consumers by enforcing the Federal Food, Drug, and Cosmetic Act and several related public health laws. The FDA employs 1100 investigators located in district and local offices in 157 cities who cover approximately 95,000 FDA-regulated businesses. Investigators and inspectors visit more than 15,000 facilities a year to oversee production and labeling. The FDA examines about 80,000 domestic and imported product samples for label checks. If a company violates any of the laws that the FDA enforces, the FDA encourages the firm to voluntarily correct the problem or to recall a faulty product from the market. The FDA can ask the courts to force a company to stop selling a product and to have items already produced seized and destroyed. Criminal penalties—including prison sentences—can be sought against manufacturers and distributors. About 3000 products a year are declared unfit for consumers and withdrawn from the marketplace (voluntarily or by court-ordered seizure). The FDA detains about 30,000 import shipments a year at the port of entry because the goods appear unacceptable. The FDA employs 2100 scientists who work in 40 laboratories around the country. These include evaluation of products seeking agency approval such as drugs, vaccines, food additives, coloring agents, and medical devices. The FDA also monitors the safety of the nation's blood supply and routinely examines blood bank operations, from record keeping to testing for contaminants. The FDA ensures the purity and effectiveness of biologicals (medical preparations made from living organisms and their products) such as insulin and vaccines. The FDA collects and analyzes tens of thousands of reports each year on drugs and devices for any unexpected adverse reactions after they become commercially available. In a recent report (Feb. 28, 2003: http://www.fda.gov/bbs/topics/NEWS/ephedra/factsheet.html), the FDA announced a series of actions to protect Americans from potentially serious risks of dietary supplement products containing ephedra. The announcement cited recent studies and provided additional evidence that ephedra may be associated with important health risks. The report concluded there are reasons for heightened concern that dietary supplements containing ephedra may present a significant and unreasonable risk of illness and injury. The report reviewed approximately 16,000 adverse event reports including two deaths, four heart attacks, nine strokes, one seizure, and five psychiatric cases involving ephedra in which the records appeared thorough and no other contributing factors were identified. The specifics of the role of the FDA in regulating dietary supplements can be found in the posted website: http//www.cfsan.fda.gov/dms/ds-oview.html. A comprehensive, encyclopedic source that reviews hundreds of supplement ingredients with frequent updates can be found online at the subscription-based *Natural Medicines Comprehensive Database* (www.naturaldatabase.com).

[c] Kurtzwell, P. Center for food safety and applied nutrition. FDA Consumer April 27, 1997. Internet site for CFSAN: http://vm.cfsan.fda.gov/list.html

ceuticals. Marketing of dietary supplements does not require such approval because they are considered foods. In contrast to medicines, which must meet safety and efficacy requirements before they come to market, legislation places the burden on the FDA to prove that a supplement is harmful before it can remove it from the market. Marketing a supplement can progress with *only* the manufacturer's assurance of safety as long as the supplement does not claim disease-fighting benefits. Since DSHEA passage, dietary supplements in the United States have skyrocketed, jumping to nearly $12 billion in 1997 from more than $8 billion in 1994. Of this total amount, consumers spend nearly $1 billion on dietary supplements related to "sports nutrition."

A manufacturer of an iron-containing supplement cannot make a specific unsubstantiated health claim about a product such as "This product cures anemia." However, more generalized "structure and function" claims are permissible, such as: "Iron is important in the synthesis of hemoglobin in red blood cells." The frightening aspect of lessened control over the supplement industry means that many supplements consumed in excess mimic the harmful effects of illegally obtained chemicals and drugs.

Rules for Dietary Supplements

To add strength to the 1994 DSHEA, the FDA approved a dietary supplement bill in September 1997. The FDA published final rules that provided consumers with somewhat more complete information in the labeling of dietary supplement products. These rules implement some of the major provisions of the DSHEA of 1994 designed to facilitate public access to "natural" medicines. The act requires the FDA to develop labeling requirements specifically designed for products containing ingredients such as vitamins, minerals, herbs, or amino acids intended to supplement the diet.

The new rules require these products to be labeled as dietary supplements (e.g., "Vitamin C Dietary Supplement") and to carry a "Supplement Facts" panel with information similar to the "Nutrition Facts" panel that appears on most processed foods. The rules also set parameters for use of the terms "high potency" and "antioxidant" when used in the labeling of dietary supplements. *Despite this attempt by the government to upgrade standards in this industry, consumers must recognize that quality control does not exist for dietary supplements.*

The rules also require that the labels of products containing botanical ingredients identify the part of the plant used. In addition, the source of the dietary ingredient may either follow the name or be listed in the ingredient statement below the "Supplement Parts" panel.

The following guidelines apply for use of the terms "high potency" and "antioxidant" on food labels:

- **High potency** may be used to describe a nutrient in a food product including dietary supplements, at 100% or more of the Reference Daily Intake (RDI)

REQUIRED INFORMATION ON THE "SUPPLEMENT FACTS" PANEL

- An appropriate serving size

- Information on 14 nutrients, including sodium, vitamin A, vitamin C, calcium, and iron, when present at significant levels

- Other vitamins and minerals if added or part of a nutritional claim on the label

- Dietary ingredients with no established Reference Daily Intakes (RDIs; see page 263)

- If the product contains a proprietary blend of ingredients, the total amount of the blend and the identity of each dietary ingredient in the blend (amounts of individual ingredients in the blend are not required)

---

established for that vitamin or mineral. High potency can be used with multiingredient products if two-thirds of the product's nutrients occur at levels more than 100% of the RDI.

- **Antioxidant** may be used in conjunction with currently defined claims for "good source" and "high" to describe a nutrient for which scientific evidence shows that following absorption of a sufficient quantity, the nutrient (e.g., vitamin C) inactivates free radicals or prevents free radical-initiated chemical reactions.

User Beware. Because dietary supplements need not meet the same quality control for purity and potency as pharmaceuticals, considerable variation exists in the concentration of marker compounds.[9] So-called all natural pills and powders sold as dietary supplements have caused lead poisoning, impotence, lethargy and "unarousable" sleep, nausea, vomiting, diarrhea, and abnormal heart rhythms (from the presence of powerful pesticides, herbs, toxic contaminants, or potent prohibited drugs and hormones) in persons trying to self-treat diverse ailments or improve physical function.[1]

Advertisements for "health food" preparations containing natural herbs often promise weight loss, muscle growth, increased endurance capacity, and a drug-free "herbal high." Unfortunately, many of these concoctions have contained the now-banned ephedrine, a drug linked to heart attacks, stroke, angina, arrhythmias, seizures, and at least 17 deaths. As one government official said: "Some of these products are nothing more than street drugs masquerading as diet supplements." To compound matters, the preparations appear as dietary supplements and thus escape the FDA's rigid control over pharmaceuticals. Many compounds fail to conform to labeling requirements of the DSHEA in terms of proper and correct identification of the strength of the product's ingredients.[4,5] Simply stated, supplement manufacturers need not guarantee that all ingredients are on its label. In this regard, independent organizations such as ConsumerLab (http://www.Consumer-Lab.com) provide their "seal of approval" as to purity and quality control and the safety, effectiveness, and potential for adverse effects for numerous dietary and sport nutrition supplements. These include herbal, vitamin, and mineral supplements that affect health, wellness, and nutrition.

United States Department of Agriculture (USDA)[d]

The USDA deals with farm and foreign agricultural services, food, nutrition, and consumer services, food safety, marketing and regulatory programs, natural resources and environment, research, education, economics, marketing and regulatory programs, and rural development. The Center for Nutrition Policy and Promotion coordinates nutrition policy in the USDA and provides overall leadership in nutrition education for consumers. The goals of the program include providing needy individuals with access to a more nutritious diet, improving the eating habits of American children, and helping America's farmers find an outlet for distributing food purchased under farmer assistance authorities. The Center serves as the link between basic science and the consumer. The Center coordinates with the DHHS the review, revision, and dissemination of the *Dietary Guidelines for Americans*. This represents the federal government's statement of nutrition policy, formed by a consensus of professionals in science and medicine. The USDA regulates food labels for poultry and meat products.

---

[d] USDA Internet site: http://www.usda.gov. The Food and Nutrition Information Center, as part of the USDA, Agricultural Research Service, the National Agricultural Library, maintains an Internet presence (http://www.nal.usda.gov/fnic/) where users may read, download, or print information. The site links to other sites, including the Healthy School Meals Resource System (http://schoolmeals.nal.usda.gov:8001). Individuals can access full texts of the Food and Nutrition Information Center's (FNIC) bibliographies, resource lists, and fact sheets covering nutrition education, human nutrition, food service management, and others. Databases available include Food and Nutrition Software and Multimedia Programs, Foodborne Illness Educational Materials, and Hazard Analysis Critical Control Points (HACCP) Training Programs and Resources. Government publications include *Dietary Guidelines for Americans*, Healthy Eating Index, USDA's Food Composition data, Food Guide Pyramid publications and images, and Food and Nutrition Research Briefs. Individuals can search the database of food and nutrition software and multimedia programs. (http://www.nal.usda.gov/fnic/software/software.html). Thirteen distinguished professionals from academia serve on the Dietary Guidelines Advisory Committee, the group responsible for reviewing the *Dietary Guidelines for Americans* report published every 5 years. A broad-based nutrition policy guide, the *Guidelines* uses the latest scientific and medical knowledge to advise the general public on ways to improve overall health through proper nutrition. The Committee reviews and updates the most recent scientific literature in preparation for the release of the 2005 version of *Dietary Guidelines for Americans*.

Bureau of Alcohol, Tobacco and Firearms (ATF)[e]

The ATF, a law enforcement organization within the United States Department of Treasury, came into existence in 1972 after separating from the Internal Revenue Service (Alcohol, Tobacco and Firearms Division). The ATF has responsibilities dedicated to reducing violent crime, collecting revenue, and protecting the public. It enforces federal laws and regulations relating to alcohol, tobacco, firearms, explosives, and arson.

THE FOOD LABEL

The FDA and the Food Safety and Inspection Service (FSIS) of the USDA issued new regulations concerning nutritional information about food labels to *(a)* help consumers choose more healthful diets and *(b)* offer an incentive to food companies to improve the nutritional qualities of their products.[f] Also, the Nutrition Labeling and Education Act (NLEA) of 1990 (including 1993–1998 updates to the regulations) now requires food manufacturers to strictly adhere to regulations about what can and cannot be printed on food labels. The key provisions of food label reform include

- Nutrition labeling for almost all foods to assist consumers in making more healthful food choices
- Information on the amount per serving of saturated fat, cholesterol, dietary fiber, and other nutrients considered of major health concern to consumers. In light of mounting evidence that *trans* fatty acids increase heart disease risk, food processors must also include, by the year 2006, the amount of *trans* fatty acids on nutrition labels
- Nutrient reference values, expressed as % Daily Values, to help consumers determine how a food fits into an overall daily diet
- Uniform definitions for terms that describe a food's nutrient content, such as "light," "low-fat," and "high-fiber," to ensure that such terms have the same meaning for any product on which they appear
- Substantiating claims about the relationship between a nutrient or food and a disease or health-related

---

[e] The ATF (http://www.atf.treas.gov) regulates the qualification and operation of distilleries, wineries, breweries, importers, and wholesalers. The ATF National Laboratory founded in 1886 tests new products coming onto the market and whether any products currently on the market pose a health risk to consumers. In 1996, the ATF laboratories analyzed 8400 alcohol and tobacco samples, processed over 3134 forensic cases, spent 342 days giving expert court testimony, 360 days at crime scenes, and 101 days training federal, state, and local investigators and examiners. To ensure that alcohol beverage labels do not contain misleading information and adhere to regulatory mandates, ATF examines all label applications for approval. The ATF maintains statistics about domestic alcohol and tobacco production.

[f] Reprints of Federal Register documents on FDA food labeling rules are available by contacting the National Technical Information Service, (703) 487-4650 (ask for #PB-93-139905).

CASE STUDY/PERSONAL HEALTH AND EXERCISE NUTRITION 9–1

To Use the Term *Organically Grown*

William and Cathy have three small children. They live in a rural northeastern community where they operate a small farm stand to supplement their income. They always have sold their products as "organically grown" because they believe that pesticides and other traditional additives produce products "not as healthy" as their organic fruits and vegetables. On a recent visit to the vegetable department of a large supermarket in a nearby city, they questioned the produce manager about the market's organically labeled products. William believed the market was using deceptive advertising to get customers to buy the products, so he consulted the manager who arranged for William to meet with the local food inspector. To William's surprise, here is what he learned about organically grown products, not only for foods purchased at the supermarket but for his own farm stand.

Q: Are there regulations about organically grown foods?

A: Yes. The USDA supervises the National Organic Program (NOP).

Q: Where can I obtain information about this agency?

A: On the Internet at http://www.ams.usda.gov/nop

Q: When did the NOP regulations come into existence?

A: Beginning on October 21, 2002, producers and handlers must be certified by a USDA-accredited certifying agent to sell, label, or represent their products as "100% organic," "organic," or "made with organic (specified ingredients or food group(s)."

Q: I run a small farm that sells what I call "organically grown foods." Am I subject to the NOP rules and regulations?

A: It depends. If your gross agricultural income from organic sales total $5,000 or less annually, you are exempt from certification (for specifics, refer to the NOP regulations).

Q: I sell less than $5,000 worth of organic product. Can I be certified?

A: Yes. Any qualified agricultural production or handling operation may be certified as an organic production and handling operation. This includes all qualified production and handling operations eligible for exemption or exclusion under section 205.101 of the NOP regulations.

Q: Can noncertified companies use the word "organic?"

A: Producers and handlers that qualify for exemption or exclusion from certification may use the term "organic" in compliance with the labeling requirements specific to their exemption or exclusion (again, refer to section 205.101 of the NOP regulations).

Q: Who may use the term "organic" and how the term is to be used?

A: Any production or handling operation certified according to the provisions of regulations may use the term "organic." Production or handling operations that are exempted under the regulations may use the term "organic" according to the regulations

provided they comply with the production and handling requirements of the national standards.

Q: What are the penalties for misuse of the term "organic"?

A: Any operation that knowingly sells or mislabels a product as "organic," may be subject to a civil penalty of not more than $10,000 per violation.

Q: Who will be responsible for the enforcement of the National Organic Program?

A: USDA, accredited certifying agents, and where applicable, approved state organic programs will be responsible for enforcement of the national regulations.

Q: When a retail establishment markets products supplied from a certified producer, in the event the producer is found noncompliant, will the retailer be subject to any legal recourse from the NOP? Do the same rules apply (to the retailer) for products produced by exempt and nonexempt producers?

A: If a provider of product to a retail food establishment is found to be in violation of the national organic standards and the retail food establishment is not a party to that violation, there will be no action by the NOP against the retail food establishment. This holds true for certified producers and handlers as well as those claiming exemption under section 205.101.

Any person, including a retail food establishment, who knowingly sells or labels a product as organic, except in accordance with the OFPA and the national organic standards, shall be subject to a civil penalty of not more than $10,000 per violation.

Products that have entered the channels of commerce before the certified operation's suspension or revocation will not result in a product recall, unless the noncompliance involves a food safety issue.

Q: If my farm becomes certified as organic and I wish to purchase compost from a commercial compost operation, does this compost have to be certified organic?

A: No. Although a commercial compost operation may become USDA certified, there is no requirement for it to do so, and there is no requirement for you to use certified organic compost. However, any compost you use must meet all the requirements of the NOP regulations. The burden of proving that compost used on a certified organic operation meets all the NOP requirements rests with the certified organic operation that uses the compost. That operation must show in its organic systems plan, and be able to prove to its certifying agent, that the compost it uses meets the NOP requirements.

Q: Do fields have to meet any size requirements to produce crops certified as organic?

A: No. There are no field-size requirements relative to whether or not an operation can be certified organic.

Q: Is the feed that is fed to organic livestock and poultry "vegetarian" feed?

A: Not necessarily. "The producer of an organic operation must not feed mammalian or poultry slaughter byproducts to mammals or poultry." There is no restriction against organic livestock feed containing appropriate fish products.

Q: Must manure used to fertilize organic crops come from an organic source, that is, from an animal that has been raised in accordance with the organic standards?

A: No. There are no restrictions as to the source of manure.

Q: Is it safe to say that using organic fertilizers and other or-

ganic farming practices is better for the soil and less of a threat to ground and surface water than commercial methods?

A: USDA's National Organic Program is a marketing program and makes no claims that organic farming is "better" in any respect than conventional farming.

condition, such as calcium and osteoporosis, and fat and cancer
- Standardized serving sizes to make nutritional comparisons among similar products easier
- Declaration of total percentage of juice in juice drinks so consumers can determine a product's juice content
- Voluntary nutrition information for many raw foods

Nutrition Panel Title

The new food label displayed in FIGURE 9.1 features a revamped nutrition panel. It has a new title, "Nutrition Facts," which replaced "Nutrition Information Per Serving." The new title signals that the product contains a label according to the new regulations. For the first time, requirements include type size, style, spacing, and contrast to ensure a more distinctive, easy-to-read label.

Serving Sizes

The serving size remains the basis for reporting each food's nutrient contents. Prior to the new regulations, the food manufacturer determined the criteria for serving size. Serving sizes now must reflect the amounts that persons actually eat at one time and must express quantities in both common household measures (cup, tablespoon, piece, slice, fraction) and metric measures (g and mL).

Nutrition Information

The nutrition panel contains a new set of dietary components. The mandatory (boldface type) and optional (normal type) components and the order in which they must appear are as follows:

- **Total calories**
- **Calories from fat**
- Calories from saturated fat
- **Total fat**
- **Saturated fat**
- Polyunsaturated fat
- Monounsaturated fat
- **Cholesterol**
- **Sodium**
- Potassium

- **Total carbohydrate**
- **Dietary fiber**
- Soluble fiber
- Insoluble fiber
- **Sugars**
- Sugar alcohol (e.g., the sugar substitutes xylitol, mannitol, and sorbitol)
- Other carbohydrate (the difference between total carbohydrate and the sum of dietary fiber, sugars, and sugar alcohol if declared)
- **Protein**
- **Vitamin A**
- Percentage of vitamin A present as β-carotene
- **Vitamin C**
- **Calcium**
- **Iron**
- Other essential vitamins and minerals

Nutrition information for optional components or for foods fortified or enriched with them becomes mandatory if claims are made about any of these components. The nutrition panel can contain only these mandatory and optional components.

The listing of single amino acids, maltodextrin, calories from polyunsaturated fats, and calories from carbohydrates may not appear as part of the Nutrition Facts on the label. Order of appearance reflects the priority of current dietary recommendations. Thiamin, riboflavin, and niacin are no longer required in nutrition labeling (although they can be listed voluntarily), because deficiencies of each are no longer considered of public health significance.

Nutrition Panel Format

The format for showing nutrient content per serving must be declared as percentages of the Daily Values—the new label reference values. The amount of nutrients (expressed in g or mg) such as fat, cholesterol, sodium, carbohydrates, and protein must be listed to the immediate right of each named nutrient. A column headed "% Daily Value" also must appear on the label.

Declaring nutrients as a percentage of the Daily Values should prevent misinterpretations that arise with quantitative values. For example, one could mistake a food with 140 mg of sodium as a high-sodium food because the number 140 seems

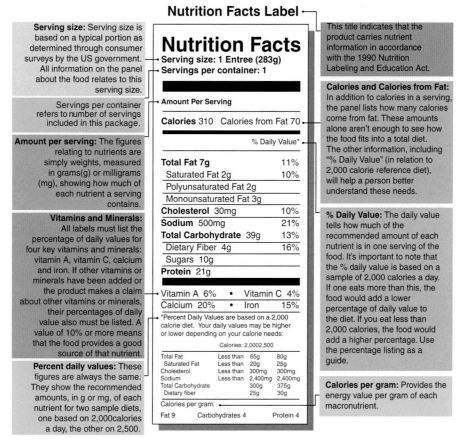

Nutrition Facts Label

Serving size: Serving size is based on a typical portion as determined through consumer surveys by the US government. All information on the panel about the food relates to this serving size.

Servings per container refers to number of servings included in this package.

Amount per serving: The figures relating to nutrients are simply weights, measured in grams(g) or milligrams (mg), showing how much of each nutrient a serving contains.

Vitamins and Minerals: All labels must list the percentage of daily values for four key vitamins and minerals: vitamin A, vitamin C, calcium and iron. If other vitamins or minerals have been added or the product makes a claim about other vitamins or minerals, their percentages of daily value also must be listed. A value of 10% or more means that the food provides a good source of that nutrient.

Percent daily values: These figures are always the same. They show the recommended amounts, in g or mg, of each nutrient for two sample diets, one based on 2,000calories a day, the other on 2,500.

Nutrition Facts

Serving size: 1 Entree (283g)
Servings per container: 1

Amount Per Serving

Calories 310   Calories from Fat 70

% Daily Value*

Total Fat 7g	11%
Saturated Fat 2g	10%
Polyunsaturated Fat 2g	
Monounsaturated Fat 3g	
Cholesterol 30mg	10%
Sodium 500mg	21%
Total Carbohydrate 39g	13%
Dietary Fiber 4g	16%
Sugars 10g	
Protein 21g	

Vitamin A 6%	•	Vitamin C	4%
Calcium 20%	•	Iron	15%

*Percent Daily Values are based on a 2,000 calorie diet. Your daily values may be higher or lower depending on your calorie needs:

Calories: 2,000   2,500

Total Fat	Less than	65g	80g
Saturated Fat	Less than	20g	25g
Cholesterol	Less than	300mg	300mg
Sodium	Less than	2,400mg	2,400mg
Total Carbohydrate		300g	375g
Dietary fiber		25g	30g

Calories per gram:

Fat 9   Carbohydrates 4   Protein 4

This title indicates that the product carries nutrient information in accordance with the 1990 Nutrition Labeling and Education Act.

Calories and Calories from Fat: In addition to calories in a serving, the panel lists how many calories come from fat. These amounts alone aren't enough to see how the food fits into a total diet. The other information, including "% Daily Value" (in relation to 2,000 calorie reference diet), will help a person better understand these needs.

% Daily Value: The daily value tells how much of the recommended amount of each nutrient is in one serving of the food. It's important to note that the % daily value is based on a sample of 2,000 calories a day. If one eats more than this, the food would add a lower percentage of daily value to the diet. If you eat less than 2,000 calories, the food would add a higher percentage. Use the percentage listing as a guide.

Calories per gram: Provides the energy value per gram of each macronutrient.

Figure 9.1 Reading the nutrition facts panel. Food labels help one make informed choices. Foods that contain only a few of the nutrients required on the standard label have a shorter label format. What is on the label depends on what is in the food. Small- and medium-sized packages with limited label space also can use the short form.

relatively large. In actuality, this amount represents less than 6% of the 2400-mg Daily Value for sodium. On the other hand, a food with 5 g of saturated fat could be construed as being low in that nutrient. However, that food provides one-fourth the total 20-g Daily Value for saturated fat based on a 2000-kcal diet. (The % Daily Value listing carries a footnote declaring that percentages are based on a 2000-kcal diet.)

DAILY REFERENCE VALUE (DRV)

The new label reference value, referred to as Daily Value, comprises two sets of dietary standards: Daily Reference Values (DRVs) and Reference Daily Intakes (RDIs). Only the DRV term appears on the label to make label reading less confusing. DRVs established for macronutrients include sources of energy (fat, carbohydrate [including fiber], and protein) and for non-calorie-contributing cholesterol, sodium, and potassium. A daily intake of 2000 calories serves as the reference number of calories for determining the DRVs for the energy-producing nutrients. The 2000-calorie level was chosen, in part, because it approximates the caloric requirements for postmenopausal women, the group with the highest risk for excessive intake of calories and fat.

DRVs for the energy-producing nutrients are calculated as follows:

- Fat based on 30% of calories
- Saturated fat based on 10% of calories
- Carbohydrate based on 60% of calories
- Protein based on 10% of calories (the DRV for protein applies only to adults and children above age 4)
- Fiber based on 11.5 g of fiber per 1000 calories; because of current public health recommendations, DRVs for some nutrients represent the uppermost limit considered desirable

The DRVs for fats and sodium include

- Total fat: less than 65 g
- Saturated fat: less than 20 g
- Cholesterol: less than 300 mg
- Sodium: less than 2400 mg

REFERENCE DAILY INTAKE (RDI)

The RDI replaces the term "U.S. RDA," introduced in 1973 as a label reference value for vitamins, minerals, and protein in voluntary nutrition labeling. The name change was sought because of confusion over "U.S. RDA," the values determined by FDA and used on food labels, and "RDA" (Recommended Dietary Allowance), the values determined by the National Academy of Sciences for various population groups and used by the FDA to determine the U.S. RDAs. As of mid-1988, the values for the new RDIs remain the same as the old U.S. RDAs.

NUTRIENT CONTENT DESCRIPTORS

The new food labeling regulations explain what terms to use to describe the level of a nutrient in a food and proper use of these terms. Core terms include the following:

- **Free.** A product contains no amount of, or only trivial or "physiologically inconsequential" amounts of, one or more of these components: fat, saturated fat, cholesterol, sodium, sugars, and calories. For example, "calorie-free" means fewer than 5 calories per serving and "sugar-free" and "fat-free" both mean less than 0.5 g per serving. Synonyms for "free" include "without," "no," and "zero."
- **Low.** Foods that can be eaten frequently without exceeding dietary guidelines for one or more of these components: fat, saturated fat, cholesterol, sodium, and calories. Thus, descriptors are defined as follows:
  - **low fat:** 3 g or less per serving
  - **low saturated fat:** 1 g or less per serving
  - **low sodium:** 140 mg or less per serving
  - **very low sodium:** 35 mg or less per serving
  - **low cholesterol:** 20 mg or less and 2 g or less of saturated fat per serving
  - **low calorie:** 40 calories or less per serving

Synonyms for low include "little," "few," and "low source of."

- **Lean and extra lean.** These terms can be used to describe the fat content of meat, poultry, seafood, and game meats.
  - **lean:** less than 10 g of fat, 4.5 g or less of saturated fat, and less than 95 mg of cholesterol per serving and per 100 g
  - **extra lean:** less than 5 g of fat, less than 2 g of saturated fat, and less than 95 mg of cholesterol per serving and per 100 g
- **High.** This term can be used if the food contains 20% or more of the Daily Value for a particular nutrient in a serving.
- **Good source.** This term means that one serving of a food contains 10 to 19% of the Daily Value for a particular nutrient.
- **Reduced.** This term means that a nutritionally altered product contains at least 25% less of a nutrient or of calories than the regular, or reference, product.

However, a reduced claim cannot be made for a product if its reference food already meets the requirement for a "low" claim.

- **Less.** This term means that a food, whether altered or not, contains 25% less of a nutrient or of calories than the reference food. For example, pretzels that have 25% less fat than potato chips could carry a "less" claim. "Fewer" is an acceptable synonym.
- **Light.** This descriptor can mean two things: First, that a nutritionally altered product contains one-third fewer calories or one-half the fat of the reference food. If the food derives 50% or more of its calories from fat, the reduction must be 50% of the fat. Second, that the sodium content of a low-calorie, low-fat food has been reduced by 50%. In addition, "light in sodium" may be used on food in which the sodium content has been reduced by at least 50%. The term "light" still can describe such properties as texture and color, as long as the label explains the intent, for example, "light brown sugar" and "light and fluffy."
- **More.** This term means that a serving of food, whether altered or not, contains a nutrient with at least 10% more of the Daily Value than the reference food. The 10% of Daily Value also applies to "fortified," "enriched," and "added" claims, but in those cases, the food must be altered. Alternative spelling of these descriptive terms and their synonyms are allowed, for example, "hi" and "lo," as long as the alternatives do not mislead.

Additional Definitions

The labeling regulations also provide guidelines for additional definitions:

- **Percent fat free.** A product bearing this claim must be a low-fat or a fat-free product. In addition, the claim must accurately reflect the amount of fat present in 100 g of the food. Thus, if a food contains 2.5 g fat per 50 g, the claim must be "95% fat free."
- **Implied.** These types of claims are prohibited when they wrongfully imply that a food contains or does not contain a meaningful level of a nutrient. For example, a product claiming to be made with an ingredient known as a source of fiber (such as "made with oat bran") is prohibited unless the product contains enough of that ingredient (e.g., oat bran) to meet the definition for "good source" of fiber. As another example, a claim that a product contains "no tropical oils" is allowed, but only for foods that are "low" in saturated fat, because consumers have come to equate tropical oils with high saturated fat.
- **Meals and main dishes.** Claims that a meal or main dish is "free" of a nutrient, such as sodium or cholesterol, must meet the same requirements as those for individual foods. Other claims can be used under spe-

cial circumstances. For example, "low-calorie" means the meal or main dish contains 120 kcal or less per 100 g. "Low-sodium" means the food has 140 mg or less per 100 g. "Low-cholesterol" means the food contains 20 mg of cholesterol or less per 100 g and no more than 2 g of saturated fat. "Light" means the meal or main dish is low fat or low calorie.

- **Standardized foods.** Any nutrient content claim, such as "reduced fat," "low calorie," and "light," may be used in conjunction with a standardized term if the new product has been specifically formulated to meet FDA's criteria for that claim, if the product is not nutritionally inferior to the traditional standardized food, and the new product complies with certain compositional requirements set by the FDA. A new product bearing a claim also must have performance characteristics similar to those of the referenced traditional standardized food. If the product does not and the differences materially limit the product's use, its label must state the differences (e.g., not recommended for baking) to inform consumers.

- **Healthy**: A "healthy" food must be low in fat and saturated fat and contain limited amounts of cholesterol and sodium. In addition, if it is a single-item food, it must provide at least 10% of one or more of vitamins A or C, iron, calcium, protein, or fiber. A meal-type product such as frozen entrees and multi-course frozen dinners must provide 10% of two or three of the above vitamins, minerals, protein, or fiber, in addition to meeting the other criteria. Limits on sodium have been phased in. Since January 1996, FDA-regulated individual foods labeled "healthy" must provide no more than 480 mg of sodium per serving. After January 1, 1998, the sodium limit for FDA-regulated foods decreased to 360 mg per serving for individual foods and 480 mg per serving for meal-type products that carry the "healthy" claims. Effective dates for the sodium phase-in for USDA-regulated products were November 1995 and November 1997. The sodium limits match the FDA's limits for this mineral.

What Does "Fresh" Mean?

Although not mandated by labeling regulations, the FDA has issued directions for use of the term "fresh." The agency took this step because of concern over possible misuse of this term on some food labels. The regulation defines "fresh" to suggest that a food is raw or unprocessed. In this context, "fresh" can describe a raw food, a food that has never been frozen or heated, and one that contains no preservatives (irradiation at low levels is allowed). "Fresh frozen," "frozen fresh," and "freshly frozen" can describe foods quickly frozen while still fresh. Blanching (brief scalding before freezing to prevent nutrient breakdown) is allowed. Other uses of the term "fresh," as in "fresh milk" or "freshly baked bread," are not affected.

FOOD ADDITIVES

A manufacturer wishing to include an additive in a food must follow specific FDA guidelines. The manufacturer must test to ensure the additive meets its claims. The FDA also requires that the additive be detected and measured in the product and that it produces no undesirable health effects (e.g., cancer or birth defects) when given in large doses to animals. Strict guidelines exist once the FDA approves an additive.

Approximately 700 additives were initially included on a list of additives **generally recognized as safe (GRAS)**. An expanded GRAS list currently includes about 2000 flavoring agents and 200 coloring agents. These substances do not receive permanent approval but face review periodically. Additives include emulsifiers, stabilizers, thickeners (to provide texture, smoothness, and consistency), nutrients such as vitamin C added to fruit juice or potassium iodide added to salt (to improve nutritive value), flavoring agents (to enhance taste), leavening agents (to make baked goods rise, or to control acidity or alkalinity), preservatives, antioxidants, sequestrants, and antimycotic agents (to prevent spoilage, rancidity of fats, and microbial growth), coloring agents (to increase attractiveness), bleaches (to whiten foods and speed up the maturing of cheese), and humectants and anticaking agents (to retain moisture and keep products like salts and powders free flowing).

BABY FOODS

The FDA does not allow the broad use of nutrient claims on infant and toddler foods. The agency may propose later claims specifically for these foods. The terms "unsweetened" and "unsalted" can be used on these foods because they relate to taste and not nutrient content.

HEALTH CLAIMS

Current regulations now permit claims for relationships between intake of a nutrient or a food and the risk of disease or health-related condition. They can be made in several ways: through third-party references, such as the National Cancer Institute or the American Heart Association; statements; symbols, such as a heart; and vignettes or descriptions. Whatever the case, the claim must meet requirements for authorized health claims. For example, a claim cannot state the degree of risk reduction; it can only use "may" or "might" in discussing the nutrient–or food–disease relationship. In addition, claims must state that other factors play a role in that disease. Health claims also must be phrased so that consumers can understand the relationship between the nutrient and the disease, and the nutrient's importance to a daily diet. The following exemplifies an appropriate health claim: "While many factors affect heart disease, diets low in saturated fat and cholesterol may reduce the risk of this disease."

Nutrient–disease relationship claims are as follows:

Approved health claims
- Soluble fiber and heart disease
- Dietary fat and cancer
- Saturated fat/cholesterol and heart disease
- Calcium and osteoporosis
- Fiber-containing grain products, fruits, and vegetables and cancer
- Folate and neural tube defects
- Dietary sugar alcohols and dental caries
- Whole oats, psyllium, and heart disease
- Soy protein and heart disease
- Calcium and hypertension

Approved authoritative health claim statements
- Whole grains and heart disease and cancer (first health claim approved under the FDA Modernization Act of 1997)
- Potassium and high blood pressure

Qualified Health Claims (supportive but not conclusive research)
- Heart-healthy benefits of omega-3 fatty acids
- Eating 1.5 ounces of walnuts a day may reduce coronary heart disease risk
- Eating two tablespoons (23 g) of olive oil daily may reduce the risk of coronary heart disease due to the monounsaturated fat in olive oil

Health claims denied approval
- Dietary fiber and cancer (wheat bran and colon cancer)
- Dietary fiber and cardiovascular disease
- Antioxidant vitamins and cancer
- Zinc and immune function and the elderly

Possible future health claims (1–5 years)
- Folic acid/B_6/B_{12} and heart disease
- Low-fat dairy products and hypertension

TABLE 9.2 presents rules for the use of allowable health claims and an example of an accompanying label statement.

LABELING OF INGREDIENTS

The list of ingredients has undergone changes in terms of labeling requirements. Chief among them includes a requirement for full ingredient labeling on previously exempt "standardized foods." Foods with more than one ingredient now require ingredient declaration. The ingredient list includes, when appropriate:

- FDA-certified color additives identified by name
- Sources of protein hydrolysates, used in many foods as flavors and flavor enhancers

- Declaration of caseinate as a milk derivative in the ingredient list of foods that claim to be nondairy, such as coffee whiteners

By including these new labeling requirements, people with allergies to additives can avoid food containing them. Beverages that claim to contain juice now must declare the total percentage of juice on the information panel. In addition, the regulation establishes criteria for naming juice beverages. For example, when the label of a multijuice beverage states one or more, but not all of the juices present, and the predominantly named juice occurs in minor amounts, the product's name must state that the beverage is flavored with that juice or declare the amount of the juice in a 5% range (e.g., "raspberry-flavored juice blend," or "juice blend, 2 to 7% raspberry juice").

ECONOMIC IMPACT

The new food label initially cost FDA-regulated food processors an estimated $1.4 billion; this increases to $2.3 billion through the year 2014. However, public health benefits should exceed the monetary costs. According to the FDA, the potential health benefits of honest and more complete labeling include decreased rates of coronary heart disease, cancer, osteoporosis, obesity, high blood pressure, and allergic reactions to food.

DETERMINING THE NUTRIENT PERCENTAGE IN A FOOD

Food labels must indicate the amount of a nutrient in packaged foods, yet no requirement exists to list nutrient composition in foods sold over-the-counter or in restaurants. Such information becomes quite revealing and often embarrassing to manufacturers who extol their "commitment to consumers" by providing "healthful" products. Consider several popular franchise chains that tout their hamburgers for providing quality nutrition: McDonald's informs consumers that a "Big Mac" contains *only* 35 g of fat; Burger King lists the fat content of a "Whopper" at 42 g, and Roy Rogers' cheeseburger contains 37.3 g of fat. But these food retailers conceal important information about the food's lipid content, expressed as a percentage of total calories. For the Big Mac, 35 g of fat amounts to 315 kcal from fat ($35 \text{ g} \times 9 \text{ kcal·g}^{-1}$). Because a Big Mac contains a total of 570 kcal, the percentage calories from fat ($[315 \div 570] \times 100$) translates to 55.2% fat! Burger King's "Whopper" contains a whopping 57.7% fat, and the cheeseburger from Roy Rogers tops the list at 59.6%.

Not surprisingly, manufacturers downplay such information. TABLE 9.3 illustrates the importance of understanding the information in a product's label, particularly its lipid

Table 9.2	REQUIREMENTS FOR APPROVED HEALTH CLAIMS WITH AN EXAMPLE OF LABEL STATEMENT
Nutritional Requirements for Claims	*Example of Label Statement*

Dietary Fat and Cancer
The food must meet the criteria for "low-fat."

Development of cancer depends on many factors. A diet low in total fat may reduce the risk of some cancers.

Saturated Fat/Cholesterol and Heart Disease
The food must meet the criteria for "low-fat," "low saturated fat," and "low cholesterol."

Although many factors affect heart disease, diets low in saturated fat and cholesterol may reduce the risk of this disease.

Calcium and Osteoporosis
The food must meet the criteria for "high in calcium."
The calcium in the product must be bioavailable.
The food shall not contain more phosphorus than calcium on a weight basis.

(For foods containing more than 40% recommended dietary intake of calcium, special requirements exist.)

Regular exercise and a healthy diet with enough calcium helps teens and young adults and white and Asian women maintain good bone health and may reduce their high risk of osteoporosis later in life.

Fiber-Containing Grain Products, Fruits, Vegetables, and Cancer
The claim is limited to foods that are or that contain a fruit, vegetable, or grain product.
The food must meet the criteria for "low-fat" and "good source of fiber."

Low-fat diets rich in fiber-containing grain products, fruits, and vegetables may reduce the risk of some types of cancer, which is associated with many factors.

Fruit and Vegetables and Cancer
The claim is limited to foods that are or that contain a fruit or vegetable.
The food must meet the criteria for "low-fat."
The food must meet the criteria for "good source" of vitamins A or C or dietary fiber (prior to fortification).

Low-fat diets rich in fruits and vegetables (foods that are low in fat and may contain dietary fiber, vitamins A and C) may reduce the risk of some types of cancer, which is associated with many factors.

Folate and Neural Tube Defects
The food must meet the criteria for a "good source of folic acid."

Healthful diets with adequate folate may reduce a woman's risk of having a child with a brain or spinal cord birth defect.

Dietary Sugar and Dental Caries
The food must meet the criteria for "sugar-free."
Sugar alcohol in the food must be a xylitol, sorbitol, mannitol, maltitol, isomalt, lactitol, hydrogenated starch hydrolysates, hydrogenated glucose syrups, or a combination of these.

Frequent between-meal consumption of foods high in sugars and starches promotes tooth decay. The sugar alcohols in [name of food] do not promote tooth decay.

Oats and Psyllium and Heart Disease
The food must meet the criteria for "low-fat," "saturated fat," and "low-cholesterol."
The food must contain at least 0.75 g of soluble fiber from beta glucan or 7 g of soluble fiber from *psyllium* (prior to fortification)

[#] grams of soluble fiber daily from [source of soluble fiber] such as [name of product] as part of a diet low in saturated fat and cholesterol, may reduce the risk of heart disease. [Name of product] provides [#] grams per [#] cup.

Soy Protein and Heart Disease
The food must meet the criteria for "low fat," "saturated fat" and "low-cholesterol."
The food must contain at least 6.25 g of soy protein.

Diets low in saturated fat and cholesterol that include 25 g of soy protein may reduce the risk of heart disease. A serving of [name of food] provides [#] g of soy protein.

Whole Grains and Heart Disease and Cancer
Whole grain must contain all portions of the kernel: bran, germ, and endosperm.
The food must contain at least 51% whole-grain ingredients by weight.
The food must meet the criteria for "low-fat"

Low-fat diets rich in whole-grain foods and other plant foods may reduce the risk of heart disease and certain cancers.

Potassium and High Blood Pressure
The food must meet criteria for "good source of potassium" and "low in sodium."

Diets containing foods that are good sources of potassium and low in sodium may reduce the risk of high blood pressure and stroke.

CASE STUDY/PERSONAL HEALTH AND EXERCISE NUTRITION 9–2

Nutritional Quagmire— The Devil Is in the Details

In 1991, one in eight Americans was obese. In 1999, the number had skyrocketed to one in five. The meteoric rise of obesity has not been overlooked by the $115 billion fast-food industry. Powerful and influential fast-food chains have added new entries in what they tout in their advertising as more healthful and nutritious foods. Millions of people are looking to upgrade their food choices in the hope of trimming their waistlines and improving their health. The following case study of a 24-year-old male fitness enthusiast (Frank) shows the difficulty in balancing daily exercise with sound nutritional choices.

The fitness consultant at Frank's health club often told clients to eat "well" and carefully plan their daily meals. He advocated eating a wide variety of fruits, vegetables, and salads. He also recommended specific fast-food eateries that now offered more nutritious meal choices.

Frank took the "expert's" advice to heart; he visited McDonald's, Arby's, Taco Bell, Wendy's, and Jack in the Box to scout out their new offerings. He then surfed their web sites or read their promotional literature to determine the nutritional content of selected "healthy" foods on their menus (Table 1). He listed the cost of the item, the total calories, and the fat content. He also calculated the percentage of fat in the item. Frank was surprised that although the ingredients in the different foods seemed like "healthy" ingredients, the devil is in the details. Check out the separate ingredients for each of the food selections—then assess the accompanying factual information in the table.

THOUGHT QUESTIONS

1. Why do you think Frank was surprised at the results?
2. What practical conclusion can you draw about the listing of apparently healthy food items and the nutritional analysis of the food product?
3. What advice should Frank give to others like him about the latest efforts of fast-food chains to promote more "healthful" choices?
4. What strategies are available to general consumers and individuals like Frank concerning food advertising and the rising prevalence of obesity in the United States.

Table 1   COMPARISON OF NUTRITIONAL INFORMATION FOR MORE "HEALTHY" CHOICES FROM FIVE FAST-FOOD CHAINS

Food Selection	Ingredients	Cost	kcal	Fat (g)	Fat (%)
McDonald's Grilled Chicken California Cobb Salad	White-meat chicken chunks, mixed greens, shaved carrots, blue cheese, chopped egg, grape tomatoes, and bacon bits; includes packet of Newman's Own Cobb dressing	$3.99	400	23	51.8
Arby's Philly Beef Supreme Sandwich	Baguette, mayonnaise, roasted red and green bell peppers and onions, Swiss-style cheese, and shaved roast beef	$5.99	730	40	49.3
Taco Bell Southwestern Steak Bowl	Refried beans, green onions, rice, grilled beef, tomato and yellow and white cheeses, topped with creamy jalapeno sauce	$3.49	700	32	41.1
Wendy's Mandarin Chicken Salad	Diced white-meat chicken, mixed greens and Mandarin orange slices; includes packets of sliced almonds, rice noodles, and Oriental sesame dressing	$3.99	630	35	50
Jack in the Box Turkey Jack Sandwich	Turkey patty, cheese, lettuce, tomatoes, red onion, pickles, ketchup, and mayo–onion sauce on toasted sesame bun	$3.39	700	32	41.4

To calculate % fat, multiply fat (g) × 9, then divide by total calories. Example for McDonald's Grilled Chicken California Cobb Salad: 23 g × 9 = 207 calories from fat; 207 ÷ 400 × 100 = 51.8%.

Table 9.3   **READING BETWEEN THE LINES: (A) COMPARISON OF THE PERCENTAGE OF TOTAL CALORIES FROM LIPID IN FIVE GRANOLA CEREALS (ONE LOW-FAT) WITH WHEATIES AND CHEERIOS AND (B) MACRONUTRIENT CONTENT AS WEIGHT AND PERCENTAGE OF TOTAL CALORIES IN ONE LARGE SERVING OF MCDONALD'S FRENCH FRIES**

A. Granola Cereals: Source of Hidden Fat

Type	Total kcal	Lipid (g)	kcal from Lipid (lipid, g·9)	% kcal from Lipid
Erewhon Honey Almond	130	6.0	54.0	41.5
Good Morning Pecan Splendor	130	6.0	54.0	41.5
Quaker 100% Natural	130	5.0	45.0	34.6
Homemade with nuts, raisins	138	7.7	69.0	50.0
Kellogg's Low-Fat	120	2.0	18.0	15.0
Wheaties	99	0.5	4.5	4.5
Cheerios	110	1.8	14.7	15.0

B. Food Weight versus Number of Calories (Food: McDonald's french fries, large; weight: 122.3 g [4.3 oz])

Nutrient	Weight (g)	Kcal	% of Weight	% of kcal
Protein	6	24	4.9	6.0
Carbohydrate	45.9	183.6	37.5	45.7
Lipid	21.6	194.4	17.7	48.3
Ash	3.2	0	2.6	0
Water	45.6	0		0
Total	122.3	402	100	100

Conversion factors: protein and carbohydrate, 4 kcal per g; lipid, 9 kcal per g
Source of nutrient information: McDonald's Nutrition Information Center, McDonald's Corporation, Oak Brook, IL 60521

content. For example, most regular granola-type cereals contain a variety of nutritious whole grains; but they also contain considerable fat (Table 9.3A). Similarly, the number of fat grams in McDonald's French fries represents only 17.7% of the food's weight, but the percentage of total calories as fat jumps to 48.3% (Table 9.3B) Thus, fat contributes the largest percentage of this serving's 402 kcal. This occurs in spite of McDonald's commendable decision to replace the

trans fatty acid component of the fries with a less harmful form of unsaturated fatty acid.

Learn to Read Food Labels

To illustrate the importance of understanding the components of a food label, TABLE 9.4 compares four popular products from the Hershey Foods company for protein,

Table 9.4   **CONSUMER BEWARE. LEARN TO INTERPRET THE NUTRITIONAL LABEL TO DETERMINE THE PERCENTAGE OF A PARTICULAR NUTRIENT IN RELATION TO A FOOD'S TOTAL ENERGY CONTENT**

Item	Amount	Total kcal	Protein (g)	Protein % kcal[a]	Carbohydrate (g)	Carbohydrate % kcal[a]	Lipid (g)	Lipid % kcal[a]
Hershey's Chocolate milk (2% low fat)	1 cup (8 oz)	190	8	16.8	29	61.0	5	23.7
Hershey's Chocolate Kisses	9 pieces (1.5 oz)	220	3	5.5	23	41.8	13	53.0
Hershey's Reese's Peanut Butter Cup	2 cups (1.8 oz)	280	6	8.6	26	37.1	17	54.6
Hershey's New Trail Granola Snack Bars, chocolate covered cocoa crème	1.3 oz	190	2	4.2	24	50.5	9	42.6

Data from Nutrition Information for Consumers. Hershey Foods, Consumer Relations Department, P.O. Box 815, Hershey, PA 17033-0815. The percentage values were computed from the nutrient information listed in the table provided by Hershey's; data on percentages were not included as part of their table.
[a] This column, which represents the percentage of total calories for each of the macronutrients, was not provided by the manufacturer. To compute the percentage contribution of a particular nutrient, multiply the caloric value for the nutrient (protein and carbohydrate = 4 kcal/g; lipid = 9 kcal/g) times the number of grams. Express the value in relation to the total number of calories. For example, to compute the percentage of lipid in Hershey's Chocolate Kisses (last column), multiply 9 (kcal/g) × 13 (number of grams) to obtain 117 kcal. Then (117 ÷ 220) × 100 = 53%, which is the percentage of total calories supplied by lipid!

carbohydrate, and lipid content. The comparison includes the caloric value (kcal) and amount (g) of the nutrient, information provided by the manufacturer. Reading the table's footnote easily uncovers the percentage of a nutrient in relation to the product's total caloric content (not provided by the manufacturer). In Hershey's nutrition brochure widely distributed to consumers, a common question concerning their chocolate products states: "How many calories does a Hershey's Miniature Bar contain?" The manufacturer's answer: "There are 40 calories in a Hershey's Miniature Bar. This same calorie count applies for all the Hershey's Miniature Bars—Milk Chocolate, Special Dark, Mr. Goodbar, and Krackel." The brochure fails to reveal that the chocolate bars contain approximately 50% lipid, whether they are small or large size! A consumer does not need the skills of Sherlock Holmes to revel in such discoveries. This applies to any food; just perform the same computations as done for the chocolate products listed in Table 9.4.

NUTRIENT DENSITY

Determining a food's **nutrient density** provides useful information about its nutritional quality. Nutrient density refers to the quantity of a specific nutrient (protein, vitamins, and minerals) per 100 g of the food or per 1000 kcal of that food. In essence, comparing foods for nutrient density conveniently determines the better food source for a particular nutrient. Computing a food's **Index of Nutritional Quality (INQ)** makes this practical. Usually, the numerator of the INQ refers to the nutrient amount per 100 g of food divided by the RDA for that nutrient. The denominator represents the number of kcal per 100 g divided by the population average for energy intake (3000 kcal for men and 2000 kcal for women). An INQ greater than 1.0 means the food provides an adequate source of that nutrient; an INQ less than 1.0 indicates an inadequate nutritional source. For convenience in classification, a food considered "good" has an INQ between 2 and 6, while an INQ above 6 denotes an excellent source of the nutrient.

> INQ = (Amount of nutrient per 100 g ÷ RDA for that nutrient) ÷ (kcal in 100 g ÷ Population average for energy intake)

Let's determine which food provides the best source of protein: whole milk, 1 and 2% low-fat milk, a raw egg, regular vanilla ice cream, chocolate chip cookies, or a McDonald's Big Mac hamburger. The calculations apply to an adult male (age 25–50) with an average daily energy intake of 3000 kcal.

First, refer to Appendix A for the protein content for 100 g (3.52 oz) of each of the six foods. The following example illustrates how to compute the INQ for protein in one raw egg:

Step 1. Compute the amount of protein in 100 g of egg. Appendix A presents the values in 1 oz, or 28.4 g. Since there is 3.52 g of protein per 28.4 g (0.124 per gram of egg), 100 g of egg yields 12.4 g of protein.

Step 2. Divide the step 1 result by 63 g (protein RDA for adult males, age 25–50); 12.4 g ÷ 63 g = 0.197.

Step 3. Compute the number of calories in 100 g of egg. Because 1 oz yields 40 (1.41 calories per g of egg), then 100 g of egg yields 141 calories.

Step 4. Divide the step 3 result by 3000 (energy expenditure for average adult male): 141 calories ÷ 3000 calories = 0.047.

Step 5. Divide the step 2 result by the step 4 result to obtain the INQ for the protein in egg: 0.197 ÷ 0.047 = 4.2.

The other food items have the following protein INQ values: whole milk, 2.67; 2% milk, 3.24; 1% low-fat milk, 3.75; chocolate chip cookies, 0.61; Big Mac, 0.525. The inescapable conclusion: the egg ranks first and 1% low-fat milk second as best protein sources per quantity of food compared with the other food items.

A food's excellent INQ rating for a single nutrient does not reflect an equivalent rating for other nutrients. No single food ranks excellent for all of its nutrients. *In essence, no perfect food exists; some foods are just more nutritious than others per amount of a particular nutrient consumed.*

WHAT AMERICANS EAT

The panels in FIGURE 9.2 display patterns of eating in the United States over a 20-year period for red meat, fish, and poultry; whole, low-fat, and nonfat milk; eggs; fats and oils from animal and vegetable sources; and refined sugars, corn sweeteners, honey, and low-calorie sweeteners. For some classes of foods, the scorecard on a health basis rates as improved; most other items have a considerable way to go. For example, beef, mostly as hamburger, still maintains a prime position on the menus of American restaurants. Still, this popularity has failed to stem the decline in beef consumption. Twenty years ago, Americans consumed about 77 lb of beef per person and 51 lb of chicken, whereas in 2001 this figure changed to 66 lb of beef and 76 lb of chicken.

The meaningful trends in the data summarize as follows:

- An inverse relation exists between red meat consumption and consumption of poultry and fish. On a yearly per person basis over the 20-year period, Americans now consume 8.2 kg less red meat, 13.2 kg more poultry, and about 1 kg more fish and shellfish. The relatively small increase in fish consumption may relate to fear of contamination. Unlike red meat and poultry, seafood does not require federal inspection. The United States ranks twenty-seventh in fish and shellfish consumption among 45 other countries surveyed by the Food and Agricultural Organization of the United Nations. For example, the per capita yearly fish intake in Japan (86.2 kg) and Iceland (180.5 kg) far exceeded that in the United States (16.6 kg).

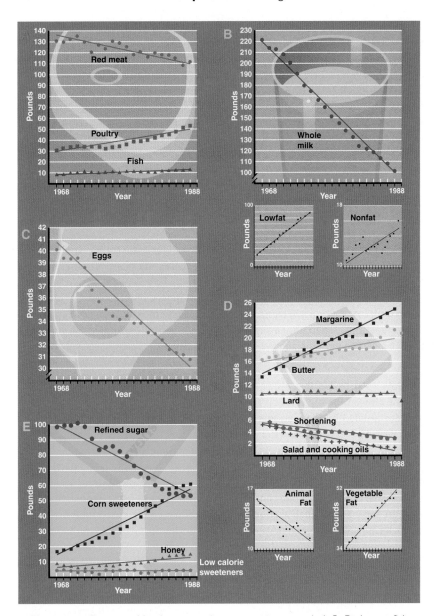

■ **Figure 9.2** Patterns of food consumption over a 20-year period. **A.** Red meat, fish, and poultry. **B.** Whole, lowfat, and nonfat milk. **C.** Eggs. **D.** Fats and oils from animal and vegetables. **E.** Refined sugars, corn sweeteners, honey, and low-calorie sweeteners. (Data from Putnam JJ. Food consumption, prices, and expenditures, 1967–1988. Unites States Department of Agriculture. Commodity Economics Division. Economic Research Service. statistical bulletin no. 804. Washington, D.C., May 1990.)

- A marked increase occurred in drinking low-fat and nonfat milk compared with whole milk. This represents a 54% decline in consumption of whole milk and more than a 300% increase in low-fat and skim milk consumption (from 18.6 kg to 56.2 kg per person) over the study period.
- Americans consume fewer eggs purchased in shells (285 per capita in 1968 vs. 184 in 1990), but eggs consumed in products such as pasta have correspondingly increased by 40.6% (14.5 kg in 1968 vs. 20.5 kg in 1989). The steady decline in shell egg consumption

relates to media attention concerning dietary cholesterol and its link to coronary heart disease.
- Since 1968, fat and oil consumption increased 19.5% from 23.1 kg to 27.6 kg per person yearly. The 4.77 ratio of vegetable to animal fats consumed in 1989 (22.9 kg ÷ 4.8 kg) averaged tenfold higher than the 0.475 ratio in 1968 (7.45 kg ÷ 15.7 kg). Animal fat accounted for 17% of total lipid intake in 1989, compared with 32% in 1968. Vegetable fat and oil represented 68% of total lipid consumption in 1968, compared with 83% in 1989. The shift from

animal to vegetable sources of lipids reflects the consumer's health preference for reduced cholesterol and increased intake of unsaturated rather than saturated fatty acids. Of potential concern is the increase in total lipid consumption from (a) a greater intake of fried foods from various food outlets, particularly fast-food restaurants, and (b) the increased consumption of salad oils. Salad and cooking oil use has doubled, and shortening use has increased by one third, yet decreases occurred for whole-lard shortening, butter, and margarine. Of the total 6.6 billion kg of oils consumed in 1988, 4% (250 million kg) consisted of the highly saturated palm, palm kernel, and coconut tropical oils.

- Per capita yearly consumption of sweeteners increased steadily from 56.8 kg in 1968 to 69.5 kg in 1988. Since 1968, intake of high-fructose corn syrup increased from 0.23 kg to 22.2 kg per person in 1990! The dramatic rise in low-calorie sweeteners reflects the 1981 introduction of aspartame, a sugar substitute almost 200 times sweeter than sucrose.

Findings from a review of eating habits in the United States between 1965 and 1989–1991 reveal that fewer than 25% of the people surveyed followed the eight recommendations for healthful eating formulated by the National Research Council (see Fig. 7.3).[8] This represented the first study to evaluate dietary trends based on economic, racial, and socioeconomic status.

TABLE 9.5 shows the percentage change in dietary patterns over the study period between blacks and whites and the poor and affluent. Contrary to the conventional wisdom in 1965 (and perhaps presently), an apparent convergence exists between blacks and whites and across socioeconomic groups. The wealthier whites in 1965 had the lowest score for a healthful diet, while the poorer blacks consumed a diet rated more healthful, a difference attributed to inability of blacks to afford more "unhealthful" food choices of meat and other foods high in saturated fatty acids. In the 1991 analysis, affluent Americans ate more like their low-income counterparts. A higher percentage of both blacks and whites (the most dramatic gain among the wealthier whites) ate health-promoting diets; they reduced consumption of saturated fats and cholesterol and reduced total fat intake to 35% of total calories (down from 40%). An increase occurred in skim milk or low-fat milk consumption, yet negative trends persisted for both groups for increased intake of "hidden" fats in pizza, tacos, and pasta dishes. Intake of dietary fiber changed little.

Despite positive gains of all groups in nutrient intake, less than 25% of any group met four of the recommendations for dietary improvement. This resulted partly from the sharp increase in consuming packaged and restaurant food—foods high in lipid, saturated fatty acids, salt, and calories and low in fiber.

Thirty-Year Increase in Calorie Intake: More Food and More of It Carbohydrates

A 30-year study by the Centers for Disease Control and Prevention of Americas' eating habits shows that the amount of fat people eat has remained relatively steady while total energy has increased, particularly energy derived from increased carbohydrate intake. FIGURE 9.3 indicates that from 1971 to 2000, women increased caloric intake by 22%, while men increased intake by 7%. While the percentages of calories from fat has remained deceivingly stable over the 30-year period, the amount of fat eaten has actually gone up, because of the steadily rising increase in caloric intake. In 1971, women consumed 1542 kcal on average compared with the year 2000 value of 1887 kcal (+22%), while men increased from 2450 kcal to 2618 kcal (+7%).

Portion Size Distortion

Changing trends in eating behaviors coincide with the current classification by the Centers for Disease Control and Prevention of more than 44 million Americans as obese. Part of this upswing in the body weight relates to the nearly 300% increase between 1977 and 1996 in the proportion of foods that children consume from restaurants and fast-food outlets. Also, soft drink consumption in young consumers currently accounts for an additional 188 kcal per day beyond the energy intake of children that do not consume these beverages.[10] Supersized servings of French fries and sodas are often two to five times larger than when they were first introduced. In 1954 a hamburger at Burger King averaged 2.9 ounces and contained 202 kcal while the 2004 version weighs 4.3 ounces and contains 310 kcal. Likewise, the 1955 McDonald's French fries weighed 2.4 ounces with 210 kcals while in 2004 the weight has increased to 7 ounces with 610 kcal. The 1950s 3-cup version of movie

Table 9.5	PERCENTAGE CHANGES IN HIGH-FAT AND LOW-FAT FOOD CONSUMPTION AMONG AMERICANS OF DIFFERENT RACES AND INCOME LEVELS FROM 1965 TO 1991

	Poorer Respondents		Wealthier Respondents[a]
	Whites	*Blacks*	*Whites*
High fat			
Milk	−92	−66	−99
Cheese	+130	+271	+72
Egg items	−45	−24	−62
Red meat	−71	−89	−89
Low fat			
Milk	+607	+92	+256
Poultry	+77	−26	+157
Noncitrus fruits	−4	−24	−25
Dark green or orange vegetables	+21	+3	+44
Soy products and legumes	0	−24	+156

From Popkin BM, et al. A comparison of dietary trends among the racial and socioeconomic groups in the United States. N Engl J Med 1996;335:716.
[a] Blacks of high socioeconomic status are not listed because of the small number of respondents in the 1965 survey.

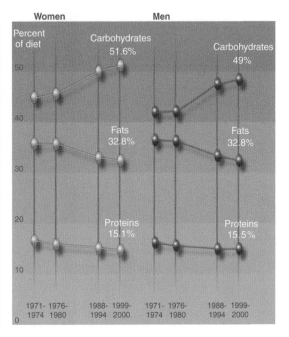

Figure 9.3 Patterns of macronutrient and energy intake of men and women over a 30-year period (Centers for Disease Control and Prevention).

popcorn contained 174 kcal while the contemporary 21-cup buttered version contains 1700 kcal. Americans do not just supersize their portions in fast-food restaurants but they are doing it in their own kitchens. FIGURE 9.4 shows the progressive increase in portion size of such foods as hamburgers, burritos, tacos, French fries, sodas, ice cream, pie, cookies, and salty snacks between 1970s and the 1990s, regardless of whether people ate out or at home.[6] The size of hamburgers made at home increased from 5.7 oz in 1977 to 8.4 oz in 1996. Over the same time, fast food hamburgers increased from 6.1 to 7.2 oz. For Mexican food, a person consumed an average of 408 calories in one sitting in 1977 compared with 541 calories in 1996. Entrée size increase has also affected eating behaviors of preschool children. The large, fixed size of these portions may constitute an "obesigenic" environmental influence that contributes to excessive caloric intake at meals.[3] The U.S. Department of Agriculture considers 2 to 3 oz of cooked lean meat a serving and suggests consuming between 1600 and 2800 kcal per day, depending on a person's age, gender, and physical activity level. These findings point up the need to evaluate not just what we eat but also the size of the portions we eat when assessing and modifying energy intake.

Increases in portion size and fat content of typical dietary items have not been limited to the United States. For example, on June 9, 2003, the British Medical Association proposed a 17.5% "fat-tax" on high-fat foods (e.g., biscuits and processed meats) to combat obesity-related problems, which cost the National Health Service approximately 500 million pounds ($825 million in U.S. currency) a year. Ex-

cess weight has reached epidemic proportions in Britain, where one in five men and one in four women classify as obese. The Australian Medical Association is also considering such a fat tax as one of several fat-fighting ideas for consideration by the country's health ministers.

ACTIVE PEOPLE ON THE GO—EATING AT FAST-FOOD RESTAURANTS

Athletes and other physically active men and women who follow prudent guidelines for food consumption still must choose from a plethora of foods. Like the typical person, these individuals endure a continual stream of advertising to lure them to consume a particular brand of food, or to "take a break" and eat at a favorite restaurant. Many athletes eat their meals at sport-specific "training tables" during the competitive season. However, the off season and summer months provide a unique challenge to maintain an optimal food intake that minimizes total fat intake and emphasizes unrefined complex carbohydrates, while ensuring adequate vitamins and minerals from the main food groups.

An occasional trip to a fast-food eatery may temporarily disrupt the recommended intake of higher-carbohydrate, lower-fat foods. On the other hand, regular visits to franchise establishments can wreak havoc on consuming the recommended nutrients from the major food groups. Many physically active individuals often stray from planned nutritional regimens. Attending parties, going out to dinner with friends, and "hanging out" often include eating foods that provide nonnutritious or "empty" calories, high in saturated fatty acids.

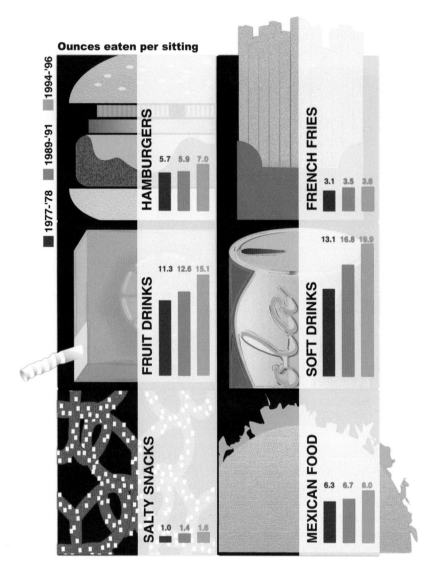

Ounces eaten per sitting

1977-'78 | 1989-'91 | 1994-'96

HAMBURGERS 5.7 5.9 7.0

FRENCH FRIES 3.1 3.5 3.8

FRUIT DRINKS 11.3 12.6 15.1

SOFT DRINKS 13.1 16.8 19.9

SALTY SNACKS 1.0 1.4 1.6

MEXICAN FOOD 6.3 6.7 8.0

■ **Figure 9.4** Portion size distortion. Trends in the portion size, shown as ounces consumed per sitting, of some common foods that Americans eat.

Ethnic Sources for Poor Nutrition

The nongovernmental, watchdog organization, Center for Science in the Public Interest (CSPI; http://www.cspinet. org), publishes information about a variety of food–health related topics including analyses of menu items from different ethnic eateries. Consider the nutritional consequences of eating at Chinese and Mexican restaurants. For the analysis of typical foods from Chinese restaurants, CSPI bought dinner-size takeout portions of 15 popular dishes from 20 midpriced Chinese restaurants in Washington, D.C., Chicago, and San Francisco. For the Mexican dishes, they purchased takeout portions of 15 popular appetizers and main dishes at 19 midpriced Mexican restaurants (including large and medium-sized chains, e.g., Chi-Chi's, El Torito, Chevys, El Chico) in Chicago, Dallas, San Francisco, and Washington, D.C. The CSPI constructed a "composite" from nine samples of each dish (e.g., equal portions of nine restaurants' chicken tacos were mixed together). An independent laboratory analyzed the food for total calories, lipid, saturated fat, cholesterol, and sodium. TABLE 9.6 provides examples of the lipid content of typical Chinese and Italian food, including appetizers, entrees, and side dishes from noted theme restaurants (Chili's, T.G.I. Friday's, Bennigan's, Hard Rock Cafe, and Planet Hollywood). The high fat content of such popular food items should serve as a beacon that the nutritional quality of many foods at popular ethnic and chain restaurants remains a nutritional quagmire. Consult Appendix A to compare the lipid content of foods in Table 9.6 with the lipid content of foods at 11 popular fast-food restaurants.

The following conclusions from the CSPI food analyses illustrate that "eating out" regularly at ethnic restaurants does not qualify as more healthful eating than eating at popular fast-food restaurants such as Arby's, Burger King, Kentucky Fried Chicken, McDonald's, Taco Bell, Roy Rogers, or Wendy's.

- The average Chinese dinner contains more sodium than the daily requirement. It also has 70% of a

Table 9.6 LIPID CONTENT OF FOODS FROM CHINESE AND ITALIAN EATERIES AND APPETIZERS, MAIN DISHES, AND SIDE DISHES AT POPULAR "THEME" (CHAIN) RESTAURANTS

Food	Total Calories	Lipid (g)	Lipid (kcal)	Lipid (%)
Chinese [a]				
Kung pao chicken	1275	75	675	53
Egg roll	190	75	99	52
Moo shu pork	1220	64	576	47
Sweet & sour pork	1635	71	639	39
Beef with broccoli	1180	46	414	35
General Tso's chicken	1607	59	531	33
Orange (crispy) beef	1798	66	594	33
Hot and sour soup	109	4	36	32
House lo mein	1048	36	324	31
House fried rice	1498	50	450	30
Chicken chow mein	1067	32	288	28
Hunan tofu	931	28	252	27
Shrimp with garlic sauce	972	27	243	25
Stir fried vegetables	778	19	171	22
Szechwan shrimp	949	19	171	18
Italian				
Fettucini Alfredo	1505	97	873	58
Lasagna	954	53	477	50
Cheese manicotti	697	38	342	49
Eggplant parmigiana	1212	62	558	46
Cheese ravioli	615	26	234	38
Veal parmigiana	1070	44	396	37
Spaghetti with sausage	1025	39	351	34
Chicken marsala with side of spaghetti	1155	39	351	30
Spaghetti with meatballs	1170	39	351	30
Spaghetti with meat sauce	900	25	225	25
Linguini with red clam sauce	899	23	207	23
Spaghetti with tomato sauce	850	17	153	18
Olive Garden (Italian chain restaurant)				
Garlic bread, 8 oz	818	40	360	44
Fried calamari	1032	70	630	61
Antipasto (assorted meats, cheeses, marinated vegetables, dressings, tomato, lettuce)	631	47	423	67
Hot artichoke spinach dip with garlic crisps	266	15	135	51
Bread sticks & dipping sauce, 1 stick	116	2.6	23	20
Chicken giardino	484	11	99	20
Capellini primavera	281	4.7	42	15
Appetizers				
Chili, 1 cup	350	16	144	41
Buffalo wings, 12 pieces (13 oz)	700	48	432	62
Fried mozzarella sticks, 9 pieces (8 oz)	830	51	459	55
Stuffed potato skins, 8 pieces (12 oz)	1120	79	711	64
Entrée & side dishes				
Grilled chicken, 6 oz	270	8	72	27
with baked potato + 1 Tbsp sour cream + 1 cup vegetable	640	14	126	20
with loaded potato + 1 cup vegetable	950	42	378	40
Sirloin steak, 7 oz	410	20	180	44
with baked potato + 1 Tbsp sour cream + 1 cup vegetable	780	26	234	30
with 2 cups french fries + 1 cup vegetable	1060	54	486	46
with loaded baked potato + 1 cup vegetable	1090	54	486	45
Chicken Caesar salad with dressing	660	46	414	63
Bacon & cheese grilled chicken sandwich	650	30	270	42
with 2 cups French fries	1230	61	549	45
with 11 onion rings	1550	94	846	55

(continues)

Table 9.6 **LIPID CONTENT OF FOODS FROM CHINESE AND ITALIAN EATERIES AND APPETIZERS, MAIN DISHES, AND SIDE DISHES AT POPULAR "THEME" (CHAIN) RESTAURANTS** *(continued)*

Food	Total Calories	Lipid (g)	Lipid (kcal)	Lipid (%)
Steak fajitas with 4 tortillas	860	31	279	32
with guacamole, sour cream, pico de gallo, diced cheese	1190	63	567	48
Chicken fajitas with 4 tortillas	840	24	216	26
Oriental chicken salad with dressing	750	49	441	59
Chicken fingers, 5 pieces (9 oz)	620	34	306	49
with 2 cups French fries + 1 cup cole slaw + 4 Tbsp dressing	1640	106	954	58
Hamburger with trimmings	660	36	324	49
with 2 cups French fries	1240	67	603	49
with 11 onion rings	1550	101	909	59
BBQ baby back ribs, 14 ribs (16 oz)	770	54	486	63
Fudge brownie sundae (10 oz)	1130	57	513	45
Philly cheese steak sandwich (6 inch)	680	35	315	46
with 2 cups French fries	1270	66	594	47
Chicken pot pie	680	37	333	49
Turkey club sandwich (13 oz)	740	34	306	41
Subway steak & cheese sub (6 inch)	370	13	117	32
Lobster, shrimp, scallop pasta	536	23	207	39

a Food portions without rice.

day's lipid, 80% of a day's cholesterol, and almost one-half day's saturated fatty acid recommendation.

- An order of lo mein contains as much salt as a whole Pizza Hut cheese pizza.
- An order of kung pao chicken (52% lipid) contains as much lipid as four McDonald's Quarter Pounders.
- An order of beef and cheese nachos contains the lipid in 10 glazed doughnuts from Dunkin' Donuts.
- A chicken burrito dinner yields one day's worth of sodium.
- A chile relleno dinner contains as much saturated fatty acid as 27 slices of bacon.
- An oriental chicken salad contains more fat than a foot-long Subway cold-cut sub washed down with a Dunkin' Donuts Bavarian Kreme donut.
- Nine fried mozzarella sticks contain as much lipid as one-half stick of butter (1/4 cup or 4 tablespoons).

Beware of Theater Popcorn. In addition to revelations about the high lipid content of popular foods at ethnic restaurants, the CSPI in 1994 evaluated the lipid content of movie theater popcorn. Popcorn samples came from 12 theaters from six chains in San Francisco, Chicago, and Washington, D.C. The CSPI combined the popcorn into three "composites" (coconut oil, coconut oil with topping, and canola shortening) for analysis by an independent laboratory for total calories from lipid, including artery-clogging saturated fatty acids. The results for popcorn's lipid content were as revealing as for Chinese and Mexican foods and in some cases worse.

Without adding butter, a large popcorn contained 80 g of lipid (720 kcal from using hydrogenated soybean oil, canola oil, or coconut oil-based fats during popping). More than 450 kcal (50 g) of these calories came from saturated fatty acids—the equivalent saturated fatty acid content of six McDonald's Big Macs! Buttering the popcorn boosted the

total lipid content 50 more grams to 130 g or a whopping 1170 lipid kcal, equivalent to the saturated fatty acid content in eight McDonald's Big Macs (or the 4-day limit for the recommended amount of saturated fatty acids in the diet).

What can one do to avoid such high-fat "treats?" Become an activist consumer. Let theater managers know you want them to do the following: *(a)* Substitute liquid corn oil (it contains minimal saturated fatty acids and no harmful *trans* fatty acids) for hydrogenated and partially hydrogenated oils and shortenings. *(b)* Switch to air-popped popcorn, which eliminates any oil in the preparation and reduces total lipid content by over 95%! If the theater cannot switch, make your own popcorn and bring it with you. Also, making popcorn without salt spares an additional 300 to 700 mg of salt per bag.

Ice Cream Is Also in the Crosshair. Even the most cherished of American staples, ice cream, has not escaped the close scrutiny of CSPI's calorie sleuths (http://www.cspinet.org/new/200307231.html). Some of CSPI's findings—published in the July/August 2003 issue of its *Nutrition Action Healthletter*—include

- **Ben & Jerry's** *empty Waffle Cone Dipped in Chocolate* has 320 kcal and a half-day's worth of saturated fat—the equivalent of a half-pound rack of BBQ baby back ribs. Fill it with a regular scoop of Chunky Monkey Ice Cream and the cone becomes worse (820 kcal and 30 g of saturated fat) than a full 1-lb rack of ribs.
- **Cold Stone Creamery's** *regular Mud Pie Mojo*—a mixture of coffee ice cream, roasted almonds, fudge, Oreos, peanut butter, and whipped topping—is the equivalent of two Pizza Hut Personal Pan Pepperoni Pizzas (1180 kcal and 26 g saturated fat).
- **Häagen-Dazs'** *Mint Chip Dazzler* is a portable sundae with three scoops of mint chip ice cream, hot

fudge, Oreos, chocolate sprinkles, and whipped cream. Nutritionally, it's like eating a T-bone steak, Caesar salad, and a baked potato with sour cream (1270 kcal and 38 g saturated fat).

Summary

1. The past 55 years have witnessed a tremendous increase in public awareness of the health benefits of good nutrition. Concurrently, advertisers have linked many food products to health maintenance and enhancement. However, new regulations from the Food and Drug Administration (FDA) under the aegis of the United States Department of Agriculture's (USDA) Food Safety and Inspection Service now require manufacturers to adhere to guidelines when linking a nutrient(s) to medical or health benefits.

2. Four governmental agencies create the rules, regulations, and legal requirements concerning advertising, packaging, and labeling of foods and alcoholic beverages.

3. The Federal Trade Commission (FTC) regulates food product advertising in various media (TV, radio, and newsprint) and pursues legal action against manufacturers who advertise unsubstantiated claims or deceptive ads.

4. The FDA regulates *(a)* what manufacturers state on food labels, *(b)* safety of cosmetics, medicines, medical devices, feed and drugs for pets and farm animals, and *(c)* what additives manufacturers can add to foods, including potential hazards with food additives (contaminants), food-borne infections, toxicants, artificially constituted foods, and pesticide residues.

5. The USDA deals with farm and foreign agricultural services, food, nutrition and consumer services, food safety, marketing and regulatory programs, natural resources and environment, research, education, economics, marketing and regulatory programs, and rural development.

6. The Bureau of Alcohol, Tobacco and Firearms enforces federal laws and regulations relating to alcohol, tobacco, firearms, explosives, and arson.

7. Prior to 1990, the law did not require manufactures (and their advertising agencies) to adhere to rules and regulations to describe foods. The Nutrition Labeling and Education Act (NLEA) of 1990 (including 1993–1998 updates to the regulations) now requires food manufactures to strictly comply to regulations about what can and cannot be printed on food labels.

8. The format for the nutrition panel on foods must declare the nutrient content per serving as percentages of the Daily Values—the new label reference values.

9. The new "% Daily Value" comprises two sets of dietary standards: Daily Reference Values (DRVs) and Reference Daily Intakes (RDIs).

10. DRVs established for macronutrients include sources of energy (lipid, carbohydrate [including fiber], and protein) and non-calorie contributors (cholesterol, sodium and potassium).

11. The RDI replaces the term "U.S. RDA." The new RDIs remain the same as the old U.S. RDAs.

12. Food labels must indicate the amount of a particular nutrient, but no requirement exists to list its relative percentage in a food. Consequently, a food may be advertised as "low fat" (absolute quantity) when, in reality, its percentage of fat might exceed 50%! The NLEA requires manufacturers to list on the food label the percentage of fat in relation to the DRV for total calorie intake for most food items.

13. A manufacturer wishing to include an additive in a food must follow specific FDA guidelines to ensure the additive's effectiveness (i.e., it meet its claims). A list of additives that are generally recognized as safe (GRAS) currently includes about 2000 flavoring agents and 200 coloring agents.

14. Many factors influence the amount, type, and quality of food consumed by a particular group or individual in the group. These include level of income and education, racial and ethnic background, and geographic locale and personal interests.

15. Significant changes have occurred in patterns of food consumption over the past 35 years. Partly this reflects heightened public awareness of the relationship between diet and health. Unfortunately, increased reliance on "eating out" at restaurants has a negative impact on nutrition quality.

16. The nongovernmental watchdog organization, Center for Science in the Public Interest, raises public awareness about the nutritional content of favorite foods and meals, often with alarming results about high fat content (particularly saturated fat) and excessive calorie content.

TEST YOUR KNOWLEDGE **ANSWERS**

1. False The Food and Drug Administration (FDA) is not required to provide adequate scientific data to support claims for food or chemicals classified as dietary supplements. They only intervene when a supplement causes documented injury or illness. Consequently, consumers must remain continually aware of advertising hype in the various media that promote the health and fitness benefits of products. Far too few "watchdog" organizations and adequately staffed and funded governmental agencies exist to patrol overzealous promoters whose products often pledge longer life, improved bodily functions, and instant cure for every possible ailment and misfortune.

2. True The Federal Trade Commission (FTC) regulates food product advertising in various media (TV, radio, newsprint) and pursues legal action against manufacturers who advertise unsubstantiated claims or deceptive ads. The FTC has authority to remove a product from the marketplace if the product's claims cannot be verified.

3. False The FDA stands for Food and Drug Administration. This federal agency represents one of 13 agencies within the Department of Health and Human Services (DHHS). With the exception of poultry and meat products, the FDA regulates what manufacturers state on food labels and the safety of cosmetics, medicines, medical devices, and feed and drugs for pets and farm animals. The FDA also decides what additives manufacturers can add to foods, including potential hazards with food additives (contaminants), food-borne infections, toxicants, artificially constituted foods, and pesticide residues.

4. False The marketing of dietary supplements requires no government approval because supplements are considered foods and not drugs. In contrast to medicine, which must meet many safety and efficacy requirements before coming to market, legislation places the burden on the FDA to prove that a supplement is harmful before it can be removed from the market. Supplement marketing can progress with only the manufacturer's assurance of safety as long as the supplement does not claim disease-fighting benefits.

5. True New rules in 1997 require supplements to be labeled as dietary supplements (e.g., "Vitamin C Dietary Supplement") and to carry a "Supplement Facts" panel with information similar to the "Nutrition Facts" panel that appears on most processed foods. Included on the facts panel must be an appropriate serving size; information on 14 nutrients, including sodium, vitamin A, vitamin C, calcium and iron, when present at significant levels; other vitamins and minerals if added or part of a nutritional claim on the label; dietary ingredients with no established Reference Daily Intakes; if the product contains a proprietary blend of ingredients the total amount of the blend and the identity of each dietary ingredient in the blend (although amounts of individual ingredients in the blend are not required). The rules also require that the labels of products containing botanical ingredients identify the part of the plant used.

6. True The Bureau of Alcohol, Tobacco and Firearms (ATF) is a law enforcement organization within the United States Department of Treasury. It came into existence in 1972 after separating from the Internal Revenue Service (Alcohol, Tobacco and Firearms Division). The ATF has responsibilities dedicated to reducing violent crime, collecting revenue, and protecting the public. It enforces the federal laws and regulations relating to alcohol, tobacco, firearms, explosives, and arson.

7. False A daily intake of 2000 kcal serves as the reference number of calories for determining Daily Reference Values for the energy-producing nutrients. The 2000-kcal level was chosen, in part, because it approximates the caloric requirements for postmenopausal women, the group with the highest risk for excessive intake of calories and fat.

8. False A "healthy" food must be low in fat and saturated fat and contain limited amounts of cholesterol and sodium. In addition, a single-item food must provide at least 10% of one or more of vitamins A or C, iron, calcium, protein, or fiber. A meal-type product, such as frozen entrees and multicourse frozen dinners, must provide 10% of two or three of these vitamins or minerals or of protein or fiber in addition to meeting the other criteria. Sodium content must be less than 360 mg per serving for individual foods and 480 mg per serving for meal-type products that carry the "healthy" claim.

9. False Nutrient density refers to the quantity of a specific nutrient (protein, vitamins, and minerals) per 100 g of the food, or per 1000 kcal of that food. In essence, comparing foods for nutrient density conveniently determines the better food source for a particular nutrient. Computing a food's Index of Nutritional Quality (INQ) makes this practical. Usually, the numerator of the INQ refers to the nutrient amount per 100 g of food divided by the RDA for that nutrient. The denominator represents the number of kcal per 100 g divided by the population average for energy intake (3000 kcal for men and 2000 kcal for women). For convenience in classification, a food considered "good" has an INQ between 2 and 6, while an INQ above 6 denotes an excellent source of the nutrient.

10. False Significant trends have taken place in eating behaviors. For example, Americans are not just supersizing their portions in fast-food restaurants but also in their own kitchens. A progressive increase has occurred in portion size of hamburgers, burritos, tacos, French fries, sodas, ice cream, pie, cookies, and salty snacks between 1970s and the 1990s, regardless of whether people ate out or at home. The size of hamburgers made at home increased from 5.7 oz in 1977 to 8.4 oz in 1996. Over the same time, fast-food hamburgers increased from 6.1 oz to 7.2 oz. Entrée size increase also has affected the eating behaviors of preschool children. The large, fixed size of these portions may constitute an "obesigenic" environmental influence that contributes to excessive caloric intake at meals.

References

1. Angell M, Kassirer JP. Alternative medicine—the risks of untested and unregulated remedies. N Engl J Med 1998;339:831.
2. Caspersen CJ, et al. Changes in physical activity patterns in the United States, by sex and cross-sectional age. Med Sci Sports Exerc 2000;32:1601.
3. Fisher JO, et al. Children's bite size and intake of an entrée are greater with large portions than with age-appropriate or self-selected portions. Am J Clin Nutr 2003;77:1164.
4. Green GA, et al. Analysis of over-the-counter dietary supplements. Clin J Sports Med 2001;11:254.
5. Kamber M, et al. Nutritional supplements as a source for positive doping cases? Int J Sport Nutr Exerc Metab 2001;11:258.
6. Nielsen SJ, Popkin BM. Patterns and trends in food portion sizes, 1977-1998. JAMA 2003;289:450.
7. Physical activity trends—United States, 1990-1998. MMWR 2001;March 9:166.
8. Popkin BM, et al. A comparison of dietary trends among racial and socioeconomic groups in the United States. N Engl J Med 1996;335:716.
9. Sarubin A. Government regulation of dietary supplements. Chapter 1 in The health professional's guide to dietary supplements, Chicago: The American Dietetic Association, 1999.
10. U.S. Department of Health and Human Services. Healthy people 2000 midcourse review and 1995 revisions. Washington, DC: U.S. Government Printing Office, 1996.

Additional Readings

Burton A. Fewer colds with increased Vitamin E intake. Lancet Infect Dis 2004;4:600.

Conway JM, et al. Commercial portion-controlled foods in research studies: How accurate are label weights? J Am Diet Assoc 2004;104:1420.

Eigenmann PA, Haenggeli CA. Food colourings and preservatives—allergy and hyperactivity. Lancet 2004;364:823.

Jacobson MF. High-fructose corn syrup and the obesity epidemic. Am J Clin Nutr 2004;80:1081.

Mehlman MJ, Binstock RH, Juengst ET, Ponsaran RS, Whitehouse PJ. Anti-aging medicine: can consumers be better protected? Gerontologist 2004;44:304.

Leary TB. The ongoing dialogue between the Food and Drug Administration and the Federal Trade Commission. Food Drug Law J 2004;59:209.

Licence K. Promoting and protecting the health of children and young people. Child Care Health Dev 2004;30:623.

Lin CT, et al. Do dietary intakes affect search for nutrient information on food labels? Soc Sci Med 2004;59:1955.

Macon JF, et al. Food label use by older Americans: Data from the Continuing Survey of Food Intakes by Individuals and the Diet and Health Knowledge Survey 1994-1996. J Nutr Elder 2004;24:35.

Perls TT. Anti-aging quackery: Human growth hormone and tricks of the trade—more dangerous than ever. J Gerontol A Biol Sci Med Sci 2004;59:682.

Roefs A, Jansen A. The effect of information about fat content on food consumption in overweight/obese and lean people. Appetite 2004;43:319.

Sitzman K. Expanding food portions contribute to overweight and obesity. AAOHN J 2004;52:356.

Vos E. Nuts, omega-3s and food labels. CMAJ 2004;171:829.

Section IV
Thermoregulation and Fluid Balance During Heat Stress

Outline

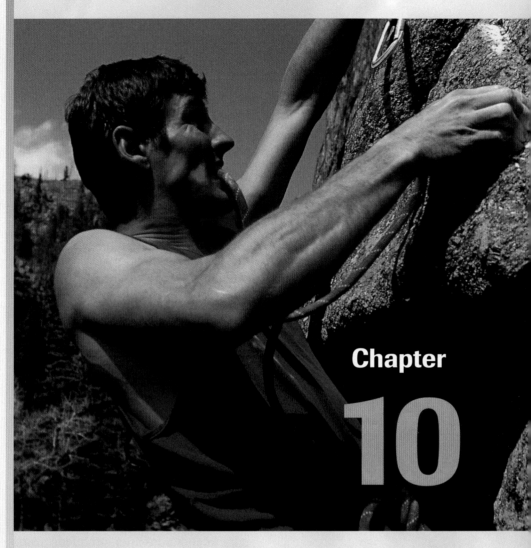

Chapter

10

Exercise Thermoregulation, Fluid Balance, and Rehydration

TEST YOUR KNOWLEDGE

Answer these ten statements about exercise thermoregulation, fluid balance, and rehydration during heat stress. Use the scoring key at the end of the chapter to check your results. Repeat this test after you have read the chapter and compare your results.

1. **T F** Core body temperature remains stable despite significant changes in environmental temperature.

2. **T F** The hypothalamus contains the central coordinating center for temperature regulation.

3. **T F** The body loses heat primarily via the physical mechanism of radiation.

4. **T F** Relative humidity refers to how dry the environment becomes in the warm weather.

5. **T F** ADH is a major heat conserving hormone.

6. **T F** Exercising while dehydrated significantly increases the risk for heat injury.

7. **T F** The thirst mechanism provides a precise gauge to replenish water lost during exercise.

8. **T F** You can never consume too much water.

9. **T F** Air temperature primarily determines the potential physiologic strain produced by environmental heat.

10. **T F** Oral temperature provides the most rapid and reliable estimate of core temperature after strenuous exercise.

The requirements for thermoregulation are considerable—the price of failure is death. A person can tolerate a drop in deep body temperature of 10°C but an increase of only 5°C. The latter condition of **hyperthermia** occurred more than 100 times over the past 25 years in football players who died from excessive heat stress during practice or competition. Hyperthermia and dehydration were linked to the deaths of three collegiate wrestlers in the latter part of 1997. Heat injury also commonly occurs during military operations and longer-duration athletic events. Athletes who illegally use erythropoietin, a hormone that boosts production of red blood cells, experience an even greater risk of heat injury. Their increased blood viscosity from increased hematocrit magnifies as dehydration progresses while exercising in the heat.

The decision to hold the 1996 Summer Olympics in Atlanta (average summer temperature between 21 and 31°C, relative humidity between 50 and 90%) refocused interest in temperature regulation during exercise. Particular emphasis was placed on understanding *(a)* the challenges from environmental heat and humidity on the exercising individual and *(b)* the appropriate means of diminishing the adverse effects of heat stress on participants and spectators. Knowledge of thermoregulation and the most effective ways to support its mechanisms significantly reduces heat-related tragedies. Coaches, athletes, race and event organizers, and those who provide overall nutritional advice must use strategies based on factors that contribute to heat gain and dehydration during exercise in a hot environment. Concern also must focus on the most effective behavioral approaches (e.g., prudent scheduling of events, acclimatization, proper clothing, and fluid and electrolyte replacement before, during, and after exercise) to blunt the potential for negative effects on performance and safety. Water becomes the most important performance-enhancing nutrient when exercise and heat stress combine. The exercise nutritionist must apply knowledge of the basic physics and physiology of thermoregulation to defend effectively against the potentially lethal challenge of heat stress.

➤ Mechanisms of Thermoregulation

THERMAL BALANCE

FIGURE 10.1 shows body temperature (more specifically, the temperature of the deeper tissues or **core**) in dynamic equilibrium between factors that add and subtract body heat. This balance results from integrating mechanisms that:

- Alter heat transfer to the periphery **(shell)**
- Regulate evaporative cooling
- Vary the rate of heat production

Core temperature rises quickly when heat gain exceeds heat loss during vigorous exercise in a warm environment.

TABLE 10.1 presents thermal data for heat production (oxygen consumption) and heat loss from sweating at rest and during maximal exercise. The body gains considerable heat from the reactions of energy metabolism, particularly from active muscle. From shivering alone, the total metabolic rate increases three- to fivefold. During sustained exercise by aerobically fit men and women, metabolic rate often increases 20 to 25 times above the resting level to 20 kcal·min^{-1}; heat production of this magnitude could theoretically increase core temperature 1°C (1.8°F) every 5 to 7 minutes! The body also absorbs heat from the environment by solar radiation and from objects warmer than the body. Heat loss occurs by the physical mechanisms of radiation, conduction, and convection. However, water vaporization (evaporation) from the skin and respiratory passages provides the most important avenue for heat loss. Evaporative cooling under optimal conditions accounts for a heat loss of about 18 kcal·min^{-1}.

Circulatory adjustments provide "fine tuning" for temperature regulation. Heat conservation occurs by rapidly shunting blood deep to the cranial, thoracic, and abdominal cavities and portions of the muscle mass. This optimizes insulation from subcutaneous fat and other areas of the body's shell. Conversely, excessive internal heat buildup dilates peripheral vessels that channel warm blood

Figure 10.1 Factors that contribute to heat gain and heat loss to regulate core temperature at about 37°C.

to the cooler periphery. During exercise in the heat, the strong drive for thermal balance can increase sweat rate to as high as 3.5 L·h^{-1}.

HYPOTHALAMIC REGULATION OF CORE TEMPERATURE

*The **hypothalamus** contains the central coordinating center for temperature regulation.* This group of specialized neurons at the floor of the brain serves as a "thermostat" (usually set and carefully regulated at 37°C ± 1°C) that makes thermoregulatory adjustments to deviations from a temperature norm. Unlike a thermostat in a building, however, the hypothalamus cannot "turn off" the heat; it only initiates responses to protect the body from heat gain or heat loss.

Table 10.1 THERMODYNAMICS AT REST AND DURING EXERCISE		
Body's heat production	**Rest**	**Maximal exercise**
(1 L O$_2$ uptake = ~4.82 kcal)	~0.25 L O$_2$·min^{-1}	~4.0 L O$_2$·min^{-1}
	~1.2 kcal·min^{-1}	~20.0 kcal·min^{-1}
Body's capacity for evaporative cooling		**Maximal sweating**
(Each 1 mL sweat evaporation = ~0.6 kcal body heat loss)		30 mL·min^{-1} = ~18 kcal · min^{-1}
Core temperature increase	No increase	~1°C every 5–7 min

Heat-regulating mechanisms become activated in two ways:

1. Temperature changes in blood perfusing the hypothalamus directly stimulate this thermoregulatory control center.
2. Thermal receptors in the skin provide input to modulate hypothalamic activity.

THERMOREGULATION IN HEAT STRESS: HEAT LOSS

The body's thermoregulatory mechanisms primarily protect against overheating. Defense against a rise in core temperature becomes particularly crucial during exercise in hot weather. Here, competition exists between mechanisms that maintain a large muscle blood flow to deliver oxygen and nutrients and remove waste products and mechanisms that provide for adequate regulation of body temperature. FIGURE 10.2 illustrates the potential avenues for heat exchange in an exercising human. Body heat loss occurs in four ways: *(a)* **radiation**, *(b)* **conduction**, *(c)* **convection**, and *(d)* **evaporation**.

Heat Loss by Radiation

Objects continually emit electromagnetic heat waves. Because our bodies are usually warmer than the environment, the net exchange of radiant heat energy occurs from the body through the air to solid, cooler objects around us. This form of heat transfer, similar to how the sun's rays warm the earth, does not require molecular contact between objects. Despite subfreezing temperatures, a person can remain warm by absorbing sufficient radiant heat energy from direct sunlight (or reflected from the snow, sand, or water). The body absorbs radiant heat energy when the temperature of objects in the environment exceeds skin temperature.

Heat Loss by Conduction

Heat loss by conduction transfers heat directly through a liquid, solid, or gas from one molecule to another. The circulation transports most of the body heat to the shell, but a small amount continually moves by conduction directly through the deep tissues to the cooler surface. Conductive heat loss then involves the warming of air molecules and cooler surfaces in contact with the skin.

The rate of conductive heat loss depends on the temperature gradient between the skin and surrounding surfaces and their thermal qualities. Warm-weather hikers gain considerable heat from their physical activity and the environment. Some relief comes from lying on a cool rock shielded from the sun. Conductance between the rock's cold surface and the hiker's warmer surface facilitates favorable loss of body heat.

Heat Loss by Convection

The effectiveness of heat loss by conduction via air depends on how rapidly air near the body exchanges once it warms. With little or no air movement or convection, the warmed air

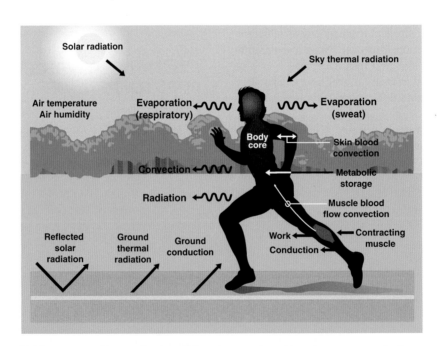

■ **Figure 10.2** Heat production within active muscle and its subsequent transfer from the core to the skin. Under appropriate environmental conditions, excess body heat dissipates to the environment and core temperature stabilizes within a narrow range. (From Gisolfi CV, Wenger CB. Temperature regulation during exercise: old concepts, new ideas. Exerc Sport Sci Rev 1984;12:339.)

next to the skin acts as a zone of insulation, minimizing further conductive heat loss. Conversely, if cooler air continuously replaces the warmer air surrounding the body (as occurs on a breezy day, in a room with a fan, or during running), heat loss increases because convective currents carry the heat away. For example, air currents at 4 miles per hour cool twice as effectively as air moving at 1 mile per hour.

Heat Loss by Evaporation

Evaporation of sweat provides the major physiologic defense against overheating. Water vaporization from the respiratory passages and skin surface continually transfers heat to the environment. Each liter of water that vaporizes transfers 580 kcal of heat energy from the body to the environment.

In response to heat stress, 2 to 4 million sweat (eccrine) glands secrete large quantities of hypotonic saline solution (0.2–0.4% NaCl). Cooling occurs when sweat evaporates from the skin surface. The cooled skin then cools blood shunted from the interior to the surface. Along with heat loss through sweating, approximately 350 mL of water seeps through the skin (called *insensible perspiration*) each day and evaporates to the environment. Also, approximately 300 mL of water vaporizes daily from the respiratory passages' moist mucous membranes. In cold weather, this source of evaporation appears as "foggy breath."

Evaporative Heat Loss at High Ambient Temperatures

Increased ambient temperature reduces the effectiveness of heat loss by conduction, convection, and radiation. When ambient temperature exceeds body temperature, these three mechanisms of thermal transfer actually contribute to heat gain. When this occurs (or when conduction, convection, and radiation cannot adequately dissipate a large metabolic heat load), sweat evaporation from the skin and water vaporization from the respiratory tract provide the only avenue to dissipate heat. Sweating rate increases directly with ambient temperature. For someone relaxing in a hot, humid environment, the normal 2-L daily fluid requirement doubles or even triples from evaporative fluid loss.

Heat Loss in High Humidity

Figure 10.3 illustrates the influence of exercise intensity and environmental conditions on sweating rate. Sweat evaporation from the skin depends on three factors: *(a)* surface exposed to the environment, *(b)* temperature and relative humidity of ambient air, and *(c)* convective air currents around the body. *By far, relative humidity exerts the greatest impact on the effectiveness of evaporative heat loss.*

Relative humidity refers to the percentage of water in ambient air at a particular temperature compared with the total quantity of moisture that the air could carry. For example, 40% relative humidity means that ambient air con-

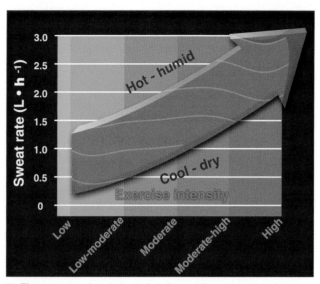

Figure 10.3 Approximate hourly sweating rates related to environmental conditions and exercise intensity.

tains only 40% of the air's moisture-carrying capacity at that specific temperature. With high humidity, ambient air's vapor pressure approaches that of the moist skin (approximately 40 mm Hg). Consequently, evaporative heat loss becomes thwarted, even though a large quantity of sweat beads on the skin and eventually rolls off. This represents a useless water loss that can lead to dehydration and overheating.

Continually drying the skin with a towel before sweat evaporates also thwarts evaporative cooling. *Sweat does not cool the skin; rather, skin cooling occurs only when sweat evaporates.* One can tolerate relatively high environmental temperatures as long as humidity remains low. For this reason, people prefer the comfort of hot, dry desert climates to "cooler" but more humid tropical climates.

Integration of Heat-Dissipating Mechanisms

Circulation

The circulatory system serves as the "workhorse" to maintain thermal balance. At rest in hot weather, heart rate and blood flow from the heart (cardiac output) increase while superficial arterial and venous blood vessels dilate to divert warm blood to the body's shell. This manifests as a flushed or reddened face on a hot day or during vigorous exercise. With extreme heat stress, 15 to 25% of the cardiac output passes through the skin, greatly increasing the thermal conductance of peripheral tissues. Increased peripheral blood flow favors radiative heat loss, particularly from the hands, forehead, forearms, ears, and tibial area of the lower legs.

Evaporation

Sweating begins within several seconds of the start of vigorous exercise and, after about 30 minutes, reaches equilibrium directly related to exercise load. A large cutaneous blood flow coupled with evaporative cooling generally produces an effective thermal defense. The cooled peripheral blood then returns to the deeper tissues and picks up additional heat as it returns to the heart.

Hormonal Adjustments

Heat stress initiates hormonal adjustments to conserve the loss of salts and fluid in sweat. During heat exposure, the pituitary gland releases **antidiuretic hormone (ADH)**. ADH increases water reabsorption from the kidney tubules, causing urine to become more concentrated. Concurrently, during a single bout of exercise or with repeated days of exercise in hot weather, the adrenal cortex releases the sodium-conserving hormone **aldosterone**, which increases the renal tubules' reabsorption of sodium. Aldosterone also decreases sodium concentration in sweat (i.e., reduces sweat osmolality); this aids in additional electrolyte conservation.

EFFECTS OF CLOTHING ON THERMOREGULATION IN THE HEAT

Different materials absorb water at different rates. Cottons and linens readily absorb moisture. In contrast, heavy "sweat shirts" and rubber or plastic garments produce high relative humidity close to the skin and retard the vaporization of moisture. This significantly inhibits or even prevents evaporative cooling. Moisture-wicking fabrics (e.g., polypropylene, Coolmax, Drylite) worn close to the skin provide optimal transfer of heat and moisture from the skin to the environment, particularly during high-intensity exercise in hot weather. These fabrics wick moisture away from the skin. They offer great benefits during exercise in cold environments because dry clothing (in contrast to sweat-drenched clothing) greatly reduces the risk for hypothermia. Color also plays an important role; dark colors absorb light rays and add to radiant heat gain, whereas clothing of lighter color reflects heat rays away from the body.

Football Uniforms

Football uniforms and equipment present a significant barrier to heat dissipation during environmental heat exposure.[27] Even with loose-fitting porous jerseys, the wrappings, padding (with plastic covering), helmet, and other objects of "armor" effectively seal off 50% of the body's surface from the benefits of evaporative cooling. Just wearing the 6 to 7 kg of football equipment significantly increases the metabolic load, not to mention the thermal challenge from a hot artificial playing surface and the body heat-retaining qualities of the equipment. The large body size of these athletes further magnifies the heat load, particularly for offensive and defensive linemen. They possess a relatively small body surface area-to-body

mass ratio and a higher percentage of body fat than players at other positions.

The Modern Cycling Helmet Does Not Thwart Heat Dissipation

Wearing a commercial cycling helmet provides considerable protection against possible head injury, but does the helmet impede thermoregulatory processes in a hot–dry or hot–humid environment? Because the head provides an important avenue for heat loss during exercise,[34] many competitive cyclists believe that not wearing a helmet reduces thermal strain and physical discomfort. This belief persists even though the design of current commercial helmets remains aerodynamic and lightweight, with ventilation ports for convective and evaporative cooling. To evaluate the physiologic and perceptual responses to wearing a helmet, male and female competitive cyclists pedaled for 90 minutes at 60% peak oxygen uptake in both hot–dry (35°C, 20% relative humidity) and hot–humid (35°C, 70% relative humidity) environments with and without a protective helmet.[39] Measurements included oxygen uptake, heart rate, core, skin, and head skin temperatures, rating of perceived exertion, and perceived thermal sensations of the head and body. Results showed that exercising in a hot–humid environment produced significantly greater thermal stress, yet wearing the helmet during exercise did not increase the riders' level of heat strain or perceived heat sensation of the head or body.

Summary

1. Humans tolerate relatively small variations in internal (core) temperature. Consequently, exposure to heat or cold initiates thermoregulatory mechanisms that generate and conserve heat at low ambient temperatures and dissipate heat at high temperatures.

2. The hypothalamus serves as the "thermostat" for temperature regulation. This coordination center initiates adjustments from thermal receptors in the skin and changes in hypothalamic blood temperature.

3. Warm blood diverts from the body's core to the shell in response to heat stress. Heat loss occurs by radiation, conduction, convection, and evaporation. Evaporation provides the major physiologic defense against overheating at high ambient temperatures and during exercise.

4. Warm, humid environments dramatically decrease the effectiveness of evaporative heat loss. This increases one's vulnerability to a dangerous state of dehydration and spiraling core temperature.

5. The ideal warm-weather clothing consists of lightweight, loose-fitting, and light-color clothes. Moisture-wicking fabrics against the skin optimize heat and moisture transfer from the skin to the environment.

6. Football uniforms impose a significant barrier to heat dissipation because they effectively seal off about 50% of the body's surface from the benefits of evaporative cooling. They also add to the metabolic load imposed by exercise.

7. During exercise in hot–humid environments, the modern cycling helmet does not increase the level of heat strain or perceived heat sensation of the head or body above that with the no-helmet condition.

➤ Thermoregulation During Exercise in the Heat

Cardiovascular adjustments and evaporative cooling dissipate metabolic heat during exercise, particularly in hot weather. A tradeoff occurs, because the fluid lost in thermoregulation often creates a relative state of dehydration. Excessive sweating leads to more serious fluid loss with accompanying reductions in plasma volume. This end result produces circulatory failure, and core temperature rises to lethal levels. During near-maximal exercise in the heat, with accompanying dehydration, relatively less blood diverts to peripheral areas for heat dissipation. Reduced peripheral blood flow reflects the body's attempt to maintain cardiac output despite a diminishing plasma volume caused by sweating.

CORE TEMPERATURE DURING EXERCISE

Heat generated by active muscles can raise core temperature to fever levels that incapacitate a person if caused by external heat stress alone. However, champion distance runners show no ill effects from rectal temperatures as high as 41°C (105.8°F) recorded at the end of a 3-mile race.[19] Within limits, an increased core temperature with exercise does not reflect a failure of heat-dissipating mechanisms. To the contrary, a well-regulated rise in core temperature occurs even during exercise in the cold. *More than likely, a modest rise in core temperature reflects a favorable internal adjustment that creates an optimal thermal environment for physiologic and metabolic functions.*

WATER LOSS IN THE HEAT: DEHYDRATION

Dehydration refers to an imbalance in fluid dynamics when fluid intake does not replenish water loss from either hyperhydrated or normally hydrated states. A moderate exercise workout generally produces a moderate 0.5 to 1.5 L sweat loss over a 1-hour period. Significant water loss occurs during several hours of heavy exercise in a hot environment. Even with exercise performed in less challenging thermal environments (e.g., swimming and cross-country skiing), significant sweating occurs. For the swimmer, immersion in water per se stimulates body water loss through cold-induced increased urine production. Non-exercise-induced water loss also occurs when power athletes (wrestlers, boxers, weight lifters, and rowers) aggressively attempt to "make weight" through rapid weight loss induced by common dehydration techniques (e.g., heat exposure via sauna, steam room, hot whirlpool or shower; fluid and food restriction; diuretic and laxative drugs; or vomiting). These individuals often combine techniques, hoping to achieve even faster weight loss.

Intracellular and extracellular compartments contribute to the fluid deficit (dehydration), which can rapidly reach levels that impede heat dissipation, reduce heat tolerance, and severely compromise cardiovascular function and exercise capacity. *The risk of heat illness greatly increases when a person begins exercising in a dehydrated state.* Dehydration associated with a 3% decrease in body weight also slows gastric emptying rate, thus increasing epigastric cramps and feelings of nausea.[47] Thus, avoiding dehydration not only optimizes exercise performance but also reduces the feelings of gastrointestinal discomfort associated with body fluid loss. Because sweat is hypotonic with other body fluids, the reduced plasma volume caused by sweating correspondingly increases blood plasma osmolality.

In a practical sense, rapid weight loss through dehydration does not impair maximal exercise performance of short durations up to 60 seconds. When exercise exceeds 1 minute, dehydration profoundly impairs physiologic function and compromises optimal ability to train and compete.

Magnitude of Fluid Loss

Water loss by sweating in an acclimatized person peaks at about 3 L per hour during intense exercise in the heat and averages nearly 12 L (26 lb) on a daily basis. Several hours of intense sweating can cause sweat-gland fatigue, which ultimately impairs core temperature regulation. Elite marathon runners frequently experience fluid losses in excess of 5 L during competition; this represents between 6 and 10% of body mass. For slower-paced marathons or ultramarathons, average fluid loss rarely exceeds 500 mL per hour.[31] Even in a temperate climate, an average fluid loss of 2 L takes place in soccer players during a 90-minute game played at about 10°C (50°F).[23]

A large sweat output and subsequent fluid loss occurs in sports other than distance running; football, basketball, and hockey players also lose large quantities of fluid during a contest. High school wrestlers often lose 9 to 13% of their preseason body mass before certification. The greatest portion of this weight loss comes from voluntary water restriction and excessive sweating before weigh-in. Collegiate wrestlers, excluding heavyweights who have no weight restriction, regain an average of 3.7 kg (8.1 lb) during the 20-hour period between weigh-in and competition.[38] This means that high school and collegiate wrestlers usually compete in a dehydrated state in their desire to "make weight."

Significant Physiologic Consequences

Just about any degree of dehydration impairs the capacity of circulatory and temperature-regulating mechanisms to adjust to exercise demands. As dehydration progresses and plasma volume decreases, peripheral blood flow and sweating rate diminish and thermoregulation becomes progressively more difficult. Cumulatively, this contributes to larger increases in heart rate, perception of effort, and core temperature, and premature fatigue than under normal hydration. A fluid loss of only 1% of body mass increases rectal temperature above that with the same exercise performed when fully hydrated. Preexercise dehydration equivalent to 5% of body mass (common among high school wrestlers) increases rectal temperature and heart rate during exercise, while decreasing sweating rate, $\dot{V}O_2$max, and exercise capacity compared with values under fully hydrated conditions. The 5 hours available to wrestlers between weigh-in and match time does not adequately ensure complete rehydration and electrolyte balance.

Considerable Fluid Loss in Winter Environments. The risk for dehydration increases during vigorous cold-weather exercise. For one thing, colder air contains less moisture than air at warmer temperature, particularly at higher altitudes. Consequently, greater fluid volumes leave the respiratory passages as the incoming cold, dry air becomes fully humidified and warmed to body temperature. This air-conditioning process can create a 1-L daily fluid loss. Cold stress also increases urine production, which adds to total body fluid loss. Furthermore, many people overdress for outdoor winter activities. As exercise progresses and body heat production increases, heat gain exceeds body heat loss, which initiates sweating. All of these factors become magnified, in that many individuals consider it unimportant to consume fluids before, during, and in recovery from prolonged exercise in cold weather. FIGURE 10.4 illustrates a back-mounted hydration system to provide ready access to water *during* such prolonged winter activities as Nordic or alpine skiing, serious outdoor winter trekking including ice and mountain climbing at high altitudes, or distance cycling or running. In the military, back-mounted hydration systems are often attached to load-bearing equipment. Many different styles and configurations of hydration systems are available at sporting goods or cycling shops and through sports equipment mail-order catalogues.

Diuretic Use

Athletes who use diuretics to lose body water to rapidly "make weight" place themselves at a distinct performance disadvantage because a disproportionate reduction in plasma volume occurs, which negatively affects thermoregulation and cardiovascular function. In addition, Diuretic drugs also can markedly impair neuromuscular function not noted when comparable fluid loss occurs by exercise. Athletes who use vomiting and diarrhea to lose weight not only produce dehydration, but also cause excessive mineral loss with accompanying muscle weakness and impaired neuromuscular function. This clearly gives a competitive "edge" to the opponent—a result entirely opposite that anticipated.

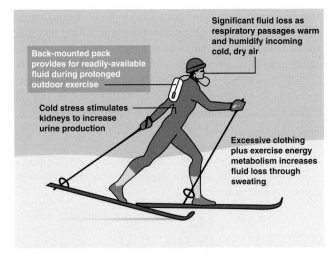

■ **Figure 10.4** Factors that increase the potential for dehydration during cold-weather exercise. The illustration depicts a back-mounted hydration system to provide ready access to water during continuous exercise in the outdoor environment.

CASE STUDY/PERSONAL HEALTH AND EXERCISE NUTRITION 10–1

How To Assess and Upgrade The Lipid Quality of Your Diet

The typical Western diet contains too much total lipid, too much saturated fat, and too much cholesterol. Dietary lipids represent about 36% of total caloric intake, with the average person consuming 15% of total calories as saturated fatty acids. Health professionals recommend that lipid intake should not exceed 30% of the diet's total energy content, and consuming less (about 20%) may confer even greater health benefits. Unsaturated fatty acids should account for at least 70% of the total lipid intake, equally distributed between polyunsaturates and monounsaturates, with cholesterol intake below 300 mg per day.

ESTIMATING THE PERCENTAGE OF TOTAL CALORIES CONSUMED FROM FAT

Based on research correlating food intake from a diary with data from a simple questionnaire it is possible to estimate the percentage of total calories from fat.

CHOOSING AMONG THE DIFFERENT FATS IN YOUR DIET

Lipids (fats) not only provide fuel for energy but also aid in the absorption of fat-soluble vitamins, are an integral part of the plasma membrane, provide for hormone synthesis (steroids), and aid in insulation and protection of vital organs. Most lipids store in adipose tissue for subsequent release into the bloodstream as free fatty acids (FFAs), which. broadly classify as monounsaturated, polyunsaturated, and saturated. Each exerts different effects on cholesterol and lipoprotein deposition in arteries and subsequent coronary heart disease risk.

CHOOSING THE PROPER DIETARY FAT

Table 1 shows the available food choices for different types of lipids based on how they affect total cholesterol and the different lipoprotein fractions.

CASE STUDY/PERSONAL HEALTH AND EXERCISE NUTRITION 10–1 (*continued*)

QUESTIONNAIRE

HOW MUCH FAT DO YOU CONSUME? THINK OF YOUR DIET OVER THE PAST 3 MONTHS AND ANSWER THE FOLLOWING QUESTIONS.

Choices: 1 = Usually/always; 2 = Often; 3 = Sometimes; 4 = Rarely/never

1. _____ When I eat bread, rolls, muffins, or crackers, I eat them without butter or margarine.

2. _____ When I eat cooked vegetables, I eat them without butter, margarine, salt pork, or bacon fat.

3. _____ When I eat cooked vegetables, they are cooked by a method other than frying.

4. _____ When I eat potatoes, they are cooked by a method other than frying.

5. _____ When I eat boiled or baked potatoes I eat them without butter, margarine, or sour cream.

6. _____ When I eat green salads, I eat them without dressing.

7. _____ When I eat dessert, I eat it without cream or whipped-cream topping.

8. _____ When I eat spaghetti or noodles, I eat it plain or use a meatless sauce.

9. _____ My main meal for the day is usually meatless.

10. _____ When I eat fish, it is broiled, baked, or poached.

11. _____ When I eat chicken, it is broiled or baked.

12. _____ When I eat chicken, I remove the skin.

13. _____ When I eat red meat, I trim off all visible fat.

14. _____ When I eat ground beef, I choose extra lean.

15. _____ When I drink milk I choose skim or 1% fat milk instead of 2% fat or whole milk.

16. _____ When I eat cheese, it is the reduced fat variety.

17. _____ When I eat a frozen dessert, it is sherbet, ice milk, or nonfat versions of ice cream or yogurt.

18. _____ When I eat green salads with dressing, I use a low-fat or nonfat dressing.

19. _____ When I sauté or pan fry food I use a nonstick spray instead of oil, margarine, or butter.

20. _____ When I use mayonnaise or a mayonnaise-type dressing, I usually use a low-fat or nonfat variety.

21. _____ When I eat dessert, I usually eat fruit.

22. _____ When I eat snacks, I usually eat raw vegetables.

23. _____ When I eat snacks, I usually eat fresh fruit.

SCORING

Total your score and divide by 23

Your average	Percentage kcal from fat
1.0 to <1.5	Less than 25%
1.5 to <2.0	25% to 29%
2.0 to <2.5	30 to 34%
2.5 to <3.0	35 to 39%
3.0 to <3.5	40 to 44%
3.5 to <4.0	45+%

CASE STUDY/PERSONAL HEALTH AND EXERCISE NUTRITION 10-1 (continued)

Table 1   **CHOOSE THE RIGHT FAT FOR YOUR DIET**

Best Choice Monounsaturated Fatty Acids	Good Choice Polyunsaturated Fatty Acids	Occasional Choice Saturated/ Hydrogenated Fatty Acids
Effects on Cholesterol and Lipoproteins		
• Decreases total cholesterol	• Decreases total cholesterol	• Increases total cholesterol
• Decreases LDL-cholesterol	• Decreases LDL-cholesterol	• Increases LDL-cholesterol
• No effect on HDL-cholesterol	• Decreases HDL-cholesterol	• Decreases HDL-cholesterol
Food Examples		
Vegetable oils: avocado, canola, olive, peanut	**Vegetable oils:** corn, safflower, sesame, soybean, sunflower, *trans*-fat-free margarine, mayonnaise, Miracle Whip	**Tropical vegetable oils:** coconut, palm, palm kernel, cocoa butter
		Hydrogenated oils: margarine, shortening
Nuts: acorns, almonds, beechnuts, cashews, chestnuts, hazelnuts, hickory, macadamia, natural peanut butter, peanuts, pecans, pistachios	**Nuts:** Brazil, butternuts, pine, walnuts	**Animal fats:** bacon, beef fat, chicken fat, egg yolk, fatty meats, lamb fat, lard, pepperoni, pork fat, salt pork, sausage, kielbasa
Other: fish fat (omega-3 fatty acids)	**Seeds:** sesame, pumpkin, sunflower	**Dairy products:** butter, cheese (regular, light, low fat), cream cheese, half & half, ice cream, sour cream, whole milk, 2% milk

Hutchinson Cancer Research Center, Seattle, WA. www.shcrc.org

WATER REPLACEMENT: REHYDRATION

Adequate fluid replacement sustains the exceptional potential for evaporative cooling of acclimatized humans. Although glycogen depletion during exercise impairs high-intensity endurance performance, failure to replenish this energy reserve does not impose a risk to health and safety. In contrast, inadequate water replenishment not only impairs exercise capacity but also creates life-threatening disturbances in fluid balance and core temperature. *Properly scheduling fluid replacement maintains plasma volume so circulation and sweating progress optimally.* Strictly following an adequate water replacement schedule prevents dehydration and its consequences, particularly hyperthermia. This replenishment is often "easier said than done" because some coaches and athletes still believe water consumption hinders performance. Left on their own, most individuals voluntarily replace only about one-half of the water lost (less than 500 mL·h^{-1}) during exercise.[30]

For wrestlers, dehydration represents a "way of life" to compete in a lower weight category. This also pertains to ballet dancers and female gymnasts who continually strive to maintain a thin appearance. The enlightened exercise nutritionist must remain vigilant about the key role of hydration in thermoregulation and its impact on exercise performance and safety. The competitive wrestler (and others who dehydrate to compete in a specific weight class) and athletes who engage in more than one event or training session on a given day must optimize fluid replenishment practices.

"Cold treatments"—periodic application of cold towels to the forehead and abdomen during exercise, or taking a cold shower before exercising in a hot environment—do not facilitate heat transfer at the body's surface compared with the same exercise without skin wetting. Adequate hydration provides the most effective defense against heat stress by balancing water loss with water intake, not by pouring water over the head or body. No evidence exists that restricting fluid intake during training prepares a person to perform better in the heat. *A well-hydrated individual always functions at a higher physiologic and performance level than a dehydrated one.*

Preexercise Hydration

Ingesting "extra" water (**hyperhydration**) before exercising in a hot environment protects to some extent against heat stress because it delays dehydration, increases sweating during exercise, and diminishes the rise in core temperature. These outcomes contribute to enhanced exercise performance and the participant's overall safety. In addition to increasing fluid intake 24 hours before strenuous exercise in the heat, we recommend consuming 400 to 600 mL (13–20 oz) of cool water about 20 minutes before such exercise. Preexercise fluid intake increases the stomach's volume, a major factor that optimizes gastric emptying (see Chapter 8). A systematic regimen of hyperhydration (4.5 L fluid per day) 1 week prior to soccer competition by acclimated elite young players in Puerto Rico increased body water reserves (despite greater urine output) and improved temperature regulation during the soccer match in warm weather.[36] This structured sequence of preexercise hyperhydration produced a body fluid volume 1.1 L greater than that produced when the players consumed their normal daily fluid volume of 2.5 L. In Chapter 12, we discuss the role of glycerol supplementation to augment preexercise hyperhydration.

Preexercise hyperhydration does not replace the need to continually replace fluid during exercise. In intense endurance activities in the heat, matching fluid loss with fluid intake often becomes impossible, because only about 1000 mL of fluid each hour empties from the stomach. This volume does not match a sweat loss that averages nearly 2000 mL per hour. Even individuals with unlimited access to water should be carefully monitored during exercise in the heat.

Adequacy of Rehydration

Body weight changes indicate the extent of water loss from exercise and adequacy of rehydration during and after exercise or athletic competition. Voiding small volumes of dark yellow urine with a strong odor provides a qualitative indication of inadequate hydration. Well-hydrated individuals typically produce urine in large volumes, light in color, and without a strong smell. For team athletes, assign each player a squeeze bottle for fluids to emphasize the importance of fluid replacement and to monitor the fluid consumed. TABLE 10.2 recommends fluid intake with weight loss during exercise. Although these standards were developed for a 90-minute football practice, they easily adapt to most exercise situations. Menstrual cycle variations do not adversely affect rehydration.[25]

Coaches often require athletes to weigh-in before and after practice (following urination) to monitor fluid balance; each 1-pound weight loss represents 450 mL (15 fl oz) of dehydration. FIGURE 10.5 gives a practical illustration to determine quantity and rate of fluid loss from exercise. To properly match fluid loss with intake, partition the estimated hourly fluid loss from a workout or competition into 10- or 15-minute periods and ingest that amount of fluid at those intervals. For example, we recommend fluid intake every 15 minutes for hourly losses up to 1000 mL, whereas fluid ingestion at 10-minute intervals optimizes replenishing a fluid loss in excess of 1000 mL per hour. Make water available

---

Table 10.2 RECOMMENDED FLUID AVAILABILITY AND INTAKE FOR A STRENUOUS 90-MINUTE ATHLETIC PRACTICE[a]

Weight Loss		Minutes Between Water Breaks	Fluid per Break		Fluid Availability for an 11-Member Squad	
lb	kg		oz	mL	gal	L
8	3.6	No practice recommended	–	–		
7.5	3.4		–	–		
7	3.2	10	8–10	266	6.5–8	27.4
6.5	3.0	10	8–9	251	6.5–7	25.5
6	2.7	10	8–9	251	6.5–7	25.5
5.5	2.5	15	10–12	325	5.5–6.5	22.7
5	2.3	15	10–11	311	5.5–6	21.8
4.5	2.1	15	9–10	281	5–5.5	19.9
4	1.8	15	8–9	251	4.5–5	18.0
3.5	1.6	20	10–11	311	4–4.5	16.1
3	1.4	20	9–10	281	3.5–4	14.2
2.5	1.1	20	7–8	222	3	11.4
2	0.9	30	8	237	2.5	9.5
1.5	0.7	30	6	177	1.5	5.7
1	0.5	45	6	177	1	3.8
0.5	0.2	60	6	177	0.5	1.9

[a] Based on 80% replacement of weight loss.

Name	Date	Body weight		DBW (A-B)	Drink volume	Urine volume*	Sweat loss C+D-E	Exercise time	Sweat rate
		Before exercise (A)	After exercise (B)						
Mackinzie	9/15								
		61.7 kg	60.3 kg	1400 g	420 mL	90 mL	1730 mL	90 min	19.2 mL·min^{-1}
								1.5 h	1153 mL·h^{-1}

*Weight of urine should be subtracted if urine was excreted prior to postexercise body weight
DBW, difference in body weight
Sweat loss = total fluid loss during exercise
Sweat rate = fluid loss per unit time

Sweat rate		Fluid intake		Rehydration intervals min
mL·h^{-1}	lb·h^{-1}	mL	oz	
500	1.1	125	4	15
750	1.7	190	6.5	15
1000	2.2	250	8.5	15
1500	3.3	250	8.5	10
2000	4.4	330	11	10
2500	5.5	415	14	10
3000	6.6	500	17	10

Figure 10.5 Computing the magnitude of sweat loss and rate of sweating in exercise. In this example, Mackinzie should drink about 1000 mL (32 oz) of fluid during each hour of activity (250 mL every 15 min) to remain well hydrated. (Modified from Gatorade Sports Science Institute, 9:(4 suppl 63), 1996.)

(and consumed) during practice and competition. Urge individuals to rehydrate themselves, because the thirst mechanism imprecisely indicates water needs, particularly in children and the elderly. The elderly generally require longer time to achieve rehydration after dehydration.[20] If rehydration were left entirely to a person's thirst, it could take several days after severe dehydration to reestablish fluid balance. *Drink at least 125 to150% of the existing fluid loss (body weight loss) as soon as possible after exercising. The 25 to 50% "extra" water accounts for that portion of ingested water lost in urine.*[41]

Flavored Drinks Can Help

Consuming highly palatable flavored beverages with added salt facilitates voluntary rehydration in children and adults.[20,22] After exercise, dehydration, and heat exposure, boys voluntarily consumed one of three beverages: *(a)* plain water, *(b)* grape-flavored water, or *(c)* grape-flavored water containing 6% carbohydrate (14 g per 8 oz) and 18 mmol·L^{-1} NaCl (110 mg per 8 oz).[48] The flavored carbohydrate–electrolyte drink elicited the largest total voluntary fluid intake (1157 mL), followed by the flavored drink (1112 mL), with the smallest volume recorded for plain water (610 mL).

Aging Affects Rehydration

Older men and women require particular attention when evaluating rehydration following exercise in the heat. These individuals do not recover from dehydration as effectively as younger adults, probably because of a depressed thirst drive. This increases susceptibility to chronic hypohydration, which creates a suboptimal plasma volume and diminished thermoregulatory capacity.

Sodium Facilitates Rehydration

In Chapter 8, we pointed out that a moderate amount of sodium added to a rehydration beverage provides more complete rehydration than plain water.[35,40] Restoring water and electrolyte balance in recovery occurs most effectively by *(a)* adding moderate to high amounts of sodium (100 mmol·L^{-1}, an amount exceeding that in commercial beverages) to the rehydration drink or *(b)* combining solid food (with appropriate sodium content) with plain water.[22,24,26] In addition, a small amount of potassium (2–5 mmol·L^{-1}) enhances water retention in the intracellular space and may diminish any extra potassium loss that results from sodium retention by the kidneys.[8]

The kidneys continually form urine, so the volume of ingested fluid following exercise should exceed exercise sweat loss by 25 to 50% to restore fluid balance. Unless the beverage has a sufficiently high sodium content, excess fluid intake merely increases urine output with *no benefit* to rehydration.[42] Pure water absorbed from the gut rapidly dilutes plasma sodium concentration. A decrease in plasma osmolality, in turn, stimulates urine production and blunts the normal sodium-dependent stimulation of the thirst mechanism. Maintaining a relatively high plasma concentration of sodium (by adding sodium to ingested fluid) sustains the thirst drive, promotes retention of ingested fluids (less urine output), and more rapidly restores lost plasma volume during rehydration.

FIGURE 10.6 illustrates the effect of adding sodium to a rehydration beverage on retention of ingested fluid in recovery. Six healthy men exercised in a warm, humid environment until sweating produced a 1.9% loss of body mass. They then ingested 2045 mL of one of four test drinks containing sodium in a concentration of either 2, 26, 52, or 100 mmol·L^{-1} over a 30-minute period beginning 30 minutes after exercise stopped. (Typical "sports drinks" contain between 10 and 25 mmol of sodium·L^{-1}; normal plasma sodium concentration ranges between 138 and 142 mmol·L^{-1}.) From the 1.5-hour urine sample onward, urine volume inversely related to the rehydration beverage's sodium content. At the end of the study period, a difference in total body water content of 787 mL existed between trials using drinks with the lowest and highest sodium content. The drink containing sodium at a concentration of 100 mmol·L^{-1} contributed to the greatest fluid retention.

With prolonged exercise in the heat, sweat loss can deplete the body of 13 to 17 g of salt (2.3–3.4 g per L of sweat), about 8 g more than typically consumed daily in the diet. It seems prudent in this situation to replace the lost sodium by adding about one-third teaspoon of table salt to 1 L of water. The ACSM recommends that sports drinks contain 0.5 to 0.7 g of sodium per liter of fluid consumed during exercise lasting more than one hour. Moderate exercise produces negligible losses of potassium in sweat. Even at intense physical activity levels, potassium lost in sweat ranges between 5 and 18 mEq, which poses no immediate danger. One can replace potassium lost with heavy sweating by increasing intake of potassium-rich foods (citrus fruits and bananas). A glass of orange juice or tomato juice replaces almost all the potassium, calcium, and magnesium excreted in 3 L of sweat. Except in unusual cases, minor adjustments in food intake and electrolyte conservation by the kidneys compensate adequately for mineral loss through sweating. TABLE 10.3 gives examples of drinks from five major sports-beverage categories including their carbohydrate and calorie content per 8-ounce serving. Beverages in the recovery drink and energy drink categories most effectively facilitate glycogen replenishment because of their high carbohydrate content.

■ **Figure 10.6** Cumulative urine output during recovery from exercise-induced dehydration. The oral rehydration beverages consisted of four test drinks (equivalent to 1.5 times the body mass loss, or approximately 2045 mL) containing sodium (and matching anion) in a concentration of either 2 (trial A), 26 (trial B), 52 (trial C), or 100 (trial D) mmol·L^{-1}.(From Maughan J, Leiper JB. Sodium intake and post-exercise rehydration in man. Eur J Appl Physiol 1995;71:311.)

| Table 10.3 | HOW THE DRINKS STACK UP. FIVE MAJOR SPORTS DRINK CATEGORIES INCLUDING THEIR CALORIE AND CARBOHYDRATE CONTENT PLUS NUTRITIONAL "EXTRAS" PER 8-OZ SERVING |

	Calories	*Carbohydrate (g)*	*Extras*
Waters			
Tap water	0	0	Minerals—vary by source
Dasani	0	0	Spring source
Fiji	0	0	Artesian source
Penta	0	0	Purified
Fitness waters			
ChampionLyte	0	0	Electrolytes
Life O_2	0	0	10 times O_2 of tap water
Propel	10	3	Electrolytes, vitamins
Reebok	12	3	Electrolytes, vitamins, trace minerals
Sports drinks			
All Sport	70	20	No longer carbonated, vitamins B and C
G-Push (G^2)	70	18	Electrolytes, vitamins
Gatorade	50	14	Electrolytes
GU_2O	50	14	Electrolytes
Powerade	72	19	Electrolytes, vitamins
Simple Sports Drink	80	21	Electrolytes, vitamin C
Recovery drinks			
Endurox R^4	180	35	Electrolytes, vitamins
G-Push (G^4)	110	27	Electrolytes, vitamins, trace minerals
Gatorade Energy Drink	207	41	Vitamins
Energy Drinks			
Red Bull	109	27	Taurine, caffeine, vitamins
SoBe Adrenaline Rush	135	35	Taurine, ribose, caffeine

HYPONATREMIA: REDUCED SODIUM CONCENTRATION IN BODY FLUIDS

Major concerns in hot-weather exercise include the following:

- Dehydration
- Decreased plasma volume and resulting hemoconcentration
- Impaired physical performance and thermoregulatory capacity
- Increased risk of heat injury (especially heat stroke)

The exercise physiology literature contains more than ample information about the need to consume fluid before, during, and after exercise. In many instances the recommended beverage remains plain, hypotonic water. However, we now know that excessive water intake under certain exercise conditions can produce potentially serious medical complications from the syndrome termed **hyponatremia** or "water intoxication." Hyponatremia exists when serum sodium concentration falls below 135 mEq·L^{-1}; a serum sodium concentration below 125 mEq·L^{-1} triggers severe symptoms. A sustained low plasma sodium concentration creates an osmotic imbalance across the blood–brain barrier that causes rapid water influx into the brain. The resulting swelling of brain tissue produces a cascade of symptoms that range from mild (headache, confusion malaise, nausea, cramping) to severe (seizures, coma, pulmonary edema, cardiac arrest, and death).[2,14]

More Prevalent Than Previously Thought

The exercise scenario conducive to the development of hyponatremia involves water overload during continuous high-intensity, ultramarathon-type exercise of 6- to 8-hours duration, particularly in hot weather.[4,5,16,18,29] It can also occur in events lasting less than 4 hours, such as standard marathons.[45] In a large study of more than 18,000 ultraendurance runners (including triathletes), approximately 9% of collapsed individuals presented with symptoms of hyponatremia.[32] The athletes, on average, drank fluids with low sodium chloride content (less than 6.8 mmol·L^{-1}). The runner with the most severe hyponatremia (serum sodium level of 112 mmol·L^{-1}) excreted more than 7.5 L of dilute urine during the first 17 hours of hospitalization.

Researchers monitored changes in body mass and blood sodium concentration in 95 competitors receiving medical care and 169 competitors not requiring care in the 1996 New Zealand Ironman Triathlon (swim 3.8 km, cycle 180 km, run 42 km).[43] For individuals with clinical evidence of fluid or electrolyte disturbance, body mass declined 2.5 kg (−2.9 kg in competitors without medical care). Hyponatremia accounted for 9% of medical abnormalities (identical to that reported above[32]). One person with hyponatremia (Na = 130 mEq·L^{-1}) drank 16 L of fluid over the course of the race, with a weight gain of 2.5 kg (consistent with the hypothesis that fluid overload causes hyponatremia). An inverse relationship existed between postrace sodium concentration and percentage change in body mass; individuals who lost less weight tended to have a higher serum sodium concentration.

In an ultradistance multisport triathlon (kayak 67 km, cycle 148 km, run 23.8 km), body mass declined 2.5 kg or 3% of initial body mass.[44] None of the competitors gained weight, six weighed the same, and one became hyponatremic (serum Na = 134 mEq·L) maintained weight, and did not seek medical attention. Serum sodium concentration for 47 athletes at the end of the race averaged 139.3 mEq·L^{-1}.

Level of acclimatization affects sodium loss. For example, sodium concentration in sweat ranges from 5 to 30 mmol·L^{-1} (115–690 mg·L^{-1}) in individuals fully acclimatized to the heat to 40 to 100 mmol·L^{-1} (920–2300 mg·L^{-1}) in the unacclimatized. In addition, some individuals produce relatively highly concentrated sweat regardless of their degree of acclimatization. *Development of hyponatremia requires extreme sodium loss through prolonged sweating coupled with dilution of existing extracellular sodium (and accompanying reduced osmolality) from consuming large fluid volumes containing low or no sodium* (FIG. 10.7A). A

■ **Figure 10.7 A.** Factors that contribute to the development of hyponatremia. AVP, arginine vasopressin; CFTR, cystic fibrosis transmembrane regulatory gene. **B.** Physiologic consequences of hyponatremia. CNS, central nervous system. (Modified from Montain SJ, et al. Hyponatremia associated with exercise: risk factors and pathogenesis. Exerc Sport Sci Rev 2001;2:113.)

PREDISPOSING FACTORS TO HYPONATREMIA

- Prolonged high-intensity exercise in hot weather
- Large sodium loss associated with sweat containing high sodium concentration; particularly prevalent in relatively unfit individuals
- Beginning physical activity in a sodium-depleted state owing to "salt-free" or "low-sodium" diet
- Use of diuretic medication for hypertension
- Frequent intake of large quantities of sodium-free fluid prior to, during, and after prolonged exercise

reduced extracellular solute concentration promotes movement of water into the cells (Fig. 10.7B). Water movement of sufficient magnitude congests the lungs, swells brain tissue, and adversely affects central nervous system function.

Several hours of exercise in the heat can cause considerable sodium loss. Exercise in hot, humid weather produces a sweat rate of more than 1 L per hour, with a sweat-sodium concentration ranging between 20 and 100 mEq·L^{-1}. Also, frequently ingesting large volumes of plain water draws sodium from the extracellular fluid compartment into the unabsorbed intestinal water, further diluting serum sodium concentration. Exercise compounds the problem because urine production decreases during exercise owing to a significantly reduced renal blood flow. This reduces the body's ability to excrete excess water.

Competitive athletes, recreational participants, and occupational workers should be aware of the dangers of excessive hydration and that fluid intake should not exceed fluid loss. To reduce risk of overhydration and hyponatremia in prolonged exercise, we recommend the following four steps:

1. Two to three hours before exercise drink 400 to 600 mL (14–22 oz) of fluid.
2. Drink 150 to 300 mL (5–10 oz) of fluid about 30 minutes before exercise.
3. Drink no more than 1000 mL·h^{-1} (33 oz) of plain water spread over 15-minute intervals during or after exercise.
4. Add a small amount of sodium (approximately 1/4 to 1/2 teaspoon per 32 oz) to the ingested fluid. Commercial sports drinks are also effective in providing water, carbohydrate fuel, and electrolytes.
5. Do not restrict salt in your diet.

Including some glucose in the rehydration drink facilitates intestinal water uptake via the glucose–sodium transport mechanism (see Chapters 3 and 8).

FACTORS THAT IMPROVE HEAT TOLERANCE

Acclimatization

Relatively moderate exercise performed in cool weather becomes taxing if attempted on the first hot day of spring. The early stages of spring training can present a hazard for heat injury because thermoregulatory mechanisms have not adjusted to the dual challenge of exercise and environmental heat. *Repeated exposure to hot environments, particularly when combined with physical activity, improves capacity for exercise with less discomfort upon heat exposure.*

Heat acclimatization refers to the physiologic adaptations that improve heat tolerance. FIGURE 10.8 shows that the

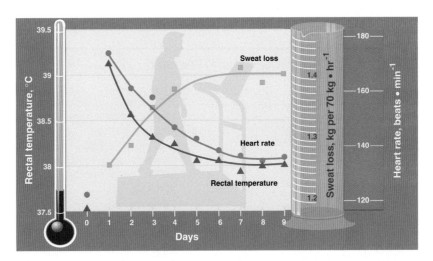

■ **Figure 10.8** Average rectal temperature (▲), heart rate (●), and sweat loss (■) during 100 minutes of daily heat-exercise exposure for 9 consecutive days. On day 0, the men walked on a treadmill at an exercise intensity of 300 kcal·h^{-1} in a cool climate. Thereafter, the same daily exercise took place in the heat at 48.9°C (26.7°F wet bulb). (From Lind R, Bass DE. Optimal exposure time for development of acclimatization to heat. Fed Proc 1963;22:704.)

major acclimatization to heat stress occurs during the first week of heat exposure (2–4 h each day) with essentially complete acclimatization after 10 days. In practical terms, use 15 to 20 minutes of light-intensity exercise during the first several exercise sessions in a hot environment. Thereafter, exercise sessions can increase systematically to reach the normal duration and intensity for training.

Increased Production of a More Dilute Sweat

TABLE 10.4 summarizes the main physiologic adjustments during heat acclimatization. As acclimatization progresses, larger quantities of blood shunt to cutaneous vessels to facilitate heat transfer from the core to the periphery during exercise. More effective cardiac output distribution maintains blood pressure during exercise; a lowered threshold (earlier onset) for sweating complements this cardiovascular acclimatization. An earlier onset of sweating initiates cooling before internal temperature increases too markedly. After 10 days of heat exposure, sweating capacity nearly doubles, and sweat becomes dilute (less salt lost) and more evenly distributed on the skin surface. Increased sweat loss in an acclimatized individual creates a greater need to rehydrate during and following exercise. Adjustments in circulatory function and evaporative cooling enable a heat-acclimatized person to exercise with lower skin and core temperatures and heart rate than an unacclimatized individual. Optimal acclimatization necessitates adequate hydration. Also, one loses the major benefits of heat acclimatization within 2 to 3 weeks upon return to a more temperate climate.

Full Acclimatization Requires Hot-Weather Training

As one might expect, exercise "heat conditioning" in cool weather produces less effective results than acclimatization from similar exercise training in the heat. *Full heat acclimatization cannot take place without exposure to environmental heat stress.* Individuals who train and compete in hot weather show a distinct thermoregulatory advantage over those who train in cooler climates and only periodically compete in hot weather.

Children

Prepubescent children have a greater number of heat-activated sweat glands per unit skin area than adolescents and adults, yet they sweat less and achieve higher core temperatures during heat stress.[6,11] These thermoregulatory differences probably last through puberty but only limit exercise capacity during extreme environmental heat stress.[10] Sweat composition differs between children and adults; adults have higher concentrations of sodium and chloride, but lower lactate, H^+, and potassium concentrations.[11,28] Children also take longer to acclimatize to heat than adolescents and young adults. *From a practical standpoint, children exposed to environmental heat stress should exercise at reduced intensity and receive more time to acclimatize than more mature competitors.*

Male/Female Differences

Early comparisons between men and women showed that men had greater tolerance to environmental heat stress during exercise. However, the research was flawed because women consistently exercised at higher intensities relative to their aerobic capacity. When comparing men and women of equal fitness, the sex differences in thermoregulation became much less pronounced.[15,17] *Generally, women tolerate the physiologic and thermal stress of exercise as well as men of comparable fitness and level of acclimatization; both sexes acclimatize to a similar degree.*[1,46]

Table 10.4 PHYSIOLOGIC ADJUSTMENTS DURING HEAT ACCLIMATIZATION	
Acclimatization Response	*Effect*
• Improved cutaneous blood flow	• Transports metabolic heat from deep tissues to the body's shell
• Effective distribution of cardiac output	• Appropriate circulation to skin and muscles to meet demands of metabolism and thermoregulation; greater stability of blood pressure during exercise
• Lowered threshold for start of sweating	• Evaporative cooling begins early during exercise
• More effective distribution of sweat over skin surface	• Optimum use of effective surface for evaporative cooling
• Increased sweat output	• Maximizes evaporative cooling
• Lowered salt concentration in sweat	• Dilute sweat preserves electrolytes in extracellular fluid
• Lower skin and core temperature and heart rate for standard exercise	• Frees greater portion of cardiac output for distribution to active muscles
• Less reliance on carbohydrate catabolism during exercise	• Carbohydrate-sparing effect

Sweating

A distinct sex difference in thermoregulation exists for sweating. Women possess more heat-activated sweat glands per unit skin area than men, yet they sweat *less* prolifically. Women begin sweating at higher skin and core temperatures; they also produce less sweat for a similar heat–exercise load, even with acclimatization comparable to that of men.

Evaporative Versus Circulatory Cooling

Despite a lower sweat output, women show heat tolerance similar to that of men of equal aerobic fitness at the same exercise level. *Women rely more on circulatory mechanisms for heat dissipation, whereas a greater evaporative cooling occurs in men.* Clearly, less sweat production to maintain thermal balance protects women from dehydration during exercise at high ambient temperatures.

Ratio of Body Surface Area to Body Mass

Women possess a relatively large body surface area-to-body mass ratio, a favorable dimensional characteristic for heat dissipation. Stated differently, the smaller female has a larger external surface per unit of body mass exposed to the environment. Consequently, under identical conditions of heat exposure, women cool at a faster rate than men through a smaller body mass across a relatively large surface area. In this regard, children also possess a "geometric" advantage during heat stress, because boys and girls have larger surface areas per unit body mass than adults.

Level of Body Fat

Excess body fat negatively affects exercise performance in hot environments. Because body fat's specific heat exceeds that of muscle tissue, fat increases the insulatory quality of the shell to retard heat conduction to the periphery. The relatively large, obese person also possesses a relatively small body surface area-to-body mass ratio for sweat evaporation compared to a leaner, smaller person.

Excess body fat directly adds to the metabolic cost of weight-bearing activities in addition to retarding effective heat exchange. The additional demands of equipment weight (such as football gear), intense competition, and a hot, humid environment compound these effects. Thus, a fat person experiences considerable difficulty in temperature regulation and exercise performance.[13] Fatal heat stroke occurs 3.5 times more frequently in obese young adults than in individuals whose body mass falls within reasonable limits.

EVALUATING ENVIRONMENTAL HEAT STRESS

Factors other than air temperature that determine the physiologic strain imposed by heat include *(a)* body size and fatness, *(b)* level of training, *(c)* acclimatization, *(d)* adequacy of hydration, and *(e)* external factors (convective air currents; radiant heat gain; intensity of exercise; amount, type, and color of clothing; and most importantly relative humidity). Several football deaths from hyperthermia occurred when air temperature dipped below 75°F (23.9°C) but relative humidity exceeded 95%.

The most effective way to control heat-stress injuries involves prevention. Acclimatization greatly reduces the chance for heat injury. Another defense involves use of the **wet bulb-globe temperature (WB-GT)** to evaluate the environment for its potential thermal challenge. This index of environmental heat stress, developed by the United States military, incorporates ambient temperature, relative humidity, and radiant heat in its calculations as follows:

$$\text{WB-GT} = 0.1 \times \text{DBT} + 0.7 \times \text{WBT} + 0.2 \times \text{GT}$$

where

DBT = dry-bulb (air) temperature in the shade recorded by an ordinary mercury thermometer that measures air temperature.

WBT (accounts for 70% of the index) = temperature recorded by an ordinary mercury thermometer and a thermometer with a wet wick that surrounds the mercury bulb (wet bulb) exposed to rapid air movement in direct sunlight. With high relative humidity, little evaporative cooling occurs from the wetted bulb, so the temperature of this thermometer remains similar to that of the dry-bulb. On a dry day, significant evaporation occurs from the wetted bulb. This maximizes the difference between the two thermometer readings. A small difference between readings indicates high relative humidity, whereas a large difference indicates little air moisture and a high rate of evaporation.

GT = globe temperature in direct sunlight recorded by a thermometer with a black metal sphere surrounding the bulb. The black globe absorbs radiant energy from the surroundings to provide a measure of radiant heat gain.

FIGURE 10.9 illustrates the apparatus to measure WB-GT. The top portion of the inset table presents WB-GT guidelines for athletic activities to reduce the chance of heat

---

AMERICAN COLLEGE OF SPORTS MEDICINE WB-GT RECOMMENDATIONS FOR CONTINUOUS ACTIVITIES SUCH AS ENDURANCE RUNNING AND CYCLING

- **Very high risk:** Above 28°C (82°F)—postpone race

- **High risk:** 23 to 28°C (73–82°F)—heat-sensitive individuals (e.g., obesity, low physical fitness, unacclimatized, dehydrated, previous history of heat injury) should not compete

- **Moderate risk:** 18 to 23°C (65–73°F)

- **Low risk:** Below 18°C (65°F)

| WB-GT Range | | Recommendations |
°F	°C	
80–84	26.5–28.8	• Use discretion, especially if unconditioned or unacclimated
85–87	29.5–30.5	• Avoid strenuous activity in the sun
> 88	> 31.2	• Avoid exercise training

| WBT Range | | Recommendations |
°F	°C	
60	15.5	• No prevention necessary
61–65	16.2–18.4	• Alert all participants to problems of heat stress and importance of adequate hydration
66–70	18.8–21.1	• Insist that appropriate quantity of fluid be ingested
71–75	21.6–23.8	• Rest periods and water breaks every 20 to 30 minutes; limits placed on intense activity
76–79	24.5–26.1	• Practice curtailed and modified considerably
> 80	> 26.5	• Practice cancelled

▓ **Figure 10.9** Wet bulb-globe temperature (WB-GT) for outdoor activities and wet-bulb temperature (WBT) guide. (Modified from Murphy RJ, Ashe WF. Prevention of heat illness in football players. JAMA 1965;194:650.)

injury. These standards apply to lightly clothed humans; they do not consider the specific heat load imposed by football uniforms or other types of equipment. For football, the lower end of each temperature range serves as a more prudent guide.

An indication of ambient heat load also comes from the wet-bulb thermometer because this reading reflects both air temperature and relative humidity. Purchase an inexpensive wet-bulb thermometer at most industrial supply companies. The bottom portion of the inset table of Figure 10.9 presents heat stress recommendations based on the wet-bulb temperature. Without the WBT, but knowing relative humidity via local meteorological stations' media reports and the Internet (www.weather.com), the **Heat Index** (FIG. 10.10) devised by the U.S. National Weather Service also evaluates the relative heat stress. Sometimes referred to as the "apparent temperature," the index provides an accurate measure of how hot it feels when the relative humidity combines with the air temperature. The heat index values were determined for shady, light wind conditions, so exposure to full sunshine increases values by up to 15°F. In addition, strong winds (particularly with hot, dry air) present an extreme hazard. Determine the index close to the race site to eliminate potential error from using meteorological data some distance from the event. Data collected for the 24-hour trend of ambient temperature and relative humidity justified changing the race time for the 1996 Olympic Marathon run in Atlanta from 6:30 PM to 7:00 AM to reduce heat injury risk.

HEAT ILLNESS: COMPLICATIONS FROM EXCESSIVE HEAT STRESS

From the perspective of health and safety, it is far easier to prevent heat injury than remedy it. However, if one fails to heed the normal signs of heat stress—thirst, tiredness, grogginess, and visual disturbances—cardiovascular decompensation triggers a series of disabling complications termed **heat illness**. Heat-related disabilities become more apparent among overweight and poorly conditioned individuals, including those who exercise when dehydrated.[12,33] Heat illness, in order of increasing severity, includes heat cramps, heat exhaustion, and exertional heat stroke. No clear-cut demarcation exists between these maladies because symptoms usually overlap. When serious heat illness occurs, only immediate corrective action can reduce heat stress using rehydration until medical help arrives.[9]

Heat Cramps

Heat cramps (involuntary muscle spasms) occur during or after intense physical activity, usually in the specific muscles exercised. Cramping most likely occurs from an imbalance in hydration level and electrolyte concentrations. During heat exposure, sweating augments salt loss. If electrolytes are not replenished, this increases the chance for muscle pain and spasm (most commonly in the muscles of the abdomen and extremities). Crampers tend to have high sweat rates and/or high sweat sodium concentrations. With heat cramps,

Figure 10.10 How hot is too hot? The Heat Index.

body temperature does not necessarily increase. Prevention involves two factors: *(a)* providing copious amounts of water that contains salt (e.g., Gatorade or GatorLytes) and *(b)* increasing daily salt intake (e.g., adding salt to foods at mealtime) several days before heat stress.

Heat Exhaustion

Heat exhaustion, the most common heat illness among the physically active, usually develops in dehydrated, untrained, and unacclimatized people; it mainly occurs during the first summer heat wave or first hard training session on a hot day. Exercise-induced heat exhaustion occurs because of ineffective circulatory adjustments compounded by depletion of extracellular fluid (plasma volume) from excessive sweating. Blood pools in the dilated peripheral vessels. This drastically reduces the central blood volume required to maintain cardiac output. Characteristics of heat exhaustion include weak,

rapid pulse; low blood pressure in the upright position; headache; nausea; dizziness; "goose bumps;" and general weakness. Sweating may decrease somewhat, but body temperature does not rise to dangerous levels (i.e., above 104°F or 40°C). A person experiencing heat exhaustion symptoms should stop exercising and move to a cooler environment; administer fluids orally or via intravenous therapy with 5% dextrose sugar in either 0.45% NaCl or 0.9% NaCl.[1,3]

Exertional Heat Stroke

Exertional heat stroke, the most serious and complex heat-stress malady, requires immediate medical attention. Heat stroke syndrome reflects a failure of the heat-regulating mechanisms induced by excessively high body temperature. With thermoregulatory failure, sweating usually ceases, the skin becomes dry and hot, body temperature rises to 41.5°C or higher, and the circulatory system becomes excessively strained.

Subtle symptoms often confound the complexity of exertional hyperthermia. Sweating can occur during intense exercise (e.g., 10-km running race) in young, hydrated, and highly motivated individuals. However, the body's heat gain greatly exceeds avenues for heat loss because of the high metabolic heat production. If left untreated, the disability becomes fatal from circulatory collapse and damage to the central nervous system and other organs. Heat stroke represents a medical emergency! *While awaiting medical care, only aggressive treatment to rapidly lower elevated core temperature can avert death; the magnitude and duration of hyperthermia determine organ damage and mortality risk.* Immediate treatment includes alcohol rubs and application of ice packs. Whole-body cold or ice water immersion remains the most effective treatment for a collapsed hyperthermic individual.[7] Individuals most susceptible to heat stroke include larger individuals, especially those who are unfit, poorly acclimatized to the heat, and excessively fat.

Don't Rely on Oral Temperature

Oral temperature does not accurately measure deep body (core) temperature following strenuous exercise. Large and consistent differences exist between oral and rectal temperatures; rectal temperature following a 14-mile race in a tropical climate averaged 103.5°F, while oral temperature remained normal at 98°F.[37] Part of this discrepancy lies in the lowering effect on oral temperature of evaporative cooling in the mouth and airways during high levels of exercise and recovery pulmonary ventilation.

Summary

1. Cutaneous and muscle blood flow increase during exercise in the heat, while other tissues temporality compromise their blood supply.

2. Core temperature normally increases in exercise; the relative stress of exercise determines the magnitude of the increase. A well-regulated temperature increase creates a more favorable environment for physiologic and metabolic functions.

3. Increased sweating strains fluid reserves, creating a relative state of dehydration. Excessive sweating without fluid replacement decreases plasma volume and core temperature rises precipitously.

4. Exercise in a hot, humid environment poses a thermoregulatory challenge because a large sweat loss in high humidity contributes little to evaporative cooling.

5. Fluid loss in excess of 5% of body mass impedes heat dissipation, compromises cardiovascular function, and diminishes exercise capacity.

6. Adequate fluid replacement maintains plasma volume so circulation and sweating progress at optimal levels. The ideal replacement schedule during exercise matches fluid intake with fluid loss. This is effectively monitored by changes in body weight.

7. Each hour, the small intestine absorbs about 1000 mL of water. Prime factors that affect absorption rate include stomach volume and the osmolality of the oral rehydration beverage.

8. Excessive sweating plus ingesting large volumes of plain water during prolonged exercise sets the stage for hyponatremia (water intoxication). A decrease in extracellular sodium concentration causes this potentially dangerous malady.

9. A small amount of electrolytes in the rehydration beverage facilitates fluid replenishment more than drinking plain water.

10. Repeated heat stress initiates thermoregulatory adjustments that improve exercise capacity and reduce discomfort on subsequent heat exposure. Heat acclimatization triggers favorable redistribution of cardiac output and increases sweating capacity. Full acclimatization generally occurs in about 10 days of heat exposure.

11. Aging affects thermoregulatory function, yet acclimatization to moderate heat stress does not appreciably deteriorate with age.

12. When controlling for fitness and acclimatization levels, women and men show equal thermoregulatory efficiency during exercise. Women produce less sweat than men do at the same core temperature.

13. Various practical heat-stress indices (e.g., Heat Stress Index) use ambient temperature and relative humidity to evaluate the environment's potential thermal challenge to an exercising person.

14. Heat cramps, heat exhaustion, and heat stroke are the major forms of heat illness. Heat stroke represents the most serious and complex of these maladies

15. Oral temperature underestimates core temperature following strenuous exercise. This discrepancy results from evaporative cooling of the mouth and airways during high levels of pulmonary ventilation.

TEST YOUR KNOWLEDGE **ANSWERS**

1. False Core temperature (the temperature of deep tissues) remains in dynamic equilibrium between factors that add and subtract body heat. This balance results from integrating mechanisms that alter heat transfer to the periphery (shell), regulate evaporative cooling, and vary the rate of heat production

2. True The hypothalamus contains the central coordinating center for temperature regulation. This group of specialized neurons at the floor of the brain serves as a "thermostat" (usually set and carefully regulated at 37°C±1°C) for making thermoregulatory adjustments to deviations from a temperature norm. Unlike a thermostat in a building, the hypothalamus cannot "turn off" the heat; it only initiates responses to protect the body from heat gain or heat loss.

3. False Body heat loss occurs in four ways: radiation, conduction, convection, and evaporation. Evaporation of sweat provides the major physiologic defense against overheating. Water vaporization from the respiratory passages and skin surface continually transfers heat to the environment. For each liter of water that vaporizes, 580 kcal of heat energy transfers from the body to the environment.

4. False Sweat evaporation from the skin depends on three factors: *(a)* surface exposed to the environment, *(b)* temperature and relative humidity of ambient air, and *(c)* convective air currents around the body. By far, relative humidity exerts the greatest impact on the effectiveness of evaporative heat loss. Relative humidity refers to the percentage of water in ambient air at a particular temperature compared with the total quantity of moisture that the air could carry. For example, 40% relative humidity means that ambient air contains only 40% of the air's moisture-carrying capacity at that specific temperature.

5. True During heat stress, the pituitary gland releases antidiuretic hormone (ADH). ADH increases water reabsorption from the kidney tubules, causing urine to become more concentrated during heat stress. This action of ADH helps to protect against dehydration during heat stress.

6. True Dehydration refers to an imbalance in fluid dynamics when fluid intake does not replenish water loss from either hyperhydrated or normally hydrated states. A moderate exercise workout generally produces a moderate 0.5- to 1.5-L sweat loss over a 1-hour period. Significant water loss occurs during several hours of heavy exercise in a hot environment. The risk of heat illness greatly increases when a person begins exercising in a dehydrated state. Dehydration associated with a 3% decrease in body mass also slows the rate of gastric emptying thus increasing epigastric cramps and feelings of nausea.

7. False Urge individuals to rehydrate themselves, because the thirst mechanism imprecisely indicates water needs, particularly in children and the elderly. If left to depend on thirst, most individuals voluntarily replace only about one-half of the water lost during exercise. It could take several days after severe dehydration to reestablish fluid balance. Drink at least 125 to 150% of the existing fluid loss (body weight loss) as soon as possible after exercising. The 25 to 50% "extra" water accounts for that portion of ingested water lost in urine.

8. False Excessive water intake under certain exercise conditions produces potentially serious medical complications from the syndrome termed *hyponatremia* (water intoxication). Hyponatremia exists when serum sodium concentration falls below 136 mEq·L^{-1} and serum sodium concentrations below 130 mEq·L^{-1}. A sustained low plasma sodium concentration creates an osmotic imbalance across the blood–brain barrier, which causes rapid water influx into the brain. The resulting swelling of brain tissue produces a cascade of symptoms that range from mild (headache, confusion malaise, nausea, cramping) to severe (seizures, coma, pulmonary edema, cardiac arrest, and death).

9. False Factors other than air temperature determine the physiologic strain imposed by heat. These include *(a)* body size and fatness, *(b)* level of training, *(c)* acclimatization, *(d)* adequacy of hydration, and *(e)* external factors (convective air currents; radiant heat gain; intensity of exercise; amount, type, and color of clothing; and most importantly the relative humidity of ambient air).

10. False Oral temperature underestimates core temperature after strenuous exercise. This discrepancy largely results from evaporative cooling of the mouth and airways during high levels of pulmonary ventilation.

References

1. American College of Sports Medicine: American College of Sports Medicine position stand on heat and cold illnesses during distance running. Med Sci Sports Exerc 1996;28(12):1.
2. Androgué HJ, Madias NE. Hyponatremia. N Engl J Med 2000;342:1581.
3. Armstrong LE, Pandolf KB. Physical training, cardiorespiratory physical fitness and exercise-heat tolerance. In: Pandolf KB, et al., eds. Human performance physiology and environmental medicine at terrestrial extremes. Indianapolis, IN: Benchmark Press, 1988.
4. Armstrong L.E, et al.: Symptomatic hyponatremia during prolonged exercise in heat. Med Sci Sports Exerc 1993;25:543.
5. Ayus JC, et al. Hyponatremia, cerebral edema, and noncardiogenic pulmonary edema in marathon runners. Ann Intern Med 2000;132:711.
6. Bar-Or O. Temperature regulation during exercise in children and adolescents. In: Gisolfi CV, Lamb DR, eds. Perspectives in exercise science and sports medicine. Vol. 2. Indianapolis, IN: Benchmark Press, 1989.
7. Costrini A. Emergency treatment of exertional heatstroke and comparison of whole body cooling techniques. Med Sci Sports Exerc 1990;22:15.
8. Cunningham JJ. Is potassium needed in sports drinks for fluid replacement during exercise? Int J Sport Nutr 1997;7:154.
9. Donaldson GC, et al. Cardiovascular responses to heat stress and their adverse consequences in healthy and vulnerable human populations. Int J Hyperthermia 2003;19:225.
10. Falk B. Exercise in the pediatric population—effects of thermal stress. In: Doubt T, ed. Environmental and exercise physiology. Champaign, IL: Human Kinetics, 1997.
11. Falk B, et al. Thermoregulatory responses of pre-, mid-, and late pubertal boys to exercise in dry heat. Med Sci Sports Exerc 1992;24:688.
12. Frye AJ, Kamon E. Responses to dry heat of men and women with similar capacities. J Appl Physiol 1981;50:65.
13. Gardner JW, et al. Risk factors predicting exertional heat illness in male Marine Corps recruits. Med Sci Sports Exerc 1996;28:939.

14. Gardner JW. Death by water intoxication. Milit Med 2002;5:432.
15. Haymes EM. Physiological responses of female athletes to heat stress: a review. Phys Sportsmed 1984;12:45.
16. Hew TD, et al. The incidence, risk factors, and clinical manifestations of hyponatremia in marathon runners. Clin J Sports Med 2003;13:41.
17. Horstman DH, Christensen E. Acclimatization to dry heat: active men vs. active women. J Appl Physiol 1982;52:825.
18. Hsieh M, et al. Hyponatremia in runners requiring on-site medical treatment at a single marathon. Med Sci Sports Exerc 2002;34:185.
19. Irving RA, et al. Evaluation of renal function and fluid homeostasis during recovery from exercise induced hyponatremia. J Appl Physiol 1991;70:342.
20. Kenney WL, Chiu P. Influence of age on thirst and fluid intake. Med Sci Sports Exerc 2001;332:1524.
21. Kenney WL, Ho C-W. Age alters regional distribution of blood flow during moderate-intensity exercise. J Appl Physiol 1995;79:1112.
22. Maughan RJ, Leiper JB. Post-exercise rehydration in man: effects of voluntary intake of four different beverages. Med Sci Sports Exerc 25(suppl):S2, 1993.
23. Maughan RJ, Leiper JB. Fluid replacement requirements in soccer. J Sports Sci 1994;12(special issue):S29.
24. Maughan R.J, Lieper JB. Sodium intake and post-exercise rehydration in man. Eur J Appl Physiol 1995;71:311.
25. Maughan RJ, et al. Influence of menstrual status on fluid replacement after exercise dehydration in healthy young women. Br J Sports Med 1996;30:41.
26. Maughan RJ, et al. Restoration of fluid balance after exercise-induced dehydration: effect of food and fluid intake. Eur J Appl Physiol 1996;73:317.
27. McCullough EA, Kenney WL. Thermal insulation and evaporative resistance of football uniforms. Med Sci Sports Exerc 2003;35:832.
28. Meyer F, et al. Sweat electrolyte loss during exercise in the heat: effects of gender and maturation. Med Sci Sports Exerc 1992;24: 776.
29. Montain SJ, et al. Hyponatremia associated with exercise: risk factors and pathogenesis. Exerc Sport Sci Rev 2001;2:113.
30. Noakes D. Fluid replacement during exercise. Exerc Sports Sci Rev 1993;21:297.
31. Noakes TD, et al. The danger of an inadequate water intake during prolonged exercise. A novel concept re-visited. Eur J Appl Physiol 1988;57:210.
32. Noakes TD, et al. The incidence of hyponatremia during prolonged ultraendurance exercise. Med Sci Sports Exerc 1990;22:165.
33. Porter AM. Collapse from exertional heat illness: implications and subsequent decisions. Milit Med 2003;168:76.
34. Rasch W, Cabanac M. Selective brain cooling is affected by wearing headgear during exercise. J Appl Physiol 1993;74:1229.
35. Rehrer NJ. The maintenance of fluid balance during exercise. Int J Sports Nutr 1996;15:122.
36. Rico-Sanz J, et al. Effects of hyperhydration on total body water, temperature regulation and performance of elite young soccer players in a warm climate. Int J Sports Med 1996;17:85.
37. Rozycki TJ. Oral and rectal temperatures in runners. Phys Sportsmed 1984;12:105.
38. Scott JR, et al. Acute weight gain in collegiate wrestlers following a tournament weigh-in. Med Sci Sports Exerc 1994;26:1181.
39. Sheffield-Moore M, et al. Thermoregulatory responses to cycling with and without a helmet. Med Sci Sports Exerc 1997;29:755.
40. Shi X, et al. Effects of carbohydrate type and concentration and solution osmolality on water absorption. Med Sci Sports Exerc 1995;27:1607.
41. Shirreffs SM, Maughan RJ. Rehydration and recovery of fluid balance after exercise. Exerc Sport Sci Rev. 2000;28:27.
42. Shirreffs SM, et al. Post-exercise rehydration in man: effects of volume consumed and drink sodium content. Med Sci Sports Exerc 1996;28:1260.
43. Speedy DB, et al. Hyponatremia and weight changes in an ultradistance triathlon. Clin J Sport Med 1997;7:180.
44. Speedy DB, et al. Weight changes and serum sodium concentrations after an ultradistance multisport triathlon. Clin J Sport Med 1997;7:100.
45. Speedy DB, et al. Hyponatremia in ultradistance triathletes. Med Sci Sports Exerc 1999;31:809.
46. Stephenson LA, Kolka MA. Thermoregulation in women. Exerc Sport Sci Rev 1993;21:231.
47. van Niewenhoven MA, et al. Effect of dehydration on gastrointestinal function at rest and during exercise in humans. Eur J Appl Physiol 2000;83:578.
48. Wilk B, Bar-Or O. Effect of drink flavor and NaCl on voluntary drinking and hydration in boys exercising in the heat. J Appl Physiol 1996;80:1112.

Additional Readings

Charkoudian N, Joyner MJ. Physiologic considerations for exercise performance in women. Clin Chest Med 2004;25:247.

Coyle EF. Fluid and fuel intake during exercise. J Sports Sci 2004;22:39.

Fowkes Godek S, et al. Thermal responses in football and cross-country athletes during their respective practices in a hot environment. J Athl Train 2004;39:235.

Hue O, et al. Effects of 8 days acclimation on biological and performance response in a tropical climate. J Sports Med Phys Fitness 2004;44:30.

Kilduff LP, et al. The effects of creatine supplementation on cardiovascular, metabolic, and thermoregulatory responses during exercise in the heat in endurance-trained humans. Int J Sport Nutr Exerc Metab 2004;14:443.

Levine JA. Nonexercise activity thermogenesis (NEAT): Environment and biology. Am J Physiol Endocrinol Metab 2004;286:E675.

Maughan RJ, et al. Fluid and electrolyte intake and loss in elite soccer players during training. Int J Sport Nutr Exerc Metab 2004;14:333.

Morgan RM, et al. Acute effects of dehydration on sweat composition in men during prolonged exercise in the heat. Acta Physiol Scand 2004;182:37.

Murray B, Eichner ER. Hyponatremia of exercise. Curr Sports Med Rep 2004;3:117.

Passe DH, et al. Palatability and voluntary intake of sports beverages, diluted orange juice, and water during exercise. Int J Sport Nutr Exerc Metab 2004;14:272.

Shirreffs SM, et al. Fluid and electrolyte needs for preparation and recovery from training and competition. J Sports Sci 2004;22:57. Review.

Von Duvillard SP, et al. Fluids and hydration in prolonged endurance performance. Nutrition 2004;20:651.

Walsh NP, et al. Saliva parameters as potential indices of hydration status during acute dehydration. Med Sci Sports Exerc 2004;36:1535.

Waterhouse J, et al. Thermoregulation during mild exercise at different circadian times. Chronobiol Int 2004;21:253.

Section V
Purported Ergogenic Aids

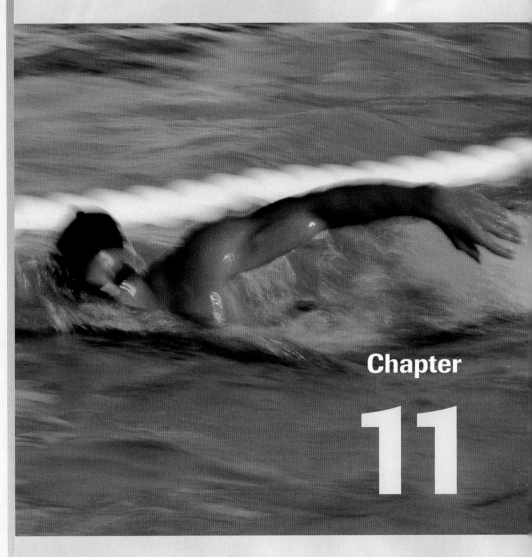

Chapter

11

Pharmacologic and Chemical Ergogenic Aids Evaluated

TEST YOUR KNOWLEDGE

Answer these ten statements about pharmacologic and chemical ergogenic aids. Use the scoring key at the end of the chapter to check your results. Repeat this test after you have read the chapter and compare "before and after" results.

1. **T F** Use of ergogenic drugs by athletes reportedly began with the modern era (after 1900) and coincides with the ability to create "new" laboratory chemicals.

2. **T F** The term "placebo effect" in exercise research refers to the ability of a treatment or a compound to affect a person psychologically in manner that improves physical performance independent of any real physiologic effect.

3. **T F** Because anabolic steroids mimic the function of the hormone testosterone, there is little chance for harmful side effects.

4. **T F** Androstenedione, an intermediate or precursor hormone between DHEA and testosterone, significantly increases endurance performance.

5. **T F** Amphetamines (pep pills) are dangerous and should not be taken by athletes.

6. **T F** Caffeine exerts no ergogenic effect other than to increase alertness in some persons.

7. **T F** The term *functional food* relates to the effects specific foods exert on muscular function and responsiveness to resistance training.

8. **T F** The herbal remedy ephedrine provides safe and positive effects for sports participants, particularly as a substance to facilitate fat loss.

9. **T F** Consuming a light-to-moderate amount of alcohol (e.g., a beer or two) after exercise speeds rehydration and replenishes depleted carbohydrate stores.

10. **T F** β-Hydroxy-β-methylbutyrate (HMB), a bioactive metabolite generated from the breakdown of the essential branched-chain amino acid leucine, decreases protein loss during stress by inhibiting protein catabolism.

Many men and women at all levels of physical prowess use pharmacologic and chemical agents, believing that a specific drug positively influences skill, strength, power, endurance, or responsiveness to training. In our drug-oriented, competitive culture, drug use for ergogenic[a] purposes continues to be on the upswing among high school and even junior high school athletes. Among older, more highly competitive athletes, illegal drug use is a cancer infecting the very foundation of sports competition. Prior to the 1996 Atlanta Olympic Games, only women's field hockey and gymnastics remained free from detection of anabolic steroids. When winning becomes all-important, cheating to win becomes pervasive. Often, one can do little to prevent the use *and* abuse of drugs by athletes, despite scant "hard" scientific evidence indicating a performance-enhancing effect of many of these compounds. Ironically, ath-

[a] Ergogenic ("work producing") refers to the application of a nutritional, physical, mechanical, psychologic, physiologic, or pharmacologic procedure or aid to improve exercise capacity, athletic performance, and responsiveness to training. Included are aids that prepare an individual to exercise, improve exercise efficiency, or facilitate the recovery process.

letes go to great lengths to promote all aspects of their health. They train hard, eat well-balanced meals, receive medical attention even for minor injuries, yet they purposely ingest synthetic agents, many of which trigger negative health effects ranging from nausea, hair loss, itching, and nervous irritability to an array or potential life-threatening conditions.

Considerable information exists concerning possible ergogenic effects of nutritional and pharmacologic aids on exercise performance and training. These include testimonials and endorsements from sports professionals and organizations, media publicity, television infomercials, and Internet home pages for untested products. This also includes research studies that extol potential performance benefits from alcohol, amphetamines, hormones, carbohydrates, amino acids (either consumed singularly or in combination), fatty acids, caffeine, buffering compounds, wheat-germ oil, vitamins, minerals, catecholamine agonists, steroid hormone precursors and stimulants, and even marijuana and cocaine[b] TABLE 11.1 gives examples of ingredients and the frequently *unsubstantiated* (largely incorrect) claims advertised by makers of nutritional supplements in the physical fitness marketplace. Active individuals routinely use many of these compounds, believing that they enhance the response to exercise. The general population considers supplementation a way to improve physical appearance; in this regard, products aggressively marketed to reduce fat and increase muscle mass become "best sellers." Sports nutrition supplements are the largest growing segment of the $18 billion dietary supplement industry.

AN AREA OF INCREASING COMPLEXITY AND CONTROVERSY

Several explanations account for heightened interest in factors other than innate physical ability and commitment to training that might enhance capacity for exercise and training. First, more persons participate in high-level competitive amateur and professional athletics. Second, competitive success brings significant personal recognition and approval, but also more tangible rewards ranging from valuable college scholarships to lucrative professional contracts and commercial endorsements. Concurrently, exercise science continues to produce research about how pharmacologic agents and nutritional modification and supplementation affect energy supply, muscle metabolism, physiologic function, and growth and development.

In Use Since Antiquity

Ancient athletes of Greece reportedly used hallucinogenic mushrooms plant seeds and ground dog testicles for ergogenic

purposes, while Roman gladiators ingested the equivalent of "speed" to enhance performance in the Circus Maximus. Athletes of the Victorian era routinely used caffeine, alcohol, nitroglycerine, heroin, cocaine, and the rat poison strychnine for a competitive edge. For today's exercise enthusiast, dietary supplements consist of nonprescription plant extracts, vitamins, minerals, enzymes, and hormonal products. To positively influence overall health and exercise performance, these supplements must provide a nutrient undersupplied in the diet or exert a druglike influence on cellular function.

In today's technological society, little demarcation exists between diet, nutrient supplements (often at exposure levels greater than in foods), and chemical agents used to enhance training and gain a competitive edge. For example, vitamin intake in megadose quantities often exerts druglike effects once these chemicals saturate tissues, while the trace minerals chromium, vanadium, copper, and iron become harmful chemicals with potentially lethal side effects in excess. One could ask: "Does an inordinate intake of a particular amino acid, fatty acid, pyruvate salt, leucine metabolite, or other 'natural' chemical simply reflect manipulation of one's normal diet or an abnormal pharmacologic intervention of a potentially harmful compound?"

Not Without Risk

The indiscriminate use of alleged ergogenic substances increases the likelihood of adverse side effects ranging from relatively benign physical discomfort to life-threatening episodes.[8] Many of these compounds fail to conform to labeling requirements to correctly identify the strength of the product's ingredients.[98,124] Results from a study at the Institute of Biochemistry at the German Sports University of Cologne (www.dopinginfo.de) and supported by the Medical Commission of the International Olympic Committee (IOC) indicate that up to 20% of the nutritional supplements sampled contain substances that produce a positive result for doping, including nandrolone, testosterone, and other steroids not declared on the label. The supplements analyzed included vitamins and minerals, protein supplements, and creatine. These findings raise the real possibility that cross contamination occurs in laboratories that produce both prohormone products and nutrient supplements. Use of a dietary supplement contaminated with the prohibited anabolic substance 19-norandrosterone was the explanation offered by a member of the United States Olympic bobsled team for his disqualification just prior to the start of the Salt Lake City Winter Games. This is particularly ironic because the Unites States Olympic Committee and Salt Lake City Olympic organizers signed a $20 million deal through 2004 with Nu Skin, a Utah-based company, to supply Olympic training centers with dietary supplements.

ON THE HORIZON

The day may not be far off when individuals born lacking certain "lucky" genes that augment growth and development and exercise performance will simply add them, dop-

---

[b] Well-documented evidence exists about the addictive nature of cocaine and potential for significant health risks. Research has never shown that cocaine provides an ergogenic effect. Studies have been limited to animals (for obvious reasons), and results show that cocaine triggers an exaggerated catecholamine response during submaximal exercise, augments glycogen depletion in skeletal muscle, and causes lactate to rapidly accumulate in the blood.[24,25,48,130] These effects all impair exercise performance.

Table 11.1   INGREDIENTS COMMONLY ADVERTISED BY NUTRITIONAL SUPPLEMENT MANUFACTURERS (THE DEFINITION/ALLEGED ATTRIBUTES ARE VERBATIM FROM LITERATURE SUPPLIED BY MANUFACTURERS, PRODUCT LABELS, PROMOTIONAL MATERIAL ABOUT THE PRODUCT ON THE INTERNET, AND ADVERTISEMENTS IN MUSCLE AND BODY BUILDING MAGAZINES.)

American ginseng. Restores energy after great fatigue. Reported to have invigorating and stimulating power. Acts as a general tonic. A booster.

Barley Green. Used by athletes for energy. Extremely nutritious and loaded with vitamins, proteins, minerals, chlorophyll, and enzymes.

BCAAs. Branched-chain amino acids that assist the muscles in synthesizing other amino acids to aid muscle growth. Help muscles absorb blood sugar for energy.

Chromium (picolinate). Activates enzymes involved in glucose and protein for burning and increasing lean body mass. Builds stamina.

Cinnamon. Promotes internal energy and strengthens the body. Strong tonic that promotes good circulation.

Codonopsis. Restores energy, balances metabolism, and stimulates the production of blood.

Colostrum. Increases strength and lean body mass.

CoQ$_{10}$. Plays a role in energy production. Powerful antioxidant. Enhances the body's total systems.

Cordyceps. Renown as a supertonic. Builds physical power and mental energy.

Creatine monohydrate. Enhances energy and athletic performance and significantly increases muscle mass and strength.

Dendrobium. Quickly and effectively restores spent energy. A tonic and longevity herb.

DHEA. Regulates metabolism and increases muscle mass while burning fat. Strengthens and maintains the immune system and enhances energy. Increases physical well-being. A wonder supplement.

Digestive enzymes. Break down food particles for storage in the liver and muscles for energy. Help to construct new muscle tissue.

Epemedium. A powerful tonic and stimulant. Helps strengthen bones and joints.

Eucommia. Superb energy tonic. Often used by athletes to strengthen the joints and the body.

Guarana extract. Increases energy and alertness. Increases fat-burning process.

Ho Shu Wu (FoTi). Increases and builds essential energy and cleanses the blood. Oriental wonder.

Kola nut. Increases energy and alertness. Increases fat-burning process.

L-Carnitine. Controls increases in body-fat stores by converting nutrients into energy. Burns body fat and improves athletic performance.

L-Glutamine. Promotes protein and glycogen synthesis in muscles and liver. Prevents muscle catabolism. Helps buffer lactic acid buildup while training. Alleviates fatigue. Promotes recovery.

Licorice root. Strengthens muscles. Regulates blood sugar levels. Strongest detoxifier known to man without side effects.

Lipoic acid. Key compound for producing energy in muscles and normalizing blood sugar levels. Lipoic acid combats free radical formation.

L-Lysine. Essential building block for all proteins. Uses fatty acids required in energy production. Important for recovery from sports injuries.

Lycii fructus. Nourishes the blood and liver. Excellent energy and blood tonic. Pain reliever.

Magnesium carbonate. Essential for vital enzymes. Aids in transmitting nerve and muscle impulses. Prevents muscle weakness.

Mexican wild yam. Increases physical well-being, enhances energy, and decreases body fat. Improves ability to deal with stressful situations. Clears the mind.

Muirapuama. Stimulant to enhance sports performance because of the rush it produces. Increases energy.

NAC. Reduces fatigue in muscles and improves liver metabolism. Aids the main antioxidant enzyme, glutathione peroxidase.

Nettle root. Rich in vitamins, lipids, and chlorophyll. Increases aerobic power and muscle strength. Mild antiinflammatory and diuretic.

Orchic. Main source of natural testosterone production. Helps the body retain more protein and nitrogen to increase muscle mass and strength.

PAK. Significantly improves aerobic and anaerobic performance by increasing energy production. Reduces lactic acid.

Peony. Nourishes the blood. Helps detoxify the liver and improve blood circulation.

Phosphatidyl serine. Stops exercise-induced increase in cortisol, which has an anticatabolic effect in muscles and tissues.

Plant sterols. Improve physical performance. Have general anabolic activity within muscle cells. Allow athletes to adapt to harder training loads.

Potassium chloride. Essential in maintaining fluid balance within the muscles. Aids in muscle contraction and transmission of glucose into glucogen for energy.

Quebracho bark. Highly effective stimulant. Known to elevate mood and increase energy. Builds overall strength and power. Great for endurance.

Radix angelicae. Used as a muscle building tonic. Nourishes the blood and activates blood circulation.

Radix astragali. Strengthens muscle and improves metabolic function. Potent immune system tonic. Fabulous for fighting injuries.

RNA–DNA. Increases cell energy and protein synthesis. Helps rebuild cells to ensure postworkout repair and growth. A good protein.

Royal jelly. High concentration of nutrients, especially B-complex vitamins. High concentration of vitamins, minerals, enzymes, and amino acids.

Saw palmetto. Contains plant sterols that improve physical performance and has profound effects on testosterone metabolism.

(continues)

Table 11.1   **INGREDIENTS COMMONLY ADVERTISED BY NUTRITIONAL SUPPLEMENT MANUFACTURERS (THE DEFINITION/ALLEGED ATTRIBUTES ARE VERBATIM FROM LITERATURE SUPPLIED BY MANUFACTURERS, PRODUCT LABELS, PROMOTIONAL MATERIAL ABOUT THE PRODUCT ON THE INTERNET, AND ADVERTISEMENTS IN MUSCLE AND BODY BUILDING MAGAZINES.)** *(CONTINUED)*

Schizandra. Increases endurance and strengthens the whole body. A powerful tonic that improves memory.

Selenium. Boosts immunity and neutralizes many free radicals and carcinogens. Vital antioxidant.

Siberian ginseng. Helps one adapt to all kinds of stresses. Improves the blood oxygen-carrying capacity. Promotes mental and physical vigor, metabolism, stamina, and endurance under stressful conditions. "Gets the body going."

Silica. Excellent for building strong bones and connective tissue.

Smilax. Increases muscle strength and size. Augments the body's natural production of its own testosterone.

Sumac. High in nutrients. Contains 19 different amino acids and electrolytes. Helps oxygenate the system and build and maintain lean muscle mass.

Vanadyl sulfate. Helps increase muscle growth and development and reduces body fat stores.

Vitamin C. Powerful antioxidant required for tissue growth and repair. Protects against infection and enhances immunity.

Vitamin E. A powerful antioxidant. Improves oxygen use. Enhances immune response and improves athletic performance.

Wild oats. Aids digestion and increases testosterone levels. Increases aerobic power and muscle strength. A great muscle builder.

Yerba mate. Helps to relieve fatigue and stress. Cleanses the blood and stimulates the mind. A fat-burner in vital body areas.

Yohimbe bark. Male athletes use this herb because of its reputed muscle-building effects. It improves sports performance and increases energy.

Zinc aspartate. Helps protein synthesis and collagen formation. Essential to athletes for growth and development, and to increase performance.

ing undetectably with DNA not drugs. In these instances, the use of "gene doping" misappropriates the medical applications of gene therapy that treats atherosclerosis, cystic fibrosis, and other diseases and uses them to increase the size, speed, and strength of healthy humans. For example, genes that cause muscles to enlarge would be ideal for sprinters, weightlifters, and other power athletes. On the other hand, endurance athletes would benefit from genes that boost the production of red blood cells (e.g., gene for erythropoietin) or stimulate the development of blood vessels (e.g., gene for vascular endothelial growth factor).

An increasing belief in the potential for selected foods to promote health has led to coining of the term **functional food** (see Case Study 6.1, page 172). Beyond meeting three basic nutrition needs for survival, hunger satisfaction, and preventing adverse effects, functional foods comprise those foods and their bioactive components (e.g., olive oil, soy products, n-3 fatty acids) that promote well being, health, and optimal body function or reduce disease risk (FIG. 11.1).[154,164,201,225] Examples include many polyphenolic substances (simple phenols and flavinoids found in fruits, vegetables, and nuts), carotinoids, soy isoflavones, fish oils, and components of nuts that possess antioxidant and other properties that decrease risk of vascular diseases and cancers. Primary targets for this expanding branch of food science include gastrointestinal functions, antioxidant systems, and macronutrient metabolism. Clearly, enormous implications exist for society from a greater understanding of nutrition's role in optimizing an individual's genetic potential, resistance to disease, and overall performance. Unfortunately, the science base generated by research in this valid field of human nutrition often falls prey to nutritional hucksters and scam artists.

Biotechnology also has created the emerging field of **transgenic nutraceuticals**—modifying a biochemical path-

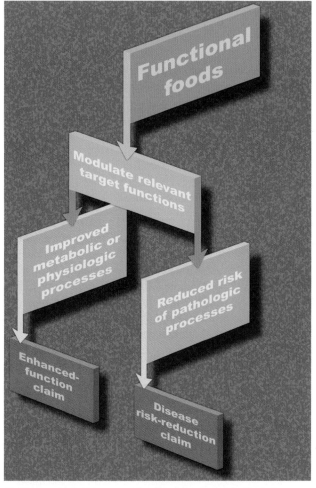

Figure 11.1 Strategy of functional food science. Basis for enhanced structure–function or disease risk-reduction claims. (From Roberfroid MB. Concepts and strategy of functional food science: the European perspective. Am J Clin Nutr 2000;71(suppl):1163S.)

way by use of genes introduced into a host plant or animal. This produces a new class of "natural" bioactive components of food in a nonfood matrix with physiologic and therapeutic functions (e.g., pharmaceutical proteins such as vaccines and monoclonal antibodies) to promote disease prevention and treatment. Nutraceuticals differ from functional foods that deliver their active ingredients within the food matrix. By definition, nutraceutical compounds fall along the continuum from food to food supplements to drugs. Examples of such genetic engineering of nutrients include remodeling of mammary gland milk of cows (adding or deleting specific milk proteins or adding oligosaccharides) to provide medical benefits, and development of novel food oils that do not require chemical hydrogenation (and thus no harmful *trans* fatty acids). Through genetic tinkering, scientists can dramatically augment the vitamin C levels in the leaves and seeds of crop plants by increasing expression of a gene that causes recycling of vitamin C within the plant. Undoubtedly, some of these biotechnology products will make their way into the exercise enthusiast's nutritional armamentarium to form the next wave of alleged performance enhancers.

A NEED TO CRITICALLY EVALUATE

Companies expend considerable money and effort, often illegally, to show a beneficial effect of an "aid." Often, however, a **"placebo effect"** improves performance because of psychological factors—the individual performs at a higher level because of the suggestive power of believing that a substance or procedure should work. Sports nutritionists must evaluate the scientific merit of articles and advertisements about nutrition products. To separate marketing "hype" from scientific fact, we pose five areas for questioning the validity of research claims concerning the efficacy of chemical, pharmacologic, and nutritional ergogenic aids:

I. **Justification**
    - **Scientific rationale:** Does the study represent a "fishing expedition" or is there a sound rationale that the specific treatment should produce an effect? For example, a theoretical basis exists to believe that ingesting creatine elevates intramuscular creatine and phosphocreatine to possibly improve short-term power output capacity. In contrast, no rationale exists to hypothesize that hyperhydration, breathing hyperoxic gas, or ingesting medium-chain triglycerides should enhance 100-m dash performance.
II. **Subjects**
    - **Animals or humans:** Many diverse mammals exhibit similar physiologic and metabolic dynamics, yet significant species differences exist, which often limit generalizations to humans. For example, the models for disease processes, nutrient requirements, hormone dynamics, and growth and development often differ markedly between humans and different animal groups.

- **Sex:** Sex-specific responses to the interactions between exercise, training, and nutrient requirements and supplementation limit generalizability of findings to the sex studied.
- **Age:** Age often interacts to influence the outcome of an experimental treatment. Effective interventions for the elderly may not apply to growing children or young and middle-aged adults.
- **Training status:** Fitness status and training level can influence the effectiveness (or ineffectiveness) of a particular diet or supplement intervention. Treatments that benefit the untrained (e.g., chemicals or procedures that enhance neurologic disinhibition) often have little effect on elite athletes who practice and compete routinely at maximal arousal levels.
- **Baseline level of nutrition:** The research should establish the subjects' nutritional status prior to experimental treatment. Clearly, a nutrient supplement administered to a malnourished group typically improves exercise performance and training responsiveness. Such nutritional interventions fail to demonstrate whether the same effects occur if subjects received the supplement with their baseline nutrient intake at recommended levels. It should occasion little surprise, for example, that supplemental iron enhances aerobic fitness in a group with iron-deficiency anemia. One cannot infer, however, that iron supplements provide such benefits to all individuals.
- **Health status:** Nutritional, hormonal, and pharmacologic interventions profoundly affect the diseased and infirmed yet offer no benefit to those in good health. Research findings from diseased groups should not be generalized to healthy populations.

III. **Research sample, subjects, and design**
    - **Random assignment or self-selection:** Apply research findings only to groups similar to the sample studied. If subject volunteers "self-select" into an experimental group, does the experimental treatment produce the results or did a change occur from the individual's motivation to take part in the study? For example, desire to enter a weight loss study may elicit behaviors that produce weight loss independent of the experimental treatment per se. Great difficulty exists in assigning truly random samples of subjects into an experimental group and a control group. When subjects volunteer to take part in an experiment they must be randomly assigned to a control or experimental condition, a process termed **randomization**. When all subjects receive the experimental supplement and the placebo treatment (see below), supple-

ment administration is counterbalanced, and half the subjects receive the supplement first, while the other half takes the placebo first.

- **Double-blind, placebo-controlled:** The ideal experiment to evaluate performance-enhancing effects of an exogenous supplement requires that experimental and control subjects remain unaware or "blinded" to the substance administered. To achieve this goal, subjects should receive a similar quantity and/or form of the proposed aid. In contrast, control group subjects receive an inert compound or placebo. The placebo treatment evaluates the possibility of subjects performing well or responding better simply because they receive a substance they believe should benefit them (psychological or placebo effect). To further reduce experimental bias from influencing the outcome, those administering the treatment and recording the response must not know which subjects receive the treatment or placebo. In such a **double-blinded** experiment both investigator and subjects remain unaware of the treatment condition.

- **Control of extraneous factors:** Under ideal conditions, experiences should be similar for both experimental and control groups, except for the treatment variable. Random assignment of subjects to control or experimental groups goes a long way to control factors that could influence the study's outcome.

- **Appropriateness of measurements:** Reproducible, objective, and valid measurement tools must evaluate research outcomes. For example, a step test to predict aerobic capacity, or infrared interactance to evaluate components of body composition represent imprecise tools to answer meaningful questions about the efficacy of a proposed ergogenic aid.

IV. Conclusions

- **Findings should dictate conclusions:** The conclusions of a research study must logically follow from the research findings. Frequently, investigators who study ergogenic aids extrapolate conclusions beyond the scope of their data. The implications and generalizations of research findings must remain within the context of the measurements made, the subjects studied, and the magnitude of the response. For example, increases in anabolic hormone levels in response to a dietary supplement reflect just that; they do not necessarily indicate an augmented training responsiveness or an improved level of muscular function. Similarly, significant improvement in brief anaerobic power output capacity with creatine supplementation does not justify the conclusion that exogenous creatine improves overall "physical fitness."

- **Appropriate statistical analysis:** Appropriate inferential statistical analysis must be applied to quantify the potential that chance caused the research outcome. Other statistics must objectify averages, variability, and degree of association between variables.

- **Statistical versus practical significance:** The finding of statistical significance of a particular experimental treatment only means a high probability exists that the result did not occur by chance. One must also evaluate the magnitude of an effect for its real impact on physiology and/or performance. A reduced heart rate of 3 beats per minute during submaximal exercise may reach statistical significance, yet have little practical effect on aerobic fitness or cardiovascular function.

V. Dissemination of findings

- **Published in peer-reviewed journal:** High-quality research withstands the rigors of critical review and evaluation by colleagues with expertise in the specific area of investigation. Peer review provides a measure of quality control over scholarship and interpretation of research findings. Publications in popular magazines or quasi-professional journals do not undergo the same rigor of evaluation as peer-review. In fact, self-appointed "experts" in sports nutrition and physical fitness pay eager publishers for magazine space to promote their particular viewpoint. In some cases, the expert owns the magazine!

- **Findings reproduced by other investigators:** Findings from one study do not necessarily establish scientific fact. Conclusions become stronger and more generalizable when support emerges from the laboratories of other independent investigators. Consensus reduces the influence of chance, flaws in experimental design, and investigator bias.

TABLE 11.2 summarizes recommendations for future research on performance-enhancing products put forth at the Conference on the Science and Policy of Performance-Enhancing Products held in January 2002.

SUPPLEMENT USE AND ABUSE AMONG ELITE ATHLETES

Based on the latest survey of college student–athletes by the National Collegiate Athletic Association (NCAA) in 2001, 29% of the respondents used nutritional supplements during the previous year.[99] The most popular supplement was creatine (26%), followed by amino acids (10%), with androstenedione, chromium, and ephedra each used by about 4% of the

Table 11.2	RESEARCH-BASED RECOMMENDATIONS FOR INVESTIGATING THE OPTIMAL DOSING, HEALTH RISKS, AND EFFICACY OF ALLEGED PERFORMANCE-ENHANCING PRODUCTS

- Evaluation of the risks and benefits of performance-enhancing supplements among subpopulations with diverse dietary patterns and nutrient intakes, such as adolescents, body builders, military personnel, and the elderly
- Monitoring and surveillance of the effects of chronic, prolonged use of performance-enhancing supplements, particularly androstenedione, ephedrine, and creatine
- Identification and characterization of mechanism(s) of action of performance-enhancing ingredients
- Characterization of the patterns of use (e.g., type of product, frequency) and psychosocial behavioral aspects of use among various subpopulations in the United States
- Characterization of dose-response curves for performance-enhancing supplements, particularly those containing ephedrine, alkaloids, and steroid hormone precursors such as androstenedione
- Characterization of the endocrine effects of performance-enhancing supplements, especially those containing hormonal ingredients such as androstenedione and dehydroepiandrosterone (DHEA), according to age, gender, and physiological life stage (e.g., female athletes with amenorrhea or disordered eating or at high risk for osteoporosis)
- Comparative studies of analytical grade dietary supplement ingredients (particularly caffeine and ephedrine) with formulations currently in the marketplace
- Evaluation of the effects of combining performance-enhancing ingredients as in "stacking formulas" or the simultaneous use of multiple sports supplements
- Comparative studies that examine the effect of frequency and timing of supplementation on physical performance
- Determining targeted approaches to communicate the risks and benefits of performance-enhancing products to various segments of the U.S. population (professional and lay audiences)
- Determining whether other stimulant and thermogenic ingredients might serve as substitutes for ephedrine alkaloids

From Fomous CM, et al. Symposium: conference on the science and policy of performance-enhancing products. Med Sci Sports Exerc 2002;34:1685.

athletes. The IOC initiated drug testing for stimulants in Olympic competition in the 1968 Mexico City games following the death of a famed Tour de France British cyclist from amphetamine overdose a year earlier. Testing has consistently expanded, with the initiation of random unannounced drug testing in track and field in 1989 to the administration of 3500 tests before the opening ceremonies of the 2002 Winter Games in Salt Lake City. The following broad categories encompass substances and methods banned by the IOC as of 2005:

- Stimulants
- Narcotic analgesics
- Androgenic anabolic steroids
- β-Blockers and alcohol
- β-2 agonists
- Diuretics and other masking agents
- Agents with anti-estrogenic activity
- Peptide hormones and analogues
- Substances that alter the integrity of urine samples
- Enhancers of oxygen transport, chemical and physical manipulation, and gene doping
- Cannabinoids
- Glucocorticosteroids

Testing of urine samples provides the primary method for drug detection. The urine sample is cleaned, dried, stabilized, and vaporized. The standard testing procedure adds chemicals to the dried urine, vaporizes it with heat, and then blows the vapor through an absorbent column and an electric or magnetic field (gas chromatography-mass spectrometry). The pattern made by the molecules deflected by the field is compared with patterns made by known chemicals.

The following quote from the February 27, 1997, edition of the *New York Times* sadly points up the state of affairs concerning the risks and extremes for performance enhancement that even the world's best athletes go to gain the competitive advantage:

> *Lyubov Egorova, a six-time Olympic champion from Russia, failed a drug test during the World Nordic Ski Championships and likely will be banned from her sport for two years. It is believed to be the first time a cross-country skier tested positive for banned drugs in the competition since it began in 1925. Egorova, 31, won the 5K classical style race Sunday, three years after winning the same distance in the Lillehammer Olympics, south of Trondheim. She will be stripped of her medal and barred from these championships.*

Seventeen months later on July 16, 1998, the international governing body of bicycle racing suspended the coach of the top-ranked Festina team of France in a drug scandal that threatened to overwhelm the 85th Tour de France, bicycle racing's most prestigious and financially rewarding competition. The suspension resulted after the team car was found to contain large quantities of illicit drugs. These drugs included amphetamines, steroids, masking drugs (frequently diuretics to prevent steroid detection), and the blood-boosting epoetin, a genetically engineered copy of a kidney hormone erythropoietin linked to more than a dozen heart attacks among competitive cyclists. The following day, after the sixth stage of the Tour, all nine members of Festina were suspended after its coach admitted supplying illegal drugs to his riders. One week later, four Chinese swimmers were suspended from all meets for 2 years for using triamterene (a banned diuretic than can mask anabolic steroid use) during the world championships in January.

On August 6, 1998, the International Swimming Federation, the swimming world's governing body, banned from competition for 4 years the Irish swimmer who won three gold medals at the 1996 Summer Olympics. They accused her of manipulating a drug test by spiking her urine sample with alcohol in an attempt to mask forbidden performance-enhancing drugs. Germany's leading Paralympian became the first athlete ejected from a Winter Paralympics for a doping scandal. He was stripped of two gold medals (biathlon and 5-km cross-country skiing) on March 12, 2002, and ejected from the Salt Lake Winter Games after testing positive for methenolone, a muscle-building steroid. On January 8, 2003, the third place finisher in the 2002 New York City Marathon was disqualified and stripped of her prize money after a positive drug test result indicated she used ephedrine, a stimulant in dietary supplements. Also in January 2003, a member of the United States Pan American Games swim team tested positive for 19-norandrosterone (a prohibited steroid), for which the swimmer received a 4-year ban from competition by the United States Anti-Doping Agency (USADA: www.usantidoping.org/). On its web site, the USADA sends a clear message to athletes:

> THE USE OF DIETARY/NUTRITIONAL SUPPLEMENTS IS COMPLETELY AT THE ATHLETE'S OWN RISK, EVEN IF THE SUPPLEMENTS ARE "APPROVED" OR "VERIFIED."

> If you take dietary/nutritional supplements you may test positive for a prohibited substance, which is not disclosed on the product label. This would result in a doping violation.

According to documents released in 2003 by Dr. Wade Exum, the USOC's former director for drug control, United States athletes tested positive for drugs more than 100 times from 1988 to 2000. These allegations were contained in 30,000 documents made available to *Sports Illustrated* about drug abuse that included Olympic standout Carl Lewis and tennis player Mary Joe Fernandez and others. Only a handful of athletes were barred from competing and 19 went on to win medals. A December 3, 2004 news report indicates that N.Y. Yankee baseball player Jason Giambi admitted to a federal grand jury to using performance enhancing drugs, including testosterone, human growth hormone, and a liquid (tetrahydrogestrinone, or THG) and cream (testosterone-based lotion) anabolic steroid for at least three seasons. The competitive athlete should consult with the IOC Medical Commission, national governing bodies, international federations, and the USDA Drug Reference Line (1-800-233-0393) for the most up-to-date list of banned substances[c] and other timely information about drugs and enforcement policies and sanctions. Interestingly, many attention deficit disorder (ADD) and attention deficit hyperactivity disorder (ADHD) medications classify as banned substances. The

drug Straterra is a permitted medication for in-competition and out-of-competition events. A physician should be consulted about the drug's effects and how Straterra may be effective to treat the ADD and ADHD competitor instead of the stimulant drugs most often prescribed.

In this chapter we discuss common pharmacologic agents purported to enhance exercise performance, increase the quality and quantity of training, and augment the body's adaptation to regular exercise. Chapter 12 discusses the role of nutritional supplementation for ergogenic purposes. The following chart presents five mechanisms by which such foods, food components, and pharmacologic agents might enhance exercise performance:[115]

MECHANISM FOR HOW PURPORTED ERGOGENIC AIDS MIGHT WORK

- Act as central or peripheral nervous system stimulant (e.g., caffeine, choline, amphetamines, alcohol)

- Increase storage and/or availability of a limiting substrate (e.g., carbohydrate, creatine, carnitine, chromium)

- Act as supplemental fuel source (e.g., glucose, medium-chain triglycerides)

- Reduce or neutralize performance-inhibiting metabolic byproducts (e.g., sodium bicarbonate or sodium citrate, pangamic acid, phosphate)

- Facilitate recovery (e.g., high-glycemic carbohydrates, water)

ANABOLIC STEROIDS

Anabolic steroids for medical use became prominent in the early 1950s to treat patients deficient in natural androgens or with muscle-wasting diseases (muscular dystrophies). Other legitimate steroid uses include treatment for osteoporosis and severe breast cancer in women and to counter the excessive decline in lean body mass and increase in body fat often observed among elderly men, HIV patients, and individuals undergoing kidney dialysis.

Anabolic steroids have become an integral part of the high-technology scene of competitive American sports beginning with the U.S. weightlifting team (1955) who used Dianabol (modified, synthetic testosterone molecule, methandrostenolone). From the early 1960s until the fall of the Berlin Wall, a new era ushered in the systematic "drugging" of East German competitive athletes with formulation of other anabolic steroids.[78,239] An estimated one to three million athletes (90% of male and 80% of female profes-

---

[c] The United States Olympic Committee (USOC) provides background information about prohibited substances and methods on their Web site <http://test.olympic-usa.org/insiide/in_1_1_4_6_5.html#TOC> with links to different sport organization web sites (NGB) and International Federations (IF). Contact the USOC Drug Control Program in Colorado Springs to obtain the most recent *"Guide to Prohibited Substances and Methods."*

sional body builders) currently use androgens, often combined with stimulants, hormones, and diuretics, to facilitate the training response.[40,56]

Screening for exogenous anabolic steroid use among athletes includes a measure of the urinary ratio of testosterone to luteinizing hormone (T/LH) or the urinary ratio of testosterone to epitestosterone (T/E). A urinary T/LH ratio of 30 or above provides a more sensitive marker of anabolic steroid use than a T/E ratio of 6 or above.[191]

Structure and Action

Anabolic steroids function in a manner similar to the chief male hormone testosterone. By binding with special receptor sites on muscle and other tissues, testosterone contributes to male secondary sex characteristics. These include sex differences in muscle mass and strength that develop at the onset of puberty. Testosterone production takes place mainly in the testes (95%), with the remainder produced by the adrenal glands. One can minimize the hormone's androgenic or masculinizing effects by synthetically manipulating the steroid's chemical structure to increase muscle growth from nitrogen retention and anabolic tissue building. Nevertheless, the masculinizing effect of synthetically derived steroids still occurs despite chemical alteration, particularly in females.

Athletes who take these drugs typically do so during the active years of their athletic careers. They combine supraphysiologic dosages of multiple steroid preparations in oral and injectable form (combined because they believe the various androgens differ in physiologic action)—a practice called **"stacking"**—progressively increasing drug dosage **("pyramiding")** usually during 4- to 18-week cycles. A drug-free period is included between cycles. The drug quantities far exceed the recommended medical dose, often up to 200 times or more the therapeutic amounts. The athlete then progressively reduces the dosage in the months prior to competition to reduce risk of detection during drug testing. The difference between dosages in research studies and the excess typically abused by athletes has largely contributed to credibility gap between scientific findings (often, no effect

of steroids) and what most in the athletic community "know" to be true. TABLE 11.3 lists examples of oral and injectable anabolic steroids, including typical retail cost and black market prices, which vary considerably in different domestic regions and internationally.

Designer Drug Unmasked

Researchers in the Department of Molecular and Medical Pharmacology at UCLA's IOC-accredited Olympic Analytical Laboratory have unmasked a potentially illegal "designer" compound that mimics the chemical structure similar to the prohibited steroids gestrinome and trenbolone. The researchers called the discovery a new standalone steroid chemical entity, not a "pro-steroid" or "precursor steroid" like many performance-boosting substances on the market—a drug with no prior record of manufacture or existence. The U.S. Anti-Doping Agency (USADA: www.usantidoping.org), which oversees drug testing for all sports federations under the U.S. Olympic umbrella, said an anonymous tipster provided a syringe sample of a steroid identified as tetrahydrogestrinone, or THG. The researchers painstakingly developed a new test to detect THG, apparently taken not by injection but in droplets under the tongue, and then reanalyzed 350 urine samples from participants at the U.S. track and field championships in June 2003, and 100 samples from random out-of-competition tests. Each urine sample is divided in two and stored for future reference. The athletes whose "A" samples revealed THG were notified, with their "B" samples yet to be tested to confirm the positive "A" tests. Remarkably, a half dozen athletes tested positive. A positive test result prompts a review process to ensure that proper antidoping procedures were followed. Athletes who test positive face 2-year suspensions that would prohibit participation in international meets. As of October 17, 2003, the National Football League began testing players for THG to avoid the scandal that has embarrassed track and field. Professional basketball and baseball may also follow suit. USADA's mission is to fight doping through drug testing, research, and education. The USADA con-

Table 11.3 EXAMPLES OF ANABOLIC STEROIDS (GENERIC AND COMMERCIAL NAME), INCLUDING TYPICAL RETAIN COSTS AND BLACK MARKET PRICES[a]

Generic Name	Commercial Name	Form	Retail Price	Black Market Price
Oxymetholone	Anadrol	Oral	$90/100 tabs	$300/100 tabs
Testosterone cypionate	Testosterone	Injectable	$35/10 ml	$200/10 mL
Stanazolol	Winstrol V	Injectable	$250/30 mL	$400/30 mL
Boldenone	Equipoise	Injectable	$150/30 mL	$450/30 mL
Oxandrolone	Anavar	Oral	$75/100 tabs	4150/100 tabs
Methandrostenolone	Dianabol	Oral	$100/100 tabs	$200/100 tabs

[a] 2005 estimated prices in the Detroit, Michigan area. Prices vary depending on location. Black market price reflects typical prices from various sources.

ducts nearly 6500 drug tests on top-level athletes annually. These tests take place both in-competition and out-of-competition without notice at the athletes' training sites and homes.

On October 23, 2003, the **American College of Sports Medicine (ACSM)**, the largest sports medicine and exercise science organization in the world (http://www.acsm-msse.org), issued a statement that called for increased vigilance in identifying and eradicating steroid use. They condemned the development and use of new "designer" steroids such as THG that are cloaked to avoid detection by doping tests. ACSM considers the use of these chemicals "serious threats to the health and safety of athletes, as well as detriments to the principle of fair play in sports. Any effort to veil or disguise steroid use in sports through stealth, designer, or precursor means, puts elite, amateur and even recreational athletes at risk."

A Drug With a Considerable Following

Anabolic steroid use usually combines with resistance training and augmented protein intake to improve strength, speed, and power. The image of the steroid abuser often pictures massively developed body builders; abuse also occurs frequently among athletes in road cycling, tennis, track and field, baseball, American collegiate and professional football, and swimming. Surveys of U.S. Powerlifting Team members indicate that up to two thirds use androgenic–anabolic steroids.[52,253] In the United States, more than 300,000 men and women took anabolic steroids between 1992 and 1993.[269] These statistics, now more than 10 years old, are probably a conservative estimate, with a likely increase of at least 10% above the 1993 data. Federal authorities conservatively estimate that the business of illegal trafficking in steroids exceeds $100 million yearly.

Increasingly Prevalent Among Young Athletes and Nonathletes

Because many competitive and recreational athletes obtain steroids on the "black market" or the legal equivalent, androstenedione, from mall nutrition stores, misinformed individuals take massive and prolonged dosages without medical monitoring for possible harmful alterations in physiologic function. Particularly worrisome is steroid abuse among boys and girls as young as 10 and high school students who do not play team sports.[5,71,88,263] Accompanying risks including extreme virilization and irreversible premature cessation of bone growth in children who would otherwise continue to develop. One report indicated that 1 of 15 high school students or about one-half million adolescents (250,000 high school seniors) have used steroids—these same youngsters likely abuse other illicit drugs and share needles.[66,147,148] Those teenagers who use steroids cite improved athletic performance as the most common reason for

taking them, although 25% acknowledged enhanced appearance—simply wanting to look good—as the main reason.[31] In this struggle for self-image, a disturbance in body image (dissatisfaction/unhappiness with upper and lower body parts, facial features) contributes to anabolic steroid abuse among teenagers and young men.[264] The latest survey for federal drug agencies indicates that nearly half a million teenagers in the United States use anabolic steroids, with a 50% increase in use among high school seniors over the previous year. The National Institutes of Drug Abuse, an arm of the National Institutes of Health, claims that steroid use among high school sophomores more than doubled nationwide between 1992 and 2000. A Blue Cross/Blue Shield national survey noted a 25% increase in steroid and similar drug use from 1999 to 2000 among boys ages 12 to 17 (FIG. 11.2). Twenty percent of these teenagers took steroids to improve their looks, not to enhance sports performance. These findings certainly run counter to the Healthy People 2010 report indicating a decline in steroid use of 2.8% for male and 0.3% for female high school seniors based on data obtained in 1998.[240]

A bright side to this relatively gloomy picture has emerged. Research sponsored by the National Institute on Drug Abuse showed that student–athletes subject to random drug testing at an Oregon high school were almost three

Figure 11.2 On the upswing: percentage of adolescent students claiming to have used anabolic steroids at least once. (Source: University of Michigan.)

times less likely to use performance-enhancing substances such as steroids (nearly four times less likely to use drugs in general) than counterparts at a similar school that did not test.[89] The issue of drug testing of high school students remains controversial. In June 2002, the U.S. Supreme Court ruled that public schools could require students to participate in drug testing if they join any competitive after-school activity.

Effectiveness Questioned

For nearly five decades, researchers and athletes have debated the true effect of anabolic steroids on human body composition and exercise performance. Much of the confusion about anabolic steroids' ergogenic effectiveness stems from variations in experimental design: poor selection of controls; differences in specific drugs, dosages, treatment duration, accompanying nutritional supplementation, training intensity, evaluation techniques; and individual variation in response.[35,105,106] The relatively small residual androgenic effect of the steroid also may augment central nervous system function to make the athlete more aggressive (so-called "roid" rage), competitive, and fatigue resistant. Such facilitatory effects allow the athlete to train harder for a longer time or to believe that training improvement actually occurred. Abnormal alterations in mood and psychiatric dysfunction also are associated with androgen use.[227,230]

Research with animals suggests that anabolic steroid treatment, when combined with exercise and adequate protein intake, stimulates protein synthesis and increases a muscle's protein content (myosin, myofibrillar, and sarcoplasmic factors).[203] In contrast, other data show no benefit from steroid treatment on the leg muscle weight of rats subjected to functional overload by surgically removing the synergistic muscle.[157] In this study, treatment with anabolic steroids did not complement functional overload to stimulate muscle development.

The response of humans is often difficult to interpret. Some studies show augmented body mass gains and reduced body fat with steroid use in men who train, while other studies show no effects on strength and power or body composition, even with sufficient energy and protein intake to support an anabolic effect.[75,105] When steroid use produced body mass gains, the compositional nature of these gains (water, muscle, fat) remains unclear.

Patients receiving dialysis and those infected with the HIV commonly experience malnutrition, reduced muscle mass, and chronic fatigue. For dialysis patients, a 6-month supplement with the anabolic steroid nandrolone decanoate significantly increased lean body mass and the level of daily function.[120] Similarly, a moderate supraphysiologic androgen regimen that included the anabolic steroid oxandrolone substantially facilitated lean tissue accrual and muscle strength gains from resistance training in men with HIV compared with testosterone replacement alone.[228]

Dosage Is an Important Factor

Variations in drug quantity may account for confusion (and create a credibility gap between scientist and steroid abuser) about the true ergogenic effectiveness of anabolic steroids. Research focused on 43 healthy men with some resistance training experience. Diet (energy and protein intake) and exercise (standard weight lifting, three times weekly) were controlled, and steroid dosage (600 mg testosterone enanthate injected weekly or placebo) exceeded that in previous human studies. FIGURE 11.3 illustrates changes from baseline average values for fat-free body mass (FFM), triceps and quadriceps cross-sectional muscle areas, and muscle strength (1-RM) after 10 weeks of treatment. The men who received the hormone while continuing to train gained about 0.5 kg (1 lb) of lean tissue weekly, with no increase in body fat over the relatively brief 10-week treatment period. Even the group receiving the drug and not training significantly increased muscle mass and strength compared with men receiving the placebo, but their increases were less than those of men who trained while taking testosterone. The researchers emphasized they did not design their study to justify or endorse steroid use for athletic purposes because of the health risks (see next section). Their data indicated the potential for medically supervised anabolic steroid treatment to restore and enhance muscle mass from tissue-wasting diseases.

Do Risks Exist?

Debate exists about the health risks of anabolic steroids used by the athletic population because much of the research on steroid risk comes from medical observations.[229] *In our opinion, the infrequent but distinct possibility of harmful side effects from anabolic steroid treatment, particularly orally administered steroids, greatly outweighs any potential ergogenic effect.* Prolonged high dosages of steroids often impair normal testosterone endocrine function. Twenty-six weeks of steroid administration to male power athletes reduced serum testosterone to less than one half the level when the study began; this effect lasted throughout a 12- to 16-week steroid-free follow-up.[75] Infertility, reduced sperm concentrations (azoospermia), and decreased testicular volume pose additional problems for the steroid abuser.[85] Gonadal function usually returns to normal after several months of steroid cessation.

Other hormonal alterations that accompany steroid use in men include a sevenfold increase in estradiol concentration, the major female hormone. The higher estradiol level represents the average value for normal females and possibly explains the **gynecomastia** (excessive development of the male mammary glands, sometimes secreting milk) noted in men who take anabolic steroids. Steroid use with exercise training also causes connective tissue damage that decreases the tensile strength and elastic compliance of tendons.[139,145] Furthermore, steroids use causes the following four worri-

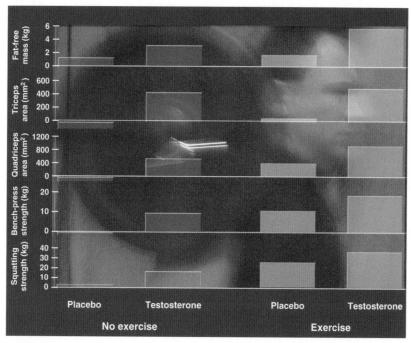

■ **Figure 11.3** Changes from baseline in mean fat-free body mass, triceps and quadriceps cross-sectional areas, and muscle strength in bench press and squatting exercises over 10 weeks of treatment. (From Bhasin S, et al. The effects of supraphysiological doses of testosterone on muscle size and strength in normal men. N Engl J Med 1996;335:1.)

some responses: *(a)* chronic stimulation of the prostate gland (may increase prostate size), *(b)* injury and alterations in cardiovascular function and myocardial cell cultures, *(c)* possible pathologic ventricular growth and dysfunction when combined with resistance training, and *(d)* impaired cardiac microvascular adaptation to exercise training, and increased blood platelet aggregation.[3,59,72,112,163,208,233] Increased blood platelet aggregation and impaired myocardial blood supply could increase risk of stroke and acute myocardial infarction.

Steroid Use and Life-Threatening Disease

Dramatic life-shortening effects of steroids occurred in adult rats exposed to the type and relative levels of steroids taken by physically active humans. One year after terminating the 6-month steroid exposure, 52% of the mice given the high dosage had died compared with 35% of the mice given the low dosage and only 12% of the control animals not given the exogenous hormone (FIG. 11.4). Autopsy of steroid-treated mice revealed a broad array of pathologic effects that did not appear until long after cessation of steroid use. Most prevalent pathologies included liver and kidney tumors, lymphosarcomas, and heart damage, frequently in combinations. A 6-month exposure period represents about one fifth of a male mouse's life expectancy, a relative duration considerably longer than exposures of most humans to steroid use. However, several of the pathologies, particularly liver damage, are typically seen in humans on steroids. These findings, if applicable to humans, indicate that it may require several decades before the true negative effects of anabolic steroid use emerge.

TABLE 11.4 lists the undesirable side effects and medical risks of anabolic steroid use. Concern centers on evidence about possible links between androgen abuse and abnormal liver function.[223] Because the liver almost exclusively metabolizes androgens, it becomes susceptible to damage from long-term steroid use and toxic excess. One of the serious effects of androgens on the liver occurs when it (and at times splenic tissue) develops localized blood-filled lesions, a condition called **peliosis hepatis**. In the extreme, the liver eventually fails and the patient dies. We present these data to emphasize the potentially serious side effects, even when a physician prescribes the drug in the recommended dosage. Although patients often take steroids for a longer duration than athletes, some athletes take steroids on and off for years, with daily doses exceeding typical therapeutic levels (5–20 mg vs. 50–200 mg used by athletes).

Steroid Use and Plasma Lipoproteins

Anabolic steroid use, particularly the orally active 17-alkylated androgens, in healthy men and women rapidly reduces high-density lipoprotein cholesterol (HDL-C), elevates both low-

Control Low dose High dose

Figure 11.4 Life-shortening effects of exogenous anabolic steroid use in mice. (Modified from Bronson FH, Matherne CM. Exposure to anabolic–androgenic steroids shortens life span of male mice. Med Sci Sports Exerc 1997;29:615.)

density lipoprotein cholesterol (LDL-C) and total cholesterol,[113,257] and reduces the HDL-C to LDL-C ratio.[46] The HDL-C of weightlifters who used anabolic steroids averaged 26 mg·dL^{-1} compared with 50 mg·dL^{-1} for weightlifters not taking the drug.[125] Reduced HDL-C at this level significantly increases a steroid user's coronary artery disease risk. HDL-C remained low among weightlifters, even after abstaining from steroid use for at least 8 weeks between consecutive steroid cycles.[209] The long-term effects of steroid use on cardiovascular morbidity and mortality remain undetermined.

Position Statement on Anabolic Steroids

As part of their long-range educational program, the ACSM has taken a stand on the use and abuse of anabolic–androgenic steroids.[7] We endorse their position, which follows.

Table 11.4 SIDE EFFECTS AND MEDICAL RISKS OF ANABOLIC STEROIDS

Males		Females	
Increase	*Decrease*	*Increase*	*Decrease*
Testicular atrophy	Sperm count	Voice change	Breast tissue
Gynecomastia	Testosterone levels	Facial hair	
		Menstrual irregularities	
		Clitoral enlargement	

Males and Females		
Increase	*Decrease*	*Possible*
LDL-C	HDL-C	Hypertension
LDL-C/HDL-C		Connective tissue damage
Potential for neoplastic disease of the liver		Myocardial damage
Aggressiveness, hyperactivity, irritability		Myocardial infarction
Withdrawal and depression upon stopping steroid use		Impaired thyroid function
Acne		Altered myocardial structure
Peliosis hepatitis		

LDL-C, low-density lipoprotein cholesterol; HDL-C, high-density lipoprotein cholesterol.

Steroid Side Effects in Females

Besides the broad range of side effects from anabolic steroid use, females have additional concerns about their dangers. These include virilization (more apparent than in men), disruption of normal growth pattern by premature closure of the plates for bone growth (also for boys), deepened voice, increased facial and body hair, altered menstrual function, dramatic increase in sebaceous gland size, acne, hirsutism (excessive body and facial hair), decreased breast size, and enlarged clitoris. More research is needed about the long-term effects of steroid use on reproductive function, including possible sterility.

CLENBUTEROL AND OTHER β_2-ADRENERGIC AGONISTS: ANABOLIC STEROID SUBSTITUTES?

Extensive, random testing of competitive athletes for anabolic steroid use worldwide, has ushered in a number of steroid "substitutes." These have appeared on the illicit health food, mail order, and "black market" drug network as competitors try to circumvent detection. One such drug, the sympathomimetic amine **clenbuterol** (brand names Clenasma, Monores, Novegan, Prontovent, and Spiropent) has become popular among athletes because of its purported tissue-building, fat-reducing benefits. When a body builder discontinues steroid use before competition to avoid detection and possible disqualification, the athlete substitutes clenbuterol to retard loss of muscle mass and facilitate fat burning to achieve the required "cut" look. Clenbuterol has particularly appeal to female athletes because it does not produce the androgenic side effects of anabolic steroids. Drug testing by use of gas chromatography coupled to high-resolution mass spectrometry introduced in the 1996 Atlanta Olympic Games detects most anabolic steroid use as far back as 18 months.

Clenbuterol, one of a group of chemical compounds (albuterol, clenbuterol, salbutamol, salmeterol, terbutaline) classified as a β_2-adrenergic agonist, facilitates responsiveness of adrenergic receptors to circulating epinephrine, norepinephrine, and other adrenergic amines. A review of the available studies of animals (no human studies) indicates that when fed to sedentary, growing livestock in dosages in excess of those prescribed in Europe for human use for bronchial asthma, clenbuterol increases skeletal and cardiac muscle protein deposition and slows fat gain (enhanced lipolysis). It also increases FFM and decreases fat mass when administered long term at therapeutic levels to thoroughbred racehorses.[127] Clenbuterol has been used experimentally in animals to counter the effects on muscle of aging, immobilization, malnutrition, and pathological tissue-wasting conditions. In these situations, the β_2-agonists show specific growth-promoting actions on skeletal muscle.[65,265,270] In rats, clenbuterol altered muscle fiber type distribution, inducing an enlargement and increased proportion of type II muscle fibers.[51] Decreased protein breakdown and increased protein synthesis accounted for the animals' increased muscle size from clenbuterol treatment.[1,21,150]

Potential Negative Effects on Muscle, Bone, and Cardiovascular Function

Female rats treated with clenbuterol ($2 \text{ mg} \cdot \text{kg}^{-1}$) injected subcutaneously or sham injected with the same volume of fluid carrier each day for 14 days significantly increased *(a)* muscle mass, *(b)* absolute maximal force-generating capacity, and *(c)* hypertrophy of fast- and slow-twitch muscle fibers.[62] A negative finding showed hastened fatigue during short-term, intense muscle actions. Others have noted similar positive and negative effects. For example, regular exercise and regular exercise combined with clenbuterol decreased the progression of muscular dystrophy in *mdx* mice as reflected by increases in muscle force-generating capacity.[270] The group receiving clenbuterol experienced increased muscle fatigability and cellular deformities not noted in the exercise-only group. This negative effect on muscle structure and function may explain findings that clenbuterol treatment negated the beneficial effects of exercise training on endurance performance of animals, despite increases in muscle protein content.[114] Clenbuterol treatment induced muscular hypertrophy in young male rats, but it concomitantly inhibited the longitudinal growth of bones.[132] This effect may relate to clenbuterol's acceleration of epiphyseal closure in the bones of growing animals, and certainly would contraindicate its use for prepubescent and adolescent humans.

Recent echocardiographic evaluations from Standardbred mares indicate that chronic clenbuterol administration, even at low therapeutic levels, changes the heart's structural dimensions in a manner that negatively alters cardiac function.[222] Effects occurred whether the animals exercised or remained inactive. Furthermore, clenbuterol caused the aorta to enlarge after exercise to a degree indicating increased risk of aortic rupture and sudden death. Clenbuterol treatment when combined with aerobic training also blunts the normal training-induced increase in plasma volume in Standardbred mares; this related to a decrease in aerobic exercise performance and ability to recover.[126]

Clenbuterol, not approved for human use in the United States, is commonly prescribed abroad as an inhaled bronchodilator for treating obstructive pulmonary disorders. Reported short-term side effects in humans accidentally "overdosing" from eating clenbuterol-tainted meat include skeletal muscle tremor, agitation, palpitations, dizziness, nausea, muscle cramps, rapid heart rate, and headache. Despite such negative side effects, supervised use of clenbuterol may benefit humans in treating muscle wasting in disease, forced immobilization, and aging. Unfortunately, no data exist for potential toxicity level or its efficacy and safety in long-term use. Clearly, clenbuterol cannot be justified or recommended for use as an ergogenic aid.

Other β₂-Adrenergic Agonists

Research has focused on possible strength-enhancing effects of sympathomimetic β₂-adrenergic agonists other than clenbuterol. Men with cervical spinal-cord injuries took 80 mg of metaproterenol daily for 4 weeks in conjunction with physical therapy. Significant increases occurred in estimated muscle cross-sectional area and strength of the elbow flexors and wrist extensors compared with the placebo condition.[219] Albuterol administration (16 mg per day for 3 weeks) without exercise training improved muscular strength 10 to 15%.[152] Therapeutic doses of albuterol also facilitated isokinetic strength gains from slow-speed concentric/eccentric isokinetic training.[34]

Training State Makes a Difference

Animals

Untrained skeletal muscle responds to the effects of β₂-adrenergic agonists. The increase in muscle mass with clenbuterol treatment plus exercise training becomes more pronounced in animals without prior training experience than in trained animals that continue training and then receive this β₂-adrenergic agonist.[172]

Humans

Some research shows augmented muscle power output with albuterol administration.[218] No ergogenic effect on short-term performance emerged from salbutamol administration in two 10-minute cycling trials.[47] Similarly, no effect on power output during a 30-second Wingate test occurred in nonasthmatic trained cyclists who received 360 μg (twice normal dose administered by inhaler in 4 measured doses of 90 μg each) 20-minutes before testing.[142] In other research, twice the recommended dose of salbutamol (albuterol; 400 μg administered in four inhalations 20 minutes before exercising) did not enhance anaerobic power output, endurance performance, ventilatory threshold, or dynamic lung function of trained endurance cyclists.[179] The researchers maintained that competitive athletes should not be prohibited from using these compounds because they provide no ergogenic benefit, yet they "normalize" individuals with obstructive pulmonary disorders. Differences in the groups' training status may explain discrepancies among studies concerning albuterol's effect on short-term power output.

Albuterol's ergogenic benefit supposedly comes from its stimulating effects on skeletal muscle β₂-receptors to increase muscle force and power. With exercise training, the muscle β₂-receptors undergo downregulation (become less sensitive to a given stimulus) from long-term exposure to training-induced elevations in blood catecholamine levels. This makes the trained athlete *less responsive* to a sympathomimetic drug than an untrained counterpart. More research must verify any ergogenic benefit of exogenous β₂-adrenergic agonists, elucidate possible mechanisms for action, and determine their influence on muscle mass.

GROWTH HORMONE: GENETIC ENGINEERING COMES TO SPORTS

Human growth hormone (GH or hGH), also known as *somatotropin*, now competes with anabolic steroids in the illicit market of alleged tissue-building, performance-enhancing drugs. The adenohypophysis of the pituitary gland produces GH, which serves as a potent anabolic and lipolytic agent for tissue building and growth and increasing fat catabolism. Specifically, GH stimulates bone and cartilage growth, enhances fatty acid oxidation, and slows glucose and amino acid breakdown. Reduced GH secretion (about 50% less at age 60 than age 30) accounts for some of the decreases in FFM and increases in fat mass that accompany aging. Exogenous recombinant GH supplements produced by genetically engineered bacteria can reverse these negative changes in body composition. Such results have led to a dramatic rise in the number of antiaging clinics throughout the country that provide GH to thousands of older persons looking to "turn back the clock," at a cost of $1000 or more a month.

Research has produced equivocal results concerning the true benefits of GH supplementation to counter the effects of aging—loss of muscle mass, thinning bones, increase in body fat, particularly abdominal fat, and a depressed energy level. For example, healthy men 70 to 85 years old who received GH supplements increased FFM by 4.3% and decreased fat mass by 13.1%.[187] Supplementation did not reverse the negative effects of aging on functional measures of muscular strength and aerobic capacity. Furthermore, men receiving the supplement experienced hand stiffness, malaise, arthralgias, and lower-extremity edema. One of the largest studies to date determined the effects of GH on changes in the body composition and functional capacity of healthy men and women ranging in age from mid-60s to late 80s.[22] Men who took GH gained 7 pounds of lean body mass and lost a similar amount of fat mass. Women gained about 3 pounds of lean body mass and lost 5 pounds of body fat compared with counterparts who received a placebo. The subjects remained sedentary and did not change their diet over the 6-month study period. Unfortunately, serious side effects afflicted between 24 and 46% of the subjects. These included swollen feet and ankles, joint pain, carpal tunnel syndrome (swelling of tendon sheath over a nerve in the wrist), and development of a diabetic or prediabetic condition. As in previous research, no effects were noted for GH treatment on measures of muscular strength or endurance capacity despite increased lean body mass.

Excessive GH production during the growth period produces **gigantism**, an endocrine and metabolic disorder that triggers abnormal size or overgrowth of the entire body or any of its parts. Excessive GH production following cessation of growth produces the irreversible disorder **acromegaly**. Enlarged hands, feet, and facial features characterize this malady. Medically, children who suffer from kidney failure or GH deficiency receive thrice-weekly injections of this hormone until adolescence, at a cost of about $20,000 to $40,000 yearly

to help them achieve near-normal size.[109] In young adults with hypopituitarism, GH replacement therapy improves muscle volume, isometric strength, and exercise capacity.

Disagreement Concerning Ergogenic Effects

At first glance, GH use seems appealing to the strength and power athlete because at physiologic levels this hormone stimulates amino acid uptake and muscle protein synthesis while enhancing lipid breakdown and conserving glycogen reserves. However, few well-controlled studies have examined how GH supplements affect healthy subjects who undertake exercise training. In one study, well-trained men maintained a high-protein diet while taking either biosynthetic GH or a placebo.[50] During 6 weeks of standard resistance training with GH, percentage body fat decreased and FFM increased. No changes in body composition occurred for the group training with the placebo. Subsequent investigations have not supported these findings.[58,268] Previously sedentary young men who participated in a 12-week resistance-training program received daily recombinant human GH supplements (40 $\mu g \cdot kg^{-1}$) or a placebo.[267] FFM, total body water, and whole body protein synthesis increased more in the GH recipients. No significant differences emerged between groups in fractional rate of protein synthesis in skeletal muscle and torso and limb circumferences. TABLE 11.5 shows equivalent effects of control and experimental treatments on muscle function in dynamic and static strength measures. The authors attributed the greater increase in whole body protein synthesis in the group receiving GH to a possible increase in nitrogen retention in lean tissue other than skeletal muscle (e.g., connective tissue, fluid, and noncontractile proteins).

Until fairly recently, healthy persons could only obtain GH on the black market and often in an adulterated form. Human cadaver-derived GH (used until May 1985 by U.S. physicians to treat children of short stature) greatly increases the risk for contracting Creutzfeldt-Jakob disease, an infec-

Table 11.5	MAXIMAL FORCE PRODUCTION OF KNEE EXTENSOR AND FLEXOR MUSCLE GROUPS BEFORE AND AFTER TRAINING WITH OR WITHOUT GROWTH HORMONE (GH) SUPPLEMENTS					
	Exercise plus Placebo			**Exercise plus GH**		
	Initial[a]	Final[a]	% Change	Initial[a]	Final[a]	% Change
Concentric						
Knee extensors	212 ± 13	248 ± 10	+17	191 ± 11	214 ± 9	+12
Knee flexors	137 ± 11	158 ± 7	+15	122 ± 12	143 ± 6	+17
Isometric						
Knee extensor	220 ± 13	252 ± 13	+14	198 ± 15	207 ± 7	+5
Knee flexors	131 ± 8	158 ± 8	+20	127 ± 13	140 ± 16	+10

From Yarasheski KF, et al. Effect of growth hormone and resistance exercise on muscle growth in young men. Am J Physiol 1992;262:E261.
[a] Values are mean ± SE. Maximum force (N) determined using a Cybex dynamometer. Concentric force measured at 60° · s^{-1} angular velocity. Isometric force measured at 135° of knee extension. The maximum concentric force production of the knee flexor and extensor muscles increased significantly in both groups (P < .05), but these increments and the increments in maximum isometric force production were not greater in the exercise plus GH group.

tious, incurable brain-deteriorating disorder. Currently, a synthetic form of GH (Protoropin and Humantrope) produced by genetic engineering is approved for treating GH-deficient children. But once a drug reaches market, doctors can prescribe it at their discretion. For example, over a 4-year period from 1997 to 2001, prescriptions for growth hormone have more than tripled from 6000 to 21,000. Men's fitness magazines currently advertise growth hormone, providing telephone numbers to call for a list of doctors who prescribe it. Undoubtedly, child athletes who take GH believing they gain a competitive edge will suffer increased incidence of gigantism, while adults will develop acromegalic syndrome. Additional less visual side effects include insulin resistance that leads to type 2 diabetes, water retention, and carpal tunnel compression.

DHEA: A WORRISOME TREND

Increased use of synthetic **dehydroepiandrosterone (DHEA)** by exercise enthusiasts and the general population has raised concerns about its safety and effectiveness among sports medicine personnel and the medical community in general. DHEA (and its sulfated ester, DHEA sulfate or DHEAS), a relatively weak steroid hormone, is synthesized from cholesterol, primarily by the adrenal cortex. A small amount of DHEA (commonly referred to as "mother hormone") and other related **prohormone compounds** are naturally derived precursors to testosterone or other anabolic steroids. FIGURE 11.5 outlines the major pathways for synthesizing DHEA, androstenedione, and related compounds. The quantity of DHEA the body produces surpasses all other known steroids with its largest concentrations in the brain. Its chemical structure closely resembles that of the sex hormones testosterone and estrogen. News reports and advertisements tout DHEA as a "superhormone," a "Holy Grail" that increases testosterone production, preserves youth, invigorates sex life, and counters the debilitating effects of aging. Home pages on the World Wide Web regularly extol its benefits.

Because DHEA occurs naturally, the Food and Drug Administration (FDA) has no control over its distribution or claims for its action and effectiveness. The lay press, mail order companies, and health food industry describe DHEA as

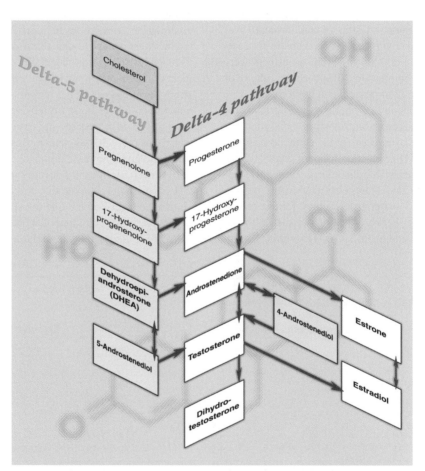

■ **Figure 11.5** Outline of metabolic pathways for dehydroepiandrosterone (DHEA), androstenedione, and related compounds. *Directional arrows* signify one-way and two-way conversions. Compounds in *bold print* are products currently available on the market.

Figure 11.6 Generalized trend for plasma levels of dehydroepiandrosterone (DHEA) for men and women during a lifetime.

a pill (even available as a chewing gum, each piece containing 25 mg) to cure just about any bodily ill. Advocates claim that it extends life; protects against cancer, heart disease, diabetes, and osteoporosis; enhances sexual drive; facilitates lean tissue gain and body fat loss; enhances mood and memory; improves muscular capacity; and boosts immunity against a variety of infectious diseases including AIDS. The hormone's detractors consider it "snake oil." The IOC and USOC have placed DHEA on their banned substance lists at zero tolerance levels.

FIGURE 11.6 illustrates the generalized trend for plasma DHEA levels during a lifetime. For boys and girls, DHEA levels are substantial at birth and then decline sharply. A steady increase in DHEA production occurs from age 6 to 10 years, an occurrence that some researchers feel contributes to the beginning of puberty and sexuality. Peak production occurs between ages 18 and 25 (higher in males than in females). In contrast to the glucocorticoid and mineralocorticoid adrenal steroids whose plasma levels remain relatively high with aging, a long, slow decline in DHEA begins after age 30. By age 75, the plasma level decreases to only about 20% of the value in young adulthood. This fact has fueled speculation that plasma DHEA levels might serve as a marker of biologic aging and disease susceptibility. Popular reasoning concludes that supplementing with DHEA blunts the negative effects of aging by raising plasma levels to more "youthful" concentrations.[190] Many persons supplement with this "natural" hormone just in case it proves beneficial, without considering the potential for harm.

An Unregulated Compound with Uncertain Safety

In 1994, the FDA reclassified DHEA (along with many other "natural" chemicals under the Dietary Supplement and Education Act) from the category of unapproved new drug (prescription required) to a dietary supplement for sale over the counter without a prescription. Pharmaceutical companies synthesize DHEA from chemicals found in soybeans and wild yams. In this process, other compounds such as androstenedione may be produced that contaminate the DHEA. Many consider the current unregulated and unmonitored use of DHEA by healthy men and women (daily dosage varies from 5 to 10 mg to as much as 2000 mg) a disaster waiting to happen. Despite its quantitative significance as a hormone, researchers know little about DHEA, particularly with respect to the following:

- Health and aging
- Cellular or molecular mechanism(s) of action
- Possible receptor sites (although its sulfate interacts with brain receptors for the neurotransmitter γ-aminobutyric acid [GABA])
- Potential for adverse effects from exogenous dosage, particularly among young adults with normal DHEA levels

The appropriate DHEA dosage for humans has not been determined. Concern exists about possible harmful effects on blood lipids, glucose tolerance, and prostate gland health. The major reason is because medical problems associated with hormone supplementation often do not appear until years after initiation of use. A number of over-the-counter supplements contain DHEA (and other prohormones). One can readily purchase DHEA through mainstream grocery chains, drug and nutrition stores, health clubs, mail-order catalogs, and the Internet.

Early support for DHEA came from studies of rodents fed daily supplements of this hormone.[54,68,91,213] Treatment indicated beneficial effects in preventing cancer, atherosclerosis, viral infections, obesity, and diabetes; enhancing immune function; and even extending life span. Scientists have argued that the findings from research on rats and mice—who produce little, if any, DHEA—do not necessarily apply to healthy humans. Cross-sectional observations relating levels of DHEA to risk of death from heart disease provided the early indirect evidence for a possible beneficial effect in humans. A high DHEA level conferred protection in men, while women with a high DHEA level increased their heart disease risk. Subsequent research showed only a moderate protective association for men and no association for women. Studies also suggested that DHEA supplements might provide a cardioprotective effect with aging (more beneficial in men than in women),[118] boost immune function in disease,[203] and provide antioxidant protection during aging.[12]

In other research on humans, middle-aged men and women received either 100 mg of DHEA or a placebo daily for 3 months, and the other treatment for the next 3 months.[169] Both groups exhibited a slight increase of 1.2%

in lean body mass during DHEA supplementation. Fat mass decreased in the men, but a small increase occurred for the women. Chemical markers also indicated improved immune function. These findings suggest some possible positive effects of exogenous DHEA on muscle mass and immune system function in middle-aged men and women. Subsequent research in young men evaluated short-term ingestion of 50 mg of DHEA daily on serum steroid hormones and the effect of 8 weeks of supplementation (150 mg daily) on resistance-training adaptations.[26] Short-term DHEA supplementation rapidly increased serum androstenedione concentrations (see FIG. 11.5 and next section), although it exerted *no effect* on serum testosterone and estrogen concentrations. Furthermore, longer-term DHEA supplementation raised serum androstenedione levels, but had *no effect* on anabolic hormones, serum lipids, liver enzymes, muscular strength, and lean body mass compared with a placebo given to men undergoing similar training. These and similar results of other investigators indicate that relatively low dosages of DHEA do not increase serum testosterone levels, enhance muscular strength or change muscle and fat cross-sectional areas, or facilitate adaptations to resistance training.[190,254]

Concern exists about the effect of unregulated long-term DHEA supplementation (particularly in doses >50 mg daily) on body function and overall health. Converting DHEA into potent androgens like testosterone in the body promotes facial hair growth in females and alters normal menstrual function. As with exogenous anabolic steroids, DHEA lowers HDL-cholesterol, which increases heart disease risk. Limited, conflicting data exist concerning its effects on breast cancer risk. Clinicians have expressed fear that elevated plasma DHEA through supplementation might stimulate growth of otherwise dormant prostate gland tumors or cause benign hypertrophy of the prostate gland itself. If cancer is present, DHEA may accelerate its growth. On a positive note, recent data show that supplements of DHEA for elderly men and women decreased abdominal (visceral) fat and improved the body's use of insulin.[249] Such findings indicate a potential for DHEA in treating components of the metabolic syndrome.

Despite its popularity among exercise enthusiasts, no data exist concerning ergogenic effects of DHEA supplements on young adult men and women. On a brighter side, DHEA supplementation may reduce the required dose of corticosteroid medication required by patients with the autoimmune disease lupus. This effect would certainly reduce side effects such as accelerated osteoporosis that accompany steroid therapy.

ANDROSTENEDIONE: BENIGN PROHORMONE NUTRITIONAL SUPPLEMENT OR POTENTIALLY HARMFUL DRUG?

Many physically active individuals now use the so-called legal over-the-counter "nutritional" supplement androstenedione (and androstenediol and norandrostenediol), believing that these steroid products *(a)* directly stimulate endogenous testosterone production or form androgen-like derivatives (as shown in Fig 11.5) and *(b)* enable them to train harder, build muscle mass, and repair injury more rapidly. Found naturally in meat and extracts of some plants, the World Wide Web touts androstenedione as "a prohormone, a metabolite only one step away from the biosynthesis of testosterone." The National Football League, NCAA, Men's Tennis Association, and the IOC ban its use because they believe it provides unfair competitive advantage and may endanger health. The IOC banned the 1996 Olympic shot-put gold medallist for life because he used androstenedione. Presently, Major League Baseball, the National Basketball Association, and the National Hockey League do not forbid its use. Despite the ban by certain sports governing bodies, supplements containing androstenedione and its derivatives remain readily available in a number of retail outlets to the millions of recreational and competitive athletes.

Originally developed by East Germany in the 1970s to enhance performance of their elite athletes, androstenedione was first commercially manufactured and sold in the United States in 1996. By calling the substance a supplement and avoiding any claims of medical benefits, the 1994 FDA rules enable androstenedione to be marketed as a food ($800 million in yearly sales on the Internet and over-the-counter). Because many countries consider androstenedione a controlled substance, individuals travel to the United States to purchase it, further contributing to the supplement industry's yearly sales. Currently available are an androstenedione-containing chewing gum and a steroid lozenge that dissolves under the tongue.

Androstenedione, an intermediate or precursor hormone between DHEA and testosterone, aids the liver in synthesizing other biologically active steroid hormones. Normally produced by the adrenal glands and gonads, it converts to testosterone enzymatically by 17β-hydroxysteroid dehydrogenase, found in diverse body tissues. Androstenedione also serves as an estrogen precursor.

Little scientific evidence supports claims about the effectiveness or anabolic qualities of andro-type compounds.[55,197] One study showed that oral treatment with 200 mg of 4-androstene-3,17-dione or 200 mg of 4-androstene-3β,17β-diol increased peripheral plasma total and free testosterone concentrations compared with a placebo.[67] Androstenedione dosages as high as 300 mg per day have elevated testosterone levels by 34%.[140] However, chronic androstenedione administration also elevates serum estradiol and estrone in men and women. This response could offset any potential anabolic effect.

A two-phase investigation systematically evaluated whether short- or long-term androstenedione supplementation elevates blood testosterone concentrations or enhances muscle size and strength gains during resistance training.[131] In one phase, young-adult men received either a single 100-mg dose of androstenedione or a placebo containing 250 mg of rice flour. FIGURE 11.7A shows that serum androstenedione rose 175% during the first 60 minutes following in-

■ **Figure 11.7 A.** Effect of short-term (single dose) exogenous supplementation with 100 mg of androstenedione or placebo on serum concentrations of androstenedione and free and total testosterone. **B.** Serum free and total testosterone, and **(C)** serum estradiol and estrone with 300-mg daily supplementation and androstenedione (n = 9) during 8 weeks of resistance training. (From King DS, et al. Effect of oral androstenedione on serum testosterone and adaptations to resistance training in young men. JAMA 1999;281:2020.)

gestion and then increased further to 350% above baseline values between minutes 90 and 270. On the other hand, short-term supplementation did not affect serum concentrations of either free or total testosterone.

In the experiment's second phase, young men received either 300 mg of androstenedione or 250 mg of a rice flour placebo daily during weeks 1, 2, 4, 5, 7, and 8 of an 8-week whole-body resistance-training program. Serum androstenedione levels increased 100% in the androstenedione-supplemented group and remained elevated throughout training. Although serum testosterone levels (FIG.11.7B) remained significantly higher in the androstenedione-supplemented group than in the placebo group before and after supplementation, they remained unaltered for both groups during the supplementation–training period. Serum estradiol and estrone concentrations increased significantly during training in the group receiving the supplement. This suggested increased aromatization of the ingested androstenedione to estrogens (FIG. 11.7C). While resistance training increased muscle strength and lean body mass and reduced body fat for both groups, no synergistic effect emerged with androstenedione supplementation. Instead, the supplement caused a 12% HDL-C *reduction* after only 2 weeks, which remained lower for the 8-week training period.[27,131] Serum liver enzyme concentrations remained within normal limits for both groups throughout the experimental period.

These findings indicate *no effect* of androstenedione supplementation on *(a)* basal serum concentrations of testos-

terone or *(b)* training response in terms of muscle size and strength and body composition. Worrisome are the potentially negative effects of a lowered HDL-C on overall heart disease risk and the elevated serum estrogen level on risk of gynecomastia and possibly pancreatic and other cancers. The findings must be viewed within the context of this specific study because test subjects took far smaller dosages of androstenedione (≤ 300 mg per day) than those routinely taken by body builders and other athletes.

RESEARCH FINDINGS CONCERNING ANDROSTENEDIONE

- Little or no elevation of plasma testosterone concentrations
- No favorable effect on muscle mass
- No favorable effect on muscular performance
- No favorable alterations in body composition
- Elevates a variety of estrogen subfractions
- No favorable effects on muscle protein synthesis or tissue anabolism
- Impairs the blood lipid profile in apparently healthy men
- Increases likelihood of testing positive for steroid use

Questions concerned the legal use of androstenedione by professional baseball players during the 1998 season in their attempt to break the home run records of Babe Ruth and Roger Maris. The sport-related issues focus on *(a)* whether supplementation increases muscular strength and power and *(b)* whether any fitness increase transfers performance improvements in the diverse, precise motor skills required in baseball, basketball, ice and field hockey, soccer, and golf. If positive effects occur then scientists should be able to objectively assess any improvements in such tasks. As far as we know, no reliable evidence demonstrates such sport-specific benefits. Further studies in larger groups of men and women for longer time periods must determine what dosage consistently raises testosterone to high enough levels long enough to provide ergogenic effects and whether such use causes harm. Currently, some athletes supplement with a daily dose of androstenedione in the range of 500 to 1200 mg.

A Modified Version. Norandrostenedione and norandrostenediol are norsteroid compounds available over-the-counter in the United States. They are chemically similar to androstenedione and androstenediol, respectively, with slight chemical modification that supposedly enhances anabolic properties without converting to testosterone but to the steroid nandrolone. These modifications should theoretically confer anabolic effects via the compounds' direct activation of the androgen receptors in skeletal muscle. To test this hypothesis, research evaluated 8 weeks of low-dose norsteroid supplementation on body composition, girth measures, muscular strength, and mood states of young adult, resistance-trained men.[243] The men received either 100 mg of 19-nor-4-androstene-3,17-dione plus 56 mg of 19-nor-4-androstene-3,17-diol (156 mg total norsteroid per day) or a multivitamin placebo. Each subject also resistance-trained 4 days a week for the duration of the study. Norsteroid supplementation provided *no additional effect* on any of the body composition or exercise performance variables measured.

Competitive Athletes Beware

Of great concern to the athletic community is that consuming trace amounts (as low as 10 μg) of 19-norandrostenedione daily (levels common in over-the-counter androstenedione) cause many users to test positive for 19-norandrosterone, the standard marker for the banned anabolic steroid nandrolone.[39] Because many nutritional supplements may be tainted with 19-norandrostenedione (and undisclosed by product labeling), the caveat "buyer beware" is all too apropos! Many androstenedione preparations are grossly mislabeled. Analysis of nine different 100-mg doses indicated wide fluctuations in overall content, ranging from 0 to 10 μg of 19-norandrostenedione, with one brand also containing testosterone. In summary, while androgen prohormone supplements taken in large dosages *may* transiently increase serum testosterone, available data indicate no ergogenic effects on muscular strength, no favorable changes in body composition, and no enhancement of overall health profile.

AMPHETAMINES

Amphetamines, or "pep pills," consist of pharmacologic compounds that exert a powerful stimulating effect on central nervous system function. Athletes most frequently use amphetamine (Benzedrine) and dextroamphetamine sulfate (Dexedrine). Amphetamines are sympathomimetic because their effects mimic actions of the sympathetic hormones epinephrine and norepinephrine. These hormones increase blood pressure, pulse rate, cardiac output, breathing rate, metabolism, and blood sugar. Taking 5 to 20 mg of amphetamine usually produces an effect for 30 to 90 minutes after ingestion, although the drug's influence persists for much longer. Besides arousing sympathetic function, amphetamines supposedly increase alertness and wakefulness and augment work capacity by depressing sensations of muscle fatigue. The deaths of two famed cyclists in the 1960s during competitive road racing were attributed to amphetamine use for just such purposes. In one of these deaths in 1967, British Tour de France rider Tom Simpson overheated and suffered a fatal heart attack during the ascent of Mont Ventoux. Soldiers in World War II commonly used amphetamines to increase alertness and reduce feelings of fatigue. Consequently, it should come as little surprise that athletes use amphetamines believing they gain an ergogenic edge; ironically, little or no performance advantage exists.

Dangers of Amphetamines

The following facts argue against amphetamine use:

- Chronic use leads to physiologic or emotional drug dependency. This often causes cyclical use of "uppers" (amphetamines) and "downers" (barbiturates)—the barbiturates reduce or tranquilize the "hyper" state brought on by amphetamines.
- General side effects include headache, tremulousness, agitation, insomnia, nausea, dizziness, and confusion, all of which negatively affect sports performance requiring rapid reaction and judgment and a high level of steadiness and mental concentration.
- Taking larger doses eventually requires more drug to achieve the same effect because drug tolerance increases with prolonged use; this may aggravate or even precipitate cardiovascular and mental disorders.
- The drugs suppress normal mechanisms for perceiving and responding to pain, fatigue, or heat stress; this effect severely jeopardizes health and safety.
- Prolonged intake of high doses produces weight loss, paranoia, psychosis, repetitive compulsive behavior, and nerve damage.

Amphetamine Use and Athletic Performance

TABLE 11.6 summarizes the results of seven experiments on amphetamine use and physical performance. In almost all instances, amphetamines produced little or no affect on exercise capacity or the performance of simple psychomotor skills.

Athletes take amphetamines to get "up" psychologically for competition. On the day or evening before a contest, competitors often seem nervous, irritable, and have difficulty relaxing. Under these circumstances, they take a barbiturate to induce sleep. They then regain the "hyper" condition by popping an "upper." This cycle of depressant-to-stimulant becomes potentially dangerous because the stimulant acts abnormally following barbiturate intake. The IOC, American Medical Association, and most sport-governing groups have rules that disqualify athletes for amphetamine use. Ironically, most research indicates that amphetamines do *not* enhance exercise performance. Perhaps their greatest influence pertains to the psychologic realm where naive athletes believe that taking any supplement contributes to a superior performance. A placebo containing an inert substance often produces identical results.

CAFFEINE

Caffeine represents a compound whose classification and prior regulatory status depends on its use as either a drug (over-the-counter migraine products), food (in coffee and soft drinks), or dietary supplement (alertness products).[74] Caffeine represent possible exception to the general rule against taking stimulants.[9,44,95,116,134,2**] The most widely consumed behaviorally active substance in the world, caffeine belongs to a group of lipid-soluble compounds called *purines* (chemical name, 1,3,7-trimethylxanthine) found naturally in coffee beans, tea leaves, chocolate, cocoa beans, and cola nuts and often added to carbonated beverages and nonprescription medicines. Sixty-three plant species contain caffeine in their leaves, seeds, or fruits. In the United States, 75% (14 million kg) of caffeine intake comes from coffee (3.5 kg per person per year), 15% from tea, and the remainder from the items listed in TABLE 11.7. Depending on preparation, one cup of brewed coffee contains 60 to 150 mg of caffeine, instant coffee about 100 mg, brewed tea between 20 and 50 mg, and caffeinated soft drinks about 50 mg. For comparison, 2.5 cups of percolated coffee contain 250 to 400 mg of caffeine or between 3 and 6 mg per kg of body mass. This produces urinary caffeine concentrations within the pre-

Table 11.6	SUMMARY OF RESULTS ON THE EFFECTS OF AMPHETAMINES ON ATHLETIC PERFORMANCE		
Study	*Dose (mg)*	*Type of Experiment*	*Effect of Amphetamines*
1	10–20	Two all-out treadmill runs with 10-min rest between runs	None
		Consecutive 100-yd swims with 10-min rest intervals	None
		220- to 440-yd swims for time	None
		220-yd track runs for time	None
		100-yd to 2-mile track runs for time	None
2	10	Bench stepping to fatigue carrying weights equal to 1/3 body mass, 3 times with 3-min rest intervals	None
3	5	100-yd swim for speed	None
4	10	All-out treadmill runs	None
5	10	Stationary cycling at work rates of 275–2215 kg-m·min^{-1} for 25–35 min followed by treadmill run to exhaustion	None on submaximal or maximal oxygen uptake, heart rate, ventilation volume, or blood lactic acid; work time on the bicycle and treadmill increased significantly
6	20	Reaction and movement time to a visual stimulus	None; subjective feelings of alertness or lethargy unrelated to reaction or movement time
7	5	Psychomotor performance during a simulated airplane flight	Enhanced performance and lessened fatigue, but if preceded by secobarbital (barbiturate), decreased performance

[1] Karpovich PV. Effect of amphetamine sulfate on athletic performance. JAMA 1959;170:558.
[2] Foltz EE, et al. The influence of amphetamine (Benzedrine) sulfate and caffeine on the performance of rapidly exhausting work by untrained subjects. J Lab Clin Med 1943;28:601.
[3] Haldi J, Wynn W. Action of drugs on efficiency of swimmers. Res Q 1959;17:96.
[4] Golding LA, Barnard RJ. The effects of *d*-amphetamine sulfate on physical performance. J Sports Phys Med Fitness 1963;3:221.
[5] Wyndham CH, et al. Physiological effects of the amphetamines during exercise. S Afr Med J 1971;45:247.
[6] Pierson WR, et al. Some psychological effects of the administration of amphetamine sulfate and meprobamate on speed of movement and reaction time. Med Sci Sports 1961;12:61.
[7] McKenzie RE, Elliot LL. Effects of secobarbital and D-amphetamine on performance during a simulated air mission. Aerospace Med 1965;36:774.

Table 11.7   CAFFEINE CONTENT (MG) OF SOME COMMON FOODS, BEVERAGES, AND OVER-THE-COUNTER AND PRESCRIPTION MEDICATIONS

Substance	Caffeine content (mg)	Substance	Caffeine content (mg)
Beverages and Foods		Pepsi Cola	38
Coffee[a]		Diet Pepsi, Pepsi Light, Diet RC, RC Cola, Diet Rite	36
Coffee, Starbucks, grande, 16 oz	550		
Coffee, Starbucks, tall, 12 oz	375	**Frozen Desserts**	
Coffee, Starbucks, short, 8 oz	250	Ben and Jerry's no fat coffee fudge frozen yogurt, 1 cup	85
Caffe, Starbucks, Americano, grande, 16 oz	105	Starbucks coffee ice cream, assorted flavors, 1 cup	40–60
Caffe, Starbucks, Americano, tall, 12 oz	70	Haagen-Dazs coffee ice cream, 1 cup	58
Caffe, Starbucks, Americano, short, 8 0z	35	Haagen-Dazs coffee frozen yogurt, fat-free, 1 cup	42
Caffe, Starbucks, latte or cappucinno, grande, 16 oz	70	Haagen-Dazs coffee fudge ice cream, low-fat, 1 cup	30
Caffe Mocha, Starbucks, short (8 oz) or tall (12 oz)	35	Starbucks frappuccino bar, 1 bar (2.5 oz)	15
Espresso, Starbucks, 8 oz	280	Healthy Choice cappuccino chocolate chunk or cappuccino mocha fudge ice cream, 1 cup	8
Brewed, drip method	110–150		
Brewed, percolator	64–124		
Instant	40–108	**Over-the-counter Products**	
Expresso	100	**Cold remedies**	
Decaffeinated, brewed or instant; Sanka	2–5	Dristan, Coryban-D, Triaminicin, Sinarest	30–31
Tea, 5 oz cup[a]		Excedrin	65
Brewed, 1 min	9–33	Actifed, Contac, Comtrex, Sudafed	0
Brewed, 3 min	20–46	**Diuretics**	
Brewed, 5 min	20–50	Aqua-ban	200
Iced tea, 12 oz; instant tea	12–36	Pre-Mens Forte	100
Chocolate		**Pain remedies**	
Baker's semi-sweet, 1 oz; Baker's chocolate chips, 1/4 cup	13	Vanquish	33
		Anacin; Midol	32
Cocoa, 5 oz cup, made from mix	6–10	Aspirin, any brand; Bufferin, Tylenol, Excedrin P.M.	0
Milk chocolate candy, 1 oz	6		
Sweet/dark chocolate, 1 oz	20	**Stimulants**	
Baking chocolate, 1 oz	35	Vivarin tablet, NoDoz maximum strength caplet, Caffedrine	200
Chocolate bar, 3.5 oz	12–15	NoDoz tablet	100
Jello chocolate fudge mousse	12	Enerjets lozenges	75
Ovaltine	0	**Weight control aids**	
Soft Drinks		Dexatrim, Dietac	200
7-Eleven Big Gulp Cola, 64 oz	190	Prolamine	140
Jolt	100	**Pain drugs**[b]	
Sugar Free Mr. Pibb	59	Cafergot	100
Mellow Yellow, Mountain Dew	53–54	Migrol	50
Tab	47	Fiorinal	40
Coca Cola, Diet Coke, 7-Up Gold	46	Darvon compound	32
Shasta-Cola, Cherry Cola, Diet Cola	44		
Dr. Pepper, Mr. Pibb	40–41		
Dr. Pepper, sugar free	40		

Data from product labels and manufacturers, and National Soft Drink Association, 1997.
[a] Brewing tea or coffee for longer periods slightly increases the caffeine content.
[b] Prescription, 1 oz ; 30 mL.
Caffeinism refers to caffeine intoxication characterized by restlessness, tremulousness, nervousness, excitement, insomnia, flushed face, dieresis, gastrointestinal complaints, rambling flow of thought and speech, tachycardia or cardiac arrhythmia, periods of inexhaustibility, and/or psychomotor agitation.

viously established IOC acceptable limit of 12 μg·mL^{-1} and NCAA limit of 15 μg·mL^{-1}. In January 2004, the IOC removed caffeine from its list of restricted substances.

The intestinal tract absorbs caffeine rapidly. with peak plasma concentration reached within 1 hour. Caffeine also clears from the body fairly rapidly, taking about 3 to 6 hours for blood caffeine concentrations to decrease by one half. As

a frame of reference, it requires about 10 hours for other stimulants like methamphetamine.

Ergogenic Effects

Drinking 2.5 cups of regularly percolated coffee 1 hour before exercising significantly extends endurance in strenuous aerobic exercise under laboratory conditions, as it also does in higher-intensity, shorter-duration effort.[29,63,220] An ergogenic effect even occurs with caffeine ingestion in the minutes just prior to exercising. Elite distance runners who consumed 10 mg of caffeine per kg of body mass immediately before a treadmill run to exhaustion improved performance time by 1.9% compared with placebo or control conditions.[79] Ergogenic effects during exhaustive exercise at 80% $\dot{V}O_2$max that follows a 5-mg·kg^{-1} caffeine dose is maintained 5 hours later during a subsequent exercise challenge.[17] Thus, there is no need to ingest a smaller additional caffeine dose to preserve high blood caffeine levels to sustain the ergogenic effect during subsequent exercise within 5 hours.

FIGURE 11.8 shows that subjects exercised for 90.2 minutes with 330 mg of preexercise caffeine compared with 75.5 minutes without it. Despite similar heart rate and oxygen uptake values during the two trials, the caffeine made the work "feel easier." Consuming caffeine 60 minutes before exercise increased exercise fat catabolism and reduced carbohydrate oxidation as assessed by plasma glycerol and free fatty acid levels and the respiratory quotient. The ergogenic effect of caffeine on endurance performance also applies to similar exercise performed at high ambient temperatures.[45]

Caffeine provides an ergogenic benefit during maximal swimming for durations less than 25 minutes. In a double-blind, crossover research design, competent male and female distance swimmers (<25 min for 1500-m swims) consumed caffeine (6 mg·kg body mass^{-1}) 2.5 hours prior to swimming 1500 m. FIGURE 11.9 illustrates that split times improved significantly with caffeine for

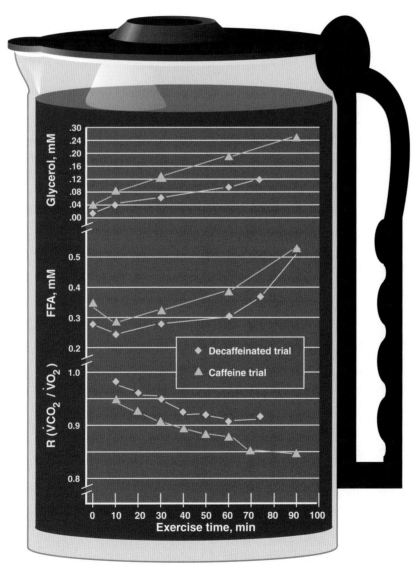

■ **Figure 11.8** Average values for plasma glycerol, free fatty acids *(FFA),* and the respiratory exchange ratio *(R)* during endurance exercise trials after ingesting caffeine and decaffeinated liquids. (From Costill DL, et al. Effects of caffeine ingestion on metabolism and exercise performance. Med Sci Sports 1978;10:155.)

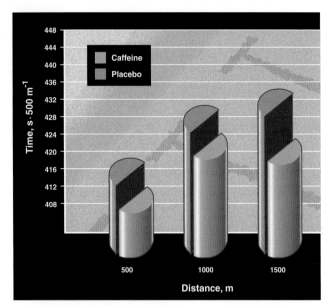

■ **Figure 11.9** Split times for each 500-m of a 1500-m for caffeine *(light purple)* and placebo *(dark purple)* time trials. Caffeine produced significantly faster split times. (From MacIntosh BR, Wright BM. Caffeine ingestion and performance of a 1,500-metre swim. Can J Appl Physiol 1995;20:168.)

each 500-m of the swim. Total swim time averaged 1.9% faster with caffeine than without it (20:58.6 vs. 21:21.8). Enhanced performance associated with lower plasma potassium concentration prior to exercise and higher blood glucose levels at the end of the trial. These responses suggest a possible caffeine effect on electrolyte balance and glucose availability.

No Dose-Response Relationship

FIGURE 11.10 illustrates the effects of preexercise caffeine on endurance time of well-trained male cyclists. Subjects received a placebo or a capsule containing 5, 9, or 13 mg of caffeine per kg of body mass 1 hour before cycling at 80% of maximal power output on a $\dot{V}O_2$max test. All caffeine trials improved exercise performance by 24%. No greater benefit occurred for quantities above 5 mg·kg body mass^{-1}.

Proposed Mechanism for Ergogenic Action

A precise explanation for the ergogenic boost from caffeine remains elusive.[92,93,149,188] *Most likely, the ergogenic effect of caffeine (or related methylxanthine compounds) in high-intensity, endurance exercise results from the facilitated use of fat as an exercise fuel, thus sparing the limited glycogen reserves.* Caffeine most likely acts in either of two ways: *(a)* directly on adipose and peripheral vascular

tissues[93,245] or *(b)* indirectly from stimulating epinephrine release by the adrenal medulla; epinephrine then acts to inhibit adipocyte cell adenosine receptors that normally repress lipolysis.[61,177]

Caffeine's inhibition of adenosine receptors on adipocyte cells increases cellular levels of cyclic-3',5'-adenosine monophosphate (cyclic-AMP). Cyclic-AMP, in turn, activates hormone-sensitive lipases to promote lipolysis, which releases free fatty acids into the plasma. Increased levels of free fatty acids contribute to increased fat oxidation, thus conserving liver and muscle glycogen. Sparing glycogen reserves benefits prolonged high-intensity exercise; diminished glycogen in active muscles coincides with reduced capacity to sustain a high rate of power output.

Some investigators have found the ergogenic effect to be unrelated to general hormonal or metabolic changes with

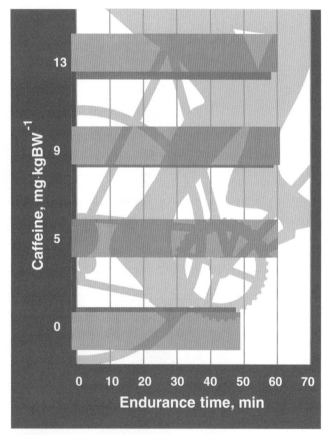

■ **Figure 11.10** Endurance performances following preexercise dosages of caffeine in different concentrations. The cycling time (min) represents the average for the nine male cyclists. All of the caffeine trials were significantly better than the placebo condition. No dose-response relationship occurred between caffeine concentration and endurance performance. The 5 mg per kg body mass dosage produced the only treatment that passed the IOC's doping standards for urinary caffeine concentrations. (From Pasman WJ, et al. The effect of different dosages of caffeine on endurance performance time. Int J Sports Med 1995;16:225.)

caffeine.[237] This suggests possible caffeine action on specific tissues including those of the central nervous system. Caffeine and its metabolites readily cross the blood–brain barrier to produce analgesic effects on the central nervous system. This effect would reduce the perception of effort during exercise. Caffeine also enhances motoneuronal excitability, thus facilitating motor unit recruitment. The stimulating effects of caffeine do not result from its direct action on the central nervous system. Rather, caffeine indirectly stimulates the nervous system by blocking another chemical neuromodulator, adenosine, which calms brain and spinal cord neurons. Four factors likely interact to produce caffeine's facilitating effect on neuromuscular activity:

1. Lowered threshold for motor unit recruitment
2. Altered excitation/contraction coupling
3. Facilitated nerve transmission
4. Increased ion transport within the muscle itself

Conflicting evidence concerns the effect of preexercise caffeine on $\dot{V}O_2$max.[61,236] Little effect has been noted for caffeine on repeated 20-m sprint running performance for team-sport female athletes.[189]

Effects Are Often Inconsistent

Prior nutrition partly accounts for the variation frequently observed among individuals in their exercise response after consuming caffeine. While caffeine generally elicits group improvements in endurance, individuals who normally consume a high-carbohydrate diet show little effect of caffeine on free fatty acid mobilization.[259] Individual differences in caffeine sensitivity, tolerance, and hormonal response from short- and long-term patterns of caffeine consumption also affect this drug's ergogenic qualities.[36,60] Interestingly, the ergogenic effects on endurance occur less for caffeine in coffee than for an equivalent dose from a caffeine capsule in water.[94] Apparently, components in coffee antagonize caffeine's actions. Beneficial effects do not consistently occur among habitual caffeine users;[234,244,246] thus, an athlete must consider "caffeine tolerance" before assuming it provides a consistent benefit to all persons. *From a practical standpoint, the individual should omit caffeine-containing foods and beverages 4 to 6 days before competition to optimize caffeine's potential for ergogenic effects.*

Effects on Muscle

Caffeine acts directly on muscle to enhance exercise capacity.[165,205,231] A double-blind research design evaluated voluntary and electrically stimulated muscle actions under "caffeine-free" conditions and following oral administration of 500 mg of caffeine.[146] Electrically stimulating the motor nerve enabled the researchers to remove central nervous system control and quantify caffeine's direct effects on skeletal muscle. Caffeine produced no effect on maximal muscle force during voluntary or electrically stimulated muscle actions. For submaximal effort, however, caffeine increased force output for low-frequency electrical stimulation before and after muscle fatigue. In addition, caffeine extended time to exhaustion on short-term tests of anaerobic power.[19] Preexercise caffeine administration also increased by 17% repeated submaximum isometric muscular endurance.[192] Caffeine probably exerts a direct and specific effect on skeletal muscle and its sensory processes during repetitive stimulation. Perhaps caffeine increases the sarcoplasmic reticulum's permeability to Ca^{2+}, thus making this mineral readily available for contraction. Caffeine could also influence the myofibril's sensitivity to Ca^{2+} to augment excitation–contraction coupling. In Chapter 12, we discuss how caffeine diminishes the ergogenic effect of creatine supplementation on short-term muscular power.[242]

Warning About Caffeine

Individuals who normally avoid caffeine can experience undesirable side effects when they consume it. Caffeine stimulates the central nervous system and in quantities greater than 1.5 g per day, can produce typical symptoms of caffeinism: restlessness, headaches, insomnia, and nervous irritability, muscle twitching, tremulousness, psychomotor agitation, and elevated heart rate and blood pressure and trigger premature left ventricular contractions. From the standpoint of temperature regulation, caffeine's effect as a potent diuretic could cause unnecessary preexercise loss of fluid that negatively affects thermal balance and exercise performance in a hot environment. This dehydrating effect is probably minimal when consumed in fluids during exercise because *(a)* an exercise-induced catecholamine release greatly reduces renal blood flow (and thus urine production) and *(b)* enhanced renal solute reabsorption in exercise facilitates water conservation (osmotic effect).[260]

Normal caffeine intake generally poses no significant health risk, yet death from caffeine overdose can occur. The LD_{50} (lethal oral dose required to kill 50% of the population) for caffeine is estimated at 10 g (150 mg·kg body mass^{-1}). Thus, for a 50-kg woman, significant acute health risk occurs at a caffeine intake of 7.5 g. Moderate caffeine toxicity has been reported in small children consuming 35 mg·kg body mass^{-1}. Such observations provide clear indication of the *inverted U-shaped relationship* between certain exogenous chemicals and exercise performance (and health and safety). For caffeine, if ingesting small-to-moderate quantities produces desirable effects, consuming significant excess can wreak havoc.

GINSENG AND EPHEDRINE

The popularity of herbal and botanical remedies to improve health, control body weight, and better exercise performance has soared. In 2001 alone, Americans spent $4.2 billion on such products. Ginseng and ephedrine are commonly marketed as nutritional supplements to "reduce tension," "revitalize," "burn calories," and "optimize mental and physical performance," particularly during times of fatigue and stress. The herb ginseng also plays a role as an alternative therapy to treat diabetes, stimulate immune function, and treat male impotence. Clinically, 1 to 3 g of ginseng administered 40 minutes before an oral glucose challenge reduces postprandial glycemia in nondiabetic subjects.[252] As with caffeine, ephedrine and ginseng occur naturally and for years have been used in folk medicine to enhance "energy."

Ginseng

Currently used in Asian medicine to prolong life, strengthen and restore sexual functions, and invigorate the body, the ginseng root (*Panax ginseng* C.A., Meyer), often sold as Panax or Chinese or Korean ginseng, currently serves no recognized medical use in the United States except as a soothing agent in skin ointments. Commercial ginseng root preparations generally take the form of powder, liquid, tablets, or capsules; widely marketed foods and beverages also contain various types and amounts of ginsenosides. Because dietary supplements need not meet the same quality control for purity and potency as pharmaceuticals do, considerable variation exists in the concentrations of marker compounds for ginseng as well as levels of potentially harmful impurities and toxins like pesticide and heavy metal contamination.[104] Neither the FDA nor other state or federal agencies routinely test ginseng-containing products or other nutritional supplements for quality or purity.

A common claim for ginseng in the Western world is its ability to boost energy and diminish the negative effects of overall stress on the body. Reports of an ergogenic effect often appear in nontraditional journals.[30] A review of the research literature provides little objective evidence to support the effectiveness of ginseng as an ergogenic aid.[4,15] For example, volunteers consumed either 200 or 400 mg of the standardized ginseng concentrate each day for 8 weeks in a double-blind research protocol.[70] Neither treatment significantly affected submaximal or maximal exercise performance, ratings of perceived exertion, or physiologic parameters of heart rate, oxygen consumption, or blood lactate concentrations. Similarly, no ergogenic effects emerged on diverse physiologic and performance variables following a 1-week treatment with a ginseng saponin extract administered in two doses of either 8 or 16 mg per kg of body mass.[168] When effectiveness has been demonstrated, the research has failed to use adequate controls, placebos, or double-blind testing protocols.[76] At present, no compelling scientific evidence exists that ginseng supplementation offers any ergogenic benefit for physiologic function or exercise performance.[143,250]

Ephedrine

Unlike ginseng, Western medicine recognizes the potent amphetamine-like alkaloid compound ephedrine (with sympathomimetic physiologic effects) found in several species of the plant ephedra (dried plant stem called ma huang [ma wong; *Ephedra sinica*]). The ephedra plant contains two major active components first isolated in 1928, ephedrine and pseudoephedrine, which exerts weaker effects than ephedrine. The medicinal role of this herb has included use to treat asthma, symptoms of the common cold, hypotension, and urinary incontinence and as a central stimulant to treat depression. Physicians in the United States discontinued using ephedrine as a decongestant and asthma treatment in the 1930s in favor of safer medications; pseudoephedrine occurs in over-the-counter decongestant preparations. The milder pseudoephedrine remains common in nonprescription cold and flu medications and has been clinically used to treat mucosal congestion that accompanies hay fever, allergic rhinitis, sinusitis, and other respiratory conditions. Ephedrine exerts both central and peripheral effects, with the latter reflected in increased heart rate, cardiac output, and blood pressure. Owing to its β-adrenergic effect, ephedrine produces bronchodilation in the lungs. High ephedrine dosages can produce hypertension, insomnia, hyperthermia, and cardiac arrhythmias. Other possible side effects include dizziness, restlessness, anxiety, irritability, personality changes, gastrointestinal symptoms, and difficulty concentrating.

Despite the legal and scientific categorizations of ephedrine as a potent drug, one could legally sell it as a dietary supplement. Its claim for accelerated metabolism and enhanced exercise performance greatly increased ephedrine's popularity as a nutritional supplement. Sales of $1.4 billion in the year 2002 included an array of products in capsule, drink, and chewing gum form. The botanical source of ephedra alkaloids had popularity as a weight-loss dietary supplement.[266] Many commercial weight-loss products contained combinations of ephedrine and caffeine designed to speed up metabolism. No credible evidence exists, however, that the initial weight loss obtained with high doses of ephedrine plus caffeine lasts beyond 6 months.[214]

The potent physiologic effects of ephedrine have led researchers to investigate its potential as an ergogenic aid—sold commercially (prior to its December 2003 ban by the FDA) as *Ripped Fuel, Metabolift, Xenadrine RFA-1, Hyrocut,* and *ThermoSpeed.* No effect of a 40-mg dose of ephedrine occurred on indirect indicators of exercise performance or ratings of perceived exertion (RPE).[57] The less concentrated pseudoephedrine also produced no effect on $\dot{V}O_2$max, RPE, aerobic cycling efficiency, anaerobic power output (Wingate test), time to exhaustion on a bicycle ergometer[110,232] and a 40-km cycling trial,[86] or physiologic and performance measures during 20 minutes of running at 70% of $\dot{V}O_2$max followed by a 5000-m time trial.[42] Conversely, a series of double-blind, placebo-controlled studies by the Canadian Defense and Civil Institute of Environmental Medicine using relatively high preexercise ephedrine dosage (0.8–1.0 mg·kg body mass^{-1}), either alone or combined with caffeine, produced small but statistically significant effects on endurance performance[16,18,20] and anaerobic power output during the early phase of the Wingate test.[19] Also, ephedrine supplementation increased muscular endurance during the first set of traditional resistance-training exercise.[117] Whether central mechanisms that increase arousal and tolerance to discomfort, peripheral mechanisms that influence substrate metabolism and muscle function, or the combined effect of both account for the ergogenic effect remains undetermined.

Numerous anecdotal reports exist of adverse effects from ephedra-containing compounds, but a cause-and-effect relationship between use and untoward responses, including death, remains hotly debated. On February 28, 2003, the FDA (www.fda.gov) ordered that a prominent warning label be emblazoned on the front of all ephedra products, listing death, heart attack, or stroke as possible consequences of use. Published reports indicate nearly 1400 adverse effects from ephedra use reported to the FDA from January 1993 to February 2000.Incidents included 81 deaths, 32 heart attacks, 62 cases of cardiac arrhythmia, 91 cases of increased blood pressure, 69 strokes, and 70 seizures. A recent evaluation of more than 16,000 adverse reactions showed "five deaths, five heart attacks, 11 cerebrovascular accidents, 4 seizures, and 8 psychiatric cases as 'sentinel events' associated with prior consumption of ephedra or ephedrine."[214] During 2001, 1178 adverse reactions were reported to American poison control centers. In general, the cardiovascular toxic effects of ephedra (increased heart rate and blood vessel constriction) are not limited to massive doses but rather to the amount recommended by the manufacturer. In 2002, an Alabama jury awarded $4.1 million to four persons who suffered strokes or heart attacks after taking an ephedra-based appetite suppressant produced by Metabolite International. In addition, the supplement maker Twin Laboratories Inc. has been sued by the families of a 28-year-old bodybuilder and a 27-year-old Marine Corps officer, blaming the men's deaths on the ephedra supplement called Ripped Fuel. For additional information on the untoward effects of ephedra, visit the web site of the Centers for Disease Control and Prevention (www.cdc.gov).

The IOC and NCAA currently ban ephedrine use, and the National Football League (NFL) represents the first professional sports league to do so. Although professional baseball discourages ephedrine use it does not ban its use. As of July 1, 2002, the NFL tested for this stimulant under the league's Policy on Anabolic Steroids and Related Substances. Any player who tests positive for ephedra is subject to a four- game suspension. Many players have acknowledged using the herbal stimulant seeking to lose weight or get a "quick burst of energy." The rationale for testing put forth by the NFL and the NFL Players Association was the growing evidence linking ephedrine-containing products to life-threatening strokes, seizures, thermoregulatory disorders that predispose to heat stroke, and heart arrhythmia. In spring training of 2003, ephedrine use was implicated in the death from organ failure complications in heat stroke of Baltimore Orioles pitcher Steve Bechler. He allegedly used the ephedrine-containing supplement Xenadrine RFA-1 to facilitate weight loss. Based on risk–benefit assessment, physicians have recently declared ephedra use unsafe, even when taken in recommended doses. Although products containing ephedra represent less than 1% of sales of all herbal supplements, they account for 64% of the adverse reactions. Consequently, ephedra poses a 200-fold greater risk than all other herbal supplements combined. Based on an analysis of existing data, including commissioning a safety study by independent research group (the Rand Corporation), the FDA announced on December 31, 2003 a ban on ephedra, the first time this federal agency has moved to ban a dietary supplement.

ALCOHOL

Alcohol, more specifically ethyl alcohol or ethanol (a form of carbohydrate), classifies as a depressant drug. Alcohol provides 7 kcal of energy per gram (mL) of pure (100% or 200 proof) substance. Adolescents and adults, athletes and nonathletes, abuse alcohol more than any other drug in the United States.[102,103] The 2001 National Household Survey on Drug Abuse by the U.S. Department of Health and Human Services Substance Abuse and Mental Health Services Administration summarizes alcohol consumption in the United States as follows:

- Almost half of Americans aged 12 or older reported being current drinkers of alcohol in the 2001 survey (48.3%). This translates to an estimated 109 million persons.
- Approximately one fifth (20.5%) of persons aged 12 or older participated in binge drinking at least once in the 30 days prior to the survey.
- Heavy drinking was reported by 5.7% of the population aged 12 or older, or 12.9 million persons.

- The prevalence of current alcohol use in 2001 increased with increasing age for youths, from 2.6% at age 12 to a peak of 67.5% for persons 21 years old. For persons aged 21 to 25 and those aged 26 to 34, the rates of current alcohol use in 2001 were 64.3 and 59.9%, respectively. Past-month drinking was reported by 45.6% of respondents aged 60 to 64, and 33.0% of persons 65 or older.

- The highest prevalence of both binge and heavy drinking in 2001 was for young adults aged 18 to 25, with the peak rate occurring at age 21. The rate of binge drinking was 38.7% for young adults and 48.2% at age 21. Heavy alcohol use was reported by 13.6% of persons aged 18 to 25 and by 17.8% of persons aged 21. Binge and heavy drinking were relatively rare among persons aged 65 or older, with reported rates of 5.8 and 1.4%, respectively.

- Of all youths, 10.6% were binge drinkers, and 2.5% were heavy drinkers.

Alcohol Use Among Athletes

Statistics remain equivocal about alcohol use among athletes compared with the general population. In a study of athletes in Italy, 330 male high school nonathletes consumed more beer, wine, and hard liquor and had greater episodes of heavy drinking (including greater cigarette smoking rates) than 336 athletes.[64] Interestingly, the strongest predictor of the participants' alcohol consumption was their best friend and girlfriend's drinking habits. In other research, physically active men drank less alcohol than sedentary counterparts.[101] Some athletes possess a more negative attitude about drinking than the general population,[185] but collegiate athletes generally drink more heavily and are more likely to drive while intoxicated than their nonathletic peers.[173] In a sample of former world-class Finnish athletes who competed between 1920 and 1965, the current alcohol consumption of the endurance athletes (average age, 57.5 years) was less than that of an age-matched control group.[73] A study of the relationship between athletic participation and depression, suicidal ideation, and substance use among high school students in Kentucky reported no greater alcohol consumption for 823 athletes than for the school's general student body.[182] Athletes also reported less depression, thoughts about suicide, and cigarette smoking and marijuana use than nonathletes. Teenage male athletes also drank 25.5% less beer and 39.9% less wine and whiskey than nonathletes.[77]

Several studies indicate that athletes are more likely to engage in binge drinking.[133,141,174] A self-reported questionnaire assessed alcohol intake of randomly selected students in a representative national sample of 4-year colleges in the United States.[175] Compared with nonathletic students, athletes were at high risk for binge drinking (≥5 alcoholic drinks on at least one occasion in the past

2 weeks for men and ≥4 for women), heavier alcohol use, and a greater number of drinking-related harms. Athletes were also more likely than nonathletes to surround themselves with (*a*) others who binge drink and (*b*) a social environment conducive to excessive alcohol consumption. These findings support the position that future alcohol prevention programs targeted to athletes should address the unique social and environmental influences that affect the current athletes' heavier alcohol use.

TABLE 11.8 compares serious male and female recreational runners and matched controls on responses to the Michigan Alcoholism Screening Test (MAST).[100] Male runners drank more (14.2 vs. 5.4 drinks per week) and felt guiltier about their drinking behavior (26.6%) than nonexercising controls (3.8%). Male and female runners drank more frequently than controls (2.8 vs. 2.3 times per week), while runners with MAST scores suggesting a history of problems with alcohol drank significantly less than nonathletic controls with a similar score. Men also consumed more alcohol and drank more frequently (including binge drinking) than women. While the controls reported that drinking alcohol did not interfere with sports participation and performance, the runners reported that they were unsure of alcohol's affect on their running and race performance. This study illustrates that problems associated with alcohol consumption do not exclude adult runners. However, running may serve as a healthy substitute for those runners prone to alcoholic behavior.

Alcohol's Action and Effect on Athletic Performance

Levels of Alcohol in Beverages and in the Body

One alcoholic drink contains 1.0 oz (28 g or 28 mL) of 100 proof (50%) alcohol.[181] This translates into 12 ounces of regular beer (about 4% alcohol by volume) or 5 ounces of wine (11–14% alcohol by volume). The stomach absorbs between 15 and 25% of the alcohol ingested. The small intestine rapidly takes up the remainder for distribution throughout the body's water compartments, particularly the water-rich tissues of the central nervous system. The absence of food in the digestive tract facilitates alcohol absorption. The liver, the major organ for alcohol metabolism, removes alcohol at a rate of about 10 g per hour, equivalent to the alcohol content of one drink. Consequently, consuming more than one drink per hour significantly increases blood alcohol concentration, expressed in grams per deciliter ($g \cdot dL^{-1}$).

Consuming two alcoholic drinks in 1 hour produces a blood alcohol concentration between 0.4 and 0.5 $g \cdot dL^{-1}$. However, factors such as age, body mass, body fat content, and gender influence blood alcohol level. Depending on the state, the legal limit for alcohol intoxication generally ranges between a blood alcohol concentration of 0.11 and 0.16 $g \cdot dL^{-1}$. Blood alcohol concentration above 0.40 (19

Table 11.8   RESPONSES FROM MALE AND FEMALE RECREATIONAL RUNNERS AND MATCHED CONTROLS TO THE SHORTENED[a] AND BRIEF[b] VERSIONS OF THE MICHIGAN ALCOHOLISM SCREENING TEST (MAST)

MAST Item	Men (N = 536)		Women (N = 262)	
	Runners, % (N)	Controls, % (N)	Runners, % (N)	Controls, % (N)
1. I am not a normal drinker.[a, b]	19.1 (75)	22.8 (31)	12.1 (17)	13.9 (16)
2. My friends and relatives think I'm not a normal drinker.[a, b]	14.5 (56)	22.8 (31)	10.1 (14)	13.0 (15)
3. Attended Alcoholics Anonymous for drinking.[a, b]	4.5 (18)	8.9 (12)	2.1 (3)	4.3 (5)
4. Lost friends because of drinking.[a]	6.1 (24)	7.9 (11)	1.4 (2)	4.3 (5)
5. Trouble at work because of drinking.[a, b]	3.8 (15)	5.0 (7)	0.7 (1)	3.4 (4)
6. Feel guilty about drinking.[b]	26.6 105)	13.8 (19)	16.7 (24)	15.5 (18)
7. Neglected obligations, family, work for 2 or more days in a row due to drinking.[a, b]	4.8 (19)	5.0 (7)	1.4 (2)	0.9 (1)
8. Experienced delirium tremens.[a]	4.3 (17)	2.9 (4)	0.7 (1)	3.4 (4)
9. Unable to stop drinking when desired.[b]	5.4 (21)	7.2 (10)	4.3 (6)	3.4 (4)
10. Sought help for drinking.[a, b]	5.3 (21)	7.2 (10)	2.1 (3)	6.0 (7)
11. Hospitalized for drinking.[a, b]	1.5 (6)	4.3 (6)	0.7 (1)	3.4 (4)
12. Drinking caused problems with spouse, parent, or other relative.[b]	20.6 (81)	21.0 (29)	2.8 (4)	8.5 (10)
13. Arrested for drunk driving.[a, b]	9.4 (37)	11.5 (16)	2.8 (4)	2.6 (3)
14. Arrested for drunken behavior.[b]	5.5 (22)	5.8 (8)	0.7 (1)	1.7 (2)

Adapted from Gutgesell M, et al. Reported alcohol use and behavior in long-distance runners. Med Sci Sports Exerc 1996;28:1063.
[a] Shortened MAST; from Binokur A, VanRooijen I. A self-administered short Michigan Alcoholism Screening Test (SMAST). J Stud Alcohol 1975;36:117.
[b] Brief MAST; from Pokorny AD, et al. The brief MAST: a shortened version of the Michigan Alcoholism Screening Test. Am J Psychiatry 1972;129:342.

drinks or more in 2 hours) leads to coma, respiratory depression, and eventual death.

Psychologic and Physiologic Effects

Athletes use alcohol to enhance performance because of its psychologic and physiologic effects. In the psychologic realm, some have argued that alcohol before competition reduces tension and anxiety (**anxiolytic effect**), enhances self-confidence, and promotes aggressiveness. It also facilitates neurological "disinhibition" because of its initial, though transitory, stimulatory effect. Thus, the athlete believes that alcohol facilitates physical performance at or close to physiologic capacity, particularly for activities requiring maximal strength and power. *Research does not substantiate any ergogenic effect of alcohol on muscular strength, short-term anaerobic power, or longer-term aerobic activities.*

Initially acting as a stimulant, alcohol's ultimate effect produces generalized neurologic depression (memory, visual perception, speech, motor coordination). These effects relate directly to blood alcohol concentration. Damping of psychomotor function causes the antitremor effect of alcohol ingestion. Consequently, alcohol use has been particularly prevalent in rifle and pistol shooting and archery, which require steadiness and accuracy. Achieving an antitremor effect also provides the primary rationale for using drugs called β-blockers such as propranolol, which diminish the arousal effect of sympathetic stimulation. Most research indicates that alcohol at best provides no ergogenic benefit; at worst, it precipitates undesirable side effects that impair performance (**ergolytic effect**). For example, alcohol's depression of nervous system function profoundly impairs just about all sports performances requiring balance, hand–eye coordination, reaction time, and overall need to process information rapidly. While these effects may vary considerably among individuals, they become apparent in a dose-response relationship at blood alcohol levels above 0.05 g·dL^{-1}.[170,180] In the extreme, it seems unlikely that a legally intoxicated person or team could perform optimally in competitive sports such as ping pong, volleyball, baseball, tennis, gymnastics, diving, soccer, or figure skating.

From a physiologic perspective, alcohol impairs cardiac function.[128,129] In one study, ingesting 1 g of alcohol per kg of body mass during 1 hour raised blood alcohol level to just over 0.10 g·dL^{-1}.[138] This level, often observed among "social drinkers," acutely depresses myocardial contractility. In terms of metabolism, alcohol blunts the liver's capacity to synthesize glucose from noncarbohydrate sources via gluconeogenesis. Each of these effects impairs performance in high-intensity aerobic activities that rely heavily on cardiovascular capacity and energy from carbohydrate catabolism. Alcohol provides no benefit as an energy substrate and does not favorably alter the metabolic mixture in endurance exer-

Alcohol Metabolism and Use: The Correct Approach

BACKGROUND

Abraham Lincoln, who enjoyed whiskey every now and then, once said, "It is true that many were injured by intoxicating drink, but none seemed to think the injury arose from the use of a bad thing, but from the abuse of a very good thing." President Lincoln most likely knew little about the medicinal benefits of "lighter drinking;" he simply enjoyed an occasional drink, like many persons in present-day society.

Alcohol abuse among college students, however, remains a persistent problem, representing the leading cause of death among individuals between ages 15 and 24. In America, more than 100,000 people die each year from alcohol-related deaths (mostly related to driving). Recently, advertisers have touted the health benefits of "light" drinking. Many individuals have used this as justification to increase alcohol consumption.

Much confusion exists regarding *(a)* alcohols' metabolic effects, *(b)* defining levels of intake, *(c)* determining safe intake limits, and *(d)* the role of alcohol as a nutrient.

ALCOHOL CHEMISTRY AND METABOLISM

Some alcohol metabolizes in the cells lining the stomach, while most breaks down in the liver. About 10% is directly eliminated by diffusion through the kidneys or the lungs. From a structural standpoint, ethanol contains a hydroxyl group (OH^-) and therefore resembles a carbohydrate. Because it converts directly to acetyl-CoA during catabolism, it does not proceed through glycolysis, in contrast to glucose and glycogen breakdown. Consequently, ethanol cannot provide substrate for glucose synthesis (gluconeogenesis). In metabolic terms, alcohol metabolizes more like a lipid than a sugar.

Alcohol concentration varies with the type of beverage. "Proof" value indicates its concentration, which equals two times the percentage concentration. For example, an 80-proof beverage contains 40% alcohol. When discussing alcohol consumption, "one drink" refers to a 12-oz bottle of beer, a 5-oz glass of table wine, or a cocktail with 1.5 oz of 80-proof liquor. Each of these drinks contains about 0.6 oz of alcohol by weight.

Alcohol Metabolism With Low Blood Alcohol Levels

At low consumption and correspondingly low blood levels, alcohol reacts with nicotinamide adenine dinucleotide (NAD) in the cell's cytosol to form acetaldehyde and NADH under the influence of the zinc-requiring enzyme alcohol dehydrogenase. Acetaldehyde then converts to acetyl-CoA (see Chapter 4) to yield more NADH. Acetyl-CoA enters the citric acid cycle; the NADH, $FADH_2$, and GTP molecules produced in acetaldehyde and acetyl-CoA formation and in the citric acid cycle provide energy to synthesize ATP (see Figure below)

Alcohol Metabolism With High Blood Alcohol Levels

When blood alcohol levels increase with high alcohol intake, alcohol dehydrogenase cannot sustain the metabolism of all

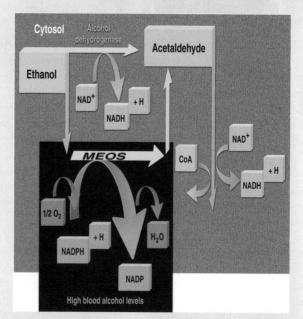

■ Alcohol metabolism. With low blood alcohol levels, the alcohol dehydrogenase pathway in the cytosol is used primarily. With high blood alcohol levels, the microsomal ethanol-oxidizing system (MEOS) in the cytosol is used. MEOS uses rather than yields energy.

CASE STUDY/PERSONAL HEALTH AND EXERCISE NUTRITION 11-1

alcohol into acetaldehyde. In this situation, an alternative metabolic pathway, the microsomal ethanol-oxidizing system (MEOS), becomes activated. MEOS uses considerable energy to break down alcohol, in contrast to the simpler alcohol dehydrogenase pathway that readily produces useful energy as ATP. Normally, the MEOS metabolizes drugs and other "foreign" substances in the liver. Under the stress of excessive alcohol intake, the liver "registers" alcohol as a foreign substance for breakdown by the MEOS. Chronic MEOS activation increases alcohol tolerance because high alcohol intake proportionally increases its rate of breakdown.

Rather than forming NADH by use of alcohol dehydrogenase (as occurs with moderate alcohol intake), the MEOS uses nicotinamide adenine dinucleotide phosphate (NADPH), a compound similar to NADH. However, instead of yielding potential ATP molecules via formation of NADH from the first step in alcohol breakdown, the MEOS uses potential ATP energy (in the form of NADPH) as NADPH converts to NADP. The use of different pathways to catabolize alcohol, depending on intake level, helps to explain why alcoholics do not gain the weight expected based on the alcohol-derived energy consumed. High alcohol use damages liver function in a manner that hampers other metabolic pathways. This cascading effect also contributes to the reduced energy yield associated with high alcohol use. In addition, alcohol increases metabolic rate to further contribute to an alcoholic's increased weight loss.

DETERMINING A SAFE LIMIT OF ALCOHOL INTAKE

Arbitrary limits define a "safe" alcohol intake, but "light," "moderate," and "heavy" represent the most common classifications. Historically, Anstie's rule (attributed to the British neurologist Sir Francis Edmund Anstie [1833–1874]), provided a frequently used operational definition, based on a person's ability to safely "handle" alcohol. At the time, the safe level for a typical male amounted to about three standard drinks daily (over 8 hours).

We now know that three factors—age, sex, and body weight (size)—determine a person's ability to "handle" alcohol. For a standard alcohol intake, blood alcohol levels inversely relate to body weight; the lower the weight, the greater the effect. Blood alcohol levels below 0.01% almost never impair function; levels from 0.01 to 0.04% sometimes impair function; 0.05 to 0.07% usually impair function; and levels of 0.08% and above always impair function. For most individuals who weigh less than 170 pounds blood alcohol levels achieve the usually impaired level with only two drinks over 2 hours. For those who exceed 170 pounds, three drinks in 2 hours impair function. Consequently, consuming no more than two drinks daily classifies as light-to-moderate drinking.

Benefits and Risks of Light-to-Moderate Drinking

For adults older than 18 years, light-to-moderate drinking associates with a lower risk of coronary heart disease, decreased incidence of ischemic stroke, and reduced occurrence of gallstones compared with alcohol abstinence. Moderate drinking is

not risk free, however. Obviously, any level of drinking increases addiction risk, particularly for individuals with a family history of alcoholism. Links exist between light-to-moderate drinking and female breast cancer risk, harm to the fetus, and increased colon cancer risk in men and women.

Risks of Heavy Drinking

Heavy drinkers experience the highest overall risk of morbidity (contracting illness) and mortality, compared with nondrinkers or to those who drink moderately. Heavy drinking associates with diverse health problems including cirrhosis of the liver, inflammation of the pancreas and stomach, certain cancers, high blood pressure, diseases of the heart muscle, heart arrhythmias, hemorrhagic stroke, and increased accidents and suicide.

GENERAL GUIDELINES FOR ALCOHOL USE

Neither the Surgeon General's office, the National Academy of Science, nor the U.S. Department of Agriculture/Department of Health and Human Services recommends drinking alcohol. All groups caution that if adults consume alcohol, it should be in moderation and with meals (no more than two drinks a day for men and one for women). Avoid drinking any alcohol before or while driving, operating machinery, taking medications, or engaging in other activity requiring sound judgment; no alcohol should be consumed while pregnant.

DO YOU HAVE A PROBLEM?

Asking a person about the quantity and frequency of alcohol consumption provides an important means to detect abuse and dependence. The following CAGE questionnaire is popular for use in routine health care.

CAGE QUESTIONNAIRE TO SCREEN FOR ALCOHOL ABUSE

C: Have you ever felt you ought to CUT down on drinking?

A: Have people ANNOYED you by criticizing your drinking?

G: Have you ever felt bad or GUILTY about your drinking?

E: Have you ever had a drink first thing in the morning to steady your nerves or get rid of a hangover (EYE-OPENER)?

More than one positive response to the GAGE questionnaire suggests an alcohol problem.

Marks DB, et al. Basic medical biochemistry. Baltimore: Williams & Wilkins, 1996.
Mayfield D, et al. The CAGE questionnaire: validation of a new alcoholism instrument. Am J Psychiatry 1974;131:1121.
Suter PM. Effects of alcohol on energy metabolism and body weight regulation: is alcohol a risk factor for obesity. Nutr Rev 55:157, 1997.

cise. In addition, substituting alcohol for high glycemic carbohydrates in the postexercise replenishment period decreases optimal glycogen storage in recovery.[32]

Alcohol and Fluid Replacement

Alcohol exaggerates the dehydrating effect of exercise in a warm environment; it acts as a potent diuretic by depressing antidiuretic hormone release from the posterior pituitary and blunting the arginine–vasopressin response.[210] Both of these effects impair thermoregulation during heat stress, thus placing the athlete at greater risk for heat injury during exercise.

Because many athletes consume alcohol-containing beverages after exercising and/or sports competition, one question concerns the degree to which alcohol impairs rehydration in recovery. Alcohol's effect on rehydration has been studied following exercise-induced dehydration of about 2% of body mass.[155,216,217] Subjects consumed rehydration fluid volumes equivalent to 150% of fluid lost and containing 0, 1, 2, 3, or 4% alcohol. Urine volume produced during the 6-hour study period directly related to the beverage's alcohol concentration—greater alcohol consumption produced more urine. Increases in plasma volume in recovery compared with the dehydrated state averaged 8.1% when the rehydration fluid contained no alcohol, but only 5.3% for the beverage with 4% alcohol content. The bottom line: *Alcohol-containing beverages impede rehydration.*

Alcohol acts as a peripheral vasodilator, so it should not be consumed during cold exposure or to facilitate recovery from hypothermia. A good "stiff drink" just won't warm you up! Current debate exists as to whether moderate alcohol intake exacerbates body cooling during mild cold exposure.[121]

The major conclusions of a position statement of the American College of Sports Medicine on alcohol use in sports remain as germane today as when first published in 1982.[6] Two main conclusions emerged: *(a)* acute alcohol ingestion impairs psychomotor skill, including reaction time, balance, accuracy, hand–eye coordination, and complex coordination and *(b)* alcohol does not improve and may even decrease strength, power, speed, local muscular endurance, and cardiovascular endurance.

Perhaps of Some Benefit

A moderate daily alcohol intake—2 oz or 30 mL of 90-proof alcohol, three 6-oz glasses of wine, or slightly less than three 12-oz beers—reduces a healthy person's risk of heart attack and stroke, independent of physical activity level,[14,207,262] and improves the likelihood of surviving a myocardial infarction.[171] The heart-protective benefit of moderate alcohol consumption also applies to individuals with type 2 diabetes.[241,256] The mechanism for benefit remains elusive, yet moderate alcohol intake increases HDL-C, particularly its subfractions HDL_2 and HDL_3.[84] In addi-

tion, certain components of red wine (e.g., polyphenols) may inhibit LDL-C oxidation, thus blunting a critical step in arterial plaque formation.[176,200] Moderate wine intake also associates with more "heart-healthy" dietary choices that positively affect plasma lipids.[235] For nondiabetic postmenopausal women, consuming 30 g (2 drinks) of alcohol each day benefited insulin and triacylglycerol concentrations and insulin sensitivity.[53] In contrast, excessive alcohol consumption offers no lipoprotein benefit and increases liver disease and cancer risk.[80]

PANGAMIC ACID

Some athletes tout pangamic acid, commonly known as "vitamin" B_{15}, for its alleged ergogenic benefits in aerobic exercise. Proponents argue that studies conducted in Russia showed that pangamic acid increased cellular oxygen use, reduced lactate buildup, and enhanced endurance performance. As with many proposed ergogenic aids, testimonials from athletes abound about the effectiveness of pangamic acid as a training aid and performance enhancer. Careful scrutiny of the early studies of pangamic acid raises questions concerning the validity of the findings owing to significant flaws in experimental design and research methods. Research in the United States failed to show any benefit of this compound for aerobic capacity, endurance performance, or circulating levels of blood glucose and lactate.[87,97] From a nutritional perspective, pangamic acid has no vitamin or provitamin properties; it serves no particular purpose in the body. In fact, synthetic mixtures sold as B_{15} may harm humans. FDA guidelines make it illegal to sell pangamic acid as a dietary supplement or drug.

BUFFERING SOLUTIONS

Dramatic alterations occur in the acid–base balance of the intracellular and extracellular fluids during maximal exercise of between 30- and 120-seconds duration because the muscle fibers rely predominantly on anaerobic energy transfer. As a result, significant quantities of lactate accumulate, with a concurrent fall in intracellular pH. Increased acidity inhibits the energy transfer and contractile capabilities of active muscle fibers, thereby causing exercise performance to decline.

The bicarbonate aspect of the body's buffering system provides a major line of defense against increased intracellular H^+ concentration (see Chapter 3). Maintaining high levels of extracellular bicarbonate rapidly releases H^+ from the cells and delays the onset of intracellular acidosis. Increasing bicarbonate (alkaline) reserves might enhance anaerobic exercise performance because increased H^+ concentration in intense exercise reduces the calcium sensitivity of the contractile proteins, which impairs muscle function.[43] Research in this area has produced conflicting results, perhaps from

| Table 11.9 | PERFORMANCE TIME AND ACID–BASE PROFILES FOR SUBJECTS UNDER CONTROL (PLACEBO) AND INDUCED PREEXERCISE ALKALOSIS CONDITIONS IMMEDIATELY BEFORE AND AFTER AN 800-M RACE | | | |

Variable	Condition	Pretreatment	Preexercise	Postexercise
pH	Control	7.40	7.39[a]	7.07[b]
	Placebo	7.93	7.40[a]	7.09[b]
	Alkalosis	7.40	7.49[a]	7.18[b]
Lactate (mmol·L^{-1})	Control	1.21	1.15[a]	12.62[b]
	Placebo	1.38	1.23[a]	13.62[b]
	Alkalosis	1.29	1.31[a]	14.29[b]
Standard HCO$_3^-$ (mEq·L^{-1})	Control	25.8	24.5[a]	9.90[b]
	Placebo	25.6	26.2[a]	11.00[b]
	Alkalosis	25.2	33.5[a]	14.30[b]

	Control	Placebo	Alkalosis
Performance Time (min)	2:05.8	2:05.1	2:02.9[c]

From Wilkes D, et al. Effects of induced metabolic alkalosis on 800-m racing time. Med Sci Sports Exerc 1983;15:277.
[a] Preexercise values significantly higher than pretreatment values.
[b] Alkalosis values significantly higher than placebo and control values after exercise.
[c] Alkalosis time significantly faster than control and placebo times.

variations in the preexercise sodium bicarbonate dose and the type of exercise to evaluate the effects of preexercise alkalosis.[96,161,226,258]

To improve experimental design, one early study evaluated the effects of acute induced alkalosis on short-term fatiguing exercise that greatly increased anaerobic metabolites. Trained middle-distance runners ran an 800-m race under normal (control) conditions or after ingesting either a sodium bicarbonate solution (300 mg per kg body mass) or a similar quantity of calcium carbonate placebo. TABLE 11.9

shows that the alkaline drink raised pH and standard bicarbonate levels before exercise. Subjects ran an average of 2.9 seconds faster under alkalosis and achieved higher postexercise values for blood lactate, pH, and extracellular H$^+$ concentration than those under placebo or control conditions.

The ergogenic benefit of preexercise alkalosis also occurs in women (FIG. 11.11). Moderately trained women performed one bout of maximal cycle ergometer exercise for 60 seconds on separate days in a double-blind research design under the following conditions: (a) control, no treatment,

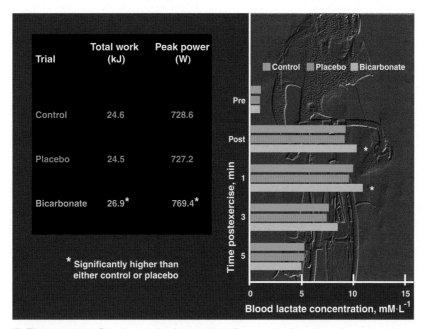

Figure 11.11 Bicarbonate loading and its effects on total work, peak power output, and postexercise blood lactate levels in moderately trained women. (From McNaughton LR, et al. Effect of sodium bicarbonate ingestion on high intensity exercise in moderately trained women. J Strength Cond Res 1997;11:98.)

(b) 300 mg·kg body mass^{-1} dose of sodium bicarbonate in 400 mL of low-calorie flavored water 90 minutes prior to testing, and *(c)* placebo of equimolar dose of sodium chloride (to maintain intravascular fluid status as in bicarbonate condition) 90 minutes prior to testing. Exercise capacity represented total work accomplished during the ride. The figure's inset box shows that total work performed and peak power output reached higher levels with preexercise bicarbonate treatment than with either control or placebo conditions. The bicarbonate treatment also produced a higher level of blood lactate in the immediate and 1-minute postexercise periods, which explained the greater anaerobic exercise capacity. Similar benefits of induced alkalosis occur in short-term anaerobic performance using exogenous **sodium citrate** as the alkalinizing agent.[107,159]

Augmented anaerobic energy transfer during exercise probably explains the ergogenic effect of preexercise alkalosis.[111,194,196] More than likely, increased extracellular buffering from exogenous bicarbonate or citrate facilitates coupled transport of lactate and H$^+$ across the muscle cell membrane during anaerobic exercise.[123] This delays the fall in intracellular pH and its subsequent negative effects on muscle function. Nearly 3 seconds represents a dramatic improvement in 800-m race time; it transposes to a distance of about 19 m at race pace, bringing a last place finisher to first place!

Effects Related to Dosage and Degree of Exercise Anaerobiosis

The interaction between bicarbonate dosage and the cumulative anaerobic nature of the exercise influences the ergogenic effects of preexercise alkalosis. Doses of at least 0.3 g per kg body mass (ingested about 1 to 2 h precompetition) facilitate H$^+$ efflux from the cell. This significantly enhances a single maximal effort of 1 to 2 minutes duration,[90,153,160] including longer-term arm or leg exercise that exhausts within 6 to 8 minutes.[202] Even long-term bicarbonate ingestion (0.5 g per kg body mass) for 5 days added to the normal diet raised plasma pH and increased performance in a 60-second maximal effort. No ergogenic effect emerges for typical resistance training exercises (e.g., squat, bench press), perhaps because of the generally lower absolute anaerobic metabolic load compared with continuous, maximal whole-body activities.[258] Bicarbonate loading with all-out effort of less than 1 minute improves performance *only* with repetitive exercise bouts that produce high intracellular H$^+$ concentrations.[49]

Inconsistencies in the research literature cloud the issue concerning the effectiveness of preexercise alkalosis. For example, despite dose-dependent changes in pH, base excess, and HCO$_3^-$ after ingestion of sodium citrate, no effect occurred on measures of performance in a bicycling time trial, even when the simulated race contained a multiple-sprint component.[211]

High-Intensity Endurance Performance

Preexercise alkalosis does not benefit low-intensity, aerobic exercise (because pH and lactate remain near resting levels), but some research indicates benefits in prolonged aerobic exercise of higher intensity.[162] More specifically, race times of trained male cyclists were better after consuming sodium citrate (0.5 g per kg body mass) prior to a 30-km time trial than in placebo trials.[193] Despite the relatively small anaerobic component in high-intensity aerobic exercise (compared with short-term, all-out exercise), ingesting buffer before exercise facilitates lactate and hydrogen ion efflux. This maintains pH closer to normal resting levels to improve muscle function in prolonged effort.

Although the IOC does not ban alkalinizing agents, more research must clarify the ergogenic benefits (and possible dangers) of short-term induced alkalosis. Individuals who bicarbonate-load often experience abdominal cramps and diarrhea about 1 hour after ingestion. This adverse effect would surely minimize any potential ergogenic benefit. Substituting the buffering agent sodium citrate (0.4–0.5 g per kg body mass) for sodium bicarbonate can reduce or eliminate adverse gastrointestinal effects.[144,158]

PHOSPHATE LOADING

The rationale concerning preexercise phosphate supplementation ("phosphate loading") focuses on increasing the levels of extracellular and intracellular phosphate. This may in turn *(a)* increase the potential for ATP phosphorylation, *(b)* increase aerobic exercise performance and myocardial functional capacity, and *(c)* augment peripheral oxygen extraction in muscle tissue by stimulating red blood cell glycolysis and subsequent elevation of erythrocyte 2,3-diphosphoglycerate (2,3-DPG). The compound 2,3-DPG, produced within the red blood cell during the anaerobic reactions of glycolysis, binds loosely with subunits of hemoglobin, thus reducing its affinity for oxygen. Additional oxygen then releases to the tissues for a given decrease in the cellular oxygen pressure.

Despite the theoretical rationale for ergogenic effects with phosphate loading, benefits have not consistently emerged.[2,83,151] Some studies show improvement in maximal oxygen uptake ($\dot{V}O_2$max)[135,136] and arteriovenous oxygen difference following phosphate loading, whereas others report no effects on aerobic metabolism and cardiovascular function.[2,151]

There are major reasons for the inconsistencies in research findings; these include variations in exercise mode and intensity, dosage and duration of supplementation, standardization of pretest diets, and subjects' fitness level. In one study, subjects with low and high aerobic capacities consumed a drink containing either 22.2 g of dibasic calcium phosphate or a calcium carbonate placebo.[83] Each subject then pedaled a cycle ergometer for 20 minutes at an exercise intensity equivalent to 70% $\dot{V}O_2$max, followed by a

30-minute rest and then an incremental ride to exhaustion. For high- and low-fitness groups, no differences occurred for any of the variables measured, including erythrocyte 2,3-DPG, submaximal or maximal oxygen uptake, exercise time to exhaustion, and plasma lactate in submaximal exercise.

Little reliable scientific evidence exists to recommended exogenous phosphate as an ergogenic aid. On the negative side, excess plasma phosphate stimulates secretion of **parathormone**, the parathyroid hormone. Excessive production of this hormone accelerates the kidneys' excretion of phosphate and facilitates reabsorption of calcium salts from bones to cause loss of bone mass. Research has not yet determined whether short-term phosphate supplementation poses a risk to normal bone dynamics

ANTICORTISOL COMPOUNDS: GLUTAMINE AND PHOSPHATIDYLSERINE

The hypothalamus secretes corticotrophin-releasing factor as a normal response to emotional stress, trauma, infection, surgery, and physical exertion such as resistance training. This releasing factor, in turn, stimulates the anterior pituitary gland to secrete adrenocorticotropic hormone (ACTH), which induces the adrenal cortex to release the glucocorticoid hormone cortisol (hydrocortisone). Cortisol decreases amino acid transport into the cell; this depresses anabolism and stimulates protein breakdown to its building-block amino acids in all cells except liver cells. The circulation delivers these "liberated" amino acids to the liver for synthesis to glucose (gluconeogenesis). Cortisol also serves as an insulin antagonist by inhibiting glucose uptake and oxidation.

A prolonged, elevated serum concentration of cortisol (usually from therapeutic exogenous glucocorticoid intake in drug form) leads to excessive protein breakdown, tissue wasting, and negative nitrogen balance. The potential catabolic effect of cortisol has convinced many bodybuilders and other strength and power athletes to use supplements thought to inhibit the body's normal cortisol release. They believe that blunting cortisol's normal rise following exercise augments muscular development with resistance training by attenuating catabolism. In this way, muscle tissue synthesis progresses unimpeded in recovery. Glutamine and phosphatidylserine are two supplements used to produce an anticortisol effect.

Glutamine

Glutamine, a nonessential amino acid, is the most abundant amino acid in plasma and skeletal muscle. It accounts for more than one half of the muscles' free amino acid pool. Glutamine exerts many regulatory functions, one of which provides an anticatabolic effect and augments protein synthesis.[119,156,261] Glutamine supplementation effectively

counteracts the decline in protein synthesis and muscle wasting from repeated glucocorticoid use. In one study of female rats, infusing glutamine for 7 days inhibited the downregulation of myosin (muscle contractile protein) synthesis and atrophy in skeletal muscle that normally accompanies chronic glucocorticoid administration.[108]

Data also indicate that infusing glutamine following exercise promotes muscle glycogen accumulation in human muscle in recovery, perhaps by serving as a gluconeogenic substrate in the liver.[248] The practical application of these findings for promoting glycogen replenishment in recovery or enhancing glycogen accumulation in the preexercise period requires further research. The potential anticatabolic and glycogen- synthesizing effects of exogenous glutamine have promoted speculation that glutamine supplementation might benefit responses to resistance training.[11] However, daily glutamine supplementation (0.9 g per kg lean tissue mass) during 6 weeks of resistance training in healthy young adults did not affect muscle performance, body composition, or muscle protein degradation compared with a placebo.[33]

Immune Response

Glutamine plays an important role in normal immune function. Through its use as metabolic fuel by disease-fighting cells that defend against infection.[199,255] Glutamine plasma concentrations decrease following prolonged high-intensity exercise, so a glutamine deficiency has been linked to the immunosuppression caused by strenuous exercise.[23,198,204]

Chapter 7 discusses glutamine and the immune response, particularly in regards to supplementation and the incidence and severity of upper respiratory tract infections.

Phosphatidylserine

Phosphatidylserine (PS) is a glycerophospholipid typical of a class of natural lipids that constitute the structural components of biologic membranes, particularly the internal layer of the plasma membrane that surrounds all cells. Through its potential for modulating functional events in the plasma membrane (e.g., number and affinity of membrane receptor sites), PS might modify the neuroendocrine response to stress. In one study, healthy men consumed 800 mg of PS derived from bovine cerebral cortex daily for 10 days.[167] Three 6-minute intervals of cycle ergometer exercise of increasing intensity induced physical stress. Compared with the placebo condition, the PS treatment significantly diminished ACTH and cortisol release without affecting growth hormone release. These results confirmed earlier findings by the same researchers that a single intravenous PS injection counteracted hypothalamic–pituitary–adrenal axis activation with exercise.[166] Soybean lecithin provides most PS used for supplementation by athletes, yet research showing physiologic effects have used bovine-derived PS. Subtle differences in the chemical structure of these two forms of PS may create differences in physiologic action, including the potential for ergogenic effects.

Is Cortisol Release Really "Bad"?

Research must determine if the normal release and rise in serum cortisol with heavy training actually counteracts muscular growth and development and recovery and repair. One could argue that cortisol release with exercise represents an appropriate and beneficial response to physiologic function and overall good health. It also remains unclear whether a supplement-induced decrease in cortisol output with resistance training translates into greater improvements in muscular strength and size.

β-HYDROXY-β-METHYLBUTYRATE

β-Hydroxy-β-methylbutyrate (HMB), a bioactive metabolite generated from the breakdown of the essential branched-chain amino acid leucine, may decrease protein loss during stress by inhibiting protein catabolism. A marked decrease in protein breakdown and a slight increase in protein synthesis occurred in muscle tissue of rats and chicks (in vitro) exposed to HMB.[183] Data also suggest an HMB-induced increase in fatty acid oxidation in vitro in mammalian muscle cells exposed to HMB.[41] Depending on the amount of HMB contained within foods—relatively rich sources include catfish, grapefruit, breast milk—the body synthesizes between 0.3 and 1.0 g daily, of which about 5% derives from dietary leucine catabolism. Because of its possible nitrogen-retaining effects, many resistance-trained athletes supplement directly with HMB to prevent or slow muscle damage and depress muscle breakdown (proteolysis) associated with intense physical effort.

Research has studied the effects of exogenous HMB on skeletal muscle's response to resistance training.[81,122,137,178,186,221] For example, young adult men participated in two randomized trials. In *study 1*, 41 subjects received 0, 1.5, or 3.0 g of HMB (calcium salt of HMB mixed with orange juice) daily at two protein levels, either 115 g or 175 g per day for 3 weeks. The men lifted weights during this time for 1.5 hours, 3 days a week for 3 weeks. In *study 2*, subjects consumed either 0 or 3.0 g of HMB per day and weight lifted for 2 to 3 hours, 6 days a week for 7 weeks. In the first study, HMB supplementation significantly depressed the exercise-induced rise in muscle proteolysis as reflected by urine 3-methylhistidine and plasma creatine phosphokinase (CPK) levels during the first 2 weeks of training. These biochemical indices of muscle damage ranged between 20 and 60% lower in the HMB-supplemented group. In addition, this group lifted more total weight than the unsupplemented group during each training week (FIG. 11.12A), with the greatest effect in the group receiving the largest HMB supplement. Specifically, muscular strength in-

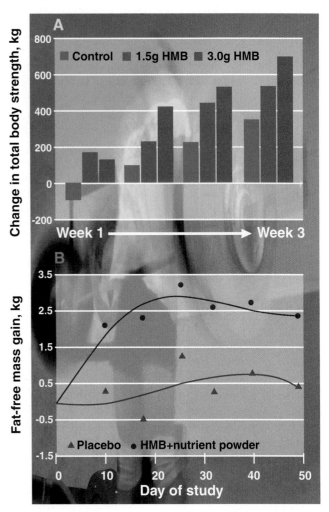

■ **Figure 11.12** A. Change in muscle strength (total of upper- and lower-body exercises) during *study 1* from week 1 to week 3 in subjects supplemented with HMB (β-hydroxy-β-methylbutyrate). Each grouping of bars represents one complete set of upper- and lower-body workouts. B. Total body electrical conductivity assessed change in fat-free body mass during *study 2* for a control group that received a carbohydrate drink *(placebo)* and an HMB group that received 3 g Ca-HMB per day mixed in a nutrient powder *(HMB + nutrient powder)*. (From Nissen S, et al. Effect of leucine metabolite β-hydroxy-β-methylbutyrate on muscle metabolism during resistance-exercise training. J Appl Physiol 1996;81:2095.)

creased 8% for the unsupplemented group, whereas it increased 13% for the 1.5-g HMB per day group and 18.4% for the 3.0-g HMB per day group. Additional protein (not indicated in graph) provided no augmenting effect on any of the measurements. The lack of effect with additional protein should be viewed in proper context because the group consuming the "lower" protein quantity (115 g per day) received the equivalent of about twice the protein RDA.

In *study 2*, subjects who received the HMB supplement had significantly higher FFM than unsupplemented subjects at 2 and 4–6 weeks of training (Fig. 11.12B). However, at the last measurement during training the difference between groups decreased to the point at which no statistical significance between pretraining baseline values occurred.

The mechanism for HMB's action on muscle metabolism, strength improvement, and body composition remains unknown. Researchers speculate that this metabolite inhibits normal proteolytic processes that accompany intense muscular overload. While the results appear to demonstrate an ergogenic effect of HMB supplementation, it remains to be shown just what component of the FFM (protein, bone, water) HMB affects. Furthermore, the data in Figure 11.12B indicate potentially transient body-composition benefits of supplementation that tend to revert toward the unsupplemented state as training progresses. Additional studies must verify the present findings and assess the long-term effects of HMB supplements on body composition, training responsiveness, and overall health and safety.

Not all research shows beneficial effects of HMB supplementation with resistance training.[81,195,221] One study evaluated the effects of varied amounts of HMB (approximately 3 vs. 6 g·d^{-1}) on muscular strength during 8 weeks of resistance training in untrained, young men.[81] The study's primary finding indicated that HMB supplementation, regardless of dosage, produced *no difference* in most of the strength data (including 1-RM strength) compared with placebo treatment. Increases in training volume remained similar among groups. Significantly lower levels of CPK in both HMB-supplemented groups in recovery indicate some potential effect of HMB in inhibiting muscle breakdown with resistance training. HMB supplementation with a dosage as high as 6 g·d^{-1} during 8 weeks of resistance training does not appear to cause adverse effects on hepatic enzyme function, blood lipid profile, renal function, or immune function.[82] Age does not affect responsiveness to HMB–supplementation.[251]

A NEW TWIST: HORMONAL BLOOD BOOSTING

To eliminate the cumbersome and lengthy process of blood doping, endurance athletes now use recombinant **epoietin (EPO)**, a. synthetic form of **erythropoietin**. This hormone, produced by the kidneys, regulates red blood cell production within the marrow of the long bones. Exogenous epoetin, commercially available since 1988, has proven clinically useful in combating anemia in patients with severe renal disease. Normally, a decrease in red blood cell concentration or decline in the pressure of oxygen in arterial blood—as in severe pulmonary disease or on ascent to high altitude—releases EPO to stimulate erythrocyte production. The 5 to 12% increase in hemoglobin and hematocrit (% red blood cells in 100 mL blood) that typically occurs following a 6-week EPO treatment significantly improves endurance-exercise performance.[69,206] Unfortunately, if self-administered in an unregulated and unmonitored manner—simply injecting the hormone requires much less sophistication than procedures for blood doping—hematocrit can increase by more than 60%. This dangerously high hemoconcentration (and corresponding increase in blood viscosity) increases the likelihood for stroke, heart attack, heart failure, and pulmonary edema.

EPO use has become particularly prevalent in cycling competition and allegedly has contributed to at least 18 deaths (attributed to heart attacks) among competitive bicyclists. EPO cannot be detected in urine, so blood hematocrit level serves as a surrogate marker. During the 1997 and 1998 competitive seasons, Tour de France officials spot-checked the hematocrits of riders, suspending for 2 weeks any rider with an abnormally high value. This resulted in suspension of 12 riders during 1997 and 6 riders midway through the 1998 competitive season. The International Cycling Union has set a hematocrit threshold of 50% for males and 47% for females, while the International Skiing Federation uses a hemoglobin concentration of 18.5 g·dL^{-1} as the disqualification threshold. Hematocrit cutoff values of 52% for men and 48% for women (roughly 3 standard deviations above the mean normal value) represents "abnormally high" or extreme values in triathletes.[184] Of course, use of a hematocrit level cutoff raises the unanswered question concerning the number of disqualified "clean" cyclists. Estimates place this number at between 3 and 5%, due mainly to factors that affect normal variation in hematocrit such as genetics, posture, altitude training, and hydration level.[13,28]

The 2002 Olympics did not escape controversy; the Russian Olympic Committee threatened to withdraw from the Salt Lake City Winter Games. One of four incidents cited as the basis of their complaint concerned disqualification of the 20-km cross-country ski relay team because of an elevated hemoglobin concentration of one of its members, a nine-time Olympic medalist. The Russians claimed a false-positive test result. Additionally, the IOC stripped two cross-country skiers from Spain and Russia of gold medals (and banished them from future Olympic competition) after they tested positive for darbepoietin, a blood-boosting analogue of erythropoietin.

Current concern by the medical community centers on an anomaly in iron metabolism frequently observed among elite international cyclists. Large numbers of these athletes typically show serum iron levels in excess of 500 ng·L^{-1} (normal iron level, 100 ng·L^{-1}) with some values as high as 1000 ng·L^{-1}. The elevated iron level results from regular injections of supplemental iron to support the increased synthesis of red blood cells induced by repeated EPO use. Chronic iron overload increases the risk of liver dysfunction among these athletes.

Other Means to Enhance Oxygen Transport

New classes of substances may emerge to enhance aerobic exercise performance.[212] These doping threats include perfluorocarbon emulsions and solutions formulated from either bovine or human hemoglobin that improve oxygen transport and delivery to muscle. Despite their potential benefits in clinical use, these substances exhibit potentially lethal side effects that include increased systemic and pulmonary blood pressure, renal toxicity, and impaired immune function.

IN THE FUTURE

As we envision the future, we see many physically active individuals, particularly athletes, with medicine chests containing an array of pharmaceutics that guarantee "even more fantastic" benefits than today's armamentarium of natural and synthetic "aids." As long as winning remains the priority, individuals will experiment with substances to improve exercise and sports performance and the response to training. Realistically, we see little hope for curbing this trend. We wish for optimism and decry presenting a negative perspective, but at this time we can offer little in constructive comment on how to stem the onslaught of commercial exploitation. The quest for an ergogenic boost in athletics had its roots 2500 years ago in the ancient Olympic Games. Perhaps the new generation of testing equipment can stay one step ahead of the abusers, but this seems doubtful. Increased legal statutes and penalties can curb the abuse, but drug enforcement remains difficult. Maintaining stricter laws at the local, state, and national levels may provide some relief, but thus far, additional vigilance by law enforcement has not curbed the problem. Perhaps a clearer identification of the characteristics of at-risk athletes and a vigorous education about drug abuse (coupled with a focus on improving the individual's decision-making skills and substituting more healthful alternatives) beginning in the early school years and continuing through college offers some limited hope for future generations.[10,238] We certainly hope so.

Summary

1. Ergogenic aids consist of substances or procedures that improve physical work capacity, physiologic function, or athletic performance.

2. Anabolic steroids, pharmacologic agents commonly used as ergogenic aids, function similarly to the hormone testosterone. Research findings often are inconsistent, and the precise mechanism(s) of action unclear.

3. Negative side effects of anabolic steroid use in males include infertility, reduced sperm concentrations, decreased testicular volume, gynecomastia, connective tissue damage that decreases the tensile strength and elastic compliance of tendons, chronic stimulation of the prostate gland, injury and functional alterations in cardiovascular function and myocardial cell cultures, possible pathologic ventricular growth and dysfunction, and increased blood platelet aggregation that can compromise cardiovascular system health and function and increase risk of stroke and acute myocardial infarction.

4. Unique negative side effects of anabolic steroid use in females include virilization (more apparent than in men), deepened voice, increased facial and body hair (hirsutism), altered menstrual function, dramatic increase in sebaceous gland size, acne, decreased breast size, and enlarged clitoris. The long-term effects of steroid use on reproductive function remain unknown.

5. The β_2-adrenergic agonists clenbuterol and albuterol increase skeletal muscle mass and slow fat gain in animals to counter the effects of aging, immobilization, malnutrition, and tissue-wasting pathology. A negative finding showed hastened fatigue during short-term, intense muscle actions.

6. Debate exists as to whether administration of exogenous growth hormone to normal, healthy people augments increases in muscle mass when combined with resistance training.

7. DHEA levels decrease steadily throughout adulthood, prompting many individuals (including large numbers of athletes) to supplement with this hormone in the hope of optimizing training and countering the effects of aging.

8. No data support the ergogenic effects of DHEA supplements on young adult men and women.

9. Research findings generally indicate *no effect* of androstenedione supplementation on basal serum concentrations of testosterone or training response in terms of muscle size and strength and body composition. Worrisome are the potentially negative effects of a lowered HDL-C on overall heart disease risk and the elevated serum estrogen level on risk of gynecomastia and possibly pancreatic and other cancers

10. Little credible evidence exists that amphetamines ("pep pills") aid exercise performance or psychomotor skills any better than an inert placebo. Side effects of amphetamines include drug dependency, headache, dizziness, confusion, and upset stomach.

11. Caffeine can exert an ergogenic effect in extending aerobic exercise duration by increasing fat use for energy, thus conserving glycogen reserves. These effects become less apparent in individuals who (a) maintain a high-carbohydrate diet or (b) habitually use caffeine

12. No compelling scientific evidence exists to conclude that ginseng supplementation offers positive benefit for physiologic function or performance during exercise. Accumulating evidence indicates significant health risk accompany ephedrine use.

13. Consuming ethyl alcohol produces an acute anxiolytic effect because it temporarily reduces tension and anxiety, enhances self-confidence, and promotes aggression. Other than the antitremor effect, alcohol conveys no ergogenic benefits and likely impairs overall athletic performance (ergolytic effect).

14. Increasing the body's alkaline reserve before anaerobic exercise by ingesting buffering solutions of sodium bicarbonate or sodium citrate improves performance. Buffer dosage and the cumulative anaerobic nature of the exercise interact to influence the ergogenic effect of bicarbonate (or citrate) loading.

15. Little scientific evidence exists to recommend exogenous phosphates or pangamic acid as ergogenic aids.

16. An objective decision about the potential benefits and risks of glutamine, phosphatidylserine, and β-hydroxyl-β-methyl butyrate to provide a "natural" anabolic boost with resistance training for healthy individuals awaits further research.

17. Erythropoietin (EPO), a hormone produced by the kidneys that regulates red blood cell production within the marrow of the long bones, increases hemoglobin and hematocrit to improve endurance performance. Significant risks accompany its unsupervised use.

TEST YOUR KNOWLEDGE ANSWERS

1. False Ancient athletes of Greece reportedly used hallucinogenic mushrooms for ergogenic purposes, while Roman gladiators ingested the equivalent of "speed" to enhance performance in the Circus Maximus. Athletes of the Victorian era routinely used chemicals such as caffeine, alcohol, nitroglycerine, heroin, cocaine, and the rat poison strychnine for a competitive edge.

2. True A "placebo effect" refers to improved performance due to psychologic factors in that the individual performs at a higher level simply because of the suggestive power of believing that a substance or procedure should work.

3. False Anabolic steroids function in a manner similar to testosterone, the chief male hormone. Prolonged high dosages of anabolic steroids often impair normal testosterone endocrine function, cause infertility, reduce sperm concentrations (azoospermia), decrease testicular volume, induce connective tissue damage, increase prostate size, cause injury and alterations in cardiovascular function and myocardial cell cultures, produce possible pathologic ventricular growth and dysfunction when combined with resistance training, impair cardiac microvascular adaptations, and diminish myocardial blood supply, leading to stroke and acute myocardial infarction.

4. False Little scientific evidence supports claims about the effectiveness or anabolic qualities of andro-type compounds. Research findings show that androstenedione (a) elevates plasma testosterone concentrations, (b) exerts no favorable effect on muscle mass, (c) does not favorably affect muscular performance, (d) does not favorably alter body composition, (e) provides no beneficial effects on muscle protein synthesis or tissue anabolism, and (f) impairs the blood lipid profile in apparently healthy men.

5. True The following reasons argue against amphetamine use by athletes: it leads to physiologic or emotional drug dependency; induces headache, tremulousness, agitation, insomnia, nausea, dizziness, and confusion, all of which negatively affect sports performance requiring rapid reaction and judgment; taking larger doses eventually requires more of the drug to achieve the same effect because drug tolerance increases with prolonged use; aggravates or even precipitates cardiovascular and mental disorders; or suppresses normal mechanisms for perceiving and responding to pain, fatigue, or heat stress; and it can produce unwanted weight loss, paranoia, psychosis, repetitive compulsive behavior, and nerve damage.

6. False Drinking 2.5 cups of regularly percolated coffee about 1 hour before exercising significantly extends endurance in strenuous aerobic exercise under laboratory conditions, as it does in higher-intensity, shorter-duration effort. An ergogenic effect even occurs with caffeine ingestion in the minutes just prior to exercising. Elite distance runners who consume 10 mg of caffeine per kg of body mass immediately before a treadmill run to exhaustion improve performance time by 1.9% compared with placebo or control conditions.

7. False An increasing belief in the potential for selected foods to promote health has led to coining the term *functional food*. Beyond meeting three basic nutrition needs (survival, hunger satisfaction, and preventing adverse effects), functional foods comprise those foods and their bioactive components (e.g., olive oil, soy products, n-3 fatty acids) that promote well being, health, and optimal body function or reduce disease risk. Examples include many polyphenolic substances (simple phenols and flavinoids found in fruits and vegetables), carotenoids, soy isoflavones, fish oils, and components of nuts that possess antioxidant and other properties that decrease risk of vascular diseases and cancers. Primary targets for this expanding branch of food science include gastrointestinal functions, antioxidant systems, and macronutrient metabolism.

8. False Many commercial weight-loss products contain combinations of ephedra and caffeine, supposedly designed to accelerate metabolism. No evidence exists that the initial weight loss obtained with high doses of ephedrine plus caffeine lasts beyond 6 months. In 2003, the FDA ordered that a prominent warning label be emblazoned on the front of all ephedra products listing death, heart attack, or stroke as possible consequences of use. In addition, a recent evaluation of more than 16,000 adverse reactions showed "five deaths, five heart attacks, 11 cerebrovascular accidents, four seizures, and eight psychiatric cases as 'sentinel events' associated with prior consumption of ephedra or ephedrine." In December 2003 the FOA banned the use of ephedra as a dietary supplement.

9. False Alcohol's effect on rehydration has been studied following exercise-induced dehydration of about 2% of body mass. Increases in plasma volume in recovery compared with the dehydrated state averaged 8.1% when the rehydration fluid contained no alcohol, but only 5.3% for the beverage with 4% alcohol content. The bottom line: Alcohol-containing beverages impede rehydration.

10. True Many resistance-trained athletes supplement directly with HMB to prevent or slow muscle damage and depress muscle breakdown (proteolysis) associated with intense physical effort. Subjects who received an HMB supplement showed significantly higher fat-free body mass than unsupplemented subjects. However, not all research has shown beneficial effects of HMB supplementation with resistance training. Furthermore, available data indicate potentially transient body-composition benefits of supplementation that revert toward the unsupplemented state as training progresses. Additional studies must verify beneficial findings, and assess the long-term effects of HMB supplements on body composition, training responsiveness, and overall health and safety.

References

1. Agbenyega ET, Warham AC. Effect of clenbuterol on normal and denervated muscle growth and contractility. Muscle Nerve 1990;13:199.
2. Ahlberg A, et al. Effect of phosphate loading on cycle ergometer performance. Med Sci Sports Exerc (abstr) 1986;18:S11.
3. Ajayi AAL, et al. Testosterone increases human platelet thromboxane A_2 receptor density and aggregation responses. Circulation 1995;91:2742.
4. Allen JD, et al. Ginseng supplementation does not enhance healthy young adults peak aerobic exercise performance. J Am Coll Nutr 1998;17:462.
5. American Academy of Pediatrics. Adolescents and anabolic steroids: a subject review. Pediatrics 1997;99:904.
6. American College of Sports Medicine. The use of alcohol in sports. Med Sci Sports Exerc 1982;14:481.
7. American College of Sports Medicine. The use of anabolic-androgenic steroids in sports. Sports Med Bull 1984;19:13.
8. Angell M, Kassirer JP. Alternative medicine—the risks of untested and unregulated remedies. N Engl J Med 1998;339:831.
9. Anselme F, et al. Caffeine increases maximal anaerobic power and blood lactate concentration. Eur J Appl Physiol 1992;65:188.
10. Anshel MH, Russel KG. Examining athletes' attitudes toward using anabolic steroids and their knowledge of the possible effects. J Drug Educ 1997;27:121.
11. Antonio J, Street C. Glutamine: a potentially useful supplement for athletes. Can J Appl Physiol 1999;24:1.
12. Araghiniknam M, et al. Antioxidant activity of dioscorea and dehydroepiandrosterone (DHEA) in older humans. Life Sci 1996; 59:11.
13. Audran M, et al. Effects of erythropoietin administration in training athletes and possible indirect detection in doping control. Med Sci Sports Exerc 1999;31:639.
14. Baer DJ, et al. Moderate alcohol consumption lowers risk factors for cardiovascular disease in postmenopausal women fed a controlled diet. Am J Clin Nutr 2002;75:593.
15. Bahrke M, Morgan WP. Evaluation of the ergogenic properties of ginseng. Sports Med 2000;29:113.
16. Bell DG, Jacobs I. Combined effects of caffeine and ephedrine ingestion improves run times of Canadian Forces Warrior Test. Aviat Space Environ Med 1999;70:325.
17. Bell DG, McLellan TM. Effect of repeated caffeine ingestion on repeated exhaustive exercise endurance. Med Sci Sports Exerc 2003;35:1348.
18. Bell DG, et al. Effects of caffeine, ephedrine and their combination on time to exhaustion during high-intensity exercise. Eur J Appl Physiol 1998;778:427.
19. Bell DG, et al. Effect of caffeine and ephedrine ingestion on anaerobic performance. Med Sci Sports Exerc 2001;33:1399.
20. Bell DG, et al. Effect of ingesting caffeine and ephedrine on 10-km run performance. Med Sci Sports Exerc 2002;34:344.
21. Benson DW, et al. Decreased myofibrillar protein breakdown following treatment with clenbuterol. J Surg Res 1991;50:1.
22. Blackman MR, et al. Growth hormone and sex steroid administration in healthy aged women and men: a randomized controlled trial. JAMA 2002;288:2282.
23. Blanchard MA, et al. The influence of diet and exercise on muscle and plasma glutamine concentrations. Med Sci Sports Exerc 2001;33:69.
24. Bracken ME, et al. The effect of cocaine on exercise endurance and glycogen use in rats. J. Appl Physiol 1988;64:884.
25. Braiden RW, et al. Effects of cocaine on glycogen metabolism and endurance during high intensity exercise. Med Sci Sports Exerc 1994;26:695.
26. Brown GA, et al. Effect of oral DHEA on serum testosterone and adaptations to resistance training in young men. J Appl Physiol 1999;87:2274.
27. Brown GA et al. Endocrine response to chronic androstenedione intake in 30- to 56-year-old men. J Clin Endocrinol Metab 2000;85:4074.
28. Browne A, et al. The ethics of blood testing as an element of doping control in sport. Med Sci Sports Exerc 1999;31:497.
29. Bruce CR, et al. Enhancement of 2000-m rowing performance after caffeine ingestion. Med Sci Sports Exerc 2000;32:1958.
30. Bucci LR. Selected herbals and human exercise performance. Am J Clin Nutr 2000:72(suppl):624S.
31. Buckley WE, et al. Estimated prevalence of anabolic steroid use among male high school seniors. JAMA 1988;260:3441.
32. Burke LM, et al. Effect of alcohol intake on muscle glycogen storage after prolonged exercise. J Appl Physiol 2003 95:983.
33. Candow DG, et al. Effect of glutamine supplementation combined with resistance training in young adults. Eur J Appl Physiol 2001;86:142.

34. Caruso JF, et al. The effects of albuterol and isokinetic exercise on the quadriceps muscle group. Med Sci Sports Exerc 1995;27:1471.

35. Casaburi R, et al. Androgen effects on body composition and muscle performance. In: Bhasin S, et al., eds. Pharmacology, biology, and clinical applications of androgens: current status and future prospects. New York: Wiley-Liss, 1996.

36. Casal DC, Leon AS. Failure of caffeine to affect substrate utilization during prolonged exercise. Med Sci Sports Exerc 1985;17:174.

37. Deleted.

38. Castell LM, et al. Some aspects of the acute phase response after a marathon race, and the effects of glutamine supplementation. Eur J Appl Physiol 1997;75:47.

39. Catlin DH, et al. Trace contamination of over-the-counter androstenedione and positive urine test results for nandrolone metabolite. JAMA 2000;285:2618.

40. Catlin P, et al. Assessing the threat of anabolic steroids. Phys Sportsmed 1993;21(8):37.

41. Cheng W, et al. Beta-hydroxy-beta-methyl butyrate increases fatty acid oxidation by muscle cells. FASEB J 1997;11(3):A381.

42. Chester N, et al. Physiological, subjective and performance effects of pseudoephedrine and phenylpropanolamine during endurance running exercise. Int J Sports Med 2003;24:3.

43. Chin ER, Allen DG. The contribution of pH-dependent mechanisms to fatigue at different intensities in mammalian single muscle fibres. J Physiol (Lond) 1998;512:831.

44. Clarkson P. Nutritional ergogenic aids: caffeine. Int J Sports Nutr 1993;3:103.

45. Cohen BS, et al. Effects of caffeine ingestion on endurance racing in heat and humidity. Eur J Appl Physiol 1996;73:358.

46. Cohen LI, et al. Lipoprotein (a) and cholesterol in body builders using anabolic androgenic steroids. Med Sci Sports Exerc 1996;28:176.

47. Collomp K, et al. Effects of salbutamol and caffeine ingestion on exercise metabolism and performance. Int J Sports Med 2002;23:549.

48. Conlee RK, et al. Effect of cocaine on plasma catecholamine and muscle glycogen concentrations during exercise in the rat. J Appl Physiol 1991;70:1323.

49. Costill DL, et al. Acid-base balance during repeated bouts of exercise: influence of HCO_3. Int J Sports Med 1984;5:228.

50. Crist DM, et al. Body composition response to exogenous GH during training in highly conditioned adults. J Appl Physiol 1988;65:579.

51. Criswell DS, et al. Clenbuterol-induced fiber type transition in the soleus of adult rats. Eur J Appl Physiol 1996;74:391.

52. Curry LA, et al. Qualitative description of the prevalence and use of anabolic androgenic steroids by United States powerlifters. Percept Mot Skills 1999;88:224.

53. Davis MJ, et al. Effects of moderate alcohol intake on fasting insulin and glucose concentrations and insulin sensitivity in postmenopausal women: a randomized controlled trial. JAMA 2002;287:2559.

54. Daynes RA, Araneo BA. Prevention and reversal of some age-associated changes in immunologic responses by supplemental dehydroepiandrosterone sulfate therapy. Aging Immunol Infect Dis 1992;3:135.

55. DeCree C. Androstenedione and dehydroepiandrosterone for athletes. Lancet 1999;354:779.

56. Delbeke FT, et al. The abuse of doping agents in competing body builders in Flanders (1988–1993). Int J Sports Med 1995;16:60.

57. DeMeersman R, et al. Sympathomimetics and exercise enhancement: all in the mind? Pharmacol Biochem Behav 1987;28:361.

58. Deyssig R, et al. Effect of growth hormone treatment on hormonal parameters, body composition and strength in athletes. Acta Endocrinol 1993;128:313.

59. Dickerman RD, et al. Echocardiography in fraternal twin body-builders with one abusing anabolic steroids. Cardiology 1997;88:50.

60. Dodd SL, et al. The effects of caffeine on graded exercise performance in caffeine naive versus habituated subjects. Eur J Appl Physiol 1991;62:424.

61. Dodd SL, et al. Caffeine and exercise performance. Sports Med 1993;15:14.

62. Dodd SL, et al. Effects of clenbuterol on contractile and biochemical properties of skeletal muscle. Med Sci Sports Exerc 1996;28:669.

63. Doherty M, et al. Caffeine is ergogenic after supplementation of oral creatine monohydrate. Med Sci Sports Exerc 2002;34:1785.

64. Donato T. Alcohol consumption among high school students and young athletes in north Italy. Rev Epidemiol Sante Publique 1994;42:198.

65. Dupont-Versteegdn EE. Exercise and clenbuterol as strategies to decrease progression of muscular dystrophy in mdx rats. J Appl Physiol 1995;80:734.

66. Durant RH, et al. Use of multiple drugs among adolescents who use anabolic steroids. N Engl J Med 1993;328:922.

67. Earnst DP, et al. In vivo 4-androstene-3,17-dione and 4-androstene-3β,17β-diol supplementation in young men. Eur J Appl Physiol 2000;81:229.

68. Eich DM, et al. Inhibition of accelerated coronary atherosclerosis with dehydroepiandrosterone in the heterotropic rabbit model of cardiac transplantation. Circulation 1993;87:261.

69. Ekblom B, Berglund B. Effect of erythropoietin administration on maximal aerobic power in man. Scand J Med Sci Sports 1991;11:88.

70. Engels HJ, et al. No ergogenic effects of ginseng (Panax ginseng C.A. Meyer) during graded maximal aerobic exercise. J Am Diet Assoc 1997;97:1110.

71. Faigenbaum A, et al. Anabolic androgenic steroid use by 11- to 13-yearold boys and girls: knowledge, attitudes, and prevalence. J Strength Cond Res (abstr) 1996;10:285.

72. Ferenclick GS, Adelman S. Myocardial infarction associated with anabolic steroid use in a previously healthy 37-year-old weightlifter. Am Heart J 1992;124:507.

73. Fogelholm M, et al. Healthy lifestyles of former Finnish world class athletes. Med Sci Sports Exerc 1994;26:224.

74. Fomous CM, et al. Symposium: conference on the science and policy of performance-enhancing products. Med Sci Sports Exerc 2002;34:1685.

75. Forbes GB, et al. Sequence of changes in body composition induced by testosterone and reversal of changes after drug is stopped. JAMA 1992;267:397.

76. Forgo I, Kirchdorfer AM. The effect of different ginsenoside concentrations on physical work capacity. Notabene Medici 1982;12:721.

77. Forman ES, et al. High-risk behaviors in teenage male athletes. Clin J Sports Med 1995;5:36.

78. Franke WW, Berendonk B. Hormonal doping and androgenization of athletes: a secret program of the German Democratic Republic government. Clin Chem 1997;43:1262.

79. French C, et al. Caffeine ingestion during exercise to exhaustion in elite distance runners. J Sports Med Phys Fitness 1991;31:425.

80. Fuchs GS, et al. Alcohol consumption and mortality among women. N Engl J Med 1995;332:1245.

81. Gallagher PM, et al. β-Hydroxy-β-methylbutyrate ingestion. Part I: effects on strength and fat free mass. Med Sci Sports Exerc 2000;32:2116.

82. Gallagher PM, et al. β-Hydroxy-β-methylbutyrate ingestion. Part II: effects on hematology, hepatic and renal function. Med Sci Sports Exerc 2000;32:2116.

83. Galloway SDR, et al. The effects of acute phosphate supplementation in subjects of different aerobic fitness levels. Eur J Appl Physiol 1996;72:224.

84. Gaziano JM, et al. Moderate alcohol intake, increased levels of high-density lipoprotein and its subfractions, and decreased risk of myocardial infarction. N Engl J Med 1993;329:1829.

85. Gazvani M, et al. Conservative management of azoospermia following steroid abuse. Hum Reprod 1997;12:1706.

86. Gillies H, et al. Pseudoephedrine is without ergogenic effects during prolonged exercise. J Appl Physiol 1996;81:2611.

87. Girondola RN, et al. Effects of pangamic acid (B_{15}) ingestion on metabolic response to exercise. Biochem. Med 1980;24:218.

88. Goldberg L, et al. Effects of a multidimensional anabolic steroid prevention intervention: the Adolescents Training and Learning to Avoid Steroids (ATLAS) Program. JAMA 1996;276:1555.

89. Goldberg L, et al. Drug testing athletes to prevent substance abuse: background and pilot study results of the SATURN (Student Athlete Testing Using Random Notification) Study. J Adolesc Health 2003;32:16.

90. Goldfinch J, et al. Induced metabolic alkalosis and its effects on 400-m racing time. Eur J Appl Physiol 1988;57:45.

91. Gordon GB, et al. Reduction of atherosclerosis by administration of DHEA. J Clin Invest 1988;82:712.

92. Graham TE, Spriet LL. Performance and metabolic responses to a high caffeine dose during exercise. J Appl Physiol 1991;71:2292.

93. Graham TE, Spriet LL. Metabolic, catecholamine and exercise performance responses to varying doses of caffeine. J Appl Physiol 1996;78:867.

94. Graham TE, et al. Metabolic and exercise endurance effects of coffee and caffeine ingestion. J Appl Physiol 1998;85:883.

95. Graja TE, Spirit LL. Metabolic, catecholamine, and exercise performance responses to various doses of caffeine. J Appl Physiol 1995;78:867.

96. Granier PL, et al. Effect of NaHCO$_3$ on lactate kinetics in forearm muscles during leg exercise in man. Med Sci Sports Exerc 1996;28:692.

97. Gray ME, Titlow LW. B$_{15}$: myth or miracle? Phys Sportsmed 1982;10(1):107.

98. Green GA, et al. Analysis of over-the-counter dietary supplements. Clin J Sports Med 2001;11:254.

99. Green GA, et al. NCAA study of substance use and abuse habits of college student-athletes. Clin J Sports Med 2001;11:56.

100. Gutgesell M, et al. Reported alcohol use and behavior in long-distance runners. Med Sci Sports Exerc 1996;28:1063.

101. Hallfrisch J, et al. Physical conditioning status and diet intake in active and sedentary older men. Nutr Res 1994;14:817.

102. Harburg E, et al. Using the Short Michigan Alcoholism Screening Test to study social drinkers: Tecumseh, Michigan. J Stud Alcohol 1988;49:522.

103. Harburg E, et al. Psychosocial factors, alcohol use and hangover signs among social drinkers: a reappraisal. J Clin Epidemiol 1993;46:413.

104. Harkey MR, et al. Variability in commercial ginseng products: an analysis of 25 preparations. Am J Clin Nutr 2001;73:1101.

105. Hartgens F, et al. Body composition and anthropometry in body-builders: regional changes due to nandrolone deconate administration. Int J Sports Med 2001;22:235.

106. Hartgens F, et al. Misuse of androgenic-anabolic steroids and human deltoid muscle fibers: differences between polydrug regimes and single drug administration. Eur J Appl Physiol 2002;86:233.

107. Hausswirth C, et al. Sodium citrate ingestion and muscle performance in acute hypobaric hypoxia. Eur J Appl Physiol 1995;71:362.

108. Hickson RC, et al. Glutamine prevents down-regulation of myosin heavy-chain synthesis and muscle atrophy from glucocorticoids. Am J Physiol 1995;31:E730.

109. Hintz RL, et al. Effect of growth hormone treatment on adult height of children with idiopathic short stature. N Engl J Med 1999;340:502.

110. Hodges AN, et al. Effects of pseudoephedrine on maximal cycling power and submaximal cycling efficiency. Med Sci Sports Exerc 2003;35:1316.

111. Hollidge-Horvat MG, et al. Effect of induced metabolic alkalosis on human skeletal muscle metabolism during exercise. Am J Physiol 2000;278:E316.

112. Huie MJ. An acute myocardial infarction occurring in an anabolic steroid user. Med Sci Sport Exerc 1994;26:408.

113. Hurley BF, et al. High density lipoprotein cholesterol in body builders vs. power-lifters. Negative effects of androgen use. JAMA 1984;252:4.

114. Ingalls CP, et al. Interaction between clenbuterol and run training: effects on exercise performance and MLC isoform control. J Appl Physiol 1996;80:795.

115. Ivy JL. Food components that may optimize physical performance: an overview. In: Marriott BM, ed. Food components to enhance performance. Committee on Military Nutrition Research. Washington, DC: National Academy Press, 1994.

116. Jackman MP, et al. Metabolic, catecholamine and endurance responses to caffeine during intense exercise. J Appl Physiol 1996;81:1658.

117. Jacobs I, et al. Effects of ephedrine, caffeine, and their combination on muscular endurance. Med Sci Sports Exerc 2003;35:987.

118. Jakaubowicz D, et al. Effect of dehydroepiandrosterone on cyclic-guanosine monophosphate in men of advancing age. Ann NY Acad Sci 1995;774:312.

119. Jepson MM, et al. Relationship between glutamine concentration and protein synthesis in rat skeletal muscle. Am J Physiol 1988;255(Endocrinol Metab 18):E166.

120. Johansen KL, et al. Anabolic effects of nandrolone decanoate in patients receiving dialysis. A randomized controlled trial. JAMA 1999;281:1275.

121. Johnson CE, et al. Alcohol lowers the vasoconstriction threshold in humans without affecting core cooling rate during mild cold exposure. Eur J Appl Physiol 1996;74:293.

122. Jowko E, et al. Creatine and beta-hydroxy-beta-methylbutyrate (HMB) additively increase lean body mass and muscle strength during a weight training program. Nutrition 2001;17:558.

123. Juel C. Lactate-proton cotransport in skeletal muscle. Physiol Rev 1997;77:321.

124. Kamber M, et al. Nutritional supplements as a source for positive doping cases? Int J Sport Nutr Exerc Metab 2001;11:258.

125. Kantor MA, et al. Androgens reduce HDL$_2$-cholesterol and increase hepatic triglyceride lipase activity. Med Sci Sports Exerc 1985;17:462.

126. Kearns CF, McKeever J. Clenbuterol diminishes aerobic performance in horses. Med Sci Sports Exerc 2002;34:1976.

127. Kearns CF, et al. Chronic administration of therapeutic levels of clenbuterol acts as a repartitioning agent. J Appl Physiol 2001;91:2064.

128. Kelbaek H, et al. Acute effects of alcohol on left ventricular function in healthy subjects at rest and during upright exercise. Am J Cardiol 1985;55:164.

129. Kelbaek H, et al. Left ventricular function during alcohol intoxication and autonomic nervous blockade. Am J Cardiol 1987;59:685.

130. Kelly KP, et al. Cocaine and exercise: physiological responses of cocaine-conditioned rats. Med Sci Sports Exerc 1995;27:65.

131. King DS, et al. Effect of oral androstenedione on serum testosterone and adaptations to resistance training in young men. JAMA 1999;281:2020.

132. Kitaura T, et al. Inhibited longitudinal growth of bones in young male rats by clenbuterol. Med Sci Sports Exerc 2002;34:267.

133. Kokotailo PK, et al. Substance use and other health risk behaviors in collegiate athletes. Clin J Sport Med 1996;6:183.

134. Kovacs EM, et al. The effect of ad libitum ingestion of caffeinated carbohydrate-electrolyte solution on urinary caffeine concentration after 4 hours of endurance exercise. Int J Sports Med 2002;23:237.

135. Kreider RB, et al. Effects of phosphate loading on oxygen uptake, ventilatory anaerobic threshold, and run performance. Med Sci Sports Exerc 1990;22:250.

136. Kreider R.B, et al. Effects of phosphate loading on metabolic and myocardial responses to maximal and endurance exercise. Int J Sports Nutr 1992;2:20.

137. Kreider RB, et al. Effects of calcium beta-hydroxy-beta-methylbutyrate (HMB) supplementation during resistance training on markers of catabolism, body composition, and strength. Int J Sports Med 1999;20:503.

138. Lang RM, et al. Adverse cardiac effects of alcohol ingesting in young adults. Ann Intern Med 1985;102:742.

139. Laseter JT, Russell JA. Anabolic steroid-induced tendon pathology: a review of the literature. Med Sci Sports Exerc 1991;23:1.

140. Leder BZ, et al. Oral androstenedione administration and serum testosterone concentrations in young men. JAMA 2000;283:779.

141. Leichliter JS, et al. Alcohol use and related consequences among students with varying levels of involvement in college athletics. J Am School Health 1998;46:257.

142. Lemmer JT, et al. The effects of albuterol on power output in non-asthmatic athletes. Int J Sports Med 1995,16:243.

143. Lieberman HR. The effects of ginseng, ephedrine, and caffeine on cognitive performance, mood and energy. Nutr Rev 2001;50:91.

144. Linossier M-T, et al. Effect of sodium citrate on performance and metabolism of human skeletal muscle during supramaximal cycling exercise. Eur J Appl Physiol 1998;76:48.

145. Liow RYL, Tavares S. Bilateral rupture of the quadriceps tendon associated with anabolic steroids. Br J Sports Med 1995;29:77.

146. Lopes JM, et al. Effect of caffeine on skeletal muscle function before and after fatigue. J Appl Physiol 1983;54:1303.

147. Lukas SE. CNS effects and abuse liability of anabolic-androgenic steroids. Annu Rev Pharmacol Toxicol 1996;36:333.

148. Lutekemeier MJ, et al. Anabolic-androgenic steroids: prevalence, knowledge, and attitudes in junior and senior high school students. J Health Educ 1995;26:4.

149. MacIntosh BR, Wright BM. Caffeine ingestion and performance of a 1500-meter swim., Can J Appl Physiol 1995;20:168.

150. MacLennan PA, Edwards RHT. Effects of clenbuterol and propranol on muscle mass. Biochem J 1989;264:573.

151. Mannix ET, et al. Oxygen delivery and cardiac output during exercise following oral glucose phosphate. Med Sci Sports Exerc 1990;22:341.

152. Martineau L, et al. Salbutamol, a β-agonist, increases skeletal muscle strength in young men. Clin Sci 1992;83:615.

153. Matson LG, Tran ZV. Effects of sodium bicarbonate ingestion on anaerobic performance: a meta-analytic review. Int J Sports Nutr 1993;3:2.

154. Matvienko OA, et al. A single dose of soybean phytosterols in ground beef decreases total serum cholesterol and LDL cholesterol in young, mildly hypercholesterolemic men. Am J Clin Nutr 2002;76:57.

155. Maughan RJ, et al. Rehydration and recovery after exercise. Sports Sci Exchange, Gatorade Sports Science Institute 1996;9(3).

156. Max SR. Glucocorticoid-mediated induction of glutamine synthetase in skeletal muscle. Med Sci Sports Exerc 1990;22:325.

157. Max SR, Rance NE. No effect of sex steroids on compensatory muscle hypertrophy. J Appl Physiol 1984;56:1589.

158. McNaughton LR. Sodium citrate and anaerobic performance: implications of dosage. Eur J Appl Physiol 1990;61:392.

159. McNaughton LR, Cedaro R. Sodium citrate ingestion and its effects on maximal anaerobic exercise of different durations. Eur J Appl Physiol 1992;64:36.

160. McNaughton LR, et al. Effect of sodium bicarbonate ingestion on high intensity exercise in moderately trained women. J Strength Cond Res 1997;11:98.

161. McNaughton L, et al. Effects of chronic bicarbonate ingestion on the performance of high-intensity work. Eur J Appl Physiol 1999;80:333.

162. McNaughton L, et al. Sodium bicarbonate can be used as an ergogenic aid in high-intensity, competitive cycle ergometry of 1 h duration. Eur J Appl Physiol 1999;80:64.

163. Melchert RB, Lelder AA. Cardiovascular effects of androgenic-anabolic steroids. Med Sci Sports Exerc 1995;27:1252.

164. Milner JA. Functional foods: the US perspective. Am J Clin Nutr 2000;71 (suppl):1654S.

165. Mohr T, et al. Caffeine ingestion and metabolic responses of tetraplegic humans during electrical cycling. J Appl Physiol 1998;85:979.

166. Monteleone P, et al. Effects of phosphatidylserine on the neuroendocrine response to physical stress in humans. Neuroendocrinology 1990;52:243.

167. Monteleone P, et al. Blunting by chronic phosphatidylserine administration of the stress-induced activation of the hypothalmo-pituitary-adrenal axis in healthy men. Eur J Clin Pharmacol 1992;41:385.

168. Morris AC, et al. No ergogenic effects of ginseng ingestion. Int J Sport Nutr 1996;6:263.

169. Mortola J, Yen SSC. The effects of oral dehydroepiandrosterone on endocrine-metabolic parameters in postmenopausal women. J Clin Endocrinol Metab 1990;71:696.

170. Moskowitz H, et al. Skills performance at low blood alcohol levels. J Stud Alcohol 1995;46:482.

171. Mukamal KJ. Prior alcohol consumption and mortality following acute myocardial infarction. JAMA 2001;285:1965.

172. Murphy RJ, et al. Clenbuterol has a greater influence on untrained than previously trained skeletal muscle in rats. Eur J Appl Physiol 1996;73:304.

173. Nativ A, Puffer JC. Lifestyles and health risks of collegiate athletes. J Fam Pract 1991;33:585.

174. Nativ A, et al. Lifestyle and health risks of collegiate athletes: a multi-center study. Clin J Sport Med 1997;7:262.

175. Nelson TF, Wechsler H. Alcohol and college athletes. Med Sci Sports Exerc 2001;33:43.

176. Nigdikar SV, et al. Consumption of red wine polyphenols reduces susceptibility of low-density lipoproteins to oxidation in volunteers. Am J Clin Nutr 1998;68:258.

177. Nishijima Y, et al. Influence of caffeine ingestion on autonomic nervous system activity during endurance exercise in humans. Eur J Appl Physiol 2002;87:475.

178. Nissen S, et al. Effect of leucine metabolite β-hydroxy-β-methylbutyrate on muscle metabolism during resistance-exercise training. J Appl Physiol 1996;81:2095.

179. Norris SR, et al. The effect of salbutamol on performance in endurance cyclists. Eur J Appl Physiol 1996;73:364.

180. Nuotto EJ, Korttila KT. Evaluation of a new computerized psychomotor test battery: effects of alcohol. Pharmacol Toxicol 1991;68:360.

181. Nutrition and Your Health: Dietary Guidelines for Americans. 4th ed. Washington, DC: U.S. Department of Agriculture and U.S. Department of Health and Human Services, 1995.

182. Oler M.J, et al. Depression, suicidal ideation, and substance use among adolescents. Are athletes at less risk? Arch Fam Med 1994;3:791.

183. Ostaszewksi P, et al. The effect of the leucine metabolite 3-hydroxy 3-methyl butyrate (HMB) on muscle protein synthesis and protein breakdown in chick and rat muscle. J Anim Sci 1996;74(suppl):138A.

184. O'Toole M., et al. Hematocrits of triathletes: is monitoring useful? Med Sci Sports Exerc 1999;31:372.

185. Overmann SJ, Terry T. Alcohol use and attitudes: a comparison of college athletes and non-athletes. J Drug Educ 1991;2:107.

186. Panton LB, et al. Nutritional supplementation of the leucine metabolite beta-hydroxy-beta-methylbutyrate (HMB) during resistance training. Nutrition 2000;16:734.

187. Papadakis MA, et al. Growth hormone replacement in healthy older men improves body composition but not functional ability. Ann Inter Med 1996;124:708.

188. Pasman WJ, et al. The effect of different dosages of caffeine on endurance performance time. Int J Sports Med 1995;16:225.

189. Paton CD, et al. Little effect of caffeine ingestion on repeated sprints in team-sport athletes. Med Sci Sports Exerc. 2001;33:822.

190. Percheron G, et al. Effect of 1-year oral administration of dehydroepiandrosterone to 60- to 80-year-old individuals on muscle function and cross-sectional area: a double-blind placebo-controlled trial. Arch Intern Med 2003;163:720.

191. Perry PJ, et al. Detection of anabolic steroid administration: ratio of urinary testosterone to epitestosterone vs the ratio of urinary testosterone to luteinizing hormone. Clin Chem 1997;43:731.

192. Plaskett CJ, Cafarelli E. Caffeine increases endurance and attenuates force sensation during submaximal isometric contractions. J Appl Physiol 2001;91:1535.

193. Potteiger JA, et al. Sodium citrate ingestion enhances 30 km cycling performance. Int J Sports Med 1996;17:7.

194. Price M, et al. Effects of sodium bicarbonate ingestion on prolonged intermittent exercise. Med Sci Sports Exerc 2003:35:1303.

195. Ransone J, et al. The effect of beta-hydroxy beta-methylbutyrate on muscular strength and body composition in collegiate football players. J Strength Cond Res 2003; 17:34.

196. Raymer GH, et al. Metabolic effects of induced Alkaloids during progressive forearm exercise to fatigue. J Appl Physiol 2004;96:2050.

197. Rasmussen BB, et al. Androstenedione does not stimulate muscle protein anabolism in young healthy men. J Clin Endocrinol Metab 2000;85:55.

198. Rhode T, et al. Competitive sustained exercise in humans, lymphokine activated killer cell activity, and glutamine—an intervention study. Eur J Appl Physiol 1998;78:448.

199. Rhode T, et al. Effect of glutamine supplementation on changes in the immune system induced by repeated exercise. Med Sci Sports Exerc 1998;30:856.

200. Rifici VA, et al. Red wine inhibits the cell-mediated oxidation of LDL and HDL. J Am Coll Nutr 1999;18:137.

201. Roberfroid MB. Concepts and strategy of functional food science: the European perspective. Am J Clin Nutr 2000;71(suppl):1660S.

202. Robertson RJ, et al. Effect of induced alkalosis on physical work capacity during arm and leg exercise. Ergonomics 1987;30:19.

203. Rogozkin V. Metabolic effects of anabolic steroids on skeletal muscle. Med Sci Sports 1979;11:160.

204. Rowbottom DG, et al. The emerging role of glutamine as an indicator of exercise stress and overtraining. Sports Med 1996;21:80.

205. Roy BD, et al. An acute oral dose of caffeine does not alter glucose kinetics during prolonged dynamic exercise in trained endurance athletes. Eur J Appl Physiol 2001;85:280.

206. Russell G, et al. Effects of prolonged low dosage of recombinant human erythropoietin during submaximal and maximal exercise. Eur J Appl Physiol 2002;86:442.

207. Sacco RL, et al. The protective effect of moderate alcohol consumption on ischemic stroke. JAMA 1999;28:913.

208. Sachtleben TR, et al. The effects of anabolic steroids on myocardial structure and cardiovascular fitness. Med Sci Sports Exerc 1993;25:1240.

209. Sachtleben TR, et al. Serum lipoprotein patterns in long-term anabolic steroid users. Res Q Exerc Sport 1997;68:110.

210. Saini J, et al. Influence of alcohol on the hydromineral hormone responses to exercise in a warm environment. Eur J Appl Physiol 1995;72:32.

211. Schabort EJ, et al. Dose-related evaluations in venous pH with citrate ingestion do not alter 40-km cycling time-trial performance. Eur J Appl Physiol 2000;83:320.

212. Schumacher YO, et al. Artificial oxygen carriers—the new doping threat in endurance sport? Int J Sports Med 2001;22:566.

213. Schwartz AG, et al. A new class of cancer chemo-preventive agents. Adv Cancer Res 1988;51:391.

214. Shekelle PG, et al. Efficacy and safety of ephedra and ephedrine for weight loss and athletic performance: a meta-analysis. JAMA 2003;289:1463.

215. Deleted.

216. Shirreffs SM, Maughan RJ. The effect on alcohol consumption on fluid retention following exercise-induced dehydration in man. J Physiol 1995;489:33P.

217. Shirreffs SM, Maughan RJ. The effect of alcohol consumption on the restoration of blood and plasma volume following exercise-induced dehydration in man. J Physiol 1996;491:64P.

218. Signorile JF, et al.: Effects of acute inhalation of the bronchodilator, albuterol, on power output. Med Sci Sports Exerc 1992;24:638.

219. Signorile JF, et al. The effects of the chronic administration of metaproterenol on muscle size and function. Arch Phys Med Rehab 1995;76:55.

220. Sinclair CI, Geiger JD. Caffeine use in sports. J Sports Med Phys Fitness 2000;40:71.

221. Slater B, et al. Beta-hydroxy-beta-methylbutyrate (HMB) supplementation does not affect changes in strength or body composition during resistance training in trained men. Int J Sport Nutr Exerc Metab 2001;11:384.

222. Sleeper MM, et al. Chronic clenbuterol, administration negatively alters cardiac function. Med Sci Sports Exerc 2002;34:643.

223. Soe LJ, et al. Liver pathology associated with the use of anabolic-androgenic steroids. Liver 1992;12:73.

224. Spriet LL, et al. Caffeine ingestion and muscle metabolism during prolonged exercise in humans. Am J Physiol 1992;262:E891.

225. Stark AH, Madar Z. Olive oil as a functional food: epidemiology and nutritional approaches. Nutr Rev 2002;60:170.

226. Stephens TJ, et al. Effect of sodium bicarbonate on muscle metabolism during intense endurance cycling. Med Sci Sports Exerc 2002;34:614.

227. Strauss RH, et al. Anabolic steroid use and perceived effects in ten weight-trained women athletes. JAMA 1985;253:2871.

228. Strawford A, et al. Resistance exercise and supraphysiologic androgen therapy and supraphysiologic androgen therapy in eugonadal men with HIV-related weight loss. A randomized controlled trial. JAMA 1999;281:1282.

229. Street C, et al. Androgen use by athletes: a reevaluation of the health risks. Can J Appl Physiol 1996;21:421.

230. Su TP, et al. Neuropsychiatric effects of anabolic steroids in male normal volunteers. JAMA 1993;269:2760.

231. Supinski GS, et al. Caffeine effect on respiratory muscle endurance and sense of effort during loaded breathing. J Appl Physiol 1986;60:2040.

232. Swain RA, et al. Do pseudoephedrine or phenylpropanolamine improve maximum oxygen uptake and time to exhaustion? Clin J Sports Med 1997;7:168.

233. Tagarakis CV, et al. Anabolic steroids impair the exercise-induced growth of the cardiac capillary bed. Int J Sports Med 2000; 21:412.

234. Tarnopolsky MA, et al. Physiological responses to caffeine during endurance running in habitual caffeine users. Med Sci Sports Exerc 1989;21:418.

235. Tjønneland A, et al. Wine intake and diet in a random sample of 48,763 Danish men and women. Am J Clin Nutr 1999;69:49.

236. Toner MM, et al. Metabolic and cardiovascular responses to exercise with caffeine. Ergonomics 1982;25:1175.

237. Trice I, Haymes EM. Effects of caffeine ingestion on exercise-induced changes during high-intensity, intermittent exercise. Int J Sports Nutr 1995;5:37.

238. Tricker R, Connolly D. Drugs and the college athlete: an analysis of the attitudes of student athletes at risk. J Drug Educ 1997;27:105.

239. Ungerleider S. Faust's gold. New York: St. Martin's Press, 2001.

240. US Department of Health and Human Services: Healthy People 2010 (conference ed, 2 vol). Washington, DC: Department of Health and Human Services, 2000.

241. Valmadrid CT, et al. Alcohol intake and risk of coronary heart disease mortality in persons with older-onset diabetes mellitus. JAMA 1999;282:239.

242. Vandenberghe K, et al. Caffeine counteracts the ergogenic action of creatine loading. J Appl Physiol 1996;80:452.

243. Van Gammeren D, et al. The effects of supplementation with 19-nor-4-androstene-3,17-dione and 19-nor-4-androstene-3,17-diol on body composition and athletic performance in previously weight-trained male athletes. Eur J Appl Physiol 2001;84:426.

244. Van Soeren MH, et al. Caffeine metabolism and epinephrine responses during exercise in users and nonusers. J Appl Physiol 1994;75:805.

245. Van Soeren MH, et al. Acute effects of caffeine ingestion at rest in humans with impaired epinephrine responses. J Appl Physiol 1996;80:999.

246. Van Soeren MH, Graham TE. Effect of caffeine on metabolism, exercise endurance, and catecholamine responses after withdrawal. J Appl Physiol 1998;85:1493.

247. Van Vollenhoven RF, et al. An open study of dehydroepiandrosterone in systemic lupus erythematosus. Arthritis Rheum 1994;37:1305.

248. Varnier M, et al. Stimulatory effect of glutamine on glycogen accumulation in human skeletal muscle. Am J Physiol 1995;269:E309.

249. Villareal DT, Holloszy JO. Effect of DHEA on abdominal fat and insulin action in elderly women and men. JAMA 2004;292:2243.

250. Vogler BK, et al. The efficacy of ginseng. A systematic review of randomized clinical trials. Eur J Clin Pharmacol 1999;55:567.

251. Vukovich MD, et al. Body composition in 70-year-old adults responds to dietary beta-hydroxy-beta-methylbutyrate similarly to that of young adults. J Nutr 2001;131:2049.

252. Vuksan V, et al. American ginseng (*Panex quinquefolius* L.) attenuates postprandial glycemia in a time-dependent but not dose-dependent manner in healthy individuals. Am J Clin Nutr 2001;73:753.

253. Wagman DF, et al. An investigation into anabolic androgenic steroid use by elite U.S. powerlifters. J Strength Cond Res 1995;9:149.

254. Wallace MB, et al. Effects of dehydroepiandrosterone vs androstenedione supplementation in men. Med Sci Sports Exerc 1999;31:1788.

255. Walsh NP, Blannin AK. Effect of oral glutamine supplementation on human neutrophil lipopolysaccharide-stimulated degranulation following prolonged exercise. Int J Sport. Nutr Exerc Metab 2000; 1:39.

256. Wannamethee SG, et al. Alcohol and diabetes risk. Arch Intern Med 2003;163:1329.

257. Webb OL, et al. Severe depression of high density lipoprotein cholesterol levels in weight lifters and body builders by self-administered exogenous testosterone and anabolic-androgenic steroids. Metabolism 1984;33:11.

258. Webster MJ, et al. Effect of sodium bicarbonate ingestion on exhaustive resistance exercise performance. Med Sci Sports Exerc 1993;25:960.

259. Weir J, et al. A high carbohydrate diet negates the metabolic effects of caffeine during exercise. Med Sci Sports Exerc 1987;19:100.

260. Wemple R.D, et al. Caffeine vs caffeine-free sports drinks: effects on urine production at rest and during prolonged exercise. Int J Sports Med 1997;18:40.

261. Wernerman J, et al. Glutamine and ornithine-α-ketoglutarate but not branched-chain amino acids reduce the loss of muscle glutamine after surgical trauma. Metabolism 1989;38(suppl1):63.

262. Williams PJ. Interactive effects of exercise, alcohol, and vegetarian diet on coronary artery disease risk factors in 9242 runners: The National Runners' Health Study. Am J Clin Nutr 1997;66:1197.

263. Windsor R, Dumitrv D. Prevalence of anabolic steroid use by male and female adolescents. Med Sci Sports Exerc 1989;21:494.

264. Wroblewska A-M. Androgenic-anabolic steroids and body dysmorphia in young men. J Psychosom Res 1997;42:225.

265. Yang YT, McElligott MA. Multiple actions of β-adrenergic agonists on skeletal muscle and adipose tissue. Biochem J 1989;261:1.

266. Yanovski SZ, Yanovski JA. Drug therapy: Obesity. N Engl J Med 2002;346:591.

267. Yarasheski KE, et al. Effect of growth hormone and resistance exercise on muscle growth in young men. Am J Physiol 1992;262:E261.

268. Yarasheski KE, et al Short-term growth hormone treatment does not increase muscle protein synthesis in experienced weight lifters. J Appl Physiol 1993;74:3073.

269. Yesalis CE, et al. Anabolic-androgenic steroid use in the United States. JAMA 1993;270:1217.

270. Zeman RJ, et al. Clenbuterol, a β_2-agonist, retards wasting and loss of contractility in irradiated dystrophic *mdx* muscle. Am J Physiol 1994;267:C865.

Additional Readings

Bahrke MS, Yesalis CE. Abuse of anabolic androgenic steroids and related substances in sport and exercise. Curr Opin Pharmacol 2004;4:614.

Dalgaard M, et al. Effects of one single bout of low-intensity exercise on postprandial lipaemia in type 2 diabetic men. Br J Nutr 2004;92:469.

Doherty M, et al. Caffeine lowers perceptual response and increases power output during high-intensity cycling. J Sports Sci 2004;22:637.

Fiala KA, et al. Rehydration with a caffeinated beverage during the nonexercise periods of 3 consecutive days of 2-a-day practices. Int J Sport Nutr Exerc Metab 2004;14:419.

Foster ZJ, Housner JA. Anabolic-androgenic steroids and testosterone precursors: Ergogenic AIDS and sport. Curr Sports Med Rep 2004;3:234.

Hartgens F, Kuipers H. Effects of androgenic-anabolic steroids in athletes. Sports Med 2004;34(8):513.

Hunter AM, et al. Caffeine ingestion does not alter performance during a 100-km cycling time-trial performance. Int J Sport Nutr Exerc Metab 2002;12:438.

Magkos F, Kavouras SA. Caffeine and ephedrine: Physiological, metabolic and performance-enhancing effects. Sports Med 2004;34:871.

Minuto F, et al. Indirect evidence of hormone abuse. Proof of doping? J Endocrinol Invest 2003;26:919.

Morrison LJ, et al. Prevalent use of dietary supplements among people who exercise at a commercial gym. Int J Sport Nutr Exerc Metab 2004;4:481.

Motl RW, et al. Effect of caffeine on perceptions of leg muscle pain during moderate intensity cycling exercise. J Pain 2003;4:316.

Noakes TD. Tainted glory-doping and athletic performance. N Engl J Med 2004;351:847–849.

Stafford SJ, Jenkins MG. The hidden dangers of dietary supplements. Emerg Med J 2004;21:754.

Tokish JM, et al. Ergogenic AIDS: A review of basic science, performance, side effects, and status in sports. Am J Sports Med 2004;32:1543.

Trout GJ, Kazlauskas R. Sports drug testing—an analyst's perspective. Chem Soc Rev 2004; 33:1.

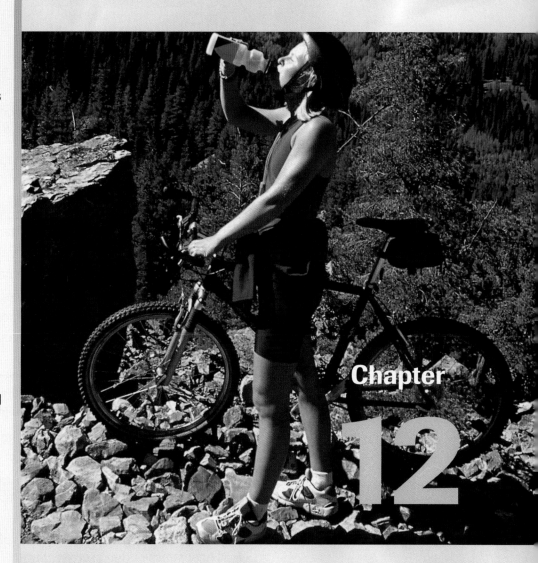

Chapter

12

Nutritional Ergogenic Aids Evaluated

TEST YOUR KNOWLEDGE

Answer these ten statements about nutritional ergogenic aids. Use the scoring key at the end of the chapter to check your results. Repeat this test after you have read the chapter and compare your results.

1. **T F** A reduced level of muscle glycogen precipitates fatigue in high-intensity aerobic exercise.

2. **T F** It is possible to modify nutrition to "superpack" muscle with glycogen and thereby delay the onset of fatigue in prolonged high-intensity marathon running.

3. **T F** Amino acid supplements provide distinct benefits for augmenting muscular strength and size in response to resistance training.

4. **T F** L-Carnitine supplementation aids endurance athletes by enhancing fat burning and sparing liver and muscle glycogen; it also promotes fat loss in body builders.

5. **T F** Chromium, the second largest selling mineral supplement in the United States (used by more than 10 million people), is a well-documented "fat burner" and "muscle builder."

6. **T F** Creatine supplementation improves performance in short-duration, high-intensity exercise.

7. **T F** Limited research indicates a potential for exogenous pyruvate, as a partial replacement for dietary carbohydrate, to augment endurance exercise performance and to promote fat loss.

8. **T F** The hyperhydra tion effect of glycerol supplementation reduces overall heat stress during exercise, lowers heart rate and core temperature, and enhances endurance performance under heat stress.

9. **T F** Bee pollen contains special sugars in natural form that enhance exercise performance.

10. **T F** Because of its role in electron transport–oxidative phosphorylation, athletes supplementing with coenzyme Q_{10} (CoQ_{10}) improve aerobic capacity and cardiovascular dynamics in healthy individuals.

Chapter 11 highlighted that physically active individuals often resort to using banned pharmacologic and chemical agents to augment training and gain a competitive edge. They also focus on gaining a performance-enhancing advantage from specific foods and food components consumed in the diet.

MODIFICATION OF CARBOHYDRATE INTAKE

Exercise performance benefits from increased carbohydrate intake before and during high-intensity aerobic exercise and heavy training. Vigilance and mood also improve with a carbohydrate beverage administered during a day of sustained aerobic activity interspersed with rest periods.[108] Carbohydrate loading represents one of the more popular nutritional modifications to increase glycogen reserves. Judicious adherence to this dietary technique improves specific exercise performance, yet some aspects of carbohydrate loading could prove detrimental.

Nutrient-Related Fatigue in Prolonged Exercise

Glycogen stored in the liver and active muscle supplies most of the energy for intense aerobic exercise. Prolonging such exercise reduces glycogen reserves and allows fat catabolism to supply a progressively greater percentage of energy from fatty acid mobilization from the liver and adipose tissue. Exercise that severely lowers muscle glycogen precipitates fatigue, even though active muscles have sufficient oxygen and unlimited potential energy from stored fat. Ingesting a glucose and water solution near the point of fatigue allows exercise to continue, but for all practical purposes the muscles' "fuel tank" reads empty. A corresponding decrease in exercise power output occurs from the slower rate of fat's mobilization and catabolism compared with carbohydrate. Marathon runners use the term **"hitting the wall"** (endurance cyclists use *bonking*) to describe sensations of fatigue and discomfort in the active muscles associated with severe glycogen depletion.

In the late 1930s, Nordic scientists reported a startling discovery—athletes' endurance performance improved markedly when they consumed a carbohydrate-rich diet in the days prior to exercising. Conversely, switching to a high-fat diet drastically reduced endurance capacity. Modifying the diet's macronutrient composition alters carbohydrate stores and profoundly affects subsequent performance in high-intensity aerobic exercise (see Fig. 5.6 and Chapters 1 and 5). In a classic series of experiments, endurance capacity tripled for subjects fed a high-carbohydrate diet compared with a high-fat diet of similar energy content.[10] Because carbohydrate represents the important energy substrate during 1 to 2 hours of high-intensity exercise, researchers began to investigate additional relatively "simple" ways to elevate the body's glycogen reserves.

Enhanced Glycogen Storage: Carbohydrate Loading

Combining a specific dietary regimen with exercise produces significant "packing" of muscle glycogen, a procedure termed **carbohydrate loading**, or **glycogen supercompensation**. Endurance athletes often use carbohydrate loading before competition because it increases muscle glycogen even more than a high-carbohydrate diet. Normally, each 100-g of muscle contains about 1.7 g of glycogen; carbohydrate loading packs up to 5 g of glycogen in 100 g of skeletal muscle.

Classic Loading Procedure

TABLE 12.1 indicates that the classic procedure for achieving the supercompensation effect first reduces the muscle's glycogen content with prolonged exercise about 6 days before competition. Because glycogen supercompensation occurs *only* in the specific muscles depleted by exercise, athletes must use the muscles involved in their sport in the depletion phase. Preparing for a marathon requires a 15- or 20-mile run, whereas for swimming and bicycling, approximately 90 minutes of moderately intense submaximal exercise in each activity takes place. The athlete then maintains a low-carbohydrate diet (about 60–100 g per day) for several days to further deplete glycogen stores. Glycogen depletion causes increased formation of intermediate forms of the glycogen-storing enzyme **glycogen synthetase** in the muscle fiber. Moderate training continues during this time. Then, at least 3 days before competing, the athlete switches to a high-carbohydrate diet (400–700 g per day) and maintains this regimen up to the precompetition meal. The supercompensation diet should also contain adequate protein, minerals, and vitamins and abundant water. For athletes who follow the classic loading procedure, the supercompensated muscle glycogen levels remain stable in a resting, nonexercising individual for at least 3 days if the diet contains 60% of calories from carbohydrate.[61]

Exercise training facilitates both the rate and magnitude of glycogen replenishment.[123] For sports competition and exercise training, a diet containing between 60 and 70% of calories as carbohydrates generally provides adequate

---

Table 12.1 TWO-STAGE DIETARY PLAN FOR INCREASING MUSCLE GLYCOGEN STORAGE

Stage 1—Depletion
  Day 1: Exhausting exercise performed to deplete muscle glycogen in specific muscles
  Days 2, 3, 4: Low-carbohydrate food intake (high percentage of protein and lipid in the daily diet)

Stage 2—Carbohydrate loading
  Days 5, 6, 7: High-carbohydrate food intake (normal percentage of protein in the daily diet)

Competition day
  Follow high-carbohydrate precompetition meal.

muscle and liver glycogen reserves. This diet ensures about twice the level of muscle glycogen obtained with consumption of a typical diet. For well-nourished, physically active individuals, the supercompensation effect remains relatively small. During intense training, however, individuals who do not increase daily caloric and carbohydrate intakes to meet increased energy demands may experience chronic muscle fatigue and staleness.[38]

Individuals should learn all they can about carbohydrate loading before trying to manipulate diet and exercise habits to achieve a supercompensation effect. If a person decides to supercompensate, after weighing the pros and cons (see page 361), the new food regimen should progress in stages during training, not for the first time before competition. For example, a runner should start with a long run followed by a high-carbohydrate diet. Keep a detailed log of how the dietary manipulation affects performance. Note subjective feelings during exercise depletion and replenishment phases. With positive results, then try the entire series of depletion, low-carbohydrate diet, and high-carbohydrate diet but maintain the low-carbohydrate diet for only 1 day. If no adverse effects appear, the low-carbohydrate diet should gradually extend to a maximum of 4 days.

Sample Diets to Achieve the Supercompensation Effect. TABLE 12.2 gives meal plans for carbohydrate depletion (*stage 1*) and carbohydrate loading (*stage 2*) preceding an endurance event.

Limited Applicability

Carbohydrate loading only benefits intense aerobic activities lasting more than 60 minutes, unless the person begins competing in a relative state of glycogen depletion. In contrast, less than 60 minutes of intense exercise requires only normal carbohydrate intake and glycogen reserves. For example, carbohydrate loading did not benefit trained runners in a 20.9-km (13-mile) run compared with a run following a low-carbohydrate diet. Similarly, no ergogenic effect emerged in time trial performance, heart rate, and rating of perceived exertion (RPE) for endurance-trained cyclists in a 100-km trial that simulated continuous changes in exercise intensity typical of competition.[22] In addition, ingesting 40 g of carbohydrate immediately before exercise did not benefit a 30-minute maximal cycling performance by trained cyclists.[130] Variations in the carbohydrate percentage between 40 and 70% for an isocaloric diet produced no effect on intense exercise of either 10 or 30 minutes duration.[132] Furthermore, anaerobic power output for 75 seconds did not improve when preexercise dietary manipulation increased muscle glycogen above normal levels.[71] A 2-day maintenance on a high-carbohydrate diet (61% carbohydrate) or a low–moderate carbohydrate diet (31% carbohydrate) produced no effect on intermittent anaerobic exercise consisting of five 20-second bouts interspersed with a 100-second recovery period followed by a sixth 30-second bout to exhaustion.[110] Ergogenic benefits did emerge for high-carbohydrate versus low-carbohydrate intakes when performing *multiple bouts* of short-term sprints.[6]

Table 12.2	SAMPLE MEAL PLAN FOR CARBOHYDRATE DEPLETION AND CARBOHYDRATE LOADING DIETS PRECEDING AN ENDURANCE EVENT	
Meal	*Stage 1–Depletion*	*Stage 2–Carbohydrate Loading*
Breakfast	0.5 cup fruit juice 2 eggs 1 slice whole-wheat toast 1 glass whole milk	1 cup fruit juice 1 bowl hot or cold cereal 1 to 2 muffins 1 Tbsp butter Coffee (cream/sugar)
Lunch	6 oz hamburger 2 slices bread Salad (normal size) 1 Tbsp mayonnaise and salad dressing 1 glass whole milk	2–3 oz hamburger with bun 1 cup juice 1 orange 1 Tbsp mayonnaise Pie or cake (1 8-inch slice)
Snack	1 cup yogurt	1 cup yogurt, fruit, or cookies
Dinner	2–3 pieces of chicken, fried 1 baked potato with sour cream 0.5 cup vegetables Iced tea (no sugar) 2 Tbsp butter	1–1.5 pieces of chicken, baked 1 baked potato with sour cream 1 cup vegetables 0.5 cup sweetened pineapple Iced tea (sugar) 1 Tbsp butter
Snack	1 glass whole milk	1 glass chocolate milk with 4 cookies

During *stage 1*, the intake of carbohydrate approaches approximately 100 g, 400 kcal; in *stage 2*, the carbohydrate intake increases to 400 to 625 g or about 1600 to 2500 kcal.

Negative Aspects of Carbohydrate Loading

The addition of 2.7 g of water with each gram of glycogen stored makes this a heavy fuel compared with equivalent energy stored as fat. The added body mass in the carbohydrate loaded state often makes the person feel "heavy" and uncomfortable; any extra load also directly adds to the energy cost of running, racewalking, or cross-country skiing, all weight-bearing activities. This effect of extra weight may negate the potential benefits from increased glycogen storage. On the positive side, water liberated during glycogen breakdown aids in temperature regulation, which provides benefits during exercise in the heat.

The classic model for supercompensation poses a potential hazard for individuals with specific health problems. A severe long-term carbohydrate overload, interspersed with periods of high lipid or high protein intake, can increase blood cholesterol and urea nitrogen levels. This could negatively affect individuals susceptible to type 2 diabetes and heart disease or those with muscle enzyme deficiencies (e.g., McArdle's disease) or renal disease. High lipid intake causes gastrointestinal distress, plus poor recovery from the exercise depletion sequence of the loading procedure. During the low-carbohydrate phase, marked ketosis can occur among individuals who exercise while carbohydrate-depleted. Failure to eat a balanced diet often produces mineral and vitamin deficiencies, particularly of the water-soluble vitamins, which then require supplementation. The glycogen-depleted state certainly reduces one's capability to train hard, possibly resulting in a detraining effect during the loading period. Adverse alterations in mood state also appear in individuals who train while consuming low-carbohydrate diets. Dramatically reducing dietary carbohydrate for 3 or 4 days sets the stage for lean tissue loss because muscle protein serves as gluconeogenic substrate to maintain blood-glucose levels in the glycogen-depleted state.

Modified Loading Procedure

Following the less stringent modified dietary protocol outlined in FIGURE 12.1 eliminates many of the negative outcomes of the classic glycogen-loading sequence. This 6-day protocol does not require prior exercise to exhaustion. The athlete exercises at about 75% of $\dot{V}O_2max$ (85% HR_{max}) for 1.5 hours and then on successive days, gradually reduces or tapers exercise duration. During the first 3 days, carbohydrates supply about 50% of total calories. Three days before competition, the diet's carbohydrate content then increases to 70% of total energy intake. This causes glycogen reserves to accumulate to about the *same level* as with the classic protocol. The modified approach to carbohydrate loading increases the glycogen-storing enzyme (glycogen synthetase), without requiring the dramatic glycogen depletion with exercise and diet required by the classic loading procedure.[198]

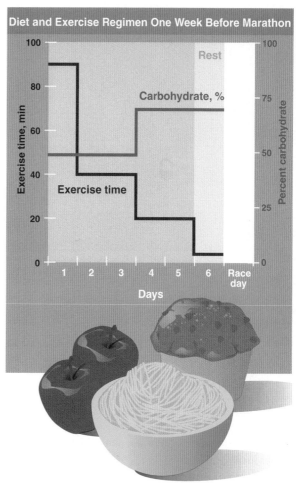

■ **Figure 12.1** The modified carbohydrate-loading approach. Recommended combination of diet and exercise for overloading muscle glycogen stores in the week before an endurance contest. Time devoted to exercise becomes gradually reduced during the week, while the diet's carbohydrate content increases for the last 3 days. (From Sherman WM, et al. Effect of exercise-diet manipulation on muscle glycogen and its subsequent utilization during performance. Int J Sports Med 1981;2:114.)

Rapid Loading Procedure: A One-Day Requirement

The 2 to 6 days required to achieve supranormal muscle glycogen levels represent a limitation of typical carbohydrate loading procedures. Research has evaluated whether a shortened time period that combines a relatively brief bout of high-intensity exercise with only 1 day of high-carbohydrate intake achieves the desired loading effect.[51] Endurance-trained athletes cycled for 150 seconds at 130% of $\dot{V}O_2max$ followed by 30 seconds of all-out cycling. In the recovery period, the men consumed 10.3 g·kg body mass^{-1} of high glycemic carbohydrate foods. Biopsy data presented in FIGURE 12.2 indicated that carbohydrate levels increased in all fiber types of the vastus lateralis muscle from a 109.1 mmol·kg^{-1} preloading average to 198.3 mmol·kg^{-1} after only 24 hours. This 82% increase in glycogen storage

■ **Figure 12.2** Muscle glycogen concentration of the vastus lateralis before (preloading) and after 180 seconds of near-maximal intensity cycling exercise followed by 1 day of high carbohydrate intake (postloading). (From Fairchild TJ, et al. Rapid carbohydrate loading after short bout of near maximal-intensity exercise. Med Sci Sports Exerc 2002;34:980.)

equaled or exceeded values reported by others using a 2- to 6-day regimen. The short-duration loading procedure benefits individuals who do not wish to disrupt normal training with the time required and potential negative aspects of other loading protocols.

Gender Differences in Glycogen Supercompensation and Glucose Catabolism in Exercise

Gender-related differences in muscle glycogen supercompensation remain controversial. One study reported a relatively small 13% increase in the muscle glycogen content of women when they switched from a mixed diet to a high-carbohydrate diet.[186] Other research also indicated that women stored less glycogen than men when dietary carbohydrate increased from 60 to 75% of total energy intake.[164] However, this increase in carbohydrate intake as a percentage of total calories represents *significantly less total carbohydrate intake* relative to lean body mass for women than for men. FIGURE 12.3 illustrates that equalizing daily carbohydrate intake for endurance-trained men and women at 12 g per kg of lean body mass for 3 consecutive days produced no gender differences in glycogen loading.[85] These and other findings[165] support the notion that men and women possess an equal capacity to accumulate muscle glycogen when fed comparable amounts of carbohydrate relative to their lean body mass.

Significant gender differences exist in carbohydrate metabolism during exercise before and after endurance training. During submaximal exercise at equivalent percentages of $\dot{V}O_2max$ (same relative workload), women derive a

smaller proportion of total energy from carbohydrate oxidation than men.[87] This gender difference in substrate oxidation does not persist into recovery.[78]

With similar endurance-training protocols, both women and men decrease glucose flow for a given submaximal power output.[32,56] However, at the same relative workload after training, women show an exaggerated shift toward fat catabolism, whereas men do not.[87] This suggests that endurance training induces greater glycogen-sparing at a given percentage of maximal effort for women. Gender differences in exercise substrate metabolism may reflect sympathetic nervous system adaptation to training with a more-diminished catecholamine response for women. A glycogen-sparing metabolic adaptation could benefit a woman's performance during high-intensity endurance competition.

Muscle Glycogen Supercompensation Enhanced by Prior Creatine Supplementation

A synergy exists between glycogen storage and creatine supplementation. For example, preceding a glycogen loading protocol with a 5-day creatine loading protocol (20 g per day) produced 10% more glycogen packing in the vastus lateralis muscle than was achieved with glycogen loading alone.[148] More than likely, increases in creatine and cellular volume with creatine supplementation facilitate subsequent storage of muscle glycogen.

■ **Figure 12.3** Muscle glycogen concentrations pre- and post-carbohydrate loading in exercise-trained men and women. (From James AP, et al. Muscle glycogen supercompensation: absence of a gender-related difference. Eur J Appl Physiol 2001;85:533.)

CASE STUDY/PERSONAL HEALTH AND EXERCISE NUTRITION 12–1

How to Identify the Metabolic Syndrome

In addition to lowering LDL-cholesterol, modification of other risk factors greatly reduce the likelihood of coronary heart disease (CHD). Specifically, a major target of therapy includes a constellation of lipid and nonlipid risk factors of metabolic origin known as the *Metabolic syndrome*. This syndrome closely links to the generalized metabolic disorder of *insulin resistance*, in which the normal actions of insulin are impaired. Excess body fat (particularly abdominal obesity) and physical inactivity promote the development of insulin resistance. In addition, some individuals are genetically predisposed to this condition.

The risk factors for the metabolic syndrome are highly concordant; in aggregate they enhance risk for CHD at any given LDL-cholesterol level. Diagnosis of the metabolic syndrome is made when three or more of the risk determinants shown in Table 1 are present. These determinants include a combination of categorical and borderline risk factors that can be readily measured.

Table 1	CLINICAL IDENTIFICATION OF THE METABOLIC SYNDROME
Risk Factor	*Defining Level*
Abdominal obesity[a]	**Waist girth**[b]
Men	>102 cm (>40 in.)
Women	>88 cm (>35 in.)
Triacylglycerols	≥ 150 mg $\cdot$ dL^{-1}
HDL-cholesterol	
Men	<40 mg $\cdot$ dL^{-1}
Women	<50 mg $\cdot$ dL^{-1}
Blood pressure	$\geq 130/\geq 85$ mm Hg
Fasting glucose	≥ 110 mg $\cdot$ dL^{-1}

From Third Report of the National Cholesterol Education Program (NCEP) Expert Panel on Detection, evaluation, and treatment of high blood cholesterol in adults (Adult Treatment Panel III). National Heart, Lung, and Blood Institute. NIH publ. no. 01-3670, May 2001.

[a] Overweight and obesity are associated with insulin resistance and the metabolic syndrome. However, the presence of abdominal obesity is more highly correlated with the metabolic risk factors than is an elevated body mass index (BMI). Therefore, the simple measure of waist girth is recommended to identify the body weight component of the metabolic syndrome.

[b] Some males can develop multiple metabolic risk factors when the waist girth is only marginally increased, e.g., 94 to 102 cm (37–39 in.). Such patients may have a strong genetic contribution to insulin resistance. They would benefit from changes in life habits, similar to men with larger increases in waist girth.

MANAGEMENT OF UNDERLYING CAUSES OF THE METABOLIC SYNDROME

Weight reduction and increased physical activity represent the first-line therapy for the metabolic syndrome. Weight reduction facilitates the lowering of LDL-cholesterol and reduces all of the risk factors of the syndrome. Regular physical activity reduces very low density lipoprotein (VLDL) levels, raises HDL-cholesterol, and in some persons lowers LDL-cholesterol. It also can lower blood pressure, reduce insulin resistance, and favorably influence overall cardiovascular function.

AMINO ACID SUPPLEMENTS AND OTHER DIETARY MODIFICATIONS FOR AN ANABOLIC EFFECT

Chapter 11 focused on anabolic–androgenic steroid use by an alarming number of male and female athletes in diverse sports. Coincidentally, an emerging trend involves using nutrition as a legal alternative for activating the body's normal anabolic mechanisms. Highly specific dietary changes supposedly create a hormonal milieu to facilitate protein synthesis in skeletal muscle. More than 100 companies in the United States market such alleged ergogenic stimulants. Weightlifters, body builders, and fitness enthusiasts use amino acid supplements believing they boost the body's natural production of the anabolic hormones testosterone, growth hormone (GH), insulin, or insulin-like growth factor I (IGF-I) to increase muscle size and strength and decrease body fat. The rationale for trying nutritional ergogenic stimulants comes from the clinical use of amino acid infusion or ingestion in protein-deficient patients to regulate anabolic hormones.

Research on healthy subjects does not provide convincing evidence for an ergogenic effect of a general dietary increase of oral amino acid supplements on hormone secretion, training responsiveness, or exercise performance. For example, in studies with appropriate design and statistical analysis, supplements of arginine, lysine, ornithine, tyrosine, and other amino acids, either singly or in combination, produced no effect on GH levels,[54,163] insulin secretion,[20,54] diverse measures of anaerobic power,[53] or all-out running performance at $\dot{V}O_2$max.[161] Furthermore, elite junior weightlifters who supplemented regularly with all 20 amino acids did not improve physical performance or resting or exercise-induced responses of testosterone, cortisol, or GH.[58] The indiscriminate use of amino acid supplements at dosages considered pharmacologic rather than nutritional increases risk of direct toxic effects or creation of an amino acid imbalance.[113]

Prudent Means to Possibly Augment an Anabolic Effect

Manipulation of exercise and nutritional variables in the immediate pre- and postexercise periods can impact the responsiveness to resistance training via mechanisms that alter nutrient availability, circulating metabolites and hormonal secretions and interactions with receptors on target tissues, and gene translation and transcription.[180] With resistance training, muscle enlargement (hypertrophy) occurs from a shift in the body's normal dynamic state of protein synthesis and degradation to greater tissue synthesis. The normal hormonal milieu (e.g., insulin and GH levels) in the period following resistance exercise stimulates the muscle fiber's anabolic processes while inhibiting muscle protein degradation. Specific dietary modifications that increase amino acid transport into muscle, raise energy availability, or increase anabolic hormone levels would theoretically augment the training effect by increasing the rate of anabolism and/or depressing catabolism. Either effect should create a positive body protein balance for improved muscular growth and strength.

Carbohydrate–Protein Supplementation Immediately in Recovery Augments Hormonal Response to Resistance Exercise

Studies of hormonal dynamics and protein anabolism indicate a transient but potential ergogenic effect (up to 4-fold increase in protein synthesis[139]) of carbohydrate and/or protein supplements consumed *prior to,*[168,195] or *immediately following,* resistance exercise workouts.[13,48,119,138,144,151,189] This effect of supplementation in the immediate postexercise period of resistance exercise may also prove effective for repair and synthesis of muscle proteins following aerobic exercise.[106,107]

Drug-free male weightlifters with at least 2 years of resistance training experience consumed carbohydrate and protein supplements immediately following a standard resistance-training workout.[29] Treatment included either *(a)* placebo of pure water, or a supplement of *(b)* carbohydrate

(1.5 g per kg body mass), *(c)* protein (1.38 g per kg body mass), or *(d)* carbohydrate/protein (1.06 g carbohydrate plus 0.41 g protein per kg body mass) consumed immediately following and then 2 hours after the training session. Compared with the placebo condition, each supplement produced a hormonal environment in recovery conducive to protein synthesis and muscle tissue growth (elevated plasma concentrations of insulin and GH). Subsequent research from the same laboratory showed that protein–carbohydrate supplementation before and after resistance training favorably altered metabolic and hormonal responses to three consecutive days of heavy resistance training.[99] Changes in the immediate recovery period included increased concentrations of glucose, insulin, GH, and IGF-I and decreased blood lactate concentration. Such data provide indirect evidence for a possible training benefit of increasing carbohydrate and/or protein intake immediately after a resistance-training workout.

Postexercise Glucose Augments Protein Balance After Resistance Training. Research with postexercise glucose ingestion complements the previously described studies of carbohydrate/protein supplementation following resistance training.[150] Healthy men familiar with resistance training performed unilateral knee extensor exercise consisting of eight sets of 10 repetitions at 85% of maximum strength (1-RM) in a placebo-controlled, randomized, double-blind trial. Immediately following the exercise session and 1 hour later, subjects received either a carbohydrate supplement (1.0 g per kg body mass) or a placebo (NutraSweet). Measurements consisted of *(a)* urinary 3-methylhistidine excretion (3-MH) to indicate muscle protein degradation, *(b)* vastus lateralis muscle incorporation rate for the amino acid leucine (L-[l-^{13}C]) to indicate protein synthesis, and *(c)* urinary nitrogen excretion to reflect protein breakdown. FIGURE 12.4 shows that glucose supplementation reduced myofibrillar protein breakdown reflected by decreased excretion of both 3-MH and urinary urea. Although not statistically significant, glucose supplementation also increased leucine incorporation into the vastus lateralis over the 10-hour postexercise period. All of these alterations indicated a more positive protein balance after exercise in the supplemented condition. The beneficial effect of glucose supplementation immediately following resistance exercise most likely resulted from increased insulin release. This hormone would enhance a positive muscle protein balance in recovery.

Although of possible significance as a "natural" means to stimulate anabolic processes and augment protein accretion, the effects of immediate postexercise carbohydrate and/or protein supplementation must be viewed in perspective. The question awaiting an answer is the degree to which any transient (albeit positive) change in hormonal milieu favoring anabolism and net protein synthesis caused by postexercise dietary maneuvers contributes to long-term muscle growth and strength enhancement. In this regard, recent research failed to show any effect of immediate postexercise ingestion of an amino

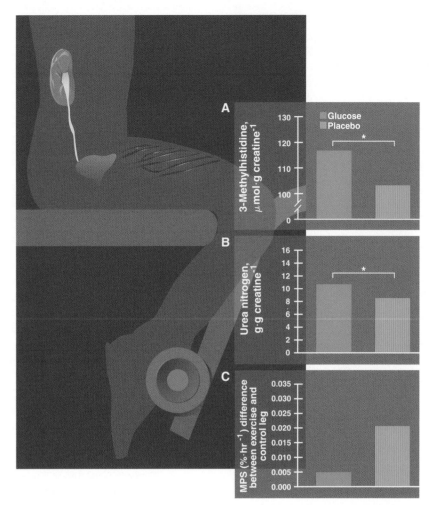

Figure 12.4 The effects of glucose (1.0 g per kg body mass) versus NutraSweet placebo ingested immediately after exercise and 1 hour later on protein degradation reflected by 24-hour urinary output of **(A)** 3-methylhistidine and **(B)** urea nitrogen, and **(C)** the rate of muscle protein synthesis *(MPS)* measured by vastus lateralis muscle incorporation rate for the amino acid leucine (L-[I-^{13}C]). *Bars* for MPS indicate difference between exercise and control leg for glucose and placebo conditions. *Significantly different from placebo condition. (From Roy BD, et al. Effect of glucose supplement timing on protein metabolism after resistance training. J Appl Physiol 1997;82:1882.)

acid–carbohydrate mixture on muscular strength or size gains of older men undergoing 12-weeks of knee extensor resistance training.[60] Differences in study population, criterion variables, specific amino acid mixtures, diet composition, and subjects' age may account for future discrepancies in research findings.

Dietary Lipid Affects Hormonal Milieu

The diet's lipid content modulates resting neuroendocrine homeostasis in a direction that may modify tissue synthesis. Research evaluated the effects of an intense resistance exercise bout on postexercise plasma testosterone, an anabolic and anticatabolic hormone released by the Leydig cells of the testes.[182] In agreement with prior research, testosterone levels significantly increased 5-minutes postexercise. A more impressive finding revealed a close association between the individual's regular dietary nutrient composition and resting plasma testosterone levels. TABLE 12.3 shows that dietary macronutrient amount and composition (protein, lipid, saturated fatty acids, monounsaturated fatty acids, polyunsaturated unsaturated fatty acid/saturated fatty acid ratio, and protein-to-carbohydrate ratio) correlated significantly with preexercise testosterone concentrations. More specifically, dietary lipid and saturated and monounsaturated fatty acid levels best predicted testosterone concentrations at rest—lower levels of each of these dietary components related to lower testosterone levels. These findings agree with previous studies that showed a low-fat diet of about 20% fat produced lower testosterone levels than a diet with a higher 40% lipid content.[137,143,166]

Table 12.3	CORRELATION COEFFICIENTS BETWEEN PRE-EXERCISE TESTOSTERONE CONCENTRATION AND SELECTED NUTRITIONAL VARIABLES

Nutrient	Correlation with testosterone[a]
Energy, kJ	−0.18
Protein, %[b]	−0.71*
CHO, %	−0.30
Lipid, %	0.72*
SFA, g·1000 kcal^{-1}·day^{-1}	0.77†
MUFA, g·1000 kcal^{-1}·day^{-1}	0.79†
PUFA, g·1000 kcal^{-1}·day^{-1}	0.25
Cholesterol, g·1000 kcal^{-1}·day^{-1}	0.53
PUFA/SFA	−0.63‡
Dietary fiber, g·1000 kcal^{-1}·day^{-1}	−0.19
Protein/CHO	−0.59‡
Protein/lipid	0.16
CHO/lipid	0.16

From Volek JS, et al.: Testosterone and cortisol in relationship to dietary nutrients and resistance exercise. J Appl Physiol 1997;82:49.
[a] Correlation coefficients, Pearson product-moment correlations.
[b] Nutrient percentage values expressed as percentage of total energy per day.
*$P \leq .01$. †$P \leq .005$. ‡$P \leq .05$.
SFA, saturated fatty acids; MUFA, monounsaturated fatty acids; PUFA, polyunsaturated fatty acids; CHO, cholesterol.

Interestingly, the data in Table 12.3 also show that the diet's protein percentage correlated *inversely* with testosterone levels in that higher protein levels related to *lower* testosterone levels. Because many resistance-trained athletes consume considerable dietary protein, the implications of this association for exercise training remain unresolved. Also, if low dietary lipid levels decrease resting levels of testosterone, then individuals consuming low-fat diets (e.g., vegetarians, and many dancers, gymnasts, and wrestlers) may experience a diminished training response. Furthermore, athletes who show reduced plasma testosterone with overtraining might benefit from changing their diet's macronutrient composition in the direction of higher lipid intake. Whether or not this proves correct awaits further prospective trials that assess the effects of manipulating diet composition on hormonal balance and training responsiveness.

Nutrient Timing to Optimize Muscle Response to Resistance Training. An evidence-based nutritional approach has been proposed to enhance the quality of resistance training and facilitate muscle growth and strength development.[82] This easy-to-follow new dimension to sports nutrition emphasizes not only the specific type and mixture of nutrients but also the timing of nutrient intake. Its goal is to blunt the catabolic state (release of hormones glucagon, epinephrine, norepinephrine, cortisol) and activate the natural muscle-building hormones (testosterone, growth hormone, IGF-1,

insulin) to facilitate recovery from exercise and maximize muscle growth. Three phases for optimizing specific nutrient intake are proposed:

(1) The *energy phase* enhances nutrient intake to spare muscle glycogen and protein, enhance muscular endurance, limit immune system suppression, reduce muscle damage, and facilitate recovery in the post-exercise period. Consuming a carbohydrate/protein supplement in the immediate pre-exercise period and during exercise extends muscular endurance; the ingested protein promotes protein metabolism thus reducing demand for amino acid release from muscle. The carbohydrates consumed during exercise suppress the release of cortisol. This blunts the suppressive effects of exercise on immune system function and lessens the use of branched-chain amino acids generated by protein breakdown for energy.

The recommended energy phase supplement profile contains the following nutrients: 20–26 g of high-glycemic carbohydrates (glucose, sucrose, maltodextrin), 5–6 g whey protein (rapidly digested, high-quality protein separated from milk in the cheese-making process), 1 g leucine; 30–120 mg vitamin C, 20–60 IU vitamin E, 100–250 mg sodium, 60–100 mg potassium, and 60–220 mg magnesium.

(2) The *anabolic phase* consists of the 45-minute post-exercise metabolic window—a period of enhanced insulin sensitivity for muscle glycogen replenishment and the repair and synthesis of muscle tissue. This shift from catabolic to anabolic state occurs largely by blunting the action of the catabolic hormone cortisol and increasing the anabolic, muscle-building effects of the hormone insulin by consuming a standard high-glycemic carbohydrate/protein supplement in liquid form (e.g., whey protein and high-glycemic carbohydrates). In essence, the high-glycemic carbohydrate consumed post exercise serves as a nutrient activator to stimulate the release of insulin, which, in the presence of amino acids, increases muscle tissue synthesis and decreases protein degradation.

The recommended anabolic phase supplement profile contains the following nutrients: 40–50 g of high-glycemic carbohydrates (glucose, sucrose, maltodextrin), 13–15 g whey protein, 1–2 g leucine; 1–2 g glutamine, 60–120 mg vitamin C, and 80–400 IU vitamin E.

(3) The *growth phase* extends from the end of the anabolic phase to the beginning of the next workout. It represents the time period to maximize insulin sensitivity and maintain an anabolic state to accentuate gains in muscle mass and muscle strength. The first several hours (rapid segment)

of this phase is geared to maintaining increased insulin sensitivity and glucose uptake to maximize glycogen replenishment. It also aims to speed the elimination of metabolic wastes via an increase in blood flow and stimulate tissue repair and muscle growth. The next 16 to 18 hours (sustained segment) maintains a positive nitrogen balance. This occurs with a relatively high daily protein intake (between 0.91 and 1.2 g of protein per pound of body weight) that fosters sustained but slower muscle tissue synthesis. An adequate carbohydrate intake emphasizes glycogen replenishment.

The recommended growth phase supplement profile contains the following nutrients: 14 g whey protein, 2 g casein, 3 g leucine, 1 g glutamine, and 2–4 g of high-glycemic carbohydrates.

L-CARNITINE

L-Carnitine (L-3-hydroxytrimethylamminobutanoate), a short-chain carboxylic acid containing nitrogen, is a vitamin-like compound with well-established functions in intermediary metabolism. It is found mostly in meat and dairy products. (*Note:* DL-carnitine is toxic and should never be consumed.) The liver and kidneys synthesize L-carnitine from methionine and lysine, with about 95% of the 20-g (120 mmol) total of carnitine located within muscle cells. Vital to normal metabolism, carnitine facilitates the influx of long-chain fatty acids into the mitochondrial matrix as part of the carnitine–acyl-CoA transferase system. The system causes activated acyl groups to reversibly transfer between coenzyme A and carnitine (see Chapter 4). The fatty acid components then enter β-oxidation during mitochondrial energy metabolism as follows:

$$\text{Carnitine} + \text{acyl-CoA} \leftrightarrow \text{acylcarnitine} + \text{CoA}$$

The reaction enables the acyl components of long-chain fatty acyl-CoA (carbon chain lengths ≥ 10) to cross the mitochondrial membrane as substrate for oxidation. This carnitine-dependent process is probably an important rate-limiting step in fatty acid oxidation.[17,117]

Intracellular carnitine helps to maintain the acetyl-CoA/CoA ratio within the cell. Optimizing this ratio augments skeletal muscle energy metabolism by limiting inhibition of the pyruvate dehydrogenase enzyme; this effect facilitates conversion of pyruvate (and lactate) to acetyl-CoA, particularly in the type I, slow-twitch muscle fibers.[27,57] Theoretically, enhanced carnitine function could inhibit lactate accumulation and enhance exercise performance.[35,169] TABLE 12.4 outlines the potential mechanisms by which carnitine supplementation could enhance exercise performance.

Table 12.4	**POTENTIAL MECHANISMS FOR A BENEFICIAL EFFECT OF CARNITINE SUPPLEMENTATION ON EXERCISE PERFORMANCE IN HEALTHY HUMANS**

- Enhance muscle fatty acid oxidation
- Decrease muscle glycogen depletion rates
- Shift substrate use in muscle from fatty acid to glucose
- Replace muscle carnitine redistributed into acylcarnitine
- Activate pyruvate dehydrogenase via lowering of acetyl-CoA content
- Improve muscle fatigue resistance
- Replace carnitine lost during training

From Brass EP. Supplemental carnitine and exercise. Am J Clin Nutr 2000;72(suppl):618S.

Rate of Fatty Acid Oxidation Affects Aerobic Exercise Intensity

During prolonged aerobic exercise, plasma free fatty acids (FFAs) often rise to a greater extent than required by the actual energy expenditure. The plasma lipid elevation could result from inadequate mitochondrial fatty acid uptake and oxidation because of insufficient L-carnitine concentration. Thus, increasing intracellular L-carnitine levels through dietary supplementation should elevate aerobic energy transfer from fat breakdown while conserving limited glycogen reserves. Supplementation should prove most beneficial under conditions of glycogen depletion, which places the greatest demand on fatty acid oxidation. Consequently, L-carnitine marketing targets endurance athletes who believe this "metabolic stimulator" enhances fat burning and spares glycogen. Not surprisingly, the alleged fat-burning benefits of carnitine also appeal to body builders as a practical way to reduce body fat.

While patients with progressive muscle weakness have benefited from carnitine administration, few data suggest that healthy adults require carnitine above levels in a well-balanced diet. *Research shows no ergogenic benefits, positive metabolic alterations (aerobic or anaerobic), or body fat-reducing effects from L-carnitine supplementation.*[18,34,185] For example, no difference exists in muscle carnitine levels between young and middle-aged men who consume a normal carnitine intake of about 100 to 200 mg daily. For these individuals, typical variations in carnitine levels do not reflect capacity for aerobic metabolism.[159] Furthermore, no L-carnitine deficit occurs during long-term exercise or heavy training.[40,86,129] The low bioavailability and rapid renal excretion of oral carnitine make it highly unlikely that supplementation affects muscle carnitine stores in healthy subjects. Taking up to 2000 mg of L-carnitine, either orally or intravenously, during aerobic exercise does not affect the fuel mixture catabolized or endurance performance, aerobic capacity, or the exercise level for the onset of blood lactate accumulation (OBLA).[18,185,197]

Short-term administration of 2000 mg of L-carnitine to endurance athletes 2 hours before a marathon and after 20-km of the run increased plasma concentrations of all carnitine fractions.[34] The carnitine increases did not affect running performance, alter metabolic mixture during the run, or enhance recovery. Even with exercise prolonged and intense enough to deplete glycogen reserves, L-carnitine supplements did not alter substrate metabolism to indicate enhanced fat oxidation.[41] Carnitine supplementation also exerts no effect on repetitive short-term anaerobic exercise. Lactate accumulation, acid–base balance, or performance in five, 100-yard swims with 2-minute rest intervals did not differ between competitive swimmers who consumed 2000 mg of L-carnitine in a citrus drink twice daily for 7 days and swimmers who only consumed the citrus drink.[169]

Perhaps of Some Benefit

L-Carnitine acts as a vasodilator in peripheral tissues, thus possibly enhancing regional blood flow and oxygen delivery. In one study, subjects took either L-carnitine supplements (3000 mg per day for 3 weeks) or an inert placebo to evaluate the effectiveness of L-carnitine supplementation on delayed-onset muscle soreness (DOMS).[59] They then performed eccentric muscle actions to induce muscle soreness. Compared with placebo conditions, subjects receiving L-carnitine experienced less postexercise muscle pain and tissue damage as indicated by lower plasma levels of the muscle enzyme creatine kinase. The vasodilation property of L-carnitine might improve oxygen supply to injured tissue and promote clearance of muscle damage byproducts, thus reducing DOMS.

BEE POLLEN

Bees gather pollen, the material from the fine, powderlike reproductive substance produced by flowering plants. Bee pollen's allure as a nutrient supplement for physically active individuals lies in its relatively rich mixture of vitamins, minerals, and amino acids required for energy-producing reactions. It also has the appeal of a compound directly synthesized in nature, making it an advertiser's dream as a cancer-preventing, life-prolonging "perfect food." Unfortunately, no reliable data attest to its effectiveness as an ergogenic aid. In one study, highly trained runners who received bee pollen supplements showed no improvement in recovery rate from repeated maximal treadmill runs to exhaustion.[194] Furthermore, no effects of bee pollen supplementation occurred for maximal oxygen uptake, endurance performance, or other physiologic responses to exercise.[28] In addition to a lack of scientific evidence to justify its use as an ergogenic aid, supplementing with bee pollen does not lack risk. Individuals allergic to specific pollens may experience extreme reactions when taking this supplement.

BORON

The precise biochemical function of the trace mineral boron remains unclear, although it appears in high concentrations in bone and tissues of the spleen and thyroid gland. Boron deprivation significantly depresses bone tissue synthesis. Studies of postmenopausal women previously deprived of dietary boron showed that supplementing with boron augmented calcium and magnesium metabolism and increased testosterone levels.[124] The promise of increased testosterone output tempts weightlifters and body builders to consume excess boron to promote an anabolic effect. Mail-order advertisements extol boron-containing supplements as a safe replacement for anabolic steroids, without harmful side effects.

Limited information indicates that boron supplements do not affect testosterone levels in individuals adequately nourished for this mineral. For individuals undergoing resistance training, daily 6-mg supplements of boron (plus 800 μg of chromium picolinate) did not enhance lean tissue accretion or promote fat loss compared to a maltodextrin placebo.[1] Until more research becomes available, we recommend that an individual's total intake of boron not exceed 10 mg daily.

CHROMIUM

Chromium occurs widely in soil as chromite at a concentration that averages 250 μg per kg of soil. Its distribution in plants ranges between 100 and 500 μg per kg and in foodstuffs between 20 and 590 μg per kg. This trace mineral serves as a cofactor (as trivalent chromium) for a low-molecular-weight protein that potentiates insulin function, although chromium's precise mechanism of action remains unclear. Insulin promotes glucose transport into cells, augments fatty acid metabolism, and triggers cellular enzyme activity to facilitate protein synthesis. Chronic chromium deficiency increases blood cholesterol and decreases sensitivity to insulin, thus increasing the chance for type 2 diabetes. Some adult Americans consume less than the 50 to 200 μg of chromium each day considered the estimated safe and adequate daily dietary intake (ESADDI). This occurs largely because chromium-rich foods—brewer's yeast, broccoli, wheat germ, nuts, liver, prunes, egg yolks, apples with skins, asparagus, mushrooms, wine, and cheese—do not usually form part of the regular diet. Processing also removes significant chromium from foods. In addition, strenuous exercise and associated high carbohydrate intake promote urinary chromium losses, thus increasing the potential for chromium deficiency. For athletes with chromium-deficient diets, modifications to increase chromium intake or prudent use of chromium supplements seem appropriate. Touted as a "fat burner" and "muscle builder," chromium represents the largest selling mineral supplement in the United States (second only to calcium) in today's health food/fitness literature.[125] Used by more than 10 million people, it commands annual sales of roughly $500 million. Poor intestinal absorption of chromium in its inorganic form (chromium chloride) provides a main hindrance to effective oral chromium supplementation. Supplement intake of chromium, usually as **chromium picolinate** (picolinic acid, an organic compound in breast milk that helps transport minerals), often reaches 600 μg daily. This chelated picolinic acid combination supposedly improves chromium absorption. A 2-month supply of 500-μg chromium pills retails for about $10. Millions of Americans believe the unsubstantiated claims of health food faddists, television infomercials, and exercise zealots that additional chromium promotes muscle growth, curbs appetite, fosters body fat loss, and lengthens life. Advertising targets chromium to body builders and other resistance-trained individuals as a safe alternative to anabolic steroids to favorably change body composition. Chromium supplements supposedly potentiate insulin's action, thus increasing skeletal muscle's amino acid anabolism. This belief persists despite current scientific belief that chromium supplements exert no effect on glucose or insulin concentrations in non-diabetic individuals.[2]

Generally, studies suggesting beneficial effects of chromium supplements on body fat and muscle mass inferred body composition modifications from changes in body weight (or unvalidated anthropometric measurements) instead of a more appropriate assessment by hydrostatic weighing or dual energy x-ray absorptiometry (DXA). One study observed that supplementing daily with 200 μg (3.85 μmol) of chromium picolinate for 40 days produced a small increase in fat-free body mass (FFM; estimated from skinfold thickness) and a decrease in body fat in young men undergoing 6 weeks of resistance training.[49] However, the researchers presented no data to show increased muscular strength. Another study reported increased body mass without changes in muscular strength or body composition in previously untrained female college students (no change in males) receiving daily chromium supplements of 200 μg during a 12-week resistance training program compared with unsupplemented controls.[74]

Other research evaluated the effects of a daily 200-μg chromium supplement on muscle strength, body composition, and chromium excretion in untrained men during 12 weeks of resistance training.[70] Muscular strength improved 24% for the supplemented group and 33% for the placebo group. No changes occurred in any of the body composition variables. The group receiving the supplement did show significantly higher chromium excretion than the controls after 6 weeks of training. The researchers concluded that chromium supplements provided *no ergogenic effect* on any of the measured variables. Furthermore, a daily supplement of 800 μg of chromium picolinate (plus 6 mg of boron) produced no greater effects than a maltodextrin placebo on lean tissue gain or fat loss during resistance training.[1]

Daily supplementation of 400 μg of chromium picolinate for 9 weeks did not promote weight loss for sedentary obese women, but actually caused significant weight gain during the treatment period.[63] In support of chromium supplementation, greater body fat loss (no increase in FFM) occurred in subjects "recruited from a variety of fitness and athletic clubs" who consumed 400 μg daily over 90 days than in subjects receiving a placebo.[95] Hydrostatic weighing and DXA assessed body composition. However pre- versus posttest body composition data from hydrostatic weighing were not presented, and the DXA-derived analysis indicated average percentage body fat values of 42% for both control and experimental subjects, a seemingly extraordinary level of obesity for fitness club members.

Collegiate football players who received daily supplements of 200 μg of chromium picolinate for 9 weeks showed no changes in body composition and muscular strength from intense weight-lifting training compared with a control group who received a placebo.[31] Similar findings of no benefit on body composition and exercise performance variables emerged from a 14-week study of NCAA division I wrestlers who combined chromium picolinate supplementation with a typical preseason training program, compared with identical training without supplementation.[187]

Because loss of muscle mass commonly affects older individuals, any potential benefit on muscle from chromium supplementation should readily emerge in this group. This did not occur for older men involved in high-intensity resistance training. A daily high dose of 924 μg of chromium picolinate did not augment gains in muscle size, strength, or power or FFM compared with the no-supplement condition.[24] Among obese personnel enrolled in the U.S. Navy's mandatory remedial physical conditioning program, consuming additional 400 μg of chromium picolinate daily caused no greater loss in body weight and percentage body fat or increase in FFM than occurred in a group receiving a placebo.[170]

A comprehensive double-blind research design studied the effect of a daily chromium supplement (3.3–3.5 μmol either as chromium chloride or chromium picolinate) or a placebo for 8 weeks during resistance training in young men.[109] For each group, dietary intakes of protein, magnesium, zinc, copper, and iron equaled or exceeded recommended levels during training; subjects also maintained adequate baseline chromium intakes. Supplementation increased serum chromium concentration and urinary chromium excretion equally, regardless of its ingested form. TABLE 12.5 shows that compared with placebo treatment, chromium supplementation did not affect training-related changes in muscular strength, physique, FFM, or muscle mass. In November 1996, the Federal Trade Commission ordered three makers of chromium supplements to cease promoting unsubstantiated weight loss and health claims (reduced body fat, increased muscle mass, increased energy level) for chromium picolinate. Under the settlement, the companies could no longer claim benefit unless reliable research data substantiated such a claim.

Not without a Potential Down Side

Chromium competes with iron for binding to transferrin, a plasma protein that transports iron from ingested food and damaged red blood cells and delivers it to tissues in need. The chromium picolinate supplements for the group whose data appear in Table 12.5 did reduce serum transferrin (a measure of current iron intake) compared with chromium chloride or placebo treatments. However, other researchers have observed that giving middle-aged men 924 μg of supplemental chromium picolinate daily for 12 weeks did not affect hematologic measures or indices of iron metabolism or iron status.[23] Further research must determine whether chromium supplementation above recommended values adversely affects iron transport and distribution within the body. Furthermore, no studies have evaluated the safety of long-term supplementation with chromium picolinate or the ergogenic efficacy of supplementation in individuals with suboptimal chromium status. Concerning the bioavailability of trace minerals in the diet, excessive dietary chromium inhibits zinc and iron absorption. At the extreme, this could induce iron-deficiency anemia, blunt the ability to train intensely, and negatively affect exercise performance requiring a high level of aerobic metabolism.

Further potential bad news emerges from studies in which human tissue cultures that received extreme doses of chromium picolinate showed eventual chromosomal damage. Critics contend that such high laboratory dosages would not occur with supplement use in humans. Nonetheless, one could argue that cells continually exposed to excessive chromium (e.g., long-term supplementation) accumulate this mineral and retain it for years. Further research must determine the possible ill effects of long-term chromium supplementation at the considerable excess ingested by some athletes.[88]

COENZYME Q10 (UBIQUINONE)

Coenzyme Q_{10} (CoQ_{10}, ubiquinone in oxidized form and ubiquinol when reduced), found primarily in meats, peanuts, and soybean oil, functions as an integral component of the mitochondrion's electron transport system of oxidative phosphorylation. This lipid-soluble natural component of all cells exists in high concentrations within myocardial tissue. CoQ_{10} has been used therapeutically to treat cardiovascular disease because of (a) its role in oxidative metabolism and (b) its antioxidant properties that promote scavenging of free radicals that damage cellular components.[89,178] Owing to its

| Table 12.5 | EFFECTS OF TWO DIFFERENT FORMS OF CHROMIUM SUPPLEMENTATION ON AVERAGE VALUES FOR ANTHROPOMETRIC, BONE, AND SOFT TISSUE COMPOSITION MEASUREMENTS BEFORE AND AFTER WEIGHT TRAINING |

	Placebo		Chromium chloride		Chromium picolinate	
	Pre	Post	Pre	Post	Pre	Post
Age (years)	21.1	21.5	23.3	23.5	22.3	22.5
Stature (cm)	179.3	179.2	177.3	177.3	178.0	178.2
Weight (kg)	79.9	80.5[a]	79.3	81.1[a]	79.2	80.5
Σ4 skinfold thickness (mm)[b]	42.0	41.5	42.6	42.2	43.3	43.1
Upper arm (cm)	30.9	31.6[a]	31.3	32.0[a]	31.1	31.4[a]
Lower leg (cm)	38.2	37.9	37.4	37.5	37.1	37.0
Endomorphy	3.68	3.73	3.58	3.54	3.71	3.72
Mesomorphy	4.09	4.36[a]	4.25	4.42[a]	4.21	4.33[a]
Ectomorphy	2.09	1.94[a]	1.79	1.63[a]	2.00	1.88[a]
FFMFM (kg)[c]	62.9	64.3[a]	61.1	63.1[a]	61.3	62.7[a]
Bone mineral (g)	2952	2968	2860	2878	2918	2940
Fat-free mass (kg)	65.9	67.3[a]	64.0	65.9[a]	64.2	66.1[a]
Fat (kg)	13.4	13.1	14.7	15.1	14.7	14.5
Fatness (%)	16.4	15.7	18.4	18.2	18.4	17.9

From Lukaski HC, et al. Chromium supplementation and resistance training: effects on body composition, strength, and trace element status of men. Am J Clin Nutr 1996;63:954.
[a] Significantly different from pretraining value.
[b] Measured at biceps, triceps, subscapular, and suprailiac sites.
[c] Fat-free, mineral-free mass.

positive effect on oxygen uptake and exercise performance in cardiac patients, some consider CoQ_{10} a potential ergogenic nutrient for endurance performance. Based on the belief that supplementation could increase the flux of electrons through the respiratory chain and thus augment aerobic resynthesis of adenosine triphosphate (ATP), the popular literature touts CoQ_{10} supplements to improve "stamina" and enhance cardiovascular function.

Although CoQ_{10} supplementation increases serum CoQ_{10} levels, it does not improve aerobic capacity, endurance performance, plasma glucose or lactate levels at submaximal workloads, or cardiovascular dynamics, compared with a placebo.[19,146,200] One study evaluated oral supplements of CoQ_{10} on the exercise tolerance and peripheral muscle function of healthy, middle-aged men. Measurements included $\dot{V}O_2max$, lactate threshold, heart rate response, and upper-extremity exercise blood flow and metabolism.[134] For 2 months, subjects received either CoQ_{10} (150 mg per day) or a placebo. Blood levels of CoQ_{10} increased significantly during the treatment period and remained unchanged in the controls. No differences occurred between groups for any of the physiologic or metabolic variables. Similarly, for trained young and older men, CoQ_{10} supplementation of 120 mg per day for 6 weeks did not benefit aerobic capacity or lipid peroxidation, a marker of oxidative stress.[104] More recent data also indicate that CoQ_{10} supplements (60 mg daily combined with vitamins E and C) did not affect lipid peroxidation during exercise in endurance athletes.[178] On the other hand, rats supplemented with CoQ_{10} (10 mg per day for 4 days), showed marked suppression of exercise-induced lipid peroxidation in liver, heart, and gastrocnemius muscle tissues.[50]

Future research must elucidate any potential benefits from exogenous CoQ_{10} supplementation. If benefits result, do they depend on the health status of one's cardiovascular system? On a negative note, CoQ_{10} supplementation may induce harmful effects. Increased cell damage (increased plasma CK) occurred during intense exercise in subjects receiving 60 mg of CoQ_{10} twice daily for 20 days.[114] Researchers speculate that under conditions of high proton concentrations as occur in high-intensity aerobic exercise, CoQ_{10} supplementation augments free radical production.[43,114] If this proves true, supplementation could trigger plasma membrane lipid peroxidation and eventual cellular damage. This is indeed paradoxical in light of CoQ_{10}'s wide use as an oral antioxidant supplement.

CREATINE

Meat, poultry, and fish provide rich sources of creatine; they contain approximately 4 to 5 g per kg of food weight. The body synthesizes only about 1 to 2 g of this nitrogen-containing organic compound daily, primarily in the kidneys, liver, and pancreas, from the amino acids arginine,

glycine, and methionine. Thus, adequate dietary creatine usually becomes important for obtaining required amounts of this compound.[196] Because the animal kingdom contains the richest creatine-containing foods, vegetarians experience a distinct disadvantage in obtaining ready sources of exogenous creatine.

Creatine supplements, sold as **creatine monohydrate (CrH_2O)**, come as a powder, tablet, capsule, and stabilized liquid. The trade publication *Nutrition Business Journal* estimated sales of creatine at about $260 million in 2000, with continued growth through 2004. A person can purchase creatine over-the-counter or via mail order as a nutritional supplement (without guarantee of purity). Ingesting a liquid suspension of creatine monohydrate at the relatively high dosage of 20 to 30 g a day for up to 2 weeks increases intramuscular concentrations of free creatine and phosphocreatine by 10 to 30%. These levels remain high for weeks after only a few days of supplementation.[66,73,79,116] An athlete can supplement with creatine in international competition because governing bodies (including the IOC) do not consider creatine an illegal substance.

Important Component of High-Energy Phosphates

The precise physiologic mechanisms underlying the potential ergogenic effectiveness of supplemental creatine remain poorly understood. Creatine passes through the digestive tract unaltered for absorption into the bloodstream by the intestinal mucosa. Just about all ingested creatine incorporates within skeletal muscle (120–150 g total with average concentration of 125 mM [range, 90–160 mM] per kg dry muscle) via insulin-mediated active transport. About 40% of the total exists as free creatine; the remainder combines readily with phosphate (in the creatine kinase reaction shown below) to form phosphocreatine, or PCr. Type II, fast-twitch muscle fibers store about 4 to 6 times more PCr than ATP.[26] As emphasized in Chapter 4, PCr serves as the cells' "energy reservoir" to provide rapid phosphate-bond energy to resynthesize ATP (more rapid than ATP generated in glycogenolysis[67]) in the reversible creatine kinase reaction:

$$PCr + ADP \xrightarrow{\text{creatine kinase}} Cr + ATP$$

PCr may also function to "shuttle" intramuscular high-energy phosphate between the mitochondria and the cross-bridge sites that initiate muscle action. Maintaining a high sarcoplasmic ATP/ADP ratio by energy transfer from PCr becomes important in all-out effort lasting up to 10 seconds. Such short-duration exercise places significant demands on the rate of ATP resynthesis, the breakdown of which greatly exceeds energy transfer from the intracellular macronutrients.[15,171] Improved energy transfer capacity from PCr also lessens reliance on energy transfer from anaerobic glycolysis with its associated increase in intramuscular H^+ and decrease in pH from lactate accumulation. Owing to limited amounts of intramuscular PCr, it seems reasonable that any increase in PCr availability should have the following four effects:[15,25,68,175]

1. Accelerating ATP turnover rate to maintain power output during short-term muscular effort
2. Delaying PCr depletion
3. Diminishing dependence on anaerobic glycolysis with subsequent lactate formation
4. Facilitating muscle relaxation and recovery from repeated bouts of an intense, brief effort via increased rate of ATP and PCr resynthesis; rapid recovery allows continued high-level power output

Individuals involved in power-type physical activities believe that creatine supplementation at recommended levels exerts the following three effects:

1. Improves repetitive performance in muscular strength and short-term power activities
2. Augments short bursts of muscular endurance
3. Provides for greater muscular overload to enhance training effectiveness

Documented Benefits Under Certain Exercise Conditions

Creatine received notoriety as an ergogenic aid when used by British sprinters and hurdlers in the 1992 Barcelona Olympic Games. Creatine supplementation at the recommended level exerts ergogenic effects in short-duration, high-intensity exercise (5–10% improvement) without producing harmful side effects (TABLE 12.6). However, anecdotes indicate a possible association between creatine supplementation and cramping in multiple muscle areas during competition or lengthy practice by football players. This effect may result from (a) altered intracellular dynamics from increased free creatine and PCr levels or (b) an osmotically induced enlarged muscle cell volume (greater cellular hydration) caused by the increased creatine content. Gastrointestinal tract disturbances such as nausea, indigestion, and difficulty absorbing food have also been linked to exogenous creatine ingestion.

FIGURE 12.5 clearly illustrates the significant ergogenic effects of creatine loading on total work accomplished during repetitive sprint cycling performance. Physically active but untrained males performed sets of maximal 6-second bicycle sprints interspersed with various recovery periods

Table 12.6	SELECTED STUDIES SHOWING INCREASE IN EXERCISE PERFORMANCE FOLLOWING CREATINE MONOHYDRATE SUPPLEMENTATION		
Reference	Exercise	Protocol	Exercise Performance
d	Isokinetic, unilat. knee extensions ($180°·s^{-1}$)	5 bouts of 30 ext. w/ 1-min rest periods	Reduction in decline of peak torque production during bouts 2, 3, and 4
e	Running	Four 300 m w/ 4-min rest periods; four 1000 m w/ 3-min rest periods	Improved time for final 300- and 1000-m runs; improved total time for four 1000-m runs; reduction in best time for 300- and 1000-m runs
a	Cycle ergometry (140 rev·min^{-1})	Ten 6-s bouts w/ 1-min rest periods	Better able to maintain pedal frequency during 4–6 s of each bout
f	Cycle ergometry (140 rev·min^{-1})	Five 6-s bouts w/ 30- s recovery followed by one 10-s bout	Better able to maintain pedal frequency near end of 10-s bout
b	Cycle ergometry (80 rev·min^{-1})	Three 30-s bouts w/ 4-min rest periods	Increase in peak power during bout 1 and increase in mean power and total work during bouts 1 and 2
c	Bench press	1-RM bench press and total reps at 70% of 1-RM	Increase in 1-RM; increase in reps at 70% of 1-RM
g	Bench press	5 sets bench press w/ 2-min rest periods	Increase in reps completed during all 5 sets
	Jump squat	5 sets jump squat w/ 2-min rest periods	Increase in peak power during all 5 sets

From Volek JS, Kraemer WJ. Creatine supplication: its effect on human muscular performance and body composition. J Strength Cond Res 1996;10:200.
[a] Balsom PD, et al. Creatine supplementation and dynamic high-intensity intermittent exercise. Scand J Med Sci Sports 1993;3:143.
[b] Birch R, et al. The influence of dietary creatine supplementation on performance during repeated bouts of maximal isokinetic cycling in man. Eur J Appl Physiol 1994; 69:268.
[c] Earnest CP, et al. The effect of creatine monohydrate ingestion on anaerobic power indices, muscular strength and body composition. Acta Physiol Scand 1995;153:207.
[d] Greenhaff PL, et al. Influence of oral creatine supplementation on muscle torque during repeated bouts on maximal voluntary exercise in man. Clin Sci 1993;84:565.
[e] Harris RC, et al. The effect of oral creatine supplementation on running performance during maximal short-term exercise in man. J Physiol 1993;467:74P.
[f] Soderlund K, et al. Creatine supplementation and high-intensity exercise: influence on performance and muscle metabolism. Clin Sci 1994;87(suppl.):120.
[g] Volek JS, et al. Creatine supplementation enhances muscular performance during high-intensity resistance exercise. J Am Diet Assoc 1997;97:765.

Figure 12.5 Effects of creatine loading versus placebo on total work accomplished during long-term (80-min) repetitive sprint-cycling performance. (From Preen CD, et al. Effect of creatine loading on long-term sprint exercise performance and metabolism. Med Sci Sports Exerc 2001;33:814.)

(24, 54, or 84 s) between sprints to simulate sport conditions. Performance evaluations took place under creatine-loaded (20 g per day for 5 days) or placebo conditions. Supplementation significantly increased muscle creatine (48.9%) and PCr (12.5%) over the placebo levels. Increased intramuscular creatine produced a 6% increase in total work accomplished (251.7 kJ presupplement vs. 266.9 kJ creatine loaded) compared with that of the group that consumed the placebo (254.0 kJ presupplement vs. 252.3 kJ placebo). Creatine supplements have also benefited an on-court "ghosting" routine of simulated positional play of competitive squash players.[149] It also augments repeated sprint cycle performance after 30 minutes of constant load, submaximal exercise in the heat, without adversely affecting thermoregulatory dynamics.[184] These benefits to muscular performance also occur in normally active older men.[62]

FIGURE 12.6 outlines mechanisms of how elevating intramuscular free creatine and PCr with creatine supplementation might enhance exercise performance and the training response. Besides benefiting weight lifting and body building, improved immediate anaerobic power output capacity also aids sprint running, swimming, kayaking, and cycling, and in jumping, football, and volleyball. Increased intramuscular PCr concentrations should also enable individuals to increase training intensity.

Ergogenic effects of creatine supplementation also occur in animals. Specifically, supplementation combined with exercise training enhanced repetitive high-intensity running performance of rats to a greater extent than only training or only supplementing.[16] In addition, in vitro preparations of myogenic satellite cells obtained from young adult sheep showed increased proliferation or differentiation when exposed to creatine.[179] In humans, oral creatine supplementation combined with heavy resistance training affected cellular functional processes in a manner that increased protein deposition within the muscle's contractile mechanism.[192] This response could possibly explain any increase in muscle size and strength associated with creatine supplementation in vivo. From a clinical perspective, exogenous creatine may reduce damage when administered after traumatic head injury, although the protective mechanism remains unknown.

Oral supplements of creatine monohydrate (20–25 g per day) significantly increase muscle creatine and performance in high-intensity exercise, particularly repeated intense muscular effort.[14,36,126,135,174] The ergogenic effect does not vary between vegetarians or meat eaters.[152] Even daily doses as low as 6 g for 5 days promote significant improvements in repeated power performance.[47] Other research evaluated the effects of a 6-day creatine supplement of 30 g daily on the exercise performance of trained runners under two conditions: *(a)* four repeated 300-m runs with 4-minute recovery and *(b)* four 1000-m runs with 3-minute recovery.[72] Compared with placebo treatment, creatine supplementation improved performance in both running events. The most impressive improvements occurred in the repeated 1000-m runs. Supplementing 20 g of creatine daily for 4 days also benefited anaerobic capacity on three 30-second bicycle ergometer Wingate tests with a 5-minute rest between trials.

For division I football players, creatine supplementation with resistance training increased body mass, lean body mass, cellular hydration, and muscular strength and performance.[8] Similarly, supplementation augmented muscular strength and size increases during 12-weeks of resistance training.[191] The enhanced hypertrophic response with supplementation and resistance training possibly resulted from accelerated myosin heavy chain synthesis. For resistance-trained men classified as "responders" to creatine supplementation, (i.e., an increase of ≥ 32 mmol·kg dry wt muscle^{-1}), 5 days of supplementation increased body weight and FFM and peak force and total force during repeated maximal isometric bench-presses.[97] For men classified as "nonresponders" to supplementation (i.e., increase of ≤ 21 mmol·kg dry wt muscle^{-1}), no ergogenic effect occurred.

Creatine supplementation does *not* improve exercise performance that requires a high level of aerobic energy transfer,[4,5,47] or cardiovascular and metabolic responses during continuous incremental treadmill running.[64] It also exerts little effect on isometric muscular strength or dynamic muscle force measured during a brief single movement.[7,55,140,141]

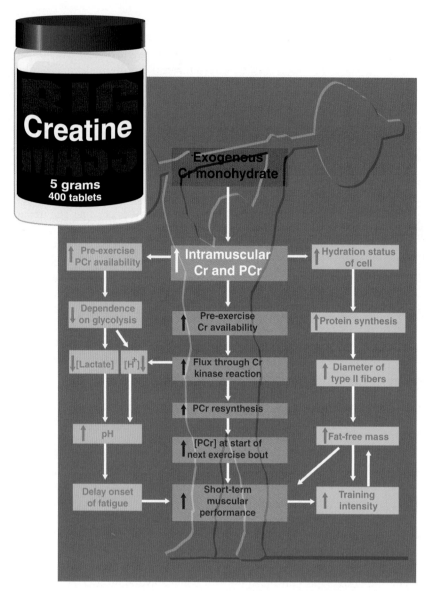

Age Effects Uncertain

Whether or not creatine supplementation augments the training response in older individuals remains equivocal. For 70-year old men, a creatine supplementation loading phase (0.3 g per kg body mass for 5days) followed by a daily maintenance phase (0.07 g per kg body mass) increased lean tissue mass, leg strength, muscular endurance, and average power of the legs during resistance training to a greater extent than a placobo.[30] Additional research shows no enhancement in resistance training response to creatine ingestion among sedentary and weight-trained older adults.[11] The investigators attributed their results to an age-related decline in creatine transport efficiency. Short-term creatine supplementation per se, without resistance training, does not increase muscle protein synthesis or FFM.[131]

Metabolic Reloading of High–Energy Phosphates

A large dose of creatine helps to replenish muscle creatine levels following heavy exercise.[26,68] Such metabolic "reloading" should facilitate recovery of muscle contractile capacity, thus enabling athletes to sustain repeated efforts of intense exercise. Whether this potential to maintain "quality" workouts enhances the training response for strength athletes and power athletes awaits further research.

Are There Risks?

Limited research exists about the potential dangers of creatine supplementation in healthy individuals, particularly the effects on cardiac muscle and kidney function (creatine degrades to creatinine before excretion in urine). Short-term use (e.g., 20 g per day for 5 consecutive days) in healthy men produced no detrimental effect on blood pressure, plasma creatine, plasma CK activity, or the renal response as measured by glomerular filtration rate and total protein and albumin excretion rates.[94,102,118] In addition, no differences emerged in healthy subjects in plasma contents and urine excretion rates for creatinine, urea, and albumin between control subjects and those who consumed creatine for between 10 months and 5 years.[133] Glomerular filtration rate, tubular reabsorption, and glomerular membrane permeability also remained normal with chronic creatine use. Individuals with suspected renal malfunction should refrain from creatine supplementation because of the potential for exacerbating the disorder.[136] As a nutritional supplement, creatine requires less stringent regulations governing its manufacturing standards, purity, and reporting of adverse side effects than if classified as a drug.

Effects on Body Mass and Body Composition

Body mass increases of between 0.5 and 2.4 kg often accompany creatine supplementation,[45,68,83,93,120] *independent of short-term changes in testosterone or cortisol concentrations.*[181] In fact, short-term creatine supplementation exerts no effect on the hormonal response to resistance training.[127] It remains unclear how much of the weight gain occurs from *(a)* the anabolic effect of creatine on muscle tissue synthesis, *(b)* osmotic retention of intracellular water from increased creatine stores, or *(c)* other factors.

Research has determined the effect of creatine supplementation plus resistance training on body composition, muscle fiber hypertrophy, and exercise performance adaptations. In one study of young adult women, creatine intake during resistance training (4 days pretraining dose of 20 g a day followed by 5 g a day during training) caused greater increases in muscle strength (20–25%), maximal intermittent exercise capacity of the arm flexors (10–25%), and FFM (6%) than the placebo condition.[173] Part of the FFM increase resulted from muscle water content. Data also indicate that a 2.42-kg body mass gain with creatine supplementation plus resistance/agility training partly resulted from increases in fat/bone-free body mass that did not relate to an increase in total body water.[100]

In other research, resistance-trained men, matched on physical characteristics and maximal strength, randomly received either a placebo or a creatine supplement. Supplementation consisted of 25 g daily followed by maintenance with 5 g daily. Both groups engaged in heavy resistance training for 12 weeks. FIGURE 12.7 shows the greater training-induced increase in body mass (6.3%) and FFM (6.3%)

Figure 12.7 Effects of 12 weeks of creatine supplementation plus heavy resistance training on changes in **(A)** body mass *(BM)*, fat-free body mass *(FFM)*, and body fat, **(B)** muscular strength in the squat and bench press, and **(C)** cross-sectional areas of specific muscle fiber types. The placebo group underwent identical training and received an equivalent quantity of powdered cellulose in capsule form. *Change significantly greater than in placebo group. (From Volek JS, et al. Performance and muscle fiber adaptations to creatine supplementation and heavy resistance training. Med Sci Sports Exerc 1999;31:1147.)

for the creatine-supplemented group than for controls (3.6% increase body mass and 3.1% increase FFM). Maximum bench press (+24%) and squat strength (+32%) increases were greater in the creatine group than in controls (+16% bench press; +24% squat; Fig. 12.7B). Creatine supplementation also induced a greater muscle fiber hypertrophy as indicated by enlargement in types I (35 vs. 11%), IIA (36 vs. 15%), and IIAB (35 vs. 6%) muscle fiber cross-sectional areas (Fig. 12.7C). The larger average volume of weight lifted in the bench press during weeks 5 to 8 for the creatine supplement group suggests that a higher quality of training mediated more favorable adaptations in FFM, muscle morphology, and strength.

Creatine Loading

Many creatine users pursue a "loading" phase by ingesting 20 to 30 g of creatine daily (usually in tablet from or as powder added to liquid) for 5 to 7 days. A maintenance phase follows the loading phase, in which the person supplements daily with as little as 2 to 5 g of creatine. Individuals who consume vegetarian-type diets show the greatest increase in muscle creatine because of the already low creatine content of their diets. Large increases also characterize "responders," that is, individuals with normally low basal levels of intramuscular creatine.[66]

Practical questions for the person desiring to elevate intramuscular creatine with supplementation concern *(a)* the magnitude and time course of intramuscular creatine increase, *(b)* the dosage necessary to maintain a creatine increase, and *(c)* the rate of creatine loss or "washout" following cessation of supplementation. To provide insight into these questions, researchers studied two groups of men.[79] In one experiment, the men ingested 20 g of creatine monohydrate (approximately 0.3 g per kg of body mass) for six consecutive days, at which time supplementation ceased. Muscle biopsies were taken before supplement ingestion and at days 7, 21, and 35. Similarly, another group of men took 20 g of creatine monohydrate daily for six consecutive days. Instead of discontinuing supplementation, they reduced dosage to 2 g daily (approximately 0.03 g per kg body mass) for an additional 28 days. FIGURE 12.8A shows that after 6 days, muscle creatine concentration increased by approximately 20%. Without continued supplementation, muscle creatine content gradually declined to baseline in 35 days. The group that continued to supplement with reduced creatine intake for an additional 28 days maintained muscle creatine at the increased level (Fig. 12.8B).

For both groups, the increase in total muscle creatine content during the initial 6-day supplement period averaged 23 mmol per kg of dry muscle, which represented about 20 g (17%) of the total creatine ingested. Interestingly, a similar 20% increase in total muscle creatine concentration occurred with only a 3-g daily supplement. This increase progressed more gradually and required 28 days in contrast to only 6 days with the 6-g supplement.

A rapid way to "creatine load" skeletal muscle requires ingesting 20 g of creatine monohydrate daily for 6 days; then switching to a reduced dosage of 2 g per day keeps levels elevated for up to 28 days. If rapidity of "loading" is not a consideration, supplementing 3 g daily for 28 days achieves the same high levels.

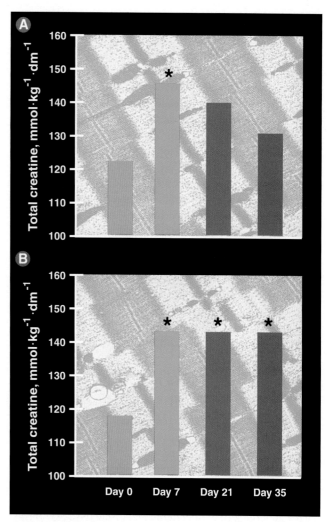

Figure 12.8 A. Muscle total creatine concentration in six men who ingested 20 g of creatine for 6 consecutive days. Muscle biopsy samples were obtained before ingestion (day 0) and on days 7, 21, and 35. **B.** Muscle total creatine concentration in nine men who ingested 20 g of creatine for 6 consecutive days and thereafter ingested 2 g of creatine daily for the next 28 days. Muscle biopsy samples taken before ingestion (day 0) and on days 7, 21, and 35. Values refer to averages per dry mass (dm). *Significantly different from day 0. (From Hultman E, et al. Muscle creatine loading in men. J Appl Physiol 1996;81:232.)

Carbohydrate Ingestion Augments Creatine Loading

Research supports the common belief among athletes that consuming creatine with a sugar-containing drink increases creatine uptake and storage in skeletal muscle (FIG. 12.9).[65,153] For 5 days, subjects received either 5 g of creatine four times daily, or a 5-g supplement followed 30 minutes later by 93 g of a high glycemic simple sugar four times daily. For the creatine-only supplement group, significant increases occurred for muscle PCr (7.2%), free creatine (13.5%), and total creatine (20.7%). However, much larger increases took place for the creatine plus sugar-supplemented group (14.7% for muscle PCr, 18.1% in free creatine, and a 33.0% in total creatine). Creatine supplementation alone did not affect insulin secretion, whereas adding sugar elevated plasma insulin. More than likely, augmented creatine storage with a creatine plus sugar supplement results from insulin-mediated glucose absorption by skeletal muscle, which also facilitates transport of creatine into muscle fibers.

Stop Caffeine When Using Creatine

Caffeine diminishes the ergogenic effect of creatine supplementation. To evaluate the effect of preexercise caffeine ingestion on intramuscular creatine stores and high-intensity exercise performance, subjects consumed either a placebo, a daily creatine supplement (0.5 g per kg body mass), or the same daily creatine supplement plus caffeine (5 mg per kg body mass) for 6 days.[172] Under each condition, they performed maximal intermittent knee extension exercise to fatigue on an isokinetic dynamometer. Creatine supplementation, with or without caffeine, increased intramuscular PCr by between 4 and 6%. Dynamic torque production also increased by 10 to 23% with creatine-only treatment compared with the placebo. Consuming caffeine *totally negated* creatine's ergogenic effect.

The researchers initially speculated that caffeine, through its action as a sympathomimetic agent, might facilitate the up-

take and trapping of exogenous creatine by skeletal muscle. However, no enhanced retention occurred. From a practical standpoint, caffeine supplements totally counteracted any ergogenic effect of muscle creatine loading. *Thus, athletes who load creatine should refrain from caffeine-containing foods and beverages for several days prior to competition.*

Some Research Shows No Benefit

Not all research reports ergogenic results from standard creatine supplementation. For example, no effects on exercise performance, fatigue resistance, and recovery appeared for untrained subjects performing a single 15-second bout of sprint cycling,[36] trained subjects performing sport-specific physical activities such as swimming, cycling, and running,[21,52,120,142] trained and untrained older adults,[84,193] resistance-trained individuals,[162] or trained rowers[44] or when short-term supplementation failed to significantly increase muscle PCr.[52,120] The reason for these discrepancies could include variations in subject population, length of exercise and recovery intervals, training methods, inadequate statistical power, inappropriate or unreliable performance measures, and the degree that supplementation increases intramuscular creatine and PCr concentrations.

RIBOSE: THE NEXT CREATINE ON THE SUPPLEMENT SCENE?

Ribose has emerged as a competitor to creatine as a supplement to increase power and replenish high-energy compounds after intense exercise. The body readily synthesizes ribose, and the diet provides small amounts through ripe fruits and vegetables. Metabolically, this 5-carbon sugar serves as an energy substrate for ATP resynthesis. Because of this role in energy metabolism, exogenous ribose ingestion has been touted as a means to quickly restore the body's limited amount ATP. To maintain optimal ATP levels and thus provide its ergogenic effect, recommended ribose doses range from 10 to 20 g per day. Clearly, any compound that either increases ATP levels or facilitates its resynthesis would benefit short-term, high-power physical activities. However, only limited experimentation exists to assess this potential for ribose. A double-blind randomized study evaluated the effects of oral ribose supplementation (4 doses per day at 4 g per dose) on repeated bouts of maximal exercise and ATP replenishment after intermittent maximal muscle contractions.[128] No significant difference in any measure (e.g., intermittent isokinetic knee extension force, blood lactate, and plasma ammonia concentration) emerged between ribose and placebo trials. Although the exercise significantly decreased intramuscular ATP and total adenine nucleotide content immediately after exercise and 24 hours later, ribose supplementation proved ineffective in facilitating recovery of these compounds. Other researchers have also demonstrated no ergogenic effects of ribose supplementation in healthy untrained or trained groups.[9,101]

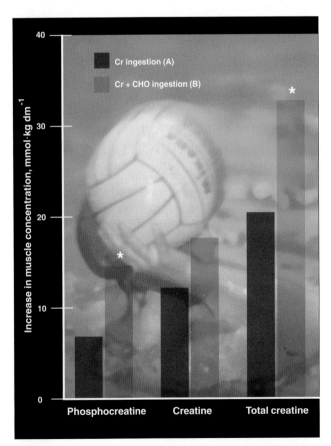

Figure 12.9 Increases in dry muscle (dm) concentrations of phosphocreatine, creatine *(Cr)*, and total creatine in group A after 5 days of Cr supplementation and in group B after 5 days of Cr plus carbohydrate *(CHO)* supplementation. Values represent averages. *Significantly greater than creatine-only supplementation. (From Green AL, et al.: Carbohydrate ingestion augments skeletal muscle creatine accumulation during creatine supplementation in humans. Am J Physiol 1996;E821.)

INOSINE AND CHOLINE

Inosine

Many popular articles and advertisements tout inosine as an amino acid, when in fact it is a nucleic acid derivative found naturally in brewer's yeast and organ meats. Inosine (and choline) are not considered essential nutrients. The body synthesizes inosine from precursor amino acids and glucose. Metabolically, inosine participates in forming purines such as adenine, one of the structural components of ATP. Strength and power athletes supplement with inosine believing that it increases ATP stores to improve training quality and competitive performance. Some also theorize that inosine supplementation augments synthesis of red blood cell 2,3-diphosphoglycerate, thus facilitating oxygen release from hemoglobin at the tissue level. Others suggest that inosine plays an ergogenic role by *(a)* stimulating insulin release to speed glucose delivery to the myocardium, *(b)* augmenting cardiac contractility, or *(c)* acting as a vasodilating agent. These theoretical considerations, including anecdotal claims, provide the basis for popular marketing themes that extol inosine as a supplement to boost anaerobic and aerobic exercise performance.

Objective data do not support an ergogenic role for inosine supplementation. Highly trained young and older men and women who supplemented daily with 6000 mg of inosine for 2 days failed to improve 3-mile treadmill run time, peak oxygen uptake, blood lactate level, heart rate, or RPE.[190] Interestingly, subjects could not exercise as long on a test for aerobic capacity when supplemented with inosine as in the unsupplemented state. In another study, male competitive cyclists received either a placebo or a 5000-mg per day oral inosine supplement for 5 days.[160] They then performed a Wingate bicycle test, a 30-minute self-paced bicycle endurance test, and a constant load, supramaximal cycling sprint to fatigue. FIGURE 12.10 shows the results for maximal anaerobic power output on the 30-second Wingate test *(A)* and heart rate *(B)*, RPE *(C)*, and total work accomplished *(D)* during segments of the 30-minute endurance ride. No significant differences occurred in any of the criterion variables between placebo and supplemented conditions. In agreement with the ergolytic effect of inosine noted above,[190] cyclists fatigued nearly 10% faster on the supramaximal sprint test when they consumed inosine than without it. Additionally, serum uric acid levels increased nearly twofold following 5 days of inosine supplementation—a level normally associated with gout, an inherited metabolic disorder characterized by recurrent acute arthritis and deposition of crystalline urate in connective tissues and articular cartilage. *Clearly, these findings alone contraindicate any use of inosine supplements for possible ergogenic effects.*

Choline

All animal tissues contain choline, an important compound for normal cellular functioning. Although humans synthe-size choline, it (like inosine) also must be obtained in the diet. Lecithin, a structural component of the lipoproteins and the cells' phospholipid plasma membrane, and the neurotransmitter acetylcholine (which controls skeletal muscle activation at the myoneural junction) incorporate choline into their chemical structures. Choline functions as a lipotrophic agent as part of the lecithin molecule either to depress accumulation of fat in the liver or to increase fatty acid uptake by the liver. Very low density lipoproteins (the major transporting vehicle of triacylglycerols synthesized in the liver) also contain choline. A subpar choline intake increases the triglyceride content of the liver. Many foods contain ample choline; top food sources include eggs (yolk), brewer's yeast, liver (beef, pork, lamb), wheat germ, soybeans, dehydrated potatoes, oatmeal, and vegetables in the cabbage (cucurbit) family.

Inositol and choline supplements depress fat accumulation in the liver when given to animals deficient in these compounds. However, supplements did not affect percentage carcass fat of aerobically trained rats, although the supplemented animals gained less weight during the training period.[96] Body builders frequently take choline- and inositol-containing "metabolic optimizing powders" and "fat-burning tablets" prior to competition, hoping to increase their muscle mass/fat mass ratio to achieve the "cut" look. We are unaware of any research on humans that supports supplementation with inositol–choline products for such purposes.

LIPID SUPPLEMENTATION WITH MEDIUM-CHAIN TRIACYLGLYCEROLS

Do high-fat foods or supplements elevate plasma lipid levels to make more energy available during prolonged aerobic exercise? One must consider several factors to achieve such an effect. For one thing, consuming triacylglycerols composed of predominantly long-chain fatty acids (12 to 18 carbons) significantly *delays* gastric emptying. This negatively affects the rapidity of exogenous fat availability and also fluid and carbohydrate replenishment. Both are crucial factors in high-intensity endurance exercise. In addition, following digestion and intestinal absorption (normally 3 to 4 hours), long-chain triacylglycerols reassemble with phospholipids, fatty acids, and a cholesterol shell to form fatty droplets called chylomicrons. Chylomicrons then travel slowly to the systemic circulation via the lymphatic system. Once in the bloodstream, the tissues remove the triacylglycerols bound to chylomicrons. Consequently, the relatively slow rate of digestion, absorption, and oxidation of long-chain fatty acids make this energy source undesirable as a supplement to augment energy metabolism in active muscle during exercise.[42,46]

Medium-chain triacylglycerols (MCTs) provide a more rapid source of fatty acid fuel. MCTs are processed oils, frequently produced for patients with intestinal malabsorption and tissue-wasting diseases. Marketing for the

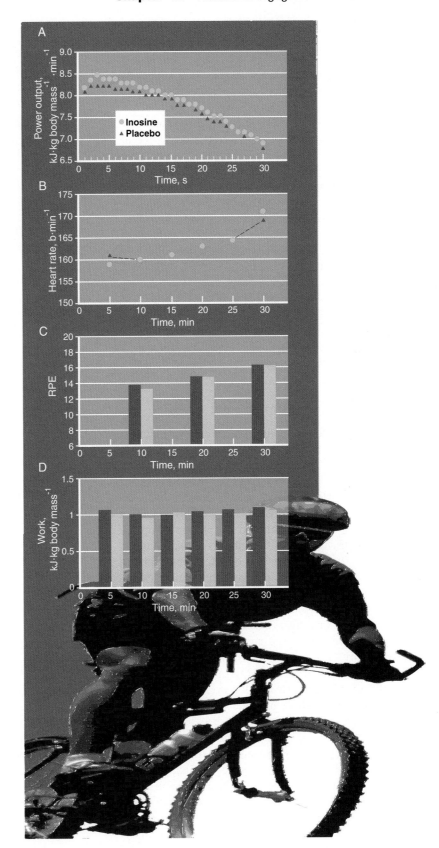

Figure 12.10 Maximal anaerobic power output on the 30-second Wingate test **(A)** and for heart rate **(B)**, ratings of perceived exertion *(RPE)* **(C)**, and total work accomplished **(D)** during segments of the 30-minute endurance ride for inosine and placebo trials for 10 male competitive cyclists. (From Starling RD, et al. Effect of inosine supplementation on aerobic and anaerobic cycling performance. Med Sci Sports Exerc 1996;28:1193.)

sports enthusiast hypes MCT as a "fat burner," "energy source," "glycogen sparer," and "muscle builder." Unlike longer-chain triacylglycerols, MCTs contain saturated fatty acids with 8 to 10 carbon atoms along the fatty acid chain. During digestion (see Chapter 3), they hydrolyze by lipase action in the mouth, stomach, and intestinal duodenum to glycerol and medium-chain fatty acids (MCFAs). The water-solubility of MCFAs enables them to move across the intestinal mucosa directly into the bloodstream (portal vein) without the necessity of slow transport in chylomicrons by the lymphatic system as required for long-chain triacylglycerols. Once at the tissues, MCFAs readily move through the plasma membrane, where they diffuse across the inner mitochondrial membrane for oxidation. They pass into the mitochondria largely independent of the carnitine–acyl-CoA transferase system; which contrasts with the relatively slower transfer and mitochondrial oxidation rate of long-chain fatty acids. Owing to their relative ease of oxidation, MCTs do not usually store as body fat. Because ingesting MCTs elevates plasma FFAs rapidly, some speculate that supplements of these lipids might spare liver and muscle glycogen during high-intensity aerobic exercise.[115]

Exercise Benefits Inconclusive

Consuming MCTs does not inhibit gastric emptying, as does common fat, but conflicting research exists about their use in exercise.[3,92,177] In early studies, subjects consumed 380 mg of MCT oil per kg of body mass an hour before exercising 1 hour at between 60 and 70% of aerobic capacity.[39] Plasma ketone levels generally increased with MCT ingestion, but the exercise metabolic mixture did not change compared with a placebo trial or a trial after subjects consumed a glucose polymer. By consuming 30 g of MCTs (an estimated maximal amount tolerated in the gastrointestinal tract) before exercising, MCT catabolism contributed only between 3 and 7% of the total exercise energy cost.[90]

Research has investigated the metabolic and ergogenic effects of consuming a large quantity of 86 g of MCTs (surprisingly well tolerated by subjects). Endurance-trained cyclists rode for 2 hours at 60% $\dot{V}O_2$peak; they then immediately performed a simulated 40-km cycling time trial.[177] During each of three rides they drank 2 L containing either10% glucose, 4.3% MCT emulsion, or 10% glucose plus 4.3% MCT emulsion. FIGURE 12.11 shows the effects of the beverages on average speed in the 40-km trials. Replacing the carbohydrate beverage with only the MCT emulsion impaired exercise performance by approximately 8% (in agreement with another study[92]). However, the combined carbohydrate plus MCT solution consumed repeatedly during exercise produced a significant 2.5% improvement in cycling speed. This small ergogenic effect occurred with (a) reduced total carbohydrate oxidation at a given level of oxygen uptake, (b) higher final circulating FFA and ketone levels, and (c) lower final glucose and lactate concentrations. The

Figure 12.11 Effects of carbohydrate (*CHO;* 10% solution), medium-chain triglyceride (*MCT;* 4.3% emulsion), and carbohydrate + MCT ingestion during exercise on simulated 40-km time-trial cycling speeds after 2 hours of exercise at 60% of peak oxygen uptake. *Significantly faster than 10% CHO trials; **significantly faster than 4.3% MCT trials. (From Van Zyl CG, et al. Effects of medium-chain triglyceride ingestion on fuel metabolism and cycling performance. J Appl Physiol 1996;80:2217.)

small endurance enhancement with MCT supplementation probably occurred because this exogenous fatty acid source contributed to the total exercise energy expenditure and total fat oxidation.[91]

Consuming MCT does not stimulate the release of bile, the fat-emulsifying agent from the gall bladder. Thus, cramping and diarrhea often accompany excess intake of this lipid form. Additional research must validate the ergogenic claims for MCT, including the tolerance level for these lipids during exercise. In general, relatively small alterations in substrate oxidation occur by increasing the availability of FFAs during exercise at 65 to 90% of aerobic capacity; this likely accounts for its small effect on exercise capacity.[75]

(−)-HYDROXYCITRATE: A POTENTIAL FAT BURNER?

(—)-Hydroxycitrate (HCA), a principal constituent of the rind of the fruit of *Garcinia cambogia* used in Asian cuisine, is the latest compound promoted as a "natural fat burner" to facilitate weight loss and enhance endurance performance. Metabolically, HCA operates as a competitive inhibitor of citrate lyase, which catalyzes breakdown of citrate to oxaloacetate and acetyl-CoA in the cytosol. Inhibition of this enzyme limits the pool of two-carbon acetyl compounds and thus reduces cellular ability to synthesize fat. Because inhibition of citrate catabolism also slows carbohydrate breakdown, HCA supplementation should provide a means to conserve glycogen and increase lipolysis during exercise.

Research has evaluated short-term effects of HCA ingestion on (a) HCA availability in the plasma and (b) fat oxidation rates at rest and during moderate-intensity exercise.[176] Endurance-trained cyclists received either a 3.1 mL per kg of body mass HCA solution (19 g·L^{-1}; 6 to 30 times the dosage in weight-loss studies) or a placebo at 45 and 15 minutes before starting exercise (resting measure) and 30 and 60 minutes after a 2-hour exercise bout at 50% maximal working capacity. Plasma concentrations of HCA increased at rest and during exercise after supplementation, but no difference occurred between trials in energy expenditure or in fat and carbohydrate oxidation. These findings indicate that increasing plasma HCA availability with supplementation exerts no effect on skeletal muscle fat oxidation during rest or exercise, at least in endurance-trained humans. In addition, no effects of HCA supplementation occurred for resting or postexercise energy expenditure and markers of lipolysis in healthy men[103] or weight or fat loss in obese subjects.[76] Taken together, these findings cast serious doubt on the usefulness of large quantities of HCA as an antiobesity agent or ergogenic aid—claims frequently made by supplement purveyors.

VANADIUM

Vanadium, a trace element widely distributed in nature, comes from the bluish salt of vanadium acid and was named in 1831 for the Norse goddess of beauty (Vanadis) because of how it forms multicolored compounds. This important element (without an RDA) exhibits insulin-like properties by facilitating glucose transport and use in skeletal muscle, stimulating glycogen synthesis, and activating glycolytic reactions.[33] In animals, vanadium supplements attenuated the effects of diabetes, perhaps by augmenting the action of available insulin.[12,122,167] In humans, administering 50 mg of vanadium twice daily for 3 weeks improved hepatic and skeletal muscle insulin sensitivity in type 2 diabetics, partly by enhancing insulin's inhibitory effect on fat breakdown. No altered insulin sensitivity occurred in nondiabetic subjects.[69] Optimal iodine metabolism and thyroid function may also require adequate vanadium intake. The best "natural" sources of vanadium include cereal and grain products and dietary oils, although meat, fish, and poultry also contain moderate amounts of this element.

Body builders ingest vanadium supplements, usually in its oxidized form as vanadyl sulfate, often combined with additional minerals or coatings, or as bis-maltolato-oxovanadium (BMOV).[199] Enthusiasts believe that vanadium provides the "pumped look" to give the appearance of muscular hypertrophy (hardness, density, and size) because of enhanced muscle glycogen storage and amino acid uptake. No research supports an ergogenic role for vanadium supplements. Individuals should use extreme care when supplementing with this element because an extreme excess of vanadium becomes toxic (particularly to the liver) in mammals.

PYRUVATE

Ergogenic effects have been extolled for pyruvate, the three-carbon end product of the cytoplasmic breakdown of glucose in glycolysis. Exogenous pyruvate, as a partial replacement for dietary carbohydrate, allegedly augments endurance exercise performance and promotes fat loss. Pyruvic acid, a relatively unstable chemical, causes intestinal distress. Consequently, various forms of the salt of this acid (sodium, potassium, calcium, or magnesium pyruvate) are provided in capsule, tablet, or powder form. Supplement manufacturers recommend taking 2 to 4 capsules daily. One capsule usually contains 600 mg of pyruvate, at a cost of approximately $40 for 120 capsules. The calcium form of pyruvate contains approximately 80 mg of calcium with 600 mg of pyruvate. Some advertisements recommend a dose of one capsule per 20 pounds of body weight. Manufacturers also combine creatine monohydrate and pyruvate; 1 g of creatine pyruvate provides about 80 mg of creatine and 400 mg of pyruvate. Recommended pyruvate dosages range from 5 to 20 g per day. Pyruvate content in the normal diet ranges from 100 mg to 2000 mg daily. The largest dietary amounts occur in fruits and vegetables, particularly red apples (500 mg each), with smaller quantities in dark beer (80 mg per 12 oz) and red wine (75 mg per 6 oz).

Effects on Endurance Performance

Several reports indicate beneficial effects of exogenous pyruvate on endurance performance. Two double-blind, crossover studies by the same laboratory showed that 7 days of daily supplementation of a 100-g mixture of pyruvate (25 g) plus 75 g of dihydroxyacetone (DHA; another three-carbon compound of glycolysis) increased upper- and lower-body aerobic endurance by 20% compared with exercise with a 100-g supplement of an isocaloric glucose polymer.[155,156] The pyruvate–DHA mixture increased cycle ergometer time to exhaustion of the legs (lower body) by 13 minutes (66 vs. 79 min), while upper-body arm-cranking exercise time increased by 27 minutes (133 vs. 160 min). Local muscle and overall body ratings of perceived exertion were also lower when subjects exercised with the pyruvate–DHA mixture than with the placebo condition.[147] Dosage recommendations range between a total of 2 and 5 g of pyruvate spread throughout the day and taken with meals.

Proponents of pyruvate supplementation maintain that elevations in extracellular pyruvate augment glucose transport into active muscle. Enhanced "glucose extraction" from blood provides the important carbohydrate energy source to sustain high-intensity aerobic exercise while at the same time conserving intramuscular glycogen stores.[81] When the individual's diet contains a normal level of carbohydrate (approximately 55% of total energy), pyruvate supplementation also increases preexercise muscle glycogen levels.[156] Both of these effects, higher preexercise glycogen levels and facilitated glucose uptake and oxidation by active muscle, benefit high-intensity endurance exercise in much the same way as preexercise carbohydrate loading and glucose feedings during exercise exert their ergogenic effects. The question awaiting research concerns whether pyruvate ingestion provides any greater ergogenic benefit than carbohydrate loading and/or carbohydrate consumption during exercise.

Body Fat Loss

Subsequent research by the same investigators who showed ergogenic effects of pyruvate supplementation indicates that exogenous pyruvate intake also augments body fat loss when accompanied by a low-energy diet. Obese women in a metabolic ward maintained a liquid 1000-kcal daily energy intake (68% carbohydrate, 22% protein, 10% lipid). Adding 20 g of sodium pyruvate plus 16 g of calcium pyruvate (13% of energy intake) daily for 3 weeks induced greater weight loss (13.0 vs. 9.5 lb) and fat loss (8.8 vs. 5.9 lb) than in a control group on the same diet who received an equivalent amount of extra energy as glucose.[157] These findings complement the researchers' previous study with obese subjects that showed that adding DHA and pyruvate (substituted as equivalent energy for glucose) to a severely restricted low-energy diet facilitated weight and fat loss (without increased nitrogen loss).[158] The inhibition of weight and fat gain through dietary substitution with three-carbon compounds, originally observed in growing animals, indicated that pyruvate might cause a greater effect than DHA.[37,154] The precise role of pyruvate in facilitating weight loss remains unknown. Taking pyruvate may stimulate small increases in futile metabolic activity (metabolism not coupled to ATP production) with a subsequent wasting of energy.

Adverse side effects of a 30- to 100-g daily pyruvate intake include diarrhea as well as gastrointestinal gurgling and discomfort. *Until additional studies from independent laboratories reproduce existing findings for exercise performance and body fat loss, one should view the effectiveness of pyruvate supplementation with caution.*

GLYCEROL

Glycerol is a component of the triacylglycerol molecule, a gluconeogenic substrate, an important constituent of the cells' phospholipid plasma membrane, and an osmotically active natural metabolite. The two-carbon glycerol molecule achieved clinical notoriety (along with mannitol, sorbitol, and urea) for helping to produce an osmotic diuresis. The capacity for influencing water movement within the body makes glycerol effective in reducing excess accumulation of fluid (edema) in the brain and eye. Glycerol's effect on water movement occurs because extracellular glycerol enters the tissues of the brain, cerebrospinal fluid, and eye's aqueous humor at a relatively slow rate; this creates an osmotic effect that draws fluid from these tissues.

Ingesting a concentrated mixture of glycerol plus water increases the body's fluid volume and glycerol concentrations in plasma and interstitial fluid compartments. This sets the stage for fluid excretion from increased renal filtrate and urine flow. The proximal and distal tubules reabsorb much of this glycerol, so a large fluid portion of renal filtrate also becomes reabsorbed, which averts a marked diuresis. Renal reabsorption does not occur with tissue dehydrators like mannitol and sorbitol, which produce a true osmotic diuresis.

The kidneys generally reabsorb from the renal filtrate almost all of the glycerol from food and metabolism. Normal plasma glycerol concentration at rest averages 0.05 $mmol \cdot L^{-1}$; it often rises to 0.5 $mmol \cdot L^{-1}$ during prolonged exercise with accompanying carbohydrate depletion and elevated fat catabolism. Exaggerated increases in urine glycerol concentration most likely indicate the use of exogenous glycerol, usually ingested at quantities of 1.2 g per kg of body mass.

When consumed with 1 to 2 L of water, glycerol facilitates water absorption from the intestine and causes extracellular fluid retention, mainly in the plasma fluid compartment.[98,145,188] The hyperhydration effect of glycerol supplementation reduces overall heat stress during exercise as reflected by increased sweating rate; this lowers heart rate and body temperature during exercise and enhances endurance performance under heat stress.[77,111] Reducing heat stress with hyperhydration using glycerol plus water supplementation prior to exercise increases safety for the exercise participant. The typically recommended preexercise glycerol dosage of 1.0 g of glycerol per kg of body mass in 1 to 2 L of water lasts up to 6 hours.

Not all research demonstrates meaningful thermoregulatory or exercise performance benefits of glycerol hyperhydration over preexercise hyperhydration with plain water.[105,112] For example, exogenous glycerol diluted in 500 mL of water consumed 4 hours before exercise failed to promote fluid retention or ergogenic effects.[80] Also, no cardiovascular or thermoregulatory advantages occurred when consuming glycerol with small volumes of water during exercise.[121] Side effects of exogenous glycerol ingestion include nausea, dizziness, bloating, and light-headedness. Proponents of glycerol supplementation argue that any ban on glycerol use only increases the risk of elite athletes to heat injury, including potentially fatal heat stroke. Clearly, this area requires further research.

Summary

1. Carbohydrate loading generally increases endurance in prolonged submaximal exercise. A modification of the classic loading procedure provides for the same high-level of glycogen storage without dramatic alterations in one's diet

and exercise routine. A 1-day rapid loading procedure produces nearly as high glycogen storage as the more prolonged loading techniques.

2. Men and women achieve equal supramaximal muscle glycogen levels when fed comparable amounts of carbohydrate in relation to their lean body mass.

3. Many resistance-trained athletes supplement their diets with amino acids, either singly or in combination, to create a hormonal milieu to facilitate protein synthesis in skeletal muscle. Research shows no benefit of such general supplementation on levels of anabolic hormones or measures of body composition, muscle size, or exercise performance.

4. Carbohydrate–protein supplementation immediately in recovery from resistance training produces a hormonal environment conducive to protein synthesis and muscle tissue growth (elevated plasma concentrations of insulin and GH). Such data provide indirect evidence for a possible training benefit of increasing carbohydrate and/or protein intake immediately after a resistance-training workout. The question awaiting answer is the degree to which any transient change in hormonal milieu favoring anabolism and actual net protein synthesis caused by postexercise dietary maneuvers contributes to long-term muscle growth and strength enhancement.

5. Long-term exercise or heavy training does not adversely affect intracellular carnitine levels. This explains why most research with carnitine supplementation fails to show an ergogenic effect, positive metabolic alterations, or body fat reductions.

6. Bee pollen contains many important nutrients but it does not provide ergogenic effects compared with a well-balanced diet. On the negative side, bee pollen produces an extreme allergic reaction in individuals sensitive to specific pollens.

7. Boron, a trace mineral important in bone development and metabolism, increases testosterone levels in boron-deprived, postmenopausal women. Boron supplements have no effect on anabolic hormone levels in individuals with adequate boron intake.

8. Many tout chromium supplements (usually as chromium picolinate) for their fat- burning and muscle-building properties. For individuals with adequate dietary chromium intakes, research fails to show any beneficial effect of chromium supplements on training-related changes in muscular strength, physique, fat-free body mass, or muscle mass.

9. Excess chromium can adversely affect iron transport and distribution in the body. Prolonged excess may even contribute to chromosomal damage.

10. Because of its role in electron transport-oxidative phosphorylation, athletes supplement with coenzyme Q_{10} (CoQ_{10}) to improve aerobic capacity and cardiovascular dynamics. CoQ_{10} supplements in healthy individuals provide no ergogenic effect on aerobic capacity, endurance, submaximal exercise lactate levels, or cardiovascular dynamics.

11. In supplement form, creatine significantly increases intramuscular creatine and phosphocreatine, enhances short-term anaerobic power output capacity, and facilitates recovery from repeated bouts of intense effort. Creatine loading occurs by ingesting 20 g of creatine monohydrate for six consecutive days. Reducing intake to 2 g daily then maintains elevated intramuscular levels.

12. Consuming creatine with a glucose-containing drink increases creatine uptake and storage in skeletal muscle. More than likely, this results from insulin-mediated glucose uptake by skeletal muscle, which facilitates creatine uptake.

13. Limited research indicates no effect of inosine supplements on physiologic or performance measures during aerobic or anaerobic exercise. A decidedly negative effect includes an increase in serum uric acid levels after only 5 days of supplementation.

14. Choline forms part of the cells' phospholipid plasma membrane; it is also a constituent of the neurotransmitter acetylcholine. Although body builders frequently supplement with choline to enhance fat metabolism and achieve the "cut look," research does not support such effects.

15. Owing to their relatively rapid digestion, assimilation, and catabolism for energy, some believe that consuming medium-chain triacylglycerols (MCTs) enhances fat metabolism and conserves glycogen during endurance exercise. Ingesting about 86 g of MCT enhances performance by an additional 2.5%.

16. Increasing plasma (—)-hydroxycitrate (HCA) availability via supplementation exerts no effect on skeletal muscle fat oxidation at rest or during

exercise. These findings cast serious doubt on the usefulness of HCA, even when provided in large quantities, as an antiobesity agent or ergogenic aid.

17. The trace mineral vanadium exerts insulin-like properties in humans. However, no research documents an ergogenic effect, and extreme intake produces toxic effects.

18. Pyruvate supplementation purportedly augments endurance performance and promotes fat loss. Its endurance effect appears to lie in enhanced preexercise glycogen storage and facilitated glucose transport into active muscles. Body fat loss is attributed to its small effect on increasing metabolic rate. A definitive conclusion concerning pyruvate's effectiveness requires verification by other investigators.

19. Preexercise glycerol ingestion promotes hyperhydration, which supposedly protects the individual from heat stress and heat injury during high-intensity exercise.

TEST YOUR KNOWLEDGE **ANSWERS**

1. True Glycogen stored in the liver and active muscle supplies most of the energy for intense aerobic exercise. Reduced glycogen reserves allow fat catabolism to supply a progressively greater percentage of energy from fatty acid mobilization from the liver and adipose tissue. Exercise that severely lowers muscle glycogen precipitates fatigue, even though the active muscles have sufficient oxygen and unlimited use of potential energy from stored fat. This occurs because the aerobic breakdown of FFAs progresses at about 50% the rate of glycogen breakdown. Ingesting a glucose and water solution near the point of fatigue allows exercise to continue, but for all practical purposes, the muscles' "fuel tank" reads empty.

2. True A particular combination of diet plus exercise significantly "packs" muscle glycogen, a procedure termed *carbohydrate loading* or *glycogen supercompensation*. Endurance athletes often use carbohydrate loading for competition because it increases muscle glycogen even more than a high-carbohydrate diet. Normally, each 100 g of muscle contains about 1.7 g of glycogen; carbohydrate loading packs up to 5 g of glycogen.

3. False Research on healthy subjects does not provide convincing evidence for an ergogenic effect of oral amino acid supplements on hormone secretion, training responsiveness, or exercise performance. For example, in studies with appropriate design and statistical analysis, supplements of arginine, lysine, ornithine, tyrosine, and other amino acids, either singly or in combination, produced no effect on GH levels, insulin secretion, diverse measures of anaerobic power, or all-out running performance at $\dot{V}O_2$max.

4. False Vital to normal metabolism, carnitine facilitates the influx of long-chain fatty acids into the mitochondrial matrix as part of the carnitine–acyl-CoA transferase system. Theoretically, enhanced carnitine function could inhibit lactate accumulation and enhance exercise performance. Thus, increasing intracellular L-carnitine levels through dietary supplementation should elevate aerobic energy transfer from fat breakdown while conserving limited glycogen reserves. Research shows no ergogenic benefits, positive metabolic alterations (aerobic or anaerobic), or body fat-reducing effects from L-carnitine supplementation.

5. False For individuals with adequate dietary chromium intakes, research fails to show any beneficial effect of chromium supplements on training-related changes in muscular strength, physique, fat-free body mass, or muscle mass. Excess chromium can possibly adversely affect iron transport and distribution in the body. Prolonged excess may damage chromosomes.

6. True Creatine monohydrate supplementation at the recommended level (20–25 g per day) exerts ergogenic effects in short-duration, high-intensity exercise (5–10% improvement) without producing harmful side effects. However, anecdotes indicate a possible association between creatine supplementation and cramping in multiple muscle areas during competition or lengthy practice by football players.

7. True Several reports indicate beneficial effects of exogenous pyruvate on endurance performance. Two double-blind crossover studies by the same laboratory showed that 7 days of daily supplementation of a 100-g mixture of pyruvate (25 g) plus 75 g of dihydroxyacetone (DHA; another three-carbon compound of glycolysis) increased upper- and lower-body aerobic endurance by 20% compared with exercise with a 100-g supplement of an isocaloric glucose polymer. Proponents of pyruvate supplementation maintain that elevations in extracellular pyruvate augment glucose transport into active muscle. Enhanced "glucose extraction" from blood provides the important carbohydrate energy source to sustain high-intensity aerobic exercise while at the same time conserving intramuscular glycogen stores. Subsequent research by the same investigators also indicates that exogenous pyruvate intake augments body fat loss when accompanied by a low-energy diet. Until additional studies from independent laboratories reproduce existing findings for exercise performance and body fat loss, one should view with caution conclusions about the effectiveness of pyruvate supplementation.

8. False Not all research demonstrates meaningful thermoregulatory or exercise performance benefits of glycerol hyperhydration over preexercise hyperhydration with plain water. Side effects of exogenous glycerol ingestion include nausea, dizziness, bloating, and light-headedness.

9. False Bee pollen's allure as a nutrient supplement for physically active individuals lies in its relatively rich mixture of vitamins, minerals, and amino acids required for energy-producing reactions. Bee pollen contains many important nutrients, but it does not provide ergogenic effects compared with a well-balanced diet. Individuals allergic to specific pollens may experience extreme reactions when taking this supplement.

10. False CoQ_{10} functions as an integral component of the mitochondrion's electron transport system of oxidative phosphorylation. The popular literature touts CoQ_{10} supplements to improve "stamina" and enhance cardiovascular function based on the belief that supplementation could increase the flux of electrons through the respiratory chain and thus augment aerobic resynthesis of adenosine triphosphate. Although positive benefits have been reported for cardiac patients, CoQ_{10} supplements in healthy individuals provide no ergogenic effect on aerobic capacity, endurance, submaximal exercise lactate levels, or cardiovascular dynamics On the negative side, supplementation could trigger plasma membrane lipid peroxidation and eventual cellular damage.

References

1. Almada A, et al. Effects of ingesting a nutritional supplement containing chromium picolinate & boron on body composition during resistance training. FASEB J 1995;9(4):A1015.
2. Althuis MD, et al. Glucose and insulin responses to dietary chromium supplements: a meta-analysis. Am J Clin Nutr 2002;76:148.
3. Auclair E, et al. Metabolic effects of glucose, medium chain triglyceride and long chain triglyceride feeding before prolonged exercise in rats. Eur J Appl Physiol 1988;57:126.
4. Balsom PD, et al. Creatine supplementation and dynamic high-intensity intermittent exercise. Scand J Med Sci Sports 1993;3:143.
5. Balsom PD, et al. Creatine supplementation per se does not enhance endurance exercise performance. Acta Physiol Scand 1993;149:521.
6. Balsom PD, et al. High-intensity exercise and muscle glycogen availability in humans. Acta Physiol Scand 1999;168:357.
7. Bemben MG. Effects of creatine supplementation on isometric force-time curve characteristics. Med Sci Sports Exerc 2001;33:1876.
8. Bemben MG, et al. Creatine supplementation during resistance training in college football athletes. Med Sci Sports Exerc 2001;33:1667.
9. Berardi JM, Ziegenfuss TN. Effects of ribose supplementation on repeated sprint performance in men. J Strength Cond Res 2003; 17:47.
10. Bergstrom J, et al. Diet, muscle glycogen and physical performance. Acta Physiol Scand 1967;71:140.
11. Bermon S, et al. Effects of creatine monohydrate ingestion in sedentary and weight-trained older adults. Acta Physiol Scand 1998;164:147.
12. Bhanot S, McNeil JH. Vanadyl sulfate lowers plasma insulin and blood pressure in spontaneously hypertensive rats. Hypertension 1994;24:625.
13. Biolo G, et al. An abundant supply of amino acids enhances the metabolic effect of exercise on muscle protein. Am J Physiol 1997;273:E122.
14. Birch R, et al. The influence of dietary creatine supplementation on performance during repeated bouts of maximal isokinetic cycling in man. Eur J Appl Physiol 1994;69:268.
15. Bogandis GC, et al. Contribution of phosphocreatine and aerobic metabolism to energy supply during repeated sprint exercise. J Appl Physiol 1996;80:876.
16. Brannon TA, et al. Effects of creatine loading and training on running performance and biochemical properties of rat skeletal muscle. Med Sci Sports Exerc 1997;29:489.
17. Brass EP. Supplemental carnitine and exercise. Am J Clin Nutr 2000:72(suppl):618S.
18. Brass EP, et al. Effect of intravenous L-carnitine on carnitine homeostasis and fuel metabolism during exercise in humans. Clin Pharmacol Ther 1994;55:681.
19. Braun B, et al. The effect of coenzyme Q10 supplementation on exercise performance, $\dot{V}O_2$ max, and lipid peroxidation in trained cyclists. Int J Sport Nutr 1991;1:353.
20. Bucci L, et al. Ornithine supplementation and insulin release in bodybuilders. Int J Sports Nutr 1992;2:287.
21. Burke LM, et al. Oral creatine supplementation does not improve sprint performance in elite swimmers. Med Sci Sports Exerc 1995;27:S146.
22. Burke LM, et al. Carbohydrate loading failed to improve 100-km cycling performance in a placebo-controlled trial. J Appl Physiol 2000;88:1284.
23. Campbell WW, et al. Chromium picolinate supplementation and resistive training by older men: effects on iron-status and hematologic indexes. Am J Clin Nutr 1997;66:944.
24. Campbell WW, et al. Effects of resistance training and chromium picolinate on body composition and skeletal muscle in older men. J Appl Physiol 1999;86:29.
25. Casey A, et al. Creatine ingestion favorably affects performance and muscle metabolism during maximal exercise in humans. Am J Physiol 1996;271:E31.
26. Casey A, et al. Metabolic response of type I and II muscle fibers during repeated bouts of maximal exercise in humans. Am J Physiol 1996;271:E38.
27. Cerretelli P, Marconi C. L-Carnitine supplementation in human. The effects on physical performance. Int J Sports Med 1990;11:1.
28. Chandler J, Hawkins J. The effect of bee pollen on physiological performance. Int J Biosoc Res 1984;6:107.
29. Chandler RM, et al. Dietary supplements affect the anabolic hormones after weight-training exercise. J Appl Physiol 1994;76:839.
30. Chrsuch MJ, et al. Creatine supplementation combined with resistance training in older men. Med Sci Sports Exerc 2001;33:2111.
31. Clancy S, et al. Effects of chromium picolinate supplementation on body composition, strength, and urinary chromium loss in football players. Int J Sports Nutr 1994;4:142.
32. Coggan AR, et al. Endurance training increases plasma glucose turnover and oxidation during moderate-intensity exercise in men. J Appl Physiol 1990;68:990.
33. Cohen N, et al. Oral vanadyl sulfate improves hepatic and peripheral insulin sensitivity in patients with non-insulin-dependent diabetes mellitus. J Clin Invest 1995;95:2501.
34. Colombani P, et al. Effects of L-carnitine supplementation on physical performance and energy metabolism of endurance-trained athletes—a double-blind crossover field study. Eur J Appl Physiol 1996;73:434.
35. Constantin-Teodosiu D, et al. Carnitine metabolism in human muscle fiber types during submaximal dynamic exercise. J Appl Physiol 1996;80:1061.
36. Cooke WH, et al. Effect of oral creatine supplementation on power output and fatigue during bicycle ergometry. J Appl Physiol 1995;78:670.
37. Cortez MY, et al. Effects of pyruvate and dihydroxyacetone consumption on the growth and metabolic state of obese Zucker rats. Am J Clin Nutr 1991;53:847.
38. Costill DL, et al. Effects of repeated days of intensified training on muscle glycogen and swimming performance. Med Sci Sports Exerc 1988;20:249.
39. Décombaz J, et al. Energy metabolism of medium-chained triglycerides versus carbohydrates during exercise. Eur J Appl Physiol 1983;52:9.
40. Décombaz J, et al. Muscle carnitine after strenuous endurance exercise. J Appl Physiol 1992;72:423.
41. Décombaz J, et al. Effect of L-carnitine on submaximal exercise metabolism after depletion of muscle glycogen. Med Sci Sports Exerc 1993;25:773.
42. DeLany JP, et al. Differential oxidation of dietary fatty acids in humans. Am J Clin Nutr 2000;72:905.
43. Demopoulous H, et al. Free radical pathology: Rationale and toxicology of antioxidants and other supplements in sports medicine and exercise science. In: Katch FI, ed. Sport, health, and nutrition. Champaign, IL: Human Kinetics, 1996.
44. Deutekom M, et al. No acute effects of short-term creatine supplementation on muscle properties and sprint performance. Eur J Appl Physiol 2000;82:223.
45. Earnest CP, et al. The effect of creatine monohydrate ingestion on anaerobic power indices, muscular strength and body composition. Acta Physiol Scand 1995;153:207.
46. Emken EA. Metabolism of dietary stearic acid relative to other fatty acids in human subjects. Am J Clin Nutr 1994;60(suppl):1023S.
47. Engelhardt M, et al. Creatine supplementation in endurance sports. Med Sci Sports Exerc 1998;30:1123.

48. Esmarck B, et al. Timing of postexercise protein intake is important for muscle hypertrophy with resistance training in elderly humans. J Physiol 2001;535:301.

49. Evans GW. The effect of chromium picolinate on insulin controlled parameters in humans. Int J Biosoc Med Res 1969;11:163.

50. Faff J, Frankiewicz-Józko A. Effect of ubiquinone on exercise-induced lipid peroxidation in rat tissues. Eur J Appl Physiol 1997;75: 413.

51. Fairchild TJ, et al. Rapid carbohydrate loading after a short bout of near maximal-intensity exercise. Med Sci Sports Exerc 2002;34:980.

52. Finn JP, et al. Effect of creatine supplementation on metabolism and performance in humans during intermittent sprint cycling. Eur J Appl Physiol 2001;84:238.

53. Fleck SJ, et al. Anaerobic power effects of an amino acid supplement containing no branched amino acids in elite competitive athletes. J Strength Cond Res 1995;9:132.

54. Fogelholm GM, et al. Low-dose amino acid supplementation: no effects on serum human growth hormone and insulin in male weight lifters. Int J Sports Nutr 1993;3:290.

55. Francaux M, Poortmans JR. Effects of training and creatine supplement on muscle strength and body mass. Eur J Appl Physiol 1999;80:165.

56. Friendlander AL, et al. Training induced alterations of carbohydrate metabolism in women: women respond differently than men. J Appl Physiol 1998;85:1175.

57. Friolet R, et al. Relationship between the coenzyme A and the carnitine pools in human skeletal muscle at rest and after exhaustive exercise under normoxic and acutely hypoxic conditions. J Clin Invest 1994;94:1490.

58. Fry A, et al. Endocrine and performance responses to high volume training and amino acid supplementation in elite junior weightlifters. Int J Sports Nutr 1993;3:306.

59. Giamberardino MA, et al. Effect of prolonged L-carnitine administration on delayed muscle pain and CK release after eccentric effort. Int J Sports Med 1996;17:320.

60. Godard MP, et al. Oral amino-acid provision does not affect muscle strength or size gains in older men. Med Sci Sports Exerc 2002;34:1126.

61. Goforth HW Jr, et al. Persistence of supercompensated muscle glycogen in trained subjects after carbohydrate loading. J Appl Physiol 1997;82:342.

62. Gotshalk LA, et al. Creatine supplementation improves muscular performance in older men. Med Sci Sports Exerc 2002;34:537.

63. Grant KE, et al. Chromium and exercise training: effect on obese women. Med Sci Sports Exerc 1997;29:992.

64. Green AL, et al. The influence of oral creatine supplementation on metabolism during sub-maximal incremental treadmill exercise. Proc Nutr Soc 1993;53:84A.

65. Green AL, et al. Carbohydrate ingestion augments skeletal muscle creatine accumulation during creatine supplementation in humans. Am J Physiol 1996;271:E821.

66. Greenhauf PL. Creatine and its application as an ergogenic aid. Int J Sports Nutr 1995;5:S100.

67. Greenhauf PL, Timmons JA. Interaction between aerobic and anaerobic metabolism during intense muscle contraction. Exerc Sport Sci Rev 1998;26:1.

68. Greenhaff PL, et al. Effect of oral creatine supplementation on skeletal muscle phosphocreatine resynthesis. Am J Physiol 1994;266:E725.

69. Halberstam M, et al. Oral vanadyl sulfate improves insulin sensitivity in NIDDM but not in obese nondiabetic subjects. Diabetes 1996;45:659.

70. Hallmark MA, et al. Effects of chromium and resistive training on muscle strength and body composition. Med Sci Sports Exerc 1996;28:139.

71. Hargreaves M, et al. Effect of muscle glycogen availability on maximal exercise performance. Eur J Appl Physiol 1997;75:188.

72. Harris RC, et al. The effect of oral creatine supplementation on running performance during maximal short term exercise in man. J Physiol 1993;467:74P.

73. Harris RK, et al. Elevation of creatine in resting and exercised muscle of normal subjects by creatine supplementation. Clin Sci 1992;83:367.

74. Hasten DL, et al. Effects of chromium picolinate on beginning weight training students. Int J Sports Nutr 1992;2:343.

75. Hawley JA. Effect of increased fat availability on metabolism and exercise capacity. Med Sci Sports Exerc 2002;34:1485.

76. Heymsfield SB, et al. Garcinia cambogia (hydroxycitric acid) as a po-tential antiobesity agent: a randomized controlled trial. JAMA 1998; 280:1596.

77. Hitchins S, et al. Glycerol hyperhydration improves cycle time trial performance in hot humid conditions. Eur J Appl Physiol 1999;80:494.

78. Horton TJ, et al. Fuel metabolism in men and women during and after long-duration exercise. J Appl Physiol 1998;85:1823.

79. Hultman E, et al. Muscle creatine loading in men. J Appl Physiol 1996;81:232.

80. Indner WJ, et al. The effect of glycerol and desmopressin on exercise performance and hydration in triathletes. Med Sci Sports Exerc 1998;30:1263.

81. Ivy JL. Effect of pyruvate and dehydroxyacetone on metabolism and aerobic endurance capacity. Med Sci Sports Exerc 1998;6:837.

82. Ivy JL, Portman R. Nutrient timing: the future of sports nutrition. New Jersey: Basic Health Publications, Inc., 2004.

83. Izquierdo M, et al. Effects of creatine supplementation on muscle power, endurance, and sprint performance. Med Sci Sports Exerc 2002;34:332.

84. Jakobi JM, et al. Neuromuscular properties and fatigue in older men following acute creatine supplementation. Eur J Appl Physiol 2001; 84:321.

85. James AP, et al. Muscle glycogen supercompensation: absence of a gender-related difference. Eur J Appl Physiol 2001;85:533.

86. Janssen G, et al. Muscle carnitine level in endurance training and running a marathon. Int J Sports Med 1989;10:S153.

87. Jansson E. Sex differences in metabolic response to exercise. In: Saltin B, ed. Biochemistry of exercise VI. Champaign, IL: Human Kinetics,1986.

88. Jeejeebhoy K. The role of chromium in nutrition and therapeutics and as a potential toxin. Nutr Res 1999;57:328.

89. Jenkins RR. Exercise, oxidative stress, and antioxidants: a review. Int J Sports Nutr 1993;3:356.

90. Jeukendrup AE, et al. Metabolic availability of medium-chain triglycerides coingested with carbohydrate during prolonged exercise. J Appl Physiol 1995;79:756.

91. Jeukendrup AE, et al. Effect of endogenous carbohydrate availability on oral medium chain triglyceride oxidation during prolonged exercise. J Appl Physiol 1996;80:949.

92. Jeukendrup AE, et al. Effect of medium-chain triacylglycerol and carbohydrate ingestion during exercise on substrate utilization and subsequent cycling performance. Am J Clin Nutr 1998;67:397.

93. Jowko E, et al. Creatine and beta-hydroxy-beta-methylbutyrate (HMB) additively increase lean body mass and muscle strength during a weight training program. Nutrition 2001;17:558.

94. Juhn MS, Tarnopolsky M. Potential side effects of oral creatine supplementation: a critical review. Clin J Sports Med 1998;8:298.

95. Kaats GR, et al. A randomized, double-masked, placebo-controlled study of the effects of chromium picolinate supplementation on body composition: a replication and extension of a previous study. Curr Ther Res 1998;57:747.

96. Kenney J, Carlberg KA. The effect of choline and myo-inositol on liver and carcass fat levels in aerobically trained rats. Int J Sports Med 1995;16:114.

97. Kilduff LP, et al. Effects of creatine on isometric bench-press performance in resistance-trained humans. Med Sci Sports Exerc 2002;34:1176.

98. Koenigsberg PS, et al. Sustained hyperhydration with glycerol ingestion. Life Sci 1995;57:645.

99. Kraemer WJ. et al. Hormonal responses to consecutive days of heavy-resistance exercise with or without nutritional supplementation. J Appl Physiol 1998;85:1544.

100. Kreider RB, et al. Effects of creatine supplementation on body composition, strength, and sprint performance. Med Sci Sports Exerc 1998;30:73.

101. Kreider RB, et al. Effects of oral d-ribose supplementation on anaerobic capacity and selected metabolic markers in healthy males. Int J Sport Nutr Exerc Metab 2003;13:87.

102. Kreider RB, et al. Long-term creatine supplementation does not significantly affect clinical markers of health in athletes. Mol Cell Biochem 2003;244:95.

103. Kriketos AD, et al. (-)-Hydroxycitric acid does not affect energy expenditure and substrate oxidation in adult males in a post-absorptive state. Int J Obes Relat Metab Disord 1999;23:867.

104. Laaksonen R, et al. Ubiquinone supplementation and exercise capacity in trained young and older men. Eur J Appl Physiol 1995;72:95.

105. Latzka WA, et al. Hyperhydration: tolerance and cardiovascular effects during uncompensable heat stress. J Appl Physiol 1998;84:1858.
106. Levenhagen DK, et al. Post-exercise nutrient intake is critical to recovery of leg glucose, and protein homeostasis in humans. Am J Physiol Endocrinol Metab 2001;280:E982.
107. Levenhagen DK, et al. Postexercise protein intake enhances whole-body and leg protein accretion in humans. Med Sci Sports Exerc 2002;34:828.
108. Lieberman HR, et al. Carbohydrate administration during a day of sustained aerobic activity improves vigilance, as assessed by normal ambulatory monitoring device, and mood. Am J Clin Nutr 2002;76:120.
109. Lukaski HC, et al. Chromium supplementation and resistance training effects on whole body and regional composition, strength, and trace element status of men. Am J Clin Nutr 1996;63:954.
110. Lynch NJ, et al. Effects of moderate dietary manipulation on intermittent exercise performance and metabolism in women. Eur J Appl Physiol 2000;81:197.
111. Lyons TP, et al. Effects of glycerol-induced hyperhydration prior to exercise in the heat on sweating and core temperature. Med Sci Sports Exerc 1990;22:477.
112. Magal M, et al. Comparison of glycerol and water hydration regimens on tennis-related performance. Med Sci Sports Exerc 2003;35:150.
113. Maher TJ. Safety concerns regarding supplemental amino acids: results of a study. In: Marriott BM, ed. Food components to enhance performance. Washington, DC: Committee on Military Nutrition Research. National Academy Press, 1994.
114. Malm C, et al. Supplementation with ubiquinone-10 causes cellular damage during intense exercise. Acta Physiol Scand 1996;157:511.
115. Massicotte D, et al. Oxidation of exogenous medium-chain free fatty acids during prolonged exercise: comparison with glucose. J Appl Physiol 1992;73:1334.
116. Maughan RJ. Creatine supplementation and exercise performance. Int J Sport Nutr 1995;5:94.
117. Metges CC, Wolfram G. Medium- and long-chain triglycerides labeled with ^{13}C: A comparison of oxidation after oral or parenteral administration in humans. J Nutr 1991;121:31.
118. Mihic S, et al. Acute creatine loading increases fat-free mass, but does not affect blood pressure, plasma creatine, or DK activity in men and women. Med Sci Sports Exerc 2000;32:291.
119. Miller SL, et al. Independent and combined effects of amino acids and glucose after resistance exercise. Med Sci Sports Exerc 2003;35:449.
120. Mujika I, et al. Creatine supplementation does not improve sprint performance in competitive swimmers. Med Sci Sports Exerc 1996;28:1435.
121. Murray R, et al. Physiological responses to glycerol ingestion during exercise. J Appl Physiol 1991;71:144.
122. Nakai M, et al. Mechanism of insulin-like action of vanadyl sulfate: studies on interaction between rat adipocytes and vanadium compounds. Biol Pharm Bull 1995;18:719.
123. Nakatani A, et al. Effect of endurance exercise training on muscle glycogen supercompensation in rats. J Appl Physiol 1997;82: 711.
124. Nielsen F. Facts and fallacies about boron. Nutr Today 1992;27:6.
125. Nielsen F. Controversial chromium: does the superstar mineral of the mountebanks receive appropriate attention from clinicians and nutritionists? Nutr Today 1996;31:266.
126. Odland LM, et al. Effect of oral creatine supplementation on muscle [PCr] and short-term maximum power output. Med Sci Sports Exerc 1997;29:216.
127. Op't Eijnde B, Hespel P. Short-term creatine supplementation does not alter the hormonal response to resistance training. Med Sci Sports Exerc 2001;33:449.
128. Op't Eijnde B, et al. No effects of oral ribose supplementation on repeated maximal exercise and de novo ATP resynthesis. J Appl Physiol 2001;91:2275.
129. Oyono-Enguelle S, et al. Prolonged submaximal exercise and L-carnitine in humans. Eur J Appl Physiol 1988;58:53.
130. Palmer GS, et al. Carbohydrate ingestion immediately before exercise does not improve 20 km time trial performance in well trained cyclists. Int J Sports Med 1998;19:415.
131. Parise G, et al. Effects of acute creatine monohydrate supplementation on leucine kinetics and mixed-muscle protein synthesis. J Appl Physiol 2001;91:1041.
132. Pitsiladis YP, Maughan RJ. The effects of alterations in dietary carbohydrate intake on the performance of high-intensity exercise in trained individuals. Eur J Appl Physiol 1999;79:433.
133. Poortmans JR, Francaux M. Long-term oral creatine supplementation does not impair renal function in healthy athletes. Med Sci Sports Exerc 1999;31:1108.
134. Porter DA, et al. The effect of oral coenzyme Q$_{10}$ on the exercise tolerance of middle-aged, untrained men. Int J Sports Med 1995;16:421.
135. Prevost MC, et al. Creatine supplementation enhances intermittent work performance. Res Q Exerc Sport 1997;68:233.
136. Pritchard NR, Kaira PA. Renal dysfunction accompanying oral creatine supplements. Lancet 1998;351:1252.
137. Raben AB, et al. Serum sex hormones and endurance performance after a lacto-ovo-vegetarian and mixed diet. Med Sci Sports Exerc 1992;24:1290.
138. Rasmussen BB, Phillips SM. Contractile and nutritional regulation of human muscle growth. Exerc Sport Sci Rev 2003;31;127.
139. Rasmussen BB, et al. An oral essential amino acid-carbohydrate supplement enhances muscle protein anabolism after resistance exercise. J Appl Physiol 2000;88:386.
140. Rawson ES, Clarkson PM. Acute creatine supplementation in older men. Int J Sports Med 2000;21:75.
141. Rawson ES, et al. Effects of 30 days of creatine ingestion in older men. Eur J Appl Physiol 1999;80:139.
142. Redondo D, et al. The effect of oral creatine monohydrate supplementation on running velocity. Med Sci Sports Exerc 1994;26:S23.
143. Reed MJ, et al. Dietary lipids: an additional regulator of plasma levels of sex hormone binding globulin. J Clin Endocrinol Metab 1987;64:1083.
144. Rennie MJ, Tipton KD. Protein and amino acid metabolism during and after resistance exercise and the effects of nutrition. Annu Rev Nutr 2000;20:457.
145. Riedesel ML, et al. Hyperhydration with glycerol solutions. J Appl Physiol 1987;63:2262.
146. Roberts J. The effect of coenzyme Q10 on exercise performance. Med Sci Sports Exerc 1990;22:S87.
147. Robertson RJ, et al. Blood glucose extraction as a mediator of perceived exertion during prolonged exercise. Eur J Appl Physiol 1990;61:100.
148. Robinson TM, et al. Role of submaximal exercise in promoting creatine and glycogen accumulation in human skeletal muscle. J Appl Physiol 1999;87:598.
149. Romer LM, et al. Effects of oral creatine supplementation on high intensity, intermittent exercise performance in competitive squash players. Int J Sports Med 2001;24:546.
150. Roy BD, et al. Effect of glucose supplement timing on protein metabolism after resistance training. J Appl Physiol 1997; 82:1882.
151. Roy BD, et al. Macronutrient intakes and whole body protein metabolism following resistance exercise. Med Sci Sports Exerc 2000;32:1412.
152. Shomrat A, et al. Effects of creatine feeding on maximal exercise performance in vegetarians. Eur J Appl Physiol 2000;82:321.
153. Snow RJ, Murphy RM. Factors influencing creatine loading into human skeletal muscle. Exerc Sport Sci Rev 2003;31: 154.
154. Stanko RT, et al. Inhibition of lipid accumulation and enhancement of energy expenditure by the addition of pyruvate and dihydroxyacetone to a rat diet. Metabolism 1986;35:182.
155. Stanko RT, et al. Enhanced leg-exercise endurance with a high-carbohydrate diet and dihydroxyacetone and pyruvate. J Appl Physiol 1990;69:1651.
156. Stanko RT, et al. Enhancement of arm-exercise endurance capacity with dihydroxyacetone and pyruvate. J Appl Physiol 1990; 68:119.
157. Stanko RT, et al. Body composition, energy utilization, and nitrogen metabolism with a 4.25-MJ/d low-energy diet supplemented with pyruvate. Am J Clin Nutr 1992;56:630.
158. Stanko RT, et al. Body composition, energy utilization and nitrogen metabolism with a severely restricted diet supplemented with dihydroxyacetone and pyruvate. Am J Clin Nutr 1992;55:771.
159. Starling RD, et al. Relationships between muscle carnitine, age and oxidative status. Eur J Appl Physiol 1995;71:143.
160. Starling RD, et al. Effect of inosine supplementation on aerobic and anaerobic cycling performance. Med Sci Sports Exerc 1996; 28:1193.

161. Stensrud T, et al. L-Tryptophan supplementation does not improve running performance. Int J Sports Med 1992;13:481.

162. Stevenson SW, Dudley GA. Dietary creatine supplementation and muscular adaptation to resistive overload. Med Sci Sports Exerc 2001;33:1304.

163. Suminski R, et al. The effect of amino acid ingestion and resistance exercise on growth hormone responses in young males. Med Sci Sports Exerc (abstr) 1993;25:S77.

164. Tarnopolsky MA, et al. Carbohydrate loading and metabolism during exercise in men and women. J Appl Physiol 1995;78:1360.

165. Tarnopolsky MA, et al. Gender differences in carbohydrate loading are related to energy intake. J Appl Physiol 2001;91:225.

166. Tegelman R, et al. Effects of a diet regimen on pituitary and steroid hormones in male ice hockey players. Int J Sports Med 1992;13:424.

167. Thompson KH, et al. Studies of vanadyl sulfate as a glucose-lowering agent in STZ-diabetic rats. Biochem Biophys Res Commun 1993;197:1549.

168. Tipton KD, et al. Acute response of net muscle protein balance reflects 24-h balance after exercise and amino acid ingestion. Am J Physiol 2003;284:E76.

169. Trappe SW, et al. The effects of L-carnitine supplementation on performance during swimming. Int J Sports Med 1994;15:181.

170. Trent LK, Thieding-Cancel D. Effects of chromium picolinate on body composition in a remedial conditioning program. NHRC publ 94-20, 1995.

171. Trump ME, et al. Importance of muscle phosphocreatine during intermittent maximal cycling. J Appl Physiol 1996;80:1574.

172. Vandenberghe K, et al. Caffeine counteracts the ergogenic action of creatine loading. J Appl Physiol 1996;80:452.

173. Vandenberghe K, et al. Long-term creatine intake is beneficial to muscle performance during resistance training. J Appl Physiol 1997;83:2055.

174. Vandenberghe K, et al. Phosphocreatine resynthesis is not affected by creatine loading. Med Sci Sports Exerc 1999;31:236.

175. VanLeemputte M, et al. Shortening of muscle relaxation time after creatine loading. J Appl Physiol 1999;86:840.

176. van Loon LJC, et al. Effects of acute (—)-hydroxycitrate supplementation on substrate metabolism at rest and during exercise in humans. Am J Clin Nutr 2000;72:1445.

177. van Zyl CG, et al. Effects of medium-chain triglyceride ingestion on fuel metabolism and cycling performance. J Appl Physiol 1996;80:2217.

178. Vasankari TJ, et al. Increased serum and low-density-lipoprotein antioxidant potential after antioxidant supplementation in endurance athletes. Am J Clin Nutr 1997;65:1052.

179. Vierck JL, et al. The effects of ergogenic compounds on myogenic satellite cells. Med Sci Sports Exerc 2003;35:769.

180. Volek JS. Influence of nutrition on responses to resistance training. Med Sci Sports Exerc 2004;36:689.

181. Volek JS, et al. Response of testosterone and cortisol concentrations to high-intensity resistance exercise following creatine monohydrate supplementation. J Strength Cond Res 1996;10:292.

182. Volek JS, et al. Testosterone and cortisol in relationship to dietary nutrients and resistance exercise. J Appl Physiol 1997; 82:49.

183. Volek JS, et al. Performance and muscle fiber adaptations to creatine supplementation and heavy resistance training. Med Sci Sports Exerc 1999;31:1147.

184. Volek JS, et al. Physiological responses to short-term exercise in the heat after creatine loading. Med Sci Sports Exerc 2001;33:1101.

185. Vukovich MD, et al. Carnitine supplementation: effect on muscle carnitine and glycogen content during exercise. Med Sci Sports Exerc 1994;26:1122.

186. Walker LJ, et al. Dietary carbohydrate, muscle glycogen content, and endurance performance in well-trained women. J Appl Physiol 2000;88:2151.

187. Walker LS, et al. Chromium picolinate effects on body composition and muscular performance in wrestlers. Med Sci Sports Exerc 1998;30:1730.

188. Wapnir PA, et al. Enhancement of intestinal water absorption and sodium transport by glycerol in rats. J Appl Physiol 1996;81:2523.

189. Williams AG, et al. Effects of resistance exercise volume and nutritional supplementation on anabolic and catabolic hormones. Eur J Appl Physiol 2002;86:315.

190. Williams MM, et al. Effect of inosine supplementation on 3-mile treadmill run performance and $\dot{V}O_2$ peak. Med Sci Sports Exerc 1990;22:517.

191. Willoughby DS, Rosene J. Effects of oral creatine and resistance training on myosin heavy chain expression. Med Sci Sports Exerc 2001;33:1674.

192. Willoughby DS, Rosene J. Effects of oral creatine and resistance training on myogenic regulatory factors expression. Med Sci Sports Exerc 2003;35:923.

193. Wiroth JB, et al. Effects of oral creatine supplementation on maximal pedaling performance in older adults. Eur J Appl Physiol. 2001;84:533.

194. Woodhouse M, et al. The effects of varying doses of orally ingested bee pollen extract upon selected performance variables. Athletic Training 1987;22:26.

195. Wolfe RR. Regulation of muscle protein by amino acids. J Nutr 2002;132:3219S.

196. Wyss M, Kaddurah-Daouk R. Creatine and creatinine metabolism. Physiol Rev 2000;60:1107.

197. Wyss V, et al. Effects of L-carnitine administration on $\dot{V}O_2$ max and the aerobic-anaerobic threshold in normoxia and acute hypoxia. Eur J Appl Physiol 1990;60:1.

198. Yan Z, et al. Effect of low glycogen on glycogen synthase in human muscle during and after exercise. Acta Physiol Scand 1992;145:345.

199. Yuen VG, et al. Comparison of the glucose-lowering properties of vanadyl sulfate and bis (maltolato) oxovanadium (IV) following acute and chronic administration. Can J Physiol Pharmacol 1995;73:55.

200. Zuliani U, et al. The influence of ubiquinone (CoQ10) on the metabolic response to work. J Sports Med Phys Fitness 1989;29:57.

Additional Readings

Bacurau RF, et al. Does exercise training interfere with the effects of L-carnitine supplementation? Nutrition 2003;19:337.

Branch JD. Effect of creatine supplementation on body composition and performance: A meta-analysis. Int J Sport Nutr Exerc Metab 2003;13: 198.

Brudnak MA. Creatine: Are the benefits worth the risk? Toxicol Lett 2004;150:123.

Candow DG, et al. Effect of ceasing creatine supplementation while maintaining resistance training in older men. J Aging Phys Act 2004;12:219.

Earnest CP, et al. Effects of a commercial herbal-based formula on exercise performance in cyclists. Med Sci Sports Exerc 2004;36:504.

Eckerson JM, et al. Effect of two and five days of creatine loading on anaerobic working capacity in women. J Strength Cond Res 2004;18:168.

Hellsten Y, et al. Effect of ribose supplementation on resynthesis of adenine nucleotides after intense intermittent training in humans. Am J Physiol Regul Integr Comp Physiol 2004;286:R182.

Jentjens RL, et al. High oxidation rates from combined carbohydrates ingested during exercise. Med Sci Sports Exerc 2004;36:1551.

Karlic H, Lohninger A. Supplementation of L-carnitine in athletes: Does it make sense? Nutrition 2004;20:709.

Koopman R, et al. Combined ingestion of protein and carbohydrate improves protein balance during ultra-endurance exercise. Am J Physiol Endocrinol Metab 2004;287:E712.

Mujika I, et al. Physiological changes associated with the pre-event taper in athletes. Sports Med 2004;34:891.

Paddon-Jones D, et al. Potential ergogenic effects of arginine and creatine supplementation. J Nutr 2004;134(Suppl):2888S.

Saldanha Aoki M, et al. Carnitine supplementation fails to maximize fat mass loss induced by endurance training in rats. Ann Nutr Metab 2004;48:90.

Shimomura Y, et al. Exercise promotes BCAA catabolism: effects of BCAA supplementation on skeletal muscle during exercise. J Nutr 2004;134(Suppl):1583S.

Vincent JB. The potential value and toxicity of chromium picolinate as a nutritional supplement, weight loss agent and muscle development agent. Sports Med 2003;33:213.

Watson P, et al. The effect of acute branched-chain amino acid supplementation on prolonged exercise capacity in a warm environment. Eur J Appl Physiol 2004. In Press

Section VI
Body Composition, Weight Control, and Disordered Eating Behaviors

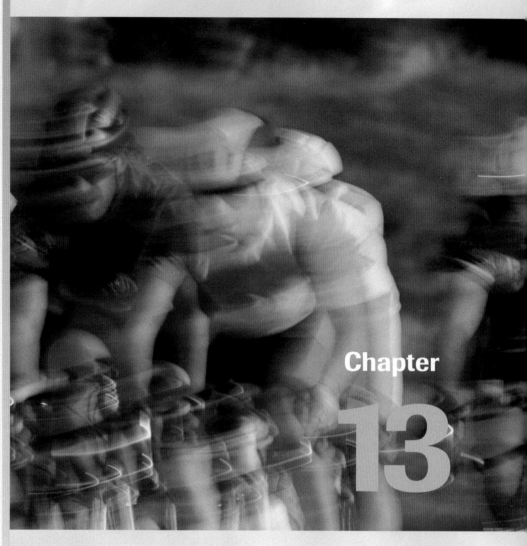

Chapter

13

Body Composition Assessment and Sport-Specific Observations

TEST YOUR KNOWLEDGE

Answer these ten statements about body composition assessment. Use the scoring key at the end of the chapter to check your results. Repeat this test after you have read the chapter and compare your results.

1. **T F** The fundamental importance of the BMI is its ability to classify individuals by level of body fat and total muscle mass.

2. **T F** A male with a stature of 175.3 cm and body mass of 97.1 kg classifies as obese.

3. **T F** Compared with women of normal body weight, obese women achieve lower economic status.

4. **T F** Total body fat exists in two storage sites called subcutaneous and intraabdominal.

5. **T F** Archimedes' fundamental discovery explained the concept of specific gravity.

6. **T F** A male with a body density of 1.0719 has a body fat content of 10% of body mass and a fat mass of 5 kg.

7. **T F** A female with a waist girth of 38 inches falls just below the threshold value for increased risk for various diseases.

8. **T F** The average percentage body fat is 15% for college age males and 25% for females.

9. **T F** A 120-kg (265-lb) shot-put athlete with 24% body fat wants to attain a body fat level of 15%. He must lose 40 pounds of fat.

10. **T F** Among female athletes, bodybuilders possess the lowest percentage body fat.

➤ Body Composition Assessment

The accurate appraisal of body composition serves an important role in a comprehensive program of total nutrition and physical fitness. Excess body fat often hinders exercise training and sports competition, particularly in activities that demand a high *relative* physiologic capacity (i.e., capacity expressed related to body mass). Men and women devote considerable time and energy to alter their body composition, hoping to increase fat-free body mass and reduce body fat to achieve an "ideal" muscularity and/or aesthetic look. There are four important reasons to assess a client's body composition:

1. Body composition assessment provides a starting point or baseline for future decisions about weight loss and weight gain.
2. Body composition assessment provides realistic goals about how to best achieve an "ideal" balance between the body's fat and nonfat compartments.
3. Body composition assessment relates to general health status and plays a vital role in the health and fitness goals of all individuals.
4. Body composition assessment monitors changes in the body's fat and lean components for tracking

progress during exercise regimens of different durations and intensities and the efficacy of rehabilitation programs using different modalities and treatment practices.

The frequently used **height–weight tables** have limited value as a standard to evaluate physique because "overweight" and "overfat" often describe different aspects of body composition for physically active men and women. Competitive athletes clearly illustrate this point, as many possess high muscularity and exceed the average weight for their sex and height but otherwise possess a lean body composition. For these individuals, attempting to lose weight can impair exercise performance.

LIMITATIONS OF HEIGHT–WEIGHT TABLES

The evaluation of body composition permits quantification of the major structural components of the body—muscle, bone, and fat. The actuarial-based height–weight tables assess the extent of "overweightness" based on sex and bony frame size, but such tables do not provide reliable information about the relative composition of the body. (Actually, the proper scientific terms [expressed in SI units] for *height* and *weight* are *stature* [cm] and *mass* [kg], respectively, and we have changed *weight* to *mass* and *height* to *stature* as long as it preserves readability.)

These tables serve as statistical landmarks based on the average ranges of body mass related to stature in which men

and women aged 25 to 59 years have the lowest mortality rate. Height–weight tables *do not* consider specific causes of death or disease status before death (morbidity). In addition, many versions of the tables recommend different "desirable" weight ranges, with some considering frame size, age, and sex, while others do not. TABLE 13.1A AND B presents examples of two height–weight standards; table A gives suggested body weights for adults, with adjustment for age. Table B presents sex-specific standards proposed by the Metropolitan Life Insurance Company with consideration for bony frame size. Table 13.1C presents a convenient method to estimate sex-specific frame size using elbow breadth and stature.

Many Overweight Elite Athletes

Many athletes weigh more than the average weight-for-height standards of life insurance company statistics—the "extra" weight due simply to additional muscle mass. According to Table 13.1A, for example, the desirable body mass for a 24-year-old professional football player 6'2" (188 cm) and 255 lb (116 kg) ranges between 148 lb (67.3 kg) and 195 lb (88.6 kg). Similarly, a young adult male of the same stature should weigh on average 187 lb (85 kg). Using either criterion, the player's "overweight" means he should reduce body mass at least 27 kg to the upper limit of the desirable weight range for a man of his stature! He must reduce an additional 3.6 kg to match his "average" American male counterpart.

If the player followed these guidelines, he certainly would jeopardize his football career and possibly overall

---

Table 13.1   HEIGHT–WEIGHT TABLES AND DETERMINATION OF FRAME SIZE

A. Suggested Body Weights for Adults, with Recommended Adjustment for Age National Institutes of Health Recommendations[a]

Height[b]	Weight (lb)[c] 19–34 years	35 years	Height[b]	Weight (lb)[c] 19–34 years	35 years
5'0"	97–128	108–138	5'10"	132–174	146–188
5'1"	101–132	111–143	5'11"	136–179	151–194
5'2"	104–137	115–148	6'0"	140–184	155–199
5'3"	107–141	119–152	6'1"	144–189	159–205
5'4"	111–146	122–157	6'2"	148–195	164–210
5'5"	114–150	126–162	6'3"	152–200	168–216
5'6"	118–155	130–167	6'4"	156–205	173–222
5'7"	121–160	134–172	6'5"	160–211	177–228
5'8"	125–164	138–178	6'6"	164–216	182–234
5'9"	129–169	142–183			

[a] The lower weights more often apply to women who have less muscle and bone.
[b] Without shoes.
[c] Without clothes.

Table 13.1   HEIGHT–WEIGHT TABLES AND DETERMINATION OF FRAME SIZE (continued)

B. 1983 Sex-Specific Standards Proposed by the Metropolitan Life Insurance Company[d]

	Men				Women		
Height (ft in.)	*Small Frame*	*Medium Frame*	*Large Frame*	*Height (ft in.)*	*Small Frame*	*Medium Frame*	*Large Frame*
5 2	128–134	131–141	138–150	4 10	102–111	109–121	118–131
5 3	130–136	133–143	140–153	4 11	103–113	111–123	120–134
5 4	132–138	135–145	142–156	5 0	104–115	113–126	122–137
5 5	134–140	137–148	144–160	5 1	106–118	115–129	125–140
5 6	136–142	139–151	146–164	5 2	108–121	118–132	128–143
5 7	138–145	142–154	149–168	5 3	111–124	121–135	131–147
5 8	140–148	145–157	152–172	5 4	114–127	124–138	134–151
5 9	142–151	148–160	155–176	5 5	117–130	127–141	137–155
5 10	144–154	151–163	158–180	5 6	120–133	130–144	140–159
5 11	146–157	154–166	161–184	5 7	123–136	133–147	143–163
6 0	149–160	157–170	164–188	5 8	126–139	136–150	146–167
6 1	152–164	160–174	168–192	5 9	129–142	139–153	149–170
6 2	155–168	164–178	172–197	5 10	132–145	142–156	152–173
6 3	158–172	167–182	176–202	5 11	135–148	145–159	155–176
6 4	162–176	171–187	181–207	6 0	138–151	148–162	158–179

From Statistical Bulletin, Metropolitan Life Insurance Company, New York City.

[d] Weights at ages 25–59 years based on lowest comparative mortality. Weight in pounds according to frame size for men wearing indoor clothing weighing 5 lb, shoes with 1-in. heels; for women, indoor clothing.

C. How to Determine Frame Size from Elbow Breadth Based on Height.

*The person's right arm extends forward perpendicular to the body, with arm bent so angle at the elbow forms 90°, with fingers pointing up and palm turned away from body. The greatest breadth across the elbow joint is measured with a sliding caliper along the axis of the upper arm. This records as **elbow breadth**. The table gives the elbow breadth measurements for medium-framed men and women of various heights. Measurements lower than those listed indicate a small frame size; higher measurements indicate a large frame size.*

	Men		Women	
	Height in 10 Heels	*Medium-Framed Elbow Breadth*	*Height in 10 Heels*	*Medium-Framed Elbow Breadth*
	5' 2"–5' 3"	2 1/2"–2 7/8"	4' 10"–4' 11"	2 1/4"–2 1/2"
	5' 4"–5' 7"	2 5/8"–2 7/8"	5' 0"–5' 3"	2 1/4"–2 1/2"
	5' 8"–5' 11"	2 3/4"–3"	5' 4"–5' 7"	2 3/8"–2 5/8"
	6' 0"–6' 3"	2 3/4"–3 1/8"	5' 8"–5' 11"	2 3/8"–2 5/8"
	>6' 4"	2 7/8"–3 1/4"	>6' 0"	2 1/2"–2 3/4"

health. Some larger-sized persons are indeed "overweight," yet they may fall within a normal range for body fat without a need to reduce weight. The football player's total fat content equaled only 12.7% of body mass (compared with 15.0% body fat for untrained young men), even though he weighed 31 kg more than the average.

In the early 1940s, Navy physician **Dr. Albert Behnke** assessed the body composition of 25 professional football players. Based on standards for height and weight, 17 players failed standards for military service because their "overweight" status incorrectly indicated excessive fatness.[10] However, carefully evaluating each player's body

composition indicated the excess weight consisted primarily of muscle mass, not fat mass. These observations clearly specified that the term "overweight" refers only to body mass greater than some standard, usually the average body mass for a given stature. Being above some "average," "ideal," or "desirable" body mass based on height–weight tables should not necessarily dictate whether someone should reduce weight. A more desirable strategy, particularly for physically active individuals, evaluates body composition by one of the techniques reviewed in this chapter.

The Body Mass Index: A Somewhat Better Use of Stature and Mass

Clinicians and researchers use the **body mass index (BMI)**, derived from body mass related to stature, to evaluate the "normalcy" of body weight. BMI has a somewhat higher, yet still moderate, association with body fat than estimates based simply on stature and mass. In addition, current classification standards for overweight and obese (see next section) assume that the relationship between BMI and percentage body fat remains independent of age, gender, ethnicity, and race. However, this is not the case. For example, at a given BMI level Asians have greater body fat content than Caucasians and thus show greater risk for fat-related illness. Recent evidence also indicates a higher body fat percentage for a given BMI among Hispanic American women than for European American and African American women.[44] Failure to consider these sources of bias alters the proportion of individuals defined as obese by measured percentage body fat.[77,120]

BMI = Body mass, kg ÷ Stature, m²

The importance of this easily obtained index illustrated in the bottom table of FIGURE 13.1 lies not in predicting obesity but rather in its curvilinear relationship to all-cause mortality ratio; as BMI increases, so does the risk for cardiovascular complications including hypertension and stroke, type 2 diabetes, and renal disease.[22,121,129] The classification schema at the bottom of the figure indicates level of risk with each 5-unit increase in BMI. The lowest health risk category occurs for individuals with BMIs between 20 and 25, and the highest risk category includes individuals whose BMIs exceed 40. For women, 21.3 to 22.1 represents the desirable BMI range; the corresponding range for men is 21.9 to 22.4. An increased incidence of high blood pressure, diabetes, and coronary heart disease occurs when BMI values exceed 27.8 for men and 27.3 for women.

Limitations of BMI for Physically Active Individuals

As with height–weight tables, the BMI fails to consider the body's proportional composition or the all-important component of body fat distribution, referred to as **fat patterning**. Specifically, factors other than excess body fat, such as bone and muscle mass and even the increased quantity of plasma volume induced by exercise training affect the numerator of the BMI equation. A high BMI could lead to an incorrect interpretation of overfatness in relatively lean individuals with excessive muscle mass because of genetic makeup or exercise training. Healthy individuals who exercise regularly may lose body fat not reflected in body weight or BMI changes because of an exercise-induced concurrent gain fat-free body mass.[54]

The possibility of misclassifying someone as overweight by BMI applies particularly to large-size field athletes, bodybuilders, weightlifters, upper-weight-class wrestlers, and professional football players, particularly offensive and defensive linemen. For example, the BMI for seven defensive linemen from a former NFL Super Bowl team averaged 31.9 (team BMI averaged 28.7), clearly signaling these professional athletes as overweight and placing them in the moderate category for mortality risk. However, their body fat content, 18.0% for the linemen and 12.1% for the team, misclassified them for fatness using BMI as the overweight standard.

Misclassification of body weight in relation to body fat also applies to the typical NFL player from 1920 to 1996. FIGURE 13.2 displays the average BMI for all NFL roster players at each five-year interval between 1920 and 1996 (53,333 players). Average body fat content during the late 1970s through the 1990s fell below the range typically associated with normal males (see Table 13.7). Body fat, evaluated by hydrostatic weighing (see page 406), for football players included teams of the New York Jets, Washington Redskins, New Orleans Saints, and Dallas Cowboys. On average, all players from 1960 forward classify as overweight (based on weight for height using insurance company statistics). Up to 1989, the BMI for the linebackers, skill players, and defensive backs represents the "low" category for disease risk, while the BMI for offensive and defensive linemen places these players at "moderate" risk. Thereafter, the BMI for linebackers changed from the low to moderate category, while the BMI for offensive and defensive linemen quickly approached "high" risk and, since 1991, remained in that category. Unfortunately, the rate of increase in BMI for the largest of the NFL players (offensive and defensive linemen) shows no sign of declining. This certainly does not bode well from a health perspective for these large-size players.

NEW STANDARDS FOR OVERWEIGHT AND OBESITY

On June 18, 1998, the 24-member expert panel convened by the National Institutes of Health and National Heart Lung and Blood Institute adopted the single standards of the World Health Organization and lowered the BMI demarca-

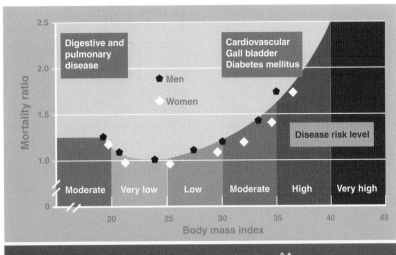

Body mass index, kg·m² *													
19	20	21	22	23	24	25	26	27	28	29	30	35	40

Height, inches	Body weight, lb													
58	91	96	100	105	110	115	119	124	129	134	138	143	167	191
59	94	99	104	109	114	119	124	128	133	138	143	148	173	198
60	97	102	107	112	118	123	128	133	138	143	148	153	179	204
61	100	106	111	116	122	127	132	137	143	148	153	158	185	211
62	104	109	115	120	126	131	136	142	147	153	158	164	191	218
63	107	113	118	124	130	135	144	146	152	158	163	169	197	225
64	110	116	122	128	134	140	145	151	157	163	169	174	204	232
65	114	120	126	132	138	144	150	156	162	168	174	180	210	240
66	118	124	130	136	142	148	155	161	167	173	179	186	216	247
67	121	127	134	140	146	153	159	166	172	178	184	191	223	254
68	125	135	138	144	151	158	164	171	177	184	190	197	230	262
69	128	135	142	149	155	162	169	176	182	189	196	203	236	270
70	132	139	146	153	160	167	174	181	188	195	202	207	243	278
71	136	143	150	157	165	172	179	186	193	200	208	215	250	286
72	140	147	154	162	169	176	183	191	199	206	213	221	258	294
73	144	151	159	166	174	182	189	197	204	212	219	227	265	302
74	148	155	163	171	178	186	194	202	210	218	225	233	272	311
75	152	160	168	176	184	192	200	208	216	224	232	240	280	319
76	156	164	172	180	189	197	205	213	221	230	238	246	287	328

*The intersection of weight and height provides the BMI (kg·m²). For an exact calculation of BMI, follow these steps:

Step 1. Multiply body weight (lb) by 0.45 to convert weight to kilograms
Step 2. Multiply height (in) by 0.0254 to convert height to meters.
Step 3. Multiply answer in step 2 by itself to obtain square meters (m²)
Step 4. Divide step 1 result (mass, kg) by step 3 result (m²).

Figure 13.1. Curvilinear relationship based on American Cancer Society data between all-cause mortality and body mass index. The classification schema proposed for very low to very high risk includes a classification relating risk to one of a number of treatments such as reduced food intake, exercise, drug therapy, and surgery. (Modified from Bray GA. Pathophysiology of obesity. Am J Clin Nutr 1992;55:488S.)

tion for "overweight" (the preobese state) for all adults from 27 to 25. FIGURE 13.3 shows the current standards for identifying obesity (defined by BMI ≥ 30.0) for six heights (from 5'6" to 6'3"). Persons with a BMI of 30 average about 30 pounds overweight. For example, a man 6'0" weighing 221 pounds and a woman weighing 186 pounds at 5'6" both have a BMI of 30, and both are about 30 pounds overweight. The revised standards place 64.5% of Americans in either

the overweight or obese categories—up from 55.9% in 1994.[50,100,177,194] For the first time in the Unites States, overweight persons (BMI above 25) outnumber those of desirable body weight. In terms of ethnicity and gender, significantly more black, Mexican, Cuban, and Puerto Rican men and women classify as overweight than their white counterparts.[49] We discuss the national prevalence of overweight and obesity more fully in Chapter 14.

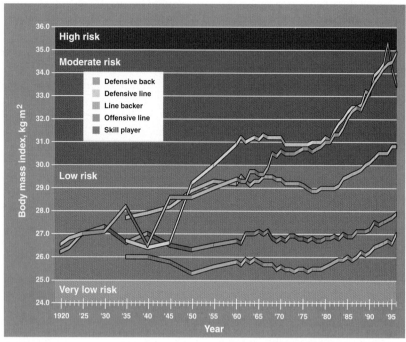

Figure 13.2. Body mass index *(BMI)* for all roster players in the National Football League between 1920 and 1996 (N = 53,333). Categories include offensive and defensive linemen, linebackers, skill players (quarterbacks, receivers, backfield), and defensive backs. The four horizontal bands of color refer to Bray's classification in Figure 13.1 for relative disease risk levels. According to the 1998 federal guidelines for identification, evaluation, and treatment of overweight and obesity, offensive and defensive linemen from 1980 to present would classify as obese. (Data compiled by K. D. Monahan in partial fulfillment for an independent research project [Professor F. Katch, advisor] in the Exercise Science Department, University of Massachusetts, Amherst [1996]).

Use the following BMI-based classification to determine adequacy of body weight:

Normal Weight: BMI ≤ 25.0
Overweight: 25.0–29.9
Obese: ≥ 30.0

Sample Computation of BMI

Male:

Stature = 175.3 cm, 1.753 m, (69 in.)
Body mass = 97.1 kg (214.1 lb)

$$BMI = 97.1 \div (1.753)^2$$
$$BMI = 31.6 \text{ kg per m}^2$$

In this example, the BMI falls above the threshold of the upper-range of BMI values and classifies the person as obese.

SPECIFIC HEALTH RISKS OF OBESITY

The June 1998 guidelines from the National Heart, Lung, and Blood Institute and the National Institute of Diabetes,

Figure 13.3. New standards for the threshold of obesity.

Digestive and Kidney Diseases labeled obesity a significant societal burden owing to the association between high levels of body weight and body fat and increased risk for adverse health consequences. Impaired glucose tolerance and overall impaired health-related quality of life emerge even among obese children and adolescents.[151,158] Obesity represents the second leading cause of preventable death in America (cigarette smoking first), with the cost of obesity-related diseases approaching $120 billion annually in the year 2000. One trip to the doctor a year made by 25% of the total obese Americans population costs more than $810 million, based on a doctor visit charge of $60. On the downside, the estimated number of annual deaths attributed to obesity per se ranges between 280,000 and 325,000.[3,22,127] Comorbidities include hypertension, elevated blood sugar, pulmonary dysfunction including asthma and sleep apnea, psychiatric problems (depression and eating disorders), postmenopausal breast cancer, pancreatic cancer (and diverse other cancers[200]), gastrointestinal disorders including gallstones, and elevated total cholesterol and low HDL-cholesterol levels. All of these heighten an overweight individual's risks of poor health at any given level of excess weight. Unfortunately, the increasing prevalence of obesity has slowed the decline in coronary heart disease among middle-aged women.[71] Obese and overweight individuals with two or more heart disease risk factors should lose weight. Overweight persons without other risk factors should at least maintain their current body weight. Even a modest weight reduction improves insulin sensitivity and the blood lipid profile and prevents or delays the onset of diabetes in high-risk individuals.[39,59] Epidemiologic evidence also indicates that excess body weight carries an independent and powerful risk for congestive heart failure.[93] In terms of cancer risk,

maintaining a BMI below 25 could prevent one of every six cancer deaths in the United States, or about 90,000 deaths each year.[23] This study, by far the largest of its kind, concluded that excess weight probably accounts for 14% of cancer deaths in men and 20% in women (FIG. 13.4).

Physical fitness interacts with obesity to lower disease risk. For example, overweight but physically fit men of all ages suffered fewer deaths by all causes than unfit but normal weight or lean men.[104,105] *Such findings support emphasizing regular physical activity to improve cardiovascular fitness of overweight men and women rather than relying solely on diet to improve health risk profile.*

Despite the current obesity epidemic that affects some 1 billion persons worldwide, weight control remains low on the list of national public health priorities; it receives far less funding from the National Institutes of Health (NIH) than other prevalent diseases.[63,74] FIGURE 13.5 illustrates that the economic cost of obesity-related medical problems in the United States equaled $56.3 billion in 1986—about 7.8% of the $715 billion cost of total illness. By 1994, obesity-related health-care costs rose to nearly $69 billion or almost 10% of the more than $1 trillion dollar cost of remaining ill! Five years later, the total health cost attributable to obesity rose to $99.2 billion dollars. Use of health care resources also increases proportionately with excess body fat.[140] Clearly, maintaining a lean body composition throughout life reduces risk for multiple diseases and the associated financial costs.

Other Than Health Risks: An Economic Burden for Mature Women

The economic cost to women of excess body weight is disproportionately high and continues to increase as a

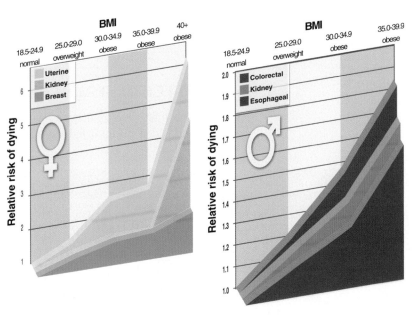

■ **Figure 13.4.** Extra weight and the risk of cancer in women and men. (From Calle EE, et al. Overweight, obesity, and mortality from cancer in a prospectively studied cohort of U.S. adults. N Engl J Med 2003;348:1625.)

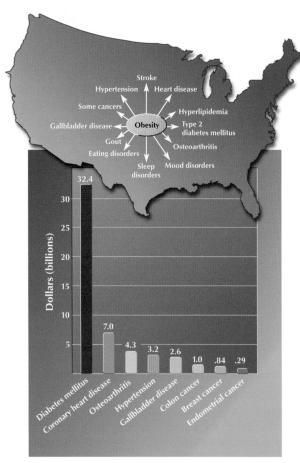

Figure 13.5. Economic cost of major obesity-related illnesses in the United States. (Modified from data in Wolf AM, Colditz GA. Current estimates of the economic costs of obesity. Obes Res 1998;6:97).

person ages. Researchers at the Institute for Social Research at the University of Michigan (University of Michigan Health & Retirement Study, Ann Arbor Michigan) studied the wealth consequences for obese and nonobese women and men between 1992 and 1998. In 1992, the net worth of a moderate to severely obese woman averaged about 40% less than that of a normal-weight female counterpart, even after controlling for health, marital status, and other demographic factors. By 1998, an obese woman reported a net worth about 60% less ($135,670 less) than a nonobese peer. No significant effect of excess body weight emerged in comparisons for men. Speculation maintains that the cultural norms of attractiveness, which stigmatize obese people in diverse ways, affect women to a greater extent than men.

COMPOSITION OF THE HUMAN BODY

One approach to body composition assessment views the human body with three major structural components— muscle, fat, and bone. Marked sex differences in the relative

amounts of these parameters make a convenient basis to compare men and women, using the concept of reference standards developed by Dr. Behnke (FIG. 13.6). The standards use the average physical dimensions from thousands of individuals measured in large-scale civilian and military anthropometric surveys to create a theoretical **reference man** and **reference woman.**[9]

Figure 13.6. Behnke's theoretical model for the reference man and reference woman. Values in parenthesis represent the specific value expressed as a percentage of total body mass.

Reference Man and Reference Woman

The reference man is taller and heavier, his skeleton weighs more, and he has a larger muscle mass and lower total fat content than the reference woman. Differences exist even when expressing the amount of fat, muscle, and bone as a percentage of body mass. This holds particularly true for body fat, which represents 15% of total body mass for the reference man and 27% for his female counterpart. The concept of reference standards does not mean that men and women should strive to achieve this body composition or that the reference man and reference woman are, in fact, "average," "normal," or "healthy." Instead, the model provides a useful frame of reference for statistical comparisons and interpretations of data from other studies of diverse groups of athletes, individuals involved in physical training programs, and the underweight and obese.

Essential and Storage Fat

In the reference model, total body fat exists in two storage sites or depots.

Essential Fat

The first depot, termed **essential fat**, consists of the fat stored in the marrow of bones, heart, lungs, liver, spleen, kidneys, intestines, muscles, and lipid-rich tissues of the central nervous system. *Normal physiologic functioning requires this fat.* In the female, essential fat includes additional **sex-specific essential fat**. Whether this fat provides reserve storage for metabolic fuel remains unclear. More than likely, sex-specific essential fat serves biologically important childbearing and other hormone-related functions. Figure 13.7 partitions the distribution of body fat for the reference woman. As part of the 5 to 9% sex-specific fat reserves, breast fat probably contributes no more than 4% of body mass for women whose body fat content varies from 14 to 35% of body mass.[91] This means that sites other than the breasts (perhaps the lower body region that includes the pelvis, hips, and thighs) furnish a large proportion of sex-specific essential fat. Essential body fat apparently represents a biologically established range limit below which encroachment impairs health status.

Storage Fat

The other major fat depot, **storage fat**, consists of fat accumulation in adipose tissue. This nutritional energy reserve contains about 83% pure fat in addition to 2% protein and 15% water within its supporting structures. Storage fat includes the **visceral fatty tissues** that protect the various internal organs within the thoracic and abdominal cavities and the larger **subcutaneous fat tissue** volume deposited beneath the skin's surface. The reference man and reference woman have similar percentages of storage fat—approximately 12% of body mass in males and 15% in females.

Fat-Free Body Mass and Lean Body Mass (Men)

The terms *fat-free body mass* and *lean body mass* refer to specific entities: **lean body mass (LBM)** contains the small percentage of essential fat stores equivalent to approximately 3% of body mass. In contrast, **fat-free body mass (FFM)** represents the body mass devoid of *all* extractable fat. Behnke points out that FFM refers to an in vitro entity appropriate to carcass analysis. In contrast, the LBM represents an in vivo entity that remains relatively constant in its content of water, organic matter, and minerals throughout the adult's life span. *In normally hydrated, healthy adults, FFM and LBM differ only in the "essential" lipid-rich stores in bone marrow, brain, spinal cord, and internal organs.* Thus, LBM calculations include the small quantity of essential fat, whereas FFM computations exclude "total" body fat (FFM = Body mass − Fat mass).

FIGURE 13.6 showed that LBM in men and the **minimal body mass** in women consist chiefly of essential fat (plus sex-specific fat for females), muscle, water, and bone. Whole-body density of the reference man with 12% storage fat and 3% essential fat equals 1.070 g·cm^{-3}, and the density of his FFM equals 1.094 g·cm^{-3}. If the reference man's total body fat percentage equals 15.0% (storage plus essential fat), the density of a hypothetical "fat-free" body attains the upper limit of 1.100 g·cm^{-3}.

Upper Limit for Fat-Free Body Mass

Considerable variation exists in the FFM of different athletes, with values ranging from a low of 48.1 kg in

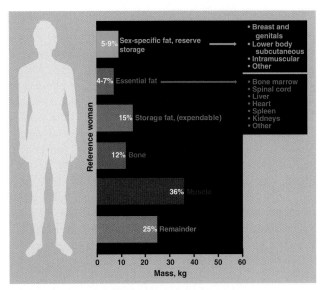

Figure 13.7. Theoretical model for body fat distribution for a reference woman whose body mass equals 56.7 kg (stature = 163.8 cm) and body fat equals 23.6%. (From Katch VL, et al. Contribution of breast volume and weight to body fat distribution in females. Am J Phys Anthropol 1980;53:93.)

some jockeys to over 100 kg in football offensive lineman and shot-putters. FFM for Japanese elite sumo wrestlers (Seki-tori) averages 109 kg. These athletes share with some American professional football players who weigh 159 kg (350 lb) the distinction of the world's largest sports participants. It seems unlikely that athletes in this weight range possess less than 15% body fat; thus, their FFM at 15% body fat corresponds to 135 kg. In reality, however, a football player with a body mass of 159 kg more likely possesses 20 to 25% body fat. At 20% body fat, FFM equals 127 kg, certainly the highest value ever attained using hydrostatic weighing to evaluate body composition. But this value remains hypothetical in the absence of reliable data. Even for an exceptionally large professional basketball player (body mass of 138.3 kg [305 lb] and stature of 210.8 cm [83 in]), percentage body fat probably does not fall below 10%, or a fat weight of 13.8 kg and FFM of 114.2 kg. This FFM seems a more likely scenario for an upper limit value for an athlete of such body dimensions.

To gain additional insight into the question of an upper limit in FFM among athletes, we reviewed over 25 years of body composition data from our laboratories to determine the largest values for FFM determined by hydrostatic weighing. Thirty-five athletes exceeded an FFM of 100 kg, the top five values being 114.3, 109.7, 108.4, 107.6, and 105.6. The three top values were larger than the two values of 106.5 kg reported for defensive football lineman from 1969–1971 data[9] and for other resistance-trained athletes.[43]

Until more data become available on the body composition of extremely large and relatively lean athletes, the FFM of 121.3 kg (267 lb) reported for one sumo wrestler remains the largest ever reported.[98] In the absence of additional data, this value represents the upper limit of FFM in athletes. Recent estimates place the upper-limit for FFM for athletic women at 80 kg (176 lb).[1]

Minimal Standards for Leanness

A biologic lower limit seems to exist beyond which a person's body mass cannot decrease without impairing health status or altering normal physiologic functions.

Men

To calculate the lower fat limit in men (the LBM), subtract storage fat from body mass. For the reference man, LBM (61.7 kg) includes approximately 3% (2.1 kg) essential body fat. Encroachment into this reserve may impair normal physiologic function and capacity for vigorous exercise.

Low body fat values exist for world-class male endurance athletes and some conscientious objectors to military service who voluntarily reduce body fat stores with prolonged semistarvation.[94] The low fat levels of marathon runners, ranging from 1 to 8% of body mass, likely reflect the combined effect of self-selection of these individuals into the sport and adaptations to the severe training for distance running. A low body fat level reduces the energy cost of weight-bearing exercise; it also provides a more effective gradient to dissipate metabolic heat generated during intense physical activity.

TABLE 13.2 presents data on the physique status and body composition of selected professional athletes classified as "underfat" and "overweight." Striking differences occur between these groups in body size, percentage body fat, FFM, lean-to-fat ratio, and various girth measures. The defensive and offensive backs in football are "underfat" compared with the reference man (or any other nonathletic standard), whereas the linemen and shot putters are clearly "overweight" for their stature. Body mass in relation to stature (mass per unit size) for these athletic men represents the 90th percentile for nonathletic males.

Women

In contrast to the lower limit of body mass for the reference man, which includes about 3% essential fat, the lower limit for the reference woman includes about 12% essential fat. This theoretical lower limit, termed **minimal body mass**, equals 48.5 kg for the reference woman. Generally, body fat percentages for the leanest women in the population do not fall below 10 to 12% of body mass. This value probably represents the lower limit of fatness for most women in good health. *Behnke's theoretical concept of minimal body mass in women, which incorporates about 12% essential fat, corresponds to the lean body mass in men that includes 3% essential fat.*

Underweight and Thin. The terms *underweight* and *thin* at times describe different physical conditions. Measurements in our laboratories have focused on the structural characteristics of apparently "thin" females.[90] Subjects were initially screened subjectively as appearing thin or "skinny." Each of the 26 women then underwent a thorough anthropometric evaluation that included measurement of skinfolds, circumferences, bone diameters, and percentage body fat and FFM from hydrostatic weighing.

Unexpectedly, the women's body fat averaged 18.2%, only about 7 percentage points below the average value of 25 to 27% typical for young adult women. Another striking finding included equivalence in four trunk and four extremity bone-diameter measurements in comparisons among the 26 thin-appearing women, 174 women who averaged 25.6% fat, and 31 women who averaged 31.4% body fat. *Thus appearing thin or skinny did not necessarily correspond to a diminutive frame size or an excessively low percentage body fat.*

Table 13.2 **PHYSIQUE AND BODY COMPOSITION OF "UNDERFAT" PROFESSIONAL FOOTBALL PLAYERS AND "OVER-WEIGHT" OFFENSIVE AND DEFENSIVE PROFESSIONAL FOOTBALL LINEMEN AND SHOT PUTTERS**

Variable	Four Defensive Backs (All-Pro)				Offensive Back, All-Pro (N = 1)	Defensive Linemen, Dallas 1977 (N = 510)	Linemen, Dallas 1977 (N = 5)	Shot-Putters, Olympics (N = 13)
	1	2	3	4				
Age, y	27.1	30.2	29.4	24.0	32	31	29	24
Stature, cm	184.7	181.9	187.2	181.5	184.7	193.8	197.6	187.0
Mass, kg	87.9	87.1	88.4	88.9	90.6	116.0	116.5	112.3
Relative fat, %	3.9	3.8	3.8	2.5	1.4	18.6	13.2	14.8
Absolute fat, kg	3.4	3.3	3.4	2.2	1.3	21.6	15.4	16.6
Fat-free body mass, kg	84.5	83.8	85.0	86.7	89.3	94.4	101.1	95.7
Lean/fat ratio	24.85	25.39	25.00	39.41	68.69	4.37	6.57	5.77
Girths, cm								
Shoulders	122.1	119.0	120.5	117.2	121.8	129.5	122.5	133.3
Chest	101.6	101.0	99.5	107.5	102.0	116.5	109.9	118.5
Abdomen, avg	81.8	85.5	81.0	82.6	81.7	102.0	97.0	100.3
Buttocks	98.0	99.0	101.9	102.0	96.5	112.8	111.5	112.3
Thigh	61.0	61.0	58.5	64.0	63.2	66.2	69.3	69.4
Knee	39.5	41.3	41.1	38.0	41.0	44.8	45.8	42.9
Calf	37.6	38.8	38.8	37.8	41.3	43.5	42.4	43.6
Ankle	21.8	23.1	23.5	22.4	22.7	25.8	25.7	24.7
Forearm	31.8	29.1	31.1	31.8	33.5	33.5	34.8	33.7
Biceps	38.0	35.8	37.1	37.7	40.4	41.5	41.7	42.2
Wrist	18.5	17.2	17.4	17.5	18.0	19.3	19.3	18.9

From Katch FI, Katch VL. The body composition profile: techniques of measurement and applications. Clin Sports Med 1984;3:30,

LEANNESS, EXERCISE, AND MENSTRUAL IRREGULARITY: AN INORDINATE FOCUS ON BODY WEIGHT

In 1967, professional models weighed only 8% less than the average American woman; today, their weight averages 23% lower. As we discuss in Chapter 15, eating disorders and unrealistic weight goals have become common among females of all ages, particularly among athletes for whom the "norm" fosters excessive leanness as a prerequisite for success.

Physically active women, particularly participants in the "low-weight" or "appearance" sports such as distance running, body building, figure skating, diving, ballet, and gymnastics increase their chances of delayed onset of menstruation (after age 16 years), an irregular menstrual cycle (oligomenorrhea), or complete cessation of menses (amenorrhea).[30,187] Amenorrhea occurs in 2 to 5% of women of reproductive age in the general population, but reaches 10 to 15% among athletes, and as high as 40% in some athletic groups. As a group, ballet dancers remain exceptionally lean with greater incidence of menstrual dysfunction, eating disorders, and a higher mean age at menarche than age-matched, nondance females.[55,190] One-third to one-half of female athletes in endurance-type sports experience some menstrual irregularity. In premenopausal women, menstrual irregularity or absence of menstrual function increases risk of bone loss and musculoskeletal injury in vigorous exercise.[7,60]

A high level of chronic physical stress may disrupt the hypothalamic–pituitary–adrenal axis to modify the output of gonadotropin-releasing hormone to alter menstrual function **(exercise stress hypothesis)**. A concurrent and more widely accepted hypothesis maintains that the body "senses" high physical stress and inadequate energy reserves to sustain a pregnancy; in such cases, ovulation ceases **(energy availability** or **energy drain hypothesis)**. Some researchers argue that at least 17% body fat represents a "critical level" for onset of menstruation, and 22% fat is the level required to maintain a normal cycle.[55,56] They reason that body fat

below these levels triggers hormonal and metabolic disturbances that affect the menses. Research with animals has identified leptin, a hormone intimately linked to both body fat levels and appetite control (see Chapter 14), as a principal chemical signal that initiates puberty.[28,170] A linkage may thus exist between the onset of sexual maturity (and perhaps continued optimal sexual function) and the level of stored energy as reflected by accumulated body fat.

Leanness Not the Only Factor

Undoubtedly, the lean-to-fat ratio plays a key role in normal menstrual function, perhaps through peripheral fat's role that converts androgens to estrogens or through leptin production in adipose tissue. *Many physically active females fall below the supposed critical level of 17% body fat, but have normal menstrual cycles and maintain a high level of physiologic and performance capacity.* Conversely, some amenorrheic athletes have average body fat levels. We evaluated menstrual cycle regularity for 30 athletes and 30 nonathletes, all with less than 20% body fat.[88] Four of the athletes and three nonathletes ranging from 11 to 15% body fat maintained regular cycles, whereas seven athletes and two nonathletes had irregular cycles or were amenorrheic. For the total sample, 14 athletes and 21 nonathletes had regular menstrual cycles. These data indicate that normal menstrual function does not *require* a critical body fat level of 17 to 22%.

Potential causes of menstrual dysfunction include the complex interplay of physical, nutritional, genetic, hormonal, fat distribution, psychosocial, and environmental factors.[72,112,204] For physically active women, an intense exercise bout triggers the release of an array of hormones, some with antireproductive properties. For example, the release of cortisol and other stress-related hormones with intense and/or prolonged exercise suggests that stimulation of the hypothalamic–pituitary–adrenal axis affects normal ovarian function.[33,114] It remains unclear whether regular intense exercise produces cumulative hormonal effects sufficient to disrupt the normal menses. In this regard, when injuries in young amenorrheic ballet dancers prevent them from exercising regularly, normal menstruation resumes, even though body weight remains low.[190] *Primary predisposing factors for reproductive endocrine dysfunction that affect physically active women include nutritional inadequacy and/or an exercise-induced energy deficit with heavy training.*[19,30,113,150] *Proper nutrition that emphasizes the maintenance of energy balance can prevent or reverse athletic amenorrhea without requiring the athlete to reduce exercise training volume or intensity.* Proponents of this "energy deficit" explanation maintain that that exercise per se exerts no deleterious effect on the reproductive system other than the potential impact of its energy cost on creating a negative energy balance.[112,197] *In all likelihood, 13 to 17% body fat represents the minimal fat level for regular menstrual function.* The effects and risks of sus-

tained amenorrhea on the reproductive system remain unknown. A gynecologist/endocrinologist should evaluate failure to menstruate or cessation of the normal cycle because it may reflect pituitary or thyroid gland malfunction or premature menopause.[6,111,157] As we point out in Chapter 2, prolonged menstrual dysfunction profoundly diminishes the density of the bone mass, which is not regained if and when menstruation resumes.

COMMON LABORATORY METHODS TO ASSESS BODY COMPOSITION

Two general approaches determine the fat and fat-free components of the human body:

1. Direct measurement by chemical analysis of the animal carcass or human cadaver.
2. Indirect estimation by hydrostatic weighing, simple anthropometric measurements, or other procedures.

Direct Assessment

One direct technique of body composition assessment literally dissolves the body in a chemical solution to determine the fat and fat-free components of the mixture. The other technique involves the physical dissection of fat, fat-free adipose tissue, muscle, and bone. Considerable research exists on the direct chemical assessment of body composition in various animal species but few studies have directly determined human fat content.[52,123] These analyses are time consuming and tedious, require specialized laboratory equipment, and involve ethical questions and legal problems in obtaining cadavers for research purposes.

Direct assessment of body composition indicates that while considerable variation exists in total body fatness, the compositions of skeletal mass and the lean and fat tissues remain relatively stable. The assumed constancy of these tissues enables researchers to develop mathematical equations to predict the body's fat percentage.

Indirect Assessment

Diverse indirect procedures commonly assess body composition. One involves **Archimedes' principle** applied to **hydrostatic weighing** (also referred to as *densitometry,* or *underwater weighing*). This method computes percentage body fat from whole-body density (the ratio of body mass to body volume). Other popular procedures to predict body fat use skinfold thickness and girth measurements, x-ray, total body electrical conductivity or impedance, near-infrared interactance, ultrasound, computed tomography, dual-energy x-ray absorptiometry, air plethysmography, and magnetic resonance imaging.

CASE STUDY/PERSONAL HEALTH AND EXERCISE NUTRITION 13-1

How to Predict Percentage Body Fat from Body Mass Index

Body weight adjusted for height squared, referred to as body mass index (BMI; in $kg \cdot m^{-2}$), in excess of 25 and 30 indicates overweight and obesity, respectively. A lower healthy BMI limit of 18.5 has also been recognized. The assumption underlying BMI guidelines lies in its supposed close association with body fatness and consequent morbidity and mortality. Several formulae predict percentage body fat (%BF) from BMI, which may provide a better indication of morbidity and mortality than BMI alone.

MEASUREMENT VARIABLES

The following variables predict %BF from BMI:
- 1.00 ÷ BMI
- Age in years
- Sex: male, female
- Race: white, African American, Asian

EQUATION

Predict percentage body fat (%BF) with the following equation:

%BF = 63.7 − 864 × (1.00 ÷ BMI) − 12.1 × sex + 0.12 × age + 129 × Asian × (1 ÷ BMI) − 0.091 × Asian × age − 0.030 × African-American × age

where sex = 1 for male and 0 for female; Asian = 1 for Asians and 0 for other races; African American = 1 for African Americans and 0 for other races; age in years; BMI = body weight in kg ÷ stature in m^2

EXAMPLES

Example 1. African American male; age 30 years; BMI = 25

%BF = 63.7 − (864 × (1÷BMI)) − (12.1 × sex) + (0.12 × age) + (129 × Asian × (1 ÷ BMI)) − (0.091 × Asian × age) − (0.030 × African American × age)
= 63.7 − (864 × 0.04) − (12.1 × 1) + (0.12 × 30) + (129 × 0 × 0.04) − (0.091 × 0 × 30) − (0.030 × 1 × 30)
= 63.7 − (34.56) − (12.1) + (3.6) + (0) − (0) − (0.9)
= 19.7%

Example 2. Asian female; age 50 years; BMI = 30

%BF = 63.7 − (864 × (1 ÷ BMI)) − (12.1 × sex) + (0.12 × age) + (129 × Asian × (1÷ BMI)) − (0.091 × Asian × age) − (0.030 × African American × age)
= 63.7 − (864 × 0.0333) − (12.1 × 0) + (0.12 × 50) + (129 × 1 × 0.0333) − (0.091 × 1 × 50) − (0.030 × 0 × 50)
= 63.7 − (28.80) − (0) + (6.0) + (4.295) − (4.55) − (0)
= 40.7%

Example 3. Asian male; age 70 years; BMI = 28

%BF = 63.7 − (864 × (1 ÷ BMI)) − (12.1 × sex) + (0.12 × age) + (129 × Asian × (1 ÷ BMI)) − (0.091 × Asian × age) − (0.030 × African-American × age)
= 63.7 − (864 × 0.03571) − (12.1 × 1) + (0.12 × 70) + (129 × 1 × 0.03571) − (0.091 × 1 × 70) − (0.030 × 0 × 70)
= 63.7 − (30.853) − (12.1) + (8.4) + (4.61) − (6.37) − (0)
= 25.4%

Example #4 White Male; Age = 55 years; BMI = 24.5

%BF = 63.7 − (864 × (1 ÷ BMI)) − (12.1 × sex) + (0.12 × age) + (129 × Asian × (1÷ BMI)) − (0.091 × Asian × age) − (0.030 × African American × age)
= 63.7 − (864 × 0.0408) − (12.1 × 1) + (0.12 × 55) + (129 × 0 × 0.0408) − (0.091 × 0 × 55) − (0.030 × 0 × 55)
= 63.7 − (35.25) − (12.1) + (6.6) + (0) − (0) − (0)
= 22.9%

ACCURACY

The correlation coefficient between predicted %BF (using the above formulae) and measured %BF (using a four-compartment model to estimate body fat) is r = 0.89, with a standard error for estimating an individual's %BF equal to ±3.9% body fat units. This compares favorably with other body fat prediction methods that use skinfolds and girths.

PREDICTED PERCENTAGE FAT AT GIVEN CRITICAL BMI VALUES

Table 1 presents predicted %BF values for different threshold BMI values for men and women of different ethnicity. These data provide an approach for developing healthy percentage body fat ranges from guidelines based on the BMI.

Table 1   **PREDICTED PERCENTAGE BODY FAT BY SEX AND ETHNICITY RELATED TO BMI HEALTHY WEIGHT GUIDELINES**

	Females			Males		
Age and BMI	*African Americans*	*Asians*	*White*	*African Americans*	*Asians*	*White*
20–39 y						
BMI <18.5	20%	25%	21%	8%	13%	8%
BMI ≥25	32%	35%	33%	20%	23%	21%
BMI ≥30	38%	40%	39%	26%	28%	26%
40–59 y						
BMI <18.5	21%	25%	23%	23%	13%	11%
BMI ≥25	34%	36%	35%	35%	24%	23%
BMI ≥30	39%	41%	42%	41%	29%	29%
60–79 y						
BMI <18.5	23%	26%	25%	11%	14%	13%
BMI ≥25	35%	36%	38%	23%	24%	25%
BMI ≥30	41%	41%	43%	29%	29%	31%

From Gallagher D, Heymsfield SB, et. al. Healthy percentage body fat ranges: an approach for developing guidelines based on body mass index. Am J Clin Nutr 2000;72:694–701.

HYDROSTATIC WEIGHING (ARCHIMEDES' PRINCIPLE)

The Greek mathematician and inventor Archimedes (287–212 BC) discovered a fundamental principle currently applied to evaluate human body composition. An itinerant scholar of that time described the interesting circumstances surrounding the event:

> King Hieron of Syracuse suspected that his pure gold crown had been altered by substitution of silver for gold. The King directed Archimedes to devise a method for testing the crown for its gold content without dismantling it. Archimedes pondered over this problem for many weeks without succeeding, until one day, he stepped into a bath filled to the top with water and observed the overflow. He thought about this for a moment, and then, wild with joy, jumped from the bath and ran naked through the streets of Syracuse shouting eureka, eureka, I have discovered a way to solve the mystery of the King's crown.

Archimedes reasoned that a substance such as gold must have a volume in proportion to its mass, and the way to measure the volume of an irregularly shaped object required submersion in water with collection of the overflow. Archimedes took lumps of gold and silver, each having the same mass as the crown, and submerged each in a container full of water. To his delight, he discovered the crown displaced more water than the lump of gold and less than the lump of silver. This could only mean the crown consisted of *both* silver and gold as the King suspected.

Essentially, Archimedes evaluated the specific gravity of the crown (ratio of the crown's mass to the mass of an equal volume of water) compared to the specific gravities of gold and silver. Archimedes probably also reasoned that an object submerged or floating in water becomes buoyed up by a counterforce equaling the weight of the volume of water it displaces. This buoyant force helps to support an immersed object against the downward pull of gravity. Thus, an object is said to lose weight in water. Because the object's loss of weight in water equals the weight of the volume of water it displaces, specific gravity refers to the ratio of the weight of an object in air divided by its loss of weight in water. The loss of weight in water equals the weight in air minus the weight in water.

> **Specific gravity = Weight in air ÷ Loss of weight in water**

In practical terms, suppose a crown weighed 2.27 kg in air and 0.13 kg less (2.14 kg) when weighed underwater (FIG. 13.8). Dividing the weight of the crown (2.27 kg) by its loss of weight in water (0.13 kg) results in a specific gravity

of 17.5. This ratio differs considerably from the specific gravity of gold, with a value of 19.3, so we too can conclude: "Eureka, the crown is a fraud!" The physical principle Archimedes discovered allows us to apply water submersion or hydrodensitometry to determine the body's volume. Dividing a person's body mass by body volume yields body density (Density = Mass ÷ Volume), and from this an estimate of percentage body fat.

Computing Body Density

For illustrative purposes, suppose a 50-kg person weighs 2 kg when submerged in water. According to Archimedes' principle, loss of weight in water of 48 kg equals the weight of the displaced water. The volume of water displaced can easily be computed because we know the density of water at any temperature. In the example, 48 kg of water equals 48 L, or 48,000 cm³ (1 g of water = 1 cm³ by volume at 39.2°F). Measuring the person at the cold-water temperature of 39.2°F requires no density correction for water. In practice,

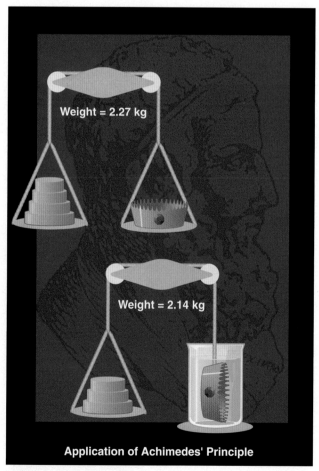

Application of Achimedes' Principle

■ **Figure 13.8.** Archimedes' principle of buoyant force to determine the volume and subsequently the specific gravity of the king's crown.

researchers use warmer water and apply the appropriate density value for water at the particular temperature. The density of this person, computed as mass ÷ volume, equals 50,000 g (50 kg) ÷ 48,000 cm^3, or 1.0417 g·cm^{-3}. The next step estimates percentage of body fat and the mass of fat and fat-free tissues.

Computing Percentage Body Fat and Mass of Fat and Fat-Free Tissues

An equation that incorporates whole-body density can estimate the body's fat percentage. This equation, derived from the premise that the densities of fat mass (all extractable lipid from adipose and other body tissues) and FFM (remaining lipid-free tissues and chemicals, including water) remain relatively constant (fat tissue, 0.90 g·cm^{-3}; fat-free tissue, 1.10 g·cm^{-3}). These consistencies remain even with large variations in total body fat and the fat-free tissue components of bone and muscle. The assumed densities for the components of the FFM at body temperature of 37°C (98.6°F) are water, 0.9937 g·cm^{-3} (73.8% of FFM); minerals, 3.038 g·cm^{-3} (6.8% of FFM); protein, 1.340 g·cm^{-3} (19.4% of FFM). The following equation, derived by Berkeley scientist Dr. William Siri, computes percentage body fat by incorporating the measured value of whole-body density:

Siri Equation
Percentage body fat = 495 ÷ Body density − 450

To estimate percentage body fat, substitute the body density value of 1.0417 g·cm^{-3} for the subject in the previous example in the Siri equation as follows:

Percentage body fat = 495 ÷ 1.0417 − 450
= 25.2

Compute mass of body fat by multiplying body mass by percentage fat:

Fat mass (kg) = Body mass (kg) × [Percentage fat ÷ 100]
= 50 kg × 0.252
= 12.6

Compute FFM by subtracting the mass of fat from body mass:

FFM (kg) = Body mass (kg) − Fat mass (kg)
= 50 kg − 12.6 kg
= 37.4

In this example, 25.2%, or 12.6 kg, of the 50 kg body mass consists of fat, with the remaining 37.4 kg representing the FFM.

Possible Limitations of the Method

The generalized density values for fat-free (1.10 g·cm^{-3}) and fat (0.90 g·cm^{-3}) tissues represent averages for young and middle-aged adults. These assumed "constants" vary among individuals and groups, particularly the density and chemical composition of the FFM. Such variation limits accuracy of predicting percentage body fat from whole-body density. More specifically, a significantly larger average density of the FFM exists for blacks (1.113 g·cm^{-3}) and Hispanics (1.105 g·cm^{-3}) than whites (1.100 g·cm^{-3}).[61,134,149,163,172] Consequently, using the existing equations formulated on assumptions for whites to calculate body composition from whole-body density of blacks or Hispanics *overestimates* the FFM and *underestimates* percentage body fat.[35,41] The following modifications of the Siri equation computes percentage body fat from body density measures for blacks.[186]

Modification of Siri equation for blacks:

Percentage body fat = [(4.858) ÷ Body density) − 4.394] × 100

Applying constant density values for the fat and fat-free tissues to growing children or aging adults also introduces errors in predicting body composition.[109] For example, the water and mineral contents of the FFM continually change during the growth period and the well-documented demineralization of osteoporosis with aging. Reduced bone density reduces the density of the fat-free tissue of young children and the elderly below the assumed constant of 1.10 g·cm^{-3}, thus *overestimating* percentage body fat. For boys and girls, researchers have modified equations to predict body fat from whole-body density to adjust for density changes in FFM during childhood and adolescence (TABLE 13.3). Alterations in the density of the fat-free component may also occur in highly trained amateur and professional football players and champion distance runners and bodybuilders and affect estimation of percentage body fat from whole-body density (see below).

Adjust for Persons with Large Musculoskeletal Development. Chronic resistance training changes the density of the FFM, thus altering body fat estimation from whole-body density determinations.[126] White male weightlifters with considerable muscular development and nontrained controls were measured for body density, total body water, and bone mineral content. Comparisons included estimations of percentage body fat using the two- compartment model (assumed densities for the fat and fat-free compartments applied in the Siri equation) and a four-compartment model using the body's fat, water, mineral, and protein content and their associated densities. Percentage body fat estimated from body density (Siri equation) produced significantly higher values than percentage body fat estimated from the four-compartment model in weight trainers, but not in the untrained controls. A *lower* FFM density in weight trainers

Table 13.3	**PERCENTAGE (%) BODY FAT ESTIMATED FROM BODY DENSITY (BD) USING AGE- AND SEX-SPECIFIC CONVERSION CONSTANTS THAT ATTEMPT TO ACCOUNT FOR CHANGES IN THE DENSITY OF THE FAT-FREE BODY MASS AS THE CHILD MATURES**	
Age, years	*Boys*	*Girls*
7–9	% Fat = (5.38/BD − 4.97) × 100	% Fat = (5.43/BD − 5.03) × 100
9–11	% Fat = (5.30/BD − 4.89) × 100	% Fat = (5.35/BD − 4.95) × 100
11–13	% Fat = (5.23/BD − 4.81) × 100	% Fat = (5.25/BD − 4.84) × 100
13–15	% Fat = (5.08/BD − 4.64) × 100	% Fat = (5.12/BD − 4.69) × 100
15–17	% Fat = (5.03/BD − 4.59) × 100	% Fat = (5.07/BD − 4.64) × 100

From Lohman T. Applicability of body composition techniques and constants for children and youth. Exerc Sports Sci Rev 1986;14:325.

than controls (1.089 vs. 1.099 $g \cdot cm^{-3}$) with the four-compartment model explained this discrepancy: it resulted from larger water and smaller mineral and protein fractions of the FFM in the resistance-trained men. For them, incorrect assumptions about density of the FFM underlying the Siri equation *overestimated* percentage body fat.

Regular weight lifting increases muscularity disproportionately to changes in bone mass. A lower FFM density occurred because the density of their fat-free muscle (1.066 $g \cdot cm^{-3}$ at 37°C) was less than the 1.1 $g \cdot cm^{-3}$ assumed in the Siri equation. Disproportionate increases in muscle mass relative to increases in bone mass reduce density of the FFM below 1.1 $g \cdot cm^{-3}$, thus *overpredicting* percentage body fat by the Siri equation.

Based on the revised densities of the FFM (1.089 $g \cdot cm^{-3}$) and fat mass (0.9007 $g \cdot cm^{-3}$), the researchers recommend modifying Siri's equation as follows for more accurate appraisal with resistance-trained white males.

Modification for Resistance-Trained White Males:

Percentage body fat = 521 ÷ Body density − 478

Measuring Body Volume by Hydrostatic Weighing

Hydrostatic weighing illustrates the most common application of Archimedes' principle to determine body volume. Body volume computes as the difference between body mass measured in air (M_a) and body weight measured during water submersion (W_w); *weight* is the correct term, since the body's mass remains unchanged under water. *Body volume equals loss of weight in water with the appropriate temperature correction for water density.*

FIGURE 13.9 illustrates the procedure for measuring body volume by hydrostatic weighing. The first step accurately assesses the subject's body mass in air, usually to the nearest ± 50 g. A diver's belt secured around the waist prevents the subject from floating toward the surface during submersion. Seated with the head out of the water, the subject makes a forced maximal exhalation while lowering the head beneath the water. The breath is held for several seconds as the underwater weight is recorded (minus the underwater weight of the divers belt and chair). The subject repeats the procedure 8 to 12 times to obtain a dependable underwater weight score. Body volume calculation requires subtraction of the buoyant effect of the air remaining in the lungs after a forced exhalation (residual lung volume) measured immediately before, during, or after the underwater weighing. Without accounting for the residual lung volume, the computed whole-body density value would decrease because the lungs' air volume contributes to buoyancy. This would indeed make a person "fatter" when converting body density to percentage body fat.

Examples of Calculations

Data for two professional football players, an offensive guard and a quarterback, illustrate the sequence of steps to compute body density, percentage body fat, mass of fat, and FFM.

	Offensive Guard	*Quarterback*
Body mass	110 kg	85 kg
Underwater weight	3.5 kg	5.0 kg
Residual lung volume	1.2 L	1.0 L
Water temperature correction factor	0.996	0.996

The loss of body weight in water equals body volume, so the body volume of the offensive guard becomes 110 kg − 3.5 kg = 106.5 kg, or 106.5 L; body volume for the quarterback (85 kg − 5.0 kg) equals 80.0 kg, or 80 L. Dividing body volume by the water temperature correction factor of 0.996 increases body volume slightly for both players (106.9 L for the guard and 80.3 L for the quarter-

Figure 13.9. Measuring body volume by underwater weighing. Prone and supine methods for underwater weighing with no difference in results, with residual lung volume measured before, during, or after the underwater weighing. Measurements taken **(A)** prone, **(B)** seated in a swimming pool, **(C)** seated in a therapy pool, and **(D)** upright in a stainless steel tank with Plexiglas front in the laboratory. For any method, subjects can use a snorkel with nose clip if apprehensive about submersion. Final calculation of underwater weight must account for these objects.

back). By subtracting residual lung volume, the body volume of the offensive guard then becomes 105.7 L (106.9 L − 1.2 L) and for the quarterback, 79.3 L (80.3 L − 1.0 L).

Body density computes as mass ÷ volume. Body density for the offensive guard becomes 110 kg ÷ 105.7 L = 1.0407 kg·L^{-1}, or 1.0407 g·cm^{-3}. The corresponding density for the quarterback equals 85.0 kg ÷ 79.3 L or 1.0719 kg·L^{-1}, or 1.0719 g·cm^{-3}.

From the Siri equation, percentage body fat computes as follows:

Offensive guard:

495 ÷ 1.0407− 450 = 25.6%

Quarterback:

495 ÷ 1.0719 − 450 = 11.8%

Total mass of body fat calculates as follows:
Offensive guard:

110 kg × 0.256 = 28.2 kg

Quarterback:

85 kg × 0.118 = 10.0 kg

FFM computes as follows:

Offensive guard:

110 kg − 28.2 kg = 81.8 kg

Quarterback:

85 kg − 10.0 kg = 75.0 kg

Body composition analysis illustrates that the offensive guard possesses more than twice the percentage body fat of the quarterback (25.6 vs. 11.8%) and almost three times as much total fat (28.2 vs. 10.0 kg). On the other hand, the guard's FFM, which largely indicates muscle mass, exceeds that of the quarterback.

SKINFOLD MEASUREMENTS

Simple anthropometric procedures validly predict body fatness. The most common of these procedures measures **skinfolds**. The rationale for using skinfolds to estimate body fat comes from the relationships among three factors: *(a)* fat in the adipose tissue deposits directly beneath the skin (subcutaneous fat), *(b)* internal fat, and *(c)* whole-body density.

The Caliper

By 1930, a special pincer-type caliper accurately measured subcutaneous fat at selected body sites. The caliper works on the same principle as a micrometer that measures distance between two points. Measuring skinfold thickness requires grasping a fold of skin and subcutaneous fat firmly with the thumb and forefingers, pulling it away from the underlying muscle tissue following the natural contour of the skinfold. The pincer jaws exert a constant tension of $10 \text{ g} \cdot \text{mm}^{-2}$ at the point of contact with the double layer of skin plus subcutaneous tissue. The caliper dial indicates skinfold thickness in millimeters, which is recorded within 2 seconds after applying the full force of the caliper. This time limitation avoids excessive skinfold compression when taking the measurement. For research purposes, the investigator should have considerable experience in taking measurements and demonstrate consistency in duplicating values for the same subject made on the same day, consecutive days, or even weeks apart. A good rule of thumb to achieve consistency requires duplicate or triplicate practice measurements on approximately 30 individuals who vary in body fat. This amount of careful attention to details usually ensures high reproducibility of measurement.

The Sites

The most common anatomic locations for skinfold measurements include the triceps, subscapular, suprailiac, abdominal, and upper thigh sites (FIG. 13.10). The tester takes a minimum of two or three measurements at each site on the right side of the body with the subject standing. The average value represents the skinfold score.

- **Triceps:** Vertical fold at the posterior midline of the upper arm, halfway between the tip of the shoulder and tip of the elbow; elbow remains in an extended, relaxed position

- **Subscapular:** Oblique fold, just below the bottom tip of the scapula
- **Suprailiac (iliac crest):** Slightly oblique fold, just above the hipbone (crest of ileum); the fold follows the natural diagonal line
- **Abdominal:** Vertical fold 1 inch to the right of the umbilicus
- **Thigh:** Vertical fold at the midline of the thigh, two thirds of the distance from the middle of the patella (kneecap) to the hip

Other sites include

- **Chest** (on men): Diagonal fold with its long axis directed toward the nipple, on the anterior axillary fold, as high as possible
- **Biceps:** Vertical fold at the posterior midline of the upper arm
- **Midaxillary:** Vertical fold on midaxillary line at the level of the xiphoid process of the sternum

Usefulness of Skinfold Scores

Skinfold measurements provide consistent and meaningful information concerning body fat and its distribution. We recommend two ways to use skinfolds. The first sums the skinfold scores to indicate relative fatness among individuals. This "sum of skinfolds" and individual skinfold values reflect with some accuracy body fat changes "before" and "after" an intervention program. Evaluate these changes on either an absolute or percentage basis.

One can draw the following conclusions from the skinfold data in TABLE 13.4, obtained from a 22-year-old female college student before and after a 16-week exercise program:

- Largest changes in skinfold thickness occurred at the suprailiac and abdominal sites.
- Triceps skinfold showed the largest percentage decrease, and the subscapular skinfold the smallest percentage decrease.
- Total skinfold reduction at the five sites equaled 16.6 mm, or 12.6% below the "before" condition.

A second use of skinfolds incorporates *population-specific* mathematical equations to predict body density or percentage body fat. The equations prove accurate for subjects similar in age, gender, training status, fatness, and race to the group for whom they were derived.[16,76,84,137,179] *When meeting these criteria, predicted percentage body fat for an individual usually ranges between 3 to 5% body fat units of the value computed using hydrostatic weighing.* The first and third skinfold equations in TABLE 13.5 accurately predict percentage body fat in men and women of diverse ages.

We have developed the following equations to predict body fat from triceps and subscapular skinfolds in young women and men:[85–87]

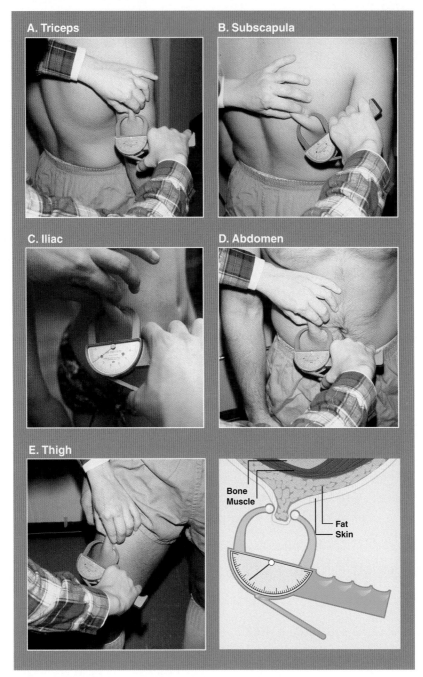

Figure 13.10 Anatomic location of five common skinfold sites: **A.** Triceps. **B.** Subscapular. **C.** Iliac (suprailiac). **D.** Abdomen. and **E.** Thigh. The *lower right* shows a schematic diagram for use of a skinfold caliper. Note the compression of a double layer of skin and underlying tissue during the measurement. Except for subscapular and suprailiac sites measured diagonally, take measurements in the vertical plane.

Table 13.4 **CHANGES IN SELECTED SKINFOLDS FOR A YOUNG WOMAN DURING A 16-WEEK EXERCISE PROGRAM**

Skinfolds	Before (mm)	After (mm)	Absolute Change	Percentage Change
Triceps	22.5	19.4	−3.1	−13.8
Subscapular	19.0	17.0	−2.0	−10.5
Suprailiac	34.5	30.2	−4.3	−12.8
Abdomen	33.7	29.4	−4.3	−12.8
Thigh	21.6	18.7	−2.9	−13.4
Sum	**131.3**	**114.7**	**−16.6**	**−12.6**

Table 13.5 **BODY COMPOSITION PREDICTION EQUATIONS FOR USE WITH ATHLETES**

Method	Sport	Gender	Equation	Ref.
Skinfolds	All	Women (18–29 y)	Db (g/cc)^a = 1.096095 − 0.0006952 (4 SKF) + 0.0000011 (4 SKF)^2 − 0.0000714 (age)	(63)
	All	Boys (14–19 y)	Db (g/cc)^a = 1.10647 − 0.00162 (subscapular SKF) − 0.00144 (abdomen SKF) 0.00077 (triceps SKF) + 0.00071 (midaxillary SKF)	(39)
	All	Men (18–29 y)	Db (g/cc)^a = 1.112 − 0.00043499 (7 SKF) + 0.00000055 (7 SKF) − 0.00028826 (age)	(62)
	Wrestling	Boys (high school)	Db (g/cc)^a = 1.0982 − 0.000815 (3 SKF) − 0.00000084 (3 SKF)^2	(149)
BIA	All	Women (NR)	FFM (kg) = 0.73 (HT^2/R) + 0.23 (X$_c$) + 0.16 (BW) + 2.0	(59)
	All	Women (college)	FFM (kg) = 0.73 (HT^2/R) + 0.116 (BW) + 0.096 (X$_c$) − 4.03	(102)
	All	Men (college)	FFM (kg) = 0.734 (HT^2/R) + 0.116 (BW) + 0.096 (X$_c$) − 3.152	(102)
	All	Men (19–40 y)	FFM (kg) = 1.949 + 0.701 (BW) + 0.186 (HT^2/R)	(117)
	All	Women (18–23 y)	FFM (kg) = 0.757 (BW) + 0.981 (neck C) − 0.516 (thigh C) + 0.79	(107)
Anthropometry (girths)	Ballet	Girls/women (11–25 y)	FFM (kg) = 0.73 (BW) + 3.0	(48)
	Wrestling	Boys (13–18 y)	Db (g/cc)^a = 1.12691 − 0.00357 (arm C) − 0.00127 (AB C) + 0.00524 (forearm C)	(73)
	Football	White men (18–23 y)	%BF = 55.2 + 0.481 (BW) − 0.468 (HT)	(55)

From Heyward VH, Stolarczyk LM. Applied body composition assessment. Champaign, IL: Human Kinetics, 1996.
Abbreviations: 4SKF (mm) = sum of four skinfolds: triceps + anterior suprailiac + abdomen + thigh; 7SKF (mm) = sum of seven skinfolds: chest + midaxillary + triceps + subscapular + abdomen + anterior suprailiac + thigh; HT, height (cm); R, resistance (Ω); Xc, reactance (Ω); BW, body weight (kg); C, circumference (cm); thigh C (cm) at the gluteal fold; AB C (cm), average abdominal circumference = [(AB$_1$ + AB$_2$)/2], where AB$_1$ (cm) = abdominal circumference anteriorly midway between the xiphoid process of the sternum and the umbilicus and laterally between the lower end of the rib cage and iliac crests, and AB$_2$ (cm) = abdominal circumference at the umbilicus level; NR, not reported.
^{a} Use the following formulas to convert body density (Db) to %body fat (BF): men %BF = [(4.95/Db) − 4.50] × 100, women %BF = [(5.01/Db) − 4.57] × 100, boys (7–12 y) %BF = [(5.30/Db) − 4.89] × 100, boys (13–16 y) %BF = [(5.07/Db) − 4.64] × 100, boys (17–19 y) %BF = [(4.99/Db) − 4.55] × 100.

Young women, ages 17 to 26 years:

Percentage body fat = 0.55(A) + 0.31(B) + 6.13

Young men, ages 17 to 26 years:

Percentage body fat = 0.43(A) + 0.58(B) + 1.47

In both equations, A = triceps skinfold (mm) and B = subscapular skinfold (mm).

We computed the "before" and "after" percentage body fat of the woman who participated in the 16-week physical conditioning program (Table 13.4). Body fat equals 24.4% by substituting the pretraining values for triceps (22.5 mm) and subscapular (19.0 mm) skinfolds into the equation.

Percentage body fat = 0.55 (A) + 0.31 (B) + 6.13
= 0.55 (22.5) + 0.31 (19.0)
+ 6.13
= 12.38 + 5.89 + 6.13
= 24.4%

Substituting the posttraining values for triceps (19.4 mm) and subscapular (17.0 mm) skinfolds produced a body fat value of 21.1%.

Percentage body fat = 0.55 (19.4) + 0.31 (17.0)
+ 6.13
= 10.67 + 5.27 + 6.13
= 22.1%

Percentage body fat determined before and after a physical conditioning or weight-loss program provides a useful means to evaluate body composition alterations, often independent of body weight changes.

Skinfolds and Age

In young adults, subcutaneous fat constitutes approximately one half of the body's total fat, with the remainder visceral and organ fat. With advancing age, a proportionately greater quantity of fat deposits internally than subcutaneously. Thus, the same skinfold score reflects *greater* total percentage body fat as one gets older. *For this reason, use age-adjusted* **generalized equations** *to predict body fat from skinfolds or girths in older men and women.*[75,76,175]

For both fatter and leaner white and African American children the following two skinfold equations best predict percentage body fat:[17]

> Percentage body fat = 9.02 + 1.09 (biceps, mm)
>   + 0.42 (calf, mm)

> Percentage body fat = 8.596 + 0.81 (biceps, mm)
>   + 0.40 (triceps, mm)
>   + 0.30 subscapular, mm)

User Beware

The person taking skinfold must develop technical expertise with the proper measurement techniques. Also, with extremely obese people skinfold thickness often exceeds the width of the caliper's jaws. The particular caliper used also contributes to measurement errors.[58] It often becomes difficult to determine which prediction equation to use because of lack of standards to judge the results of different investigators. Thus, a prediction equation developed by one researcher (that shows high validity for the sample measured) may produce large prediction errors when applied to skinfolds from a dissimilar group.

GIRTH MEASUREMENTS

Apply a linen or plastic measuring tape lightly to the skin surface so the tape remains taut but not tight. This avoids skin compression that produces lower than normal scores. Make duplicate measurements at each site and average the scores. FIGURE 13.11 displays common anatomic landmarks for taking girths for anthropometric measurement and to predict body fatness:

- **Abdomen:** 1 inch above the umbilicus
- **Buttocks:** Maximum protrusion with the heels together
- **Right thigh:** Upper thigh, just below the buttocks
- **Right upper arm (biceps):** Palm up, arm straight and extended in front of the body; taken at the midpoint between the shoulder and the elbow
- **Right forearm:** Maximum girth with the arm extended in front of the body
- **Right calf:** Widest girth midway between the ankle and knee

Usefulness of Girth Measurements

The equations and constants presented in Appendix D for young and older men and women predict an individual's body fat within ± 2.5 to 4.0% of the actual value from hydrostatic weighing, provided the person resembles the original validation group. Such relatively small prediction errors make the equations particularly useful to those without access to laboratory facilities. Do not use the equations to predict fatness in individuals who appear excessively thin or fat or who participate regularly in strenuous sports or resistance training. Along with predicting percentage body fat, girths can analyze patterns of body fat distribution, including changes in fat distribution during weight loss.[81] Specific equations based on girths also accurately estimate the body composition of obese adults.[174,192] Not surprisingly, equations that use the more labile sites of fat deposition (e.g., waist and hips instead of upper arm or thigh in females and abdomen in males) provide the greatest accuracy for predicting *changes* in body composition.[54]

Predicting Body Fat From Girths

From the appropriate tables in Appendix D, substitute the corresponding constants A, B, and C in the formula shown at the bottom of each table. This requires one addition and two subtraction steps. The following five-step example shows how to compute percentage body fat, fat mass, and FFM for a 21-year-old man who weighs 79.1 kg:

Step 1. Measure upper arm, abdomen, and right forearm girths with a cloth tape to the nearest tenth of an inch (0.24 cm): upper arm = 11.5 in. (29.2 cm); abdomen = 31.0 in. (78.7 cm); right forearm = 10.7 in. (27.3 cm).

Step 2. Determine the three constants A, B, and C corresponding to the three girths from Appendix D: constant A corresponds to 11.5 in. = 42.56; constant B corresponds to 31.0 in. = 40.68; constant C corresponds to 10.7 in. = 58.37.

Step 3. Compute percentage body fat by substituting the appropriate constants in the formula for young men shown at the bottom of Chart 1 in Appendix D.

> **Percentage fat = Constant A + Constant B**
>   **− Constant C − 10.2**
>   = 42.56 + 40.68 − 58.37 − 10.2
>   = 83.24 − 58.37 − 10.2
>   = 24.87 − 10.2
>   = 14.7%

Step 4. Calculate the mass of body fat as follows:

> **Fat mass = Body mass × (% fat ÷ 100)**
>   = 79.1 kg × (14.7 ÷ 100)
>   = 79.1 kg × 0.147
>   = 11.63 kg

Step 5. Calculate FFM as follows:

> **FFM = Body mass − Fat mass**
>   = 79.1 kg − 11.63 kg
>   = 67.5 kg

CASE STUDY/PERSONAL HEALTH AND EXERCISE NUTRITION 13–2

PREDICTING PERCENTAGE BODY FAT IN HISPANICS

Despite the fact that Hispanics represent the second largest minority population in the United States, little validated research exists on body composition prediction equations for this group. The available research suggests the density of the fat-free body mass of Hispanic women differs from that of their white counterparts, thus requiring a population-specific body density (Db)-to-percentage body fat (%BF) equation.

VARIABLES

The generalized skinfold equations of Jackson and colleagues[75,76] are appropriate for use with Hispanic men and women. The seven skinfold measurements for men and women include the following (refer to Fig. 13.10 and section entitled *The Sites* (page 412) for the specifics of measuring skinfolds at these sites):
1. Abdomen
2. Thigh
3. Triceps
4. Subscapular
5. Suprailiac
6. Midaxillary
7. Chest (women)

EQUATIONS

For both men and women: Db = body density in $g \cdot cm^{-3}$; Σ7SKF comprise chest + abdomen + thigh + triceps + subscapular + suprailiac + midaxillary skinfolds in mm.

Men (ages 18–61 years):

$$Db = 1.112 - [0.00043499 \times \Sigma7SKF] + [0.00000055 \times (\Sigma7SKF)^2] - [0.00028826 \times age]$$

To convert Db to %BF:

$$\%BF = 495 \div Db - 450$$

Women (ages 18–55 years):

$$Db = 1.0970 - [0.00046971 \times \Sigma7SKF] + [0.00000056 \times (\Sigma7SKF)^2] - [0.00012828 \times age]$$

To convert Db to %BF:

$$\%BF = 487 \div Db - 441$$

EXAMPLES

Example 1: Hispanic male, age 24 years
Skinfold data: chest = 15.0 mm; abdomen = 33.0 mm; thigh = 21.0 mm; triceps = 18 mm; subscapular = 19 mm; suprailiac = 30 mm; midaxillary = 12.0 mm

$$
\begin{aligned}
Db &= 1.112 - [0.00043499 \times \Sigma7SKF] + [0.00000055 \times (\Sigma7SKF)^2] - [0.00028826 \times age] \\
&= 1.112 - [0.00043499 \times 148] + [0.00000055 \times 21904] - [0.00028826 \times 24] \\
&= 1.112 - 0.064378 + 0.012047 - 0.0069182 \\
&= 1.0528 \ g \cdot cm^{-3}
\end{aligned}
$$

$$
\begin{aligned}
\%BF &= 495 \div Db - 450 \\
&= 495 \div 1.0528 - 450 \\
&= 20.2
\end{aligned}
$$

Example 2: Hispanic female, age 30 years
Skinfold data: chest = 12.0 mm; abdomen = 30.0 mm; thigh = 18.0 mm; triceps = 20.0 mm; subscapular = 16.0 mm; suprailiac = 30 mm; midaxillary = 15.0 mm

$$
\begin{aligned}
Db &= 1.0970 - [0.00046971 \times \Sigma7SKF] + [0.00000056 \times (\Sigma7SKF)^2] - [0.00012828 \times age] \\
&= 1.0970 - [0.00046971 \times 141 + [0.00000056 \times 19881] - [0.00012828 \times 30] \\
&= 1.0970 - 0.066229 + 0.011133 - 0.003848 \\
&= 1.0381 \ g \cdot cm^{-3}
\end{aligned}
$$

$$
\begin{aligned}
\%BF &= 487 \div Db - 441 \\
&= 487 \div 1.0381 - 441 \\
&= 28.2
\end{aligned}
$$

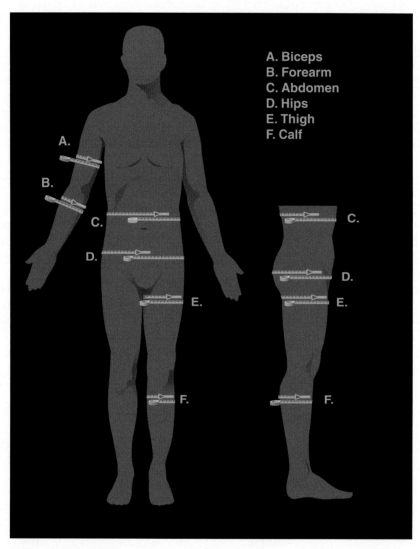

A. Biceps
B. Forearm
C. Abdomen
D. Hips
E. Thigh
F. Calf

Figure 13.11 Landmarks for measuring various girths at six common anatomic sites (see text for description).

REGIONAL FAT DISTRIBUTION: WAIST GIRTH AND WAIST/HIP RATIO

Measures of waist girth and the ratio of waist girth to hip girth provide an important indication of disease risk. However the waist/hip ratio poorly captures the specific effects of each girth measure. Waist and hip circumferences reflect different aspects of body composition and fat distribution. Each has an independent and often opposite effect on cardiovascular disease risk. Waist girth, the so-called malignant form of obesity that reflects central fat deposition, provides a reasonable indication of the accumulation of intraabdominal (visceral) adipose tissue. This currently makes waist girth the trunk measure of clinical choice in evaluating health risks associated with obesity,[64,128,156] when more precise assessments are impractical.[165] *Furthermore, waist girth independently complements BMI. Over a broad range of BMI values, men and women with high waist circumference values possess greater relative risk for cardiovascular disease, type 2 diabetes, cancer, and cataracts, the leading cause of blindness worldwide, than individuals with low waist circumference or with peripheral obesity.*[80,147] TABLE 13.6 presents classification guidelines and associated disease risk for overweight and obesity based on BMI or waist girth. Men with a 102-cm (40 in.) or larger waist and women with waist girth larger than 86 cm (35 in.) maintain a high risk for various diseases. Waist girths of 90 cm for men and 83 cm for women correspond to a BMI threshold of overweight (BMI, 25) while 100 cm (39 in.) for men and 93 cm (37 in.) for women reflect the obesity cutoff (BMI, 30).[206]

Documentation of a strong effect of regular exercise on reducing waist girth selectively in men may partially explain why physical activity reduces disease risk more effectively in men than in women. Both physical activity and energy intake selectively predict waist-to-hip ratio in men but not in women. For men, higher energy intakes and higher energy expenditures associate (independent of BMI) with higher and lower waist/hip ratios, respectively.[176]

BIOELECTRICAL IMPEDANCE ANALYSIS

A small alternating current flowing between two electrodes passes more rapidly through hydrated fat-free body tissues and extracellular water than through fat or bone tissue. This occurs because of the greater electrolyte content (lower electrical resistance) of the fat-free component. Impedance to electric current flow relates to total body water content; which in turn relates to FFM, body density, and percentage body fat.

With **bioelectrical impedance analysis (BIA)**, a person lies on a flat nonconducting surface. Injector (source) electrodes attach on the dorsal surfaces of the foot and wrist, and detector (sink) electrodes attach between the radius and ulna (styloid process) and at the ankle between the medial and lateral malleoli (FIG. 13.12). A painless, localized electric current (about 800 μA at a frequency of 50 kHz) is introduced, and the impedance (resistance) to current flow between the source and detector electrodes is determined. Conversion of the impedance value to body density—adding body mass and stature, gender, age, and sometimes race, level of fatness, and several girths to the equation—computes percentage body fat from the Siri equation or another similar density conversion equation.

Table 13.6	**CLASSIFICATIONS OF OVERWEIGHT AND OBESITY BY BMI, WAIST CIRCUMFERENCE, AND ASSOCIATED DISEASE RISK**		
		Disease Risk[a] Relative to Normal Weight and Normal Waist Circumference	
Classification	*BMI, kg·m²*	*Men ≤ 102 cm* *Women ≤ 88 cm*	*Men > 102 cm* *Women > 88 cm*
Underweight	<18.5	NR	NR
Normal[b]	18.5–24.9	NR	NR
Overweight	25.0–29.9	Increased	High
Obesity, class			
I	30.0–34.9	High	Very high
II	35.0–39.9	Very high	Very high
III (extreme obesity)	≥40	Extremely high	Extremely high

[a] Disease risk for type 2 diabetes, hypertension, and cardiovascular disease. NR indicates no risk assigned at these BMI levels.
[b] Increased waist circumference can indicate increased risk even in persons of normal weight.
From Executive summary of the clinical guidelines on the identification, evaluation, and treatment of overweight and obesity in adults. Arch Intern Med 1998;158:1855.

■ **Figure 13.12** Body composition assessment by bioelectrical impedance analysis. **A.** Four-surface electrode technique that applies current via one pair of distal (injection) electrodes while the proximal (detector) electrode pair measures electrical potential across the conducting segment. **B.** Standard placement of electrodes. **C.** Proper body position during whole-body impedance measurement.

Influence of Hydration and Ambient Temperature

Hydration level, even small changes that occur with exercise, affects BIA accuracy, and may give inaccurate information about a person's body fat content.[99,131,146] Hypohydration and hyperhydration alter normal electrolyte concentrations, which in turn affect current flow independent of a real change in body composition. For example, a loss of body water through prior exercise sweat loss or voluntary fluid restriction decreases the impedance measure. This *lowers* the estimate of percentage body fat, whereas hyperhydration produces the opposite effect (*higher* fat estimate).

Skin temperature (influenced by ambient conditions) also affects whole-body resistance and thus the BIA prediction of body fat. A *lower* predicted body fat value occurs in a warm environment (less impedance to electrical flow) than in a cold one.[5,27]

Even with normal hydration and environmental temperature, body fat predictions prove less satisfactory than hydrostatic weighing. BIA tends to *overpredict* body fat in lean and athletic subjects and *underpredict* body fat in obese subjects.[115,154] BIA often predicts body fat less accurately than girths and skinfolds.[18,40,164] Whether BIA can detect small changes in body composition during weight loss is also unclear.[102,130,138,145] In contrast to skinfold and girth measurements, conventional BIA technology cannot assess regional fat distribution.

At best, BIA provides a noninvasive, safe, and relatively easy and reliable means to assess total body water. Proper BIA use requires that experienced personnel make measurements under strictly standardized conditions,

particularly those related to electrode placement and sub-ject's body position, hydration status, previous food and beverage intake, skin temperature, and recent physical ac-tivity.[13,101,132,189] For example, ingestion of consecutive meals progressively decreases bioelectrical impedance (possibly the combined effect of increased electrolytes and a redistribution of extracellular fluid), which decreases the computed percentage body fat.[162] Level of body fatness and racial characteristics also influence predictive accu-racy.[2,167,184,203] Fatness-specific BIA equations exist for obese and nonobese American Indian, Hispanic, and white men and women.[164] With proper measurement standardiza-tion the menstrual cycle does not affect body composition assessment by BIA.[118]

Applicability of BIA in Sports and Exercise Training

Coaches and athletes need a safe, easily administered, rapid, and valid tool to assess body composition and to detect changes with caloric restriction or exercise train-ing A major limitation in achieving these goals concerns BIA's lack of sensitivity to detect small changes in body composition.[130,153] Accuracy and reliability of BIA mea-surement requires additional controls for the physically active individual. For example, sweat-loss dehydration or re-duced glycogen reserves (and associated loss of glycogen-bound water) from prior exercise increase body resistance (impedance) to electrical current flow. Increased impedance underestimates FFM and overestimates percentage body fat measured by BIA. The tendency to overestimate body fat becomes more pronounced among black athletes.[67,153] Research must also establish the validity and reliability for BIA among female athletes.

Preliminary data indicate potential use of BIA for estimating muscle volume on the basis of the electrical prop-erties of biologic tissues.[125] This type of assessment would certainly prove valuable in the exercise science area because skeletal muscle mass plays a central role in performing phys-ical activity. However, when muscle mass is relatively low (as in anorexia nervosa), the BIA technique does not provide valid estimates of muscularity.[8] Presently, computerized tomography and magnetic resonance imaging of multiple sections of the body quantify skeletal muscle volume. Limi-tations on their use in exercise studies include expense, radiation exposure, and restricted access to the appropriate instrumentation.

NEAR-INFRARED INTERACTANCE

Near-infrared interactance (NIR) applies technology developed by the U.S. Department of Agriculture to assess body composition of livestock and lipid content of various grains. The commercial versions to assess body composition in humans use principles of light absorption and reflection. A fiberoptic probe, or light "wand," emits a low-energy beam of near-infrared light into the single measuring site at the anterior midline surface of the biceps of the dominant arm. A detector within the same probe measures the intensity of the reemitted light, expressed as optical density. Shifts in the wavelength of the reflected beam as it interacts with or-ganic material in the arm, added to the manufacturer's pre-diction equation (often including variables such as subject's body mass and stature, estimated frame size, sex, and physi-cal activity level) rapidly computes percentage body fat and FFM. This safe, portable, and lightweight equipment re-quires minimal training to use and necessitates little physical contact with the subject during measurement. These test ad-ministration aspects make NIR popular for body composi-tion assessment in health clubs, hospitals, and weight-loss centers. The important question about the usefulness of NIR concerns its validity.

Questionable Validity of NIR

Early research with animals indicated a significant re-lationship between spectrophotometric measures of light interactance at various sites on the body and body composi-tion assessed by total body water.[34] Subsequent research with humans did not confirm the validity of NIR when com-pared to hydrostatic weighing and skinfold measurements. In fact, NIR may be *less accurate* than skinfolds in assessing percentage body fat.[29,62,73,180] It *overestimates* body fat in lean men and women and *underestimates* body fat in fatter subjects.[119]

FIGURE 13.13 shows that skinfold measurement more accurately predicted percentage body fat based on hydrostatic weighing than did NIR. In more than 47% of the subjects, an error greater than 4% body fat units occurred with NIR, with the greatest errors at the extremes of body fatness. Further-more, NIR produced large errors—standard error of estimate and total prediction error—when estimating percentage body fat for children[26] and youth wrestlers.[69] It significantly un-derestimated body fat in college football players.[68] *At this time, available evidence does not support NIR as a robust, valid method for assessing human body composition.*

COMPUTED TOMOGRAPHY, MAGNETIC RESONANCE IMAGING, AND DUAL-ENERGY X-RAY ABSORPTIOMETRY

Computed tomography (CT) and **magnetic resonance imaging (MRI)** produce images of body segments. Through the use of appropriate computer software, the CT scan gives pictorial and quantitative information for the total tissue area, total fat and muscle area, and thickness and volume of tissues within an organ.[57,124,183]

FIGURE 13.14A–C shows CT scans of the upper legs and a cross section at the midthigh in a professional walker

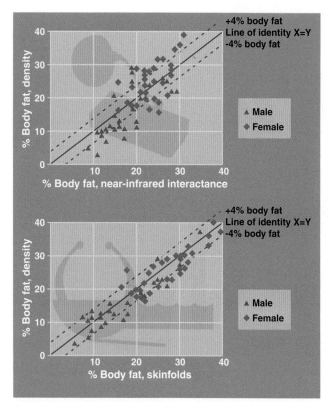

Figure 13.13 Comparison of near-infrared interactance (Futrex-5000) *(top)* and skinfolds *(bottom)* for assessing percentage body fat. (From McLean K, Skinner JS. Validity of Futrex-5000 for body composition determination. Med Sci Sports Exerc 1992;24:253.)

who completed an 11,200-mile walk through the 50 United States in 50 weeks. Total cross section of muscle increased significantly, and subcutaneous fat decreased correspondingly in the midthigh region in the "after" scans.

Studies have demonstrated the efficiency of CT scans to evaluate the relationship between simple anthropometric measures (skinfolds and girths) at the abdominal region and total adipose tissue volume measured from single or multiple pictorial "slices" through the abdominal region.[4,155] Surprisingly, almost no relationship existed between "external" (subcutaneous) abdominal fat and "internal" (visceral) abdominal fat depots in men and women.

The newer technology of MRI provides a rapid, safe technique to obtain accurate information about the body's tissue compartments.[83,106,169] Figure 13.14D displays a color-enhanced MRI transaxial image of the midthigh of a 30-year-old male middle-distance runner. Computer software subtracts fat and bony tissues *(lighter-colored areas)* to compute thigh muscle cross-sectional area *(blue area)*. With MRI, electromagnetic radiation (not ionizing radiation as in CT scans) in a strong magnetic field excites the hydrogen nuclei of the body's water and lipid molecules. The nuclei then project a detectable signal that rearranges under computer control to visually depict the body tissues. MRI effectively quantifies total and subcutaneous adipose tissue in individu-

als of varying degrees of body fatness. Combined with muscle mass analysis, MRI assesses changes in a muscle's lean and fat components following resistance training or during different stages of growth and aging,[79] including changes in muscle volume following spaceflight.[103]

Dual-energy x-ray absorptiometry (DXA), another high-technology procedure, quantifies fat and nonbone regional lean body mass, including the mineral content of the body's deeper bony structures and muscle mass.[95,97,110,143,196] It has become the accepted clinical tool to assess spinal osteoporosis and related bone disorders.[21,42] For body composition analysis, DXA does not require the assumptions about the biological constancy of the fat and fat-free components inherent with hydrostatic weighing.

With DXA, two distinct low-energy x-ray beams (short exposure with low radiation dosage) penetrate bone and soft tissue to a 30-cm depth. An entire DXA scan takes approximately 12 minutes. Computer software reconstructs the attenuated x-ray beams to produce an image of the underlying tissues and quantify bone mineral content, total fat mass, and FFM. Analyses also include selected trunk and limb regions for detailed study of tissue composition and possible relation to disease risk, including the effects of exercise training and detraining.[11,70,88,107,116,199] DXA provides a sensitive noninvasive tool to asses body composition and body composition changes in diverse populations.

BOD POD

A procedure for estimating body volume has been perfected to possibly replace densitometry to assess body volume and its changes in groups ranging from infants to the elderly to collegiate wrestlers and exceptionally large athletes like professional football and basketball players.[48,117,144,178,205] The method has adapted air displacement plethysmography first reported in the late 1800s, and in the 1950s using helium as the gas displaced. The subject sits inside a small chamber (marketed commercially as **BOD POD**, Life Measurement Instruments, Concord, CA). Measurement requires 2 to 5 minutes, and reproducibility of test scores within and across days is high ($r \geq 0.90$).

After being weighed to the nearest 5 g on an electronic scale, the subject sits comfortably in the 750-L volume, dual-chamber fiberglass shell (Fig. 13.15A). The molded front seat separates the unit into front and rear chambers. The electronics, housed in the rear of the chamber, include pressure transducers, breathing circuit, and an air circulation system. To ensure measurement accuracy, the person wears a tight-fitting swimsuit. This suit does not affect measurement reliability or accuracy compared to measurement in the nude.[182] However, wearing a hospital gown reduces estimated percentage body fat by about 9% compared with the recommended swim suit.[46] Body volume becomes the chamber's initial volume minus the reduced chamber volume with the subject inside. The subject

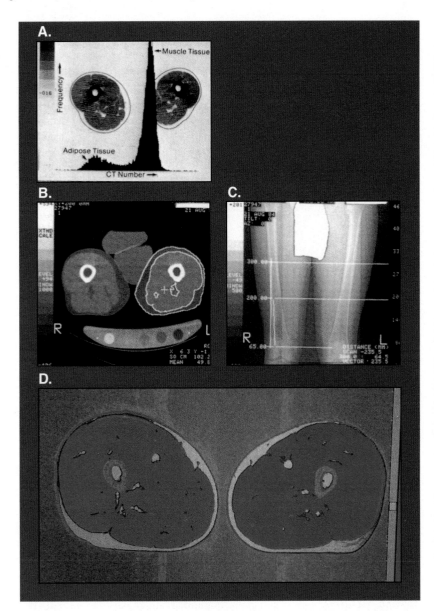

■ **Figure 13.14** Computed tomography (CT) and magnetic resonance imaging (MRI) scans. **A.** Plot of pixel elements (CT scan) illustrating the extent of adipose and muscle tissue in a thigh cross-section. The two other views show a cross section of the midthigh **B.** and an anterior view of the upper leg **C.** prior to a 1-year walk across the United States in a champion walker. **D.** MRI scan of the midthigh of a 30-year-old male middle-distance runner. (CT scans are courtesy of Dr. Steven Heymsfeld, St. Luke's Roosevelt Hospital Center, New York; MRI scan courtesy of J. Staab, Department of the Army, USARIEM, Natick, MA.)

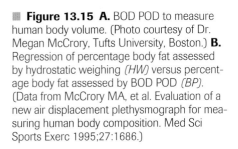

■ **Figure 13.15 A.** BOD POD to measure human body volume. (Photo courtesy of Dr. Megan McCrory, Tufts University, Boston.) **B.** Regression of percentage body fat assessed by hydrostatic weighing *(HW)* versus percentage body fat assessed by BOD POD *(BP)*. (Data from McCrory MA, et al. Evaluation of a new air displacement plethysmograph for measuring human body composition. Med Sci Sports Exerc 1995;27:1686.)

breathes into an air circuit for several breaths to assess thoracic gas volume, which when subtracted from measured body volume yields actual body volume. Body density computes as body mass (measured in air) ÷ body volume (measured in BOD POD). The Siri equation converts body density to percentage body fat. Figure 13.15B shows the relationship between percentage body fat assessed by hydrostatic weighing (HW) versus percentage body fat by BOD POD (BP). The subject pool comprised 42 men and 26 women ages 21 to 56 years who differed in ethnicity (47 non-Hispanic white, 10 Hispanic, 7 African American, 4 Asian American), body mass (52–129 kg), and stature (145–191 cm). A difference of only 0.3% (0.2% fat units) occurred between body fat determined by hydrostatic weighing and BOD POD; the validity correlation was r = 0.96 between the two methods.

More Research Required for Diverse Groups

The effect of age on BOD POD validity remains unclear. For example, BOD POD underestimated body fat of young adults compared to body fat predictions from a four-component model.[47,122] Underpredictions of body fat (–2.9% fat units) compared with DXA-derived body fat assessment also occurred in boys and girls age 10 to 18 years.[108] In contrast, for children ages 9 to 14, BOD POD precisely and accurately estimated fat mass compared with DXA, total body water, and densitometry, without introducing bias estimates.[45] Future studies must also determine BOD POD validity for groups at the extremes of fatness for young men and women (i.e., beyond 10 to 20% body fat for men and 20 to 30% for women). Available evidence indicates that compared with hydrostatic weighing, BOD POD overestimates percentage body fat among lean individuals in a heterogeneous group of adults.[181] The method can detect body composition changes from a small to moderate weight loss in overweight women and men.[193]

Assessments of collegiate football players with BOD POD, although producing reliable scores, underestimated percentage body fat compared with hydrostatic weighing and DXA.[31] Underestimation of percentage body fat also occurred in a heterogeneous sample of black men who varied considerably in age, stature, body mass, percentage body fat, and self-reported physical activity level and socioeconomic status.[185]

ESTIMATING BODY FAT AMONG ATHLETIC GROUPS

Accurate body composition assessment enhances precision in determining a competitor's appropriate body weight for sports with specific weight classifications and/or that emphasize a "required" physical appearance. Valid body composition appraisal also provides an important first step for *identifying* potential eating disorders and *formulating* and *assessing* nutritional counseling.

Skinfolds and girth measurements and BIA have estimated body density and percentage body fat for diverse groups of athletes. Table 13.5 presents (a) generalized equations using these methods for use with athletes in all sports and (b) sport-specific equations for ballet dancers, wrestlers, and football players. Additional equations for wrestlers and high school female gymnasts appear in Chapter 14. When sport-specific equations are unavailable, population-based generalized equations (accounting for age and sex) provide an acceptable alternative to estimate body fat.[29,67,75,133,161,171] The third skinfold equation in Table 13.5 estimates the body composition of adult male athletes; the second equation pertains to adolescent males, while the first equation has been recommended for adult and teenage female athletes.

AVERAGE VALUES FOR BODY COMPOSITION IN THE GENERAL POPULATION

TABLE 13.7 lists average values for percentage body fat in samples of men and women throughout the United States. Values representing ±1 standard deviation provide some indication of the variation or spread from the average; the column headed "68% Variation Limits" indicates the range for percentage body fat that includes one standard deviation, or about 68 of every 100 persons measured. As an example, the average percentage body fat of 15.0% for young men from the New York sample includes the 68% variation limits ranging between 8.9 and 21.1% fat. Interpreting this statistically, for 68 of every 100 young men measured percentage fat ranges between 8.9 and 21.1%. Of the remaining 32 young men, 16 possess more than 21.1% body fat, while 16 others have a body fat percentage below 8.9. *Percentage body fat for young adult men averages between 12 and 15%; the average fat value for women falls between 25 and 28%.* For comparative purposes, see the inset table in Figure 13.17 on page 428 for percentage body fat values for various groups of male and female athletes.

Percentage body fat usually increases in adult men and women as they age. However, individuals who maintain a vigorous physical activity profile throughout life slow the "average" or "normal" age-related fat accretion. Age-related body composition changes could occur because the aging skeleton becomes demineralized and porous, reducing body density because of decreased bone density. Regular physical activity, on the other hand, maintains or increases bone mass while preserving muscle mass. Reduced physical activity provides another reason for the relative increase in body fat with age. A sedentary lifestyle increases storage fat and reduces muscle mass, even if the daily caloric intake remains essentially unchanged.

Table 13.7 **AVERAGE VALUES OF PERCENTAGE BODY FAT FOR YOUNGER AND OLDER WOMEN AND MEN FROM SELECTED STUDIES**

Study	Age Range	Stature, cm	Mass, kg	% Fat	68% Variation Limits
Younger women					
North Carolina, 1962	17–25	165.0	55.5	22.9	17.5–28.5
New York, 1962	16–30	167.5	59.0	28.7	24.6–32.9
California, 1968	19–23	165.9	58.4	21.9	17.0–26.9
California, 1970	17–29	164.9	58.6	25.5	21.0–30.1
Air Force, 1972	17–22	164.1	55.8	28.7	22.3–35.3
New York, 1973	17–26	160.4	59.0	26.2	23.4–33.3
North Carolina, 1975		166.1	57.5	24.6	–
Army Recruits, 1986	17–25	162.0	58.6	28.4	23.9–32.9
Massachusetts, 1998	17–31	165.2	57.8	21.8	16.7–27.9
Older women					
Minnesota, 1953	31–45	163.3	60.7	28.9	25.1–32.8
	43–68	160.0	60.9	34.2	28.0–40.5
New York, 1963	30–40	164.9	59.6	28.6	22.1–35.3
	40–50	163.1	56.4	34.4	29.5–39.5
North Carolina, 1975	33–50	–	–	29.7	23.1–36.5
Massachusetts, 1993	31–50	165.2	58.9	25.2	19.2–31.2
Younger men					
Minnesota, 1951	17–26	177.8	69.1	11.8	5.9–11.8
Colorado, 1956	17–25	172.4	68.3	13.5	8.3–18.8
Indiana, 1966	18–23	180.1	75.5	12.6	8.7–16.5
California, 1968	16–31	175.7	74.1	15.2	6.3–24.2
New York, 1973	17–26	176.4	71.4	15.0	8.9–21.1
Texas, 1977	18–24	179.9	74.6	13.4	7.4–19.4
Army recruits, 1986	17–25	174.7	70.5	15.6	10.0–21.2
Massachusetts, 1998	17–31	178.1	76.4	12.9	7.8–19.0
Older men					
Indiana, 1966	24–38	179.0	76.6	17.8	11.3–24.3
	40–48	177.0	80.5	22.3	16.3–28.3
North Carolina, 1976	27–50	–	–	23.7	17.9–30.1
Texas, 1977	27–59	180.0	85.3	27.1	23.7–30.5
Massachusetts, 1993	31–50	177.1	77.5	19.9	13.2–26.5

DETERMINING A GOAL BODY WEIGHT

Excess body fat detracts from good health, physical fitness, and athletic performance. No one really knows the optimum body fat or body mass for a particular individual. Inherited genetic factors greatly influence body fat distribution and certainly affect the long-term programing of body size.[14,15] Women and men who exercise regularly have lower percentage body fat values than the population average. In contact sports and activities requiring muscular power, successful performance usually requires a large body mass with minimal body fat. In contrast, success in weight-bearing endurance activities requires a lighter body mass and less body fat. For these individuals, attaining a low body weight must not compromise lean tissue mass and energy reserves. *Proper assessment of body composition, not body weight, determines a physically active person's ideal body weight. For athletes, this* **goal body weight** *must coincide with optimizing sport-specific measures of physiologic function and exercise capacity.*

Suppose a 120-kg (265-lb) shot-put athlete, currently with 24% body fat, wishes to know how much fat weight to lose to attain a body fat composition of 15%. Compute a goal body weight based on the desired body fat level as follows:

Goal body weight = Fat-free body mass ÷ (1.00 − % fat desired)

Fat mass
= 120 kg × 0.24
= 28.8 kg

Fat-free body mass
= 120 kg − 28.8 kg
= 91.2 kg

Goal body weight
= 91.2 kg ÷ (1.00 − 0.15)
= 91.2 kg ÷ 0.85
= 107.3 kg (236.6 lb)

Desirable fat loss = Present body weight − Goal body weight
$$= 120 \text{ kg} - 107.3 \text{ kg}$$
$$= 12.7 \text{ kg } (28.0 \text{ lb})$$

If this athlete reduced 12.7 kg of body fat, his new body weight of 91.2 kg would contain fat equal to 15% of body mass. These calculations assume no change in FFM during weight loss. Moderate caloric restriction plus increased daily energy expenditure through regular exercise induce fat loss and conserve lean tissue. Chapter 14 discusses prudent yet effective approaches to lose body fat.

Summary

1. Standard "height–weight" tables reveal little about an individual's body composition. Studies of athletes clearly show that overweight does not coincide with excessive body fat.

2. Body mass index (BMI) relates more closely to body fat and health risk than simply body mass and stature. BMI fails to consider the body's proportional composition.

3. For the first time in the United States, overweight persons (BMI > 25) outnumber individuals of desirable weight.

4. Comorbidities heighten an overweight individual's risks for poor health at any given level of excess weight. These include hypertension, elevated blood sugar, pulmonary problems that include asthma and sleep apnea, psychiatric problems (depression and eating disorders), diverse cancers, gastrointestinal disorders including gallstones, and elevated total cholesterol and low HDL-cholesterol levels.

5. Total body fat consists of essential fat and storage fat. Essential fat contains fat present in bone marrow, nerve tissue, and organs; it is not a labile energy reserve, but instead an important component for normal biologic functions. Storage fat represents the energy reserve that accumulates mainly as adipose tissue beneath the skin and in visceral depots.

6. Storage fat averages 12% of body mass for men and 15% body mass for women. Essential fat averages 3% body mass for men and 12% for women. The greater essential fat for females probably relates to childbearing and hormonal functions.

7. A sumo wrestler has the largest fat-free body mass (FFM) reported in the literature (121.3 kg); this value most likely represents the upper limit for male athletes. Estimates place the upper-limit for FFM for athletic women at 80 kg (176 lb).

8. Menstrual dysfunction often occurs in athletes who train hard and maintain low body fat levels. The precise interaction among the physiologic and psychologic stress of intense training and competition, hormonal balance, energy and nutrient intake, and body fat remains unknown.

9. The most popular indirect methods to assess body composition include hydrostatic weighing and prediction methods based on skinfolds and girths. Hydrostatic weighing determines body density with subsequent estimation of percentage body fat. Subtracting fat mass from body mass yields FFM.

10. Part of the error inherent in predicting body fat from whole-body density lies in the correctness of assumptions concerning the densities of the body's fat and fat-free components. These densities differ from assumed constants because of race, age, and athletic experience.

11. Common body composition assessments use prediction equations from relationships among selected skinfolds and girths and body density and percentage fat. These equations show population specificity because they most accurately predict body fat with subjects similar to those who participated in the equations' original derivation.

12. Hydrated fat-free body tissues and extracellular water facilitate electrical flow compared with fat tissue, because of the greater electrolyte content of the fat-free component. Bioelectrical impedance analysis (BIA) applies this fact to assess body composition.

13. Near-infrared interactance should be used with caution to assess body composition because this methodology lacks verification of adequate validity.

14. Computed tomography, magnetic resonance imaging, and dual-energy x-ray absorptiometry indirectly assess body composition. Each has a unique application and special limitations for expanding knowledge of the compositional components of the live human body, and its changes with regular exercise training.

15. The BOD POD air displacement method offers promise for body composition assessment because of the high reliability of body volume scores and relatively high validity.

16. Data from healthy young adults, indicate that the average male possesses approximately 15% body

fat, and women about 25%. These values often provide a frame of reference for evaluating the body fat of individual athletes and specific athletic groups.

17. Goal body weight is computes as FFM ÷ (1.00 − desired % body fat.)

▶ Physique of Champion Athletes

Body composition differs considerably between athletes and nonathletes. Pronounced differences in physique also exist among sports participants of the same sex, including Olympic competitors, track and field specialists, wrestlers, football players, and highly proficient adolescent competitors. We now take a closer look at the physiques of elite athletes by sport category and competition level. Research may eventually discern the degree that body size and composition contribute to (and are prerequisite for) elite performance in specific sports.

THE ELITE ATHLETE

Different anthropometric methodologies have quantified physique status. Visual appraisal often describes individuals as small, medium, or large or thin (**ectomorphic**), muscular (**mesomorphic**), or fat (**endomorphic**). This approach, termed **somatotyping**, describes body shape by placing a person into a category such as thin or muscular. Visual appraisal does not quantify body dimensions such as size of the chest or shoulders, or how biceps development compares with that of the thighs or calves. While somatotyping has provided a valuable adjunct in the analysis of physique status of world-class athletes,[25,38] we focus on body fat and FFM components of body composition.

Olympic and Elite Athletes

Early studies of Olympic competitors revealed that physique related to a high level of sports achievement.[36,96] TABLES 13.8 AND 13.9 list the anthropometric characteristics of male and female competitors in the 1964 Tokyo and 1968 Mexico City Olympics.[38,65] Bone diameters and stature estimated lean body mass and percentage body fat. TABLE 13.10 lists anthropometric data (body mass, stature, and eight skinfolds) for male and female swimmers, divers, and water polo athletes at the Sixth World Championships in Perth, Australia, 1992.

Also of interest are the body size differences among different groups of athletes within a particular sport. FIGURE 13.16 (*top*) compares body mass, stature, chest girth, and upper- and lower-limb lengths for 12 male swimmers rated "best" in the 200 + 400-m free-style with measures of less successful counterparts. The bottom of the figure also compares selected body size variables between the "best" 50, 100, 200-m breaststroke female swimmers with those of the other swimmers. Little doubt exists that the best male swimmers are heavier and taller and have larger chest, upper-arm, and thigh girths and upper- and lower-limb lengths than counterparts not ranking among the top 12. The best female breaststroke swimmers are not only taller and heavier, but they also possess larger arm spans, foot and arm lengths, and hand and wrist breadth than less successful competitors.

Gender Differences

Table 13.8 indicates that male basketball players, rowers, and weight throwers were tallest and heaviest; they also possessed the largest FFM and percentage body fat. For example, weight throwers in both Olympiads averaged 30% body fat, whereas 94 marathon and 133 long-distance runners averaged an exceptionally low 1.6% body fat. The largest body composition discrepancy within a particular sports category emerged in comparisons of the Tokyo wrestlers (12.7% body fat) and wrestlers in Mexico City (1.2% body fat). Age, stature, and FFM were similar in both groups, making this difference even more remarkable.

For female Olympians (Table 13.9), a relatively low body fat is the most striking physical characteristic. Except for the weight throwers (about 31% body fat), competitors in the other sports groups approximated the 13.1% average body fat for all 676 female participants in both Olympiads.

For aquatic athletes (Table 13.10), skinfolds at most sites were larger in females than in males. Prior studies established a relationship between certain aspects of body composition and swimming performance. A swimmer's morphology

| Table 13.8 | AGE, BODY SIZE, AND BODY COMPOSITION OF MALE ATHLETES IN SELECTED EVENTS WHO COMPETED IN THE TOKYO AND MEXICO CITY OLYMPICS | | | | | | | |

Specialty	Event	Olympics	N	Age (y)	Stature (cm)	Mass (kg)	LBM[a] (kg)	Body fat[b] (%)
Sprint	100–200 m; 4 × 100 m; 110-m hurdles	Tokyo	172	24.9	178.4	72.2	64.9	10.1
		Mexico City	79	23.9	175.4	68.4	62.8	8.2
Long-distance running	3000, 5000, 10,000 m	Tokyo	99	27.3	173.6	62.4	61.5	1.4
		Mexico City	34	25.3	171.9	59.8	60.1	−0.5
Marathon	42.2 km	Tokyo	74	28.3	170.3	60.8	59.2	2.7
Decathlon		Tokyo	26	26.3	183.2	83.5	68.5	18.0
		Mexico City	8	25.1	181.3	77.5	67.1	13.4
Jump	High, long, triple jump	Tokyo	89	25.3	181.5	73.2	67.2	8.2
		Mexico City	14	23.5	182.8	73.2	68.2	6.8
Weight	Shot, discus, hammer throwing	Tokyo	79	27.6	187.3	101.4	71.6	29.4
		Mexico City	9	27.3	186.1	102.3	70.7	30.9
Swimming	Free, breast, back, butterfly, medley	Tokyo	450	20.4	178.7	74.1	65.1	12.1
		Mexico City	66	19.2	179.3	72.1	65.6	9.0
Basketball		Tokyo	186	25.3	189.4	84.3	73.2	13.2
		Mexico City	63	24.0	189.1	79.7	73.0	8.4
Gymnastics	All events	Tokyo	122	26.0	167.2	63.3	57.0	9.9
		Mexico City	28	23.6	167.4	61.5	57.2	7.0
Wrestling	Bantam, featherweight	Tokyo	29	27.3	163.3	62.3	54.4	12.7
		Mexico City	32	22.5	166.1	57.0	56.3	1.2
Rowing	Single, double skulls; pairs, fours, eights	Tokyo	357	25.0	186.0	82.2	70.6	14.1
		Mexico City	85	24.3	185.1	82.6	69.9	15.4

Adapted from De Garay, et al. Genetic and anthropological studies of Olympic athletes. New York: Academic Press, 1974, and Hirata K. Physique and age of Tokyo Olympic champions. J Sports Med Phys Fitness 1966;6:207.
[a] Calculated by Behnke's method: LBM = h × 0.204, where h = stature, dm (see ref. 9)
[b] Body fat (%) = (Body mass − LBM) ÷ Body mass × 100

| Table 13.9 | AGE, BODY SIZE, AND BODY COMPOSITION OF FEMALE ATHLETES WHO COMPETED IN THE TOKYO AND MEXICO CITY OLYMPICS IN SELECTED EVENTS | | | | | | | |

Specialty	Event	Olympics	N	Age (y)	Stature (cm)	Mass (kg)	LBM[a] (kg)	Body Fat[b] (%)
Sprint	100–200 m; 100-m hurdles	Tokyo	85	22.7	166.0	56.6	49.2	12.4
		Mexico City	28	20.7	165.0	56.8	49.0	13.7
Jump	High, long, triple jump	Tokyo	56	23.6	169.5	60.2	51.7	14.1
		Mexico City	12	21.5	169.4	56.4	51.7	8.4
Weight	Shot, discus, hammer throwing	Tokyo	37	26.2	170.4	79.0	52.3	33.8
		Mexico City	9	19.9	170.9	73.5	52.5	28.5
Swimming	Free, breast, back, butterfly, medley	Tokyo	272	18.6	166.3	59.7	49.8	16.6
		Mexico City	28	16.3	164.4	56.9	48.6	14.5
Diving	Spring, high	Tokyo	65	18.5	160.9	54.1	46.6	13.9
		Mexico City	7	21.1	160.4	52.3	46.3	11.5
Gymnastics	All events	Tokyo	102	22.7	157.0	52.0	44.4	14.7
		Mexico City	21	17.8	156.9	49.8	44.3	11.0

Adapted from De Garay, et al. Genetic and anthropological studies of Olympic athletes. New York: Academic Press, 1974, and Hirata K. Physique and age of Tokyo Olympic champions. J Sports Med Phys Fitness 1966;6:207.
[a] Calculated by Behnke's method: LBM (lean body mass) = h² × 0.18, where h = stature, dm (see ref. 9)
[b] Body fat (%) = (Body mass − LBM ÷ Body mass × 100)

Table 13.10	COMPARISON OF BODY MASS, STATURE, AND EIGHT SKINFOLDS IN MALE AND FEMALE SWIMMERS, DIVERS, AND WATER POLO ATHLETES AT THE SIXTH WORLD CHAMPIONSHIPS HELD IN PERTH, AUSTRALIA, IN 1992									
	Mass (kg)	Stature (cm)	Tri[a]	Scap	Supra	Abd	Thi	Calf	Bic	Iliac
Males										
Swimming	78.4	183.8	7.0	7.9	6.3	9.4	9.6	6.5	3.7	9.2
Diving	66.7	170.9	6.8	7.9	6.0	9.6	9.6	6.0	3.8	8.5
Water polo	86.1	186.5	9.2	9.9	8.2	14.9	12.6	7.9	4.3	13.4
Females										
Swimming	63.1	71.5	12.1	8.8	7.3	12.1	19.1	11.4	5.9	9.8
Diving	53.7	61.2	11.4	8.5	6.8	11.1	18.2	9.7	4.9	7.9
Water polo	64.8	171.3	15.3	10.5	9.6	17.6	23.4	13.5	7.1	12.1

Modified from Mazza JC, et al. Absolute body size. In: Carter JE, Ackland TR, eds. Kinanthropometry in aquatic sports. A study of world class athletes. Human Kinetics Sport Science Monograph Series, vol. 5. Champaign, IL: Human Kinetics, 1994.

[a] These abbreviations are for skinfolds (mm): Tri, triceps; Scap, subscapula; Supra, supraspinale; Abd, abdomen; Calf, midcalf; Bic, biceps; Iliac, iliac crest.

significantly influences the horizontal components of lift and drag. Selected anthropometric variables play important roles in propulsive and resistive forces acting on the swimmer that affect forward movement. The combined influence of stroke length and stroke frequency on swimming velocity also relates to a swimmer's overall body size and shape. In well-trained freestyle swimmers, arm length, leg length, and hand and foot size—factors governed largely by genetics—significantly influence stroke length and stroke frequency. TABLE 13.11 presents additional anthropometric comparisons between male and female Olympians in five different sports

(including swimming) at the 1976 Montreal Summer Olympics.

Ratio of Fat-Free Body Mass to Fat Mass. FIGURE 13.17 compares the ratios of FFM to fat mass (FFM/FM) derived from data in the world literature among male and female competitors. The *inset tables* present their average body mass, percentage body fat, fat weight, and FFM. Appendix E also presents additional body composition data from various studies of male and female athletes. These aid in evaluating typical variation in body fat within and between diverse ath-

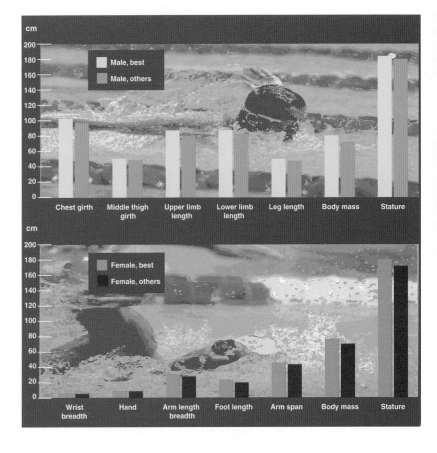

■ **Figure 13.16** *Top.* Comparison of 200- + 400-m free-style male swimmers for body mass, stature, chest girth, arm span (actual values divided by 4), and upper and lower limb lengths, categorized as best performers (top 12 ranks) with those of remaining competitors. *Bottom.* Comparison of differences in body size variables between the best 50-, 100-, and 200-m female breaststroke swimmers (top 12 ranks) and the rest of the competitors. *Y* axis in centimeters for all data except body mass (kilograms). (Modified from Mazza JC, et al. Absolute body size. In: Carter JE, Ackland TR, eds. Kinanthropometry in aquatic sports. A study of world class athletes. Human Kinetics Sport Science monograph series, vol 5. Champaign, IL: Human Kinetics, 1994.)

Table 13.11 **SELECTED ANTHROPOMETRIC MEASUREMENTS IN MALES AND FEMALES WHO COMPETED IN FIVE DIFFERENT SPORTS AT THE MONTREAL OLYMPIC GAMES**

Measurement[a]	Canoe M	Canoe F	Gymnastics M	Gymnastics F	Rowing M	Rowing F	Swimming M	Swimming F	Track M	Track F
Stature	185.4	170.7	169.3	161.5	191.3	174.3	178.6	166.9	179.1	168.5
Upper extremity L	82.4	76.0	76.0	72.2	85.2	76.0	80.2	74.7	80.9	74.8
Lower extremity L	88.0	81.8	78.9	76.5	91.7	82.3	84.1	78.1	86.9	80.3
Biacromial D	41.4	36.8	39.0	35.9	42.5	37.4	40.8	37.1	40.2	36.3
Billiac D	28.1	27.3	25.8	25.0	30.2	28.2	27.9	26.7	27.1	27.2
Arm relaxed G	32.2	27.6	30.7	24.3	31.7	27.6	30.6	27.3	29.1	24.5
Arm flexed G	35.3	29.6	33.9	25.9	34.9	29.3	33.3	28.2	32.2	26.4
Forearm G	29.3	25.4	27.5	23.2	30.3	25.5	27.4	23.9	27.9	23.3
Chest G	102.6	88.9	95.1	83.5	103.7	89.6	98.6	88.0	94.3	83.8
Waist G	80.6	69.8	72.8	63.2	84.0	70.8	79.3	69.4	77.7	67.4
Thigh G	54.6	54.0	51.0	49.9	60.2	57.5	55.4	52.8	55.0	53.9
Calf G	37.5	34.9	34.7	33.3	39.3	37.0	36.9	34.0	37.6	34.9

[a] L, length; D, diameter; G, girth; all values are in centimeters.
Adapted from Carter JE, et al. Anthropometry of Montreal Olympic athletes. In: Carter JEL, ed. Physical structure of Olympic athletes. Part 1: The Montreal Olympic Games Anthropological Project. Basal: Karger, 1982.

letic groups. Male marathon runners and gymnasts have the largest FFM/FM, while American football offensive and defensive lineman and shot putters show the smallest ratios. Among females, bodybuilders have the largest FFM/FM values (equal to those of males), while the smallest ratios emerge for field event participants. Surprisingly, female gymnasts and ballet dancers rank about intermediate compared with other female sport participants.

Percentage Body Fat Grouped by Sport Category

FIGURE 13.18 presents six classifications of sports activities based on common characteristics and performance requirements, with percentage body fat rankings within each category for male and female competitors (where applicable). This provides an overview of percentage body fat of athletes within a broad grouping of relatively similar sports.

Racial Differences. Racial differences in physique may significantly affect athletic performance.[168] Black sprinters and high jumpers, for example, have longer limbs and narrower hips than their white counterparts. From a mechanical perspective, a black sprinter with leg and arm size identical to a white sprinter would have a lighter, shorter, and slimmer body to propel. This might confer a more favorable power-to-body mass ratio at any given body size. Greater power output provides an advantage in jumping and sprint running events, where generating rapid energy for short durations is crucial to success. This advantage diminishes somewhat in the various throwing events. Compared with whites and blacks, Asian athletes have short legs relative to upper torso components, a dimensional characteristic beneficial in short and longer distance races and in weight lifting. In fact, suc-

cessful weightlifters of all races (compared with other athletic groups) have relatively short arms and legs for their stature.

Field Event Athletes

FIGURE 13.19 shows body composition obtained by densitometry and anthropometry—ranked from high to low in percentage body fat, fat weight, FFM, and lean-to-fat ratio—for the 10 top American athletes in the discus, shot put, javelin, and hammer throw 2 years before the 1980 Moscow Olympics. For comparison, data include international elite middle- and long-distance runners (average treadmill $\dot{V}O_2max = 76.9$ mL·kg^{-1}·min^{-1}) and Behnke's reference man. TABLE 13.12 lists the corresponding data for girth and skinfold anthropometry. Shot putters clearly possessed the largest overall size (body mass and girths), followed by athletes in discuss, hammer, and javelin.

Female Endurance Athletes

TABLE 13.13 presents data for body mass, stature, and body composition for 11 female long-distance runners of national and international caliber. The runners averaged 15.2% body fat (hydrostatic weighing), similar to reports of high school cross-country runners[20] and elite Kenyan female endurance runners who averaged 16.0% body fat,[12] but considerably lower than the 26% reported for sedentary females of the same age, stature, and body mass.[85] Compared with other female athletic groups, runners have relatively less fat than collegiate basketball players (20.9%),[159] competitive gymnasts (15.5%),[160] younger distance runners (18%),[96] swimmers (20.1%),[89] and tennis players (22.8%).[89]

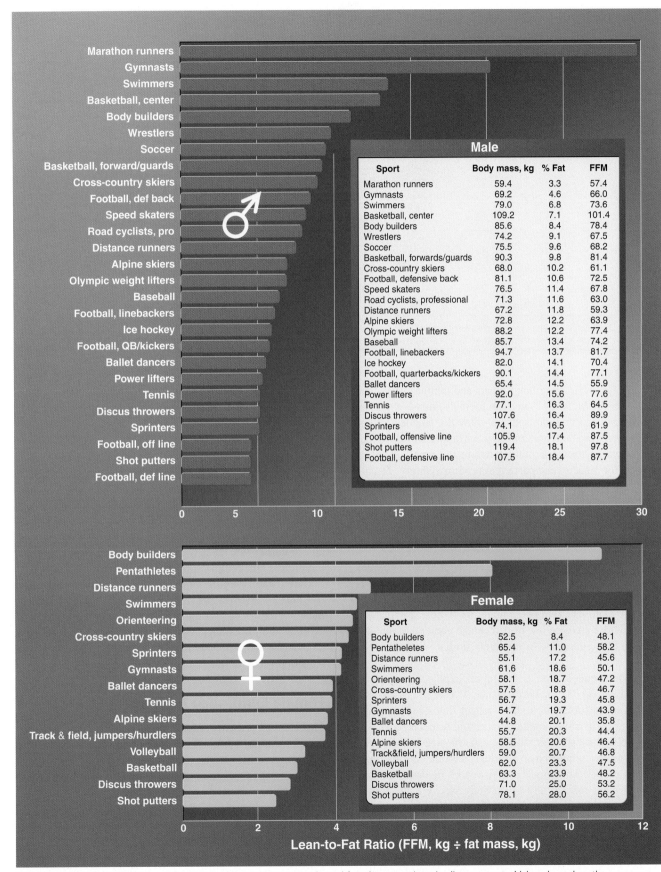

Male

Sport	Body mass, kg	% Fat	FFM
Marathon runners	59.4	3.3	57.4
Gymnasts	69.2	4.6	66.0
Swimmers	79.0	6.8	73.6
Basketball, center	109.2	7.1	101.4
Body builders	85.6	8.4	78.4
Wrestlers	74.2	9.1	67.5
Soccer	75.5	9.6	68.2
Basketball, forwards/guards	90.3	9.8	81.4
Cross-country skiers	68.0	10.2	61.1
Football, defensive back	81.1	10.6	72.5
Speed skaters	76.5	11.4	67.8
Road cyclists, professional	71.3	11.6	63.0
Distance runners	67.2	11.8	59.3
Alpine skiers	72.8	12.2	63.9
Olympic weight lifters	88.2	12.2	77.4
Baseball	85.7	13.4	74.2
Football, linebackers	94.7	13.7	81.7
Ice hockey	82.0	14.1	70.4
Football, quarterbacks/kickers	90.1	14.4	77.1
Ballet dancers	65.4	14.5	55.9
Power lifters	92.0	15.6	77.6
Tennis	77.1	16.3	64.5
Discus throwers	107.6	16.4	89.9
Sprinters	74.1	16.5	61.9
Football, offensive line	105.9	17.4	87.5
Shot putters	119.4	18.1	97.8
Football, defensive line	107.5	18.4	87.7

Female

Sport	Body mass, kg	% Fat	FFM
Body builders	52.5	8.4	48.1
Pentatheletes	65.4	11.0	58.2
Distance runners	55.1	17.2	45.6
Swimmers	61.6	18.6	50.1
Orienteering	58.1	18.7	47.2
Cross-country skiers	57.5	18.8	46.7
Sprinters	56.7	19.3	45.8
Gymnasts	54.7	19.7	43.9
Ballet dancers	44.8	20.1	35.8
Tennis	55.7	20.3	44.4
Alpine skiers	58.5	20.6	46.4
Track&field, jumpers/hurdlers	59.0	20.7	46.8
Volleyball	62.0	23.3	47.5
Basketball	63.3	23.9	48.2
Discus throwers	71.0	25.0	53.2
Shot putters	78.1	28.0	56.2

Lean-to-Fat Ratio (FFM, kg ÷ fat mass, kg)

Figure 13.17 Comparison of the lean-to-fat ratios among male and female competitors in diverse sports. Values based on the average body mass and percentage body fat for each sport from various studies in the literature. The lean-to-fat ratio equals FFM (kg) ÷ fat mass (kg). The values in the inset tables represent averages for body composition if the literature contained two or more citations about a specific sport.

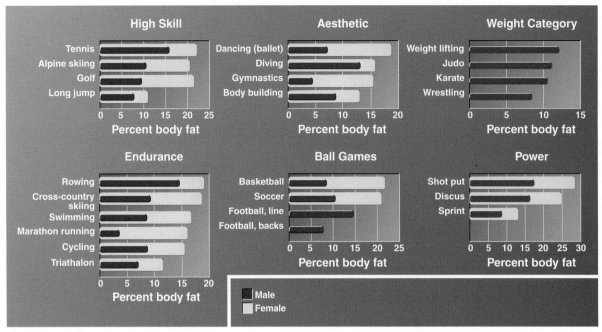

Figure 13.18 Percentage body fat in athletes grouped by sport category. Value for males displayed within the bar *(red)* when a corresponding value exists for females *(yellow)*. Values for percentage body fat represent averages from the literature.

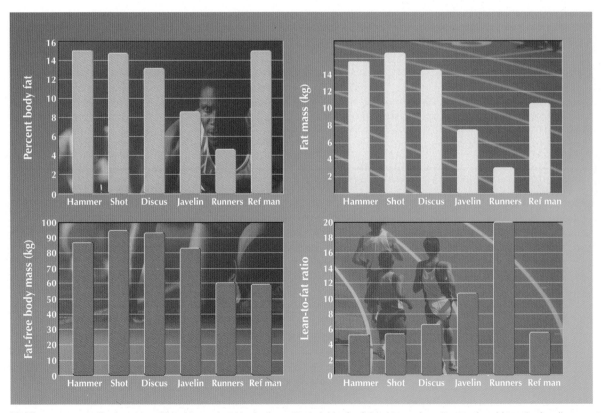

Figure 13.19 Body composition (determined by hydrostatic weighing) of the 10 top American male athletes in the discus, shot put, javelin, and hammer throw. (Data collected by two of the authors [FK and VK] at a 1978 U.S. Olympic thrower's mini-camp at the University of Houston, Houston, TX. Data include gold medalist Wilkins [discus] and world-record holder Powell [discus]. Data for the international elite middle- and long-distance runners from: Pollock ML, et al. Body composition of elite class distance runners. Ann NY Acad Sci 1977;301:361. Reference man *[Ref man]* data from Behnke model.

Table 13.12   **SKINFOLD AND GIRTH ANTHROPOMETRY OF THE TOP 10 AMERICAN ATHLETES IN THE DISCUS, SHOT PUT, JAVELIN, AND HAMMER THROW**

Measurement[a]	Discus	Shot Put	Javelin	Hammer	Runners	Ref Man
Body mass, kg	108.2	112.3	90.6	104.2	63.1	70.0
Stature, cm	191.7	187.0	186.0	187.3	177.0	174.0
Skinfolds, mm						
Triceps	13.0	15.0	11.9	12.7	5.0	—
Scapular	18.0	23.8	12.5	21.5	6.4	—
Iliac	24.5	29.6	17.0	27.4	4.6	—
Abdomen	25.6	31.4	18.4	29.1	7.1	—
Thigh	16.4	15.7	13.3	17.3	6.1	—
Girths, cm						
Shoulders	129.8	133.3	121.5	127.4	106.1	110.8
Chest	113.5	118.5	104.6	111.3	91.1	91.8
Waist	94.1	99.1	86.6	94.8	74.6	77.0
Abdomen	97.5	101.5	87.8	98.0	74.2	79.8
Hips	110.4	112.3	102.0	108.7	87.8	93.4
Thighs	66.3	69.4	61.5	67.3	51.9	54.8
Knees	41.5	42.9	40.0	41.0	36.2[b]	36.6
Calves	42.6	43.6	39.5	41.5	35.4	35.8
Ankles	25.4	24.9	24.1	24.3	21.0	22.5
Biceps	41.8	42.2	37.7	39.9	28.2	31.7
Forearms	33.1	33.7	30.8	32.4	26.4	26.4
Wrists	18.7	18.9	18.2	18.4	16.0	17.3
Diameters, cm						
Biacromial	44.5	43.8	43.2	44.8	39.5	40.6
Chest	33.1	33.7	30.8	32.6	31.3	30.0
Bi-iliac	31.3	31.2	29.6	30.4	28.0	28.6
Bitrochanter	35.5	34.9	33.7	34.8	32.2	32.8
Knee	10.2	10.5	10.0	10.2	9.5	9.3
Wrist	6.3	6.2	6.0	6.2	5.6	5.6
Ankle	7.6	7.6	7.5	7.4	—	7.0
Elbow	7.6	7.6	7.6	7.2	—	7.0

[a]Details about measurement procedures from Katch FI, Katch VL. The body composition profile: techniques of measurement and applications. Clin Sports Med, 1984;3:31. Data correspond to the athletic groups presented in Fig. 29.7.
[b]Not measured; value computed from the ratio for the reference man calf to knee.

Table 13.13   **BODY COMPOSITION OF FEMALE ENDURANCE RUNNERS**

Subjects (N)	Age (y)	Stature (cm)	Mass (kg)	FFM (kg)	Body Fat (kg)	Body Fat (%)
1[a]	24	172.7	52.6	49.5	3.1	5.9
2[b]	26	159.8	71.5	46.2	25.3	35.4
3[c]	28	162.6	50.7	47.6	3.1	6.1
4	31	171.5	52.0	47.3	4.7	9.0
5	33	176.5	61.2	50.8	10.4	17.0
6	34	166.4	52.9	44.8	8.1	15.2
7	35	168.4	55.0	48.7	6.3	11.6
8	36	164.5	53.1	44.3	8.8	16.6
9	36	182.9	61.5	50.4	11.1	18.1
10	36	182.9	65.4	55.7	9.7	14.8
11	37	154.9	53.6	44.0	9.6	18.0
Average	32.4	169.4	57.2	48.1	9.1	15.2

From Wilmore JH, Brown CH. Physiological profiles of women distance runners. Med Sci Sports 1974;6:178.
[a] World's best time in marathon (2:49:40) 1974.
[b] World's best time in 50-mile run (7:04:31); established 18 months after the body composition evaluation.
[c] Noted U.S. distance runner. Five consecutive national and international cross-country championships.

Table 13.14	**BODY COMPOSITION CHARACTERISTICS OF ELITE MALE MIDDLE- AND LONG-DISTANCE RUNNERS AND ELITE MARATHONERS**						
Group	Stature (cm)	Mass (kg)	Density (g·cm^{-3})	Body Fat (%)	FFM (kg)	Fat Mass (kg)	Sum 7 Skinfolds (mm)
Distance runners							
Brown	187.3	72.10	1.07428	10.8	64.31	7.79	53.0
Castaneda	178.6	63.34	1.09102	3.7	61.00	2.34	32.5
Crawford	171.8	58.01	1.09702	1.2	57.31	0.70	32.5
Geis	179.1	66.28	1.07551	10.2	59.52	6.76	49.0
Johnson	174.6	61.79	1.08963	4.35	9.13	2.66	35.5
Manley	177.8	69.10	1.09642	1.5	68.06	1.04	32.0
Ndoo	169.3	53.97	1.08379	6.7	50.35	3.62	33.5
Prefontaine	174.2	68.00	1.08842	4.8	64.74	3.26	38.0
Rose	175.6	59.15	1.08248	7.3	54.83	4.32	31.5
Tuttle	176.8	61.44	1.09960	0.2	61.32	0.12	31.5
Mean	170.5	60.92	1.08916	4.5	58.18	2.74	34.5
(standard deviation)	(5.0)	(5.30)	(0.00832)	(3.5)	(4.90)	(2.38)	(7.4)
Marathon runners							
Cusack	174.6	64.19	1.08096	7.9	59.12	5.07	45.5
Galloway	180.9	65.76	1.08419	6.6	61.42	4.34	43.0
Kennedy	167.0	56.52	1.09348	2.7	54.99	1.53	37.0
Moore	184.1	64.24	1.09193	3.3	62.12	2.12	37.0
Pate	179.6	57.28	1.09676	1.3	56.54	0.74	32.5
Shorter	178.4	61.17	1.09475	2.2	59.82	1.35	45.0
Wayne	172.1	61.61	1.07859	8.9	56.13	5.48	42.5
Williams	177.2	66.07	1.09569	1.8	64.88	1.19	41.5
Mean	176.8	62.11	1.08954	4.3	59.38	2.73	40.5
(standard deviation)	(5.6)	(3.66)	(0.00718)	(3.0)	(3.38)	(1.92)	(4.6)

Data from Pollock ML, et al. Body composition of elite class distance runners. Ann NY Acad Sci 1977;301:361.

Interestingly, the runners' average body fat equaled the 15% value generally reported for nonathletic males, and close to the quantity of essential fat proposed by Behnke's model for the reference woman. The 6 to 9% body fat levels of several apparently healthy runners in Table 13.13 fall within the range reported for topflight male endurance athletes. The leanest women in the population, based on Behnke's reference standards, have essential fat equal to 12 to 14% of body mass. This apparent discrepancy between estimated fat content of distance runners and the theoretical lower limit for body fat in women requires further study. Note the relatively high body fat (35.4%) of one of the best runners; other factors must override limitations to distance running imposed by excess fat.

Male Endurance Athletes

TABLE 13.14 presents the body composition of 11 male elite middle- and long-distance runners and 8 elite marathoners. The group included Steve Prefontaine, former American record holder in the 800- and 1500-m runs, and Frank Shorter, 1976 Olympic gold medalist in the marathon. A representative sample of 95 untrained college-aged men provides comparison data.

The runners maintain extremely low body fat values that average 4.5% for the distance athletes and 4.3% for the marathoners, considering that essential fat constitutes about 3% of body mass. This agrees with recent values for elite Kenyan runners whose body fat averaged 6.6% (predicted from skinfold measures).[12] Clearly, these competitors represent the lower end of the lean-to-fat continuum for topflight athletes. Such physique characteristics most likely influence success in distance running. This makes sense for several reasons: First, effective heat dissipation during running maintains thermal balance—excess fat thwarts heat dissipation. Second, excess body fat represents "dead weight"; it adds directly to exercise energy cost without providing propulsive energy.

For body dimension and structure, male distance runners generally have smaller girths and bone diameters than untrained males.[38] Structural differences, particularly bone diameters, reflect a "genetic" influence similar to the distinct anthropometric characteristics of aquatic athletes (Fig. 13.16). The best long-distance runners inherit a slight build, not only in stature but also in skeletal dimensions. Blending a genetically optimal physique profile with a lean body composition, a highly developed aerobic system, and proper psychologic attitude for prolonged, intensive training, provides the prime ingredients for a champion.

Triathletes

The triathlon combines continuous endurance performance in swimming, bicycling, and running. The extreme of triathlon requirements, the ultraendurance **Ironman competition**, requires competitors to swim 3.9 km (2.4 miles), bicycle 180.2 km (112 miles), and run a standard 42.2 km (26.2 miles) marathon. The serious triathlete's training averages nearly 4 hours daily, covering a total of 280 miles per week by swimming 7.2 miles (30:00 per mile pace), bicycling 227 miles (18.6 mph), and running 45 miles (7:42 per mile pace).[66] Percentage body fat of 6 male and 3 female participants in the 1982 Ironman Triathlon ranged between 5.0 and 11.3% for men and between 7.4 and 17.2% for women. Body fat averaged 7.1% for the top 15 male finishers, with a corresponding $\dot{V}O_2max$ value of 72.0 mL·kg^{-1}·min^{-1}. Triathletes have a body fat content and aerobic capacity comparable to those of other athletes in single endurance sports.[136] A study of 14 triathletes training for the 1984 Ironman competition concluded that the physique of male and female triathletes most resembled that of elite cyclists.[135] Male triathletes possess aerobic capacities similar to trained swimmers; $\dot{V}O_2max$ values for females cluster at the upper range for endurance runners.

Swimmers versus Runners

Male and female competitive swimmers generally have more body fat than distance runners. Speculation suggests that the cool water of the training environment produces lower core temperatures than with equivalent-intensity land exercise. A lower core temperature may prevent the decreased appetite that often accompanies heavy training on land, despite swim training's significant energy requirement.

Limited evidence indicates similar daily energy intakes for male collegiate swimmers (3380 kcal) and distance runners (3460 kcal), which balances training energy expenditure. In contrast, female swimmers averaged a higher daily energy intake of 2490 kcal, compared with 2040 kcal for their running counterparts.[78] However, the swimmers had higher estimated daily energy expenditure than did the runners. The swimmers' energy expenditure even surpassed energy intake, placing them in a slightly *negative* energy balance. Thus, a positive energy balance (intake greater than output) does not explain typically higher percentage body fat levels in male (12%) and female (20%) swimmers than in male (7%) and female (15%) runners. Subsequent research from the same laboratory evaluated energy expenditure and fuel use of swimmers and runners during each form of training (45 min at 75–80% $\dot{V}O_2max$) and 2 hours' recovery.[51] The researchers hypothesized that differences in hormonal response and substrate catabolism between the two exercise modes accounted for body fat differences between groups. The results indicated that the small differences between activities in energy expenditure, substrate use, and hormone levels could *not* account for body fat differences.

Future research must determine whether real differences in physiologic response to land and water training account for body composition differences between swimmers and runners. An alternative explanation suggests that self-selection by the participants causes individuals with higher body fat levels to compete in swimming. Excess body fat presents a liability to energy cost and thermoregulation during weight-bearing exercise on land. Conversely, it contributes importantly to buoyancy and perhaps hydrodynamic economy to forward swimming movement from reduced drag forces.

American Football Players

The first detailed body composition analyses of American professional football players in the 1940s clearly demonstrated the inadequacy of determining a person's "optimal" body mass from height–weight standards.[191] The players as a group had body fat content that averaged only 10.4% of body mass, while FFM averaged 81.3 kg (179.3 lb). Certainly these men were heavy but not fat. The heaviest lineman weighed 118 kg (260 lb, 17.4% body fat, 215 lb FFM) whereas the lineman with the most body fat (23.2%) weighed 115.4 kg (252 lb). Body mass of a defensive back with the least fat (3.3%) was 82.3 kg (182 lb) with a FFM of 79.6 kg (175 lb).

TABLE 13.15 presents a clearer picture for body mass, stature, percentage body fat, and FFM of college and professional players grouped by position.[195,198] The *Pro, older* group consists of 25 players from the 1942 Washington Redskins, the first professional players measured for body composition by hydrostatic weighing. The *Pro, modern* group consists of 164 players from 14 teams in the National Football League (NFL; 69% veterans, 31% rookies). Some 107 members of the 1976 to 1978 Dallas Cowboys and New York Jets make up the third group. Four groups of collegiate players include candidates for spring practice at St. Cloud State College in Minnesota, the University of Massachusetts (UMass), and division III Gettysburg College and teams from the University of Southern California (USC), 1973 to 1977, national champions and participants in two Rose Bowls. Body composition measurements for this data set included hydrostatic weighing with correction for measured residual lung volume.

One would generally expect modern-day professional players to have a larger body size at each position than a representative collegiate group. Although this occurred for comparison with the St. Cloud and UMass players, the USC players generally maintained a physique similar to modern professionals. With the exception of defensive linemen, the USC players at each position showed nearly the same fat content as current professionals. No USC player possessed more than 4.4 kg less FFM than that of the professionals at

Table 13.15	BODY COMPOSITIONS OF COLLEGIATE AND PROFESSIONAL FOOTBALL PLAYERS GROUPED BY POSITION					
Position[a]	Level	N	Stature (cm)	Mass (kg)	Body Fat (%)	FFM (kg)
Defensive backs	St. Cloud[b]	15	178.3	77.3	11.5	68.4
	U Mass[c]	12	179.9	83.1	8.8	76.8
	USC[d]	15	183.0	83.7	9.6	75.7
	Gettysburg[e]	16	175.9	79.8	13.6	68.9
	Pro, modern[f]	26	182.5	84.8	9.6	76.7
	Pro, older[g]	25	183.0	91.2	10.7	81.4
Offensive backs and receivers	St. Cloud	15	179.7	79.8	12.4	69.6
	U Mass	29	181.8	84.1	9.5	76.4
	USC	18	185.6	86.1	9.9	77.6
	Gettysburg	18	176.0	78.3	12.9	68.2
	Pro, modern	40	183.8	90.7	9.4	81.9
	Pro, older	25	183.0	91.7	10.0	87.5
Linebackers	St. Cloud	7	180.1	87.2	13.4	75.4
	U Mass	17	186.1	97.1	13.1	84.2
	USC	17	185.6	98.8	13.2	85.8
	Gettysburg	—	—	—	—	—
	Pro, modern	28	188.6	102.2	14.0	87.6
Offensive linemen and tight ends	St. Cloud	13	186.0	99.2	19.1	79.8
	U Mass	23	187.5	107.6	19.5	86.6
	Gettysburg	15	182.6	110.4	26.2	81.0
	USC	25	191.1	106.5	15.3	90.3
	Pro, modern	38	193.0	112.6	15.6	94.7
Defensive linemen	St. Cloud	15	186.6	97.8	18.5	79.3
	U Mass	8	188.8	114.3	19.5	91.9
	USC	13	191.1	109.3	14.7	93.2
	Gettysburg	11	178.0	99.4	21.9	77.6
	Pro, modern	32	192.4	117.1	18.2	95.8
	Pro, older	25	185.7	97.1	14.0	83.5
All positions	St. Cloud	65	182.5	88.0	15.0	74.2
	U Mass	91	184.9	97.3	13.9	83.2
	USC	88	186.6	96.6	11.4	84.6
	Gettysburg	60	178.0	90.6	18.1	73.3
	Pro, modern	164	188.1	101.5	13.4	87.3
	Pro, older	25	183.1	91.2	10.4	81.3
	Dallas-Jets[h]	107	188.2	100.4	12.6	87.7

[a] Grouping according to Wilmore JH, Haskel WL. Body composition and endurance capacity of professional football players. J Appl Physiol 1972;33:564.
[b] Data from Wickkiser JD, Kelly JM. The body composition of a college football team. Med Sci Sports 1975;7:199.
[c] UMass data from Coach Robert Stull and F Katch, University of Massachusetts. Data collected during spring practice, 1985; %fat by densitometry.
[d] USC data from Dr. Robert Girandola, University of Southern California, Los Angeles, 1978, 1993.
[e] Data courtesy of Dr. Kristin Steumple, Department of Exercise and Sport Science, Gettysburg College, Gettysburg, PA, 2000.
[f] Data from Wilmore JH, et al. Football pros' strengths—and CV weakness—charted. Phys Sportsmed 1976;4:45.
[g] Data from Dr. A. R. Behnke.
[h] Data from Katch FI, Katch, VL. Body composition of the Dallas Cowboys and New York Jets football teams, unpublished, 1978.

each position. The average defensive lineman in the NFL outweighed his USC counterpart in FFM by only 1.8 kg. Total body mass of the professional linemen significantly exceeded that of USC counterparts, primarily because professionals possessed 18.2% body fat versus the collegians 14.7%. These data suggest that elite college and professional players maintain similar body size and body composition.

As a group, professional players of 60 years ago were lower in body fat (10.4%), shorter in stature, and lighter in total body mass and FFM than modern professionals. The exceptions, defensive and offensive backs and receivers, were almost identical to more-current players in body size and composition. The biggest differences in physique emerged for defensive linemen; modern players were 6.7 cm taller, 20 kg heavier, 4.2 percentage points of body fat fatter, and had 12.3 kg more FFM. Obviously, "bigness" was not an important factor in line play during the 1940s. To illustrate this point, the *top* of FIGURE 13.20 shows the average body

weight for all roster players in the NFL (N = 51,333) over a 76-year period. From 1920 to 1985, offensive linemen were the heaviest; this changed beginning with the 1990 season, when defensive linemen achieved the same body mass as the offensive linemen and then surpassed them. While the body mass for offensive linemen appeared to level off at nearly 280 pounds, defensive linemen continued to increase in weight, particularly from 1990 to 1996 At this time, they weighed an average of 16 pounds more or double the weight gain for offensive linemen for the comparable period. On average, offensive linemen were 1.3 pounds heavier per year from 1920 to 1996. At this rate of increase, they should attain 320 pounds by the year 2007 (at an average height of 6 ft 8 in.)! At this size, their BMI equals 35.6, classifying them as high for disease risk (see Fig. 13.1). Even more eye opening is the 2003 Super Bowl football team's 28 offensive and defensive linemen (Oakland Raiders and Tampa Bay Buccaneers); their BMI averaged 37.4 (body mass, 139.2 kg;

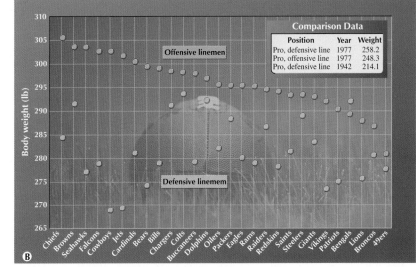

▓ **Figure 13.20 A.** Average body weights by position for all roster players in the NFL between 1920 and 1995. **B.** Average body weights of all roster offensive and defensive linemen in the NFL in 1994. Team rankings progress from the heaviest to lightest body weight for the team's offensive linemen. (From active team rosters for 28 NFL teams as of the first regular-season weekend, September 4–5, 1994.) Comparison of body weight data for the pro offensive and defensive line (1977) shown in the inset box combine data for the New York Jets and Dallas Cowboys football teams (collected by textbook's authors FK and VK). The 1942 data provided by Dr. Albert Behnke from his studies of the Washington Redskins. (Data courtesy of the National Football League public relations department.)

stature, 1.930 cm), the largest yet reported except for the 2001 Super Bowl teams (38.4 BMI) and far in excess of the projected 2007 value. Subsequent research must determine if such relatively homogenous groups of elite, physically active, overweight men experience greater morbidity and mortality than their normal-weight peers.

The body weight of offensive and defensive linemen for each of the NFL teams during the 1994 season *(bottom of figure)* ranged from heaviest (Kansas City Chiefs; Super Bowl 1970) to lightest (San Francisco 49ers; Super Bowls 1990 and 1995). For the 1994 season (the date of the comparison in the bottom figure), the average body weight of the winning Super Bowl offensive line (Dallas Cowboys) ranked fifth highest of 28 teams.

A Worrisome Trend among Less-Skilled and Younger Players

Exceptionally high BMIs also occur at less elite levels of collegiate competition. The average BMI of 33.1 for the Division III 1999 Gettysburg offensive line (N = 15) (29.9 for 2000 offensive line, N = 13)[166] and the BMI of 31.7 for other National Collegiate Athletic Association (NCAA) Division III America football linemen (N = 26; 1994–1995) raises similar concerns about potential health risks for such large young men (stature, 1.84 m; body mass, 107.2 kg).[148] At the high school level, The BMI of *Parade Magazine's* All-American football teams increased dramatically beginning in the early 1970s through 1989 and then further increased in rate of gain to the year 2000.[188] The plot in FIGURE 13.21 shows a clear shift at 1972 in the slope of the regression line *(yellow line)* relating BMI to year of competition compared with age-matched individuals from large-scale epidemiologic normative data *(red line)*. The investigators suggested this shift toward a higher BMI coincided

with either improved nutrition and training and/or the emerging prevalent use among high-school athletes of performance-enhancing drugs such as anabolic steroids. Particularly disturbing are the most recent data for high school offensive and defensive linemen, whose average BMI ranged between 31.8 and 33.5. The implications for such huge body mass in terms of the students' current health risk (e.g., insulin resistance and type 2 diabetes) and long-term outlook remain undetermined.

Other Longitudinal Trends in Body Size

To expand upon longitudinal trends in body size for elite athletes, we determined stature and body mass for two groups of professional athletes: *(a)* all National Basketball Association (NBA) players from 1970 to 1993 (number ranged from 156 to 400) and *(b)* professional major league baseball players from 28 teams during the 1986, 1988, 1990, 1992, and 1995 seasons (5031 roster players).

For the NBA players (FIG. 13.22A), average body mass increased by 3.8 pounds (1.7 kg) or 1.8% during the 23-year interval. Stature increased more slowly; it changed by only 1 inch, or less than 1%, over the same interval. The NBA players' BMI during this time remained within a narrow range of 0.8 BMI units from 23.6 to 24.4. The major league baseball players (shown in *red* in the same figure) reveal slightly higher mean values than did the basketball players. Compared with American professional and collegiate football players, baseball and basketball athletes have maintained BMIs within guidelines considered relatively healthful for minimizing mortality and disease risk.

One might question whether gross body size reflected by BMI relates to sports performance variables. For example, the graphs in Figure 13.22B show the BMI of National and American League Cy Young award winners and their

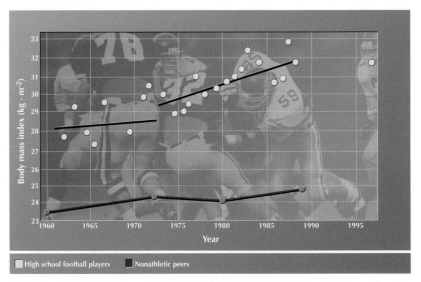

■ **Figure 13.21** Body mass index of high school football players over time compared with nonathlete counterparts.

Figure 13.22 A. BMI, body mass, and stature of professional NBA players (1970–1993) and BMI of major league baseball players (1986–1995). **B.** BMI for American League and National League Cy Young award winners (best baseball pitcher) along with corresponding earned run average (ERA). (Data for NBA players from team rosters, compiled by F. Katch; major league baseball data from team rosters courtesy of Major League Baseball.)

earned run average over the 5-year comparison period. This comparison, while of interest, fails to delineate a clear relation between BMI and performance among the best pitchers in baseball.

Wrestlers

Wrestlers represent a unique athletic group who train intensely and attempt to keep a low body weight with as high a fat-free mass as possible.[24,37,141,142,152,173,201] To discourage the prior practice among wrestlers of rapid weight loss and repeated cycles of weight loss and gain (and the potential for dramatic negative health consequences), the American College of Sports Medicine (ACSM) and NCAA recommended establishing minimal wrestling weight standards based on body fat percentage (discussed in Chapter 14). Current practice mandates a preseason determination of minimal wrestling weight based on a lower limit for body fat percentage (discussed in Chapter 14) determined prior to the start of the competitive season.

In response to the deaths of three collegiate wrestlers in 1997 from excessive weight loss (largely from dehydration), the NCAA introduced rule changes for the 1998–99 season to discourage dangerous weight-cutting practices and increase safe participation.[32] In addition to establishing a minimal wrestling weight, another rule change measures urine specific gravity (ratio of the density of urine to the density of water) to assess hydration status to ensure euhydration of wrestlers at weight certification. Athletes with a urine specific gravity of 1.020 or less are considered euhydrated while those with specific gravity in excess of 1.020 cannot have their body fat assessed to determine minimum competitive wrestling weight for the season. Urine specific gravity reflects hydration status, but it does lag behind true hydration status in periods of rapid body fluid turnover during acute dehydration. Such a scenario would fail to detect a large number of dehydrated wrestlers.[139] Table 13.16 presents recommendations for wrestlers once their appropriate and realistic wrestling weight has been established and achieved.

Table 13.16 **NUTRITION GUIDELINES FOR WRESTLERS**

- Following the Food Guide Pyramid, choose a training diet that is high in complex carbohydrates (55–60% of total energy), moderate in protein (20%), and low in fat (20–25%). Eat well-balanced meals that emphasize carbohydrate-rich fruits, vegetables, cereals, and grains.
- Energy needs depend on body size. The smallest wrestlers need at least 1700 calories per day. If body weight drops more than 2–3 pounds per week, eat more servings of fruits, vegetables, and grains.
- Maintain normal fluid intake and drink back 150% of the weight lost in practice or a match to minimize dehydration and early fatigue.
- Reduce intake of fatty foods such as butter, oils, dressings, and fried foods. Eat foods that are baked, boiled, or broiled.
- Choose fluids that rehydrate and refuel your body. Sports drinks containing carbohydrate (14–17 g per 8 oz) and a small amount of sodium chloride (salt) are formulated to meet these goals.
- After weighing in, rehydrate with sports drinks and consider well-balanced meal-replacement drinks or high-carbohydrate energy drinks to top off energy reserves without causing abdominal discomfort.

- At fast-food restaurants, choose the lower-fat items such as salads, grilled sandwiches, and low-fat yogurt.
- Eat or drink carbohydrates to replenish glycogen after practice or matches.
- Maintain strength and energy reserves by avoiding weight cycling or rapid weight loss.
- Eat small to moderate-sized meals every 3-4 hours to help maintain steady glucose levels and avoid "crashing." This helps to control appetite and reduce binge eating.
- Meal-replacement beverages can be useful in the hours before competition to minimize bulk in the gastrointestinal tract and after competition when appetite may be suppressed. High-carbohydrate supplements are helpful between competitions, especially in tournament situations, to speed restoration of glycogen stores in the body. Sports drinks can help ensure adequate bodily hydration before and during practice sessions and tournaments and can accelerate rehydration after a practice or a match.

Modified from Gatorade Sports Science Institute. Sports Science Exchange Roundtable 41. 2000;11(3).

Weightlifters and Bodybuilders

Men

Resistance-trained athletes, particularly bodybuilders, Olympic weightlifters, and power weightlifters, exhibit remarkable muscular development and FFM and a relatively lean physique. Percentage body fat from underwater weighing averaged 9.3% in bodybuilders, 9.1% in power weightlifters, and 10.8% in Olympic weightlifters.[92] Considerable leanness exists for each group of athletes, even though height–weight tables classify up to 19% of these men as overweight. Groups did not differ in skeletal frame size, FFM, skinfolds, and bone diameters. The only differences occurred for shoulders, chest, biceps (relaxed and flexed), and forearm girths with bodybuilders larger at each site. Bodybuilders exhibited nearly 16 kg more muscle than predicted for their size; power weightlifters, 15 kg; and Olympic weightlifters, 13 kg.

Women

Bodybuilding gained widespread popularity among women in the United States during the late 1970s. As women aggressively undertook the vigorous demands of resistance training, competition became more intense, and the level of achievement increased significantly. Bodybuilding success depends upon a slim and lean appearance, with a well-defined yet enlarged musculature. These requirements raise interesting questions about the women's body composition. How lean do competitors become, and does a relatively large muscle mass accompany their low body-fat levels?

Body composition of 10 competitive female bodybuilders revealed an average of 13.2% body fat (range, 8.0–18.3%) and 46.6 kg of FFM.[53] Except for champion gymnasts, who also average about 13% body fat, bodybuilders were 3 to 4% shorter, 4 to 5% lighter, and had 7 to 10% less total fat mass than other top female athletes. The bodybuilders' most striking compositional characteristic, a dramatically large FFM/FM ratio of 7:1, nearly doubles the 4.3:1 ratio for other female athletic groups. This difference presumably occurred without steroid use (assessed by questionnaire). Interestingly, 8 of the 10 bodybuilders reported normal menstrual function despite relatively low body fat.

Men Versus Women

TABLE 13.18 compares body composition, girths, and excess body mass of male and female bodybuilders. Excess body mass represents the difference between actual body mass and body mass-for-stature from the Metropolitan Life Insurance tables. Overweight for the men corresponded to a 14.8-kg (18%) excess and for the women, a 1.2- kg (2.2%) excess. Obviously, excess body mass for these lean athletes primarily reflected FFM as increased skeletal muscle mass.

Contrasting the girth data allows comparisons of individuals (or groups) who differ in body size. The analysis shows that gender differences in girths, when scaled to body size (referred to as "adjusted" in the table), do not differ as much as the uncorrected girth values. Relative to body size, females exceed the male bodybuilders in 7 of 12 body areas. *Women probably can alter muscle size to the same relative extent as males, at least when scaled to body size.* The larger hip size in women probably relates to greater fat stores in this location.

Table 13.18   **BODY COMPOSITION AND ANTHROPOMETRIC GIRTHS OF MALE AND FEMALE BODYBUILDERS**

Sex	Age, y	Mass, kg	Stature, cm	Fat, %	FFM, kg	Excess Mass,[a] kg
Male (N = 18)	27.0	82.4	177.1	9.3	74.6	14.8
Female (N = 10)	27.0	53.8	160.8	13.2	46.6	1.2

Body Girth (cm)	Males		Females		% Difference (males vs. females)	
	Raw[b]	Adjusted[c]	Raw	Adjusted	Raw	Adjusted
Shoulders	123.1	37.1	101.7	36.7	17.4	1.1
Chest	106.4	32.1	90.6	32.7	14.9	−1.9
Waist	82.0	24.7	64.5	23.3	21.3	5.7
Abdomen	82.3	24.8	67.7	25.1	15.3	−1.2
Hips	95.6	28.8	87.0	31.4	9.0	−9.0
Biceps relaxed	35.9	10.8	25.8	9.3	28.1	13.9
Biceps flexed	40.4	12.2	28.9	10.4	28.5	14.8
Forearm	30.7	9.2	24.0	8.7	21.8	5.4
Wrist	17.4	5.2	15.1	5.4	13.2	−3.8
Thigh	59.6	17.9	53.0	19.1	11.1	−6.7
Calf	37.3	11.2	32.4	11.7	13.1	−4.5
Ankle	22.8	6.9	26.3	7.3	11.0	−5.8

FFM, fat-free body mass.

[a] Body mass minus body mass estimated from height–weight tables. Abraham S, et al. Weight and height of adults 18 to 74 years of age. United States Vital and Health Statistics, series H, no. 211. Washington, DC: U.S. Government Printing Office, 1979.

[b] Actual girth measurement

[c] Girth size relative to body size using method of Behnke (9)

Summary

1. Body composition assessment reveals that athletes generally have physique characteristics unique to their specific sport. For example, field event athletes have relatively large fat-free body mass (FFM) and high percentage body fat, whereas distance runners have the lowest FFM and fat mass.

2. Champion performance blends physique characteristics with highly developed physiologic support systems.

3. Male and female triathletes possess the body composition and aerobic capacity most similar to elite bicyclists.

4. American football players are among the heaviest of all athletes, yet maintain a relatively lean body composition. At the highest levels of competition, collegiate and professional football players attain similar body size and body composition.

5. Competitive male and female swimmers generally have higher body fat levels than distance runners. The difference probably results from self-selection related to economically exercising in the different environments rather than real metabolic effects caused by the environments.

6. Wrestlers, a unique group of relatively lean athletes, undergo severe training and repeated bouts of short-term weight loss. Wrestlers should be discouraged from drastically reducing body fat, especially if it brings them below 5%.

7. The FFM/FM ratio of female bodybuilders significantly exceeds the FFM/FM ratios of other elite female athletes.

8. Female bodybuilders can probably alter muscle size to almost the same relative extent as male bodybuilders.

TEST YOUR KNOWLEDGE ANSWERS

1. False The importance of the BMI is not that it predicts body fat level (although it moderately relates to this variable) but rather its curvilinear relationship to all-cause mortality ratio. As BMI increases, so does the risk for cardiovascular complications including hypertension and stroke, diabetes, and renal disease. The lowest health risk category occurs for individuals with BMIs between 20 and 25, and the highest risk category includes individuals whose BMI exceeds 40.

2. True His BMI = 31.6 kg per m^2 [97.1 ÷ $(1.753)^2$], which exceeds the upper range of BMI values (BMI: normal weight, ≤25.0; overweight, 25.0–29.9; obese, ≥30.0). This classifies him as obese.

3. True The economic cost to women of excess body weight is disproportionately high, and that cost increases as a woman ages. In 1992, the net worth of a moderate-to- severely obese woman was about 40% less than that of a normal-weight counterpart, even after controlling for health, marital status, and other demographic factors. By 1998, an obese woman reported a net worth about 60% less ($135,670 less) than a nonobese peer. No significant economic effect of excess body weight emerged in comparisons for men.

4. False The two sites for body fat deposition are essential fat and storage fat. Essential fat comprises fat stored in the marrow of bones, heart, lungs, liver, spleen, kidneys, intestines, muscles, and lipid-rich tissues of the central nervous system. In the female, essential fat also includes additional sex-specific essential fat. Storage fat consists of fat accumulation in adipose tissue. This includes the visceral fatty tissues that protect the various internal organs within the thoracic and abdominal cavities, and the larger subcutaneous fat tissue volume deposited beneath the skin's surface.

5. True Archimedes showed that an object submerged or floating in water becomes buoyed up by a counterforce equaling the weight of the volume of water it displaces. This buoyant force helps to support an immersed object against the downward pull of gravity. Thus, an object is said to lose weight in water. Because the object's loss of weight in water equals the weight of the volume of water it displaces, specific gravity refers to the ratio of the weight of an object in air divided by its loss of weight in water.

6. False From the Siri equation, percentage body fat computes as follows: 495 ÷ 1.0719 − 450 = 11.8%. Total mass of body fat equals 85 kg × 0.118 = 10.0 kg.

7. False Men with a 102-cm (40-in.) or larger waist and women with waist girth larger than 86 cm (35 in.) maintain a high risk for various diseases. Waist girths of 90 cm for men and 83 cm for women correspond to a BMI threshold of overweight (BMI, 25), while 100 cm for men and 93 cm for women reflect the obesity cutoff (BMI, 30).

8. True Based on an average computed from data in diverse studies, percentage body fat for young adult men averages between 12 and 15%, whereas the average fat value for women ranges between 25 and 28%.

9. False Given the data, desirable fat mass loss computes as follows:

Fat mass = 120 kg × 24% (0.24) body fat = 28.8 kg

Fat-free body mass = 120 kg − 28.8 kg = 91.2 kg

Goal body weight = 91.2 kg ÷ (1.00 − 0.15) = 91.2 kg ÷ 0.85 = 107.3 kg (236.6 lb)

Desirable fat loss = Present body weight − Goal body weight = 120 kg − 07.3 kg = 12.7 kg (28.0 lb)

10. True The body composition for 10 competitive female bodybuilders averaged 13.2% body fat (range, 8.0–18.3%) and 46.6 kg of FFM. Except for champion gymnasts, who also average about 13% body fat, bodybuilders were 3 to 4% shorter, 4 to 5% lighter, and possessed 7 to 10% less total fat mass than other top female athletes. The bodybuilders' most striking compositional characteristic, a dramatically large FFM/FM ratio of 7:1, nearly double the 4.3:1 ratio for other female athletic groups.

References

1. Abe E, et al. Gender differences in FFM accumulation and architectural characteristics. Med Sci Sports Exerc 1998;30:1066.
2. Ainsworth BE, et al. Predictive accuracy of bioimpedance in estimating fat-free mass of African-American women. Med Sci Sports Exerc 1997;29:781.
3. Allison DB, et al. Annual deaths attributable to obesity in the United States. JAMA 1999;282:1530.
4. Ashwell M, et al. Obesity: new insight into the anthropometric classification of fat distribution shown by computed tomography. Br Med J 1985;290:1692.
5. Baumgartner RN, et al. Bioelectric impedance for body composition. In: Pandolf KB, Holloszy JO, eds. Exercise and sport sciences reviews. Vol 18. Baltimore: Williams & Wilkins, 1990.
6. Beals KA, Manore MM. Behavioral, psychological, and physical characteristics of female athletes with subclinical eating disorders. Int J Sport Nutr Exerc Metab 2000;10:128.
7. Beckvid Henriksson G, et al. Women with menstrual dysfunction have prolonged interruption of training due to injury. Gynecol Obstet Invest 2000;49:41.
8. Bedogni G, et al. Comparison of bioelectrical impedance analysis and dual-energy x-ray absorptiometry for the assessment of appendicular body composition in anorexic women. Eur J Clin Nutr 2003;57:1068.
9. Behnke AR, Wilmore JH. Evaluation and regulation of body build and composition. Englewood Cliffs, NJ: Prentice Hall, 1974.
10. Behnke AR, et al. The specific gravity of healthy men. JAMA 1942;118:495.
11. Bemben DA, et al. Musculoskeletal responses to high- and low-intensity resistance training in early postmenopausal women. Med Sci Sports Exerc 2000;32:1949.
12. Billat V, et al. Training and bioenergetic characteristics in elite male and female Kenyan runners. Med Sci Sports Exerc 2003;35:297.
13. Bioelectrical impedance analysis in body composition measurement: National Institutes of Health technology assessment conference statement. Am J Clin Nutr 1996;64(suppl):524S.
14. Bouchard C. Long-term programming of body size. Nutr Rev 1996;54:58.
15. Bouchard C, et al. Inheritance in the amount and distribution of human body fat. Int J Obes 1988;12:205.
16. Brandon LJ. Comparison of existing skinfold equations for estimating body fat in African American and white women. Am J Clin Nutr 1998;67:1115.

17. Bray GA, et al. Evaluation of body fat in fatter and leaner 10-y-old African American and white children: the Baton Rouge Children's Study. Am J Clin Nutr 2001;73:687.

18. Broeder CE, et al. Assessing body composition before and after resistance or endurance training. Med Sci Sports Exerc 1997;29:705.

19. Brooks-Gunn J, et al. The relation of eating problems and amenorrhea in ballet dancers. Med Sci Sports Exerc 1987;19:41.

20. Butts NK. Physiological profile of high school female cross-country runners. Phys Sportsmed 1982;10:103.

21. Cadarette SM, et al.: Evaluation of decision rules for referring women for bone densitometry by dual-energy x-ray absorptiometry. JAMA 2001;286:57.

22. Calle EE, et al. Body-mass index and mortality in a prospective cohort of U.S. adults. N Engl J Med 1999;341:1097.

23. Calle EE, et al. Overweight, obesity, and mortality from cancer in a prospectively studied cohort of U.S. adults. N Engl J Med 2003;348:1625.

24. Carey D. The validity of anthropometric regression equations in predicting percent body fat in collegiate wrestlers. J Sports Med Phys Fitness 2000;40:254.

25. Carter JEL, Ackland TR. Kinanthropometry in aquatic sports. A study of world class athletes. In: Carter JE, Ackland TR, eds. Human Kinetics Sport Science Monograph Series, vol. 5. Champaign, IL: Human Kinetics, 1994.

26. Cassady SL, et al. Validity of near infrared body composition analysis in children and adolescents. Med Sci Sports Exerc 1993;25:1185.

27. Caton JR, et al. Body composition by bioelectrical impedance: effect of skin temperature. Med Sci Sports Exerc 1988;20:489.

28. Chehab FF, et al. Early onset of reproductive function in normal female mice treated with leptin. Science 1997;275:88.

29. Clark RR, et al. A comparison of methods to predict minimal weight in high school wrestlers. Med Sci Sports Exerc 1993;25:1541.

30. Cobb KL, et al. Disordered eating, menstrual irregularity, and bone mineral density in female runners. Med Sci Sports Exerc 2003;35:711.

31. Collins MA, et al. Evaluation of the BOD POD for assessing body fat in collegiate football players. Med Sci Sports Exerc 1999;31:1350.

32. Committee refines wrestling safety rules. NCAA News 1998;35:1.

33. Constantine NW, Warren MP. Physical activity, fitness, and reproductive health in women: Clinical observations. In: Bouchard C, et al., eds. Physical activity, fitness, and health. Champaign, IL: Human Kinetics, 1994.

34. Conway JM, et al. A new approach for the estimation of body composition: infrared interactance. Am J Clin Nutr 1984;40:1123.

35. Côté KD, Adams WC. Effect of bone density on body composition estimates in young adult black and white women. Med Sci Sports Exerc 1993;25:290.

36. Cureton TK. Physical fitness of champion athletes. Urbana, IL: University of Illinois Press, 1951.

37. Dale KS, Landers DM. Weight control in wrestling: eating disorders or disordered eating? Med Sci Sports Exerc 1999;31:1382.

38. DeGaray AL, et al. Genetic and anthropological studies of olympic athletes. New York, Academic Press, 1974.

39. Diabetes Prevention Research Group. Reduction in the incidence of type 2 diabetes with lifestyle intervention or metformin. N Engl J Med 2002;346:393.

40. Eliakim A, et al. Assessment of body composition in ballet dancers: correlation among anthropometric measurements, bio-electrical impedance analysis, and dual-energy x-ray absorptiometry. Int J Sports Med 2000;21:598.

41. Ellis KJ, et al. Body composition of a young, multiethnic female population. Am J Clin Nutr 1997;65:724.

42. Engelen MP, et al. Dual-energy x-ray absorptiometry in the clinical evaluation of body composition and bone mineral density in patients with chronic obstructive pulmonary disease. Am J Clin Nutr 1998;68:1298.

43. Fahey T, et al. Body composition and $\dot{V}O_2$max of exceptional weight-trained athletes. J Appl Physiol 1975;39:559.

44. Fernández JR, et al. Is percentage body fat differentially related to body mass index in Hispanic Americans, African Americans, and European Americans. Am J Clin Nutr 2003;77:71.

45. Fields DA, Goran MI. Body composition techniques and the four-compartment model in children. J Appl Physiol 2000;89:613.

46. Fields DA, et al. Validation of the BOD POD with hydrostatic weighing: influence of body clothing. Int J Obes Relat Metab Disord 2000;24:200.

47. Fields DA, et al. Comparison of BOD POD with the four-compartment model in adult females. Med Sci Sports Exerc 2001;33:1605.

48. Fields DA, et al. Body-composition assessment via air-displacement plethysmography in adults and children: a review. Am J Clin Nutr 2002;75:453.

49. Flegal KM, Troiano RP. Changes in the distribution of body mass index of adults and children in the US population. Int J Obes Relat Metab Disord 2000;24:807.

50. Flegal KM, et al. Prevalence and trends in obesity among US adults, 1999-2000. JAMA 2002;288:1723.

51. Flynn ML, et al. Fat storage in athletes: metabolic and hormonal responses to swimming and running. Int J Sports Med 1990;11:433.

52. Forbes RM, et al. The composition of the adult human body as determined by chemical analysis. J Biol Chem 1953;203:349.

53. Freedson PS, et al. Physique, body composition, and psychological characteristics of competitive female bodybuilders. Phys Sportsmed 1983;11:85.

54. Friedl KE, et al. Evaluation of anthropometric equations to assess body-composition changes in young women. Am J Clin Nutr 2001;73:268.

55. Frisch RE, et al. Delayed menarche and amenorrhea in ballet dancers. N Engl J Med 1980;303:17.

56. Frisch RE, et al. Lower lifetime occurrence of breast cancer and cancers of the reproductive system among former college athletes. Am J Clin Nutr 1987;45:328.

57. Goodpaster BH, et al. Composition of skeletal muscle evaluated with computed tomography. Ann NY Acad Sci 2000;904:18.

58. Gore CJ, et al. Skinfold thickness varies directly with spring coefficient and inversely with jaw pressure. Med Sci Sports Exerc 2000;32:540.

59. Gower BA, et al. Effects of weight loss on changes in insulin sensitivity and lipid concentrations in premenopausal African American and white women. Am J Clin Nutr 2002;76:923.

60. Hetland ML, et al. Running induces menstrual irregularities but bone mass is unaffected, except in amenorrheic women. Am J Med 1993;95:53.

61. Heyward VH, Stolarczyk LM. Applied body composition assessment. Champaign, IL: Human Kinetics, 1996.

62. Hicks VL, et al. Validation of near-infrared interactance and skinfold methods for estimating body composition of American Indian women. Med Sci Sports Exerc 2000;32:531.

63. Hill JO, Peters JC. Environmental contributions to the obesity epidemic. Science 1998;280:1371.

64. Hiura Y, et al. Hypertriglyceridemic waist as a screening tool for CVD risk in indigenous Australian women. Ethn Dis 2003 13(1):80, 2003.

65. Hirata K. Physique and age of Tokyo Olympic champions. J Sports Med Phys Fitness 1966;6:207.

66. Holly RG, et al. Triathlete characterization and response to prolonged competition. Med Sci Sports Exerc 1986;18:123.

67. Hortobagyi T, et al. Comparison of four methods to assess body composition in black and white athletes. Int J Sports Nutr 1992;2:60.

68. Houmard JA, et al. Validity of a near-infrared device for estimating body composition in a college football team. J Appl Sport Sci Res 1991;5:53.

69. Housh TJ, et al. Validity of near-infrared interactance instruments for estimating percent body fat in youth wrestlers. Pediatr Exerc Sci 1996;8:69.

70. Houtkooper LB, et al. Comparison of methods for assessing body-composition changes over 1 y in postmenopausal women. Am J Clin Nutr 2000;72:401.

71. Hu FB, et al. Trends in the incidence of coronary heart disease and changes in diet and lifestyle in women. N Engl J Med 2000;343:530.

72. Hunter GR, et al. Fat distribution, physical activity, and cardiovascular risk factors. Med Sci Sports Exerc 1997;29:362.

73. Israel RG, et al. Validity of near-infrared spectrophotometry device for estimating human body composition. Res Q Exerc Sport 1989;60:379.

74. Istook E Jr. Research funding on major disease is not proportionate to taxpayers' needs. J NIH Res 1997;9:26.

75. Jackson AS, Pollock ML. Generalized equations for predicting body density of men. Br J Nutr 1978;40:497.

76. Jackson AS, et al. Generalized equations for predicting body density of women. Med Sci Sports 1980;12:175.

77. Jackson AS, et al. The effect of sex, age and race on estimating percentage body fat from body mass index: The Heritage Family Study. Int J Obes 2002;26:789.

78. Jang KT, et al. Energy balance in competitive swimmers and runners. J Swim Res 1987;3:19.

79. Janssen I, et al.: Skeletal muscle mass and distribution in 468 men and women aged 18-88 yr. J Appl Physiol 2000;89:81.

80. Janssen I, et al. Body mass index and waist circumference independently contribute to prediction of nonabdominal, abdominal subcutaneous, and visceral fat. Am J Clin Nutr 2002;75:683.

81. Johnston FE. Body fat deposition in adult obese women. I. Patterns of fat distribution. Am J Clin Nutr 1988;47:225.

82. Jurimae T, et al. Relationships between plasma leptin levels and body composition parameters measured by different methods in post-menopausal women. Am J Hum Biol 2003;15:628.

83. Kamba M, et al. Proton magnetic resonance spectroscopy for assessment of human body composition. Am J Clin Nutr 2001;73:172.

84. Katch FI, Katch VL. Measurement and prediction errors in body composition assessment and the search for the perfect prediction equation. Res Q Exerc Sport 1980;51:249.

85. Katch FI, McArdle WD. Prediction of body density from simple anthropometric measurements in college-age men and women. Hum Biol 1973;45:445.

86. Katch FI, McArdle WD. Validity of body composition prediction equations for college men and women. Am J Clin Nutr 1975;28:105.

87. Katch FI, Michael ED. Prediction of body density from skinfold and girth measurements of college females. J Appl Physiol 1968; 25:92.

88. Katch FI, Spiak DL. Validity of the Mellits and Cheek method for body-fat estimation in relation to menstrual cycle status in athletes and non-athletes below 22 percent fat. Ann Hum Biol 1984;11:389.

89. Katch FI, et al. Effects of physical training on the body composition and diet of females. Res Q 1969;40:99.

90. Katch FI, et al. The underweight female. Phys Sportsmed 1980;8:55.

91. Katch VL, et al. Contribution of breast volume and weight to body fat distribution in females. Am J Phys Anthropol 1980;53:93.

92. Katch VL, et al. Muscular development and lean body weight in body-builders and weightlifters. Med Sci Sports 1980;12:340.

93. Kenchaiah S, et al. Obesity and the risk of heart failure. N Engl J Med 2002;347:305.

94. Keys A, et al.: The biology of human starvation. Minneapolis, University of Minnesota Press, 1950.

95. Kim J, et al. Total-body skeletal muscle mass: estimation by a new dual-energy x-ray absorptiometry method. Am J Clin Nutr 2002;76:378.

96. Kohlraush W. Zusammenhang von Korperform und Leistung. Ergebnisse der anthropometrischen Messungen an der Athletern der Amsterdamer Olympiade. Int Z Angrew Physiol 1970;2:187.

97. Kohrt WM. Preliminary evidence that DEXA provides an accurate assessment of body composition. J Appl Physiol 1998;84:372.

98. Kondo M, et al. Upper limit of fat-free mass in humans: A study of Japanese sumo wrestlers. Am J Hum Biol 1994;6:613.

99. Koulmann N, et al. Use of bioelectrical impedance analysis to estimate body fluid compartments after acute variations of the body hydration level. Med Sci Sports Exerc 2000;32:857.

100. Kuczmarski RJ, Flegal KM. Criteria for definition of overweight in transition: background and recommendations for the United States. Am J Clin Nutr 2000;72:1074.

101. Kushner RF, et al. Clinical characteristics influencing bioelectrical impedance analysis measurements. Am J Clin Nutr 1996;64(suppl):423S.

102. Kyle UG, et al. Physical activity and fat-free and fat mass by bioelectrical impedance in 3853 adults. Med Sci Sports Exerc 2001;33:576.

103. LeBlanc A, et al. Muscle volume, MRI relaxation times (T2), and body composition after spaceflight. J Appl Physiol 2000;89:2158.

104. Lee CD, et al. Cardiorespiratory fitness, body composition, and all-cause and cardiovascular disease mortality in men. Am J Clin Nutr 1999;69:373.

105. Lee I-M, et al. U.S. weight guidelines: is it also important to consider cardiorespiratory fitness? Int J Obes 1998;22:S2.

106. Lee RC, et al. Total-body skeletal muscle mass: development and cross-validation of anthropometric prediction models. Am J Clin Nutr 2000;72:796.

107. Lehtonen-Veromaa M, et al. Influence of physical activity on ultrasound and dual-energy x-ray absorptiometry bone measurements in peripubertal girls: a cross-sectional study. Calcif Tissue Int 2000;66:248.

108. Lockner DW, et al. Comparison of air-displacement plethysmography, hydrodensitometry, and dual-energy x-ray absorptiometry for assessing body composition of children 10 to 18 years of age. Ann NY Acad Sci 2000;904:72.

109. Lohman TG, Going SB. Multicomponent models in body composition research: opportunities and pitfalls. Basic Life Sci 1993; 60:53.

110. Lohman TG, et al. Assessing body composition and changes in body composition. Another look at dual-energy x-ray absorptiometry. Ann NY Acad Sci 2000;904:45.

111. Long TD, et al. Lack of menstrual cycle effects on hypothalamic-pituitary-adrenal axis response to insulin-induced hypoglycaemia. Clin Endocrinol (Oxf) 2000;52:781.

112. Loucks AB. Energy availability, not body fatness, regulates reproductive function in women. Exerc Sport Sci Rev 2003;31:144.

113. Loucks AB. Callister R. Induction and prevention of low-T3 syndrome in exercising women. Am J Physiol 1993;264:R924.

114. Loucks AB, et al. Hypothalamic-pituitary-thyroidal function in eumenorrheic and amenorrheic athletes. J Clin Endocrinol Metabol 1992;75:514.

115. Lukaski HC. Methods for the assessment of human body composition: traditional and new. Am J Clin Nutr 1987;46:537.

116. Maddalozzo GF, Snow CM. High intensity resistance training: effects on bone in older men and women. Calcif Tissue Int 2000;66:399.

117. McCrory MA, et al. Evaluation of a new air displacement plethysmograph for measuring human body composition. Med Sci Sports Exerc 1995;27:1686.

118. McKee JE, Cameron N. Bioelectrical impedance changes during the menstrual cycle. Am J Hum Biol 1997;9:155.

119. McLean K, Skinner JS. Validity of the Futrex-5000 for body composition determination. Med Sci Sports Exerc 1992;24:253.

120. Mei Z, et al. Validity of body mass index compared with other body-composition screening indexes for the assessment of body fatness in children and adolescents. Am J Clin Nutr 2002;75:978.

121. Meyer HE, et al. Body mass index and mortality: the influence of physical activity and smoking. Med Sci Sports Exerc 2002;34:1065.

122. Millard-Stafford ML, et al. Use of air displacement plethysmography for estimating body fat in a four-component model. Med Sci Sports Exerc 2001;33:1311.

123. Mitchell HH, et al. The chemical composition of the adult human body and its bearing on the biochemistry of growth. J Biol Chem 1945;158,625.

124. Mitsiopoulos N, et al. Cadaver validation of skeletal muscle measurement by magnetic resonance imaging and computerized tomography. J Appl Physiol 1998;85:115.

125. Miyatani M, et al. Validity of bioelectrical impedance and ultrasonographic methods for estimating the muscle volume of the upper arm. Eur J Appl Physiol 2000;82:391.

126. Modlesky CM, et al. Density of the fat-free mass and estimates of body composition in male weight trainers. J Appl Physiol 1996;80:2085.

127. Must A, et al. The disease burden associated with overweight and obesity. JAMA 1999;282:1523.

128. National Institutes of Health, National Heart, Lung, and Blood Institute. Clinical guidelines on the identification, evaluation and treatment of overweight and obesity in adults—the Evidence Report. Obes Res 1998;6(suppl):51S.

129. National Task Force on the Prevention and Treatment of Obesity. Obesity, overweight and health risk. Arch Intern Med 2000;160:898.

130. Nelson ME, et al. Analysis of body composition techniques and models for detecting change in soft tissue with strength training. Am J Clin Nutr 1996;63:678.

131. O'Brien C, et al. Bioelectrical impedance to estimate changes in hydration status. Int J Sports Med 2002;23:361.

132. Oppliger RA, et al. Bioelectrical impedance prediction of fat-free mass for high school wrestlers validated. Med Sci Sports Exerc 1991;23:S73.

133. Oppliger RA, et al. Body composition of collegiate football players: Bioelectrical impedance and skinfolds compared to hydrostatic weighing. J Orthop Sports Phys Ther 1992;15:187.

134. Ortiz O, et al. Differences in skeletal muscle and bone mineral mass between black and white females and their relevance to estimates of body composition. Am J Clin Nutr 1992;55:8.

135. O'Toole ML. Training for ultraendurance triathletes. Med Sci Sports Exerc 1989;21:209.

136. O'Toole M., et al. The ultraendurance triathlete: a physiological profile. Med Sci Sports Exerc 1987;19:45.

137. Peterson MJ, et al. Development and validation of skinfold-thickness prediction equations with a 4-compartment model. Am J Clin Nutr 2003;77:1186.

138. Phillips SM, et al. A longitudinal comparison of body composition by total body water and bioelectrical impedance in adolescent girls. J Nutr 2003;133(5):1419.

139. Popowski LA, et al. Blood and urinary measures of hydration status during progressive acute dehydration. Med Sci Sports Exerc 2001;33:747.

140. Quesenberry CP, et al. Obesity, health services use, and health care costs among members of a health maintenance organization. Arch Intern Med 1998;158:466.

141. Roemmich JN, Sinning WE. Weight loss and wrestling training: effects of nutrition, growth, maturation, body composition, and strength. J Appl Physiol 1997;82:1751.

142. Sady SP, et al. Physiological characteristics of high-ability prepubescent wrestlers. Med Sci Sports Exerc 1984;16:72.

143. Salamone LM, et al. Measurement of fat mass using DEXA: a validation study in elderly adults. J Appl Physiol 2000;89:345.

144. Sardinha LB, et al. Comparison of air displacement plethysmography with dual-energy absorptiometry and 3 field methods for estimating body composition in middle-aged men. Am J Clin Nutr 1998;68:786.

145. Sartorio A, et al. Changes of bioelectrical impedance after a body weight reduction program in highly obese subjects. Diabetes Nutr Metab 2000;13:186.

146. Saunders MJ, et al. Effects of hydration changes on bioelectrical impedance in endurance trained individuals. Med Sci Sports Exerc 1998;30:885.

147. Schaumberg DA, et al. Relations of body fat distribution and height with cataract in men. Am J Clin Nutr 2000;72:1495.

148. Schmidt WD. Strength and physiological characteristics of NCAA division III American football players. J Strength Cond Res 1999;13:210.

149. Schutte JE, et al. Density of lean body mass is greater in blacks than whites. J Appl Physiol 1984;56:1647.

150. Schweiger V, et al. Caloric intake, stress, and menstrual function in athletes. Fertil Steril 1988;49:447.

151. Schwimmer JB, et al. Health-related quality of life of severely obese children and adolescents. JAMA 2003;289:1851.

152. Scott JR, et al. Acute weight gain in collegiate wrestlers following a tournament weigh-in. Med Sci Sports Exerc 1994;26:1181.

153. Segal KR. Use of bioelectrical impedance analysis measurements as an evaluation for participating in sports. Am J Clin Nutr 1996;64 (suppl):469S.

154. Segal K, et al. Lean body mass estimation by bioelectrical impedance analysis: a four-site cross-validation study. Am J Clin Nutr 1988;47:7.

155. Seidell JC, et al. Abdominal fat depots measured with computed tomography: effects of degree of obesity, sex, and age. Eur J Clin Nutr 1988;42:805.

156. Seidell JC, et al. Waist and hip circumferences have independent and opposite effects on cardiovascular disease risk factors: the Quebec Family Study. Am J Clin Nutr 2001;74:315.

157. Shangold MM, et al. Evaluation and management of menstrual dysfunction in athletes. JAMA 1990;262:1665.

158. Sinha R, et al. Prevalence of impaired glucose tolerance among children and adolescents with marked obesity. N Engl J Med 2002;346:802.

159. Sinning WE. Body composition, cardiorespiratory function, and rule changes in women's basketball. Res Q 1973;44:313.

160. Sinning WE, Lindberg GD. Physical characteristics of college age women gymnasts. Res Q 1972;43:226.

161. Sinning WE, et al. Validity of "generalized" equations for body composition analysis in male athletes. Med Sci Sports Exerc 1985;17:124.

162. Slinde F, Rossander-Hulthén L. Bioelectrical impedance effect of 3 identical meals on diurnal impedance variation and calculation of body composition. Am J Clin Nutr 2001;74:474.

163. Stolarczyk LM, et al. Predictive accuracy of bioelectrical impedance in estimating fat-free mass of Hispanic women. Med Sci Sports Exerc 1995;27:1450.

164. Stolarczyk LM, et al. The fatness-specific bioelectrical impedance analysis equations of Segal et al: are they generalizable and practical? Am J Clin Nutr 1997;66:8.

165. Stollk RP, et al. Ultrasound measurements of intraabdominal fat estimate the metabolic syndrome better than do measurements of waist circumference. Am J Clin Nutr 2003;77:857.

166. Stuempfle KJ, et al. Body composition relates poorly to performance tests in NCAA division III football players. J Strength Cond Res. 2003;17:238.

167. Sun SS, et al. Development of bioelectrical impedance analysis prediction equations for body composition with the use of a multicomponent model for use in epidemiologic surveys. Am J Clin Nutr 2003;77:331.

168. Tanner JM. The physique of the Olympic athlete. London: Allen & Unwin, 1964.

169. Thomas EL, et al. Magnetic resonance imaging of total body fat. J Appl Physiol 1998;85:1778.

170. Thong FS, et al. Plasma leptin in female athletes: relationship with body fat, reproductive, nutritional, and endocrine factors. J Appl Physiol 2000;88:2037.

171. Thorland WG, et al. Midwest wrestling study: prediction of minimal weight for high school wrestlers. Med Sci Sports Exerc 1991;23:1102.

172. Thorland WG, et al. Estimation of body composition in black adolescent male athletes. Pediatr Exerc Sci 1993;5:116.

173. Tipton C.M, Oppliger RA. Nutritional and fitness considerations for competitive wrestlers. In: Simopoulos AP, Pavlou KN, eds. Nutrition and fitness for athletes. World Rev Nutr Diet. 1993;71:84.

174. Tran ZV, Weltman A. Predicting body composition of men from girth measurements. Hum Biol 1988;60:167.

175. Tran ZV, Weltman A. Generalized equation for predicting body density of women from girth measurements. Med Sci Sports Exerc 1989;21:101.

176. Trichopoulou A, et al. Physical activity and energy intake selectively predict the waist-to-hip ratio in men but not women. Am J Clin Nutr 2001;74:574.

177. US Department of Agriculture and US Department of Health and Human Services. Nutrition and your health: dietary guidelines for America. Washington, DC: US Government Printing Office, 2000 (Home and Garden bulletin no. 232.)

178. Utter AC, et al. Evaluation of air displacement for assessing body composition of collegiate wrestlers. Med Sci Sports Exerc 2003;35:500.

179. van der Ploeg GE, et al. Use of anthropometric variables to predict relative body fat determined by a four-compartment body composition model. Eur J Clin Nutr 2003;57(8):1009.

180. Vehrs P, et al. Reliability and concurrent validity of Futrex and bioelectrical impedance. Int J Sports Med 1998;19:560.

181. Vescovi JD, et al. Evaluation of the BOD POD for estimating percentage body fat in a heterogeneous group of human adults. Eur J Appl Physiol 2001;85:326.

182. Vescovi JD, et al. Effects of clothing on accuracy and reliability of air displacement plethysmography. Med Sci Sports Med 2002;34:282.

183. von Eyben FE, et al. Intra-abdominal obesity and metabolic risk factors: a study of young adults. Int J Obes Relat Metab Disord 2003;27(8):941.

184. Wagner DR, et al. Predictive accuracy of BIA equations for estimating fat-free mass of black men. Med Sci Sports Exerc 1997;29: 969.

185. Wagner DR, et al. Validation of air displacement plethysmography for assessing body composition. Med Sci Sports Exerc 2000;32:1339.

186. Wagner DR, et al. Validity of two component models for estimating body fat of black men. J Appl Physiol 2001;90:649.

187. Walberg JL, Johnston CS. Menstrual function and eating behavior in female recreational weight lifters and competitive body builders. Med Sci Sports Exerc 1991;23:30.

188. Wang MQ, et al. Changes in body size of elite high school football players: 1963-1989. Percept Mot Skills 1993;76:379.

189. Ward IC, et al. Reliability of multiple frequency bioelectrical impedance analysis: an intermachine comparison. Am J Hum Biol 1997;9:63.

190. Warren MP. The effects of exercise on pubertal progression and reproductive function. J Clin Endocrinol Metab 1980;51:1150.

191. Welham WC, Behnke AR. The specific gravity of healthy men. JAMA 1942;118:498.

192. Weltman A, et al. Accurate assessment of body composition in obese females. Am J Clin Nutr 1988;48:1179.

193. Weyers AM, et al. Comparison of methods for assessing body composition changers during weight loss. Med Sci Sports Exerc 2002;34:497.

194. Wickelgren I. Obesity: how big a problem? Science 1998;280:1364.

195. Wickkiser JD, Kelly JM. The body composition of a college football team. Med Sci Sports 1975;7:199.

196. Williams MJ, et al. Regional fat distribution in women and risk of cardiovascular disease. Am J Clin Nutr 1997;65:855.

197. Williams NL. Lessons from experimental disruptions of the menstrual cycle in humans and monkeys. Med Sci Sports Exerc 2003;35:1564.

198. Wilmore JH, Haskell WL. Body composition and endurance capacity of professional football players. J Appl Physiol 1972;33:564.

199. Winters KM, Snow CM. Detraining reverses positive effects of exercise on the musculoskeletal system in premenopausal women. J Bone Miner Res 2000;15:2495.

200. Wolk A, et al. A prospective study of obesity and cancer risk. Cancer Causes and Control 2001;12:2001.

201. Wroble RR, Moxley DP. Acute weight gain and its relationship to success in high school wrestlers. Med Sci Sports Exerc 1998;30:949.

202. Wroble RR, Moxley DP. Weight loss patterns and success rates in high school wrestlers. Med Sci Sports Exerc 1998;30:625.

203. Yanovski JA, et al. Differences in body composition of black and white girls. Am J Clin Nutr 1996;64:833.

204. Yeager KK, et al. The female athlete triad: disordered eating, amenorrhea, and osteoporosis. Med Sci Sports Exerc 1993;25:775.

205. Yee AJ, et al. Calibration and validation of an air-displacement plethysmography method for estimating body fat in an elderly population: a comparison among compartmental methods. Am J Clin Nutr 2001;74:637.

206. Zhu S, et al. Waist circumference and obesity-associated risk factors among whites in the third National Health and Nutrition Examination Survey: Clinical action thresholds. Am J Clin Nutr 2002;76:743.

Additional Readings

Aleman Mateo H, et al. Determination of body composition using air displacement plethysmography, anthropometry and bio-electrical impedance in rural elderly Mexican men and women. J Nutr Health Aging 2004;8:344.

Aleman-Mateo H, et al. Body composition by three-compartment model and relative validity of some methods to assess percentage body fat in Mexican healthy elderly subjects. Gerontology 2004;50:366.

Bo M, et al. Body fat is the main predictor of fibrinogen levels in healthy non-obese men. Metabolism 2004;53:984.

Driscoll SD, et al. Effects of exercise training and metformin on body composition and cardiovascular indices in HIV-infected patients. AIDS 2004;18:465.

Garnett SP, et al. Relation between hormones and body composition, including bone, in prepubertal children. Am J Clin Nutr 2004;80:966.

Green JS, et al. The effects of exercise training on abdominal visceral fat, body composition, and indicators of the metabolic syndrome in postmenopausal women with and without estrogen replacement therapy: The HERITAGE family study. Metabolism 2004;53:1192.

Larssoln I, et al. Body composition in the SOS (Swedish Obese Subjects) reference study. Int J Obes Relat Metab Disord 2004;28:1317.

Lim S, et al. Body composition changes with age have gender-specific impacts on bone mineral density. Bone 2004;35:792.

Neovius MG, et al. Sensitivity and specificity of classification systems for fatness in adolescents. Am J Clin Nutr 2004;80:597.

Paillard T, et al. Effects of brisk walking on static and dynamic balance, locomotion, body composition, and aerobic capacity in ageing healthy active men. Int J Sports Med 2004;25:539.

Phares DA, et al. Association between body fat response to exercise training and multilocus ADR genotypes. Obes Res 2004;12:807.

Ruhl CE, et al. Serum leptin concentrations and body adipose measures in older black and white adults. Am J Clin Nutr 2004;80:576.

Sartorio A, et al. Body mass reduction markedly improves muscle performance and body composition in obese females aged 61–75 years: Comparison between the effects exerted by energy-restricted diet plus moderate aerobic-strength training alone or associated with rGH or nandrolone undecenoate. Eur J Endocrinol 2004;150:511.

Slattery ML, et al. Energy balance and rectal cancer: An evaluation of energy intake, energy expenditure, and body mass index. Nutr Cancer 2003;46:166

St-Onge MP, et al. Dual-energy x-ray absorptiometry-measured lean soft tissue mass: Differing relation to body cell mass across the adult life span. J Gerontol A Biol Sci Med Sci 2004;59:796.

van Marken Lichtenbelt WD, et al. Body composition changes in bodybuilders: A method comparison. Med Sci Sports Exerc 2004;36:490.

Whalley GA, et al. Association of fat-free mass and training status with left ventricular size and mass in endurance-trained athletes. J Am Coll Cardiol 2004;44:892.

Chapter

14

Energy Balance, Exercise, and Weight Control

TEST YOUR KNOWLEDGE

Answer these ten statements about energy balance, exercise, and weight control. Use the scoring key at the end of the chapter to check your results. Repeat this test after you have read the chapter and compare your results.

1. **T F** A global obesity epidemic currently exists.

2. **T F** No "racial" differences exist in the prevalence of obesity; over-fatness does not discriminate.

3. **T F** Dietary approaches offer the best defense against regaining lost body weight.

4. **T F** Weight gain is an inevitable consequence of aging.

5. **T F** The most prudent approach to weight control combines moderate food restriction with increased daily physical activity.

6. **T F** During weight loss by food restriction, the body reduces basal energy expenditure.

7. **T F** Very low calorie diets offer the best and fastest method to successfully induce weight loss.

8. **T F** Simply stated, weight gain results from excessive food intake.

9. **T F** Increasing regular physical activity improves one's health status but does little for weight control because of the small number of calories expended during most physical activities.

10. **T F** One must do aerobic exercises for weight loss; weight/resistance exercises offer little value.

Annual food intake in the United States averages about 900 kg and includes 280 eggs, 7 kg of breakfast cereal, 84 kg of meat, 91 kg of fruit, 114 kg of vegetables, 31 kg of bread, 429 soft drinks, 8 L of wine, 96 L of beer, and 8 L of liquor! Physically active men and women often consume 50% more of many of these foods. Only when calories from food exceed daily energy requirements do excess calories store as fat in adipose tissue. Slight but prolonged caloric excess produces substantial weight gain. For example, eating an extra 2 oz of roasted peanuts each day results in a weight gain of about 7.3 kg (16 lb) over a year. To prevent such a caloric disparity, energy output *must* balance energy input.

A random-digit telephone survey of nearly 110,000 U.S. adults found that nearly 70% struggle to either lose weight (29% of men and 40% of women) or just maintain it.[134] Only one fifth of the 45 to 50 million Americans trying to lose weight follow the recommended combination of eating fewer calories and engaging in at least 150 minutes of moderate physical activity weekly. Those attempting weight loss spent nearly $40 billion in the year 2000 (projected to $50 billion in 2006) on weight-reduction products and services, often using potentially harmful dietary practices and drug use while ignoring sensible approaches to weight loss.[28,126] Approximately two million Americans spend more than $125 million on over-the-counter appetite-suppressing diet pills that line the shelves of drugstores, health food and fitness centers, and supermarkets, not to mention sales via TV and radio direct marketing, mail order, and the Internet. Approximately 17.2 million Americans consumed nonprescription weight loss products between 1996 and 1998, 5.0 million used products containing phenylpropanolamine, and 2.5 million used products containing ephedra,[14] with the most common use by young obese women (>25%). Equally disturbing is the use of such products by 8% of normal-weight women. Despite the upswing in

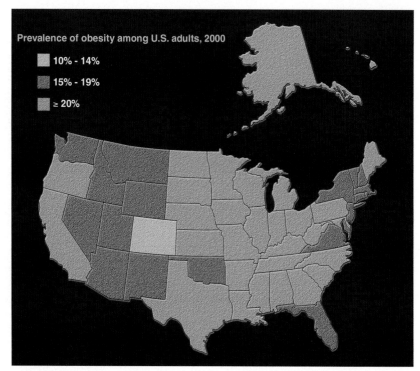

Figure 14.1 The epidemic of obesity among U.S. adults. (From Mokdad AH, et al. The continuing epidemics of obesity and diabetes in the United States. JAMA 2001;286:1195.)

attempts at weight loss, Americans have become considerably more overweight than a generation ago, with obesity increasing in all regions of the United States (Fig. 14.1).[98,99]

On a worldwide basis, the thousands of consumer books published over the past 25 years that advocate fad and bizarre diets or exercise plans for weight loss share one common thread: most claim that their easy-to-use plans guarantee results. If this were true, and a simple solution could maintain the "perfect" body size permanently, then the large number of overly fat Americans could be readily cured. Even when an advertising blitz popularizes a diet plan by "documenting" dramatic weight loss, such schemes often jeopardize the dieter's health. *An additional negative effect of inappropriate strategies for weight loss entails the increased likelihood of impaired physiologic function and exercise performance.*

WORLDWIDE EPIDEMIC

The prevalence of overweight and obesity in adult Americans has increased by 30% in the last 20 years to almost 130 million (www.obesity.org). During this time, the average national body weight has increased by about 10 pounds. A 1999–2000 estimate from a national representative survey of men and women classifies 64.5% of the U.S. population as either overweight (BMI 25.0–29.9) or obese (BMI ≥ 30). Of this total, 30.5% (59 million people) classify as obese compared with only 14.5% in 1980, a doubling of the obese condition.[42] Extreme obesity (BMI ≥ 40) also increased to 4.7% of the population. This form of severe obesity becomes especially high among African American women (6%).[46] According to a 2004 report from the Centers for Disease Control and Prevention, obesity ranks a close second to cigarette smoking as the leading cause of preventable death in America. Fourteen percent of the money spent on health care for American men ages 50 to 69 went to obesity-related complications. If the size of Americans continues to increase at the current rate, by 2020 about one in five health care dollars spent on middle-aged Americans will result from obesity.

Similar increases in obesity worldwide—contributing to the rising tide of type 2 diabetes and cardiovascular disease—has led the World Health Organization and the International Obesity Task Force to declare a global **obesity epidemic**.[105,145] FIGURE 14.2 depicts the powerful effect of excess body weight in predicting death at older age. Overweight, but not obese, nonsmoking men and women in their mid-30s to mid-40s die at least 3 years sooner than normal-weight counterparts. This risk is just as damaging to life expectancy as cigarette smoking.[108] Obese individuals can expect a about a 7-year decrease in longevity. Correctly, physicians tell us to eat less and increase the time spent exercising. In industrialized nations, economic factors operate to counter this advice: food continues to become cheaper and more fat laden, while most occupations have decreased their exertional demands.

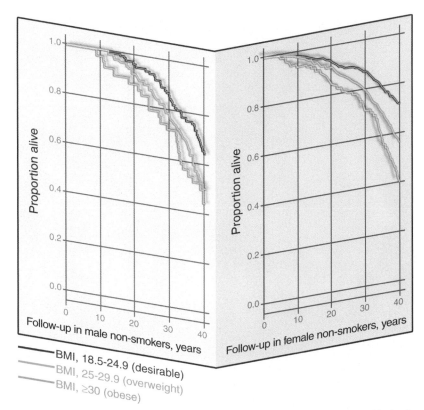

Figure 14.2 Survival estimates for groups of women and men categorized by body mass index (BMI). (From Peeters A, et al. Obesity in adulthood and its consequences for life expectancy. Ann Intern Med 2003;138:24.)

FIGURE 14.3 illustrates the results of a national survey on the prevalence of overweight (defined at the time of this 1994 publication as a BMI ≥ 27) among adults in the United States, compared with the government's objective for the year 2000. Between 1988 and 1991, one third of adults aged 20 to 74 years classified as overweight. This represents a dramatic increase from previous surveys, with obesity incidence particularly high among Hispanic, African American, and Pacific Islander females and other minority groups (*inset table*). Based on the most recent estimate, more than 50% of non-Hispanic black women aged 40 years and older are obese and more than 80% are overweight.[42]

To help stem the obesity epidemic in the United States, on December 1, 2003 the U.S. Preventive Services Task Force, a government advisory group, urged physicians to weigh and measure all patients and recommend counseling and behavior therapy for individuals found to be obese. Specifically, the group recommended that doctors prescribe intensive behavior therapy at least twice a month (in individual or group sessions) for up to three months under supervision of a health-professional team comprised of psychologists, registered dietitians, and exercise specialists. These guidelines, which usually become the standard of care for medical practice, represened a major shift in how the health

care system treats obesity, and may prompt health plans and insurers to pay for obesity treatment.

Disturbingly Prevalent Among Children

Children experience as depressing a situation as adults, because the prevalence of overweight in children (BMI > 95 percentile for age and sex) has attained grim proportions.[106,142] Among U.S. youth, the incidence of overweight has more than doubled in the last 15 years, with an ever-widening gap between the weights of individuals deemed overly fat and those considered thin. Disturbingly, data from the years 1999 and 2000 indicate that excess body fat among children continued on the upswing to claim 15.3% of children aged 6 to 11 years of age, 15.5% aged 12 to 19 years, and 10.4% aged 2 to 5 years, up from an average of 5% in the early 1970s (FIG. 14.4) The rapid rate of increase is particularly prevalent among poor and minority children, in whom excessive body fat represents the most common chronic disorder.[25,41,151] Similar results emerge from a study of Australian children aged 7 to 15 years.[15] In the period from 1985 to 1997, the prevalence of overweight and obesity combined doubled and that of obesity tripled, far greater increases than were observed over the previous 16 years.

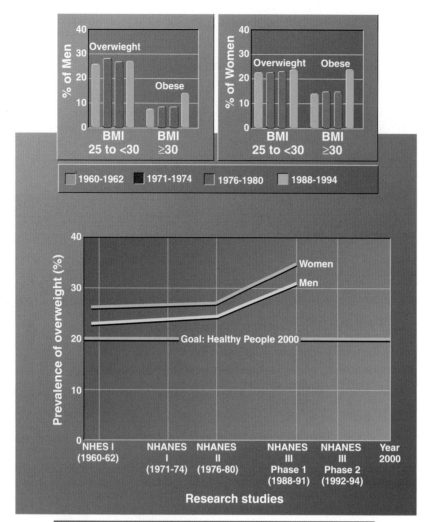

Group	Men (%)*		Women (%)*	
	Overweight	Severely overweight	Overweight	Severely overweight
White	24.4	7.8	24.6	9.6
Black	26.3	10.4	45.1	19.7
Mexican	31.2	10.8	41.5	16.7
Cuban	28.5	10.3	31.9	6.9
Puerto Rican	25.7	7.9	39.8	15.2

*Age-adjusted percentages of overweight and severely overweight persons aged 20-74 y living in the U.S.

▥ **Figure 14.3** The fattening of America. Trends in age-adjusted prevalence of overweight in the U.S. population aged 20 through 74 years, compared with the Healthy People 2000 objective for overweight. The *inset table* presents age-adjusted percentages of overweight and severely overweight persons aged 20 to 74 years from NHANES II (1976–1980) and NHANES I (1971–1974), categorized by ethnicity and gender. NHES, National Health Examination Survey; NHANES, National Health and Nutrition Examination Survey. (From Kuczmarski RJ, et al. Increasing prevalence of overweight among US adults. JAMA 1994;272:205; *inset table* from Kuczmarski RJ, et al. Prevalence of overweight and weight gain in the United States. Am J Clin Nutr 1992;55:495S.) The *inset figure* shows change in the age-adjusted prevalence of overweight and obesity in men and women aged 20 to 74 years from 1960 to 1994. (From National Task Force on the Prevention and Treatment of Obesity. Overweight, obesity, and health risk. Arch Intern Med 2000;160:898.)

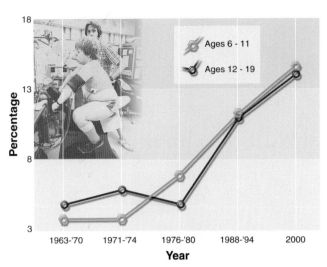

Figure 14.4 A disturbing trend in the percentage of overweight young persons from 1963 to 2000.

A child or adolescent with a high BMI percentile ranking shows a significant risk of being overweight or obese at age 35, and that risk increases with the youth's age.[53] More than 60% of children between ages 5 and 10 years have at least one risk factor for cardiovascular disease. Excessive fatness in one's youth represents even more of an adult health risk than obesity begun in adulthood. For example, overweight children and adolescents, regardless of final body weight as adults, exhibit significantly greater risk for a broad range of illnesses as adults than that of children who maintain a normal body weight.[52,158]

GENETICS PLAYS A ROLE IN BODY WEIGHT REGULATION

Body weight should be viewed as the end result of complex interactions between one's genes and environmental influences, rather than simply the consequence of psychologic factors that affect eating behaviors. Research with twins, adopted children, and specific segments of the population attribute up to 80% of the risk of becoming obese to genetic factors. For example, newborns with large body weights become fat adolescents only when the father or particularly the mother is overweight.[47] Little risk exists for an overweight toddler to grow into an obese adult if both parents are of normal weight. But if a child under age 10, regardless of current weight, has one or both obese parents, the child has more than double the normal risk of becoming an obese adult. Even among normal-weight prepubertal girls, body composition and regional fat distribution relate to the body composition characteristics of both parents.[150]

Genetic makeup does not necessarily cause excessive weight gain. However, in the presence of powerful environmental influences it lowers the *threshold* for gaining weight and contributes to variability in weight gain among individuals fed an identical daily caloric excess.[17,18] The impact of the environment on genetic predisposition largely explains the rapid increase in obesity in the U.S. over the last 25 years.

Studies of a relatively large number of different types of relatives indicate that genetic factors that affect metabolism and appetite determine about 25% of the variation among people in percentage body fat and total fat mass. A larger percentage of variation relates to a transmissible (cultural) effect (unhealthy expression patterns of preexisting genes; FIG. 14.5). *In an obesity-producing environment—sedentary,*

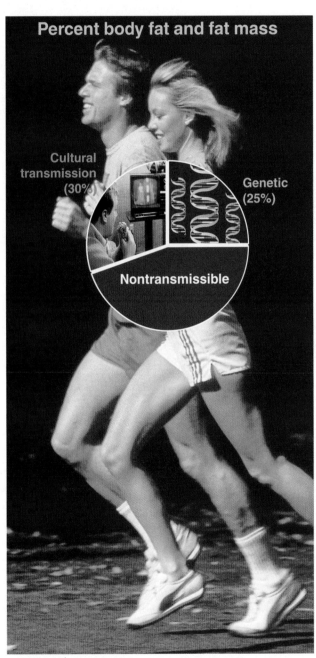

Figure 14.5 Total transmissible and genetically determined variance for body fat. (From Bouchard C, et al. Inheritance of the amount and distribution of human body fat. Int J Obes 1988;12:205.)

stressful, easy access to high-fat foods—the genetically susceptible (obesity-prone) individual gains weight and possibly lots of it.[37,50] Athletes in weight-related sports who have a genetic propensity for obesity must constantly battle to maintain an optimal body weight and body composition for competitive performance.

Racial Factors Contribute

The greater prevalence of obesity among black women (about 50%) compared with white women (33%) has frequently been attributed to racial differences in food and exercise habits and attitudes toward body weight. Studies of obese women whose weight averaged 224 pounds show that small differences in resting metabolism also contribute to the racial differences in obesity.[44,70] On average, black women burned nearly 100 fewer calories each day during rest than their white counterparts; the slower rate of processing calories persists even after adjusting for differences in body mass and body composition. The greater energy economy of black women during exercise and throughout the day reflects an inherited trait as it persists both before and after weight loss.[165] This "racial" effect, which also exists among children and adolescents,[143,149] predisposes a black female to gain weight and regain it after weight loss. A 100-kcal reduction in daily metabolism translates to nearly 1 pound of body fat gained each month. Such data suggest that black female athletes with weight problems may experience greater difficulty achieving and maintaining a goal body weight for competition than an overweight white counterpart.

Possible Mechanisms for Weight Gain

Research with a strain of mice that balloon up to five times the size of normal mice provides evidence for a genetic "destiny" to gain body fat.[175] The mutation of a gene called *obese* (or simply *ob*) disrupts hormonal signals that regulate metabolism, fat storage, and appetite. This causes the energy balance to tip toward fat accumulation.

The model in FIGURE 14.6 proposes that the *ob* gene normally becomes activated in adipose tissue to stimulate production of a body fat-signaling, hormonelike protein (***ob protein**, or **leptin**, identified by researchers at Rockefeller University in 1994) that then enters the bloodstream.[56,109] This satiety signal molecule travels to the ventromedial nucleus, the hypothalamic area of the brain that controls appetite and metabolism. Normally, leptin depresses the urge to eat when food intake maintains ideal fat stores. However, depressed leptin receptor sensitivity signals the brain that the body lacks fat reserves; which can result in overeating. Leptin may affect certain neurons in the hypothalamus to *(a)* stimulate production of chemicals that suppress appetite and/or *(b)* reduce the level of brain chemicals that stimulate appetite. These mechanisms would explain how body fat remains intimately "connected" to the brain (and

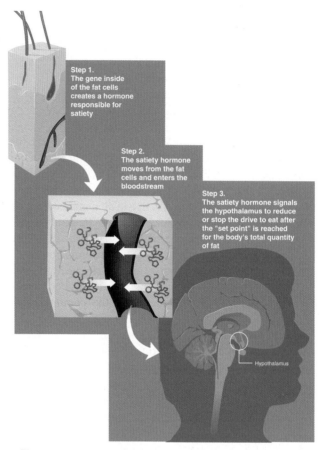

Figure 14.6 A genetic model for obesity. A malfunction of the satiety gene markedly affects production of the satiety hormone leptin (after the Greek word *leptos,* thin). This disrupts the events that occur in *step 3* in the hypothalamus, the center that adjusts body fat level. (Model is based on research conducted at Rockefeller University, New York.) Two general categories of medication treat obesity in the United States: I. Those that decrease food intake by reducing appetite or increase satiety. These medications increase availability of anorexigenic neurotransmitters such as norepinephrine, serotonin, and dopamine in the central nervous system. II. Those that decrease macronutrient absorption in the digestive tract. The fat-fighting chemicals dexfenfluramine (trade name Redux) and fenfluramine (Pondimin) promote release of serotonin thus decreasing appetite. (On Sept. 15, 1997, the FDA asked manufacturers of these drugs to remove them from the market because of their potential for causing damage to heart valves.) Sibutramine (Meridia) alters brain chemicals to trick the body into feeling full, primarily by inhibiting the reuptake of the neurotransmitters norepinephrine and serotonin; orlistat (Xenical) facilitates weight loss by inhibiting intestinal absorption of about one third of ingested lipids.

appetite) via a physiologic pathway to regulate energy balance. In a way, the adipocyte serves an endocrine-like function. With a gene defective for either adipocyte leptin production and/or hypothalamic leptin sensitivity (as probably exists in humans), the brain cannot adequately assess adipose tissue status. Thus, the urge to eat persists.

The hormone–hypothalamic control mechanism fits nicely within the set-point theory (see page 455) to explain abnormal body fat accumulation. It also accounts for the ex-

treme difficulty obese individuals have in sustaining a loss in body fat. Short- or long-term exercise alone does not appear to affect leptin levels in humans. Changes in lifestyle that combine decreased dietary fat intake *and* increased physical activity reduce plasma leptin concentrations below the reduction expected from any change in body fat mass.[110,120]

Leptin alone does not determine obesity or explain why some people eat whatever they want and gain little weight, while others become obese with the same energy intake. Besides defective leptin production, defective receptor action (via a leptin receptor molecule on brain cells) increases resistance to satiety chemicals.[29] A specific gene, the uncoupling protein-2 *(UCP2)* gene, active in all human tissue adds another piece to the obesity puzzle. The *UCP2* gene activates a protein that stimulates the burning of excess calories as heat without coupling to other energy-consuming process.[43] This **futile metabolism** blunts excess fat storage. Individual differences in gene activation and resultant alterations in metabolic activity lend credence to the common claim "Every little bit of excess I eat turns to fat." Finding a drug that turns on the *UCP2* gene to synthesize more heat-generating protein could prove a pharmacologic windfall for shedding excess body fat. Specific drugs and drug combinations that inhibit brain chemicals that stimulate appetite may ultimately provide the long-term "cure" for the overly fat condition in a way similar to drug use to manage such chronic conditions as hypertension and diabetes.

BIOCHEMICALS THAT INFLUENCE EATING BEHAVIORS: SIGNALS THAT TRAVEL AMONG THE DIGESTIVE TRACT, ADIPOSE TISSUE, AND EATING-CONTROL CENTERS

- **Leptin:** Produced by adipocytes. Normal levels signal the hypothalamus to maintain food intake so body weight remains stable. Below-normal leptin levels signal the brain to increase appetite so that body fat levels increase. Leptin also elevates metabolic rate.

- **Peptide YY3-36 (PYY):** Produced by intestinal cells in response to food intake. It then travels to the hypothalamus to inhibit the urge to eat. Overweight persons normally make less of this satiety signal than persons of normal body weight.

- **Neuropeptide Y:** A transmitter protein of the nervous system that stimulates food intake and regulates metabolism and fat synthesis.

- **Ghrelin:** Exerts effects opposite to those of leptin. A powerful appetite-stimulating hormone (also slows energy output) produced in the stomach and small intestine. Only known natural appetite stimulant made outside the brain. Drugs that block this hormone would not only stimulate weight loss but also increase energy expenditure.

- **Melanocortin-4:** Possibly supplies the signal to stop eating. About 10% of obese patients show genetic mutations in the gene that regulates this compound.

PHYSICAL ACTIVITY: A CRUCIAL COMPONENT IN WEIGHT CONTROL

The standard dietary approach to weight loss that decreases caloric intake below the requirement for current weight maintenance generally helps obese patients lose about 0.5 kg per week.[161] Success at preventing weight regain remains relatively poor, averaging between 5 and 20%. Weight loss professionals now argue that regular physical activity, through either recreation or occupation, effectively contributes to preventing weight gain and thwarts the tendency to regain lost weight.[69,80,131,168] For example, individuals who maintain weight loss over time show greater muscle strength and engage in more physical activity than counterparts who regained lost weight.[166] Variations in physical activity alone accounted for more than 75% of the regained body weight. Such findings point up the need to identify and promote strategies that increase regular physical activity. Current national guidelines by the Surgeon General and Institute of Medicine, respectively, recommend a minimum of 30 to 60 minutes of moderate physical activity daily. We endorse an increase to 80 minutes of daily exercise to combat the prevalence of obesity in the U S population.

Older men and women who maintain active lifestyles thwart the "normal" pattern of fat gain in adulthood.[82,114] Middle-aged male distance runners remain leaner than sedentary counterparts.[170] Time spent in physical activity inversely relates to body fat level in young and middle-aged men who exercise regularly.[59,96] Surprisingly, no relationship emerged between the runners' body fat level and caloric intake. Thus, the greater level of body fat among active middle-aged men compared with younger, more active counterparts resulted from less vigorous training, *not* greater energy intake.

From age 3 months to 1 year, the total energy expenditure of infants who later became overweight averaged 21% less than infants with normal weight gain.[121] For children aged 6 to 9 years, percentage body fat inversely related to physical activity level in boys but not in girls.[9] Obese preadolescent children generally spend less time in physical activity or engage in lower-intensity physical activity than normal-weight peers.[30,159] By the time young girls reach adolescence many do no leisure-time physical activity. For girls, the decline in time spent in physical activity averaged nearly 100% among blacks and 64% among whites between ages 9 or 10 and 15 or 16.[78] By age 16 or 17, 56% of the black girls and 31% of the white girls reported no leisure-time physical activity. The 24-hour energy expenditure of young-adult Native Americans inversely related to body weight changes over a 2-year period.[118] A four times greater risk of gaining more than 7.5 kg occurred in individuals with low rather than high 24-hour energy expenditures.

Increasing Energy Output May Help as One Ages

For male runners 18 years of age and older, maintaining a lifestyle that included a regular but constant level of exercise did not fully forestall the tendency to add weight through middle age. FIGURE 14.7 shows the strong inverse association between distance run and BMI and waist circumference in all age categories. Active men were leaner than sedentary counterparts for each decade. Those who ran longer distances each week weighed less than those who ran shorter distances. The typical man who maintained a constant weekly running distance through middle age added 3.3 pounds while waist size (presumably from intraabdominal fat) increased about three fourths of an inch, regardless of

distance run. Such findings suggest that by age 50, a physically active man can expect to weigh about 10 pounds more (with a 2-inch larger waist) than he weighed at age 20, despite maintaining a constant level of physical activity. The reasons for this proclivity to gain weight and girth remain unknown. Perhaps, reduced testosterone and growth hormone levels induce age-related change in physique and increase abdominal and visceral fat. The researchers advise annually increasing weekly exercise by about 1.4 miles starting at age 30 to effectively counter weight gain with aging. One can achieve the same effect without additional exercise by modestly reducing energy intake while making more nutritious food selections.

WEIGHT LOSS: A UNIQUE DILEMMA FOR THE COMPETITIVE ATHLETE

For many "overweight" athletes whose competitive careers have ended, achieving a lighter body weight and favorable body composition (combined with proper nutritional practices) offers overall health benefits. For the athlete currently competing, successful performance depends on achieving an "ideal" body mass and body composition. In figure skating, ballet dancing, diving, gymnastics, and bodybuilding, success often requires a predefined "aesthetic look." To complicate matters, the relatively low intensity of training in some of these sports contributes little to fat loss.

Reduced Body Size Affects Exercise Performance

In weight-bearing competitive sports like racewalking, running, cross-country skiing, and ice skating, energy cost relates directly to body mass. Consequently, achieving the lightest body weight without compromising physiologic function and metabolic capacity should improve performance. In weight-supported sports like swimming, body weight reduction may not have as dramatic an affect on performance, although a smaller body size should reduce the drag forces that impede movement through the water.

Drag force, the resistance created by the friction of air or water as the athlete moves forward, profoundly affects athletic performance. Drag resistance affects competitive racewalking and running, especially when advancing into a headwind. The effect becomes pronounced as forward velocity further increases, as in speed skating, ski jumping, and bicycling and in swimming, where the drag force from water becomes extreme. The body postures and specialized aerodynamic and hydrodynamic suits, equipment, and techniques (e.g., shaving the head and skin by swimmers) represent attempts to reduce drag forces and improve overall economy of effort.

A reasonable approach to enhance performance for some athletes involves reducing body weight, particularly fat

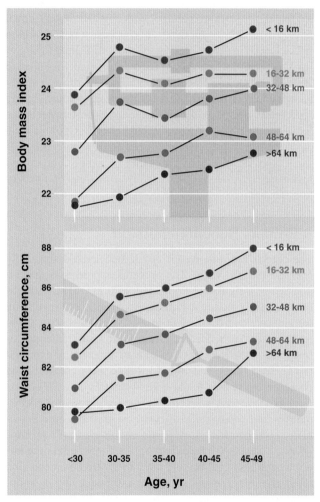

Figure 14.7 Relationship of average body mass index (BMI, kg per m²) *(top)* and waist circumference *(bottom)* and age for men who maintained constant weekly running of varying distances. Analyses of these relationships indicate that men who annually increase their distance run by 1.39 miles (2.24 km) per week compensate for the anticipated weight gain during middle age. (From Williams PT. Evidence for the incompatibility of age-neutral overweight and age-neutral physical activity standards from runners. Am J Clin Nutr 1997;65:1391.)

mass. Pole-vaulters and jumpers who reduce body weight without compromising skill and power-output capacity achieve greater ease in overcoming the force of gravity. The same holds true for runners, skaters, cyclists, and others who compete at high movement velocities. Not only does the resistance of gravity diminish with a lighter body weight, but also the impeding effects of the drag force created by air (or water) becomes less with a smaller body frontal surface area.

A Prudent Approach Most Effective

To reduce body size, a person can decrease weight in a relatively short time by restricting food and fluid intake and sweating excessively. Body weight loss in this situation occurs mainly from water loss and depletion of liver and muscle glycogen reserves. Longer-term attempts at weight loss through semistarvation increase the risk of depressing resting metabolism (making continued weight loss more difficult) and increasing lean tissue loss. For example, many adolescent wrestlers chronically restrict energy and protein intake during the wrestling season; this reduces lean tissue mass, glycogen stores, and muscular strength and power.[123] Severe dehydration in trying to "make weight" also places these individuals at risk for heat injury. *Combining moderate food restriction with additional daily physical activity offers the greatest flexibility for achieving fat loss, yet remaining well nourished for training and peak performance.*

The potential to improve competitive performance with weight loss assumes that any lost weight does not adversely affect skill, strength, or power capacity. If these important determinants of performance deteriorate, the athlete does worse not better. The weight loss program must not adversely affect daily training. One should view weight loss from a longer-term perspective, because body fat's contribution to an energy deficit increases as the duration of weight loss progresses. No more than 1 or 2 pounds (about 1% of body mass) should be lost each week to minimize adverse effects of weight loss on fat-free body mass (FFM), nutrient status, and exercise performance. Food composition tables or appropriate computer software should assess nutrient status to ensure maintenance of the predetermined daily caloric deficit and recommended carbohydrate, protein, and micronutrient intake. Concurrently, body composition evaluation can regularly assess the compositional characteristics of the weight lost.

THE ENERGY BALANCE EQUATION APPLIED TO WEIGHT LOSS

Guidelines for weight loss generally come from studies of sedentary, overly fat individuals. While precise recommendations do not exist for physically active men and women or competitive athletes, the current understanding of prudent body fat loss should also apply to these individuals. As discussed in Chapter 7 and illustrated in Figure 7 the human body functions in accord with the laws of thermodynamics. If total daily food calories exceed daily energy expenditure, excess calories accumulate as fat in adipose tissue. Conversely, if energy expenditure exceeds the energy from food intake body weight decreases.

Three methods unbalance the energy balance equation to produce weight loss:

1. Reduce caloric intake below daily energy requirements
2. Maintain daily caloric intake and increase energy expenditure through additional physical activity
3. Decrease daily caloric intake and increase daily energy expenditure

When considering the sensitivity of overall energy balance, note that if daily energy intake exceeds output by only 100 kcal, the surplus calories consumed in a year equal 36,500 kcal (365 × 100 kcal). Because each pound (454 g, or 0.45 kg) of body fat consists of about 87% lipid (454 g × 0.87 = 395 g × 9 kcal·g^{-1} = 3555 kcal (usually rounded to 3500 kcal) per 0.45 kg), this caloric excess causes a yearly gain of about 4.7 kg (10.3 lb) of body fat. In contrast, if daily food intake decreases by 100 kcal, and energy expenditure increases by 100 kcal (e.g., by jogging one extra mile each day), then the yearly caloric deficit equals about 9.5 kg (21 lb) of body fat. Whether shifting dietary composition toward higher carbohydrate content actually affects body fat gain or loss remains unresolved.[21,65,169]

A Prudent Recommendation

The objective of obesity therapy has changed dramatically over the past 10 years. The previous approach assigned a goal body weight that coincided with an "ideal" weight based on body stature and mass. Achievement of goal body weight heralded the weight-loss program's success. Currently, the World Health Organization, the Institute of Medicine of the National Academy of Sciences, and the National Heart, Lung and Blood Institute recommend that an obese person reduce initial body weight by 5 to 15%. *This more realistic weight loss diminishes weight-related comorbidities and complications from hypertension, type 2 diabetes, and abnormal blood lipids and often exerts a positive effect on social–psychologic complications.* Setting the initial weight loss goal beyond the 5 to 15% recommendation often gives patients an unrealistic and potentially unattainable target in light of current treatment methods.

DIETING TO TIP THE ENERGY BALANCE EQUATION

Many people believe that *only* calories from dietary lipids increase body fat. These individuals reduce lipid intake

(generally a good idea) but often disproportionately increase carbohydrate and protein intakes so total caloric intake remains unchanged or even increases. *Weight loss occurs whenever energy output exceeds energy intake regardless of the diet's macronutrient mixture, reaffirming the first law of thermodynamics.* A prudent dietary approach to weight loss unbalances the energy balance equation by reducing daily energy intake 500 to 1000 kcal below daily energy expenditure. Moderately reduced food intake produces greater body fat loss in relation to the energy deficit than more severe energy restriction that exacerbates loss of FFM. In addition, individuals poorly tolerate a prolonged caloric restriction of more than 1000 kcal a day; this form of semistarvation increases the chances for poor nourishment and depletion of the all-important glycogen reserves. Total energy intake, not diet composition, determines the effectiveness of weight loss with reduced-energy diets.[48]

Suppose an overly fat man who consumes 3800 kcal daily and maintains body mass of 80 kg wishes to reduce 5 kg by dieting. He maintains his activity level but decreases food intake to create a daily caloric deficit of 1000 kcal. Thus, instead of consuming 3800 kcal, he takes in only 2800 kcal daily. In 7 days, the accumulated deficit equals 7000 kcal, or the energy equivalent of 0.9 kg (2 lb) of body fat. Actually, he would lose considerably more than 0.9 kg during the first week because initially the body's glycogen stores make up a substantial portion of the energy deficit. Stored glycogen contains fewer calories per gram and considerably more water than stored fat. For this reason, short periods of caloric restriction often encourage the dieter but produce a large percentage of water and carbohydrate loss per unit weight loss, with only a small decrease in body fat. As weight loss progresses, a larger proportion of body fat supports the energy deficit created by food restriction. To reduce body fat by an additional 1.4 kg, the dieter must maintain the reduced caloric intake of 2800 kcal for another 10.5 days; at this point, body fat theoretically decreases at a rate of 0.45 kg every 3.5 days.

Weight Loss Results Not Always Predictable

The mathematics of weight loss through caloric restriction seems straightforward, but the results do not always follow. One assumes that daily energy expenditure remains relatively unchanged throughout the dieting period. However, some dieters experience lethargy (often related to depletion of the body's glycogen stores); this decreases daily energy expenditure. The energy cost of physical activity also decreases proportionally with body weight reduction. This shrinks the energy output side of the energy balance equation. As we discuss in the next section, the body also "defends" itself against a depressed caloric intake by reducing resting metabolism, which further blunts the weight loss effort.

Set-Point Theory: A Case Against Dieting

One can reduce large amounts of weight in a relatively short time simply by not eating, but success remains short-lived, and eventually the urge to eat wins out and the lost weight returns. Some argue that the reason for this failure lies in a genetically determined "set point" that differs from what the dieter would like. The proponents of a **set-point theory** maintain that all persons (fat or thin) have a well-regulated internal control mechanism located deep within the lateral hypothalamus that tightly maintains a preset level of body weight and/or body fat. In a practical sense, this represents a person's body weight when not counting calories. Exercise and drugs (e.g., fenfluramine, amphetamines, and nicotine) lower a person's set point, whereas dieting exerts no effect. Each time body fat decreases below one's preestablished set point, internal adjustments and regulatory mechanisms resist the change and attempt to conserve and/or replenish body fat. For example, resting metabolism slows, and the individual becomes obsessed with food, unable to control the urge to eat. Even when a person overeats to gain weight above the normal level, the body resists this change by increasing resting metabolism and causing the person to lose interest in food.

Resting Metabolism Decreases. *Resting metabolism often decreases when dieting progressively produces weight loss.*[39,89,100,167] This hypometabolism in response to caloric deficit often exceeds the decrease attributable to the loss of body mass or FFM. An overly reduced metabolism characterizes individuals attempting to lose weight, whether they dieted previously or whether they are fat or lean. Depressed metabolism conserves energy, causing the diet to become less effective despite a restricted caloric intake. This produces a weight-loss plateau at which further weight loss becomes considerably less than predicted from the mathematics of the restricted energy intake.

FIGURE 14.8 depicts the body's defense against deviations in body weight. This classic study carefully monitored body mass, resting oxygen uptake (minimal energy requirement), and caloric intake of six obese men for 31 days. During the prediet period, body mass and resting oxygen uptake stabilized with a daily food intake of 3500 kcal. When subjects then switched to 450-kcal low-calorie diet, body mass and resting metabolism decreased, and the percentage decline in metabolism exceeded the body mass decrease. The *dashed line* represents the expected weight loss from the 450-kcal diet. The decline in resting metabolism (*middle figure*) conserved energy, causing the diet to become progressively less effective. More than one half of the total weight loss occurred over the first 8 days of dieting; the remaining weight loss occurred during the final 16 days. A plateau in the theoretical weight-loss curve often frustrates and discourages dieters, causing them to abandon the program.

Further disconcerting news awaits those desiring permanent fat loss. When obese persons lose weight, adipocytes increase their level of the fat-storing enzyme lipoprotein li-

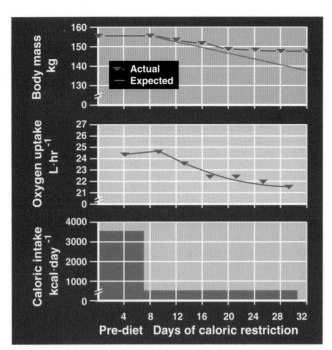

Figure 14.8 Effects of two levels of caloric intake on changes in body mass and resting oxygen uptake. Failure to lose weight at a rate predicted from food restriction leaves the dieter frustrated and discouraged. (Adapted from Bray G. Effect of caloric restriction on energy expenditure in obese subjects. Lancet 1969;2:397.)

pase.[77] Unfortunately, this adaptation facilitates body fat synthesis, and the fatter the person before weight loss the greater the lipoprotein lipase production with weight loss. This observation supports the existence of a feedback mechanism between the brain and body fat levels and helps to explain the great difficulties overweight persons encounter in maintaining weight loss.[56,65,173]

The set-point theory delivers unwelcome news to those with a set point tuned "too high." Fortunately, regular exercise may lower the set-point level. Concurrently, regular exercise conserves and even increases FFM, raises resting metabolism (if FFM increases), and alters metabolism to facilitate fat breakdown.[64,89,100,155] These healthful adaptations all augment the weight loss effort. Food intake declines initially with regular exercise for overly fat men and women. Eventually, as an active lifestyle continues and body fat reserves decrease, caloric intake balances daily energy requirements, and body mass stabilizes at a new, lower level.

Challenge to the Set-Point Proponents. Some research challenges the argument that individuals who lose weight necessarily *maintain* the initial depressed metabolism that predisposes them to weight regain.[164] Without doubt, energy restriction produces a *transient state* of hypometabolism if the dieter maintains the state of negative energy intake. This adaptive downregulation in resting metabolism does not persist when individuals lose weight but then reestablish (at their lower body weight) a balance in which energy intake equals energy expenditure. Consequently, research that fails to establish energy balance after a period of weight loss gives the inaccurate impression that individuals who lose weight necessarily battle a prolonged overcompensating reduction in resting energy expenditure until they return to their original body weight. Replication of these findings will support the contention that downregulation of resting metabolism is not a necessary characteristic of weight loss or a primary component to explain the tendency for weight regain.

Weight Cycling: Going No Place Fast

The futility of repeated cycles of weight loss and weight gain (referred to as the **yo-yo effect**) emerged from food efficiency studies that evaluated weight loss–weight gain as related to ingested calories in animals. Considerable debate exists on this subject,[12,60,72,103,116,172] but weight regain may occur more readily with repeated cycles of weight loss. For example, animals require twice the time to lose the same weight during a second period of caloric restriction and only one third the time to regain it.[22]

Obesity raises the risk of heart disease, yet failure to keep off the lost weight may pose an additional risk. Initial reports indicated that repeated bouts of weight loss–weight regain increased the likelihood of death from a heart attack. The risk averaged almost 70% more for weight regainers than for those who maintained body weight.[73] In contrast, data from 6500 originally healthy Japanese American men revealed no ill effects from a repeated cycle of weight loss and regain.[68] The periods of rapid weight loss and regain common in dieters do not increase hypertension risk any more than the increased risk from being overweight or gaining weight in the first place.[23] Furthermore, repeated cycles of dieting do not induce adverse psychologic effects for stress level, anxiety, anger, and depression.[137]

If weight cycling should pose an additional health risk, one can only speculate on the potential long-term negative effects from repeated weight cycling so common among high school and collegiate wrestlers and others that compete in sports requiring a lean and/or low body mass. From a public health perspective, however, the risks from overweight and obesity far exceed those for weight cycling. *The obese should not use the potential hazards of yo-yo dieting as an excuse to abandon efforts to reduce excess body fat. In particular, this includes efforts to increase "extra" physical activities of daily living and sports and recreational activities.*

Extremes of Dieting: Potential Negative Consequences for the Physically Active Individual

Professional organizations have voiced strong opposition to certain dietary practices, particularly extremes of fasting and low-carbohydrate, high-fat, and high-protein diets. These practices remain troublesome to professionals in sports

medicine and exercise physiology because of reports documenting that physically active individuals often exhibit bizarre and pathogenic weight-control behaviors and disordered eating patterns. Imprudent eating behaviors negatively affect body composition, energy reserves, and psychologic and physical well-being (see Chapter 15).

Low-Carbohydrate Ketogenic Diets

Low-carbohydrate ketogenic diets *emphasize carbohydrate restriction while generally ignoring total calories and the diet's protein, cholesterol, and saturated fat content.* Billed as a "diet revolution" and championed by the late Dr. Robert C. Atkins,[8] the diet was first promoted in the late 1800s and has appeared in various forms since. Long disparaged by the medical establishment, advocates maintain that restricting daily carbohydrate intake to 20 g or less for the initial 2 weeks, with some liberalization afterward, causes the body to mobilize significant fat for energy. This generates excess plasma ketone bodies—byproducts of incomplete fat breakdown from inadequate carbohydrate catabolism—that supposedly suppress appetite. Theoretically, the ketones lost in the urine represent unused energy that should facilitate further weight-loss. Proponents claim that urinary energy loss becomes so great that dieters can eat all they want provided they restrict carbohydrates. Often not considered is the fact that restricting the carbohydrate-containing foods that most people eat creates a low-calorie diet that produces weight loss.

At best, energy lost by urinary ketone excretion equals only 100 to 150 kcal daily.[2] This accounts for a small weight loss of approximately 0.45 kg per month—not appealing when lipid intake as high as 70% of total calories represents the primary food source. Initial weight loss also results from dehydration from an extra solute load on the kidneys that increases water excretion. Water loss does *not* reduce body fat. *A low-carbohydrate diet rapidly depletes glycogen reserves, which severely affects one's ability to train hard and compete.* This diet also sets the stage for significant loss of lean tissue as the body recruits amino acids from muscle to maintain blood glucose (gluconeogenesis)—an undesirable side effect for a diet designed for body fat loss.

Although an estimated 25 to 30 million Americans attempted a low-carbohydrate diet in 2003, whether the ketogenic diet facilitates fat loss more than a well-balanced, low-calorie diet remains unclear. In general, weight loss relates principally to the diet's low caloric content and diet duration rather than reduced carbohydrate content.[20] Three recent controlled clinical trials compared the Atkins-type, low-carbohydrate diet with traditional low-fat diets for weight loss.[45,130,174] The low-carbohydrate diet was more effective in achieving a modest weight loss for severely overweight people. Some measures of heart health also improved as reflected by a more favorable blood lipid profile and glycemic control in those who followed the low-carbohydrate diets for up to 1 year.[140] Such findings add a measure

of credibility to the use of low-carbohydrate diets and challenge conventional wisdom concerning the potential dangers from consuming a high-fat diet.

Importantly, Atkins-type, high-fat low-carbohydrate diets require systematic long-term evaluation (up to 5 years) for safety and effectiveness, particularly as related to the blood lipid profile. The diet, which places no limit on the amount of meat, fat, eggs, and cheese a person eats, may pose potential hazards. For example, low-carbohydrate, high-protein diets raise serum uric acid levels, potentiate the development of kidney stones, alter electrolyte concentrations to initiate cardiac arrhythmias, cause acidosis, aggravate existing kidney problems from the extra solute burden in the renal filtrate, deplete glycogen reserves to contribute to a fatigued state, decrease calcium balance and increase risk for bone loss, and cause dehydration. This diet is definitely contraindicated during pregnancy, because it retards fetal development from inadequate carbohydrate intake.

The South Beach Diet: A More Prudent Approach. In many ways, the currently popular South Beach diet, advocated by cardiologist Dr. Arthur Agatston, does not differ from the low-carbohydrate diet plan promoted successfully by Atkins. Both individuals believe that refined carbohydrates and white flour greatly contribute to the nation's climbing obesity rate. Like the Atkins diet, the South Beach diet strictly limits intake of bread, potatoes, and other carbohydrates while permitting consumption of higher-fat red meat, cheese, and eggs. Advocates argue that most carbohydrate foods in the U.S. diet are of the high glycemic variety that digest and absorb rapidly and raise blood glucose levels. This rise causes an insulin spike and rebound hypoglycemia that produces greater hunger and subsequently greater food intake that leads to weight gain. The increase in insulin stimulates greater storage of lipid within fat cells by downregulating hormone-sensitive lipase that helps to degrade lipid. In addition, the additional insulin increases the concentration of acetyl CoA carboxylase, which further promotes lipid storage. Keeping insulin levels depressed would theoretically allow more energy to be derived from lipid (and thus reduce body weight from the loss in lipid). In contrast to the Atkins diet that allows just about any fatty food with a low starch content, Dr. Agatston emphasizes moderate intake of unsaturated fats, like those in olive oil, fish, and nuts. The diet prohibits foods such as butter, margarine, bacon, or anything fried. Carbohydrates are permitted if they are of the slow-release unrefined, complex variety (relatively low glycemic index); these include multigrain bread, wild rice, lentils, and soy milk.

The first 2 weeks of the diet (phase 1) focus on stabilizing blood glucose by consuming only foods with the lowest glycemic indexes. Fiber-rich carbohydrates and unsaturated fatty acids are gradually reintroduced in phase 2 (until desired weight is reached) and phase 3 (maintenance). If weight gain occurs, the individual returns to phase 1. In

essence, the effectiveness of the South Beach diet hinges on whether it reduces caloric intake, mainly by reducing cravings induced by dramatic swings in blood insulin. With the exception of the extreme nature of phase 1 of the diet plan, the South Beach diet appears more prudent than its Atkins counterpart because it offers more variety and promotes more healthful foods. Well-controlled research must now assess the long-term effectiveness of this dietary regimen for promoting successful weight loss and markers of overall health (e.g., high-protein diets stress kidney function and bone mass). For high performance endurance athletes who train mainly above 65% of maximum effort, switching to a high fat diet is ill advised because of the body's need to maintain glucose in the bloodstream and glycogen packed in the active muscles and liver storage depots. Fatigue during high-intensity exercise for more than 60 minutes' duration occurs more rapidly when athletes have consumed high-fat meals than carbohydrate-rich meals. Refer to Chapter 12 for a thorough discussion of this topic.

High-Protein Diets

Low-carbohydrate, **high-protein diets** may shed pounds in the near term, but their long-term success remains questionable and may even pose health risks.[38] Such diets have been commercially extolled as "last-chance diets." Earlier versions consisted of protein in liquid form advertised as "miracle liquid." Unknown to the consumer, the liquid protein mixture often contained a blend of ground-up animal hooves and horns, with pigskin mixed in a broth with enzymes and tenderizers to "predigest" it. Such collagen-based blends produced from gelatin hydrolysis (supplemented with small amounts of essential amino acids) often failed to contain the highest quality amino acid mixture and lacked required vitamins and minerals, particularly copper. A negative copper balance coincides with electrocardiographic abnormalities and rapid heart rate.[40] Protein-rich foods often contain high levels of saturated fat that increase the risk for heart disease and type 2 diabetes. Diets excessively high in animal protein increase urinary excretion of oxalate, a compound that combines primarily with calcium to form kidney stones.[119] High levels of urinary calcium with these diets also indicate decreased calcium balance and increased risk for bone loss. The diet's safety improves by adding high-quality protein with ample carbohydrate, essential fatty acids, and micronutrients.[102]

Some "experts" claim that extremely high protein intake suppresses appetite through reliance on fat mobilization and subsequent ketone formation. In addition, the elevated thermic effect of dietary protein, with a relatively low coefficient of digestibility (particularly for plant protein), ultimately reduces the net calories available from ingested protein compared with a well-balanced meal of equivalent caloric value. This point has some validity, but one must consider other factors when formulating a sound weight-loss program, particularly for the physically active individual.

Important considerations include a high–protein diet's potential for (a) strain on liver and kidney function and accompanying dehydration, (b) electrolyte imbalance, (c) glycogen depletion, (d) lean-tissue loss, and (e) kidney stones and reduced calcium absorption.

Semistarvation Diets

Physically active individuals often "starve" themselves to lose weight. A therapeutic fast or **very-low-calorie diet (VLCD)** can benefit severe clinical obesity in which body fat exceeds 40 to 50% of body mass. The diet provides between 400 and 800 kcal daily as high-quality protein foods or liquid meal replacements. Dietary prescriptions usually last up to 3 months, but only as a "last resort" prior to undertaking more extreme medical approaches that include surgery. Dieting with a VLCD requires close supervision, usually in a hospital setting. Proponents maintain that severe food restriction breaks established dietary habits; this, in turn, improves prospects for long-term success. These diets also depress appetite to help compliance. Daily medications that accompany a VLCD usually include calcium carbonate or antihistamines for nausea, bicarbonate of soda and potassium chloride to maintain consistency of body fluids, mouthwash and sugar-free chewing gum for bad breath (from high ketone levels from fat catabolism), and bath oils for dry skin. Although surgical treatments such as gastric bypass (60,000 Americans in 2002 and 80,000 in 2003) induce a sustained weight loss, they are only prescribed for patients with a BMI $\geq$ 40 or a BMI of 35 to 40 accompanied by other obesity-related medical conditions.

For most individuals, semistarvation does not constitute an "ultimate diet" or the proper approach to weight control. Because a VLCD provides inadequate carbohydrate, the glycogen-storage depots in the liver and muscles deplete rapidly. This impairs physical tasks requiring either high-intensity aerobic effort or shorter-duration anaerobic power output. The continuous nitrogen loss with fasting and weight loss reflects and exacerbated lean tissue loss, which may occur disproportionately from critical organs like the heart. Finally, the success rate remains relatively poor for prolonged fasting.

TABLE 14.1 summarizes the principles and main advantages and disadvantages of popular dietary approaches to weight loss. Most diets induce weight loss during the first several weeks, but body water makes up much of the lost weight. In addition, significant lean tissue loss occurs with dieting alone, particularly in the early phase of a VLCD.

THE APPROPRIATE DIET PLAN: WELL BALANCED BUT LESS OF IT

A calorie-counting approach to weight loss should provide an appropriate dietary plan that contains all the essential nu-

| Table 14.1 | PRINCIPLES AND MAIN ADVANTAGES AND DISADVANTAGES OF SOME POPULAR WEIGHT LOSS METHODS | | | |

Method	Principle	Advantages	Disadvantages	Comments
Surgical procedure	Alteration of the gastrointestinal tract changes capacity or amount of absorptive surface	Caloric restriction less necessary	Risks of surgery and postsurgical complications can include death	Radical procedures include stapling of the stomach and removal of a section of the small intestine (a jejunoileal bypass)
Fasting	No energy input, ensures negative energy balance	Rapid weight loss (which may be a disadvantage); reduced exposure to temptation	Ketogenic; a large portion of weight lost comes from lean body mass; nutrients lacking	Medical supervision mandatory and hospitalization recommended
Protein-sparing modified fast	Same as fasting except protein or protein with carbohydrate intake presumably helps preserve lean body mass	Same as in fasting	Ketogenic; nutrients lacking; some unconfirmed deaths have been reported, possibly from potassium depletion	Medical supervision mandatory; popular presentation in Lin's "The Last Chance Diet"
One-food-centered diets	Low-caloric intake favors negative energy balance	Being easy to follow has initial psychologic appeal	Being too restrictive means that nutrients are probably lacking; repetitious nature may cause boredom	No food or food combination known to "burn off" fat; examples include grapefruit diet and egg diet
Low-carbohydrate/ high-fat diets	Increased ketone excretion removes energy-containing substances from the body; fat intake is often voluntarily decreased; a low calorie diet results	Inclusion of rich foods may have psychologic appeal; initial rapid loss of water may be an incentive	Ketogenic; high-fat intake contraindicated for heart and diabetes patients; nutrients lacking	Popular versions have been offered by Taller and Atkins; some called "Mayo," "Drinking Man's," and "Air Force" diets
Low-carbohydrate/ high-protein diets	Low caloric intake favors negative energy balance	Initial rapid water loss an incentive. Increased thermic effect of protein	Expense and repetitious nature may make diet difficult to sustain	Emphasizing meat makes the diet high in lipid; Pennington diet an example
High-carbohydrate/ low-fat diets	Low caloric intake favors negative energy balance	Wise food selections can make the diet nutritionally sound	Initial water retention may be discouraging	Pritikin diet is an example

Modified and reprinted by permission from Reed PB. Nutrition: an applied science. Copyright 1980 by West-Publishing Co. All Rights Reserved.

trients. If one maintains a caloric deficit, diet composition exerts little effect on the magnitude of weight lost. Reducing diets should contain the recommended micronutrients and protein, with reduced cholesterol and saturated and *trans* fatty acids. For the physically active person, the remainder should consist predominantly of unrefined, fiber-rich, complex carbohydrates. Calories do count; the trick lies in keeping within the daily limit specified by the rate of fat loss desired.

Two factors largely determine one's daily energy expenditure: *(a)* resting energy requirement and *(b)* energy expended in daily physical activities (see Figure 14.9). *Weight loss occurs if a true caloric deficit exists and energy output exceeds energy input.* Short periods of caloric restriction often encourage the dieter, but do not produce the desired decrease in body fat. Instead, the lost weight consists largely of water and carbohydrate per unit of body

weight lost. As weight loss progresses, a larger proportion of body fat provides energy to make up the caloric deficit created by food restriction.

MAXIMIZING CHANCES FOR SUCCESS WITH DIETING

We usually eat for two reasons. First, we consume food because of true hunger. This enables us to maintain the energy and building blocks to power the body's vital processes and sustain life. Second, we eat to satisfy appetite, which in America usually "turns on" at least three times daily. Human eating behavior intimately ties to both external (environmental) cues and internal (physiologic) cues that signal

a real need for food intake. External "food cues" include the sight of food; its packaging, display, and advertising; the time and physical environment for eating; and the taste, smell, color, texture, and size of portions, which have increased steadily over the past 20 years (see Fig.9.4).[125]

Personal Assessment: The Important First Step

Accurately assessing food intake and energy expenditure provides the framework for unbalancing the energy balance equation to favorably modify body mass and body composition.

Estimates of caloric intake from carefully obtained records of daily food intake (refer to Appendix F) usually fall within 10% of the actual number of calories consumed, an acceptable level of accuracy. For example, suppose the caloric value of daily food intake directly measured in the bomb calorimeter averages 2130 kcal. By use of a careful 3-day dietary history to estimate caloric intake, the daily value falls between about 1920 and 2350 kcal.

Careful record keeping of food intake accomplishes two things: (a) it provides the dieter with an objective list of the foods actually consumed (rather than a "guesstimate" of food intake) and (b) it triggers the awareness of current eating habits and food preferences, an important aspect of the weight control process.

Psychological Factors Influence Eating Behavior

Depression, frustration, boredom, "uptight" or anxious feelings, guilt, sadness, and anger often trigger an urge to eat. A dieter must learn to make accurate appraisals of eating behavior, not only the quantity and frequency of eating but also specific circumstances linked to food intake. Self-analysis requires keen awareness of all aspects of food consumption. Once accomplished, a new set of desirable eating responses can substitute for previously learned "undesirable" behaviors.

Behavioral Approaches Can Help: Modification of Eating Behaviors

The first step in **eating behavior modification** involves describing the various eating behaviors of the person desiring to lose weight, not immediately changing the diet. The person keeps meticulous records and answers the following questions:

- When were meals eaten?
- In what place were meals eaten?
- What was the mood, feeling, or psychological state during the meal?
- How much time was spent eating?
- What activities were engaged in during the meal (watching TV, driving a car, reading, during or after a workout)?

- Who was present during the meal?
- What food was eaten?
- How much food was eaten?

This time-consuming and often annoying record keeping provides objective information concerning one's personal eating behaviors and reveals certain recurring patterns associated with eating. For example, the dieter may discover that (a) eating candy often accompanies feelings of depression, (b) snacking occurs while watching television, (c) hunger becomes prevalent at a particular time of day or after working out, (d) an ice-cream binge usually takes place after an argument, or (e) breakfast and lunch are never eaten at the kitchen table. Based on this analysis, the next step substitutes *alternative behaviors* to replace undesirable ones.

Substituting Alternative Behaviors

Many acceptable behaviors can replace an established set of undesirable ones. The box below lists some existing behaviors associated with overeating and possible substitute behaviors. Many of these recommended substitutions have been promulgated for the general population, but they also apply to recreational and competitive athletes. The major aim of this approach creates new, more positive associations to replace inappropriate eating behavior patterns.

SUBSTITUTES FOR UNDESIRABLE EATING BEHAVIORS

Established behavior patterns

Replacement behavior

- **Eating candy while driving**

  Singing along with the radio while driving

- **Eating snacks while watching television**

  Sewing, painting, or writing letters while watching television

- **Feeling hungry at 4:00 PM**

  Going for a walk at 4:00 PM

- **Eating ice cream after an argument**

  Doing 20 repetitions of an exercise after an argument

- **Never eating breakfast or lunch at the kitchen table**

  Eating breakfast and lunch only at the kitchen table

- **Visiting the kitchen during TV commercials**

  Jogging in place; doing sit-ups

- **Food shopping on the way home before dinner**

  Do all food shopping (buying only what is on a list) after eating

UPGRADING CONTROL OF EATING BEHAVIORS

- **Make the act of eating a ritual.** Limit eating to one place in the house. No matter what foods you eat, follow a set routine. For example, use a place mat, set the table with silverware, and use the same dishes at each meal. Do this for main meals and snacks. One dieter who continually snacked between meals curbed this habit by dressing up in formal attire for each meal and snack—snacking between meals soon stopped. To discourage eating bread, take only one slice at a time and toast it before eating it. For each slice, get up from the table, unwrap the loaf and take out a slice, rewrap the loaf and replace it in the cupboard, toast the slice, and return to the table to eat it. Following an inconvenient routine to obtain some "special" food item often suppresses desire for the food.

- **Use smaller dishes.** The impetus to finish a meal may not be the food per se, but the desire to view an empty plate or glass. Also, try to always leave some food on the plate.

- **Eat slowly.** Fight the tendency to eat too rapidly by taking more time at meals. Cut food into smaller pieces and chew each piece 10 to 15 times before swallowing. Also, place the knife, spoon, or fork back on the table after each two or three bites, and allow a 1- or 2-minute rest pause between mouthfuls.

- **Reduce the lipid content of meals.** Simple modifications in food selection within the same food category dramatically affect the meal's caloric density. TABLE 14.2 presents a convenient checklist for cutting down on the intake of dietary lipid; TABLE 14.3 provides appropriate low-calorie substitutions within various food categories.

- **Follow a Food Plan.** Following a highly structured daily food plan (what, when, and where food will be eaten) reduces the risk of eating high-calorie "impulse" foods.

Developing New Techniques to Control Eating

Many useful techniques can control eating behaviors once undesirable environmental cues and associated behaviors have been identified and replaced or modified.

Other Useful Techniques. Delaying, substituting, and avoiding represent three behavioral strategies for interrupting poor eating behaviors:

- **Delaying**. Add time or steps between the links in the behavior chain:
  - Slow down the eating pace
  - Take a roundabout way to the kitchen
  - Purchase single-portion packages of snacks
  - Put off unplanned eating as long as possible— mail a letter, read a book, mow the lawn, or do sit-ups or pushups

- **Substituting**. Break the behavior chain with activities incompatible with eating:
  - Pleasant activities—read, go for a walk, listen to music, do hobbies, surf the Internet
  - Required activities—plan the budget, pay bills, do errands, clean the house

---

Table 14.2   CHECKLIST FOR CUTTING DOWN ON DIETARY LIPID

- Substitute cold cuts with 1 g of fat per 1-oz serving for regular bologna, salami, or pickled beef.
- Substitute frozen yogurt or sherbet with 4 g or less of fat per 4-oz serving for high-fat ice cream.
- Substitute air-popped popcorn and pretzels for party chips.
- Substitute whole-grain breads and crackers for croissants and corn bread.
- Substitute a variety of cereals for high-fat granola preparations.
- Substitute cheese with less than 4 to 5 g of fat per ounce for high-fat cheeses.
- Substitute egg whites for egg yolks, or use a dehydrated egg substitute.
- Substitute light or fat-free mayonnaise for regular mayonnaise.
- Substitute 2% or 1% milk for whole milk.
- Substitute a variety of herbs or use low-calorie salad dressings or salsa instead of oil-rich or creamy salad dressings.
- Avoid frozen vegetables in rich sauces.
- Buy beef and pork with words "round" or "lean" in the name.
- Buy low-fat cake mixes.
- Do not add oil or butter to water when cooking pasta, macaroni, or oatmeal.
- Make hamburgers from ground round or ground sirloin.
- Substitute two egg whites for one whole egg in baking.
- Substitute evaporated skim milk for cream in recipes.
- Replace 1/4 of the fat in your favorite recipe with applesauce.

Table 14.3 **SUBSTITUTING FOODS WITH LOWER CALORIE CONTENT**

The chart below can help you plan your meals while following the simple guidelines for healthful eating. When you select a variety of foods from those listed in the far left column, you'll be eating foods that are low in fats and/or high in dietary fiber.

Type of Food	Select Most Often	Select Moderately	Select Least Often
Animal protein	Lean cuts of beef/pork Salmon, halibut (broiled) Canned tuna in water Poultry (w/o skin) Egg Crab	Untrimmed beef and pork Canned tuna in oil Poultry (with skin) Lobster, shrimp Canadian bacon	Fatty beef, lamb, pork Luncheon meats/hot dogs Fried chicken Fried fish Liver, kidneys

Dairy	Nonfat yogurt
	
	Nonfat milk (or 1/2%)
	Nonfat dry milk
	Nonfat frozen yogurt
		Reduced fat and part-skim
		  cheeses
		Low-fat cottage cheese
		Low-fat milk
		Low-fat yogurt
		95% Fat-free frozen yogurt
			Whole-milk cheese (cheddar,
			  muenster)
			Whole milk
			Sour cream, ice cream
			Cream, half-and-half

Vegetable protein	Dried beans and peas (kidney, lima,
	  and soy beans; lentils; split peas)
	Tofu (bean curd)
		Raw or dry-roasted nuts and
		  seeds
		Peanut and other butters
		  (moderate amounts)
			Oil-processed nuts and seeds

Vegetables	Raw, fresh vegetables
	Fresh or frozen, slightly
	  cooked vegetables
		Canned vegetables
		Canned tomatoes or
		  vegetable juice
			Vegetables in cream or butter
			  sauces
			Fried vegetables

Fruits	Fresh, raw fruit Dried fruit Frozen and fresh fruit juices	Canned fruit packed in juice Canned fruit juices Frozen fruit	Fruit-flavored beverages Canned fruit packed in syrup Avocados Olives
Grain products	Shredded wheat, oats Whole-grain cereals Whole-grain breads Brown rice Wheat bran, oat bran Bagels Fig bars	Refined cereals Enriched white breads Refined pastas White rice Granolas Toast with margarine Plain cookies	Cookies, cakes, pies Sweetened cereals Tortilla chips Oil-processed crackers Cream-filled doughnuts Croissants, doughnuts
Other	Popcorn (air-popped)	Low-fat salad dressing Low-fat mayonnaise Pretzels	Fat-rich salad dressing Mayonnaise Gravies, cream sauce Potato chips

From Wardlaw GM, et al. Contemporary nutrition issues and insights. 2nd ed. St. Louis, MO: Mosby, 1992.

- **Avoiding**. Keep yourself out of situations in which food is visible or easily accessible:
  - Stay out of the kitchen or other areas associated with eating
  - Do not combine eating with other activities such as reading, TV watching, driving, or working out
  - When finished eating, remove dishes and food from the table
  - Scrape excess food directly into the garbage

EXERCISE FOR WEIGHT CONTROL

A sedentary lifestyle consistently emerges as an important factor in weight gain for children, adolescents, and adults.

Weight Gain: Not Simply a Problem of Gluttony

Conventional wisdom views excessive food intake as the prime cause of the overly fat condition. Most persons believe that the only way to reduce unwanted body fat entails caloric restriction by dieting. This overly simplistic strategy partly accounts for the dismal success in maintaining weight loss over the long term, refocusing debate on the contribution of food intake to obesity.[58,135]

In the United States, per capita caloric intake has not increased enough to account for the steady rise in the national body mass over the last century, a weight gain equivalent to 30 pounds for a 6-foot man. Only in the past decade has daily energy intake increased above the level in the early part of the 20th century. The observation that overly fat per-

sons often eat the same or even less than thinner people holds true for a large number of overly fat adults over a broad age range as they become less active and slowly add weight. *Excess weight gain often parallels reduced physical activity rather than increased caloric intake.* Current estimates indicate that 27% of U.S. adults engage in no daily physical activity and another 28% do not regularly take part in physical activity.[99] Among active endurance-trained men, body fat inversely relates to energy expenditure (low body fat, high energy expenditure and vice versa); no relationship emerges between body fat and food intake.[96] Surprisingly, physically active people who eat the most generally weigh the least and exhibit the highest levels of fitness.

Excessive food intake does not fully explain the rise in obesity among children. Obese infants do not characteristically consume more calories than recommended dietary standards. For children ages 4 to 6 years, a reduced level of physical activity primarily accounted for their daily energy expenditure 25% lower than the energy intake recommendation for this age.[24] More specifically, 50% of boys and 75% of girls in the United States fail to engage in even moderate physical activity three or more times weekly. Children ages 6 to 17 years have consumed 4% fewer calories over the past 20 years, yet the prevalence of childhood obesity continues to increase dramatically. In contrast, physically active children tend to be leaner than less active counterparts. For preschool children, no relationship emerged between total energy intake, or the fat, carbohydrate, and protein composition of the diet and percentage body fat.[7] Time-in-motion photography to document activity patterns of elementary school students showed that overweight children remained less physically active than their normal-weight peers; excess body weight did not relate to food intake. Overly fat high school girls and boys actually consumed *fewer* calories than their nonobese peers.[75,124] Excessive fatness and incidence of type 2 diabetes relate directly to the number of hours spent watching television (a consistent marker of inactivity) among individuals of all ages.[4,67] For example, 3 hours of television viewing a day led to a twofold increase in obesity and a 50% increase in diabetes.[67] Each 2-hour per day increment of TV watching coincided with a 23% increase in obesity and a 14% rise in diabetes risk. Excessive television watching, playing video games, and otherwise remaining physically inactive particularly characterizes minority teens.[49,122] Minimizing time devoted to these behaviors helps to combat childhood fat gain.

Total Daily Energy Expenditure

Total daily energy expenditure (TDEE) consists of the sum of all the anabolic and catabolic chemical reactions within the body. FIGURE 14.9 illustrates the three general factors that influence TDEE.

Factor 1. Resting metabolic rate refers to the sum of metabolic processes for maintenance of normal body function and regulatory balance during rest. It includes basal and sleeping conditions plus the added metabolic cost of arousal. Resting metabolism generally accounts for 60 to 75% of TDEE, depending on daily level of physical activity.

Factor 2. Thermogenic effect of food consumed (TEF) refers to the effect of food consumption on energy

Figure 14.9 Components of total daily energy expenditure.

metabolism. TEF (also called **dietary-induced thermogenesis**) consists of two components. One component, **obligatory thermogenesis**, results from the energy required to digest, absorb, and assimilate food nutrients. The second component, **facultative thermogenesis**, results from sympathetic nervous system activation from food ingestion and its stimulating effect on metabolism.[132]

Factor 3. Energy expended during physical activity and recovery profoundly affects variability among individuals in TDEE. World-class athletes nearly double their daily caloric output with 3 to 4 hours of arduous training. Most persons can sustain metabolic rates 10 times the resting level during "big muscle" activities like fast walking, running, cycling, and swimming. Under typical circumstances, physical activity accounts for between 15 and 30% of the TDEE.

Effectiveness of Increasing Energy Expenditure

Regular physical activity plays a central role in protecting against weight gain. *Men and women of all ages who maintain a physically active lifestyle (or become involved in regular exercise programs) maintain a more desirable level of body composition than less active counterparts.* For overweight adult women, a dose–response relationship exists between the amount of exercise and long-term weight loss.[71] Obese adolescents and adults improve body composition and visceral fat distribution from regular moderate physical activity or more vigorous exercise that improves cardiovascular fitness.[54,92,95] For obese boys and girls, the most favorable body composition changes occur with *(a)* low-intensity, long-duration exercise; *(b)* aerobic exercise combined with high-repetition resistance training; and *(c)* exercise programs combined with a behavior-modification component.[54,92] For those who lose weight, regular exercise facilitates weight-loss maintenance better than programs relying solely on dieting.[1,3,81,107,138,172] This positive effect occurs partly because regular exercise counteracts the typical postdiet decline in fat oxidation in those who lose weight by only energy restriction.[154]

Even for currently active individuals, additional exercise unbalances the energy balance equation for weight loss, favorably alters body composition and body fat distribution,[85,127,128,147] and further improves physical fitness.[13,128,152] Additional spin-off from regular physical activity includes *(a)* slowing of the age-related loss in muscle mass, *(b)* improvement in obesity-related comorbidities, *(c)* decreased mortality, and *(d)* beneficial effects on existing chronic diseases.[19,57,88,93,141,153,163]

Regular Exercise Increases Daily Energy Expenditure

Some truth exists to the notion that one must perform an extraordinary amount of exercise to lose body fat. The statistics reveal that just to lose 0.45 kg (1 lb) of body fat a person has to chop wood for 10 hours, golf for 20 hours, perform mild calisthenics for 22 hours, play ping-pong for 28 hours or volleyball for 32 hours, or run 35 miles. Understandably, such a commitment seems overwhelming to the person who plans to reduce by 10 or 15 kg or more. From a longer-term perspective, if the person walked an extra 3.5 miles (about 350 kcal) 2 days a week (700 kcal), it would take about 5 weeks, or 10 walking days, to lose 0.45 kg of body fat (3500 kcal). Assuming one continued to walk year-round, walking 2 days a week reduces body fat by 4.5 kg during the year provided food intake remains fairly constant. *Exercise produces cumulative calorie-expending effects*; *0.45-kg body fat loss occurs when the caloric deficit equals 3500 kcal, regardless of whether the deficit occurs rapidly or systematically over time.*

During low-to-moderate exercise (as performed by most persons who exercise for weight control), recovery metabolism—the so-called recovery afterglow—contributes minimally to total energy expenditure because recovery occurs rapidly. In addition, regular exercise causes faster adjustments in postexercise energetics, reducing the total recovery oxygen consumption.[136] *Calories burned during physical activity represent the most important factor in total exercise energy expenditure, not calories expended during recovery.*

The Ideal: Conserve Lean and Reduce Fat

Regular physical activity, with or without dietary restriction, protects against weight gain and favorably changes body mass and body composition.[31,32,127] This occurs because exercise training enhances fat mobilization from adipose depots and increases fat breakdown by the active muscles.[94] In addition, exercise retains skeletal muscle protein (maintains positive nitrogen balance), while simultaneously retarding protein breakdown. *The protein-sparing effect of regular exercise partly explains why more of the weight lost comes from fat in a program that uses exercise than in one using only food restriction.* Those with the largest amount of excess fat lose body weight and fat more readily with exercise than their leaner counterparts.[10] Even without dietary restrictions, exercise provides positive "spin-off" to favorably alter body composition by reducing body fat and maintaining or even increasing FFM.

Best Types of Physical Activities

When using exercise to lose weight, consider the **FITT acronym:** **F**requency, **I**ntensity, **T**ime, and **T**ype of exercise. Ideal aerobic activities having moderate-to-high caloric cost include brisk walking and hiking, running, rope skipping, stair stepping, circuit-resistance training, cycling, and swimming. TABLE 14.4 lists the "top 12" physical activities in terms of energy expenditure. Many recreational sports and games also create an effective caloric deficit for

Table 14.4	"TOP 12" EXERCISES RANKED BY RELATIVE STRENUOUSNESS (KCAL EXPENDED PER MIN)

$kcal \cdot min^{-1}$	Activity
25.9	Roller skiing, V-Skate technique, 11.2 mph, trained athletes
23.3	In-line skiing, double-pole technique, 11.2 mph, trained athletes
22.0	Skiing, cross-country, hard snow, uphill (5° grade), maximum effort, trained
19.3	Swimming, Mini-Gym Swim Bench, 45 strokes per min (freely chosen)
18.2	Rowing, mechanically braked rowing ergometer; stroke rate = 28–32 per min, 1750 kg-m·min^{-1}, athletes
18.1	Rowing, "all out" for 6 min on a rowing ergometer
18.0	Running, 10.9 mph (5.5 min per mile pace)
18.0	Race walking, competition, 8.5 mph, men
17.2	Marathon running, 5:03 min per mile pace, trained
17.1	Running, shallow water (1.3 m depth), no vest, maximal effort
17.0	Forestry, ax-chopping, fast
16.0	Skin-diving, vigorous

Data source: Katch FI, et al. Calorie expenditure charts. Fitness Technologies Press. 1132 Lincoln Avenue. Ann Arbor MI, 1996. Used by permission.

weight loss, but precise quantification and regulation of energy expenditure remain difficult with these activities. No selective effect exists for running, walking, or bicycling; each effectively burns calories and favorably alters body composition. For low-impact walking as the sole means of exercising, energy expenditure increases by adding hand, wrist, or ankle weights or using race-walking techniques. An extra 300-kcal daily caloric expenditure induced by moderate jogging daily for 30 minutes theoretically produces a 0.45-kg fat loss in about 12 days, or a yearly caloric deficit equivalent to the energy in 13.6 kg of body fat.

Resistance Training. *Resistance training provides an important adjunct to aerobic training for weight loss and weight maintenance.* The energy expended in circuit resistance training—continuous exercise using low resistance and high repetitions—averages about 9 kcal per minute. Consequently, this exercise mode burns substantial calories during a typical 30- to 60-minute workout. Even conventional resistance training that involves less total energy expenditure affects muscular strength and FFM more positively during weight loss than programs that rely solely on food restriction.[11,157] Individuals who maintain high muscular strength levels tend to gain less weight than weaker counterparts.[87] Additionally, standard resistance training performed regularly reduces coronary heart disease risk, improves glycemic control, favorably modifies the lipoprotein profile, and increases resting metabolic rate (if FFM increases).[112,113,115,144] TABLE 14.5 illustrates the effects of 12 weeks of either endurance training or resistance training on nondieting young men. Endurance training significantly reduced percentage body fat by reducing fat mass (–1.6 kg; no change in FFM), while resistance training significantly decreased body fat mass (–2.4 kg) and increased the FFM (+2.4 kg). Conserving and/or increasing FFM maintains a relatively high level of resting metabolism, independent of age.[16,34,35,90,129,171] This reduces the body's tendency to store calories, which augments the effectiveness of the weight loss program. *For athletes, maintaining FFM during weight reduction counters the potential negative effects of weight loss on exercise performance.*

A Dose–Response Relationship

Some individuals believe that light aerobic exercise induces more effective weight loss because fat contributes a greater percentage of total calories burned in exercise compared with more intense physical activity in which carbohydrate represents the primary fuel. Fat combustion does provide a greater percentage of the total energy metabolism during light versus intense aerobic exercise (see Chapter 5). However, a larger

Table 14.5	CHANGES IN BODY COMPOSITION AFTER 12 WEEKS OF EITHER RESISTANCE TRAINING OR ENDURANCE TRAINING

	Controls		Resistance Trained		Endurance Trained	
Variable	Pretreatment	Posttreatment	Pretreatment	Posttreatment	Pretreatment	Posttreatment
Relative body fat (%)	20.1±8.5	20.2±8.5	21.8±6.2	18.7±6.6[a]	18.4±7.9	16.5±6.4[a]
Fat mass (kg)	16.2±10.8	16.3±10.5	17.2±7.6	14.8±6.2[a]	14.4±7.9	12.8±7.1[a]
Fat-free body mass (kg)	64.3±5.4	64.4±6.6	61.9±8.3	64.4±9.0[a]	64.1±8.2	64.7±8.6
Total body mass (kg)	80.5±8.1	80.7±8.5	79.1±8.3	79.2±7.6	78.5±8.2	77.5±7.9

From Broeder CE, et al. Assessing body composition before and after resistance or endurance training. Med Sci Sports Exerc 1997;29:705.
[a] Significant difference between pre- and posttest measurements (P <.05).
All values means±SD.

total quantity of fat combustion occurs in higher-intensity aerobic exercise performed for an equivalent duration. *The total number of calories expended to create the exercise energy deficit, not the percentage mixture of macronutrients oxidized, determines the effectiveness of exercise in weight loss.*

A direct dose-response relationship exists between time spent exercising and weight lost. The person who exercises by walking burns considerable calories simply by extending exercise duration. Also, a proportional relationship exists between the energy cost of weight-bearing exercise like walking and body mass; thus, the overweight person expends considerably more calories walking than does someone of average body weight.

MAXIMIZING CHANCES FOR SUCCESS WITH INCREASED PHYSICAL ACTIVITY: MODIFICATION OF EXERCISE BEHAVIORS

A person burns additional calories through physical activity simply by extending exercise duration, perhaps at a lower intensity. Another effective calorie-burning strategy replaces daily periods of inactivity with additional physical activity requiring greater energy expenditure.

Describe the Behavior for Modification

Any hope of changing the profile of daily physical activity depends on an accurate appraisal of daily activities. The first step in **exercise behavior modification** determines the daily pattern of physical activity, including the minimal requirements of sleeping, eating, going to the bathroom, and bathing. The next step substitutes more strenuous activities for those that rate low in energy expenditure. Appendix F illustrates an activity profile from daily records of time spent in various activities for 3 consecutive days. The records should describe the activity, its duration, and estimated energy requirements.

Substitute Alternative Behaviors

Various options exist to increase energy expenditure within the time allotted to daily routines. The important consideration involves determining when and how to make changes with alternative exercise behaviors.

Maximize Success

Several techniques maximize success when using exercise for weight loss.

- **Progress slowly.** Add additional exercise gradually. Over time, more opportunities to add physical activity become apparent.

ALTERNATE EXERCISE BEHAVIORS

- When driving to school, work, or the gym, park one-half mile away and walk the remaining distance; brisk walking to and from the car each day, 5 days a week, burns the caloric equivalent of about 3.2 kg of body fat in 1 year.
- When taking public transportation, depart several stops early and walk the remaining distance.
- When traveling relatively short distances, walk, jog, or bicycle instead of driving.
- Skip the restaurant for lunch; instead, "brown bag" it and then participate in some form of physical activity for 15 to 30 minutes.
- Wake up an hour early and take a brisk walk, cycle, row, rollerblade, or swim before breakfast.
- Replace the cocktail hour or the evening beer with 20 minutes of exercise.
- Replace coffee breaks with exercise breaks.
- Walk up and down several flights of stairs after each hour at work or school.
- Sweep the sidewalks in front of your house, apartment, or dorm.
- Allow time for exercise when going on a family outing. Get out of the car before reaching your destination; let a friend or family member drive the rest of the way while you walk or jog.
- Instead of eating at an intermission at sporting events, walk around the stadium or arena; climb up and down stairs instead of using an elevator or escalator.
- Replace the hired help and undertake some of these tasks yourself:

    Gardening

    Mowing the lawn

    Painting

    Washing and waxing the car

    Raking leaves

    Snow shoveling

- Run in place, jump rope, jog up and down stairs, or perform vigorous calisthenics during television commercials.

- **Include variety.** Rather than performing the same exercise repeatedly in a given time, vary the exercise and number of repetitions. For a competitive athlete, the added physical activity for weight loss need not be in the specific sport.
- **Become goal oriented.** Set a specific and realistic goal for increasing physical activity. Three ways generally add additional exercise using goal-oriented behavior: *(a)* exercise for a certain length of time, *(b)*

continue to exercise until you reach a predetermined number of repetitions or distance, or *(c)* manipulate exercise duration and repetitions or distance.

- **Be systematic.** Set aside certain times during the day to exercise. Do not allow outside factors (e.g., watching television, shopping, housework) to interfere with daily physical activity.

FOOD RESTRICTION PLUS INCREASED PHYSICAL ACTIVITY

Success stories exist for those with considerable excess body fat, despite the difficulties encountered losing weight.[62,81] Among lifetime members of a commercial weight loss organization that promotes prudent caloric restriction, behavior modification, group support, and moderate physical activity, over one half maintained their original weight loss goal after 2 years, and more than one third had done so after 5 years.[97] Combinations of exercise and dietary restraint with more unrefined, low-glycemic carbohydrates and less lipids offer considerably more flexibility for achieving a negative caloric balance than either exercise alone or diet alone.[34,36,63,86,101,117,160] *Body fat losses of up to 2 pounds (0.9 kg) each week fall within acceptable limits, but a steady 0.5 to 1.0 pound a week loss may be even more desirable.*

Setting a Realistic Target Time

Suppose 20 weeks represents the target time to achieve a 9-kg (20-lb) fat loss. With this goal, the weekly energy deficit must average 3500 kcal, or a daily average of 500 kcal (3500÷7). By dieting, the person reduces daily caloric intake by 500 kcal for 5 months (3500 kcal weekly deficit) to achieve the desired 9-kg fat loss. Instead, if the dieter performed an additional one-half hour of moderate exercise equivalent to 350 "extra" kcal 3 days a week, then the weekly caloric deficit increases by 1050 kcal (3 days × 350 kcal per exercise session). Consequently, weekly food intake could decrease to only 2400 kcal (about 350 kcal a day) instead of 3500 kcal to achieve the desired 0.45-kg weekly fat loss. Increasing the number of weekly exercise days from 3 to 5 requires reducing daily food intake by only 250 kcal. If duration of the 5-day per week extra exercise lengthens from 30 minutes to 1 hour, then the desired weight loss occurs without reducing food intake because the extra physical activity produces the entire 3500-kcal deficit.

If intensity of the 1-hour exercise performed 5 days a week increased by only 10% (cycling at 22 instead of 20 mph; running a mile in 9 instead of 10 minutes; swimming each 50 yards in 54 seconds instead of 60 seconds), the number of weekly exercise calories burned increases by 350 kcal (3500 kcal per wk × 10%). This new weekly deficit of 3850 kcal, or 550 kcal per day, would then permit the "dieter" to *increase* daily food intake by 50 kcal and still lose a pound of fat each week, a clear example of "eat more, weigh less"!

The effective use of physical activity by itself or in combination with mild dietary restriction unbalances the energy balance equation to produce meaningful weight loss. This combined approach reduces feelings of intense hunger and psychologic stress more than does weight loss exclusively by caloric restriction. In addition, prolonged dieting increases the chances of developing a variety of nutritional deficiencies that hinder exercise training and competitive performance. Combining exercise with weight loss produces desirable reductions in blood pressure at rest and in situations that typically elevate blood pressure such as intense physical activity and emotional distress.[139]

SPOT REDUCTION DOES NOT WORK

The notion of **spot reduction** *comes from the belief that increasing a muscle's activity facilitates fat mobilization from the adipose tissue in close proximity to the muscle.* Exercising a specific body area should selectively reduce more fat from that area than if different muscle groups exercised at the same caloric intensity. Advocates of selective spot reduction recommend large numbers of sit-ups or side-bends for a person with excessive abdominal fat. Whereas the promise of spot reduction with exercise offers aesthetic and health-risk benefits, critical evaluation of the research evidence does not support its effectiveness.

To examine the claims for spot reduction, researchers compared the girths and subcutaneous fat stores of the right and left forearms of high-caliber tennis players.[55] As expected, the girth of the dominant or playing arm exceeded that of the nondominant arm because of modest muscular hypertrophy from the exercise overload of tennis. Measurements of skinfold thickness, indicated that years of playing tennis did not reduce subcutaneous fat in the playing arm. Another study evaluated fat biopsy specimens from the abdominal, subscapular, and buttock sites before and after 27 days of sit-up exercise training.[76] The daily number of sit-ups increased from 140 at the end of the first week to 336 on day 27. Despite this impressive amount of localized "spot" exercise, adipocytes in the abdominal region were no smaller than in unexercised buttocks or subscapular control regions.

Undoubtedly, a negative energy balance created through regular exercise reduces total body fat because exercise stimulates mobilization of fatty acids through hormones that act on fat depots throughout the body. Body areas of greatest body fat concentration and/or lipid-mobilizing enzyme activity supply the greatest amount of this energy. *Selective exercise does not cause significantly more fatty acid release from the fat pads directly over the active muscles.*

Where on the Body Does Fat Loss Occur?

Changes in body fat and fat distribution in obese females at successive 2.3-kg (5-lb) increments of weight loss over a 14-

How to Predict Percentage Body Fat for Overly Fat Men and Women from Girths

Estimating percentage body fat (%BF) in the overly fat by skinfold prediction becomes problematic because of difficulty securing accurate and repeatable measurements owing to an extensive mass of subcutaneous fat. In addition, with increasing levels of body fatness, the proportion of subcutaneous fat to total body fat changes, thereby affecting the relationship between skinfolds and body density (Db). The following factors limit skinfold use with the overly fat population:

1. Site selection and palpation of body landmarks are difficult.
2. Skinfold thickness may exceed caliper jaw aperture.
3. Variability in adipose tissue composition affects skinfold compressibility.
4. Poorer objectivity in skinfold measures as body fat increases.

Waist girth   **Abdomen girth**

CASE STUDY/PERSONAL HEALTH AND EXERCISE NUTRITION 14–1 (*continued*)

PREDICTING PERCENTAGE BODY FAT

Use the following equations to predict %BF in obese (>30%BF) women (ages 20–60 years and): men (ages 24–68 years)

Women

$$\%BF = 0.11077 \, (ABDO) - 0.17666 \, (HT) + 0.14354 \, (BW) + 51.03301$$

Men

$$\%BF = 0.31457 \, (ABDO) - 0.10969 \, (BW) + 10.8336$$

where ABDO = *(a)* waist girth (taken horizontally at the level of the natural waist—narrowest part of the torso, as seen from the anterior) and *(b)* abdomen girth (taken horizontally at the level of the greatest anterior extension of the abdomen, usually, but not always, at the level of the umbilicus). Duplicate measurements are taken and averaged. BW = body weight in kg; and HT = stature in cm.

EXAMPLES

1: Overly Fat Woman
Data: waist girth = 115 cm; abdomen girth = 121 cm; HT = 165.1 cm; BW = 97.5 kg

$$\%BF = 0.11077 \, (ABDO) - 0.17666 \, (HT) + 0.14354 \, (BW) + 51.03301$$
$$= 0.11077 \, (115+121/2) - 0.17666 \, (165.1) + 0.14354 \, (97.5) + 51.03301$$
$$= 13.07 - 29.17 + 13.995 + 51.03301$$
$$= 48.9$$

2: Overly Fat Man
Data: waist girth = 131 cm; abdomen girth = 136 cm; BW = 135.6 kg

$$\%BF = 0.31457 \, (ABDO) - 0.10969 \, (BW) + 10.8336$$
$$= 0.31457 \, (131.0+136.0/2) - 0.10969 \, (135.6) + 10.8336$$
$$= 41.995 - 14.873 + 10.8336$$
$$= 37.9$$

Weltman A, et al.: Accurate assessment of body composition in obese females. Am J Clin Nutr 1988;48:1179.
Tran ZV, Weltman A. Predicting body composition of men from girth measurements. Hum Biol 1988;60:167.

---

week period addressed the frequently asked question. "Where on the body does fat loss occur when weight is lost?" Caloric restriction and a 45-minute, 3-day per week exercise program affected weight loss.[79] FIGURE 14.10 displays the changes in body composition, skinfolds, and girths in the three subgroups that reduced body mass by 2.3, 4.5, and 9.1 kg. A 4.5-kg weight loss produced approximately twice as much change in overall body composition as a loss of 2.3 kg *(top graph)*. The corresponding change in body composition almost tripled when weight loss doubled from 4.5 to 9.1 kg. Skinfolds *(middle graph)* and girths *(bottom graph)* in the trunk region decreased about twice as much as those in the extremities. Decreases in body fat with exercise training and/or caloric restriction preferentially occur in upper-body subcutaneous fat and deep abdominal fat rather than the more "resistant" fat depots in gluteal and femoral regions.[31,33,83,104]

POSSIBLE GENDER DIFFERENCE IN EXERCISE EFFECTS ON WEIGHT LOSS

An interesting question concerns the possibility of a gender difference in the responsiveness of weight loss to regular exercise.[85,165] A meta-analysis of 53 research studies on this topic concluded that men generally respond more favorably than women to the effects of exercise on weight loss.[10] One possible explanation involves gender differences in body fat distribution. The mobilization capacity of triacylglycerols for energy depends on anatomic location. Fat distributed in the upper body and abdominal regions (central fat) shows an active lipolysis to sympathetic nervous system stimulation and preferentially mobilizes for energy during exercise.[6,133,162] The greater distribution of upper-body adipose tissue in men than in women may contribute to their greater sensitivity to lose fat with regular exercise. The final answer to this intriguing question awaits further research.

EFFECTS OF DIET AND EXERCISE ON BODY COMPOSITION DURING WEIGHT LOSS

TABLE 14.6 summarizes the benefits of exercise for weight loss. *Addition of exercise to a weight loss program favorably modifies the composition of the weight lost in the direction of greater fat loss.*[11,31,32] In a pioneering study in this area, three groups of adult women maintained a 500-kcal daily

Figure 14.10 Changes in body composition *(top)*, skinfolds *(middle)*, and girths *(bottom)* with specified amounts of weight loss. Abbreviations for girths: *Shld,* shoulders; *Umbil,* umbilicus abdomen; *Fore,* forearm SF, skinfolds. Figure 13.11 illustrates the anatomic sites. (Data from King AC, Katch FI. Changes in body density, fatfolds and girths at 2.3 kg increments of weight loss. Hum Biol 1986;58:708.)

Table 14.6	**BENEFITS OF ADDING EXERCISE TO DIETARY RESTRICTION FOR WEIGHT LOSS**

- Increases the overall size of the energy deficit.
- Facilitates fat mobilization and oxidation, especially from visceral adipose tissue depots
- Increases the relative loss of body fat by preserving the fat-free body mass
- By conserving and even increasing the fat-free body mass, blunts the drop in resting metabolism that frequently accompanies weight loss
- Requires less reliance on caloric restriction to create energy deficit
- Contributes to the long-term success of the weight loss effort
- Provides unique and significant health-related benefits
- May provide moderate suppression of appetite

caloric deficit during 16 weeks of weight loss.[176] The diet group reduced daily food intake by 500 kcal, whereas women in the exercise group maintained daily energy intake but increased energy output by 500 kcal with a supervised walking and conditioning program. The women using diet plus exercise created the daily 500 kcal deficit by reducing food intake by 250 kcal and increasing exercise energy output by 250 kcal. No significant difference emerged among the three groups for weight loss; each group lost approximately 5 kg. This finding highlights that a caloric deficit reduces body weight regardless of the method used to create the energy imbalance. An interesting observation for weight loss concerned FFM. The exercise group increased FFM by 0.9 kg, and the combination group increased FFM by 0.5 kg,

but the dieters *lost* 1.1 kg of lean tissue! *For body fat reduction, combining diet and exercise proved most effective.*

FIGURE 14.11 displays body composition changes for 40 obese women placed into one of four groups: *(a)* control, with no exercise and no diet; *(b)* diet only, no exercise (DO); *(c)* diet plus resistance exercise (D + E), and *(d)* resistance exercise only, no diet (EO). The exercise groups trained 3 days a week for 8 weeks. They performed 10 repetitions for each of 3 sets of eight strength exercises. Body mass decreased significantly for DO (–4.5 kg) and D + E (–3.9 kg) groups, compared with EO (+0.5 kg) and controls (–0.4 kg). Importantly, FFM increased significantly for EO (+1.1 kg), whereas the DO group lost 0.9 kg of FFM. Clearly, augmenting a calorie-restriction program with resistance exercise training preserves FFM compared with dietary restriction alone.

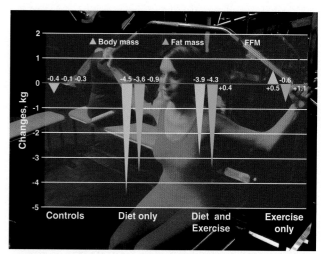

Figure 14.11 Changes in body composition with resistance exercise and diet in obese females. (From Ballor DI, et al. Resistance weight training during caloric restriction enhances lean body weight maintenance. Am J Clin Nutr 1988;47:190.)

WEIGHT LOSS RECOMMENDATIONS FOR WRESTLERS AND OTHER POWER ATHLETES

Weightlifters, gymnasts, and other athletes in sports requiring large muscular strength and power in relation to body mass often must lose body fat without negatively affecting exercise performance. For these athletes, an increase in relative muscular strength and short-term power output capacity should improve competitive performance. The following discussion focuses on wrestlers but applies to all physically active individuals who desire to reduce body fat without negatively affecting health, safety, and exercise capacity.

To reduce injury and medical complications from short- and longer-term periods of weight loss and dehydration, the American College of Sports Medicine (ACSM), National Collegiate Athletic Association (NCAA), and the American Medical Association (AMA) recommend assessing each wrestler's body composition. This assessment takes place several weeks prior to the competitive season to determine a **minimal wrestling weight** based on percentage body fat. *Five percent body fat (determined using hydrostatic weighing or population-specific skinfold equations) represents the lowest acceptable level for safe wrestling competition.*[26,146] For wrestlers under 16 years of age, 7% body fat level represents the recommended lower limit. TABLE 14.7 outlines a practical application to determine minimal wrestling weight and an appropriate competitive weight class. The ACSM also recommends that weight-loss, if warranted, should progress gradually and not exceed a 1- to 2-pound loss per week. At the same time, the athlete should continue to consume a nutritious diet.

Adolescent Female Gymnasts

As with wrestlers, coaches must establish a safe minimal competitive body weight for female gymnasts, many of whom use disordered eating behaviors to achieve weight loss (see Chapter 15). Based on an a cross-validation analyses of 11 skinfold equations for predicting percentage body fat, the following equation most accurately estimates body composition in female high school gymnasts.[66,148] This prediction equation can assess body composition in the preseason (1 standard error of estimate equals ± 2.4% body fat); for female gymnasts, body weight should contain no less than 14 to 16% body fat.

Table 14.7 USING ANTHROPOMETRIC EQUATIONS TO PREDICT A MINIMAL WRESTLING WEIGHT AND TO SELECT A COMPETITIVE WEIGHT CLASS

A. To predict body density (BD), use one of the following equations. (For each skinfold, record the average of at least three trials in mm.)
1. Lohman equation[a]
   BD = 1.0982 − (0.00815 × [triceps + subscapular + abdominal skinfolds])
   + (0.00000084 × [triceps + subscapular + abdominal skinfolds]^2)
2. Katch and McArdle equation[b]
   BD = 1.09448 − (0.00103 × triceps skinfold) − (0.00056 × subscapular skinfold) − (0.00054 × abdominal skinfold)
3. Behnke and Wilmore equation[c]
   BD = 1.05721 − (0.00052 × abdominal skinfold) + (0.00168 × iliac diameter) + (0.00114 × neck circumference)
   + (0.00048 × chest circumference) + (0.00145 × abdominal circumference)
4. Thorland equation[d]
   BD = 1.0982 − (0.000815 × [triceps + abdominal skinfolds]) + (0.00000084 × [triceps + abdominal skinfolds])

B. To determine fat percentage, use the Brožek equation:
% Fat = [4.570 ÷ BD − 4.142] × 100

C. To determine fat-free weight and to identify a minimum weight class, follow the examples below.
1. Jonathan, a 15 year-old wrestler who weighs 132 lb, has a body density of 1.075 g·cc^{-1} and hopes to compete in the 119-lb weight class.
2. Jonathan's percentage fat is (4.570 ÷ 1.075 − 4.142) × 100 = 10.9%
3. Jonathan's fat weight and fat-free weight are
   a. 132.0 lb × 0.109 = 14.4 lb fat
   b. 132.0 lb − 14.4 lb fat = 117.6 lb fat-free weight

D. To calculate a minimal wrestling weight
1. Realize that the recommended minimum body weight for those 15 years and younger contains 93% (0.93) fat-free weight and 7% fat (0.07)
2. Divide the wrestler's calculated fat-free weight by the greatest allowable fraction of fat-free weight to estimate minimal wrestling weight:
   117.6 ÷ (93/100) = 117.6 ÷ 0.93 = 126.5 lb

E. To allow for a 2% error, perform the following calculations:
1. 126.5 minimal weight × 0.02 = 2.5 lb error allowance
2. 126.5 lb − 2.5 lb = 124.0 lb minimum wrestling weight

F. Conclusion: Jonathan cannot wrestle in the 119-pound weight class; rather he must compete in the 125-pound class.

From Tipton CM. Making and maintaining weight for interscholastic wrestling. Gatorade Sports Science Exchange. 1990;2(22).
[a] Lohman TG. Skinfolds and body density and their relationship to body frames: a review. Hum Biol 1981;53:181.
[b] Katch FI, McArdle WD. Prediction of body density from simple anthropometric measurements in college-age men and women. Hum Biol 1973;l45:445.
[c] Behnke AR, Wilmore JH. Evaluation and regulation of body build and composition. Englewood Cliffs, NJ: Prentice Hall, 1974.
[d] Thorland W, et al. New equations for prediction of a minimal weight in high school wrestlers. Med Sci Sports Exerc 1989;21:S72.

Table 14.8   **RECOMMENDATIONS TO HIGH-POWER ATHLETES WHO WANT TO LOSE WEIGHT**

Many athletes will lose weight one way or another in an attempt to increase relative strength and power for their sport. These recommendations help the athlete lose weight in a way that minimizes health risks and maximizes sport performance and training.

1. Arrange for qualified personnel (exercise physiologist, nutritionist, physician, or athletic trainer) to do the following:
   a. Determine % body fat and fat-free body mass
   b. Calculate minimal weight at 5% fat (males) or 12% (females)
   The difference between present weight and minimal weight is the amount of weight that can be lost.
2. Begin weight loss early, before the competitive season begins and progress slowly to maximize fat loss and minimize muscle and water loss; maximum rate of weight loss. should be 0.5–1.0 kg (1–2 lb) per week.
3. Increase energy expenditure by doing aerobic training at least twice per week before and early in the competitive season.
4. Decrease the intake of calories by reducing dietary lipid, protein, and carbohydrate, but DO NOT totally eliminate any one of these three. Consume at least 1500 calories per day to prevent vitamin and mineral deficiencies. Specific recommendations include
   a. Cut out desserts, butter and margarine, sauces, gravy, and dressings.
   b. Eat foods high in complex carbohydrates (fruits, vegetables, whole-grain cereals).
   c. Grill, bake, broil, or boil food; do not fry.
5. Weigh in before and after each practice session to keep track of body water loss. Specifically:
   a. Do not restrict water during intense training, especially in hot training environments.
   b. Consume water, sports drinks, or other fluids after practice to restore at least 80% of the weight lost in a practice session.
   c. Drink fluids low in calories (e.g., skim milk rather than whole milk).

From Horswill CA. Does rapid weight loss by dehydration adversely affect high-power performance? Gatorade Sports Science Exchange 1991;3(30).

Female High School Gymnasts

% Body Fat = [457 ÷ 1.0987–0.00122 (Σ triceps, subscapular, suprailiac skinfolds in mm) + 0.00000263 (Σ triceps, subscapular, suprailiac skinfolds in mm)^2] − 414.2

TABLE 14.8 presents general guidelines and recommendations for athletes who wish to lose weight (specifically body fat) without jeopardizing health, safety, and exercise capacity and training responsiveness. These recommendations were originally formulated for athletes in the high-power sports, but they apply to other athletes as well.

GAINING WEIGHT: A UNIQUE DILEMMA FOR PHYSICALLY ACTIVE INDIVIDUALS

Gaining weight to enhance body composition and exercise performance in activities requiring muscular strength and power or aesthetic appearance poses a unique problem not easily resolved. Most persons focus on weight loss to reduce excess body fat and improve overall health and appearance. Weight (fat) gain per se occurs all too readily by tilting the body's energy balance to favor greater caloric intake. Weight gain for active individuals should represent muscle mass and accompanying connective tissue. Generally, this form of weight gain occurs if increased caloric intake—carbohydrates for adequate energy and protein sparing plus the amino acid building blocks for tissue synthesis—accompanies a resistance exercise program.

Individuals attempting to increase muscle mass often fall easy prey to health food and diet supplement manu-facturers who market "high-potency, tissue-building" substances—chromium, boron, vanadyl sulfate, β-hydroxy-β-methyl butyrate, and numerous protein and amino acids mixtures—none of which reliably increases muscle mass. Of the hundreds of products marketed in the health and bodybuilding literature to enhance exercise performance, most focus on augmenting muscular development.[51,111] Chapters 11 and 12 discussed the efficacy of many of these compounds and chemicals. Commercially prepared mixtures of powdered protein, predigested amino acids, or special high-protein "cocktails" do not promote muscle growth any more effectively than protein consumed in a well-balanced diet.[27] If an athlete experiences difficulty achieving the recommended protein intake through normal food intake—because of lifestyle, eating habits, and time requirements of training and competition—then high-quality protein supplements should prove beneficial.

Increase the Lean, Not the Fat

Endurance training usually increases FFM only slightly, but the overall effect reduces body weight from the calorie-burning and possible appetite depressing effects of this exercise type. In contrast, heavy muscular overload through resistance training, supported by adequate energy and protein intake (with sufficient recovery), greatly increases muscle mass and strength. Adequate energy intake during such training ensures that no catabolism of the protein available for muscle growth occurs from an energy deficit. *Intense aerobic training should not coincide with resistance training designed to increase muscle mass.*[61,84] More than likely, the added energy (and perhaps protein) demands of concurrent aerobic and resistance training impose a limit on muscle growth with resistance training. A prudent recommendation

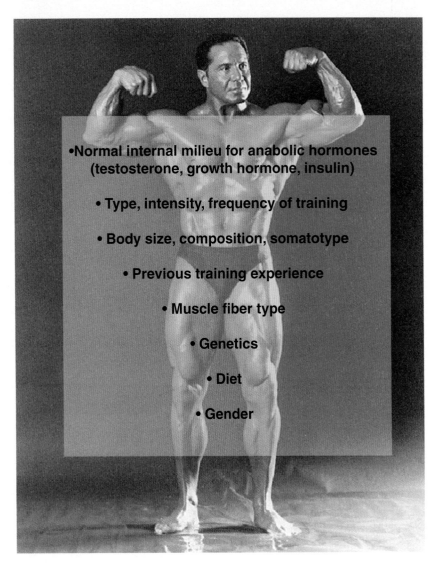

- Normal internal milieu for anabolic hormones (testosterone, growth hormone, insulin)

- Type, intensity, frequency of training

- Body size, composition, somatotype

- Previous training experience

- Muscle fiber type

- Genetics

- Diet

- Gender

Figure 14.12 Nutritional guidelines for optimizing muscle mass gains with resistance training.

increases daily protein intake to about 1.6 g per kg of body mass during the resistance-training period.[91] Diverse sources of plant and animal proteins should be consumed; relying solely on animal protein (high in saturated fatty acids and cholesterol) potentially increases heart disease risk.

If all calories consumed in excess of the energy requirement of resistance training sustained muscle growth, then 2000 to 2500 extra kcal could supply each 0.5-kg increase in lean tissue. In practical terms, 700 to 1000 kcal added to the well-balanced daily meal plan supports a weekly 0.5- to 1.0-kg gain in lean tissue plus the additional energy needs for training. The ideal situation presupposes that all extra calories synthesize lean tissue. FIGURE 14.13 gives nutritional guidelines to stimulate gains in muscle size and strength during resistance training.

How Much Lean Tissue Gain to Expect?

Many factors increase lean tissue accretion with resistance training, including energy balance, type of training program, and the individual's genetic makeup. A 1-year program of heavy resistance training for young athletic men generally increases body mass by about 20%, the major portion consisting of lean tissue. The rate of lean tissue gain rapidly plateaus as training progresses beyond the first year. For athletic women, first-year gains in lean tissue mass average 50 to 75% of the absolute values for the men, probably owing to women's smaller initial lean body mass. Individual differences in the daily amount of nitrogen incorporated into body protein (and protein incorporated into muscle) may also limit gains in muscle tissue and explain differences among people in muscle mass increases with resistance training. FIGURE 14.12 presents specific factors affecting the responsiveness of lean tissue synthesis to resistance training.

Individuals with relatively high androgen/estrogen ratios and greater percentages of fast-twitch muscle fibers probably increase lean tissue to the greatest extent in response to resistance training. Muscle mass increases occur most readily at the start of training in individuals with the largest *relative* FFM (FFM corrected for stature and body fat).[156] Regularly monitoring body mass and body fat verifies whether the combination of training and additional food intake increases lean tissue and not body fat.

Table 14.9 NUTRITIONAL SUPPLEMENTS MARKETED FOR STRENGTH-TRAINED INDIVIDUALS

Nutritional Supplement	Promoted Use/ Advertised Claim	Valid Research Data with Promoted Supplementation for Strength-Trained Individuals (STIs)
Protein supplements	Provide adequate protein to support muscle growth, weight gain	No valid data that protein supplements are more effective than natural protein sources; STIs may need 1.5–2.0 g of protein/kg body weight; easily obtained from healthful diet protein sources (e.g., lean meats, skim milk, complementary plant proteins)
Arginine, lysine, ornithine	Stimulate release of human growth hormone (hGH), insulin; promote muscle growth	May stimulate hGH release; however, hGH itself is not ergogenic to STIs; research indicates no effect on muscle growth or strength
Creatine	Increase creatine phosphate in muscles; increase energy sources and stimulate muscle growth	Preliminary research indicates increased power in short-term, high-intensity exercise; increased weight gain, either contractile protein or water
Inosine	Increase ATP synthesis; increase strength and facilitate recuperation	No valid studies document an ergogenic effect in STIs
Choline	Increase acetylcholine or lecithin to increase strength or decrease body fat, respectively	No valid studies document an ergogenic effect in STIs
Yohimbine	Increase serum testosterone levels; increase muscle growth and strength; α_2-adenoreceptor blocker; decrease body fat	No valid studies document an ergogenic effect in STIs; needs further research to document role as useful agent for weight loss in STIs
Glandulars: adrenals, pituitary, testes	Enhance function of analogous gland in humans	No valid studies document an ergogenic effect on STIs
Vitamin B_{12}	Enhance DNA synthesis; increase muscle growth	Research indicates no effect on muscle growth or strength in STIs
Antioxidant vitamins: C, E, β-carotene	Prevent muscle damage from unwanted oxidative processes following high-intensity, eccentric muscle actions	Research data inconclusive, additional research needed to document effect of antioxidants to prevent muscle damage in STIs
Carnitine	Increase transport of fatty acids into mitochondria for oxidation; promote fat loss	No valid studies document weight loss or an ergogenic effect in STIs
Chromium	Potentiate insulin action; promote muscle growth via enhanced amino acid uptake	Research data not in agreement; but more appropriately, designed studies show no effect on body composition or strength in STIs
Boron	Increase serum testosterone levels; increase muscle growth and strength	Research indicates no effect on serum testosterone levels, lean body mass, or strength in STIs
Magnesium	Increase protein synthesis or muscle contractility; increase muscle growth and strength	Research data equivocal, but generally does not support an ergogenic effect in STIs
Medium-chain triglycerides	Increase thermic effect; promote fat loss	No valid studies document body fat or weight loss in STIs
Omega-3 fatty acids	Stimulate release of hGH	No valid studies document an ergogenic effect in STIs
γ-Oryzanol	Increase serum testosterone and hGH levels; increase muscle growth	No valid studies document an ergogenic effect in STIs
Smilax	Increase serum testosterone levels; increase muscle growth and strength	No valid studies document an ergogenic effect in STIs

From Williams MH. Nutritional supplements for strength trained athletes. Gatorade Sports Science Exchange 1993;6(30); Barron R, Vanscov G. Natural products and the athlete: facts and folklore. Ann Pharmacother 1993;27:607; Grunewald K, Bailey R. Commercially marketed supplements for bodybuilding athletes Sports Med 1993;15:90; Short S, Marquart L. Sports nutrition fraud. NY State J Med 1993;93:112; Williams M. Nutrition for fitness and sport. Dubuque, IA: Brown & Benchmark, 1992.

A prudent approach to muscle building

Train Hard

Follow a strenuous resistance training program under the guidance of an expert coach or personal trainer. Depending on your training experience, you may need to begin by lifting relatively light loads for many repetitions before building up to heavier loads and fewer repetitions. An experienced supervisor can help determine what type of resistance training schedule is appropriate for you and can reduce the risk that you will injure yourself by lifting too much too soon.

Follow a sound diet

Eat a well balanced (food-guide pyramid) regular diet that contains sufficient energy (calories), protein and carbohydrate, with the balance containing mostly unsaturated fat.

Energy:

To gain 0.5 to 1.0 kilograms of body mass each week plus provide the additional energy for training, consume about 700 to 1000 kCal each day above and beyond the amount of calories that allows you to maintain a stable body weight. If you want to gain two pounds per week, consume about 1000 extra calories each day. Most athletes can consume this much extra energy simply by eating larger portions of their normal diets, but some find that it is easier if they supplement their normal foods with energy-dense protein/carbohydrate "weight gainer" products or meal-replacement drinks.

Protein:

Consume 1.6 grams of protein per kilogram of body weight on a daily basis. This protein can come from normal foods. Most athletes do not require protein supplements for optimal muscle growth.

Carbohydrate:

Each day, eat 8 - 10 grams of carbohydrate per kilogram of body weight. Emphasize cereals, fruits and vegetables as carbohydrate sources because they contain more nutrients than do sugars and sweets.

Fat:

Consume about 0.45 - 0.9 grams of fat per kilogram of body weight per day. Most of this fat should come from unsaturated sources (e.g., olive, canola and flax oils).

Don't expect miracles

Although muscle size may increase substantially in the first few months of a sound program of training and nutrition, eventually the gains in muscle mass will slow down. This is normal. You should expect to gain muscle mass gradually over years of hard training and good nutrition. There is no quick and easy way to get big and strong.

Don't rely on dietary supplements

Don't fall into the trap of spending lots of money on various "muscle builder" supplements in hopes of finding an easy road to greater muscle mass. There is no substitute for rigorous resistance training and good overall nutrition. Hundreds of supplements are marketed as muscle builders, and almost all of them have no effect whatsoever on muscle mass. Those few supplements that are supported by scientific research are noticeably effective mostly in elite athletes who have undergone many years of training. For non-elite athletes, the effects are usually trivial when compared to the much greater effects of sound training and good overall nutrition. Furthermore, some supplements have the potential to cause serious side effects.

If you are considering supplements, consult experts

Highly trained athletes who are considering the use of dietary supplements should consult regularly with a knowledgeable exercise physiologist, with a sports exercise physician who is familiar with dietary supplements or with a competent sports nutritionist or sports dietitian.

Figure 14.13 Specific factors affecting the magnitude of lean tissue synthesis with resistance training.

WEIGHT LOSS AND EXERCISE PRESCRIPTION

About 300,000 adult Americans die each year from obesity-related diseases. Heart disease, high blood pressure, and type 2 diabetes directly link to excess body weight and insufficient aerobic exercise. Regular aerobic exercise reduces risks of some diseases by 50% or more.

Exercise prescription for weight loss in overweight individuals emphasizes frequency and duration that progresses to 45 to 60 minutes each day. Exercise intensity only becomes a consideration when the individual achieves sufficient weight loss and a fitness level suitable for cardiovascular conditioning.

EXERCISE PRESCRIPTION

Initial focus of a prudent exercise prescription for weight loss centers on progressively increasing exercise volume (and caloric expenditure) with relatively low-intensity physical activity. Walking or running energy expenditure proportionally increases with speed. For example, a 70-kg person walking at 3.5 mph (17 min per mile pace) burns about 3.3 net kcal per minute, that is, calories above the resting level. If the same person runs at 7 mph (8.5 min per mile pace), net calories burn four times faster. For each mile covered, the runner burns twice as many calories as the walker and covers each mile twice as fast. This accounts for the fourfold greater rate of energy expenditure. These calculations are based on net energy expenditure values—the energy expenditure due to the exercise itself—in contrast to gross energy expenditure, which includes the resting value. The resting energy expenditure should not be counted toward weight (fat) loss, because these calories are burned whether or not the person exercises.

Interestingly, nearly the same energy expenditure occurs for running and walking a given distance (about 100 kcal per mile for a 70-kg person); this refers to the gross energy expenditure and not net values. Because walkers take longer to cover a mile than runners, they burn more calories associated with the resting component, which results in similar total kcal per mile. For weight loss purposes, however, consider only the net caloric expenditure in exercise. Thus, one must evaluate the payoff between increasing speed of walking/running and increasing exercise duration (and/or frequency) to increase total net energy expenditure. In practice, prudent exercise for the untrained, overweight individual emphasizes duration and frequency, particularly in the early stages of the program.

SUBJECT DATA AND HISTORY

Female, single with no children; cigarette smoker (10 years); secretary in big office; family history of diabetes (father, type 2 diabetes) and heart disease (mother, grandmother)

Age: 35 years
Body weight: 199 lb (90.3 kg)
Height: 5 ft 6 in. (1.676 m)
BMI: 32.1
Percentage body fat: 37%
Fat weight (FW): 73.6 lb (33.4 kg)
Fat-free body mass (FFM): 125.44 lb (56.9 kg)
Physical examination: Knee problems make walking/running difficult; no other obvious medical problems
Exercise experience: Has not exercised for past 10 years except for occasional weekend biking, which she enjoys; she dislikes walking/running/swimming; very sedentary throughout life; family of nonexercisers
Laboratory data:
• Normal lipid profile
• Normal blood glucose
• Daily caloric intake of about 3200 kcal
• High lipid intake (>38% of total kcal)
• Normal blood pressure
General impressions: Obese female with four risk factors (sedentary; obesity; smoking; family history of heart disease). Person needs lifestyle modification.

CASE QUESTIONS

1. Give a preliminary assessment
2. Recommend a body weight goal
3. Formulate a prudent exercise prescription

ANSWERS TO QUESTIONS

1. Sedentary, overly fat female (without specific symptoms) who needs to lose body fat. Individual has four heart disease risk factors that place her in a moderate-to-high risk category. She needs lifestyle modifications that include beginning an exercise program, reducing caloric intake and modifying the types of foods consumed, and starting a smoking cessation program.
2. Initially, this woman should be encouraged to lose a modest amount of weight of about 10 lb over a 5- to 10-week period. Such weight loss will favorably modify her risk profile and empower her to realize that she really can lose weight. Over the long term, a reduction in body weight to a corresponding 28% body fat level becomes a desirable goal.

$$\text{Goal body weight} = \text{FFM} \div (1.00 - \text{desired \%BF})$$
$$= 125.4 \div (1.00 - 0.28)$$
$$= 125.4 \div 0.72$$
$$= 174 \text{ lb (rounded)}$$

$$\text{Goal fat loss} = \text{Current body weight} - \text{goal body weight}$$
$$= 199 - 174 = 25 \text{ lb}$$

3. a. She should check with her physician or health care provider for clearance before beginning an exercise program. She chooses stationary bicycle riding as her primary exercise activity. After a 2-week adaptation period of shorter-duration exercise 3 to 5 days a week, exercise frequency is set at 6 days per week; the exercise duration goal is 60 minutes per session.

  b. Set intensity of exercise between 50% (lower level) and 70% (upper level) using the heart rate reserve method.

Resting heart rate determined in the morning before rising: 85 bpm

Maximum heart rate (HR_{max} [bpm]) by use of the following formula:

> **$HR_{max} = 200 - 0.5 \times$ (age in years)**
> $= 200 - 0.5 \times (35)$
> $= 183$ bpm

  c. Target heart rates using heart rate reserve method calculate as follows:

> **Target HR = (intensity percentage) (HR_{max})**
> $- HR_{rest}) + HR_{rest}$
>
> **Lower target HR** $= (0.5) (183 - 85) + 85)$
> $= 134$ bpm
>
> **Upper target HR** $= (0.7) (183 - 85) + 85)$
> $= 154$ bpm

During the first few sessions of exercise on the stationary cycle ergometer the person determines that she can exercise comfortably at a heart rate between 140 and 147 bpm at 75 watts (450 kg-m·min^{-1}). This then becomes the initial exercise intensity.

  d. Estimate the net exercise energy expenditure as follows:

Gross exercise oxygen consumption ($\dot{V}O_2$)

> Gross exercise $\dot{V}O_2$, mL·kg^{-1}·min^{-1}
> $= 7 + (1.8$ [work rate, kg·m·min^{-1}] $\div$ body weight, kg)
> $= 7 + (1.8$ [450] $\div$ 90.3)
> $= 16.1$ mL·kg^{-1}·min^{-1}

Net exercise oxygen consumption ($\dot{V}OO_2$)

> Net exercise $\dot{V}O_2$, mL·kg^{-1}·min^{-1}
> $=$ Gross exercise $\dot{V}O_2$, mL·kg^{-1}·min^{-1} $-$ Resting $\dot{V}O_2$
> $= 3.5$ mL·kg^{-1}·min^{-1}
> $= 16.1 - 3.5$
> $= 12.6$ mL·kg^{-1}·min^{-1}

Calorie conversion

Convert net exercise $\dot{V}O_2$ in mL·kg^{-1}·min^{-1} to mL·min^{-1} by multiplying by the body weight in kg
> $= 12.6 \times 90.3$
> $= 1138$ mL·min^{-1}

Divide by 1000 to convert to L·min^{-1}.
> $= 1138 \div 1000$
> $= 1.14$ L·min^{-1}

Multiply the L·min^{-1} value by 5 to convert oxygen consumption to kcal (1 L $\dot{V}O_2 = 5$ kcal)
> $= 1.14 \times 5.0$
> $= 5.7$ kcal·min^{-1}

> 5.7 kcal·min^{-1} $\times$ 60 min $= 342$ kcal per exercise session

This woman expends approximately 342 kcal per exercise session, representing about a 0.59-lb fat loss per week from exercise alone (342 kcal × 6 d = 2052 kcal; 2052 kcal ÷ 3500 kcal = 0.59). This ideally complements a dietary modification that restricts energy intake by 500 to 750 kcal daily. Combining these modifications in diet and exercise behaviors produces nearly 2 pounds of weight loss per week.

Franklin BA, et al. ACSMs guidelines for exercise testing and prescription. 6th ed. Baltimore: Lippincott Williams & Wilkins, 2000:214.

Miller WC, et al. Predicting max HR and the HR–VO₂ relationship for exercise prescription in obesity. Med Sci Sports Exerc 1993;25:1077.

Summary

1. Slight but prolonged caloric excesses produce substantial weight gain. To prevent such a caloric disparity, energy output must balance energy input.

2. Nearly 70% of Americans struggle to lose weight (29% of men and 40% of women), yet only one fifth use the recommended combination of eating fewer calories and exercising regularly.

3. Almost 65% of the U.S. population classify as either overweight (BMI 25.0–29.9) or obese (BMI ≥ 30). Of this total, 30.5% classify as obese. The obesity epidemic contributes significantly to the rising tide of type 2 diabetes, cancer, and cardiovascular disease.

4. Among U.S. youth, obesity has more than doubled in the last 15 years, with an ever-widening gap between the weights of individuals deemed overly fat and those considered thin. Excessive body fatness becomes particularly prevalent among poor and minority children.

5. Genetic factors probably account for 25 to 30% of excessive body fat accumulation.

6. Genetic predisposition does not necessarily cause obesity, but given the right environment, the genetically susceptible individual gains body fat. Substantial alterations in the population's gene pool (which requires millions of years) cannot explain the dramatic worldwide obesity epidemic.

7. A defective gene for adipocyte leptin production and/or hypothalamic leptin insensitivity (plus defects in production and/or sensitivity to other chemicals) causes the brain to assess adipose tissue status improperly. This creates a chronic state of positive energy balance.

8. The standard dietary approach to weight loss that decreases caloric intake below the requirement for current weight maintenance generally helps obese patients to lose about 0.5 kg per week. Success in preventing weight regain is relatively poor, averaging between 5 and 20% of those who lose weight. Typically, one- to two-thirds of the lost weight returns within a year, and almost all of it within 5 years.

9. Reducing body fat generally improves exercise performance because it directly increases relative (per unit body size) muscular strength and power and aerobic capacity. Reduced drag force, which impedes forward movement in air and water, also represents a positive effect of weight loss on exercise performance.

10. Three methods unbalance the energy-balance equation to produce weight loss: (a) reduce energy intake below daily energy expenditure, (b) maintain normal energy intake and increase energy output, and (c) decrease energy intake and increase energy expenditure.

11. A caloric deficit of 3500 kcal, created through either diet or exercise, represents the calories in 0.45 kg (1.0 lb) of adipose tissue.

12. Appropriate modification of eating and exercise behaviors increases one's chance for successful weight loss.

13. Prudent dieting effectively promotes weight loss. Disadvantages of extremes of semistarvation include loss of fat-free mass (FFM), lethargy, possible malnutrition, and depressed resting metabolism (as long as one maintains an energy deficit).

14. Repeated cycles of weight loss–weight regain (yo-yo effect) may increase the body's ability to conserve energy, thus making weight loss with subsequent dieting less effective. From a public health perspective, the risks from obesity far exceed those from weight cycling.

15. Daily energy expenditure consists of the sum of resting metabolism, thermogenic influences (particularly the thermic effect of food), and energy generated during physical activity. Physical activity most profoundly affects the variability among humans in daily energy expenditure.

16. The calories burned in exercise accumulate. Regular extra physical activity creates a considerable energy deficit over time.

17. The precise role of exercise in appetite suppression or stimulation remains unclear, but moderate increases in physical activity may blunt appetite and depress energy intake of a previously sedentary, overweight person. Most athletes eventually consume enough calories to counterbalance training's added caloric expenditure.

18. Combining exercise with caloric restriction offers a flexible and effective means for weight loss. Exercise enhances fat mobilization and catabolism. Regular aerobic exercise retards lean tissue loss; resistance training increases the FFM.

19. Rapid weight loss during the first few days of a caloric deficit mainly reflects loss of body water and stored glycogen; greater fat loss occurs per unit of weight lost as caloric restriction continues.

20. Selective exercise of specific body areas proves no more effective for localized fat loss than more-general physical activity. Areas of greatest fat concentration and/or lipid-mobilizing enzyme activity supply the most energy for exercise, regardless of the area exercised.

21. Differences in body fat distribution partially explain the gender difference in exercise-induced weight loss. Fat deposited in the upper body and abdominal regions (male-pattern obesity) responds readily to neurohumoral stimulation and preferentially mobilizes in exercise compared with fat deposited in gluteal and femoral regions (female-pattern obesity).

22. Physically active individuals should add weight as lean body tissue (muscle mass). This occurs most readily with a modest increase in caloric intake plus resistance training.

23. Seven hundred to 1000 extra kcal per day supports a weekly 0.5- to 1.0-kg gain in lean tissue and the energy requirements of resistance training. Individual physiologic variations and training factors affect gains in muscle mass.

TEST YOUR KNOWLEDGE ANSWERS

1. True The World Health Organization and the International Obesity Task Force have declared a global obesity epidemic. Obesity now represents the second leading cause of preventable deaths (smoking first) in the United States (300,000 deaths yearly) at a total yearly cost of $140 billion, or approximately 10% of the U.S. health care expenditures. Overweight, but not obese, nonsmoking men and women in their mid-30s to mid-40s die at least 3 years sooner than normal-weight counterparts, a risk just as damaging to life expectancy as cigarette smoking. Obese individuals can expect a about a 7-year decrease in life expectancy.

2. False There is greater prevalence of obesity among black women (about 50%) than among white women (33%). Studies of obese black and white women show small differences in resting metabolism; on average, black women burn nearly 100 fewer calories each day during rest than whites. This slower rate of processing calories persists even after adjusting for differences in body mass and body composition. The greater energy economy of black women during exercise and throughout the day most likely reflects an inherited trait, as it persists both before and after weight loss. This effect, which also exists among children and adolescents, predisposes a black female to gain weight and regain it following weight loss.

3. False The standard dietary approach to weight loss that decreases caloric intake below the requirement for current weight maintenance generally helps obese patients lose about 0.5 kg per week. Success at preventing weight regain is relatively poor, averaging between 5 and 20%. Regular physical activity, through either recreation or occupation, effectively contributes to preventing weight gain and thwarts the tendency to regain lost weight.

4. False Older men and women who maintain active lifestyles impede the "normal" pattern of fat gain observed in most adults. Research shows that time spent in physical activity inversely relates to body fat level in young and middle-aged men who exercise regularly. The greater level of body fat among active middle-aged men compared with younger, more active counterparts resulted from less vigorous training, not greater energy intake.

5. True Combining moderate food restriction with additional daily physical activity offers the greatest flexibility for achieving fat loss. This combination also enables the individual to remain well nourished for exercise training and peak performance.

6. True Resting metabolism decreases when food restriction progressively produces weight loss. This hypometabolism often exceeds the decrease attributable to the loss of body mass or fat-free body mass. Depressed metabolism conserves energy, causing the diet to become less effective despite a restricted caloric intake. This produces a weight-loss plateau at which further weight loss becomes considerably less than predicted from the mathematics of the restricted energy intake.

7. False For most individuals, semistarvation with a very low calorie diet (VLCD) does not compose an "ultimate diet" or the proper approach to weight control. Because a VLCD provides inadequate carbohydrate, the glycogen-storage depots in the liver and muscles deplete rapidly. This impairs physical tasks requiring either high-intensity aerobic effort or shorter-duration anaerobic power output. The continuous nitrogen loss with fasting and weight loss reflects and exacerbated lean tissue loss, which may occur disproportionately from critical organs like the heart. The success rate remains poor for prolonged VLCD use.

8. False Excess weight gain often parallels reduced physical activity rather than increased caloric intake. Approximately 27% of U.S. adults engage in no daily physical activity, and another 28% do not regularly take part in physical activity. Among active endurance-trained men, body fat inversely relates to energy expenditure (low body fat, high energy expenditure and vice versa); no relationship emerges between body

fat and food intake. Surprisingly, physically active people who eat the most generally weigh the least and exhibit the highest levels of fitness. Also, excessive food intake does not fully explain the rise in obesity among children. Obese infants do not characteristically consume more calories than recommended dietary standards. For children ages 4 to 6 years, a reduced level of physical activity primarily accounts for their 25% lower daily energy expenditure than the energy intake recommendation for this age.

9. False Regular physical activity plays an important role in protecting against weight gain. Men and women of all ages who maintain a physically active lifestyle (or become involved in regular exercise programs) maintain a more desirable level of body composition. For overweight adult women, a dose–response relationship exists between the amount of exercise and long-term weight loss.

10. False Resistance training provides an important adjunct to aerobic training in programs of weight loss and weight maintenance. The energy expended in circuit resistance training (continuous exercise using low resistance and high repetitions) averages about 9 kcal per minute. This exercise mode, therefore, can "burn" substantial calories during a typical 30- to 60-minute workout. Even conventional resistance training that involves less total energy expenditure affects muscular strength and fat-free body mass during weight loss more positively than programs that rely solely on food restriction.

References

1. American College of Sports Medicine: Position statement on proper and improper weight loss programs. Med Sci Sports Exerc 1993;15:9.
2. American Medical Association: A critique of low-carbohydrate ketogenic weight and reduction regimens (a review of Dr. Atkins' diet revolution). JAMA 1973;224:1418.
3. Anderson JW, et al. Long-term weight-loss maintenance: a meta-analysis of US studies. Am J Clin Nutr 2001;74:579.
4. Anderson RE, et al. Relationship of physical activity and television watching with body weight and level of fatness among children. JAMA 1998;279:938.
5. Arner P, et al. Adrenergic regulation of lipolysis in situ at rest and during exercise. J Clin Invest 1991;32:423.
6. Arner P, et al. Expression of lipoprotein lipase in different human subcutaneous adipose tissue regions. J Lipid Res 1991;32:423.
7. Atkin L-M, Davies PSW. Diet composition and body composition in preschool children. Am J Clin Nutr 2000;72:15.
8. Atkins RC. Dr Atkins' new diet revolution. New York: Avon, 1997.
9. Ball EJ, et al. Total energy expenditure, body fatness, and physical activity in children aged 6-9 Y. Am J Clin Nutr 2001;74:524.
10. Ballor DL, Keesey RE. A meta-analysis of the factors affecting changes in body mass, fat mass and fat-free mass in males and females. Int J Obes 1991;15:717.
11. Ballor DL, Poehlman ET. Exercise training enhances fat-free mass preservation during diet-induced weight loss: a meta-analytical finding. Int J Obes 1994;18:35.
12. Blackburn GL, et al. Weight cycling: the experience of human dieters. Am J Clin Nutr 1989;49:1105.
13. Blair SN, et al. Influences of cardiorespiratory fitness and other precursors on cardiovascular disease and all-cause mortality in men and women. JAMA 1996;276:205.
14. Blank HM, et al. Use of nonprescription weight loss products: results from a multistate survey. JAMA 2001;286:930.
15. Booth ML, et al. Changes in the prevalence of overweight and obesity among young Australians, 1969-1997. Am J Clin Nutr 2003;77:29.
16. Bouchard C, et al. Long-term exercise training with constant energy intake. 1: Effect on body composition and selected metabolic variables. Int J Obes 1990;14:57.
17. Bouchard C, et al. The response to long term feeding in identical twins. N Engl J Med 1990;322:1477.
18. Bouchard C, et al. The response to exercise with constant energy intake in identical twins. Obes Res 1994;2:400.
19. Boule NG, et al. Effect of exercise on glycemic control and body mass in type 2 diabetes mellitus: A meta-analysis of controlled clinical trials. JAMA 2001;286:1218.
20. Bravata DM, et al. Efficacy and safety of low-carbohydrate diets: a systematic review. JAMA 2003;289:1767.
21. Bray GA, Popkin BM. Dietary fat intake does affect obesity! Am J Clin Nutr 1998;68:1157.
22. Brownell KD, et al. The effects of repeated cycles of weight loss and regain in rats. Physiol Behav 1986;38:459.
23. Byers T, et al. Weight cycling, weight gain, and risk of hypertension in women. Am J Epidemiol 1999;150:573.
24. Carpenter WH, et al. Total energy expenditure in 4 to 6 year old children. Am J Physiol 1993;27:E706.
25. Centers for Disease Control and Prevention. Update: prevalence of overweight among children, adolescents, and adults: United States, 1988-1994. MMWR 1997;46:199.
26. Clark RR, et al. Multicomponent cross-validation of minimum weight predictions for college wrestlers. Med Sci Sports Exerc 2003;35:342.
27. Clarkson M. Dietary supplements and pharmaceutical agents for weight loss and gain. In: Lamb DR, Murray R, eds. Perspectives in exercise science and sports medicine. Vol 10. Exercise, nutrition, and weight control. Carmel, IN: Cooper Publishing, 1998.
28. Cleland R, et al. Commercial weight loss products and programs: what consumers stand to gain and lose. Washington, DC: Federal Trade Commission, Bureau of Consumer Protection, 1998.
29. Considine RV, et al. Serum immunoreactive-leptin concentrations in normal-weight and obese humans. N Engl J Med 1996;334:292.
30. DeLany JP, et al. Energy expenditure in preadolescent African American and white boys and girls: The Baton Rouge Children's Study. Am J Clin Nutr 2002;75:705.
31. Dengel DR, et al. Effects of weight loss by diet alone or combined with aerobic exercise on body composition in older obese men. Metabolism 1994;43:867.
32. Després J-P. Physical activity and adipose tissue. In: Bouchard C, et al. eds. Physical activity, fitness, and health. Champaign, IL: Human Kinetics, 1994.
33. Després J-P, et al. Loss of abdominal fat and metabolic response to exercise training in obese women. Am J Physiol 1991;261:E159.
34. DiPietro L. Physical activity, body weight, and adiposity: an epidemiologic perspective. Exerc Sport Sci Rev 1995;23:275.
35. Dolezal BA, Potteiger JA. Concurrent resistance and endurance training influence basal metabolic rate in nondieting individuals. J Appl Physiol 1998;85:695.
36. Ebbeling CB, Rodriguez NR. Effect of exercise combined with diet therapy on protein utilization in obese children. Med Sci Sports Exerc 1999;31:378.
37. Eck Clemens LH, et al. The effect of eating out on quality of diet in premenopausal women. J Am Diet Assoc 1999;99:4421.
38. Eisenstein J, et al. High-protein weight loss diets: are they safe and do they work? A review of the experimental and epidemiological data. Nutr Rev 2002;60:189.
39. Elliot DL, et al. Sustained depression of the resting metabolic rate after massive weight loss. Am J Clin Nutr 1989;49:93.
40. Fisler JS. Cardiac effects of starvation and semi-starvation diets: Safety and mechanisms of action. Am J Clin Nutr 1992;56:230S.
41. Flegal KM, Troiano RP. Changes in the distribution of body mass index of adults and children in the US population. Int J Obes Relat Metab Disord 2000;24:807.
42. Freedman CS, et al. Trends and correlates of class 3 obesity in the United States from 1990 through 2000. JAMA 2002;288:1758.
43. Fleury C, et al. Uncoupling protein-2: a novel gene linked to obesity and hyperinsulinemia. Nat Genet 1997;15:269.
44. Foster GD, et al. Resting energy expenditure in obese African American and Caucasian women. Obes Res 1997;5:1.

45. Foster GD, et al. A randomized trial of a low-carbohydrate diet for obesity. N Engl J Med 2003;348:2082.

46. French SA, et al. Predictors of weight change over two years among a population of working adults: the Healthy Worker Project. Int J Obes 1994;18:145.

47. Frisancho AR. Prenatal compared with parental origins of adolescent fatness. Am J Clin Nutr 2000;72:1186.

48. Golay A, et al. Similar weight loss with low- or high-carbohydrate diets. Am J Clin Nutr 1996;63:174.

49. Gordon-Larsen, P, et al. Adolescent physical activity and inactivity vary by ethnicity: the National Longitudinal Study of Adolescent Health. J Pediatr 1999;135:301.

50. Grundy SM. Multifactorial causation of obesity: implications for prevention. Am J Clin Nutr 1998;67(suppl):563S.

51. Grunewald K, Bailey R. Commercially marketed supplements for bodybuilding athletes. Sports Med 1993;15:90.

52. Gunnell DJ, et al. Childhood obesity and adult cardiovascular mortality: a 57-y follow-up study based on the Boyd Orr cohort. Am J Clin Nutr 1998;67:1111.

53. Guo SS, et al. Predicting overweight and obesity in adulthood form body mass index values in childhood and adolescence. Am J Clin Nutr 2002;76:653.

54. Gutin B, et al. Effect of exercise intensity on cardiovascular fitness, total body composition, and visceral adiposity of obese adolescents. Am J Clin Nutr 2002;75:818.

55. Gwinup G, et al. Thickness of subcutaneous fat and activity of underlying muscles. Ann Intern Med 1971;74:408.

56. Halaas JL, et al. Weight-reducing effects of the plasma protein encoded by the obese gene. Science 1995;269:543.

57. Hansen RD, Allen BJ. Habitual physical activity, anabolic hormones, and potassium content of fat-free mass in post menopausal women. Am J Clin Nutr 2002;75:314.

58. Harnack LJ, et al. Temporal trends in energy intake in the United States: an ecologic perspective. Am J Clin Nutr 2000;71:1478.

59. Heath GW, et al. A physiological comparison of younger and older endurance-trained athletes. J Appl Physiol 1981;51:634.

60. Heitmann BL, Garby L. Composition (lean and fat tissue) of weight changes in adult Danes. Am J Clin Nutr 2002;75:834.

61. Hennessy LC, Watson AWS. The interference effects of training for strength and endurance simultaneously. J Strength Cond Res 1994;8:12.

62. Heshka S, et al. Weight loss with self-help compared with a structured commercial program: a randomized trial. JAMA 2003;289:1792.

63. Hill JO, et al. Evaluation of an alternating-calorie diet with and without exercise in the treatment of obesity. Am J Clin Nutr 1989;50:248.

64. Hill JO, et al. Exercise and moderate obesity. In: Bouchard C, et al., eds. Physical activity, fitness, and health. Champaign, IL: Human Kinetics, 1994.

65. Hirsch J, et al. Diet composition and energy balance in humans. Am J Clin Nutr 1998;67(suppl):551S.

66. Housh TJ, et al. Validity of skinfold estimates of percent fat in high school female gymnasts. Med Sci Sports Exerc 1996;28:1331.

67. Hu F, et al. Television watching and other sedentary behaviors in relation to risk of obesity and type 2 diabetes mellitus in women. JAMA 2003;289:1785.

68. Iribarren C, et al. Association of weight loss and weight fluctuation with mortality among Japanese American men. N Engl J Med 1995;333:686.

69. Jakicic JM, Gallagher KI. Exercise considerations for the sedentary, overweight adult. Exerc Sport Sci Rev 2003;31:91.

70. Jakicic JM, Wing RR. Differences in resting energy expenditure in African American versus Caucasian overweight females. Int J Obes 1998;22:236.

71. Jakicic JM, et al. Effects of intermittent exercise and use of home exercise equipment on adherence, weight loss, and fitness in overweight women. JAMA 1999;282:1554.

72. Jeffery RW. Does weight cycling present a risk? Am J Clin Nutr 1996;63(suppl):452S.

73. Jeffrey R, et al. Weight cycling and cardiovascular risk factors in obese men and women. Am J Clin Nutr 1992;55:641.

74. Johnson MJ, et al. Loss of muscle mass is poorly reflected in grip strength performance in healthy young men. Med Sci Sports Exerc 1994;26:235.

75. Johnson ML, et al. Relative importance of inactivity and overeating in energy balance in obese high school girls. Am J Clin Nutr 1986;44:779.

76. Katch FI, et al. Effects of situp exercise training on adipose cell size and adiposity. Res Q Exerc Sport 1984;55:242.

77. Kern PA, et al. The effects of weight loss on the activity and expression of adipose-tissue lipoprotein lipase in very obese humans. N Engl J Med 1990;322:1053.

78. Kimm S, et al. Decline in physical activity in black and white girls during adolescence. N Engl J Med 2002;347:709.

79. King AC, Katch FI. Changes in body density, fatfolds and girths at 2.3 kg increments of weight loss. Hum Biol 1986;58:708.

80. King G, et al. Relationship of leisure-time physical activity and occupational activity to the prevalence of obesity. Int J Obes 2001;25:606.

81. Klem ML, et al. A descriptive study of individuals successful at long-term maintenance of substantial weight loss. Am J Clin Nutr 1997;66:239.

82. Kohrt WM, et al. Body composition of healthy sedentary and trained, young and older men and women. Med Sci Sports Exerc 1992;24:832.

83. Kohrt WM, et al. Exercise training improves fat distribution patterns in 60- to 70-year-old men and women. J Gerontol 1992;47:M99.

84. Kraemer WJ, et al. Compatibility of high-intensity strength and endurance training on hormonal and skeletal muscle adaptations. J Appl Physiol 1995;78:976.

85. Kraemer WJ, et al. Influence of exercise training on physiological and performance changes with weight loss in men. Med Sci Sports Exerc 1999;31:1320.

86. Lahti-Koski M, et al. Associations of body mass index and obesity with physical activity, food choices, alcohol intake, and smoking in the 1982-1997 Finrisk Studies. Am J Clin Nutr 2002;75:809.

87. Larew K, et al. Muscle metabolic function, exercise performance, and weight gain. Med Sci Sports Exerc 2003;35:230.

88. Lee I-M, et al. Physical activity and coronary heart disease in women: is "no pain no gain" passé? JAMA 2001;285:1447.

89. Leibel R, et al. Changes in energy expenditure resulting from altered body weight. N Engl J Med 1995;332:621.

90. Lemmer JT, et al. Effects of strength training on resting metabolic rate and physical activity: age and gender comparisons. Med Sci Sports Exerc 2001;33:532.

91. Lemon PWR. Do athletes need more dietary protein and amino acids? Int J Sports Nutr 1995;5:S39.

92. LeMura LM, Maziekas MT. Factors that alter body fat, body mass, and fat-free mass in pediatric obesity. Med Sci Sports Exerc 2002;34:487.

93. Manson JE, et al. Walking compared with vigorous exercise for the prevention of cardiovascular events in women. N Engl J Med 2002;347:716.

94. Martin WA. Effect of acute and chronic exercise on fat metabolism. Exerc Sport Sci Rev 1996;24:203.

95. Mayo MJ, et al. Exercise-induced weight loss preferentially reduces abdominal fat. Med Sci Sports Exerc 2003;35:207.

96. Meredith CN, et al. Body composition and aerobic capacity in young and middle-aged endurance-trained men. Med Sci Sports Exerc 1987;19:557.

97. Miller-Kovach K, et al. Weight maintenance among Weight Watchers lifetime members. FASEB J 1998;282:1519.

98. Mokdad AH, et al. The spread of the obesity epidemic in the United States, 1991-1998. JAMA 1999;282:1519.

99. Mokdad AH, et al. The continuing epidemics of obesity and diabetes in the United States. JAMA 2001;286:1195.

100. Molé PA, et al. Exercise reverses depressed metabolic rate produced by severe caloric restriction. Med Sci Sports Exerc 1989;21:29.

101. National Institutes of Health, National Heart, Lung, and Blood Institute. Obesity evaluation initiative, clinical guidelines and the identification, evaluation, and treatment of overweight and obesity in adults. Bethesda, MD: National Institutes of Health, June, 1998.

102. National Task Force on the Prevention and Treatment of Obesity. Very-low-calorie diets. JAMA 1993;270:976.

103. National Task Force on the Prevention and Treatment of Obesity. Weight cycling. JAMA 1994;272:1196.

104. Nicklas BJ. Effects of endurance exercise on adipose tissue metabolism. Exerc Sport Sci Rev 1997;25:77.

105. Obesity: preventing and managing the global epidemic: report of a WHO consultation. Geneva, Switzerland: World Health Organization; 2000. WHO Technical Report series, 894.

106. Ogden CL, et al. Prevalence and trends in overweight among US children and adolescents, 1999-2000. JAMA 2002;288:1728.

107. Pavlou KN, et al. Exercise as an adjunct to weight loss and maintenance in moderately obese subjects. Am J Clin Nutr 1989;49:1115.

108. Peeters A, et al. Obesity in adulthood and its consequences for life expectancy. Ann Intern Med 2003;138:24.

109. Pellymounter MA, et al. Effects of the *obese* gene product on body weight reduction in *ob/ob* mice. Science 1995;269:540.

110. Pérusse L, et al. Acute and chronic effects of exercise on leptin levels in humans. J Appl Physiol 1997;83:5.

111. Philen RD, et al. Survey of advertising for nutritional supplements in health and bodybuilding magazines. JAMA 1992;268:1008.

112. Poehlman ET, Melby C. Resistance training and energy balance. Int J Sports Nutr 1998;8:143.

113. Poehlman ET, et al. Effect of resistance training and endurance training on insulin sensitivity in nonobese, young women. J Clin Endocrinol Metab 2000;85:2463.

114. Pollock ML, et al. Twenty-year follow-up of aerobic power and body composition of older track athletes. J Appl Physiol 1997;82:1508.

115. Prabhakaran B, et al. Effect of 14 weeks of resistance training on lipid profile and body fat percentage in premenopausal women. Br J Sports Med 1999;33:190.

116. Prentice AM, et al. Effects of weight cycling on body composition. Am J Clin Nutr 1992;56:209S.

117. Racette SB, et al. Effects of aerobic exercise and dietary carbohydrate on energy expenditure and body composition during weight reduction in obese women. Am J Clin Nutr 1995;61:486.

118. Ravussin E, et al. Reduced rate of energy expenditure as a risk factor for body-weight gain. N Engl J Med 1988;318:467.

119. Reddy ST, et al. Effect of low-carbohydrate, high-protein diets on acid-base balance, stone-forming propensity, and calcium metabolism. Am J Kidney Dis 2002;40:265.

120. Reseland JE, et al. Effect of long-term changes in diet and exercise on plasma leptin concentrations. Am J Clin Nutr 2001;73:240.

121. Roberts SB, et al. Energy expenditure and intake in infants born to lean and overweight mothers. N Engl J Med 1988;318:461.

122. Robinson TN. Reducing children's television viewing to prevent obesity: a randomized clinical trial. JAMA 1999;282:1562.

123. Roemmich JN, Sinning WE. Weight loss and wrestling training: effects of nutrition, growth, maturation, body composition, and strength. J Appl Physiol 1997;82:1751.

124. Rolland-Cachera MF, Bellisle F. No correlation between adiposity and food intake: why are working class children fatter? Am J Clin Nutr 1986;44:779.

125. Rolls BJ, et al. Portion size of food affects energy intake in normal-weight and overweight men and women. Am J Clin Nutr 2002;76:1207.

126. Rosenbaum M, et al. Obesity. N Engl J Med 1997;337:396.

127. Ross R, et al. Exercise alone is an effective strategy for reducing obesity and related comorbidities. Exerc Sport Sci Rev 2000;28:165.

128. Ross R, et al. Reduction in obesity and related comorbid conditions after diet-induced weight loss or exercise-induced weight loss in men. Ann Intern Med 2000;133:92.

129. Ryan SS, et al. Resistive training increases fat-free mass and maintains RMR despite weight loss in postmenopausal women. J Appl Physiol 1995;79:818.

130. Samaha FF, et al. A low-carbohydrate as compared with a low-fat diet in severe obesity. N Engl J Med 2003;348:2074.

131. Schoeller D, et al. How much physical activity is needed to minimize weight gain in previously obese women? Am J Clin Nutr 1997;66:551.

132. Schoeller DA, et al. The importance of clinical research: the role of thermogenesis in human obesity. Am J Clin Nutr 2001;73:511.

133. Schwartz RS, et al. The effect of intensive endurance exercise training on body fat distribution in young and older men. Metabolism 1991;40:545.

134. Serdula MK, et al. Prevalence of attempting weight loss and strategies for controlling weight. JAMA 1999;282:1359.

135. Shepard TY, et al. Occasional physical inactivity combined with a high-fat diet may be important in the development and maintenance of obesity in human subjects. Am J Clin Nutr 2001;73:703.

136. Short KR, Sedlock DA. Excess postexercise oxygen consumption and recovery rate in trained and untrained subjects. J Appl Physiol 1997;83:153.

137. Simkin-Silverman L, et al. Lifetime weight cycling and psychological health in normal-weight and overweight women. Int J Eating Disord 1998;24:175.

138. Skender MI, et al. Comparison of 2-year weight loss trends in behavioral treatments of obesity: diet, exercise, and combination interventions. J Am Diet Assoc 1996;96:342.

139. Steffen PR, et al. Effects of exercise and weight loss or blood loss on blood pressure during daily life. Med Sci Sport Exerc 2001;33:1635.

140. Stern L, et al. The effects of low-carbohydrate versus conventional weight loss diets in severely obese adults: one-year follow-up of randomized trial. Arch Intern Med 2004;140:778.

141. Stewart KJ. Exercise training and the cardiovascular consequences of type 2 diabetes and hypertension: plausible mechanisms for improving cardiovascular health. JAMA 2002;288:1622.

142. Strauss RS, Pollack HA. Epidemic increase in childhood overweight, 1986–1998. JAMA 2001;286:2845.

143. Sun M, et al. A longitudinal study of resting energy expenditure relative to body composition during puberty in African American and white children. Am J Clin Nutr 2001;73:308.

144. Tanasescu M, et al. Exercise type and intensity in relation to coronary heart disease in men. JAMA 2002;288:1994.

145. Taubes G. As obesity rates rise, experts struggle to explain why. Science 1998;280:1367.

146. Tcheng T, Tipton CM. Iowa wrestling study: anthropometric measurements and the prediction of a "minimal" body weight for high school wrestlers. Med Sci Sports 1973;5:1.

147. Technology Assessment Conference Panel. Methods for voluntary weight loss and control. Technology Assessment Conference statement. Ann Intern Med 1992;116:942.

148. Thorland WG, et al. Estimation of body density in adolescent athletes. Hum Biol 1984;56:439.

149. Torshakovec AM, et al. Age, sex, ethnicity, body composition, and resting energy expenditure of obese African American children and adolescents. Am J Clin Nutr 2002;75:867.

150. Treuth MS, et al. Familial resemblance of body composition in prepubertal girls and their biological parents. Am J Clin Nutr 2001;74:529.

151. Troiano RP, Flegal KM. Overweight children and adolescents: description, epidemiology, and demographics. Pediatrics 1998;101:497.

152. Tuomilehto J, et al. Prevention of type 2 diabetes mellitus by changes in lifestyle among subjects with impaired glucose tolerance. N Engl J Med 2001;344:1343.

153. US Department of Health and Human Services. Physical activity and health: a report of the Surgeon General. Atlanta, GA: Centers for Disease Control and Prevention, 1996.

154. VanAnggel-Leijssen DPC, et al. Short term effects of weight loss with or without low-intensity exercise training on fat metabolism in obese men. Am J Clin Nutr 2001;73:523.

155. VanDale D, Saris WHM. Repetitive weight loss and weight regain: effects on weight reduction, resting metabolic rate, and lipolytic activity before and after exercise and/or diet treatment. Am J Clin Nutr 1989;49:409.

156. VanEtten LMLA, et al. Effect of body build on weight-training-induced adaptations in body composition and muscular strength. Med Sci Sports Exerc 1994;26:515.

157. VanEtten LMLA, et al. Effect of an 18-wk weight-training program on energy expenditure and physical activity. J Appl Physiol 1997;82:298.

158. VanHorn L, Greenland P. Prevention of coronary artery disease is a pediatric problem. JAMA 1997;278:1779.

159. Vincent SD, et al. Activity levels and body mass index of children in the United States, Sweden, and Australia. Med Sci Sports Exerc 2003;35:1367.

160. Wadden TA. Characteristics of successful weight loss maintenance. In: PiSunyer FX, Allison DB, eds. Obesity treatment: establishing goals, improving outcomes, and establishing the research agenda. New York: Plenum Press, 1995.

161. Wadden TA, Foster GD. Behavioral treatment of obesity. Med Clin North Am 2000;84:441.

162. Wahrenberg H, et al. Adrenergic regulation of lipolysis in human fat cells during exercise. Eur J Clin Invest 1991;21:534.

163. Wei M, et al. Relationship between low cardiorespiratory fitness and mortality in normal-weight, overweight, and obese men. JAMA 1999;282:1547.

164. Weinsier RL, et al. Do adaptive changes in metabolic rate favor weight regain in weight-reduced individuals? An examination of the set-point theory. Am J Clin Nutr 2000;72:1088.

165. Weinsier RL, et al. Energy expenditure and free-living physical activity in black and white women: comparison before and after weight loss. Am J Clin Nutr 2000;71:138.

166. Weinsier RL, et al. Free-living activity energy expenditure in women successful and unsuccessful at maintaining a normal body weight. Am J Clin Nutr 2002;75:499.

167. Weyer C, et al. Energy metabolism after 2 y of energy restriction: the Biosphere 2 experiment. Am J Clin Nutr 2000;72:946.

168. Wier L, et al. Determining the amount of physical activity needed for long-term weight control. Int J Obes 2001;25:613.

169. Willett WC. Is dietary fat a major determinant of body fat? Am J Clin Nutr 1998;67(suppl):555S.

170. Williams PT. Relationship of distance run per week to coronary heart disease risk factors in 8,283 male runners. The National Runners" Health Study. Arch Intern Med 1997;157:191.

171. Wilmore JH. Increasing physical activity: alterations in body mass and composition. Am J Clin Nutr 1996;63(suppl):456S.

172. Wing RR. Weight cycling in humans: a review of the literature. Ann Behav Med 1992;14:113.

173. Wroble RR, Moxley DP. Weight loss patterns and success rates in high school wrestlers. Med Sci Sports Exerc 1998;30:625.

174. Yancy WS Jr, et al. A low-carbohydrate, ketogenic diet versus a low-fat diet to treat obesity and hyperlipidemia: a randomized, controlled trial. Ann Intern Med 2004;140:769.

175. Zhang Y, et al. Positional cloning of the mouse obese gene and its human homologue. Nature 1994;372:425.

176. Zuti WB, Golding LA. Comparing diet and exercise as weight reduction tools. Phys Sportsmed 1976;4:49.

Additional Readings

Ardern CI, et al. Race and sex similarities in exercise-induced changes in blood lipids and fatness. Med Sci Sports Exerc 2004;36:1610.

Booth DA, et al. Patterns of eating and movement that best maintain reduction in overweight. Appetite 2004;43:277.

Datar A, Sturm R. Physical education in elementary school and body mass index: Evidence from the early childhood longitudinal study. Am J Public Health 2004;94:1501.

de Castro JM. Genes, the environment and the control of food intake. Br J Nutr 2004;92(Suppl)1:59.

Deibert P, et al. Weight loss without losing muscle mass in pre-obese and obese subjects induced by a high-soy-protein diet. Int J Obes Relat Metab Disord 2004;28:1349.

Flodmark CE, et al. New insights into the field of children and adolescents' obesity: The European perspective. Int J Obes Relat Metab Disord 2004;28:1189.

Green JS, et al. The effects of exercise training on abdominal visceral fat, body composition, and indicators of the metabolic syndrome in postmenopausal women with and without estrogen replacement therapy: The HERITAGE family study. Metabolism 2004;53:1192.

Gustafson Dr, et al. A 24-year follow-up of body mass index and cerebral atrophy. Neurology 2004;63:1876.

Gustafson Dr, et al. Body mass index and white matter lesions in elderly women: A 18-year longitudinal study. Int Psychogeriate 2004;16:327.

Hill AJ. Does dieting make you fat? Br J Nutr 2004;92(Suppl)1:15.

Hines SE. Words into action--promoting successful weight loss in overweight patients. JAAPA 2004;17:19.

Keim NL, et al. America's obesity epidemic: Measuring physical activity to promote an active lifestyle. J Am Diet Assoc 2004;104:1398.

Kruger J, et al. Attempting to lose weight: Specific practices among U.S. adults. Am J Prev Med 2004;26:402

Kruskall LJ, et al. The Yale Physical Activity Survey for older adults: Predictions in the energy expenditure due to physical activity. J Am Diet Assoc 2004;104:1251.

Linne Y, et al. Long-term weight development in women: A 15-year follow-up of the effects of pregnancy. Obes Res 2004;12:1166.

Lowe MR, Timko CA. Dieting: Really harmful, merely ineffective or actually helpful? Br J Nutr 2004;92(Suppl)1:19.

McCaffree J. What you should know about calorie restriction. J Am Diet Assoc 2004;104:1524.

Moore MS, et al. Short-term appetite and energy intake following imposed exercise in 9- to 10-year-old girls. Appetite 2004;43:127.

Prentice A, Jebb S. Energy intake/physical activity interactions in the homeostasis of body weight regulation. Nutr Rev 2004;62:S98.

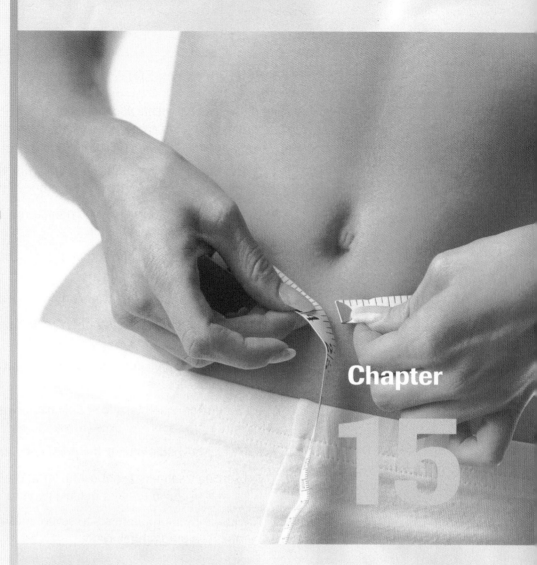

Chapter

15

Disordered Eating

AN INORDINATE FOCUS ON BODY WEIGHT

Disordered eating *refers to a broad spectrum of complex behaviors, core attitudes, coping strategies, and conditions that share a commonalty of an emotionally based, inordinate and often-pathologic focus on body shape and body weight.* Severe distortions of the eating process (ranging from calorie, protein and/or fat restriction and pathogenic weight control measures to anorexia nervosa and bulimia nervosa) remain unique to the cultural milieu of industrialized nations that focus on overindulgence with food and high priority on slimness to reflect attractiveness and interpersonal success. An estimated 8 million persons in the United States, particularly white middle-class girls and women, exhibit eating disorders, of whom females constitute about 90%.

Among 3000 middle-school children studied for body image and dietary practices, 55% of eighth-grade girls believed they were fat (13% actually were), and 50% had dieted. For the boys, 28% considered themselves fat (13% actually were), and 15% had dieted. Among 869 Australian schoolgirls ages 14 to 17 years, 335 reported at least one disordered eating behavior, while monthly bingeing occurred in 8% and vomiting in 27%.[28] TABLE 15.1 lists the prevalence of monthly unhealthy and extreme weight reduction practices of these teenage girls. Of the group, 57% practiced "unhealthy dieting," and 36% practiced dieting behaviors considered extreme—crash dieting, fasting, and use of diet pills, diuretics, laxatives, and cigarettes.

FIGURE 15.1 displays the relationship between the girls' actual body weight classification (determined by body mass index [BMI]) and perceived body weight. Regardless of objective weight categorization, 47% of all girls actively tried

to lose weight, including 19% of underweight girls and 56% of normal-weight girls. When asked to categorize their current weight, 63% considered themselves overweight, yet only 16% actually were; 28% seemed "just right" (55% were of normal weight), and 9% concluded they were underweight (30% actually were). Such findings take on additional significance because previous attempts at dieting often develop into a full-blown eating disorder.

Disordered eating behaviors generally affect females between the ages of 15 and 35, although women in their 30s, 40s, and 50s may account for up to one-third of eating disorders in the U.S. The prevalence in the general population ranges from 1 to 5% of female high school and college students to as high as 12 to 15% for females in medical and graduate schools.[16,32,33,71] Thin body preoccupation and social pressure represent important risk factors for the development of eating disorders in adolescent girls.[92] Childhood traits reflecting obsessive–compulsive personality also appear to be important risk factors.[2] Adolescent girls who experience physical and sexual dating violence show a relatively high rate of abnormal weight control behaviors such as laxative use and/or vomiting.[64,76] Contrary to the conventional belief of many health professionals, African American women are not immune from eating disorders. A survey of African American college women found a prevalence of eating disorders similar to that among white peers; 2% had a full-blown eating disorder, and 23% showed some eating disorder symptoms. Cultural differences in the view of

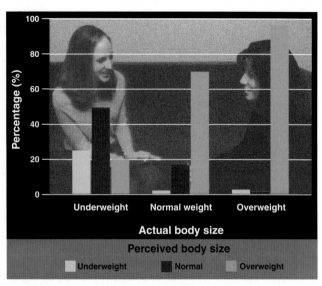

Figure 15.1 Perception of current body weight and actual body weight classification determined by BMI in 851 teenage girls. (From Grigg M, et al. Disordered eating and unhealthy weight reduction practices among adolescent females. Prevent Med 1996;25:745.)

Table 15.1	PREVALENCE OF UNHEALTHY AND EXTREME WEIGHT-REDUCTION PRACTICES AMONG TEENAGE GIRLS

Behavior (monthly)	Prevalence (%)
No dairy[a]	16
No meats[a]	18
No starchy foods[a]	13
Slimming biscuit use	15
Slimming drink use	11
Skipping meals	46
Fad dieting	14
"Crash" dieting[b]	22
Fasting[b]	21
Diet pills	5
Diuretic use[b]	2
Laxative use[b]	5
Cigarette use[b]	12

From Grigg M, et al. Disordered eating and unhealthy weight-reduction practices among adolescent females. Prevent Med 1996;25:745.

[a] These foods eliminated and not compensated for with a balanced diet (e.g., a balanced vegetarian diet).
[b] Extreme dieting defined as "crash" dieting, fasting, or use of diet pills, diuretics, laxatives, and cigarettes.

attractiveness—thin African American women are often considered unattractive—often causes some African American women to gain weight by binge eating.[55]

Miss America and BMI—Undernourished Role Models?

In 1967, only an 8% difference in body weight existed between professional models and the average American woman. Today, a model's body weight averages 23 pounds below the national average for women (5'11", 117 lb versus 5'4", 140 lb). This makes the BMI of most fashion models lower than that of all but 2% of American women. A focus on thinness has become particularly apparent among Miss America contestants.

Many consider Miss America beauty pageant contestants to possess the ideal combination of beauty, grace, and talent. Each competitor survives the rigors of state and local contests, thus satisfying judges that finalists have "ideal qualities" worthy of role-model status. To some extent, the consummate image of the Miss America physique shapes society's generalized "ideal" for female size and shape. The contest, televised worldwide to millions of viewers, reinforces this notion. However, does such an image project and/or reinforce an unhealthful message to those who attempt to emulate these women?

FIGURE 15.2 shows the BMIs of Miss America contestants from available data between 1922 and 1999 (excluding 1927–1933, when the pageant was not held). The *lower horizontal dashed line* designates the World Health Organization (WHO) cutoff for undernutrition established at a BMI of 18.5 kg·m^{-2}.[100] The *upper horizontal line* represents the

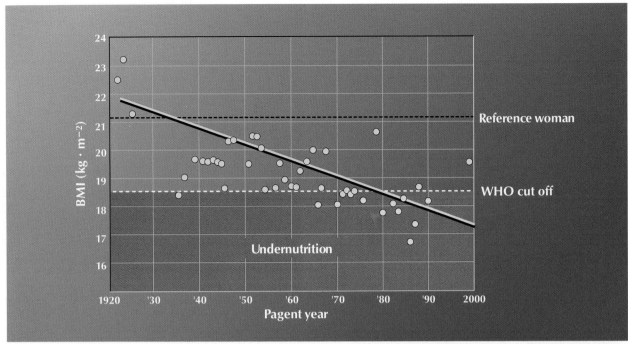

	1922–1948		
	Age	Ht	Wt
1922	18	65	135
1923	19	65	140
1924	18	66	132
1926	18	52.5	118
1936	22	66	114
1937	17	66.5	120
1939	19	67	126
1941	19	65.5	120
1942	21	65	118
1943	21	68	130
1944	21	67	125
1945	18	70	136
1946	21	68	123
1947	21	67	130
1948	18	69	138

	1951–1968		
	Age	Ht	Wt
1951	20	65.5	119
1952	25	70	143
1953	19	66.5	128
1954	20	68	132
1955	19	68.5	124
1957	19	67	120
1958	20	68.5	130
1959	21	65	114
1960	21	67	120
1961	18	66	116
1962	19	65.5	118
1964	21	66.5	124
1965	22	124	124
1966	19	115	115
1967	19	116	116
1968	19	135	135

	1970–1999		
	Age	Ht	Wt
1970	21	65.5	110
1971	21	68	121
1972	22	67	118
1973	23	68	120
1974	23	69	125
1976	18	70.5	128
1979	22	64	121
1980	22	67	114
1983	25	67	115
1984	20	66	110
1985	20	68	120
1986	21	69	114
1987	21	68.5	116
1988	24	70	131
1990	24	67.5	118
1999	24	69	133

	Girths (inches)							
	Bust	Waist	Hips	Calf	Thigh	Ankle	Biceps	Wrist
1926	33	24.5	33.5	12.5	19.5	7	—	—
1935	33	23	35.5	—	—	—	—	—
1926	34	23.5	34.5	13	19	8.5	9.5	5.5
1941	34	24	36	14	23	8	11	6
1942	34	24	34.5	—	—	—	—	—
1943	36	23	35	—	—	—	—	—
1944	36.5	25	37.5	13	19.5	8	—	—
1945	35.5	25	35	14.5	20	8.5	—	—
1946	35.5	25.5	36	13.5	22	8.5	—	—
1947	35	35	—	—	—	—	—	—
1948	37	37	—	—	—	—	—	—
1951	35	35	—	—	—	—	—	—
1952	36	24	36	—	—	—	—	—
1953	35	23	35	—	—	—	—	—
1954	37	24	36	—	—	—	—	—
1955	34.5	22	35	—	—	—	—	—
1957	35	23	35	—	—	—	—	—
1958	35	25	36	—	—	—	—	—
1959	34	22	35	—	—	—	—	—
1960	36	24	36	—	—	—	—	—
1961	35	22	35	—	—	—	—	—
1962	35	24	35	—	—	—	—	—
1964	35	23	35	—	—	—	—	—
1965	36	24	36	—	—	—	—	—
Ref W*	36.1	30.3	36.8	14.1	21.6	8.9	12.5	6.8

Ref W* = Behnke's reference woman; stature = 163.8 cm, body mass = 56.7 kg

▓ Figure 15.2 BMI of 47 Miss America pageant contestants from 1922 to 1999. The *top horizontal dashed black line* represents the BMI for Behnke's reference woman (21.1 kg·m⁻²). The *bottom horizontal dashed white line* designates the WHO's BMI demarcation for undernutrition (18.5 kg·m⁻²). The *left inset table* shows the available data for age, height (in.), and weight (lb) for the contest winners. The *right inset table* shows selected girths for 24 Miss America winners from 1926 to 1965.

BMI for Behnke's standard for the reference woman (Fig. 13.6; stature, 1.638 m; body mass, 56.7 kg; BMI, 21.1 kg·m⁻²). The downward slope of the regression line from 1922 to 1999 shows a clear tendency for relative undernutrition from the mid-1960s to approximately 1990. Using the WHO cutoff, the BMIs of 30% (N = 14) of the 47 Miss America winners fell below 18.5. Raising the BMI cutoff to 19.0 kg·m⁻² adds another 18 women, or a total of 48% of the win-

ners with undesirable values. Approximately 24% of the BMIs of contest winners ranged between 20.0 and 21.0 kg·m⁻², and no winner after 1924 had a BMI equaling that of the reference woman!

Interestingly, 1965 was the last year that we could locate girth measurements from official press releases or newspaper coverage of the contest. We compared the percentage difference between Miss America girth averages

with corresponding values for the reference woman (*bottom row* of *right inset table*). For the average bust, waist, and hip values (35.1 in., 24.0 in., 35.4 in., respectively), Miss America's bust measurement exceeded the reference woman's measurement by 2.6 inches (8%) but fell 7% below the waist value (–1.8 in.), and 5% (–1.7 in.) below the value for the hips. Unfortunately, no contemporary BMI data exist from 1966 to 2004 to compare the "modern" Miss America's physique status with historical data. If the Miss America contest indeed serves as a subtle promoter of the "ideal" female size and shape, then the more recent message delivered to impressionable teenagers overemphasizes that "thin is in," regardless of the potential negative nutritional and long-term health implications.[21]

Female Athletes at Greater Risk

Most studies documenting disordered eating behaviors among athletes rely on anonymous self-report surveys or inventories, with relatively little data from in-depth interviews. Generalizations come mainly from "snapshots" of small numbers of high school and college athletes in specific sports without considering the athletes' skill level, experience, and achievement status. Notwithstanding these limitations in research strategy, female athletes clearly face a unique set of circumstances that make them particularly vulnerable to disordered eating behaviors. These behaviors flourish when strong negative aesthetic connotations about excess body fat blend with the athlete's belief that *any* body fat dooms success. Twenty-three years ago, female gymnasts weighed about 21 pounds more than their present day counterparts. As one sports medicine physician states: "Only in gymnastics is puberty the enemy. Performance fades when girls gain fat and change shape." (Body weight of female gymnastics competitors in the 1996 Olympic games averaged as follows: US, 92.3 lb [height = 4'11 1/8"; age 17.7 years]; Russia, 84.1 lb [height 4' 10 3/4"; age 16.6 years]; China, 78.5 lb [4' 7 1/4"; age 16.0 years]). Some argue that these data indicate that the United States has made strides toward more appropriate body weights for its gymnasts, because the body weight of its 1992 Olympic gymnasts averaged only 82.9 lb [4' 9 1/2"; age 15.9 years].

Clinical observations indicate a prevalence between 15 and 60% for disordered eating patterns among athletes, with some groups at higher risk than others. More specifically, disordered eating patterns and unrealistic weight goals (and general dissatisfaction with one's body) occur most frequently among female athletes in the aesthetic sports such as ballet, bodybuilding, diving, figure skating, cheerleading, and gymnastics, in which success often coincides with extreme leanness.[9,26,30,34,37,62,69,86,95,103] An inordinate preoccupation with eating also occurs among adolescent female swimmers.[5,17] Controversy exists as to the prevalence of eating disorders among endurance runners,[12,61,96,97] but recent data show a nearly 26% prevalence of disordered eating behaviors as indicated by elevated scores on the Eating Disorders Inventory.[13]

Coaches often compound the problem.[78] Sixty-seven percent of female collegiate gymnasts reported that their coaches said they weighed too much, and 75% of these athletes used weight-loss strategies involving vomiting or laxative or diuretic use.[72] Weight reduction attempts averaged 85% in female and 93% in male weight-class athletes.[22] Between 27 and 37% of women in aesthetic, endurance, and weight-class sports experienced menstrual disorders, compared with only 5% in other sports. Unfortunately, reducing body weight significantly below normal levels also coincides with inadequate nutrient intake.[44]

Among athletes classified "at risk" for developing an eating disorder, 92% met the criteria for anorexia nervosa, bulimia nervosa, or anorexia athletica (see pp. 496, 500 and 501).[88] Eighty-five percent of the athletes dieted, compared with 27% of controls. Adolescent dancers and figure skaters exhibited more frequent patterns of disordered eating than other athletic groups and nonathletes.[8] In a survey of female college athletes, 14% of the women reported self-induced vomiting, while 16% indicated laxative use for weight control.[73] Among female college gymnasts, all were trying to diet, and 25% reported self-induced vomiting.[72] Other studies also indicate high incidence of disordered eating behaviors among female gymnasts.[57,63,65,96] However, prevalence rates did not differ from age-matched, nonathletic controls.

Risk factors for disordered eating among athletes include:[91]

- Pressure to optimize performance and/or modify appearance
- Psychologic factors, such as low self-esteem, poor coping skills, perceived loss of control, perfectionism, obsessive–compulsive traits, depression, anxiety, and history of sexual/physical abuse
- Underlying chronic diseases related to caloric use (e.g., diabetes)

On a more positive note, preoccupation with body weight and associated eating disorder symptoms among female gymnasts during college abates considerably after retirement from the sport.[5] TABLE 15.2 presents data on eating disorder symptoms from former college gymnasts approximately 15 years postcompetition. These women scored below published average values (*norms*) for each variable measured. Nonathletic controls and gymnasts scored similarly on all variables except asceticism and body dissatisfaction, on which gymnasts scored significantly lower. The former gymnasts also maintained nutrient intakes within the recommended range and possessed greater bone mineral density at multiple body sites than controls.[44] One must determine if findings from former gymnasts of 15 to 25 years ago apply to contemporary gymnasts, for whom exaggerated leanness and small body structure now seem to play an important part in competitive success.

CASE STUDY/PERSONAL HEALTH AND EXERCISE NUTRITION 15–1

How to Calculate Recommended (Ideal) Body Weight

A major objective in determining an individual's body composition relates to recommending an "ideal" body weight (IBW). Usually this refers to a recommended or optimal body weight for health considerations, occupational and sport performance requirements, or simply aesthetics (self-assessment based on appearance). IBW computation is based on comparison with an optimal or ideal percentage body fat (I%BF). Determining I%BF becomes subjective, as no absolute standards by age, fitness, ethnicity, or any other variable are available. Several body composition reference classifications can serve as guidelines for setting I%BF levels for different ages (Table 1). Selecting the I%BF should reflect the person's current %BF and his or her health/fitness objectives.

Table 1	BODY COMPOSITION CLASSIFICATION BY AGE ACCORDING TO PERCENTAGE BODY FAT FROM TYPICAL DATA IN THE RESEARCH		
Age, y	Below Average	Average	Above Average
Males			
≤19	12–17	17–22	22–27
20–29	13–18	18–23	23–28
30–39	14–19	19–24	24–29
40–49	15–20	20–25	25–30
≥50	16–20	21–26	26–31
Females			
≤19	17–22	22–27	27–32
20–29	18–23	23–28	28–33
30–39	19–24	24–29	29–34
40–49	20–25	25–30	30–35
≥50	21–26	26–31	31–36

PROCEDURES

1. Determine body weight (BW) in kilograms and %BF using an available valid technique.
2. Calculate body fat weight (FW) in kilograms.

$$FW = BW \times \%BF$$

where %BF is expressed in decimal form (e.g., 23.0% = 0.23)

3. Determine fat-free body mass (FFM) in kilograms.

$$FFM = BW - FW$$

4. Select a I%BF expressed in decimal form (e.g., 15.0% = 0.15).
5. Compute ideal (recommended) body weight (IBW) in kilograms.

$$IBW = FFM \div (1.00 - I\%BF)$$

EXAMPLE CALCULATIONS

Data: Female; age 19 years; body weight = 66.0 kg; %BF from hydrostatic weighing = 30.0% (decimal form = 0.30); I%BF chosen = 25.0% (0.25).

Calculate FW in kilograms:

$$
\begin{aligned}
FW &= BW \times \%BF \\
&= 66.0 \text{ kg} \times 0.30 \\
&= 19.8 \text{ kg (43.7 lb)}
\end{aligned}
$$

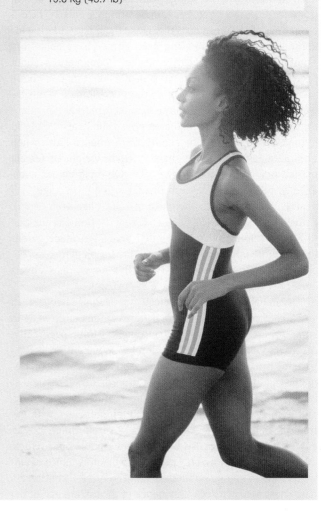

CASE STUDY/PERSONAL HEALTH AND EXERCISE NUTRITION 15-1 (*continued*)

Determine FFM in kilograms:

$$FFM = BW - FW$$
$$= 66.0 \text{ kg} - 19.8 \text{ kg}$$
$$= 46.2 \text{ kg} (101.9 \text{ lb})$$

Select I%BF expressed in decimal form:

$$I\%BF = 0.25$$

Compute IBW in kg:

$$IBW = FFM \div (1.00 - I\%BF)$$
$$= 46.2 \text{ kg} \div (1.00 - 0.25)$$
$$= 61.6 \text{ kg} (135 \text{ lb})$$

COMPUTING RECOMMENDED FAT LOSS

From the above calculations, the amount of fat loss in kilograms required to reach IBW (at the chosen %BF of 25.0%) computes as:

$$\text{Fat loss} = BW - IBW$$
$$= 66.0 \text{ kg} - 61.6 \text{ kg}$$
$$= 4.4 \text{ kg} (9.7 \text{ lb})$$

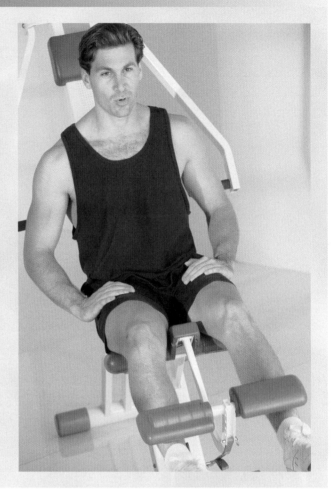

Table 15.2	EATING DISORDERS INVENTORY SCORES FOR NORMS, FORMER GYMNASTS, AND CONTROL SUBJECTS		
	Norms (N = 205)	*Gymnasts* (N = 22)	*Controls* (N = 22)
Drive for thinness	5.5	3.3	4.0
Bulimia	1.2	0.6	1.0
Body dissatisfaction	12.2	7.9	14.1*
Ineffectiveness	2.3	1.2	2.3
Perfectionism	6.2	5.0	4.3
Interpersonal distrust	2.0	1.6	2.5
Interoceptive awareness	3.0	0.9	1.4
Maturity fears	2.7	1.8	2.0
Asceticism	3.4	2.4	4.5*
Impulse regulation	2.3	0.7	0.9
Social insecurity	3.3	1.4	3.1

* Significantly different from gymnasts, $P \leq .05$.
From O'Connor PJ, et al. Eating disorder symptoms in former female college gymnasts: relations with body composition. Am J Clin Nutr 1996;64:840.

TABLE 15.3 summarizes the findings of 23 studies of eating patterns of athletes. In general, the incidence of disordered eating behaviors is greater among athletes than in nonathletic comparison groups or the general population. Future research should investigate the extent to which disordered eating behaviors permeate the competitive athletic scene among junior and senior high school female participants.

A study in conjunction with the National Collegiate Athletic Association clearly shows a greater prevalence of eating disorders among female athletes than male counterparts.[36] Among women, 1.1% met the clinical diagnostic criteria for bulimia nervosa; none met the criteria for anorexia nervosa, but 9.2% showed subclinical bulimia and subclinical anorexia. For the male athletes, none met the diagnostic criteria for anorexia, bulimia, or subclinical anorexia, and only 0.01% presented with subclinical bulimia. Further research can shed light on this gender gap in eating disorder prevalence: Does it reflect sex-related differences in sociocultural expectations and sport-specific demands or is it simply the result of an underreporting of eating disorders in males?

(*text continues on page 498*)

Table 15.3   **SUMMARY OF SELECTED STUDIES OF DISORDERED EATING BEHAVIORS IN ATHLETES**

Study (ref. #)	Sport	Subjects	Measures[a]	Outcome
6	Female and male athletes from 8 sports	695 athletes (55% female) from 8 sports. Mean age, 19 y (range, 16–25)	41-item questionnaire mailed to coaches in 21 colleges in the midwest; coaches administered it to athletes	59% lost weight by "excessive" exercise, 24% by consuming less than 600 kcal/d, 12% by fasting, 11% by using fad diets, 6% by vomiting, 4% by using laxatives, and 1% by using enemas; relatively few gender differences, but trend for males to use exercise and females to use dieting to lose weight
7	Female athletes from 7 sports	79 female athletes in sports emphasizing leanness (ballet, bodybuilding, cheerleading, gymnastics) or sports with no emphasis (swimming, track and field, volleyball); 101 nonathlete controls	EDI	No overall differences between athletes and controls; athletes in sports emphasizing leanness had a higher percentage of elevated scores than athletes in other sports
9	Ballet dancers	55 female dancers in national and regional companies	EAT-26	33% had anorexia or bulimia in the past; 50% of amenorrheic subjects reported anorexia compared with 13% of women with normal cycles
15	Various sports	64 female athletes in "thin-build" sports (e.g., gymnastics); 62 females in "normal-build" sports (e.g., volleyball); 64 female univ. student controls	EDI	Overall EDI scores not different among groups; athletes in thin-build sports had greater weight concerns, more body dissatisfaction, and more dieting than normal-build athletes and controls, even though body weights were lower
17	Swimmers	487 girls and 468 boys, ages 9–18, at a competitive swimming camp	Questionnaire on dieting and weight-control practices	15.4% of the girls (24.8% of the postmenarchal girls) and 3.6% of boys used pathogenic weight loss techniques; girls were more likely than boys to perceive themselves heavier than they were
19	Wrestlers, swimmers, Nordic skiers	26 male wrestlers, 21 male swimmers, and cross-country skiers	EAT-40, restraint questionnaire, body image assessment	Higher EAT scores in wrestlers due to higher scores on weight fluctuation and dieting; no overall differences in estimates of body size; a small subsample of wrestlers who scored high on restraint and EAT scores had distortions of body size
20	Dancers	21 female university dancers and 29 female university controls	EAT-40	33% of dancers and 14% of controls scored in the range symptomatic of anorexia on the EAT; difference in overall EAT scores not significant
23	Ballet dancers	10 female ballet dancers with stress fractures, 10 dancers without fractures, and 10 non-dancer controls	EAT-26, structured interview on DSM-III criteria for eating disorders	Nonsignificant trend for stress-fracture dancers to have higher EAT scores than other 2 groups; greater incidence of eating disorders in stress-fracture group

Table 15.3   **SUMMARY OF SELECTED STUDIES OF DISORDERED EATING BEHAVIORS IN ATHLETES** *(continued)*

Study (ref. #)	Sport	Subjects	Measures[a]	Outcome
26	Ballet dancers	35 female ballet students ages 11–14, followed 2–4 y	EDI	At follow-up, 26% of subjects had anorexia nervosa and 14% had bulimia nervosa or a "partial syndrome"; the "drive for thinness" and "body dissatisfaction" scales of the EDI predicted eating disorders at follow-up
30	Ballet dancers	55 white and 11 black female dancers in national and regional companies (mean age, 24.9 y)	EAT-26	15% of white dancers reported anorexia and 19% report bulimia; none of the black dancers reported anorexia or bulimia
31	Ballet dancers	32 female ballet dancers from 4 national US companies, 17 dancers from national company in China (mean age, 24.6 y)	Variation in EAT-26, subjects given description of eating disorders and asked if they had the problem	American dancers from less-selected companies had more eating problems, more anorectic behaviors and more female obesity than the highly-selected American or Chinese dancers
34	Majorettes	11 varsity majors	24-hour dietary recall on eating and weight practices; no standardized measures	Based on clinical observations, all subjects had distorted body image due to low weight standards. Subjects reported eating and drinking little for several days prior to weighings, high levels of exercise and using sauna, diet pills, and diuretics
Unpublished data	Runners	4551 (1911 females, 2640 males) respondents to survey in *Runners World* magazine	EAT-26 questions on eating and diet concerns	Mean EAT score = 9.0 for males, 14.1 for females; 8% of males and 24% of females scored ≥20 on EAT; 15% of males who ran ≥45 mi/wk scored ≥20, compared with 7% of males who ran less; 24% of females who ran ≥40 mi/wk scored ≥20, compared with 23% of those who ran less
41	Jockeys	10 male jockeys from England (mean age, 22.9 y; mean weight, 108.5 lb)	EDI, EAT-26	Poor response rate to full battery of tests (from 58 stables, only 10 subjects responded); mean EAT score was 14.9, higher than expected in young males; most reported food avoidance, saunas, and laxative abuse; diuretics and appetite suppressants were used; binges were common, but vomiting was unusual
45	Athletes from unspecified sports	126 female athletes from unspecified sports, 590 students from other groups (e.g., sororities, classes)	EDI questionnaire with eating disorder diagnosis questions	Athletes had generally lower scores on all eating disorders measures than other groups, but statistical tests not performed
51	Female athletes from different sports	87 female athletes from track, swimming, gymnastics, and ballet; 41 females with eating disorders, 120 female high school and junior high controls	Self-reports of dieting, vomiting, and eating disorders	Frequent dieting, vomiting, and self-reported anorexia more common in athletes than normal controls but less common than eating disorders subjects, but no statistical comparisons performed

(continued)

Table 15.3   **SUMMARY OF SELECTED STUDIES OF DISORDERED EATING BEHAVIORS IN ATHLETES** *(continued)*

Study (ref. #)	Sport	Subjects	Measures[a]	Outcome
62	Obligatory runners and weightlifters	15 males and 15 females in each of 3 groups; obligatory runners, obligatory weightlifters, and sedentary controls	Body size estimation 3 subscales on EDI	Runners and weightlifters had more eating disturbances than controls; females had more eating pathologies than males
72	Gymnasts	42 female college gymnasts	Questionnaire on dieting and weight control practices	All subjects were dieting (50% for appearance, 50% for performance); 62% used at least 1 pathogenic weight method (e.g., vomiting, diet pills, fasting); 66% were told they were too heavy by coaches
73	Varsity level female athletes from 10 sports	182 female varsity athletes	Questionnaire on dieting and weight control practices	32% engaged in at least 1 pathogenic weight-control practice; the percentages were 14% for vomiting, 16% for laxatives, 25% for diet pills, 5% for diuretics, 20% for regular binges, and 8% for excessive weight loss
74	Ice skaters	17 male (mean age, 21.1 y) and 23 female (mean age, 17.6 y) figure skaters from mid-Atlantic training facility	EAT-40	Mean EAT scores were 29.3 for women and 10 for men; 48% of the women and none of the men had EAT scores in anorectic range (>30)
80	Wrestlers	63 male college wrestlers and 378 high school wrestlers	Questionnaire on dieting and weight control practices	63% of college and 43% of high school wrestlers were preoccupied with food during the season (19% and 14% in the off-season); 41% of college and 29% of high school wrestlers reported eating out of control between matches; 52% of college and 26% of high school wrestlers reported fasting at least once a week
96	Female athletes from 7 sports	82 female athletes from gymnastics, cross-country, basketball, golf, volleyball, swimming, and tennis; 52 nonathlete controls	EAT-40, EDI	None of athletes scored in disturbed range; no overall differences between athletes and controls; cross-country runners showed less and gymnasts showed more eating disturbance than controls, but only on selected scales
97	Runners	125 female distance runners, 25 nonrunning controls	EAT-26, EDI	No greater incidence of eating problems in runners than in controls; elite runners more likely than other runners to have problems

From Brownell KD, Rodin J. Prevalence of eating disorders in athletes. In: Brownell KD, et al., eds. Eating, body weight and performance in athletes. Philadelphia: Lea & Febiger, 1992.

[a] EAT-40, Eating Attitudes Test containing 40 questions in which subjects rate how well a statement applies to them on a 6-point scale; EAT-26, 26-question modification of EAT-40; EDI, Eating Disorder Inventory containing 64 questions with 8 subscales to assess behaviors and attitudes related to body image, eating behaviors, and dieting.

Answering Questions Concerning Body Fat Prediction

A 27-year-old woman joined a local health club 1 year after the birth of her second child. Her personal trainer assessed her body composition using a three-site skinfold equation. Her results "shocked" her—the trainer said she needed to lose about 18 pounds, based on her body fat percentage of 33.4. She was told she should strive to attain a body fat percentage of about 26, with a target or goal body weight of 143 pounds. When she and her trainer met to discuss the recommended intervention strategy, she asked the following questions about her body composition assessment:

Q: How was my body fat percentage determined?

A: I used a skinfolds to predict percentage body fat. I took three measurements—one at the back of your arm called the *triceps,* one at your stomach called *abdominal,* and one on your back called *subscapular.* I then put the scores into an equation and did the calculations to predict percentage body fat.

Q: What is an equation?

A: Researchers have conducted many studies in exercise science laboratories to determine what combination of skinfold measurements best predicts a person's body fat. The equation describes the mathematical relationship between these skinfold measures and percentage body fat. Technically, it's called a *multiple regression equation.*

Q: I really don't understand how an equation that uses measures from pinched skin can predict my body fat.

A: In the experiments I mentioned, each subject has his or her skinfolds measured along with another method—the criterion variable—that gives a "true" reading of body fat. One such criterion method, called *underwater weighing,* applies a technique that the ancient Greek Archimedes discovered, based on water displacement. Fatter objects float and denser objects sink. Researchers uncovered a way to relate a person's fat content by how much they tend to sink or float when submerged in a water tank. In fact, the researchers compute the amount of water the person displaces when they are dunked underwater. By knowing how much the person weighs in air, and the weight of the water they displace, they compute body density. Someone with a low body density has more fat (tends to float), while someone with a higher density has less fat (tends to sink). This measure of whole body density then translates into a body fat percentage.

Q: I still don't understand how they go from body fat by dunking to body fat taking three skinfold measures.

A: That's what regression or prediction equations do. The researchers measure hundreds of people by both methods—a predictor method (skinfolds) and a criterion method (underwater weighing)—to develop an equation that predicts percentage body fat. It's all very scientific, but it works well for most individuals.

Q: How accurate is the equation?

A: You've asked a great question. The process is called *validation.* The researcher tests the equation on a different group of people to see how close the predicted body fat values comes to the "true" value. In general, the equations are accurate to within about ±2.5 to 4.0% body fat units of the body fat determined by the "true" or criterion method.

Q: What exactly does this mean?

A: Let's use your example of 33.4% body fat. If we use the upper "error" of 4.0% body fat units, that means *your* true body fat percentage could be as low as 33.4% minus 4% fat units or 29.4%, or you could be as high as 33.4% plus 4% fat units or 37.4%.

Q: So you mean I really am this fat?

A: I can't be absolutely sure, but I'd say the best estimate of your true fatness would put you at what the equation computed—33.4%. Even if you use the lower estimate of 29.4%, you still would be overly fat compared with the average female of your age, who averages about 26% body fat.

Q: How accurate were the skinfold measurements? Is there any possibility you made a mistake?

A: In all truthfulness, I'd have to answer "Yes." Each time I take a measurement the resulting score contains a certain amount of "error." I might not have pinched the skinfold in the exact location I was supposed to, I could have kept the caliper tips on too long and squeezed out more water from under your skin, and I may not have read the caliper dial accurately.

Q: How much could such "errors" translate too?

A: First, I would tell you than someone without experience in taking skinfolds could be in error by as much as ±100% or more at each site! Some personal trainers have little experience, so I would be leery of their results. Here is what I did to ensure my technique was as good as possible. I conducted a miniexperiment with 50 club members. I tested and retested them three times at each of the skinfold sites. Then I matched up the scores and determined that my reliability (reproducibility) of measurement was excellent. For each skinfold measure I take, on average, I'm within 1.2 mm, which is a relatively small amount of variation; this would not affect the body fat percentage when I plug those values into the body fat equation.

Q: So are you telling me I really need to lose 18 pounds?

A: Yes, I feel confident in the accuracy of these results. Even if I was off a few percentage points, I'd say your target weight loss should be a minimum of 15 pounds. My goal for you is to achieve a new body fat percentage of 26%. As you reduce weight, which will be mostly fat, particularly if you continue with your exercise program, you will progress to the 26% target. Currently, you have a total of about 54 pounds of fat, with the remaining 107 pounds called fat-free body mass. Dividing the fat-free weight by the pounds of fat you have gives the lean-to-fat ratio. For you, your ratio is 107/54 or 1.98. As you reduce your fat percentage, your ratio will increase. If you lose 15 pounds of fat, your new ratio will increase to about 2.74! That is one of the goals—to increase the lean-to-fat ratio by decreasing fat and hopefully increasing the lean tissue component.

Table 15.4 CRITERIA FOR IDENTIFYING ANOREXIA ATHLETICA

Common Features	Anorexia Athletica
Weight loss[a]	+
Delayed puberty[b]	(+)
Menstrual dysfunction[c]	(+)
GI complaints	+
Absence of medical illness or affective disorder explaining the weight reduction	+
Disturbance in body image	(+)
Excessive fear of becoming obese	+
Purging[d]	(+)
Binging[d]	(+)
Compulsive exercising[d]	(+)
Restricted caloric intake[e]	+

+, criteria that all athletes had to meet; (+), anorexia athletica athletes met one or more of the listed criteria.
[a] >5% expected body weight.
[b] No menstrual bleeding at age 16 (primary amenorrhea).
[c] Primary, secondary, or oligomenorrhea.
[d] Defined in DSM-III-R(1).
[e] Use of diets at or below 1200 kcal for unspecified durations.

Anorexia Athletica

The cluster of personality traits among athletes often shares a commonalty with patients with clinical eating disorders. The same traits that make an athlete excel in sports—compulsive, driven, dichotomous thinker, perfectionist, com-petitive, compliant and eager to please ("coachable"), and self-motivated—increase risk for developing a disordered eating pattern.[82] More than likely, the greatest risk exists for individuals whose normal, genetically determined body size and shape deviate from the "ideal" imposed by the sport. The term **anorexia athletica** describes the continuum of subclinical eating behaviors of physically active individuals who fail to meet the criteria for a true eating disorder, but who exhibit at least one unhealthy weight-control method.[57,58] This includes fasting, vomiting (termed "instrumental vomiting" when used to make weight), and use of diet pills, laxatives, or diuretics (water pills).

A study of Norwegian elite female athletes aged 12 to 35 years examined risk factors and triggers for eating disorders.[88] TABLE 15.4 lists the criteria to identify anorexia athletica. Based on the Eating Disorder Inventory (EDI), 117 of 522 athletes classified as "at risk." Follow-up with this subgroup revealed a significant incidence of anorexia nervosa (N = 7), bulimia nervosa (N = 42), and anorexia athletica (N = 43). TABLE 15.5 provides selected characteristics for sport-specific groupings from the 92 athletes with eating disorders; characteristics included weekly training volume and percentage of each athletic subgroup with high inventory scores. Interestingly, the athletes traced their eating disorder to one of three causes: *(a)* prolonged periods of dieting and fluctuations in body weight (37%), *(b)* new coach (30%), and *(c)* injury or illness (23%). All of the athletes and controls (athletes without disordered eating patterns) dieted to enhance performance. Sixty-seven percent of athletes with an eating disorder dieted on their coach's recommendation, while 75% of control athletes dieted because of a coach's influence. This latter finding reveals that most female athletes, whether or not they engaged in disordered eating behaviors, remained impressionable to an authority figure, attempting

Table 15.5 CHARACTERISTICS OF THE EATING DISORDERED ATHLETE REPRESENTING THE DIFFERENT SPORT GROUPS

Thirty control subjects represented a random sample of athletes without elevated scores on the Eating Disorder Inventory (EDI) who were matched on age, community of residence, and sport. At-risk subjects were classified by EDI scores above the mean for anorectic patients on the drive for thinness and body dissatisfaction subscales of the EDI.

Sport Groups[a]	N	Age, years[b]	BMI	Training Volume, km · wk[-1]	% with High EDI[c]
Technical sports	13	19 (14–30)	21 (17–26)	14 (12–19)	21
Endurance sports	24	22 (15–28)	20 (15–22)	21 (19–26)	20
Aesthetic sports	22	17 (12–24)	18 (15–21)	18 (17–23)	40
Weight-dependent sports	11	21 (15–23)	21 (17–23)	14 (11–16)	37
Ball game sports	21	20 (17–27)	21 (19–27)	15 (12–17)	14
Total sample	92	20 (13–28)	21 (15–27)	17 (12–26)	22
Athletic controls	30	20 (13–28)	22 (18–24)	15 (10–22)	0

From Sundgot-Borgen J. Eating disorders in female athletes. Sports Med 1994;17:176.
[a] **Technical:** alpine skiing, bowling, golf, high jump, horseback riding, long jump, rifle shooting, sailing sky diving; **Endurance:** biathlon, cross country-skiing, cycling, middle-distance and long-distance running, orienteering, race walking, rowing, speed skating, swimming: **Aesthetic:** diving, figure skating, gymnastics rhythmical gymnastics, sports dance; **Weight-dependent:** judo, karate, wrestling; **Ball games:** badminton, bandy (land hockey on ice), basketball, soccer, table tennis, team handball, tennis, volleyball, underwater rugby.
[b] Values for age, BMI, and training volume are given as means with ranges in parentheses.
[c] Based on N = 522.

to please the coach by following through on his or her recommendations.

For many athletes, disordered eating patterns coincide with the competitive season and abate when the season ends. For them, the preoccupation with body weight may not reflect true underlying pathology but rather a desire to achieve optimum physiologic function and competitive status. For a small number of athletes, the season never "ends," and they develop a clinical eating disorder.

Disordered Eating Also Afflicts Men

While most people consider disordered eating behaviors a "female problem," an increasing number of men share this affliction. The question remains unanswered whether this increased number results from an actual increase in disease incidence or because more men with the condition now seek treatment. In one New York hospital treatment center, the percentage of male patients admitted with eating disorders rose steadily from 4% in 1988 to 13% in 1995. Men currently represent 6 to 10% of individuals with eating disorders, with the greatest prevalence among models, dancers, men abused during childhood, and gays.

Body weight-dependent sports such as wrestling, horse racing, lightweight rowing, distance running, and body-building potentially create patterns of disordered eating, particularly purging.[19,41,81] Of 25 lower-weight-category collegiate wrestlers (BMI, 21.1) and 59 lightweight rowers (BMI, 21.0), 52% reported bingeing; 8% of the rowers and 16% of the wrestlers showed pathologic EDI profiles.[93] The 52% rate for bingeing behavior represents approximately twice the incidence in the normal male population. A survey of Michigan high school wrestlers showed that 72% engaged in at least one potentially harmful weight loss practice over the season, regardless of grade or success level.[42] Fasting and various dehydration methods provided the primary methods for rapid weight loss. Wrestlers who lost weight each week were the most likely to binge eat. Fifty percent of the wrestlers lost more than 5 pounds and 27% lost 10 pounds. Two percent of the wrestlers reported weekly use of laxatives, diet pills, or diuretics, and another 2% used vomiting to loose weight. With the changes in rules governing weight loss of wrestlers during the season, these practices are likely to no longer be prevalent.

MUSCLE DYSMORPHIA: CHANGING IMAGE OF THE "IDEAL" MALE

A change has taken place in the way many men view the ideal male physique. Austrian, French, and American men project the "ideal" man's body as possessing about 28 pounds more muscle than their own.[68] This mismatched perception coincides with the increased number of men who use anabolic steroids, experience eating disorders, and suffer from body obsession. An important component of body obsession relates to **muscle dysmorphia**, or the "Adonis complex," the pathologic preoccupation with muscle size and overall muscularity. These individuals view themselves as small and frail, when in reality, many are large and muscular.

In many ways, muscle dysmorphia and anorexia nervosa share common traits; these include a history of depression and anxiety, a hyperculturization of body image and unrealistic shame about one's body, and self-destructive behaviors. Both anorectic and dysmorphic groups act on their bodies for acceptance and use their bodies as a way to control their lives. They often endanger their health by excessive exercising, bingeing-and-purging rituals, steroid abuse, and inordinate reliance of nutritional and dietary supplements to alter their appearance.[4,52] A large number of these men binge eat or inordinately focus on consuming low-fat, high-protein diets. Body builders with muscle dysmorphia are likely to:[59,75]

- Respond that they are totally or mostly dissatisfied with their body
- Have higher rates of current or past major mood, anxiety, or eating disorders
- Spend more than 3 hours daily thinking about their muscularity
- Avoid activities and people because of their perceived body defect
- Report little or no control over compulsive weightlifting and dietary patterns
- Relinquish activities that were formerly enjoyable

No formal diagnostic criteria exist to identify an individual at risk for muscle dysmorphia. TABLE 15.6 proposes some characteristic features exhibited by those with the disorder.

EXCESSIVE EXERCISE—THE EXERCISE ADDICT

To some extent, cultural influences create similarities between anorexia nervosa and addictive exercise behaviors. Approximately 50% of women with eating disorders compulsively overexercise. Someone who exercises excessively—referred to as an **exercise addict** or exercise dependent—often does whatever it takes to make additional time to exercise more. A rigid daily schedule of working-out often takes place at the expense of family, career, and interpersonal relationships. Sense of worth becomes inextricably tied to the volume of exercise accomplished. Disruption of the daily exercise routine often triggers conventional withdrawal symptoms; these include anxiety, restlessness, and mood swings, traits that diminish only when exercise resumes. Typical regimens for the exercise-dependent individual include early morning and afternoon runs, an aerobics class in the evenings, and participation in

Table 15.6 **SIGNS AND SYMPTOMS OF MUSCLE DYSMORPHIA**

- The individual demonstrates a preoccupation with the idea that he is not sufficiently lean and muscular. Behaviors associated with this preoccupation include frequent weighing; constant checking of appearance in mirrors/windows, persistent criticism of body weight, size, and/or shape; wearing baggy clothing to camouflage the body; or, conversely, modifying clothing to accentuate muscularity (such as adding extra buttons to make a shirt sleeve look tighter).
- The preoccupation with muscularity causes clinically significant distress or impairment of social, occupational, or other important areas of life functioning (e.g., personal relationships), as demonstrated by at least two of the following:
    1. The individual frequently gives up important social, occupational, or recreational activities because of a compulsive need to maintain his exercise and dietary regimen.
    2. The individual avoids situations where his body would be exposed to others (e.g., at the beach or swimming pool) or endures such situations, only with marked distress or intense anxiety.
    3. The preoccupation about the inadequacy of body size of muscularity causes clinically significant distress or impairment in social, occupational, or other important areas of life.
    4. The individual continues to exercise, diet, or use performance-enhancing drugs/supplements despite knowledge of adverse physical and/or psychological consequences.
- The individual engages in excessive exercise, demonstrates preoccupation with food, follows strict dietary regimens (e.g., avoiding specific foods or groups of foods, maintaining excessively low-fat or high-protein diets), or abuses steroids and/or dietary supplements, particularly those aimed at increasing body size (e.g., creatine, HMB, DHEA, androstendione) and/or decreasing body fat (ephedrine, Ma Huang, Guarana).

From Pope HG Jr, et al. Muscle dysmorphia: an unrecognized form of body dysmorphic disorder. Psychosomatics 1997;38:548.

two or more aerobics classes on weekends. Missing a planned exercise session often produces extreme frustration, culminating in food restraint. Eventually, life becomes unmanageable from a fanatical drive to exercise or a relentless pursuit to achieve a high fitness level. Compulsive exercisers often display the same psychological characteristics as bulimics and anorectics. Some clinicians, therefore, see the need to include *exercise addiction* as a separate diagnostic category. Inclusion might help to identify potentially harmful psychological behaviors associated with an eating disorder.

FIGURE 15.3 compares scores for exercise dependence among female dancers, marathon and ultramarathon runners, and field hockey players. The key comparison variable, the negative addiction scale, reflects an inordinate level of exercise dependence. It consists of 14 equally weighted motivational, emotional, and behavioral components of running behavior. Dancers and runners scored significantly higher on exercise dependence than field hockey participants, with dancers achieving the highest scores. The researchers concluded that exercise- dependent athletes, particularly dancers, manifest a number of self-destructive behaviors. These findings highlight the need to carefully monitor females who participate in sports with above-normal levels of addictive exercise behavior (see Fig. 15.8). Compulsive exercise behavior, coupled with preoccupation to achieve an "ideal physique" for competition, should serve as a "wake-up call" to seek professional counseling or clinical intervention.

Not Simply an Athletic Problem

One of our laboratories administered the 26, six-point, forced-choice items of the Eating Attitudes Test (EAT) to evaluate eating behaviors in women (nonathletes) enrolled a university-sponsored fitness center. An EAT score of 20 or higher identifies individuals with one of the following conditions: *(a)* an eating disorder that meets strict diagnostic criteria, *(b)* a "partial syndrome" indicating marked dietary restriction, weight preoccupation, bingeing, vomiting, and other symptoms of clinical significance, but fails to meet all diagnostic criteria for an eating disorder, and *(c)* "obsessive dieters" or "weight-preoccupied" individuals who express concerns about weight and shape but do not present the abnormal concerns of those with the "partial syndrome." Of the 100 women, 24 scored higher on EAT (average score, 30.5; BMI, 22.2) than the remaining 76 women, whose score averaged 6.8 (BMI, 22.4).

FIGURE 15.4 shows significant differences in response to many of the questions on exercise habits between the high- and low-scoring groups. Women with high EAT scores focused more on extreme exercise behaviors. A disturbing aspect concerns the relatively large percentage of "nonathlete" women with either high or low EAT scores who display compulsive exercise behaviors similar to those of gymnasts, dancers, and others preoccupied with eating and weight management. The exercise addict syndrome probably affects many college-age women and is not just a characteristic unique to competitive athletes.

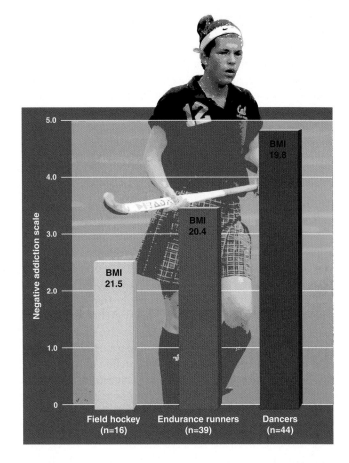

Figure 15.3 Comparison of exercise dependence scores among collegiate female ballet and modern dancers, marathon and ultramarathon (greater than 50-mile distances) runners, and field hockey athletes. The dancers scored significantly higher than the runners; the field hockey athletes scored significantly lower in exercise dependence than both of these groups. Interestingly, the dancers had the lowest mean BMI (19.8), followed by the runners (20.4) and field hockey athletes (21.5). Self-destructive behaviors included perseverance in training despite serious injury, prioritization of physical activity over other responsibilities, and significant mood disturbances. (From Sachs ML, Pearman D. Running addiction: a depth interview examination. J Sport Behav 1979;2:143.)

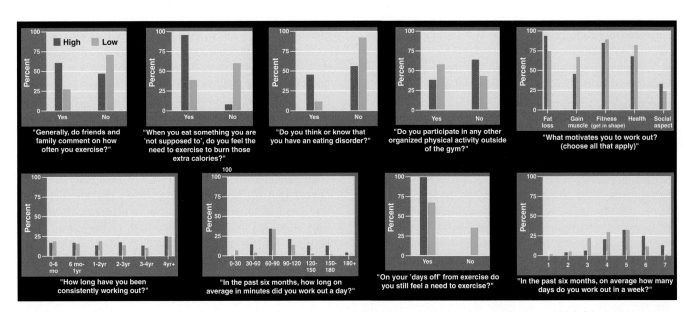

Figure 15.4 Comparison of the percentage responses to an exercise habits questionnaire by subjects who scored high (above 20; average = 30.5) on the 26-item Eating Attitudes Test (EAT) and those who scored below 20 (average = 6.8). High scores on the EAT indicate tendency toward extremes in eating behaviors. Data from University of Massachusetts, Amherst, by D. Canter, Department of Exercise Science, University of Massachusetts, Amherst.

CLINICAL EATING DISORDERS

Psychiatrists traditionally limit the definition of disordered eating to behaviors that produce negative health effects or drive a person to seek treatment. Anorexia nervosa and bulimia nervosa represent the two eating disorders included in the *Diagnostic and Statistical Manual of Mental Disorders* (DSM-IV), the American Psychiatric Association's official roster of psychiatric illnesses.

Anorexia Nervosa

Anorexia nervosa, originally described in ancient writings, represents an unhealthy physical and mental state. This "nervous loss of appetite," particularly common and increasing in prevalence among adolescent girls and young women, is characterized by four factors: *(a)* distortions of body image, *(b)* a crippling obsession with body size, *(c)* preoccupation with dieting and thinness, and *(d)* refusal to eat enough food to maintain a minimally normal body weight. A relentless pursuit of thinness (present in about 1 to 2% of the general population) culminates in severe undernutrition, altered body composition characterized by depletion of fat and fat-free body mass (FFM), and cessation of menstruation (amenorrhea) in females. Body weight decreases below normal for age and stature. Anorexia nervosa represents the third most common medical illness in girls aged 15 to 19 years. Persons with anorexia actually perceive themselves as fat despite their emaciation. Such distorted perceptions, which frequently persist into recovery, produce extreme feelings of vulnerability and personal inadequacy.[39] *Denial and secrecy become a large part of the problem.* Many anorectics do not believe they suffer from starvation—they do eat, but consume far less food than adequate to maintain energy balance.[38,43,94]

Compulsive exercise behaviors go hand-in-hand with anorexia nervosa.[11,98] Rather than starve or vomit, the anorectic fanatically expends as many calories as possible through physical activity. A common misconception about anorectics concerns their state of hunger. In reality, they often remain continually hungry; their ability to overcome the urge to eat provides a sense of self-power and control. If untreated, between 6 and 21% of anorectics die prematurely from suicide, heart disease, or infections. In about one third of patients the disease becomes chronic, marked by frequent relapses that often require hospitalization.[66] TABLE 15.7 lists the clinical criteria for diagnosing anorexia nervosa.

Weight gain becomes a primary goal in the treatment of anorexia nervosa. Interestingly, when patients regain weight through hospitalization or out-patient supervision, most of the weight is gained in the trunk region rather than the extremities, with up to 70% of the regained weight as fat.[35,60,104] For example, at the end of treatment that produced an 11.9-kg weight gain (pretreatment fat, 9.8%; post-treatment fat, 22.6%), the ratio of FFM/fat mass averaged 3.4:1, with fat representing 55% of the gained weight.[70]

Table 15.7	CLINICAL DIAGNOSTIC CRITERIA FOR ANOREXIA NERVOSA

A. Refusal to maintain body weight at or above a minimally normal weight for age and height (e.g., weight loss leading to maintenance of body weight less than 85% of that expected; or failure to make expected weight gain during period of growth, leading to body weight less than 85% of that expected).

B. Intense fear of gaining weight or becoming fat, even though underweight.

C. Disturbance in the way in which one's body weight or shape is experienced, undue influence of body weight or shape on self-evaluation, or denial of the seriousness of the current low body weight.

D. In postmenarchal females, amenorrhea. That is, the absence of at least three consecutive menstrual cycles. (A woman is considered to have amenorrhea if her periods occur only following hormone administration (e.g., estrogen).

From the American Psychiatric Association's diagnostic criteria for anorexia nervosa and bulimia. In: Diagnostic and statistical manual of mental disorders. 4th ed. (DSM-IV) Washington, DC: American Psychiatric Association, 1994:544–555.

A 9-month longitudinal study serially assessed body composition in ambulatory anorectic women.[29] Patients exhibited an abnormal body composition during times of low body weight and after weight gain compared with a control group of normal-weight women. At low body weight, anorectic women possessed trunk fat as a percentage of total body fat similar to controls, but extremity fat percentage remained lower than controls. After a modest 4.1-kg weight gain, the percentage of extremity fat changed little, but trunk fat percentage increased significantly. In contrast to results with other groups of women, estrogen therapy provided no protection against the gain in trunk fat with spontaneous weight gain in anorectic women. Researchers do not know whether anorexia nervosa patients with the most distress about weight gain in recovery (particularly abdominal fat) have the highest ratio of truncal fat to peripheral fat or gain the greatest quantity of truncal fat when they regain weight.[53]

Adolescent girls hospitalized with anorexia nervosa had significant body wasting as indicated by extremely low body fat and a low FFM as reflected by total body nitrogen (TABLE 15.8).[40] Triceps skinfold thickness provided the most significant anthropometric predictor of percentage body fat. This skinfold measure explained 68% of the variation in body fat, while body weight accurately indicated total body nitrogen and thus protein depletion in these patients.

Physical Consequences of Anorexia Nervosa

Death often results from prolonged starvation in about 7% of anorectic patients over a 10-year period; 18 to 20% die within 30 years. A range of other profound physical ailments also occur including cardiac abnormalities (e.g., arrhythmias, heart block), electrolyte disturbances, impaired kidney func-

	Age	Body Weight, kg	BMI	%Fat	%TBN	FFM, kg	Trunk fat, kg	Leg fat, kg
Anorexia nervosa	15.5	40.2	15.3	13.8	73	34.5	2.1	2.6
Healthy controls	15.1	57.3	21.2	26.3	75	41.2	6.6	7.1

Table 15.8 titled: **COMPARISON OF BODY COMPOSITIONS OF FEMALE ADOLESCENTS WITH ANOREXIA NERVOSA AND HEALTHY CONTROLS**

From Kerrvish KP, et al. Body composition in adolescents with anorexia nervosa. Am J Clin Nutr 2002;75:31.
%TBN, percentage total body nitrogen predicted for age; FFM, fat-free body mass

tion, decreased bone mineral density, gastrointestinal dysfunction (e.g., bleeding, ulceration, bloating, constipation), and anemia. Many effects such as depressed BMR and leptin concentrations, not fully explained by body composition changes,[67] reflect predictable outcomes from energy conservation as the body defends against prolonged caloric deprivation. FIGURE 15.5 depicts anorexia nervosa's potential physical and medical consequences.

Danger Signals and Indications. Anorexia nervosa usually begins with a normal attempt to lose weight through dieting. As dieting progresses, the individual continues to eat less until the person consumes practically no food. Food restriction eventually becomes an obsession, and the anorectic achieves no satisfaction with any amount of weight loss. The person denies the accompanying extreme emaciation as weight loss progresses. Some anorectic persons cannot ignore the in-

tense hunger accompanying near-total food deprivation; this causes episodes of bingeing and subsequent purging. The warning signs listed in TABLE 15.9 can help coaches and trainers identify athletes with anorexia nervosa.

Bulimia Nervosa

The term *bulimia,* literally meaning "ox hunger," refers to "gorging" or "insatiable appetite." At one time, some believed that **bulimia nervosa** reflected a manifestation of anorexia nervosa owing to similarities and overlap in the two conditions. For example, some anorectics experience bulimic episodes, while some bulimics experience episodes of anorexia. Based on more careful examination of the disorders, bulimia nervosa emerged in the late 1970s as a separate classification of eating disorder. The disease, far more common than anorexia nervosa, is characterized by frequent

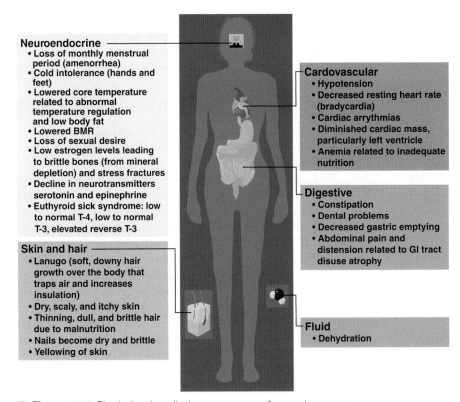

Figure 15.5 Physical and medical consequences of anorexia nervosa.

Table 15.9   **WARNING SIGNS OF ANOREXIA NERVOSA**

- Preoccupation with being "too fat" despite maintenance of a normal body weight
- Loss of menstrual cycle (amenorrhea)
- Frequently commenting about body weight or shape
- Loss of a significant amount of body weight
- Weight too low for successful athletic performance
- Ritualistic concern and preoccupation with dieting, counting calories, cooking, and eating
- Recurrent stress fractures
- Excessive concern about body weight, size, and shape, even after losing weight
- A feeling of helplessness when observing food
- Severe mood shifts
- Guilt about eating
- Compulsive need for continuous, vigorous physical activity that exceeds training requirements for their specific sport
- Maintaining a "skinny" look (body weight less than 85% of expected weight)
- Preferring to eat in isolation
- Refusal to eat to gain weight
- Wearing baggy clothes to disguise thin appearance
- Sporadic episodes of binging and purging
- Dissatisfaction with torso and extremity body parts (various areas consistently perceived as "fat" or protruding)

episodes of binge eating, followed by purging, laxative abuse, fasting, or extreme exercise and intense feelings of guilt or shame. Approximately 2 to 4% of adolescents and adults in the general population (mainly female, including about 5% of college women) are bulimic. A large percentage of the total is obese and enrolled in self-help or commercial weight loss programs. A sex difference probably exists in the emotional triggers for overindulgence in food. Compared with men, women with a weight problem exhibit greater binge eating during periods of negative emotions—anxiety, frustration, depression, or anger.[90]

Unlike the continual semistarvation with anorexia nervosa, bulimia nervosa includes binge eating of calorically dense food—often at night and usually between 1000 to 10,000 calories within several hours. Fasting, self-induced vomiting, taking laxatives or diuretics, or compulsively exercising solely to avoid weight gain takes place after the binge.[24,48] Anorectics revel in their sense of control over eating, while striving toward a perceived level of physical perfection. In contrast, bulimics lose control; they recognize their impulsive behavior as abnormal. Eating extreme quantities of food often becomes a means to reduce stress, and purging provides the only way to regain control for their inability to stop eating voluntarily. Considerable variation exists in the type of food consumed during the binge episode. Some bulimics, who often attempt dieting with healthful eating, binge on large quantities of unhealthful, "forbidden" foods (cookies, chips, and chocolates). Others binge on foods they consume regularly but only in extreme quantities. Some bulimics even overeat lower-calorie, diet-type foods, while others purge after every meal, regardless of what or how much they eat. *Bulimics span the gamut between nor-mal body weight and overweight (or a history of overweight); this represents a striking difference between anorectics and bulimics.* While obvious physical characteristics exist for anorexia nervosa, many bulimic characteristics remain behavioral.

Most patients with bulimia nervosa meet standards for major depressive disorders—loss of interest, low mood, shortened attention span, disrupted sleep patterns, and suicidal thoughts. Bulimics also abuse alcohol and drugs at a higher rate than the general population. TABLE 15.10 lists the clinical criteria for diagnosing bulimia nervosa.

Physical Consequences of Bulimia Nervosa

FIGURE 15.6 depicts the diverse physical symptoms and disorders suffered by patients with bulimia nervosa.

Danger Signals and Indications. Difficulty exists in diagnosing bulimia nervosa because many bulimics function well without noticeable signs. Bulimics remain conscious of what and how much they eat and generally never eat to excess in public. For the most part, they express feelings of perfectionist behavior, depression, low self-esteem, being out of control, and dissatisfaction with body size and shape. Often, those closest to the bulimic remain unaware of the problem. Another disturbing aspect of bulimia nervosa concerns substance abuse. In a comparison of women with anorexia nervosa and women with bulimia nervosa, the bulimics abused alcohol, amphetamines, barbiturates, marijuana, tranquilizers, and cocaine to a greater extent.[99] Independent of the diagnosis of either anorexia or bulimia, *(a)* the magnitude of caloric restriction predicted amphetamine use, *(b)* severity of

Table 15.10	**CLINICAL DIAGNOSTIC CRITERIA FOR BULIMIA NERVOSA**

A. Recurrent episodes of binge eating. An episode of binge eating is characterized by both of the following:
  (1) Eating, in a discrete period time (e.g., within any 2-hour period), an amount of food that is definitely larger than most people would eat during a similar period of time and under similar circumstances.
  (2) A sense of lack of control over eating during the episode (e.g., a feeling that one cannot stop eating or control what or how much one is eating).

B. Recurrent inappropriate compensatory behavior in order to prevent weight gain, such as self-induced vomiting, misuse of laxatives, diuretics, enemas, or other medications; fasting, or excessive exercise.

C. Binge eating and inappropriate compensatory behaviors both occur, on average, at least twice a week for 3 months.

D. Self-evaluation is unduly influenced by body shape and weight.

E. The disturbance does not occur exclusively during episodes of anorexia nervosa.

From the American Psychiatric Association's diagnostic criteria for anorexia nervosa and bulimia. In: Diagnostic and statistical manual of mental disorders. 4th ed. (DSM-IV) Washington, DC: American Psychiatric Association, 1994:544–555.

binge eating predicted tranquilizer use, and *(c)* severity of purging predicted alcohol, cocaine, and cigarette use. TABLE 15.11 lists the warning signs of bulimia nervosa.

Binge-Eating Disorder

Binge-eating disorder (BED), first described in 1959, identified specific eating behavior patterns in a subgroup of obese patients undergoing treatment to lose weight. BED is currently listed in the appendix of DSM-IV as a provisional diagnosis in need of further study. The affliction is characterized by recurrent episodes of binge eating. These occur often without subsequent purging or abusing laxatives to compensate for overeating common to bulimia nervosa and

anorexia nervosa. Psychiatrists define the disorder as episodes of binge eating at least twice a week for at least 6 months and that cause significant emotional distress. Individuals with BED eat more rapidly than normal until they can no longer consume additional food. Such high levels of food intake exceed the physiologic drive of hunger. Binge eating, undertaken in private because of embarrassment, occurs with feelings of guilt, depression, or self-disgust. Binge eaters suffer greater self-anger, shame, lack of control, and frustration than nonbingeing obese individuals.[49] They also experience relatively higher rates of sexual abuse and physical abuse and bullying by peers than the general population.[83] Studies in the early 1980s identified BED in 20 to 50% of obese patients.[27,48] Not only did these individuals

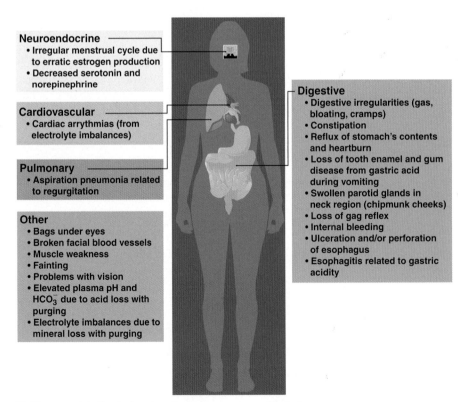

Figure 15.6 Physical and medical consequences of bulimia nervosa.

Table 15.11　**WARNING SIGNS OF BULIMIA NERVOSA**

- Excessive concern about body weight, body size, and body composition
- Frequent gains and losses in body weight
- Visits to the bathroom following meals
- Fear of not being able to control eating
- Eating when depressed
- Compulsive dieting after binge-eating episodes
- Severe shifts in mood (depression, loneliness)
- Secretive binge eating, but never overeating in front of others
- Frequent criticism of one's body size and shape
- Experiencing personal or family problems with alcohol or drugs
- Irregular menstrual cycle (oligomenorrhea)

exhibit difficulties with binge eating, but they also regained lost weight faster than obese non-binge-eaters, and they more likely failed in treatment.[50] As an outgrowth of these early clinical observations, diagnostic criteria developed in the early 1990s helped to identify BED (TABLE 15.12).

A feature distinguishing BED from anorexia nervosa and bulimia nervosa is that persons seeking treatment for BED are often overweight or obese. Approximately 2% of the U.S. population (1 to 2 million people) and about 30% of Americans treated for obesity experience BED,[56] although incidence rate decreases on the basis of personal interview rather than questionnaire to assess its prevalence.[84] Current research does not support earlier beliefs that minorities were somehow "protected" from BED.[77] For example, comparisons between Caucasian and minority females showed similar scores on measures of eating disorder symptomology and general psychopathology.[46]

Ten to 15% of mildly obese people who enroll in self-help or commercial weight loss programs meet the criteria for BED. Those with body weight in excess of 20% of ideal weight exhibit the highest prevalence of BED and develop their obesity at a younger age than their non-binge-eating obese counterparts. Women experience BED at a 50% higher rate than men do. Women also report greater binge-eating episodes in response to negative emotions such as anxiety, anger and frustration, and depression. Men and women presenting for BED treatment score similarly on measures of eating disturbance, body shape and weight concerns, interpersonal problems, and self-esteem; men experience more psychiatric disturbance and less emotional eating.[79]

The causes of BED remain unknown. Up to 50% of bingers suffer depression, which may contribute to the disorder. Individuals with BED experience higher lifetime rates of major depression, panic disorder, bulimia nervosa, borderline personality disorder, and avoidant personality disorder.[102] Moderately obese men and women with BED experience greater relative risk for psychiatric disorders than their obese counterparts without the disorder.[101]

Psychotherapy and behavioral strategies to curb binge eating help to reverse the disorder. A 1-year posttreatment follow-up of obese women with BED treated with group cognitive-behavioral therapy (CBT; see p. 508) and a weight loss program showed that those who discontinued binging maintained a 4.0-kg weight loss over 1 year.[1] In contrast, women unable to stop binging gained 3.6 kg during the same follow-up period.

Exercise Plus Behavior Therapy Intervention Helps

To investigate the role of exercise and behavior therapy in treating BED, two groups of women participated in identical exercise programs for six months.[47] One group also received behavior therapy with the exercise program. Pre- and posttreatment evaluations included exercise level, binge-eating frequency, and depressive symptoms. The results favored the group receiving exercise plus behavioral treatment for BED. At posttreatment, 81% of these subjects remained free

Table 15.12　**DIAGNOSTIC CRITERIA FOR BINGE-EATING DISORDER**

A.　Recurrent episodes of binge eating. An episode of binge eating is characterized by both of the following:
　1.　Eating, in a discrete period of time (e.g., within any two hour period), an amount of food that is definitely larger than most people would eat during a similar period of time in similar circumstances.
　2.　A sense of lack of control over eating during the episode (e.g., a feeling that one cannot stop eating or control what or how much one is eating).

B.　During most binge episodes, at least three of the following behavioral indicators of loss of control are present:
　1.　Eating much more rapidly than usual.
　2.　Eating until feeling uncomfortably full.
　3.　Eating large amounts of food when not feeling physically hungry.
　4.　Eating alone because of being embarrassed by how much one is eating.
　5.　Feeling disgusted with oneself, depressed, or feeling very guilty after overeating.

C.　The binge eating causes marked distress.

D.　The binge eating occurs, on average, at least two days a week for a six-month period.

E.　Does not currently meet the criteria for anorexia nervosa or bulimia nervosa, purging or non-purging type.

From the American Psychiatric Association's diagnostic criteria for anorexia nervosa and bulimia. In: Diagnostic and statistical manual of mental disorders. 4th ed. (DSM-IV) Washington, DC: American Psychiatric Association, 1994:731.

from binge-eating episodes. They also exercised more frequently each week and thus expended greater energy.

Future Studies

Since the early 1990s, research has expanded in areas related to BED. A multidisciplinary approach now includes aspects of pharmacology, psychiatry, psychology, sociology, and exercise intervention as discussed above.[1,18,79] Future research needs to study athletes and nonathletes regarding the influence of different modes of exercise (including frequency, duration, and intensity) on the psychologic and neurophysiologic correlates of BED.

CAUSE OR EFFECT? THE ROLE OF A SPORT IN DISORDERED EATING

Does dedication to training for a specific sport induce development of an eating disorder, or do individuals with potentially pathologic concerns about body size and shape gravi-

tate (self-select) to the sport. The **attraction to sport hypothesis** maintains that individuals with an existing eating disorder (or at high risk for developing one) find reward by participating in aesthetic-type sports that emphasize an excessively lean appearance. When training commences early in life (as in gymnastics and ballet dancing), it becomes difficult to make the case for the attraction to the sport hypothesis. This is because the young girls participated because of the sport's focus on leanness and appearance. For these girls, disordered eating behaviors probably develop progressively as the young athlete realizes an inherent incompatibility between the sport's body-type requirements and her genetic predisposition for body size and structure. Research must determine whether the inordinate focus of many athletes on food intake and leanness reflects a continuum of graded psychologic disturbance that ultimately leads to full-blown anorexia nervosa or bulimia nervosa.

TABLE 15.13 presents a brief questionnaire to evaluate the degree of restraint a person feels over issues concerning food choices, diet planning, and body-weight maintenance. Often, individuals tending toward disordered eating pat-

---

Table 15.13 HOW DO YOU RATE IN TERMS OF EATING RESTRAINT?

Circle the number that best describes your feelings or behaviors related to the question.

1. How often are you dieting?
   0 = never
   1 = rarely
   2 = sometimes
   3 = often
   4 = always

2. What is the maximum amount of weight (in pounds) that you have ever lost within one month?
   0 = 0–4
   1 = 5–9
   2 = 10–14
   3 = 15–19
   4 = 20+

3. What is the most weight (in pounds) you have ever gained within a week?
   1 = 1.1–2.0
   2 = 2.1–3.0
   3 = 3.1–5.0
   4 = 5.1+

4. In a typical week, how much does your weight fluctuate?
   0 = 0–1.0
   1 = 1.1–2.0
   2 = 2.1–3.0
   3 = 2.1–5.0
   4 = 5.1+

5. Would a weight fluctuation of 5 pounds affect the way you live your life?
   0 = not at all
   1 = slightly
   2 = moderately
   3 = very much

6. Do you eat sensibly in front of others and splurge alone?
   0 = never
   1 = rarely
   2 = often
   3 = always

7. Do you give too much time and thought to food?
   0 = never
   1 = rarely
   2 = often
   3 = always

8. Do you have feelings of guilt after overeating?
   0 = never
   1 = rarely
   2 = often
   3 = always

9. How conscious are you of what you are eating?
   0 = not at all
   1 = slightly
   2 = moderately
   3 = extremely

10. How many pounds over your desired weight were you at your maximum weight?
    0 = 0–1
    1 = 1–5
    2 = 6–10
    3 = 11–20
    4 = 21+

Add up the numbers you have circled and select the category that best describes you.
   0–15 Relatively unrestrained
   16–23 Moderately restrained
   24–35 Highly restrained

From Herman CP, Policy J. Restrained eating. In: Stunkard AJ, ed. Obesity. Philadelphia: WB Saunders, 1980.

terns exhibit extreme concern over what they eat and how it affects body weight. If they "give in" (because of a perceived lack of self-control) and eat "bad" foods believed to contribute to weight gain, they often reduce the resulting stress by purging or excessive exercise. The questions in Table 15.13 do not determine whether or not an eating disorder exists, but raise awareness about dietary restraint patterns and behaviors that ultimately may lead to disordered eating.

EATING DISORDERS AFFECT EXERCISE PERFORMANCE

An athlete with an eating disorder faces a paradox: Behavior necessary to achieve a body weight for success in certain sports—semistarvation, purging, excessive exercising—adversely affects health, energy reserves, and physiologic function and the ability to train and compete at an optimal level. In Chapter 14, we noted that athletes often reduce body fat to improve exercise power output relative to body mass and to reduce drag forces that impede forward movement through air and water. For persons with eating disorders, chronic restriction of energy intake (as in anorexia nervosa) or reduced energy availability through purging (as in bulimia nervosa) rapidly depletes glycogen reserves. As emphasized throughout this text, the normally limited quantity of muscle and liver glycogen provides rapid energy for high-intensity anaerobic and aerobic exercise. Consequently, even short periods of disordered eating deplete glycogen reserves, which profoundly affects capacity to train and recover. The reduced protein (and carbohydrate) intake with disordered eating behaviors also contributes to lean tissue loss. A subpar intake of vitamins and minerals required for energy metabolism and tissue growth and repair facilitates poor exercise performance and increases injury potential.

EATING DISORDERS AFFECT BONE MINERAL DENSITY

Dual-energy x-ray absorptiometry (DXA; see Chapter 13) has evaluated skeletal and regional body composition characteristics in anorexia nervosa. In one study, body mass averaged 44.4 kg (97.9 lb) for 10 anorectic women. FIGURE 15.7 shows an anorectic female (left two images) and a typical female whose body fat percentage averaged 25% of her 56.7-kg (125-lb) body mass. Although FFM of the anorectic women approached the normal average of 43.0 kg, body fat equaled only 7.5%, a value more than three times less than that for comparison groups of typical young women. These women were anorectic for at least 1 year, and amenorrhea duration averaged 3.1 years (range, 1–8 years). The *insert*

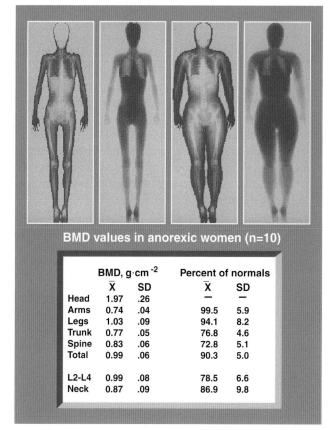

BMD values in anorexic women (n=10)

	BMD, g·cm^{-2}		Percent of normals	
	$\overline{X}$	SD	$\overline{X}$	SD
Head	1.97	.26	—	—
Arms	0.74	.04	99.5	5.9
Legs	1.03	.09	94.1	8.2
Trunk	0.77	.05	76.8	4.6
Spine	0.83	.06	72.8	5.1
Total	0.99	.06	90.3	5.0
L2-L4	0.99	.08	78.5	6.6
Neck	0.87	.09	86.9	9.8

Figure 15.7 Example of an anorectic female *(two left images)* and a typical female *(two right images)* whose body fat percentage averages 25% of body mass of 56.7 kg (125 lb). The average anorectic subject weighed 44.4 kg (97.9 lb) and had 7.5% body fat estimated by DXA from the fat percentages at the arms, legs, and trunk regions. The values in the *right column of the inset table* present percentage values for bone mineral density (BMD) for different regional body areas in the anorectic group compared to 287 normal females aged 20 to 40 years. (Photo courtesy of R. B. Mazes, Department of Medical Physics, University of Wisconsin, Madison, WI, and the Lunar Radiation Corporation, Madison, WI. Data from Mazes RB, et al. Skeletal and body composition effects of anorexia nervosa. Paper presented at the international symposium on in vivo body composition studies, June 20–23, Toronto, Ontario, Canada, 1989.)

table compares regional bone mineral densities (BMD, g·cm^{-2}) of anorectic females and 287 normal-weight females aged 20 to 40 years. The values in the *right column* represent the percentage for BMD for the anorectic group relative to the comparison group. Total-body BMD averaged 10% lower, the L2-L4 region of the lumbar spine averaged 27% less, and13% lower in the femoral neck than comparable BMDs in the normals. Spine BMD in the young anorectic group equaled the average BMD in 70-year-old women! Diminished BMD in anorexia nervosa, in addition to reducing skeletal size, may render these young women particularly vulnerable to osteoporotic fractures at a relatively young age.

MANAGEMENT OF DISORDERED EATING BEHAVIORS IN ATHLETES

Disordered eating behaviors do not just go away; there is no simple cause and no simple solution. Disordered eating not only represents a problem but an attempted solution to a problem. In its mildest aspect, the disorder often stems from poor nutritional information. Left untreated, abnormal eating behaviors often blossom into chronic eating disorders. Familial vulnerability also exists because the relatives of people with eating disorders exhibit higher risk of developing a disorder.[48] The relatives also show higher rates of depression and obsessive–compulsive disorders than the general population.

Disordered eating behaviors frequently produce nutritional problems in addition to the loss of tooth enamel from stomach acid during vomiting in bulimic patients. Effective treatment focuses primarily on the psychologic realm and attempts to reverse the negative effects of disordered eating behaviors. Depending on the patient's age, disorder severity, and its affect on health and well-being, therapy takes place either on an out-patient basis or in a hospital setting. With teenage athletes, the parents must become involved. Individuals with disordered eating patterns frequently resist outside attempts at intervention and treatment. No single approach or theory has proved helpful in treating those with eating disorders. Often treatments that appear to have a high likelihood of success give opposite results. For example, the approach to prevent eating disorders used by Stanford University—in which students who previously suffered from anorexia nervosa talked to other students—backfired. Students attending the group sessions showed more incidents of disordered eating behaviors than before. *Successful treatment usually involves a team approach using psychotherapeutic, medical, nutritional, and family support.* FIGURE 15.8 outlines an intervention model for disordered eating behaviors in an athletic setting. The process consists of four steps:

- **Step 1.** Identify and isolate the contributing factors.
- **Step 2.** Formulate appropriate goals for intervention and prevention.
- **Step 3.** Formulate long-term strategies to deal with the problem.
- **Step 4.** Initiate long-term programs to address the situation.

FIGURE 15.9 illustrates the multidisciplinary approach to manage disordered eating behaviors in athletes at the University of Texas at Austin, an early leader in confronting eating disorders among athletes. This Division I collegiate-level athletic program prohibits coaches from weighing female athletes or talking to them about body weight or body composition; these responsibilities reside with the sports medicine staff. The important components include

- *Education* to provide information concerning the eating disorder and its consequences
- *Self-monitoring* to provide a clear understanding of current eating behaviors and patterns
- *Meal planning* to help gain control of eating patterns and establish a healthful pattern of eating

COMMON SENSE GUIDELINES FOR COACHES AND TRAINERS CONCERNING EATING DISORDERS

Coaches and athletic trainers can play an important role in the lives of athletes with symptoms of disordered eating. Follow these common sense guidelines whenever possible—they can make a difference.

- Do not urge athletes to eat, do not watch them eat, refrain from discussing food, and forego discussions about body weight. Becoming involved with coaches concerning food and body weight provides a way for the athlete to "manipulate" the coaching and training staff; it refocuses attention on concerns the athlete feels about food or body weight.
- Stay free from guilt about the athlete's attitudes and behaviors toward food or body weight. Solving an eating disorder ultimately remains the athlete's responsibility; your role provides support to the athlete (and parent) and, if appropriate, encourages counseling. Coaches and trainers should not permit concerns about food and body size to go unnoticed—they must exercise professional judgment in offering advice about external counseling.
- Coaches and trainers should not counsel athletes about eating disorders. Reserve that role for a psychologist, psychiatrist, or other trained specialist in eating disorders.

■ **Figure 15.8** Model intervention for dealing with disordered eating behaviors in an athletic setting. (From Ryan R. Management of eating problems in athletic settings. In: Brownell KD, et al., eds. Eating, body weight and performance in athletes. Philadelphia: Lea & Febiger, 1992.)

- Do not focus extra attention on the athlete with an eating disorder. This exacerbates the condition and does little to resolve issues concerning food or body weight.
- Be prepared to "ignore" the athlete in matters of food or body weight; do not become so involved that teammates notice that the athletes receives "extra" attention about an eating disorder.
- Refrain from telling the athlete about "successful" athletes or friends who overcame an eating disorder. Do not ask questions such as: "How are you feeling?" "How is your weight today?" "Did you eat a good breakfast?" "Are you getting enough to eat?"
- Trust the athlete to develop her or his own standards and values rather than insisting that they emulate yours.
- Encourage the athlete to develop initiative, become self-sufficient, and make decisions. Give choices, but not solutions to problems. This encourages independence and autonomy.
- Show extreme patience when dealing with athletes who exhibit symptoms of disordered eating. No quick cures or fixes exist, so do not expect them.
- Never give up on an athlete who displays symptoms of disordered eating. Be firm but fair; be tolerant but decisive, and show respect, not contempt or disapproval.

THERAPEUTIC METHODS TO TREAT EATING DISORDERS

Various therapeutic methods treat eating disorders and give patients a sense of balance, purpose, and future. One approach, **cognitive–behavioral therapy**, particularly effective in treating bulimia nervosa, focuses on teaching the patient to identify, monitor, and modify dysfunctional attitudes, core beliefs, and eating habits to lessen binges and "retrain" normal hunger and satiety responses.[18,85,89] An important component of this therapeutic approach teaches individuals to change misconceptions and reasoning errors and develop coping strategies for modifying dysfunctional responses to stressful situations.

Interpersonal psychotherapy helps the patient and family to examine interpersonal relationships to positively affect problem areas. The therapist emphasizes the importance of body fat for the return of menses and normalization of reproductive functions. For younger patients, the therapist stresses the effects of low body weight on maturation, growth, and bone mass. Paradoxically, the therapist needs to recognize that a normalization of body fat may increase the patient's fat phobia, which initially led her to her pursue extreme thinness.[71]

Pharmacologic treatment (e.g., Prozac [fluoxetine] and other antidepressants) helps some individuals. Trials of

diverse classes of psychotropic medications to improve mood and augment weight gain in anorexia nervosa patients have generally showed little effect.[3,53] Psychiatrists have recently prescribed two drugs Zonegran and Topiramate, approved to treat epilepsy and migraine headaches, for persons whose overeating meets the criteria for binge-eating disorder. These drugs require careful use but do help to reduce the frequency of binges for a subset of patients.[54] Widespread use of such pharmacologic treatment requires further research.

No one best treatment presently exists; combined multifaceted, multidisciplinary approaches using individuals with expertise in areas of psychiatry, eating disorders, body image issues, medicine, and nutrition often work best. Improvement occurs slowly, with relapses and setbacks common. Achieving success often remains difficult for *(a)* individuals with eating disorders of long duration, *(b)* patients who have previously failed treatment, or *(c)* persons with a history of disturbed family relationships and poor individual adjustment.

Physical Activity May Prove Beneficial in Treatment of Bulimia Nervosa

A recent study evaluated16 weeks of regular physical activity versus an equivalent time of nutritional counseling or cognitive behavioral therapy in treating bulimia nervosa.[89] Normal-weight female bulimic patients randomly received either treatment or control conditions; a second control group contained healthy females. Nutritional counseling educated patients about sound principles of nutrition, nutritional needs, and the relationship between dieting and overeating. Meal-planning techniques established and maintained regular eating patterns. Cognitive behavioral therapy focused on enabling patients to *(a)* identify feelings and events related to bingeing episodes and how such episodes affected emotional status, *(b)* identify and modify core beliefs that influence bulimic behavior, *(c)* apply behavior modification techniques to combat bulimic behavior and develop more healthful strategies to deal with disturbing thoughts and emotions, and *(d)* develop general problem-solving skills. Exercise consisted of a 1-hour weekly group session of moderate physical activities to promote physical fitness, reduce feelings of fatness and bloating associated with eating, foster a more positive body image, and prevent binging and purging. These subjects were also urged to exercise at least 35 minutes twice a week on their own. FIGURE 15.10 compares the different treatments with respect to the EDI subscales of "Body dissatisfaction," "Bulimia," and "Drive for thinness" pre- and posttreatment and at 6- and 18-month follow-ups. Nutritional counseling proved no more effective than cognitive–behavioral therapy. More striking was the superior effect of regular physical activity compared with cognitive behavior therapy in reducing the pursuit of thinness, feelings of body dissatisfaction, and frequency of bingeing, purging, and laxative abuse. The augmented self-regulation with physical activity may result from

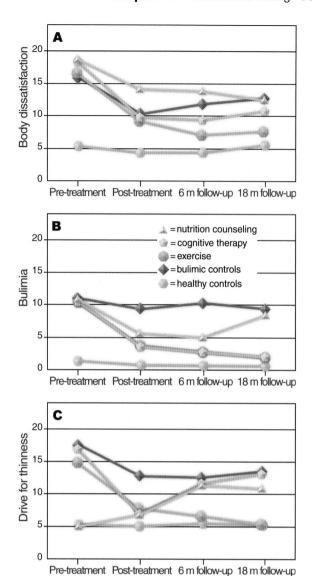

Figure 15.10 Exercise, cognitive therapy, and nutritional counseling in treating bulimia nervosa. **A.** Mean scores on the Eating Disorders Index "Body dissatisfaction" sub scale at pretreatment, post-treatment, and 6- and 18-month follow-up. **B.** Mean scores on the Eating Disorders Index "Bulimia" sub scale. **C.** Mean scores on the Eating Disorders Index "Drive for thinness" sub scale. (From Sundgot-Borgen J, et al. The effect of exercise, cognitive therapy, and nutritional counseling in treating bulimia nervosa. Med Sci Sports Exerc 2002;34:190.)

the effects of exercise on reducing bulimic patients' bodily tensions and improving stress tolerance.

ATHLETICS MUST CHANGE FROM WITHIN

The following quote highlights the proactive role professionals in exercise nutrition, sports medicine, and athletics play in affecting the negative potential for certain sports to contribute to disordered eating among participants:[25]

> *Finally, it is important to comment briefly on the need for reflection regarding the evolving aesthetic ideals for weight and shape in some sports. Particularly in those where the premium is placed on appearance and where adjudicators prevail (diving, figure skating, gymnastics and dance), questions should be raised from within the sports community regarding the potentially destructive standards for shape and weight. When these standards seriously compromise the health and well being of all but the small minority who are constitutionally gaunt, it is a matter for sincere concern for all of those involved with the sport.*

FUTURE RESEARCH

TABLE 15.14 lists 10 areas for future research about eating and weight control behaviors in athletes.[10] More focused and careful investigations with large representative samples, better measurement tools, and a longitudinal approach should provide a clearer understanding of the actual scope of disordered eating among athletes in general and specific athletic groups in particular. Appropriate research design becomes crucial in determining whether a cause-and-effect relationship exists between athletic participation and disordered eating. Better profiling of men and women with the greatest likelihood of encountering problems requires knowledge of the following factors: *(a)* role and interaction of sport-specific risk, *(b)* age risk, *(c)* gender risk, *(d)* training risk, *(e)* skill level and proficiency risk, *(f)* genetic risk, and *(g)* psychosocial risk. Intensive education must focus on upgrading the knowledge of the coaching staff. These professionals need to maintain continual vigilance for signs and symptoms of eating disorders among their athletes.

FIGURE 15.11 provides an overview of general and sport-specific factors that can lead to eating disorders in athletes. Parents, coaches, athletic trainers, and teammates should look for the seven "high-risk" factors. We recommend that coaches tilt the balance between good health and athletic success in the direction of good health. They should formulate prudent and realistic perceptions about what constitutes desirable body size and body shape. Advising an athlete without objective information about body composition (e.g., realistic target body fat levels, desirable FFM and lean/fat ratio, healthy body mass index, and appropriate appraisals of body image and current eating behaviors) often provides the blueprint for disaster. In gymnastics and classical ballet, achieving extremes of thinness should not become a goal, even when considering the participant's health and safety. Of course, this "ivory tower" but appropriate approach requires rearrangement of priorities concerning aesthetic and performance parameters. The perpetual struggle to emulate an ideal that rewards thinness, as in classical ballet, often forms the root cause of acute and chronic medical problems.

Table 15.14　RESEARCH NEEDS CONCERNING THE PREVALENCE OF EATING DISORDERS IN ATHLETES

- Carry out large-scale, epidemiologic studies using consistent measures to define the prevalence of eating disorders in various athletic populations.
- Studies on prevalence should have the proper control groups. These should include athletes from sports with equivalent training but less emphasis on weight.
- Examine both anorexia nervosa and bulimia nervosa, in addition to the range of behaviors and attitudes associated with eating disturbances.
- Identify sports that bring the greatest risk for eating and weight problems.
- Identify the psychological predisposing factors that place individual athletes at risk.
- Identify the physiological factors that place an individual athlete at risk. Examples might be genetic predisposition to be heavy, low metabolic rate, and extreme energy efficiency.
- Examine sex differences in the prevalence and development of eating disorders. This would involve studies of males and females in sports in which weight is emphasized (e.g., gymnastics, figure skating, and distance running).
- Within sports, study athletes at varying levels of training and proficiency.
- Study young athletes early in their training to identify early risk factors.
- Validate self-report measures with athletes and identify the conditions under which self-reports of eating disturbances are most likely to be accurate.

From Brownell KD, Rodin J. Prevalence of eating disorders in athletes. In: Brownell KD, et al., eds. Eating, body weight and performance in athletes. Philadelphia: Lea & Febiger, 1992.

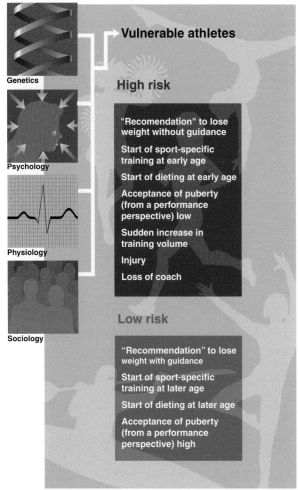

Predisposing factors

Genetics

Psychology

Physiology

Sociology

Vulnerable athletes

High risk

"Recomendation" to lose weight without guidance

Start of sport-specific training at early age

Start of dieting at early age

Acceptance of puberty (from a performance perspective) low

Sudden increase in training volume

Injury

Loss of coach

Low risk

"Recommendation" to lose weight with guidance

Start of sport-specific training at later age

Start of dieting at later age

Acceptance of puberty (from a performance perspective) high

▌ **Figure 15.11** General and sport-specific factors that lead to eating disorders in athletes. (Modified from Sundgot-Borgen J. Eating disorders in female athletes. Sports Med 1994;17: 176.)

Summary

1. Disordered eating describes a broad spectrum of complex behaviors, core attitudes, coping strategies, and conditions that share the commonalty of an emotionally based, inordinate, and pathologic focus on body shape and body weight. An estimated 8 million people in the United States exhibit eating disorders, and approximately 90% are females.

2. Miss America contestants exhibit an image of extreme thinness. Thirty percent of contestant winners fall below the World Health Organization's cutoff for undernutrition (BMI < 18.5). Raising the BMI cutoff to 19.0 adds another 18 women or a total of 48% of the winners with undesirable values. Approximately 24% of contest winners' BMIs ranged between 20.0 and 21.0, and no winner after 1924 had a BMI that equaled the BMI of the reference woman.

3. Athletes face a unique set of circumstances that makes them vulnerable to disordered eating behaviors. These behaviors flourish when the strong negative aesthetic connotations associated with excess body fat blend with the athlete's belief that any body fat spells doom for success.

4. Estimates of the prevalence of eating disorders range between 15 and 62% among female athletes, with the greatest prevalence among athletes in the aesthetic sports (ballet, bodybuilding, diving, figure skating, cheerleading, and gymnastics) in which success often coincides with extreme leanness.

5. Anorexia athletica describes the continuum of subclinical eating behaviors of physically active individuals who fail to meet the criteria for a true eating disorder but exhibit at least one unhealthy method of weight control.

6. Unhealthy weight control habits include fasting, vomiting, and use of diet pills, laxatives, or diuretics.

7. Approximately 50% of women with eating disorders compulsively overexercise. The term *exercise addict* describes someone who exercises excessively often doing "whatever it takes" to make additional time in the day to exercise more.

8. Many men project the ideal body as possessing about 28 pounds more muscle than their own. This mismatch in perception has coincided with an increase in the number of men using anabolic steroids, experiencing eating disorders, and suffering from body obsession.

9. Body obsession encompasses a broad range of body-image concerns, but an important component relates to muscle dysmorphia or a pathologic preoccupation with muscularity.

10. Anorexia nervosa, present in about 1 to 2 % of the general population, represents a crippling obsession with body size, a preoccupation with dieting and thinness, and a refusal to eat enough food to maintain a minimally normal body weight.

11. For anorectics, body weight decreases significantly below normal for age and stature, oftentimes leading to death.

12. Frequent episodes of binge eating followed by purging and intense feelings of guilt or shame characterize bulimia nervosa. Approximately 2 to 4% of all adolescents and adults in the general population suffer from bulimia nervosa.

13. Binge-eating disorder frequently occurs among obese patients undergoing treatment for weight loss.

14. Disordered eating behaviors—semistarvation, purging, excessive exercising—are used to achieve a body weight for success in certain "aesthetic" sports.

15. Four steps constitute an intervention strategy for disordered eating behaviors in athletes: (a) identify and isolate the contributing factors, (b) formulate appropriate goals for intervention and prevention, (c) formulate long-term strategies to deal with the problem, and (d) initiate a long-term program to address the situation.

16. Cognitive–behavioral therapy, interpersonal psychotherapy, and pharmacologic treatment currently treat eating disorders to give patients a sense of balance, purpose, and future. No one best treatment exists; combined approaches using individuals with expertise in psychiatry, eating disorders, body image issues, medicine, and nutrition often work best.

TEST YOUR KNOWLEDGE ANSWERS

1. False In point of fact, Miss America contestants may represent an undernourished role model. The BMI of Miss America contestants generally falls below 18.5, a cutoff below the WHO standard that characterizes relative undernutrition.

2. False Clinical observations indicate a prevalence of between 15 and 60% for disordered eating among athletes, with some groups at higher risk than others. More specifically, disordered eating patterns and unrealistic weight goals (and general dissatisfaction with one's body) occur most frequently among female athletes in the aesthetic sports such as ballet, body building, diving, figure skating, cheerleading, and gymnastics, in which success often coincides with extreme leanness. An inordinate preoccupation with eating also occurs among adolescent female swimmers. Controversy exists as to the prevalence of eating disorders among endurance runners.

3. True The term *anorexia athletica* describes the continuum of subclinical eating behaviors of physically active individuals who fail to meet the criteria for a true eating disorder, but who exhibit at least one unhealthy weight control method. This includes fasting, vomiting (termed "instrumental vomiting" when used to make weight), and use of diet pills, laxatives, or diuretics (water pills).

4. False Most persons consider disordered eating behaviors a "female problem," yet an increasing number of men share this affliction. An unanswered question concerns whether this increased number results from an increase in disease incidence or because more men seek treatment. In one New York hospital treatment center, the percentage of male patients admitted with eating disorders rose steadily from 4% in 1988 to 13% in 1995. Men currently represent about 6 to 10% of individuals with eating disorders, with the greatest prevalence among models, dancers, men abused during childhood, and gays.

5. False Anorexia nervosa, particularly common and increasing in prevalence among adolescent girls and young women, is characterized by distortions of body image, a crippling obsession with body size, a preoccupation with dieting and thinness, and a refusal to eat enough food to maintain a minimally normal body weight. A relentless pursuit of thinness culminates in severe undernutrition, altered body composition characterized by depletion of fat and fat-free body mass, and cessation of menstruation (amenorrhea) in females. Body weight decreases below normal for age and stature.

6. False Weight gain becomes a primary goal in the treatment of anorexia nervosa.

7. False Bulimia nervosa, far more common than anorexia nervosa, is characterized by frequent episodes of bingeing calorically dense food (often at night and usually between 1000 to 10,000 calories), followed within several hours by purging, laxative abuse, fasting, or extreme exercise. Intense feelings of guilt or shame accompany these behaviors.

8. False The main components in treating eating disorders include education (providing information concerning the eating disorder and its consequences); self-monitoring (providing a clear understanding of current eating behaviors and patterns); and meal planning (helping to gain control of eating patterns and establish a healthful pattern of eating).

9. True Exercise has proven useful to treat bulimia nervosa. Regular physical activity reduces the pursuit of thinness, feelings of body dissatisfaction, and the frequency of bingeing, purging, and laxative abuse. The augmented self-regulation may result from the effects of exercise to reduce bulimic patients' bodily tensions and improve stress tolerance.

10. False Muscle dysmorphia or the "Adonis complex" encompasses the pathologic preoccupation with muscle size and overall muscularity. These individuals view themselves as small and frail when in reality many are large and muscular. In many ways, muscle dysmorphia and anorexia nervosa share common traits; these include a history of depression and anxiety, a hyperculturization of body image and unrealistic shame about one's body, and self-destructive behaviors.

References

1. Agras WS. One-year follow-up of cognitive-behavioral therapy for obese individuals with binge eating disorder. J Consult Clin Psychol 1997;65:343.

2. Anderluh MB, et al. Childhood obsessive-compulsive personality traits in adult women with eating disorders: defining a broader eating disorder phenotype. Am J Psychiatry 2003;160:242.

3. Attia E, et al. Does fluoxetine augment the inpatient treatment of anorexia nervosa? Am J Psychiatry 1998;155:548.

4. Beals KA. Disordered eating among athletes: a comprehensive guide for health professionals. Human Kinetics, Champaign IL, 2004.

5. Benson J.E, et al. Eating problems and calorie intake levels in Swiss adolescent athletes. Int J Sports Med 1990;11:249.

6. Black DR, Burckes-Miller ME. Male and female college athletes: use of anorexia nervosa and bulimia nervosa weight loss methods. Res Q 1988;59:252.

7. Borgen JS, Corbin CB. Eating disorders among female athletes. Phys Sportsmed 1987;15:89.

8. Brooks-Gunn H, et al. Attitudes toward eating and body weight in different groups of female adolescent athletes. Int J Eating Disord 1988;7:748.

9. Brooks-Gunn JM, et al. The relation of eating problems and amenorrhea in ballet dancers. Med Sci Sports Exerc 1987;19:41.

10. Brownell KD, Rodin J. Prevalence of eating disorders in athletes. In: Brownell KD, et al., eds. Eating, body weight and performance in athletes. Philadelphia: Lea & Febiger, 1992.

11. Casper RC, et al. Total daily energy expenditure and activity level in anorexia nervosa. Am J Clin Nutr 1991;53:1143.

12. Clark N, et al. Nutrition education for elite female runners. Phys Sportsmed 1988;16:124.

13. Cobb KL, et al. Disordered eating, menstrual irregularity, and bone mineral density in female runners. Med Sci Sports Exerc 2003;35:711.

14. Dale KS, Landers DM. Weight control in wrestling: eating disorders or disordered eating? Med Sci Sports Exerc 1999;31:1382.

15. Davis C, Cowles M. A comparison of weight and diet concerns and personality factors among female athletes and non-athletes. J Psychosom Res 1989;33:527.

16. Drewnowski A, et al. Bulimia in college women: incidence and recovery rates. Am J Psychol 1988;145:753.

17. Dummer GD, et al. Pathogenic weight control behavior of young, competitive swimmers. Phys Sportsmed 1987;15:75.

18. Eldredge KL. The effects of extending cognitive-behavioral therapy for binge eating disorder among initial treatment nonresponders. Int J Eating Disord 1997;21:347.

19. Enns MP, et al. Body composition, body size estimation and attitudes toward eating in male college athletes. Psychosom Med 1987;49:56.

20. Evers CL. Dietary intake and symptoms of anorexia nervosa in female university dancers. J Am Diet Assoc 1987;87:66.

21. Field AE, et al. Exposure to mass media and weight concerns among girls. Pediatrics 1999;103:E36.

22. Fogelholm M, Hilloskorpi H. Weight and diet concerns in Finnish female and male athletes. Med Sci Sports Exerc 1999;31:229.

23. Frusztajer NT, et al. Nutrition and the incidence of stress fractures in ballet dancers. Am J Clin Nutr 1990;51:79.

24. Garfinkel PE. Kaplan AS. Anorexia nervosa: diagnostic conceptualizations. In: Brownell KD, Foreyt JP, eds. Handbook of eating disorders. New York: Basic Books, 1986.

25. Garner DM, Rosen LW. Eating disorders among athletes: research and recommendations. J Appl Sports Sci Res 1991;5:100.

26. Garner DM, et al. A prospective study of eating disturbances in the ballet. Psychother Psychosom 1987;48:170.

27. Gormally J, et al. The assessment of binge eating severity among obese persons. Addict Behav 1982;7:47.

28. Grigg M, et al. Disordered eating and unhealthy weight reduction practices among adolescent females. Prevent Med 1996;25:745.

29. Grinspoon S, et al. Changes in regional fat redistribution and the effects of estrogen during spontaneous weight gain in women with anorexia nervosa. Am J Clin Nutr 2001;73:865.

30. Hamilton LH, et al. Sociocultural influences on eating disorders in professional female ballet dancers. Int J Eating Disord 1985;4:465.

31. Hamilton LH, et al. The role of selectivity in the pathogenesis of eating problems in ballet dancers. Med Sci Sports Exerc 1988;20: 560.

32. Herzog DB, et al. Eating disorders and social maladjustment in female medical students. J Nerv Ment Disord 1985;173:734.

33. Herzog DB, et al. Frequency of bulimic behaviors and associated social maladjustments in female graduate students. J Psychol Res 1986; 20:355

34. Humphries LL, Gruber JJ. Nutrition behaviors of university majorettes. Phys Sportsmed 1986;14:91.

35. Iketani T, et al. Altered body fat distribution after recovery of weight in patients with anorexia nervosa. Int J Eating Disord 1999;26:275.

36. Johnson C, et al. Athletes and eating disorders: the national collegiate athletic association study. Int J Eating Disord 1999;26:179.

37. Joy E. Team management of the female athlete triad. Phys Sportsmed 1997;25:95.

38. Kaye WH, et al. Caloric intake necessary for weight maintenance in anorexia nervosa: nonbulimics require greater caloric intake than bulimics. Am J Clin Nutr 1986;44:443.

39. Kerr J. Characteristics common to females who exhibit anorexic or bulimic behavior: a review of current literature. J Clin Psychol 1991;47:846.

40. Kerrvish KP, et al. Body composition in adolescents with anorexia nervosa. Am J Clin Nutr 2002;75:31.

41. King MB, Mezey G. Eating behavior of male racing jockeys. Psychol Med 1987;17:249.

42. Kininngham RB, Gorenflo DW. Weight loss methods of high school wrestlers. Med Sci Sports Exerc 2001;33:810.

43. Kinoy BP. Eating disorders: new directions in treatment and recovery. New York: Columbia University Press, 1994.

44. Kirchner EM, et al. Bone mineral density and dietary intake of female college gymnasts. Med Sci Sports Exerc 1995;27:543.

45. Kurtzman FD, et al. Eating disorders among selected female student populations at UCLA. J Am Diet Assoc 1989;89:45.

46. Le Grange D, et al. Eating and general psychopathology in a sample of Caucasian and ethnic minority subjects. Int J Eating Disord 1997;21:285.

47. Levine MD, et al. Exercise in the treatment of binge eating disorder. Int J Eating Disord 1996;19:171.

48. Lilenfeld D, et al. A controlled family study of anorexia nervosa and bulimia nervosa: psychiatric disorders in first-degree relatives and effects of proband comorbidity. Arch Gen Psychiatry 1998;55:603.

49. Marcus MD. Binge eating in obesity. In: Fairburn CG, Wilson GT, eds. Binge eating: nature, assessment, and treatment. New York: Guilford Press, 1993.

50. Marcus MD, et al. Binge eating and dietary restraint in obese patients. Addict Behav 1985;10:163.

51. Mallick MJ, et al. Behavioral and psychological traits of weight-conscious teenagers: a comparison of eating-disordered patients and high- and low-risk groups. Adolescence 1987;22:157.

52. Marzano-Parisoli MM. The contemporary construction of a perfect body image: bodybuilding, exercise addiction, and eating disorders. Quest 2001;53:216.

53. Mayer L. Body composition and anorexia nervosa: does physiology explain psychology? Am J Clin Nutr 2001;73:851.

54. McElroy SL, et al. Topiramate in the treatment of binge eating disorder. Am J Psychiatry 2003;160:255.

55. Mulholland AM, Mintz LB Prevalence of eating disorders among African American women. J Consult Psychol 2001;48:111.

56. National Institutes of Health. Binge eating disorders. NIH Publication. no. 94-3589. Washington, DC: U.S. Department of Health and Human Services, 1993.

57. O'Conner P, et al. Eating disorder symptoms in female college gymnasts. Med Sci Sports Exerc 1995;26:550.

58. O'Connor PJ, et al. Eating disorder symptoms in former female college gymnasts: relations with body composition. Am J Clin Nutr 1996;64:840.

59. Olivardia R, et al. Muscle dysmorphia in male weightlifters: a case-control study. Am J Psychiatry 2000;157:1291.

60. Orphanidou CI, et al. Changes in body composition and fat distribution after short-term weight gain in patients with anorexia nervosa. Am J Clin Nutr 1997;65:1034.

61. Owens RG, Slade PD. Running and anorexia nervosa: an empirical study. Int J Eating Disord 1987;6:771.

62. Pasman L, Thompson JK. Body image and eating disturbance in obligatory runner, obligatory weightlifter, and sedentary individuals. Int J Eating Disord 1988;7:759.

63. Patton GC. The spectrum of eating disorder in adolescence. J Psychosom Res 1988;32:579.
64. Perkins DF, Luster T. The relationship between sexual abuse and purging: findings from community-wide surveys of female adolescents. Child Abuse Negl 1999;23:371.
65. Petrie TA, Stoever S. The incidence of bulimia nervosa and pathogenic weight control behaviors in female collegiate gymnasts. Res Quart Exerc Sport 1993;64:238.
66. Pike KM. Long-term course of anorexia nervosa: response, relapse, remission, and recovery. Clin Psychol Rev 1998;18:447.
67. Polito A, et al. Basal metabolic rate in anorexia nervosa: relation to body composition and leptin concentrations. Am J Clin Nutr 2000;71: 1495.
68. Pope HG Jr, et al. Body image perception among men in three countries. Am J Psychiatry 2000;157;1297.
69. Powers P, Johnson C. Targeting eating disorders in elite athletes. Part 1. Eating Disord Rev 1996;7:4.
70. Probst M, et al. Body composition of anorexia nervosa patients assessed by underwater weighing and skinfold-thickness measurements before and after weight gain. Am J Clin Nutr 2001;73:190.
71. Pyle RL, et al. Maintenance treatment and 6-month outcome for bulimic patients who respond to initial treatment. Am J Psychiatry 1990;147:871.
72. Rosen LW, Hough DO. Pathogenic weight control behaviors among female gymnasts. Phys Sportsmed 1988;16:140.
73. Rosen LW, et al. Pathogenic weight control behavior in female athletes. Phys Sportsmed 1986;14:79.
74. Rucinski A: Relationship of body image and dietary intake of competitive ice skaters. J Am Diet Assoc 1989;89:98.
75. Schnirring L. When to suspect muscle dysmorphia: bringing the "Adonis complex" to light. Phys Sportsmed 2000;28(12):19.
76. Silverman JG, et al. Dating violence against adolescent girls and associated substance use, unhealthy weight control, sexual risk behavior, pregnancy, and suicidality. JAMA 2001;286:572.
77. Smith DE. Binge eating in ethnic minority groups. Addict Behav 1995;20:695.
78. Sossin K. Nutrition beliefs, attitudes, and resource use of high school wrestling coaches. Int J Sport Nutr 1997;7:219.
79. Spurrell EB, et al. Age of onset for binge eating: are there different pathways to binge eating? Int J Eat Disord 1997;21:55.
80. Steen SN, Brownell KD. Current patterns of weight loss and regain in wrestlers: has the tradition changed? Med Sci Sports Exerc 1990;22:762.
81. Steen SN, McKinney S. Nutrition assessment of college wrestlers. Phys Sportsmed 1986;14:100.
82. Striegel-Moore RH. Risk factors for eating disorders. Ann NY Acad Sci 1997;817:98.
83. Striegel-Moore RH, et al. Abuse, bullying, and discrimination as risk factors for binge eating disorder. Am J Psychiatry 2002;159:1902.
84. Stunkard AJ, et al. Binge eating disorder and the night-eating syndrome. Int J Obes Relat Metab Disord 1996;20:1.
85. Sunday SR, Halmi KA. Micro- and macroanalyses of patterns within a meal in anorexia and bulimia nervosa. Appetite 1996;26:21.
86. Sundgot-Borgen J. Eating disorders among female athletes. Phys Sportsmed 1987;15:89.
87. Sundgot-Borgen J. Eating disorders in female athletes. Sports Med 1994;17:176.
88. Sundgot-Borgen J. Risk and trigger factors for the development of eating disorders in female elite athletes. Med Sci Sports Exerc 1994;26:414.
89. Sundgot-Borgen J, et al. The effect of exercise, cognitive therapy, and nutritional counseling in treating bulimia nervosa. Med Sci Sport Exerc 2002;34:190.
90. Tanofsky MB, et al. Comparison of men and women with binge eating disorder. Int J Eating Disord 1997;21:49.
91. Team Physician Consensus Statement. Female athlete issues for the team physician: a consensus statement. Med Sci Sports Exerc 2003;35:1785.
92. The McKnight Investigators. Risk factors for the onset of eating disorders in adolescent girls: Results of the McKnight Longitudinal Risk Factor Study. Am J Psychiatry 2003;160:248.
93. Thiel A, et al. Subclinical eating disorders in male athletes. A study of the low weight category in rowers and wrestlers. Acta Psychiatry Scand 1993;88:259.
94. Thompson RA, Sherman RT. Helping athletes with eating disorders. Champaign, IL: Human Kinetics Publishers, 1993.
95. Tofler IR, et al. Physical and emotional problems of elite female gymnasts. N Engl J Med 1996;335:281.
96. Warren BJ, et al. Disordered eating patterns in competitive female athletes. Int J Eating Disord 1990;9:565.
97. Weight L, Noakes T. Is running an analog of anorexia? A survey of the incidence of eating disorders in female distance runners. Med Sci Sports Exerc 1987;19:213.
98. Wichmann S, Martin DR. Eating disorders in athletes: weighing the risks. Phys Sportsmed 1993;21:126.
99. Wiederman MW, Pryor T. Substance use among women with eating disorders. Int J Eating Disord. 1996;20:163.
100. World Health Organization. Obesity: preventing and managing the global epidemic. Report of a WHO consultation presented at the World Health Organization; June 3–5, 1997; Geneva, Switzerland. Publication WHO/NUT/NCD/98.1.
101. Yannovski SV. Binge eating disorder: current knowledge and future directions. Obes Res 1993;1:306.
102. Yanovski SZ, et al. Association of binge eating disorder and psychiatric comorbidity in obese subjects. Am J Psychiatry 1993;50:1472.
103. Yeager KK, et al. The female athlete triad—disordered eating, amenorrhea and osteoporosis. Med Sci Sports Exerc 1993;25:775.
104. Zamboni M, et al. Body fat distribution before and after weight gain in anorexia nervosa. Int J Obes 1997;21:33.

Additional Readings

Becker AE, et al. Secondary prevention for eating disorders: The impact of education, screening, and referral in a college-based screening program. Int J Eat Disord 2004;36:157.

Breen HB, Espelage DL. Nutrition expertise in eating disorders. Eat Weight Disord 2004;9:120.

Chua JL, et al. Negative mood-induced overeating in obese binge eaters: An experimental study. Int J Obes Relat Metab Disord 2004;28:606.

Elliot DL, et al. Preventing substance use and disordered eating: Initial outcomes of the ATHENA (Athletes Targeting Healthy Exercise and Nutrition Alternatives) program. Arch Pediatr Adolesc Med 2004;158:1043.

Hopkinson RA, Lock J. Athletics, perfectionism, and disordered eating. Eat Weight Disord 2004;9:99.

Lantz CD, et al. Eating attitudes, exercise identity, and body alienation in competitive ultramarathoners. Int J Sport Nutr Exerc Metab 2004;14:406.

Lombardo C, et al. Internal consistency, convergent validity and reliability of a brief questionnaire on disordered eating (DEQ). Eat Weight Disord 2004;2:91.

Mathieu J. Disordered eating across the life span. J Am Diet Assoc 2004;104:1208.

Neumark-Sztainer D, et al. Are family meal patterns associated with disordered eating behaviors among adolescents? J Adolesc Health 2004;35:350.

Saules KK, et al. Effects of disordered eating and obesity on weight, craving, and food intake during ad libitum smoking and abstinence. Eat Behav 2004;5:353.

Sundgot-Borgen J. Disordered eating and exercise. Scand J Med Sci Sports 2004;14:205.

Sundgot-Borgen J, et al. Sexual harassment and eating disorders in female elite athletes—a controlled study. Scand J Med Sci Sports 2003;13:330.

Sundgot-Borgen J, Torstveit MK. Prevalence of eating disorders in elite athletes is higher than in the general population. Clin J Sport Med 2004;14:25.

Tanofsky-Kraff M, Yanovski SZ. Eating disorder or disordered eating? Non-normative eating patterns in obese individuals. Obes Res 2004;12:1361.

Thome J, L Espelage D. Relations among exercise, coping, disordered eating, and psychological health among college students. Eat Behav 2004;5:337.

Nutritive Values for Common Foods, Alcoholic and Nonalcoholic Beverages, and Specialty and Fast-Food Items

This appendix has three parts. Part 1 lists nutritive values for common foods, Part 2 lists nutritive values for alcoholic and nonalcoholic beverages, and Part 3 presents nutritive values for specialty and fast-food items. The nutritive values of foods and alcoholic and nonalcoholic beverages, expressed in 1-ounce (28.4 g) portions, allow comparisons among different food categories. Thus, for example, the protein content of 1.55 g for 1 ounce of banana nut bread can be compared directly to the protein content of 6.28 g for 1 ounce of processed American cheese.

Part 1

NUTRITIVE VALUES FOR COMMON FOODS[a]

The foods are grouped into categories and are listed in alphabetical order within each category. The categories include breads, cakes and pies, cookies, candy bars, chocolate, desserts, cereals, cheese, fish, fruits, meats, eggs, dairy products, vegetables, and typical salad bar entries. An additional section labeled *Variety* consists of food items such as soups, sandwiches, salad dressings, oils, some condiments, and other "goodies." The nutritive value for each food is expressed per ounce or 28.4 g of that food item. The specific values for each food include the caloric content (kcal) for 1 ounce, protein, total lipid, carbohydrate, calcium, iron, vitamin B_1, vitamin B_2, fiber content, and cholesterol.

---

[a]The information about the nutritive value of the foods comes from a variety of sources. This includes primarily data from Watt, B.K., and Merrill, A.L.: *Composition of Foods—Raw, Processed and Prepared,* U.S. Department of Agriculture, Washington, DC, 1963; Adams C, and Richardson, M.: *Nutritive Value of Foods.* Home and Garden Bulletin No.72, rev, Washington, DC, U.S. Government Printing Office, 1981; and Pennington JAT, and Douglass JP. Bowes & Church's food values of portions commonly used. 18th ed. Baltimore: Lippincott Williams & Wilkins, 2005. Other sources include a comprehensive database maintained by the University of Massachusetts, the consumer relations departments of manufacturers, and journal articles that evaluated specific foods items. NA *indicates data not available.*

BREADS

	kcal	Protein (g)	Lipid (g)	CHO (g)	Ca (mg)	Fe (mg)	B₁ (mg)	B₂ (mg)	Fiber (g)	Cholesterol (mg)
Banana nut	91	1.55	4.00	12.7	10.0	0.470	0.054	0.046	0.66	18.3
Boston brown—canned	60	1.26	0.39	13.2	25.8	0.567	0.038	0.025	1.34	1.9
Cornmeal muffin—recipe	91	1.89	3.15	13.2	41.6	0.567	0.069	0.069	1.00	14.5
Croutons—dry	105	3.69	1.04	20.5	35.0	1.020	0.099	0.099	0.09	0
Cracked wheat	74	2.63	0.99	14.2	18.1	0.755	0.108	0.108	1.50	0
Cracked wheat—toast	88	3.00	1.17	16.9	21.6	0.899	0.100	0.128	1.82	0
French—chunk	81	2.67	1.10	14.3	31.6	0.875	0.130	0.097	0.57	0
Italian	78	2.55	0.25	16.0	4.7	0.756	0.116	0.066	0.47	0
Mixed grain	74	2.27	1.05	13.6	30.6	0.907	0.113	0.113	1.78	0
Mixed grain—toast	80	2.47	1.15	14.8	33.3	0.986	0.099	0.123	1.97	0
Oatmeal	74	2.37	1.25	13.6	17.0	0.794	0.130	0.075	1.10	0
Oatmeal—toast	80	2.47	1.36	14.8	18.5	0.863	0.110	0.081	1.20	0
Pita pocket	78	2.94	0.42	15.6	23.2	0.685	0.129	0.061	0.45	0
Pumpernickel	71	2.60	0.98	13.6	20.4	0.777	0.097	0.147	1.67	0
Pumpernickel—toast	78	2.86	1.08	15.0	22.5	0.857	0.088	0.162	1.87	0
Raisin—	77	2.15	1.12	15.0	28.4	0.879	0.093	0.176	0.68	0
Raisin—toasted	92	2.57	1.34	17.6	33.8	1.080	0.081	0.209	0.81	0
Rye—light	74	2.40	1.04	13.6	22.7	0.771	0.116	0.090	1.87	0
Rye—light—toast	84	2.73	1.18	15.5	25.8	0.876	0.107	0.103	2.15	0
Vienna	79	2.72	1.10	14.4	31.2	0.873	0.130	0.100	0.91	0
White	76	2.35	1.10	13.8	35.7	0.806	0.133	0.088	0.54	0
White—toast	84	2.67	1.26	15.7	40.6	0.915	0.121	0.103	0.64	0
Whole wheat	69	2.84	1.22	12.9	20.2	0.964	0.100	0.059	2.10	0
Whole wheat—toasted	79	3.42	1.47	14.4	22.5	1.090	0.090	0.066	2.74	0
Bread crumbs—dry grated	111	3.69	1.42	20.7	34.6	1.160	0.099	0.099	1.15	1.4
Bread crumbs—soft	76	2.35	1.10	13.9	35.9	0.806	0.134	0.088	0.54	0
Bread sticks wo/salt	109	3.40	0.82	21.3	7.9	0.255	0.017	0.020	0.43	0
Bread sticks w/salt	86	2.67	0.89	16.4	13.0	0.243	0.016	0.024	0.41	0

CAKES AND PIES

	kcal	Protein (g)	Lipid (g)	CHO (g)	Ca (mg)	Fe (mg)	B₁ (mg)	B₂ (mg)	Fiber (g)	Cholesterol (mg)
Cakes										
Angel food cake	67	1.71	0.09	15.2	23.5	0.123	0.014	0.057	0	0
Boston cream pie	61	0.59	1.89	10.4	6.1	0.142	0.002	0.043	0	4.7
Carrot cake	103	1.05	5.32	13.2	6.9	0.304	0.030	0.035	0	14.6
Cheesecake	86	1.54	5.45	8.1	15.9	0.136	0.009	0.037	0	52.4
Choc cupcake/choc frosting	97	1.24	3.29	16.5	16.9	0.575	0.029	0.041	0	15.2
Coffee cake	91	1.78	2.70	14.8	17.3	0.480	0.054	0.059	0	18.5
Dark fruitcake	109	1.32	4.62	16.5	27.0	0.791	0.053	0.053	0	13.2
Gingerbread cake	91	1.15	2.86	15.2	12.2	0.706	0.042	0.038	0	7.8
Pound cake	113	1.89	4.72	14.2	18.9	0.472	0.047	0.057	0	30.2
Sheet cake—plain	104	1.32	3.96	15.8	18.1	0.429	0.046	0.049	0	20.1
Sheet cake—white frosting	104	0.94	3.28	18.0	14.3	0.281	0.030	0.037	0	16.4
Sponge cake	83	2.01	1.27	16.0	10.8	0.524	0.043	0.046	0	58.8
White cake/coconut	109	1.30	4.05	17.0	13.7	0.454	0.041	0.053	0	1.2

CAKES AND PIES—continued

	kcal	Protein (g)	Lipid (g)	CHO (g)	Ca (mg)	Fe (mg)	B₁ (mg)	B₂ (mg)	Fiber (g)	Cholesterol (mg)
Cakes—cont'd										
White cake/white frosting	104	1.20	3.59	16.8	13.2	0.399	0.080	0.052	0	1.2
Yellow cake/chocolate frosting	101	1.03	4.48	15.9	9.5	0.509	0.020	0.058	0	15.6
Pies										
Apple pie	73	0.66	3.14	10.7	5.0	0.300	0.031	0.023	0	0
Apple pie—fried	85	0.73	4.67	10.7	4.0	0.312	0.030	0.020	0	4.7
Banana cream pie	46	0.90	1.85	6.7	21.0	0.156	0.022	0.042	0	2.2
Blueberry pie	68	0.72	3.05	9.9	4.7	0.377	0.031	0.025	0	0
Boston cream pie	61	0.59	1.89	10.4	6.1	0.142	0.002	0.043	0	4.7
Cherry pie	74	0.77	3.19	10.9	6.6	0.569	0.034	0.025	0	0
Cherry pie—fried	83	0.68	4.74	10.7	3.7	0.233	0.020	0.020	0	4.3
Chocolate cream pie	50	1.20	2.04	6.9	25.9	0.175	0.024	0.049	0	2.4
Coconut cream pie	57	1.03	2.79	7.2	24.0	0.198	0.021	0.042	0	2.5
Coconut custard pie	66	1.69	3.85	6.3	25.0	0.304	0.029	0.055	0	31.4
Cream pie	85	0.56	4.29	11.0	8.6	0.205	0.011	0.028	0	1.5
Custard pie	55	1.43	2.65	6.3	23.1	0.269	0.026	0.050	0	27.6
Lemon meringue pie	72	0.95	2.90	10.7	5.1	0.283	0.020	0.028	0	27.7
Mincemeat pie	70	0.65	2.13	12.8	6.9	0.360	0.028	0.024	0	0
Peach pie	73	0.63	3.14	10.9	4.8	0.340	0.031	0.028	0	0
Pecan pie	120	1.30	4.87	18.9	7.2	0.380	0.045	0.034	0	28.1
Pumpkin pie	52	1.28	2.23	7.3	30.0	0.373	0.019	0.042	0	15.5
Strawberry chiffon pie	65	0.85	3.46	8.0	7.7	0.254	0.022	0.023	0	7.1

COOKIES

	kcal	Protein (g)	Lipid (g)	CHO (g)	Ca (mg)	Fe (mg)	B₁ (mg)	B₂ (mg)	Fiber (g)	Cholesterol (mg)
Animal cookies	120	1.90	2.89	22.0	3.0	0.918	0.080	0.130	0	0.1
Brownies w/nuts	135	1.84	8.93	15.6	12.8	0.567	0.070	0.070	0	25.5
Butter cookies	130	1.76	4.82	20.2	36.3	0.170	0.011	0.017	0	4.1
Fig bars	106	1.02	1.93	21.4	20.2	0.689	0.039	0.037	0	13.7
Lady fingers	102	2.19	2.19	18.3	11.6	0.515	0.019	0.039	0	101.0
Oatmeal raisin cookies	134	1.64	5.45	19.6	9.8	0.600	0.049	0.044	0	1.1
Peanut butter cookies	145	2.36	8.27	16.5	12.4	0.650	0.041	0.041	0	13.0
Sandwich type cookies	138	1.42	5.67	20.6	8.5	0.992	0.064	0.050	0	0
Shortbread cookies	137	1.77	7.09	17.7	11.5	0.709	0.089	0.080	0	23.9
Sugar cookies	139	1.18	7.09	18.3	29.5	0.532	0.053	0.035	0	17.1
Vanilla wafers	131	1.42	4.96	20.6	11.3	0.567	0.050	0.070	0	17.7

CANDY BARS

	kcal	Protein (g)	Lipid (g)	CHO (g)	Ca (mg)	Fe (mg)	B₁ (mg)	B₂ (mg)	Fiber (g)	Cholesterol (mg)
Almond Joy	151	1.69	7.82	18.5	2.0	0.778	0	0	0	0
Sugar-coated almonds	146	3.10	9.12	14.6	39.6	0.775	0.042	0.156	0	0

CANDY BARS—*continued*

	kcal	Protein (g)	Lipid (g)	CHO (g)	Ca (mg)	Fe (mg)	B₁ (mg)	B₂ (mg)	Fiber (g)	Cholesterol (mg)
Bittersweet chocolate	141	1.90	9.73	15.7	13.0	1.040	0.015	0.050	0	0
Caramel—plain or chocolate	115	1.00	2.99	22.0	41.9	0.399	0.010	0.050	0	1.0
Chocolate candy kisses	154	2.10	8.98	15.9	52.9	0.499	0.020	0.080	0	0
Chocolate-coated almonds	161	3.92	12.70	8.0	47.8	1.090	0.052	0.186	0	0
Chocolate-covered coconut	133	0.91	7.10	17.5	8.4	0.614	0.008	0.016	0	0
Chocolate-covered mints	116	0.50	2.99	23.0	16.0	0.299	0.010	0.020	0	0
Chocolate-covered peanuts	159	5.00	11.70	9.8	32.9	0.689	0.086	0.043	0	0
Chocolate-covered raisins	111	1.06	2.71	20.6	12.2	0.663	0.034	0.025	0	0
Chocolate fudge	115	0.56	2.78	21.0	22.0	0.299	0.010	0.030	0	1.0
Chocolate fudge with nuts	114	1.06	4.99	18.8	22.0	0.299	0.016	0.030	0	7.4
English toffee	195	0.89	16.90	9.8	0	0.177	0.470	0.044	0	0
Gum drops	98	0	0.20	24.8	2.0	0.100	0	0	0	0
Hard candy	109	0	0	27.6	6.0	0.100	0	0	0	0
Jelly beans	104	0	0.10	26.4	1.0	0.299	0	0	0	0
Kit Kat	138	1.98	7.25	16.5	42.9	0.369	0.020	0.073	0	0
Krackle	149	2.00	8.09	16.9	50.0	0.400	0.017	0.075	0	0
Malted milk balls	135	2.30	6.99	17.8	62.9	0	0	0	0	0
M&M's plain chocolate	140	1.95	6.08	19.5	46.7	0.449	0.015	0.073	0	0
M&M's peanut chocolate	144	3.23	7.25	16.5	35.4	0.402	0.016	0.056	0	0
Mars bar	136	2.27	6.24	17.0	48.2	0.312	0.014	0.093	0	0
Milk chocolate—plain	145	2.00	8.98	16.0	49.9	0.399	0.020	0.100	0	6.0
Milk chocolate w/almonds	150	2.90	10.40	15.0	60.9	0.559	0.030	0.130	0	4.5
Milk chocolate w/peanuts	155	4.89	11.70	10.0	31.9	0.679	0.112	0.065	0	3.0
Milk chocolate + rice cereal	140	2.00	6.99	18.0	47.9	0.200	0.010	0.080	0	6.0
Milky Way	123	1.53	4.25	20.3	40.6	0.232	0.013	0.070	0	6.6
Mr. Goodbar	151	3.62	9.05	13.9	39.2	0.567	0.030	0.072	0	4.2
Reese's peanut butter cup	151	3.65	9.07	13.9	21.7	0.430	0.020	0.032	0	1.6
Snickers	134	3.08	6.62	17.0	32.4	0.227	0.013	0.050	0	0
Vanilla fudge	118	0.70	3.15	22.0	29.9	0.030	0.006	0.025	0	10.0
Vanilla fudge with nuts	122	1.00	5.01	18.3	25.0	0.159	0.017	0.026	0	8.5

CHOCOLATE

	kcal	Protein (g)	Lipid (g)	CHO (g)	Ca (mg)	Fe (mg)	B₁ (mg)	B₂ (mg)	Fiber (g)	Cholesterol (mg)
Baking chocolate	145	3.49	15.00	7.5	22.0	1.900	0.015	0.099	0	0
Bittersweet chocolate	141	1.90	9.73	15.7	13.0	1.040	0.015	0.050	0	0
Milk chocolate—plain	145	2.00	8.98	16.0	49.9	0.399	0.020	0.100	0	6.0
Semi-sweet chocolate chips	143	1.17	10.20	16.2	8.5	0.967	0.017	0.023	0	0
Dark chocolate—sweet	150	1.00	9.98	16.0	7.0	0.599	0.010	0.040	0	0
Chocolate cupcake/ chocolate frosting	97	1.24	3.29	16.5	16.9	0.575	0.029	0.041	0	15.2
Chocolate candy kisses	154	2.10	8.98	15.9	52.9	0.499	0.020	0.080	0	0
Chocolate chip cookies	122	1.54	5.94	18.9	11.0	0.540	0.068	0.155	0	3.4

CHOCOLATE—*continued*

	kcal	Protein (g)	Lipid (g)	CHO (g)	Ca (mg)	Fe (mg)	B₁ (mg)	B₂ (mg)	Fiber (g)	Cholesterol (mg)
Chocolate coated almonds	161	3.92	12.70	8.0	47.8	1.090	0.052	0.186	0	0
Chocolate coated peanuts	159	5.00	11.70	9.8	32.9	0.689	0.086	0.043	0	0
Chocolate covered mints	116	0.50	2.99	23.0	16.0	0.299	0.010	0.020	0	0
Chocolate covered raisins	111	1.06	2.71	20.6	12.2	0.663	0.034	0.025	0	0
Chocolate cream pie	50	1.20	2.04	6.9	25.9	0.175	0.024	0.049	0	2.4
Chocolate fudge	115	0.56	2.78	21.0	22.0	0.299	0.010	0.030	0	1.0
Chocolate fudge with nuts	114	1.06	4.99	18.8	22.0	0.299	0.016	0.030	0	7.4
Cake flour-baked value	103	2.08	0.28	22.4	4.5	1.250	0.154	0.096	0	0
Reese's peanut butter cup	151	3.65	9.07	13.9	21.7	0.430	0.020	0.032	0	1.6
Chocolate pudding/recipe	42	0.88	1.25	7.3	27.3	0.142	0.005	0.039	0	4.3
Chocolate pudding instant	34	0.85	0.818	5.9	28.4	0.065	0.009	0.039	0	3.1

DESSERTS AND BREAKFAST PASTRIES

	kcal	Protein (g)	Lipid (g)	CHO (g)	Ca (mg)	Fe (mg)	B₁ (mg)	B₂ (mg)	Fiber (g)	Cholesterol (mg)
Apple brown betty	43	0.30	1.60	7.40	5.4	0.130	0.016	0.012	0	3.8
Apple cobbler	55	0.53	1.74	9.57	8.8	0.206	0.023	0.019	0	0.3
Apple crisp	53	0.33	1.93	9.09	7.4	0.278	0.018	0.013	0	0
Apple dumpling	55	0.32	2.37	8.64	7.1	0.253	0.012	0.013	0	0
Banana nut bread	91	1.60	4.00	12.70	10.0	0.470	0.054	0.046	0	18.3
Bread + raisin pudding	60	1.20	2.47	8.54	27.7	0.304	0.030	0.048	0	24.4
Cheesecake	86	1.50	5.45	8.10	15.9	0.136	0.009	0.037	0	52.4
Cherry cobbler	44	0.53	1.37	7.52	8.5	0.391	0.019	0.021	0	0.3
Cherry & cream cheese torte	79	1.28	3.96	10.00	28.5	0.266	0.015	0.052	0	11.2
Vanilla milkshake	32	0.98	0.841	5.09	34.5	0.026	0.013	0.052	0	3.2
Cream puff w/custard fill	72	1.24	4.54	6.83	16.4	0.276	0.015	0.040	0	58.8
Chocolate eclair w/custard fill	79	1.20	4.43	8.96	18.6	0.258	0.019	0.041	0	50.4
Gelatin salad	17	0.43	0	3.99	0.5	0.024	0.002	0.002	0	0
Peach cobbler	28	0.50	1.35	7.96	7.6	0.197	0.018	0.017	0	0.3
Peach crisp	34	0.31	1.06	6.18	4.8	0.203	0.010	0.010	0	0
Crepe, unfilled	49	2.06	1.32	7.07	25.0	0.475	0.045	0.070	0.21	43.0
Pancakes—plain	63	2.10	2.10	9.45	28.4	0.525	0.063	0.074	0.42	16.8
Croissant	117	2.32	6.02	13.40	10.0	1.040	0.085	0.065	0.54	6.5
Danish pastry—plain	109	1.99	5.97	12.90	29.8	0.547	0.080	0.085	0	24.4
Danish pastry w/fruit	102	1.74	5.67	12.20	7.41	0.567	0.070	0.061	0	24.4
Doughnut—cake type	119	1.33	6.75	13.90	13.0	0.454	0.068	0.068	0	11.3
Doughnut—jelly filled	99	1.48	3.84	13.00	12.2	0.349	0.052	0.044	0	0
Doughnut—yeast-raised	111	1.89	6.28	12.30	8.0	0.661	0.132	0.057	0	9.9
Chocolate pudding	42	0.88	1.25	7.28	27.3	0.142	0.005	0.039	0	4.3
Tapioca pudding	38	1.43	1.44	4.85	29.7	0.120	0.012	0.052	0	27.3
Vanilla pudding	32	0.99	1.10	4.50	33.1	0.089	0.009	0.046	0	4.1
Chocolate pudding—instant	34	0.85	0.82	5.89	28.4	0.065	0.009	0.039	0	3.1
Rice pudding	33	0.86	0.86	5.80	28.6	0.107	0.021	0.039	0	3.2
Butterscotch pudding pop	47	1.19	1.29	7.80	37.8	0.020	0.015	0.055	0	0.5
Chocholate pudding pop	49	1.34	1.34	8.20	42.8	0.179	0.015	0.055	0	0.5
Vanilla pudding pop	46	1.19	1.29	7.80	37.8	0.020	0.015	0.055	0	0.5

CEREALS (WITHOUT MILK)

	kcal	Protein (g)	Lipid (g)	CHO (g)	Ca (mg)	Fe (mg)	B₁ (mg)	B₂ (mg)	Fiber (g)	Cholesterol (mg)
All-Bran	70	3.99	0.50	21.0	23.00	4.49	0.369	0.429	8.490	0
Alpha Bits	111	2.20	0.60	24.6	7.99	1.80	0.399	0.399	0.650	0
Apple Jacks	110	1.50	0.10	25.7	2.99	4.49	0.399	0.399	0.200	0
Bran Buds	73	3.95	0.68	21.6	18.90	4.52	0.371	0.439	7.860	0
Bran Chex	90	2.95	0.81	22.6	16.80	4.51	0.347	0.150	5.200	0
Buc Wheats	110	2.00	1.00	24.0	59.90	8.09	0.674	0.764	2.000	0
C.W. Post—plain	126	2.54	4.44	20.3	13.70	4.50	0.380	0.438	0.643	0
C.W. Post w/raisins	123	2.45	4.05	20.3	14.00	4.51	0.358	0.413	0.660	0
Cap'n Crunch	120	1.46	2.60	22.9	4.60	7.53	0.506	0.544	0.709	0
Cap'n Crunchberries	118	1.46	2.35	23.0	8.91	7.32	0.478	0.543	0.324	0
Cap'n Crunch—peanut butter	125	2.03	3.64	21.5	5.67	7.37	0.486	0.567	0.324	0
Cheerios	110	4.24	1.77	19.4	47.30	4.44	0.394	0.394	3.000	0
Cocoa Krispies	109	1.50	0.39	25.2	4.73	1.81	0.394	0.394	0.354	0
Cocoa Pebbles	117	1.35	1.49	24.7	5.40	1.75	0.405	0.405	0.312	0
Corn Bran	98	1.97	1.02	23.9	32.30	9.60	0.299	0.551	5.390	0
Corn Chex	111	2.00	0.10	24.9	2.99	1.80	0.399	0.070	0.499	0
Corn flakes—Kellogg's	110	2.30	0.09	24.4	1.00	1.80	0.367	0.424	0.594	0
Corn flakes—Post Toasties	110	2.30	0.09	24.4	1.00	0.70	0.367	0.424	0.594	0
Corn grits—enriched yellow dry	105	2.49	0.33	22.5	0.55	1.10	0.182	0.107	3.270	0
Corn grits—enriched ckd	17	0.41	0.06	3.7	0.12	0.18	0.028	0.018	0.527	0
Cracklin' Oat Bran	108	2.60	4.16	19.4	18.90	1.80	0.378	0.425	4.280	0
Cream of Rice	15	0.24	0.01	3.3	0.93	0.05	0.012	0	0.163	0
Cream of Wheat	16	0.42	0.07	3.4	6.27	1.27	0.028	0.008	0.395	0
Crispy Wheat 'n Raisins	99	2.00	0.46	23.1	46.80	4.48	0.396	0.396	1.320	0
Farina—cooked	14	0.41	0.02	3.0	0.49	0.14	0.023	0.015	0.389	0
Fortified Oat Flakes	105	5.32	0.41	20.5	40.20	8.09	0.354	0.413	0.827	0
40% Bran Flakes—Kellogg's	91	3.60	0.54	22.2	13.80	8.14	0.369	0.430	0.850	0
40% Bran Flakes—Post	92	3.20	0.45	22.3	12.70	4.50	0.374	0.435	3.800	0
Froot Loops	111	1.70	1.00	25.0	2.99	4.49	0.399	0.399	0.299	0
Frosted Mini-Wheats	102	2.93	0.27	23.4	9.15	1.83	0.366	0.457	2.160	0
Frosted Rice Krispies	109	1.30	0.10	25.7	1.00	1.80	0.399	0.399	0.998	0
Fruit & Fiber w/apples	90	2.99	1.00	22.0	9.98	4.49	0.374	0.424	4.190	0
Fruit & Fiber w/dates	90	2.99	1.00	21.0	9.98	4.49	0.374	0.424	4.190	0
Fruitful Bran	92	2.50	0	22.5	8.34	6.75	0.313	0.354	4.170	0
Fruity Pebbles	115	1.10	1.50	24.4	2.99	1.80	0.399	0.399	0.226	0
Golden Grahams	109	1.60	1.09	24.1	17.40	4.50	0.363	0.436	1.670	0
Granola—homemade	138	3.49	7.69	15.6	17.70	1.12	0.170	0.072	2.970	0
Granola—Nature Valley	126	2.89	4.92	18.9	17.80	0.95	0.098	0.048	2.960	0
Grape Nuts	100	3.28	0.11	23.2	10.90	1.22	0.398	0.398	1.840	0
Grape Nuts Flakes	102	2.99	0.30	23.2	11.00	4.49	0.399	0.399	1.900	0
Honey & Nut Corn Flakes	113	1.80	1.50	23.3	2.99	1.80	0.399	0.399	0.299	0
Honey Bran	96	2.51	0.57	23.2	13.00	4.54	0.405	0.405	3.160	0
Honey Comb	111	1.68	0.52	25.3	5.15	1.80	0.387	0.387	0.387	0
Honey Nut Cheerios	107	3.09	0.69	22.8	19.80	4.47	0.344	0.430	0.790	0
King Vitamin	115	1.49	1.62	24.0	NA	17.10	0.124	1.430	0.135	0
Kix	109	2.49	0.70	23.3	34.80	8.06	0.398	0.398	0.398	0
Life	104	5.22	0.52	20.3	99.20	7.47	0.612	0.644	0.902	0
Lucky Charms	111	2.57	1.06	23.1	31.90	4.52	0.354	0.443	0.624	0
Malt-O-Meal	14	0.43	0.03	3.1	0.59	1.13	0.057	0.028	0.354	0
Maypo—cooked	1	0.02	0.01	0.1	0.52	0.04	0.003	0.003	0.012	0

CEREALS (WITHOUT MILK) — *continued*

	kcal	Protein (g)	Lipid (g)	CHO (g)	Ca (mg)	Fe (mg)	B₁ (mg)	B₂ (mg)	Fiber (g)	Cholesterol (mg)
Nutri-Grain—barley	106	3.11	0.21	23.4	7.60	1.00	0.346	0.415	1.660	0
Nutri-Grain—corn	108	2.30	0.68	24.0	0.68	0.60	0.338	0.405	1.750	0
Nutri-Grain—rye	102	2.48	0.21	24.0	5.67	0.80	0.354	0.425	2.160	0
Nutri-Grain—wheat	102	2.45	0.32	24.0	7.73	0.80	0.387	0.451	1.800	0
Oatmeal—prepared	18	0.73	0.29	3.1	2.42	0.19	0.032	0.006	0.497	0
Rolled Oats	109	4.55	1.78	19.0	14.70	1.19	0.206	0.038	3.090	0
Instant Oatmeal w/apples	26	0.74	0.30	5.0	30.00	1.15	0.091	0.053	0.552	0
Instant Oatmeal w/bran & raisins	23	0.71	0.28	4.4	25.20	1.10	0.081	0.092	0.480	0
Instant Oatmeal w/maple	30	0.84	0.35	5.8	29.60	1.16	0.097	0.059	0.530	0
Instant Oatmeal w/cinnamon & spice	31	0.85	0.34	6.2	30.30	1.17	0.099	0.60	0.510	0
Instant Oatmeal w/raisins & spice	29	0.77	0.32	5.7	29.60	1.18	0.092	0.065	0.556	0
100% Bran	77	3.57	1.42	20.7	19.80	3.49	0.687	0.773	8.380	0
100% Natural	135	3.02	6.02	18.0	48.90	0.83	0.085	0.150	3.390	0
100% Natural—w/apples	130	2.92	5.32	19.0	42.80	0.79	0.090	0.158	1.300	0
100% Natural—w/raisins & dates	128	2.89	5.23	18.7	41.20	0.80	0.077	0.165	1.080	0
Product 19	108	2.75	0.17	23.5	3.44	18.00	1.460	1.720	0.369	0
Puffed Rice	111	1.79	0.20	25.5	2.03	0.30	0.030	0.028	0.227	0
Puffed Wheat	104	4.25	0.24	22.4	7.09	1.35	0.047	0.070	5.430	0
Quisp	117	1.42	2.08	23.6	8.50	5.96	0.510	0.718	0.378	0
Raisin Bran—Kellogg's	91	3.07	0.46	21.4	14.50	13.90	0.293	0.332	3.410	0
Raisin Bran—Post	86	2.68	0.55	21.4	13.70	4.56	0.373	0.430	3.190	0
Raisins, Rice & Rye	96	1.60	0.06	24.2	6.16	3.45	0.308	0.370	0.308	0
Ralston—cooked	15	0.62	0.09	3.2	1.57	0.18	0.022	0.020	0.370	0
Rice Chex	112	1.49	1.00	25.2	3.88	1.79	0.400	0.298	1.840	0
Rice Krispies	109	1.86	0.20	24.2	3.91	1.76	0.391	0.391	0.312	0
Roman Meal—dry	91	4.07	0.60	20.4	18.40	1.31	0.142	0.069	0.905	0
Roman Meal—cooked	17	0.77	0.11	3.9	3.45	0.25	0.028	0.014	0.877	0
Shredded Wheat	102	3.09	0.71	22.5	11.00	1.20	0.070	0.080	3.100	0
Shredded wheat	97	3.06	0.45	16.4	11.20	0.89	0.082	0.075	2.900	0
Special K	111	5.58	0.10	21.3	7.97	4.48	0.399	0.399	0.266	0
Sugar Corn Pops	108	1.40	0.10	25.6	0.10	1.80	0.399	0.399	0.100	0
Sugar Frosted Flakes	108	1.46	0.08	25.7	0.81	1.78	0.405	0.405	0.446	0
Sugar Smacks	106	2.00	0.50	24.7	2.99	1.80	0.369	0.429	0.319	0
Super Golden Crisp	106	1.80	0.26	25.6	6.01	1.80	0.344	0.430	0.430	0
Team	111	1.82	0.48	24.3	4.05	1.73	0.371	0.425	0.270	0
Total	105	2.84	0.60	22.3	172.00	18.00	1.460	1.720	2.060	0
Trix	108	1.50	0.40	24.9	5.99	4.49	0.399	0.399	0.184	0
Wheat & Raisin Chex	97	2.68	0.21	22.6	NA	4.04	0.263	0.315	1.890	0
Wheat Chex	104	2.77	0.68	23.3	11.00	4.50	0.370	0.105	2.100	0
Wheat germ—toasted	108	8.25	3.09	14.0	12.50	2.19	0.474	0.233	3.910	0
Wheat germ w/brown sugar, honey	107	6.19	2.30	17.2	8.98	1.93	0.349	0.180	3.390	0
Wheatena—cooked	16	0.58	0.13	3.4	1.28	0.16	0.002	0.006	0.385	0
Wheaties	99	2.74	0.51	22.6	43.00	4.50	0.391	0.391	2.540	0
Whole wheat berries	16	0.54	0.11	3.2	1.70	0.17	0.023	0.006	0.680	0
Whole wheat cereal—cooked	18	0.58	0.11	3.9	1.99	0.18	0.020	0.014	0.457	0

CHEESE

	kcal	Protein (g)	Lipid (g)	CHO (g)	Ca (mg)	Fe (mg)	B₁ (mg)	B₂ (mg)	Fiber (g)	Cholesterol (mg)
American—processed	106	6.28	8.84	0.45	174	0.110	0.008	0.111	0	27.0
American cheese food—cold pack	94	5.23	6.78	2.36	145	0.240	0.009	0.274	0	18.0
American cheese spread	82	5.16	6.00	2.48	159	0.090	0.014	0.380	0	16.0
Blue	100	6.09	8.14	0.66	150	0.090	0.008	0.395	0	21.0
Brick	105	6.40	8.40	0.79	191	0.130	0.004	0.159	0	27.0
Brie	95	5.87	7.84	0.13	52	0.140	0.020	0.147	0	28.0
Camembert	85	5.60	6.86	0.13	110	0.094	0.008	0.138	0	20.0
Caraway	107	7.13	8.27	0.87	191	0.100	0.009	0.196	0	25.0
Cheddar	114	7.05	9.38	0.36	204	0.197	0.008	0.106	0	29.9
Cheshire	110	6.60	8.66	1.36	182	0.060	0.013	0.198	0	28.9
Colby	112	6.73	9.08	0.73	194	0.216	0.004	0.171	0	27.0
Cottage	29	3.54	1.20	0.76	17	0.040	0.006	0.115	0	4.2
Cottage—lowfat 2%	26	3.90	0.55	1.03	20	0.045	0.007	0.052	0	2.4
Cottage—lowfat 1%	21	3.51	0.29	0.77	18	0.040	0.006	0.115	0	1.3
Cottage—dry curd	24	4.89	0.12	0.52	9	0.065	0.007	0.004	0	2.0
Cottage—w/fruit	35	2.80	0.96	3.78	14	0.031	0.005	0.115	0	3.1
Cream	99	2.10	9.87	0.75	23	0.337	0.005	0.056	0	30.9
Edam	101	7.07	7.79	0.40	207	0.125	0.010	0.274	0	25.0
Feta	75	4.49	6.19	1.16	140	0.180	0.040	0.315	0	25.0
Fontina	110	7.25	8.62	0.44	156	0.060	0.006	NA	0	32.9
Gjetost	132	2.74	8.32	12.00	113	0.130	0.009	0.170	0	25.0
Gorgonzola	111	6.99	8.98	0	149	0.120	0.010	0.512	0	25.0
Gouda	101	7.06	7.72	0.63	198	0.070	0.009	0.232	0	31.9
Gruyere	117	8.44	9.05	0.10	286	0.060	0.017	0.095	0	30.9
Liederkranz	87	4.99	7.99	0	110	0.120	0.010	0.389	0	21.0
Limburger	93	5.67	7.59	0.14	141	0.040	0.023	0.227	0	26.0
Monterey jack	106	6.93	8.56	0.19	212	0.200	0.004	0.119	0	26.0
Mozzarella—skim, low moist	80	7.60	4.67	0.89	207	0.076	0.006	0.150	0	15.0
Mozzarella—whole milk, regular	80	5.50	5.75	0.63	147	0.050	0.004	0.106	0	22.0
Mozzarella—whole milk, moist	90	6.10	7.19	0.43	163	0.060	0.005	0.119	0	25.0
Muenster	104	6.40	8.42	0.32	203	0.125	0.004	0.178	0	27.0
Neufchatel	74	2.82	6.70	0.83	21	0.080	0.004	0.113	0	22.0
Parmesan—hard	111	10.00	7.30	0.91	335	0.230	0.010	0.453	0	19.0
Parmesan—grated	129	11.80	8.50	1.06	389	0.270	0.013	0.527	0	22.0
Pimento processed	106	6.26	8.82	0.49	174	0.120	0.008	0.404	0	27.0
Port du salut	100	6.73	7.99	0.16	84	0.140	0.004	0.151	0	34.9
Provolone	100	7.13	7.54	0.61	214	0.146	0.005	0.248	0	20.0
Ricotta—part skim	39	3.23	2.25	1.45	77	0.126	0.006	0.052	0	8.8
Ricotta—whole milk	49	3.19	3.68	0.86	59	0.108	0.004	0.024	0	14.3
Romano	110	9.00	7.63	1.03	301	0.230	0.010	0.339	0	28.9
Romano—grated	128	10.50	8.86	1.20	350	0.270	0.013	0.394	0	32.9
Roquefort	105	6.10	8.93	0.57	188	0.172	0.010	0.512	0	26.0
Swiss	107	8.03	7.79	0.96	272	0.050	0.006	0.074	0	26.0
Swiss processed	95	7.00	6.97	0.60	219	0.170	0.004	0.078	0	24.0

FISH

	kcal	Protein (g)	Lipid (g)	CHO (g)	Ca (mg)	Fe (mg)	B_1 (mg)	B_2 (mg)	Fiber (g)	Cholesterol (mg)
Bass—freshwater raw	32	5.36	1.05	0	22.7	0.422	0.028	0.009	0	19.3
Bluefish—baked/broiled	45	7.43	1.42	0	2.6	0.174	0.022	0.030	0	17.9
Bluefish—fried in crumbs	58	6.44	2.78	1.33	2.3	0.151	0.017	0.023	0	17
Bluefish—raw	35	5.67	1.20	0	2.0	0.136	0.016	0.023	0	16.7
Carp—raw	36	5.05	1.59	0	11.6	0.352	0.013	0.011	0	18.7
Catfish—channel—raw	33	5.16	1.20	0	11.3	0.275	0.013	0.030	0	16.4
Cod—baked w/butter	37	6.46	0.94	0	5.7	0.139	0.025	0.022	0	17.0
Cod—batter-fried	56	5.56	2.92	2.13	22.7	0.142	0.011	0.011	0	15.6
Cod—baked/broiled	30	6.46	0.24	0	4.0	0.139	0.025	0.022	0	15.6
Cod—poached	29	6.24	0.24	0	4.0	0.139	0.025	0.022	0	15.6
Cod—steamed	29	6.24	0.24	0	4.0	0.139	0.025	0.022	0	15.9
Cod—smoked	22	5.19	0.17	0	4.0	0.113	0.023	0.020	0	14.2
Cod—Atlantic—raw	23	5.05	0.19	0	4.5	0.108	0.022	0.018	0	12.2
Cod liver oil	255	0	28.40	0	0	0	0	0	0	162.0
Eel—smoked	94	5.27	7.88	0.23	26.9	0.198	0.040	0.099	0	19.8
Haddock—breaded/fried	58	5.67	3.00	2.33	11.3	0.384	0.020	0.033	0.01	18.3
Haddock—smoked	33	7.14	0.27	0	13.9	0.397	0.013	0.014	0	21.8
Haddock—raw	22	5.36	0.20	0	9.4	0.298	0.010	0.010	0	16.2
Herring—pickled	74	4.03	5.10	2.73	21.8	0.346	0.010	0.039	0	3.7
Herring—smoked/ kippered	62	6.97	3.52	0	23.8	0.428	0.036	0.090	0	22.7
Herring—canned w/liquid	59	5.64	3.86	0	41.7	0.879	0.007	0.051	0	27.5
Mackerel—fried	49	7.00	2.35	0	4.3	0.445	0.045	0.116	0	19.8
Mackerel—Atlantic— baked/broiled	74	6.78	5.05	0	4.3	0.445	0.045	0.117	0	21.3
Mackerel—Atlantic—raw	58	5.27	3.94	0	3.4	0.462	0.050	0.088	0	19.8
Mackerel—Pacific—raw	45	6.12	2.84	0	2.3	0.567	0.043	0.096	0	22.7
Northern pike—raw	25	5.47	0.20	0	16.2	0.156	0.017	0.018	0	11.0
Ocean perch—breaded/ fried	62	5.34	3.67	2.33	30.7	0.400	0.033	0.037	0.03	15.3
Pollock—baked/broiled	28	6.60	0.31	0	19.3	0.149	0.014	0.057	0	19.8
Pollock—poached	36	6.60	0.31	0	17.0	0.149	0.010	0.050	0	19.8
Salmon—broiled/baked	61	7.74	3.10	0	2.0	0.157	0.061	0.048	0	24.7
Coho salmon—steamed/ poached	52	7.77	2.14	0	8.22	0.252	0.057	0.031	0	13.9
Smoked salmon— Chinook	33	5.17	1.22	0	03.0	0.240	0.007	0.029	0	6.7
Atlantic salmon— small can	36	5.05	1.62	0	3.1	0.204	0.057	0.097	0	17.0
Pink salmon—raw	33	5.64	0.98	0	11.3	0.218	0.040	0.057	0	14.7
Sardines	59	7.00	3.24	0	108.0	0.826	0.023	0.064	0	40.4
Sea trout steelhead—raw	30	4.73	1.02	0	4.8	0.077	0.023	0.057	0	23.5
Sea trout steelhead— cooked	37	6.07	1.42	0	5.7	0.088	0.024	0.064	0	32.3
Shad—baked with bacon	57	6.58	3.20	0	6.8	0.170	0.037	0.074	0	17.0
Smelt—rainbow—raw	28	4.99	0.69	0	17.0	0.255	0.016	0.034	0	19.8
Snapper—baked or broiled	36	7.46	0.49	0	11.3	0.068	0.015	0.021	0	13.3
Snapper—raw	28	5.81	0.38	0	9.1	0.051	0.013	0.017	0	10.5
Sole/flounder—baked w/butter	40	5.34	2.00	0	5.3	0.093	0.023	0.032	0	22.7
Sole/flounder—baked/ broiled	33	6.84	0.43	0	5.3	0.093	0.023	0.032	0	19.3

FISH—*continued*

	kcal	Protein (g)	Lipid (g)	CHO (g)	Ca (mg)	Fe (mg)	B_1 (mg)	B_2 (mg)	Fiber (g)	Cholesterol (mg)
Sole/flounder—batter-fried	83	4.47	5.10	4.07	16.7	0.239	0.057	0.042	0.01	15.0
Sole/flounder—breaded/fried	53	4.96	2.55	2.54	11.3	0.128	0.037	0.034	0	15.0
Sole/flounder—steamed	26	5.67	0.33	0	4.5	0.079	0.017	0.027	0	14.7
Sole/flounder—raw	26	5.33	0.34	0	5.1	0.102	0.025	0.022	0	13.6
Lemon sole—raw	23	4.85	0.21	0	4.8	0.088	0.026	0.023	0	17.0
Lemon sole—fried w/crumbs	56	4.56	3.12	2.64	26.9	0.176	0.020	0.023	0	18.4
Lemon sole—steamed	26	5.84	0.26	0	6.0	0.147	0.026	0.026	0	17.0
Swordfish—raw	34	5.61	1.14	0	1.1	0.230	0.010	0.027	0	11.0
Swordfish—broiled/baked	44	7.20	1.46	0	1.7	0.295	0.012	0.033	0	14.2
Trout—baked/broiled	43	7.47	1.22	0	24.3	0.690	0.024	0.064	0	20.7
Tuna—oil pack	56	8.26	2.34	0	3.8	0.395	0.010	0.030	0	5.0
Tuna—water pack	37	8.38	0.14	0	3.4	0.409	0.010	0.033	0	16.0
Tuna—raw	31	6.63	0.27	0	4.5	0.207	0.123	0.013	0	12.8
Whiting—flour/bread-fried	54	5.13	1.56	1.98	11.3	0.198	0.023	0.020	0	18.4

FRUITS

	kcal	Protein (g)	Lipid (g)	CHO (g)	Ca (mg)	Fe (mg)	B_1 (mg)	B_2 (mg)	Fiber (g)	Cholesterol (mg)
Apple w/peel	16	0.055	0.100	4.31	2.05	0.051	0.005	0.004	0.709	0
Apple slices w/peel—fresh	17	0.054	0.100	4.33	2.06	0.052	0.005	0.004	0.709	0
Apple juice—canned/bottled	13	0.017	0.032	3.32	1.94	0.105	0.006	0.005	0.034	0
Apple juice—frozen concentrate	47	0.144	0.105	11.60	5.78	0.258	0.003	0.015	0.089	0
Applesauce—sweetened	22	0.052	0.052	5.67	1.11	0.111	0.003	0.008	0.397	0
Apricot—fresh halves	14	0.397	0.110	3.15	4.02	0.154	0.009	0.011	0.538	0
Apricot halves—light syrup	18	0.150	0.013	4.67	3.34	0.110	0.005	0.006	0.319	0
Apricot nectar—canned	16	0.104	0.025	4.08	2.03	0.108	0.003	0.004	0.170	0
Avocado—average	46	0.563	0.340	2.10	3.07	0.284	0.030	0.035	2.720	0
Banana—fresh slices	26	0.293	0.136	6.63	1.74	0.088	0.013	0.028	0.578	0
Blackberries—canned	26	0.370	0.040	6.54	5.98	0.184	0.008	0.011	1.011	0
Blackberries—fresh	15	0.205	0.110	3.62	9.06	0.158	0.008	0.011	1.910	0
Blackberries—frozen	18	0.334	0.122	4.45	8.26	0.173	0.008	0.013	1.460	0
Blueberries—fresh	16	0.190	0.108	4.00	1.76	0.047	0.014	0.014	0.763	0
Blueberries-frozen unsweetened	14	0.119	0.181	3.46	2.19	0.051	0.009	0.010	0.658	0
Boysenberries—frozen	14	0.314	0.075	3.46	7.73	0.240	0.015	0.010	1.100	0
Sour cherries—frozen	13	0.260	0.124	3.13	3.66	0.150	0.012	0.010	0.384	0
Sweet cherries—fresh	20	0.340	0.272	4.69	4.10	0.110	0.014	0.017	0.430	0
Sweet cherries—frozen	25	0.325	0.037	6.34	3.39	0.099	0.008	0.013	0.224	0
Cranberries—whole—raw	14	0.110	0.057	3.58	2.09	0.057	0.009	0.006	1.190	0
Cranberry/apple juice	19	0.015	0.090	4.82	2.02	0.017	0.001	0.006	0.070	0
Cranberry juice cocktail	16	0.009	0.015	4.03	0.90	0.043	0.002	0.002	0.085	0
Date—whole—each	78	0.557	0.127	20.80	9.22	0.342	0.026	0.028	2.300	0

FRUITS— *continued*

	kcal	Protein (g)	Lipid (g)	CHO (g)	Ca (mg)	Fe (mg)	B₁ (mg)	B₂ (mg)	Fiber (g)	Cholesterol (mg)
Figs—medium—fresh	21	0.215	0.085	5.44	10.20	0.102	0.017	0.014	1.050	0
Fig—dried—each	72	0.864	0.330	18.50	40.80	0.634	0.020	0.025	3.140	0
Fruit cocktail—heavy syrup	21	0.111	0.020	5.36	1.78	0.081	0.005	0.005	0.280	0
Fruit cocktail—light syrup	16	0.114	0.020	4.23	1.80	0.082	0.005	0.005	0.284	0
Grapefruit half—pink/red	9	0.157	0.028	2.18	3.00	0.034	0.010	0.006	0.369	0
Grapefruit half—white	10	0.195	0.029	2.38	3.36	0.017	0.010	0.006	0.368	0
Grapefuit sections/fresh	9	0.179	0.028	2.29	3.33	0.025	0.010	0.006	0.370	0
Grapefruit sections—canned	17	0.160	0.028	4.38	4.02	0.114	0.010	0.006	0.313	0
Grapefruit juice—fresh	11	0.142	0.029	2.60	2.53	0.056	0.011	0.006	0.113	0
Grapefruit juice—sweetened	13	0.164	0.026	3.15	2.27	0.102	0.011	0.007	0.076	0
Grapefruit juice—unsweetened	11	0.148	0.028	2.54	1.95	0.057	0.012	0.006	0.077	0
Grapefruit juice—frozen concentrate	41	0.548	0.137	9.86	7.67	0.140	0.041	0.022	0.383	0
Grapes—Thompson	20	0.188	0.163	5.03	3.01	0.073	0.026	0.016	0.333	0
Grape juice—bottled/canned	17	0.158	0.021	4.25	2.47	0.068	0.007	0.010	0.141	0
Grape juice—frozen concentrate	51	0.184	0.088	12.60	3.68	0.102	0.015	0.026	0.492	0
Grape juice—prep frozen	15	0.053	0.026	3.62	1.13	0.029	0.004	0.007	0.142	0
Kiwi fruit	17	0.280	0.127	4.22	7.46	0.112	0.007	0.015	0.962	0
Lemon—fresh wo/peel	8	0.313	0.083	2.64	7.33	0.171	0.011	0.006	0.582	0
Lemon juice—fresh	7	0.107	0.081	2.45	2.09	0.009	0.008	0.003	0.099	0
Lemon juice—bottled	6	0.114	0.081	1.84	3.02	0.036	0.012	0.003	0.085	0
Lime—fresh	9	0.199	0.055	2.99	9.30	0.169	0.008	0.006	0.228	0
Lime juice—fresh	8	0.124	0.029	2.56	2.54	0.009	0.006	0.003	0.113	0
Lime juice—bottled	6	0.115	0.115	1.84	3.46	0.069	0.009	0.001	0.099	0
Loganberries—fresh	20	0.430	0.088	3.69	8.50	0.181	0.014	0.010	1.760	0
Loganberries—frozen	16	0.430	0.089	3.68	7.33	0.181	0.014	0.010	1.760	0
Mango—fresh—slices	19	0.146	0.077	4.83	2.92	0.360	0.016	0.016	0.997	0
Mango—fresh—whole	19	0.145	0.078	4.82	2.88	0.356	0.016	0.016	1.010	0
Cantaloupe—cubes	10	0.250	0.079	2.37	3.19	0.060	0.006	0.006	0.284	0
Casaba melon—cubes	8	0.255	0.028	1.75	1.50	0.113	0.017	0.006	0.284	0
Honeydew melon—cubes	10	0.128	0.028	2.60	1.67	0.020	0.022	0.005	0.307	0
Melon balls—mixed—frozen	9	0.239	0.023	2.25	2.79	0.008	0.005	0.006	0.295	0
Mixed fruit—dried	69	0.697	0.139	18.20	10.60	0.767	0.012	0.045	1.220	0
Mixed fruit—frozen—thawed	28	0.397	0.052	6.87	2.04	0.079	0.005	0.010	0.386	0
Nectarine	14	0.267	0.129	3.34	1.25	0.044	0.005	0.012	0.554	0
Orange	13	0.266	0.035	3.33	11.30	0.029	0.025	0.011	0.680	0
Orange sections—fresh	13	0.266	0.035	3.34	11.30	0.029	0.025	0.011	0.680	0
Mandarin oranges—canned	17	0.113	0.011	4.61	2.03	0.101	0.015	0.012	0.478	0
Orange juice—fresh	13	0.199	0.057	2.95	3.09	0.057	0.025	0.008	0.113	0
Oranged juice—frozen concentrate	45	0.679	0.059	10.80	9.05	0.099	0.079	0.018	0.313	0

FRUITS—*continued*

	kcal	Protein (g)	Lipid (g)	CHO (g)	Ca (mg)	Fe (mg)	B₁ (mg)	B₂ (mg)	Fiber (g)	Cholesterol (mg)
Orange juice—frozen	13	0.191	0.016	3.05	2.50	0.031	0.023	0.005	0.057	0
Papaya—whole fresh	11	0.173	0.040	2.78	6.71	0.028	0.008	0.009	0.482	0
Papaya—slices fresh	12	0.174	0.040	2.77	6.68	0.060	0.008	0.009	0.482	0
Papaya nectar—canned	16	0.049	0.043	4.12	2.72	0.098	0.002	0.001	0.170	0
Peaches—fresh	12	0.199	0.026	3.14	1.30	0.031	0.005	0.012	0.489	0
Peach slices—frozen/ thawed	27	0.177	0.037	6.80	0.91	0.105	0.004	0.010	0.467	0
Peach halves—heavy syrup	21	0.130	0.028	5.67	1.05	0.077	0.003	0.007	0.315	0
Peach halves—light syrup	15	0.126	0.010	4.13	1.05	0.101	0.002	0.007	0.402	0
Peach halves—dried	68	0.020	0.216	17.40	8.07	1.150	0	0.060	2.330	0
Peach nectar—canned	15	0.076	0.006	3.95	1.48	0.054	0	0.004	0.170	0
Pears—Bartlett	17	0.111	0.113	4.29	3.24	0.070	0.006	0.011	0.779	0
Pear halves—heavy syrup	21	0.057	0.036	5.42	1.44	0.061	0.004	0.006	0.395	0
Pear halves—light syrup	16	0.054	0.007	4.30	1.44	0.082	0.003	0.005	0.395	0
Pear nectar—canned	17	0.030	0.003	4.47	1.25	0.073	0	0.004	0.204	0
Pineapple slices—heavy syrup	22	0.098	0.034	5.72	3.91	0.108	0.025	0.007	0.270	0
Pineapple slices—light syrup	15	0.103	0.034	3.81	3.91	0.110	0.026	0.007	0.268	0
Pineapple—frozen sweetened	24	0.113	0.029	6.29	2.55	0.113	0.028	0.009	0.496	0
Pineapple juice—frozen concentrate	51	0.369	0.029	12.60	11.00	0.255	0.065	0.017	0.255	0
Plums	16	0.223	0.176	3.69	1.29	0.030	0.012	0.027	0.550	0
Plums—canned—heavy syrup	25	0.102	0.028	6.59	2.53	0.238	0.005	0.010	0.434	0
Plums—canned—light syrup	18	0.105	0.029	4.61	2.70	0.243	0.005	0.011	0.444	0
Prunes—dried	68	0.739	0.145	17.80	14.50	0.702	0.023	0.046	2.700	0
Prune juice—bottled	20	0.172	0.009	4.95	3.43	0.334	0.005	0.020	0.310	0
Raisins—seedless	85	0.914	0.130	22.50	13.90	0.594	0.044	0.025	1.670	0
Raspberries—fresh	14	0.256	0.157	3.27	6.22	0.162	0.009	0.026	1.770	0
Raspberries—canned w/liquid	26	0.235	0.034	6.62	2.99	0.120	0.006	0.009	1.200	0
Raspberries—frozen	29	0.197	0.044	7.42	4.30	0.184	0.005	0.013	1.300	0
Rhubarb—raw—diced	6	0.253	0.056	1.29	39.50	0.062	0.006	0.009	0.737	0
Rhubarb—cooked w/sugar	33	0.111	0.013	8.85	41.10	0.060	0.005	0.006	0.624	0
Strawberries—fresh	9	0.173	0.105	2.00	4.00	0.108	0.006	0.019	0.736	0
Strawberries—frozen	10	0.120	0.030	2.59	4.38	0.213	0.006	0.010	0.736	0
Tangerine—fresh	13	0.179	0.054	3.17	4.05	0.028	0.030	0.006	0.574	0
Tangerines—canned— light syrup	17	0.127	0.028	4.61	2.03	0.105	0.015	0.012	0.453	0
Watermelon	9	0.175	0.121	2.04	2.24	0.048	0.023	0.006	0.114	0

MEATS

	kcal	Protein (g)	Lipid (g)	CHO (g)	Ca (mg)	Fe (mg)	B_1 (mg)	B_2 (mg)	Fiber (g)	Cholesterol (mg)
Beef chuck—pot roasted	108	7.20	8.64	0	3.67	0.840	0.020	0.065	0	29.0
Beef chuck—pot roasted lean	77	8.80	4.34	0	3.67	1.040	0.024	0.080	0	30.0
Beef round—pot roasted lean & fat	74	8.44	4.20	0	1.67	0.920	0.020	0.069	0	27.0
Beef round—pot roasted lean	63	8.97	2.74	0	1.33	0.980	0.021	0.074	0	27.0
Ground beef—lean	77	7.00	5.34	0	3.00	0.600	0.013	0.060	0	24.7
Ground beef—regular	82	6.67	5.94	0	3.00	0.700	0.010	0.053	0	25.3
Sirloin steak—lean	57	8.10	2.53	0	2.33	0.700	0.026	0.056	0	21.7
T-bone steak—lean & fat	92	6.80	6.97	0	2.67	0.720	0.026	0.059	0	23.7
Beef lunchmeat—thin-sliced	50	7.96	1.09	1.62	2.99	0.759	0.023	0.054	0	12.0
Beef lunchmeat—loaf/roll	87	4.06	7.42	0.82	2.99	0.659	0.030	0.062	0	18.0
Beef rib—oven roasted—lean	68	7.70	3.90	0	3.34	0.740	0.023	0.060	0	22.7
Beef round—oven roasted—lean	54	8.14	2.12	0	1.67	0.834	0.028	0.076	0	23.0
Beef rump roast—lean only	51	8.40	1.89	0	1.13	0.567	0.026	0.049	0	19.6
Beef brains—pan-fried	56	3.57	4.50	0	2.67	0.630	0.037	0.074	0	566.0
Beef heart	47	8.17	1.59	0.12	1.67	2.130	0.040	0.436	0	54.7
Beef kidney	41	7.23	0.97	0.27	5.00	2.070	0.054	1.150	0	110.0
Beef liver—fried	61	7.57	2.27	2.23	3.00	1.780	0.060	1.170	0	137.0
Beef tongue—cooked	80	6.27	5.87	0.09	2.00	0.960	0.009	0.009	0	30.4
Beef tripe—raw	28	4.14	1.12	0	36.00	0.553	0.002	0.047	0	26.9
Beef tripe—pickled	17	3.29	0.40	0	25.00	0.389	0	0.028	0	15.0
Corned beef—canned	71	7.67	4.24	0	5.67	0.590	0.006	0.042	0	24.3
Corned beef hash—canned	49	2.35	1.29	2.82	3.74	0.567	0.016	0.052	0.153	17.0
Beef—dried/cured	47	8.24	1.10	0.44	2.00	1.280	0.050	0.230	0	45.9
Beef & vegetable stew	26	1.85	1.27	1.74	3.36	0.336	0.017	0.020	0.393	8.2
Beef stew—canned	22	1.64	0.88	2.06	2.66	0.368	0.008	0.014	0.150	1.7
Burrito—beef & bean	63	3.40	2.84	6.48	26.70	0.437	0.042	0.047	0.810	8.4
Tostada w/beans & beef	49	2.72	3.06	2.98	27.50	0.319	0.012	0.036	0.583	9.1
Beef + macaroni + tomato	24	1.25	0.73	3.16	3.81	0.300	0.024	0.021	0.291	2.8
Beef enchilada	69	3.09	3.26	3.69	60.20	0.418	0.017	0.039	0.465	8.9
Frankfurter—beef	92	3.20	8.36	0.68	3.48	0.378	0.014	0.029	0	13.4
Frankfurter—beef & pork	91	3.20	8.26	0.73	2.98	0.328	0.056	0.034	0	14.4
Beef pot pie—frozen	52	1.99	2.73	4.77	2.42	0.436	0.022	0.018	0.109	5.0
Beef pie—recipe	70	2.84	4.05	5.27	3.92	0.513	0.039	0.039	0.155	5.7
Beef taco	75	4.94	4.80	3.67	30.90	0.469	0.010	0.049	0.407	16.2
Chicken meat—all-fried	62	8.67	2.59	0.48	4.86	0.383	0.024	0.056	0.002	26.5
Chicken meat—all-roasted	54	8.20	2.10	0	4.25	0.342	0.020	0.050	0	25.3
Chicken meat—all-stewed	50	7.74	1.90	0	4.05	0.330	0.014	0.046	0	23.5
Boned chicken w/broth	47	6.17	2.26	0	3.99	0.439	0.004	0.037	0	17.6
Chicken—dark meat—fried	68	8.22	3.30	0.74	5.06	0.423	0.026	0.070	0.002	27.3
Chicken—dark meat—roasted	58	7.76	2.75	0	4.25	0.377	0.020	0.064	0	26.3
Chicken—dark meat—stewed	55	7.37	2.55	0	4.05	0.385	0.016	0.057	0	24.9

MEATS—continued

	kcal	Protein (g)	Lipid (g)	CHO (g)	Ca (mg)	Fe (mg)	B₁ (mg)	B₂ (mg)	Fiber (g)	Cholesterol (mg)
Chicken—light meat—fried	54	9.31	1.57	0.12	4.45	0.322	0.020	0.036	0	25.3
Chicken—light meat—roasted	49	8.77	1.28	0	4.25	0.302	0.018	0.033	0	23.9
Chicken—light meat—stewed	45	8.18	1.17	0	3.64	0.265	0.012	0.033	0	21.7
Chicken breast—no skin	47	8.80	0.99	0	4.29	0.295	0.020	0.032	0	24.0
Chicken breast meat—stewed	43	8.20	0.86	0	3.58	0.250	0.012	0.034	0	21.8
Chicken drumstick—batter fried	76	6.22	4.45	2.36	4.73	0.382	0.032	0.061	0.008	24.4
Chicken drumstick—roasted	61	7.69	3.16	0	3.27	0.376	0.020	0.061	0	26.2
Chicken wing—batter-fried	92	5.64	6.19	3.10	5.79	0.365	0.030	0.043	0.012	22.6
Chicken wing—flour-fried	91	7.40	6.28	0.67	4.43	0.354	0.017	0.039	0.009	23.0
Chicken wing—roasted	83	7.48	5.53	0	4.17	0.359	0.012	0.037	0	24.2
Chicken gizzards—simmered	44	7.73	1.04	0.32	2.58	1.180	0.008	0.070	0	54.9
Chicken hearts—simmered	52	7.49	2.23	0.03	5.27	2.560	0.017	0.206	0	68.7
Chicken livers—simmered	44	6.90	1.55	0.25	4.05	2.400	0.043	0.496	0	179.0
Chicken roll—light meat	45	5.52	2.08	0..69	11.90	0.274	0.018	0.037	0	13.9
Chicken frankfurter	73	3.67	5.52	1.93	27.00	0.567	0.019	0.033	0	28.4
Chicken a la king	54	3.12	3.93	1.93	14.70	0.289	0.012	0.049	0.154	25.6
Chicken + noodles	43	2.60	2.13	3.07	3.07	0.278	0.006	0.020	0.142	12.2
Chicken chow mein	29	2.60	1.25	1.13	6.58	0.284	0.009	0.026	0.466	8.5
Chicken curry	26	2.21	1.53	0.64	2.52	0.170	0.009	0.019	0.033	5.3
Chicken frankfurter	72	3.67	5.52	1.93	27.00	0.567	0.019	0.033	0	28.4
Chicken pot pie—frozen	53	1.84	2.84	5.08	3.70	0.382	0.020	0.020	0.210	4.9
Chicken roll—light meat	45	5.52	2.08	0.69	11.90	0.274	0.018	0.037	0	13.9
Chicken salad w/celery	97	3.82	8.90	0.47	5.92	0.239	0.012	0.028	0.109	17.3
Chicken patty sandwich	79	4.48	4.06	6.10	7.95	0.338	0.052	0.047	0.244	12.3
Chicken broth—from dry	2	0.16	0.13	0.17	1.74	0.009	0	0.004	0.001	0.1
Chicken broth—from cube	2	0.11	0.04	0.18	0.04	0.014	0.001	0.003	0	0.1
Chicken noodle soup	9	0.48	0.29	1.10	2.00	0.092	0.006	0.007	0.085	0.8
Tostada w/beans/chicken	45	3.50	2.06	3.38	29.30	0.305	0.013	0.034	0.668	9.6
Chicken taco	63	5.60	3.03	3.67	31.60	0.237	0.014	0.043	0.407	16.5
Chicken enchilada	64	3.38	2.48	3.69	60.50	0.359	0.018	0.036	0.465	9.1
Turkey dark meat—roasted	53	8.10	2.05	0	9.11	0.662	0.018	0.070	0	24.0
Turkey white meat—roasted	44	8.48	0.91	0	5.47	0.380	0.017	0.037	0	19.6
Turkey breast—barbecued	40	6.39	1.40	0	2.00	0.120	0.010	0.030	0	16.0
Turkey gizzards	46	8.34	1.10	0.17	4.32	1.540	0.009	0.093	0	65.6
Turkey hearts	50	7.58	1.73	0.58	3.72	1.950	0.019	0.250	0	64.0
Turkey livers	48	6.80	1.69	0.97	3.02	2.210	0.015	0.404	0	177.0
Turkey loaf	31	6.38	0.45	0	2.00	0.113	0.011	0.030	0	11.6
Turkey roll	41	5.27	2.03	0.15	11.40	0.358	0.025	0.064	0	11.9
Turkey bologna	56	3.86	4.27	0.27	23.40	0.432	0.015	0.047	0	28.0
Turkey frankfurter	64	4.05	5.22	0.42	36.50	0.485	0.023	0.050	0	24.6
Turkey ham	36	5.37	1.49	0.42	2.49	0.776	0.020	0.075	0	15.9
Turkey pastrami	37	5.22	1.75	0.43	2.49	0.403	0.022	0.075	0	14.9
Turkey salami	55	4.62	3.89	0.15	5.47	0.463	0.029	0.075	0	22.9
Turkey pot pie—frozen	51	1.80	2.75	4.65	7.79	0.256	0.020	0.020	0.110	2.4

EGGS

	kcal	Protein (g)	Lipid (g)	CHO (g)	Ca (mg)	Fe (mg)	B_1 (mg)	B_2 (mg)	Fiber (g)	Cholesterol (mg)
Egg white, cooked	13	2.68	0	0.33	3.20	0.008	0.002	0.072	0	0
Egg yolk, cooked	108	4.76	8.73	0.07	44.40	1.620	0.044	0.121	0	355.0
Egg, fried in butter	56	3.54	3.45	0.38	15.70	0.536	0.018	0.148	0	129.0
Egg, hard cooked	40	3.52	2.79	0.34	13.80	0.474	0.014	0.132	0	113.0
Egg, poached	40	3.50	2.79	0.34	13.80	0.474	0.014	0.132	0	113.0
Egg, scrambled milk + butter	40	2.88	2.57	0.61	23.90	0.412	0.013	0.106	0	93.9
Egg raw—large	40	3.52	2.79	0.34	13.80	0.474	0.017	0.139	0	113.0
Egg white—raw	13	2.68	0	0.33	3.20	0.008	0.002	0.075	0	0
Egg yolk, raw	108	4.76	8.73	0.07	44.40	1.620	0.051	0.126	0	355.0
Egg substitute, frozen	45	3.20	3.15	0.91	20.80	0.562	0.034	0.110	0	0.5
Egg substitute, powder	125	15.60	3.66	6.12	90.70	0.879	0.062	0.493	0	162.0

DAIRY PRODUCTS

	kcal	Protein (g)	Lipid (g)	CHO (g)	Ca (mg)	Fe (mg)	B_1 (mg)	B_2 (mg)	Fiber (g)	Cholesterol (mg)
Milk—1% lowfat	12	0.93	0.30	1.36	34.9	0.014	0.011	0.047	0	1.16
Milk—2% lowfat	14	0.94	0.56	1.36	34.5	0.012	0.011	0.047	0	2.56
Milk—skim	10	0.97	0.05	1.38	34.9	0.012	0.010	0.040	0	0.46
Milk—whole	17	0.93	0.95	1.32	33.8	0.014	0.010	0.046	0	3.83
Buttermilk	12	0.94	0.25	1.35	33.0	0.014	0.010	0.044	0	1.04
Milk—instant nonfat dry	102	9.96	0.21	14.80	349.0	0.088	0.117	0.496	0	5.00
Canned skim milk—evaporated	22	2.11	0.06	3.22	82.0	0.078	0.013	0.088	0	1.11
Canned whole milk—evaporated	38	1.91	2.20	2.81	73.9	0.054	0.014	0.090	0	8.33
Carob flavor mix—powder	106	0.47	0.05	26.50	0	1.300	0.002	0	4.020	0
Chocolate milk—1%	18	0.92	0.28	2.96	32.5	0.068	0.010	0.047	0.425	0.79
Chocolate milk—2%	20	0.91	0.57	2.95	32.2	0.068	0.010	0.046	0.425	1.93
Chocolate milk—whole	24	0.90	0.96	2.94	31.8	0.068	0.010	0.046	0.425	3.52
Hot cocoa—with whole milk	25	1.03	1.03	2.93	33.8	0.088	0.012	0.049	0.340	3.74
Instant breakfast w/2% milk	25	1.52	0.47	3.50	31.0	0.807	0.040	0.048	0	1.82
Instant breakfast w/1% milk	23	1.51	0.25	3.50	31.3	0.807	0.040	0.048	0	1.00
Instant breakfast w/skim milk	22	1.55	0.04	3.50	31.4	0.804	0.039	0.041	0	0.40
Instant breakfast w/whole milk	28	1.51	0.82	3.47	30.4	0.807	0.040	0.047	0	3.33
Egg nog	38	1.08	2.12	3.84	36.8	0.057	0.010	0.054	0	16.60
Kefir	20	1.13	0.55	1.07	42.6	0.060	0.055	0.054	0	1.22
Malt powder—chocolate flavored	107	1.49	1.08	24.80	17.6	0.648	0.049	0.057	0.540	1.35
Malted milk powder	117	3.12	2.30	21.50	85.0	0.209	0.143	0.260	0.405	5.40
Malted milk drink—chocolate	25	1.00	0.95	3.19	32.5	0.064	0.014	0.047	0.043	3.64

DAIRY PRODUCTS—*continued*

	kcal	Protein (g)	Lipid (g)	CHO (g)	Ca (mg)	Fe (mg)	B₁ (mg)	B₂ (mg)	Fiber (g)	Cholesterol (mg)
Chocolate milkshake	36	0.96	1.05	5.80	32.0	0.088	0.016	0.069	0.035	3.70
Strawberry milkshake	32	0.95	0.80	5.35	32.0	0.030	0.013	0.055	0.024	3.10
Vanilla milkshake	32	0.98	0.84	5.09	34.5	0.026	0.013	0.052	0.019	3.20
Ovaltine powder— chocolate flavored	102	2.00	0.85	23.70	134.0	6.190	0.719	0.772	0.013	0
Ovaltine powder—malt flavored	104	2.53	0.24	23.60	106.0	5.820	0.772	1.010	0.040	0
Ovaltine drink—chocolate flavored	24	1.02	0.94	3.12	41.9	0.510	0.067	0.104	0.001	3.53
Ovaltine drink—malt flavored	24	1.06	0.89	3.10	39.7	0.480	0.072	0.124	0.003	3.53
Milk—goat	20	1.00	1.17	1.27	37.9	0.014	0.014	0.039	0	3.25
Milk—sheep	31	1.70	1.99	1.52	54.8	0.028	0.018	0.100	0	0
Milk—soybean	9	0.78	0.54	0.51	1.2	0.163	0.046	0.020	0	0
Ice cream—regular-vanilla	57	1.02	3.05	6.76	37.5	0.026	0.011	0.070	0	12.60
Ice cream—rich-vanilla	67	0.79	4.54	6.13	28.9	0.019	0.008	0.054	0	16.90
Ice cream—soft-serve	62	1.15	3.69	6.28	38.7	0.070	0.013	0.073	0	25.00
Creamsicle ice cream bar	44	0.52	1.33	7.56	19.8	0	0.009	0.034	0	0
Drumstick ice cream bar	88	1.23	4.68	10.20	31.7	0.047	0.009	0.043	0	0
Fudgesicle ice cream bar	35	1.48	0.08	7.22	50.0	0.039	0.012	0.070	0	0
Ice milk	40	1.12	1.22	6.28	38.0	0.039	0.016	0.075	0	3.90
Ice milk—soft serve— 3% fat	36	1.30	0.75	6.22	44.4	0.045	0.019	0.088	0	2.10
Yogurt—coffee-vanilla	24	1.40	0.35	3.90	48.5	0.020	0.012	0.057	0	1.42
Yogurt—lowfat with fruit	29	1.24	0.31	5.37	43.0	0.020	0.010	0.050	0	1.25
Yogurt—lowfat-plain	18	1.49	0.43	2.00	51.8	0.022	0.012	0.060	0	1.75
Yogurt—nonfat milk	16	1.62	0.05	2.17	56.5	0.025	0.014	0.066	0	0.50
Yogurt—whole milk	17	0.98	0.92	1.32	34.3	0.014	0.008	0.040	0	3.68

VEGETABLES

	kcal	Protein (g)	Lipid (g)	CHO (g)	Ca (mg)	Fe (mg)	B₁ (mg)	B₂ (mg)	Fiber (g)	Cholesterol (mg)
Alfalfa sprouts	9	1.13	0.200	1.07	9.5	0.272	0.021	0.036	1.030	0
Artichoke hearts— marinated	28	0.680	0.250	2.18	6.5	0.270	0.010	0.029	1.780	0
Asparagus—raw spears	6	0.865	0.063	1.05	6.4	0.193	0.032	0.035	0.395	0
Asparagus—canned spears	5	0.606	0.184	0.70	3.9	0.177	0.017	0.025	0.454	0
Bamboo shoots—sliced— raw	8	0.738	0.088	1.47	3.8	0.143	0.043	0.020	0.738	0
Bamboo shoots—sliced, canned	5	0.489	0.113	0.91	2.2	0.090	0.007	0.007	0.706	0
Bean sprouts—fresh raw	9	0.861	0.050	1.68	3.8	0.258	0.024	0.035	0.736	0
Bean sprouts—boiled	6	0.576	0.025	1.19	3.4	0.185	0.014	0.029	0.572	0
Bean sprouts—stir fried	14	1.220	0.059	3.00	3.7	0.549	0.040	0.050	0.777	0
Black beans—cooked	37	2.500	0.152	6.72	7.8	0.593	0.069	0.017	2.540	0

VEGETABLES—*continued*

	kcal	Protein (g)	Lipid (g)	CHO (g)	Ca (mg)	Fe (mg)	B₁ (mg)	B₂ (mg)	Fiber (g)	Cholesterol (mg)
Green beans—raw uncooked	9	0.515	0.034	2.02	10.6	0.363	0.024	0.030	0.644	0
Green beans—fresh— cooked	10	0.535	0.082	2.24	13.2	0.363	0.021	0.027	0.737	0
Green beans—frozen— cooked	8	0.386	0.038	1.73	12.8	0.233	0.014	0.021	0.880	0
Green beans—canned/ drained	6	0.326	0.028	1.28	7.6	0.256	0.004	0.016	0.378	0
Red kidney beans—dry	94	6.690	0.234	16.90	40.5	2.330	0.150	0.062	6.160	0
Lima beans—dry large	96	6.080	0.194	18.00	22.9	2.130	0.144	0.057	8.600	0
Lima beans—fresh— cooked	35	1.930	0.090	6.70	9.0	0.695	0.040	0.027	2.670	0
Lima beans—dry small	98	5.790	0.397	18.20	18.4	2.270	0.136	0.048	8.500	0
Lima beans—canned/ drained	27	1.530	0.100	5.20	8.0	0.487	0.010	0.013	2.420	0
Beans/w/franks—canned	40	1.900	1.860	4.37	13.6	0.490	0.016	0.016	1.950	1.7
Pork & beans—canned	32	1.500	0.413	5.95	17.4	0.470	0.013	0.017	1.560	1.9
Navy beans—dry, cooked	40	2.460	0.162	7.77	19.9	0.703	0.057	0.017	2.490	0
Pinto beans—dry, cooked	39	2.320	0.148	7.28	13.6	0.741	0.053	0.026	3.230	0
Refried beans—canned	30	1.770	0.303	5.24	13.2	0.500	0.014	0.016	2.470	0
Soybeans—dry	118	10.400	5.650	8.55	78.5	4.450	0.248	0.247	1.570	0
White beans—dry	95	5.990	0.334	17.70	36.0	2.190	0.210	0.059	0.766	0
White beans—dry, cooked	40	2.550	0.182	7.32	20.7	0.808	0.067	0.017	2.230	0
Yellow wax beans—raw	9	0.515	0.034	2.02	10.6	0.294	0.024	0.030	0.644	0
Yellow wax beans—raw	10	0.535	0.082	2.24	13.2	0.363	0.021	0.027	0.726	0
Yellow wax beans—frozen	8	0.386	0.038	1.73	12.8	0.233	0.014	0.021	0.880	0
Beets—cooked	9	0.300	0.014	1.90	3.1	0.176	0.009	0.004	0.539	0
Beets—pickled slices	18	0.227	0.028	4.63	3.1	0.116	0.006	0.014	0.587	0
Broccoli—raw chopped	8	0.844	0.097	1.49	13.5	0.251	0.019	0.034	0.934	0
Broccoli—raw spears	8	0.845	0.098	1.49	13.5	0.250	0.018	0.034	0.935	0
Broccoli—frozen cooked spears	8	0.879	0.034	1.51	14.5	0.173	0.015	0.023	0.826	0
Brussels sprouts—raw	12	0.960	0.084	2.54	11.6	0.396	0.039	0.026	1.260	0
Brussels sprouts—cooked	11	1.090	0.145	2.45	10.2	0.342	0.030	0.023	1.220	0
Brussels sprouts—frozen cooked	12	1.030	0.112	2.36	7.0	0.210	0.029	0.032	1.230	0
Cabbage—raw, shredded	7	0.340	0.049	1.52	13.0	0.162	0.015	0.009	0.680	0
Cabbage—cooked	6	0.272	0.070	1.35	9.5	0.110	0.016	0.016	0.661	0
Bok choy—raw, shredded	4	0.425	0.057	0.62	30.0	0.227	0.011	0.020	0.486	0
Bok choy—cooked	3	0.442	0.045	0.51	26.3	0.295	0.009	0.018	0.454	0
Red cabbage—raw	8	0.393	0.073	1.74	14.6	0.142	0.018	0.009	0.648	0
Red cabbage—cooked	6	0.299	0.057	1.32	10.6	0.102	0.010	0.006	1.567	0
Carrot—whole, raw	12	0.291	0.055	2.87	7.5	0.142	0.028	0.017	1.906	0
Carrot—grated, raw	12	0.289	0.052	2.88	7.7	0.142	0.027	0.016	0.907	0
Carrots—sliced, cooked	13	0.309	0.050	2.97	8.7	0.176	0.010	0.016	0.992	0
Carrots—frozen, cooked	10	0.338	0.031	2.34	8.2	0.136	0.008	0.010	1.050	0
Carrots—canned, drained	7	0.183	0.054	1.57	7.4	0.181	0.005	0.009	0.435	0
Carrot juice	11	0.267	0.041	2.63	6.7	0.130	0.026	0.015	0.385	0
Cauliflower—raw	7	0.561	0.051	1.39	7.9	0.164	0.022	0.016	0.720	0
Cauliflower—cooked	7	0.530	0.050	1.31	7.8	0.119	0.018	0.018	0.622	0

VEGETABLES — *continued*

	kcal	Protein (g)	Lipid (g)	CHO (g)	Ca (mg)	Fe (mg)	B₁ (mg)	B₂ (mg)	Fiber (g)	Cholesterol (mg)
Cauliflower—frozen, cooked	5	0.457	0.061	1.06	4.9	0.116	0.010	0.015	0.535	0
Celery—raw—chopped	5	0.189	0.033	1.03	10.4	0.137	0.009	0.009	0.472	0
Swiss chard—raw	5	0.510	0.057	1.06	14.5	0.510	0.011	0.025	0.512	0
Swiss chard—cooked	6	0.533	0.023	1.17	16.5	0.642	0.010	0.024	0.616	0
Collards—fresh	5	0.445	0.062	1.07	33.0	0.299	0.009	0.018	0.590	0
Collards—fresh, cooked	4	0.313	0.043	0.75	22.0	0.116	0.005	0.012	0.798	0
Collards—frozen, cooked	10	0.840	0.115	2.02	59.5	0.317	0.013	0.033	0.794	0
Corn—kernels raw	24	0.913	0.335	5.38	0.6	0.147	0.057	0.017	1.220	0
Corn on the cob—cooked	31	0.943	0.363	7.14	0.6	0.173	0.061	0.020	1.190	0
Corn—cooked from frozen	23	0.857	0.020	5.80	0.6	0.085	0.020	0.020	1.190	0
Corn—canned, drained	23	0.743	0.283	5.26	1.4	0.142	0.009	0.014	0.398	0
Corn—canned cream style	21	0.494	0.119	5.14	0.9	0.108	0.007	0.015	0.354	0
Cucumber slices w/peel	4	0.153	0.037	0.82	4.0	0.079	0.009	0.006	0.329	0
Eggplant—cooked	8	0.236	0.066	1.88	1.7	0.099	0.022	0.006	1.060	0
Escarole/curly endive—chopped	5	0.354	0.057	0.95	14.7	0.235	0.023	0.022	0.369	0
Garbanzo/chickpeas—dry	103	5.470	1.720	17.20	29.9	1.770	0.135	0.060	5.390	0
Garbanzo/chickpeas—cooked	47	2.500	0.735	7.78	13.8	0.819	0.033	0.018	1.920	0
Jerusalem artichoke—raw	22	0.567	0.004	4.95	4.0	0.964	0.057	0.017	0.369	0
Kale—fresh, chopped	14	0.935	0.198	2.84	38.0	0.482	0.031	0.037	1.650	0
Kohlrabi—raw slices	8	0.482	0.028	1.76	6.9	0.113	0.014	0.006	0.405	0
Kohlrabi—cooked	8	0.510	0.030	1.96	7.0	0.113	0.011	0.006	0.395	0
Leeks—chopped raw	17	0.425	0.085	4.00	16.7	0.594	0.017	0.008	0.668	0
Leeks—cooked, chopped	9	0.230	0.057	2.16	8.5	0.310	0.007	0.006	0.927	0
Lentils—dry	96	7.960	0.273	16.20	14.6	2.550	0.135	0.069	3.400	0
Lentils—cooked from dry	33	2.560	0.106	5.73	5.3	0.944	0.048	0.020	1.430	0
Lentils—sprouted, raw	30	2.540	0.156	6.30	7.0	0.909	0.065	0.036	1.150	0
Lettuce—butterhead	4	0.367	0.062	0.66	9.5	0.085	0.017	0.017	0.397	0
Lettuce—iceberg	4	0.286	0.054	0.59	5.4	0.142	0.013	0.009	0.347	0
Lettuce—romaine	5	0.459	0.057	0.67	10.2	0.312	0.028	0.028	0.482	0
Mushrooms—raw sliced	7	0.593	0.119	1.32	1.4	0.352	0.029	0.127	0.508	0
Mushrooms—cooked	8	0.614	0.134	1.46	1.7	0.494	0.020	0.085	0.625	0
Mushrooms—canned, drained	7	0.530	0.082	1.40	3.1	0.224	0.017	0.063	0.596	0
Mustard greens—fresh	7	0.764	0.057	1.39	29.4	0.414	0.023	0.031	0.764	0
Mustard greens—cooked	4	0.640	0.068	0.60	21.0	0.316	0.012	0.018	0.587	0
Okra pods—cooked	9	0.530	0.048	2.04	17.9	0.128	0.037	0.016	0.624	0
Okra slices—cooked	11	0.589	0.085	2.32	27.1	0.190	0.028	0.035	0.709	0
Onions—chopped, raw	10	0.335	0.074	2.07	7.1	0.105	0.017	0.003	0.454	0
Onion slices—raw	10	0.335	0.074	2.08	7.2	0.105	0.017	0.003	0.454	0
Onion—dehydrated flakes	91	2.530	0.122	23.70	72.9	0.446	0.022	0.018	2.510	0
Onion rings—frozen, heated	115	1.520	7.570	10.80	8.8	0.482	0.079	0.040	0.240	0
Parsley—freeze dried	81	8.910	1.420	11.90	40.5	15.200	0.304	0.648	22.000	0
Parsley—fresh chopped	9	0.624	0.085	1.96	36.9	1.760	0.023	0.031	1.550	0
Parsnips—sliced raw	21	0.341	0.085	5.09	10.0	0.167	0.026	0.014	1.280	0
Fresh peas—uncooked	23	1.530	0.113	4.10	7.0	0.416	0.075	0.037	1.380	0
Peas—cooked	24	1.520	0.060	4.43	7.8	0.438	0.073	0.042	1.360	0
Peas—frozen, cooked	22	1.460	0.078	4.04	6.7	0.443	0.080	0.050	1.280	0
Peas—edible pods—fresh	12	0.794	0.057	2.15	12.1	0.589	0.043	0.023	0.794	0
Split peas—dry	97	6.970	0.328	17.10	15.5	1.250	0.206	0.061	4.030	0

VEGETABLES — *continued*

	kcal	Protein (g)	Lipid (g)	CHO (g)	Ca (mg)	Fe (mg)	B₁ (mg)	B₂ (mg)	Fiber (g)	Cholesterol (mg)
Peas + carrots—frozen, cooked	14	0.875	0.120	2.87	6.4	0.266	0.064	0.020	1.170	0
Green chili pepper—raw	11	0.557	0.057	2.68	5.0	0.340	0.026	0.026	0.504	0
Red chili peppers—raw/ chopped	11	0.567	0.057	2.68	4.9	0.340	0.026	0.026	0.454	0
Jalapeno peppers—canned chopped	7	0.225	0.170	1.39	7.5	0.792	0.008	0.014	0.850	0
Baked potato with skin	31	0.653	0.028	7.16	2.8	0.386	0.030	0.009	0.660	0
Baked potato—flesh only	26	0.556	0.029	6.10	1.5	0.100	0.030	0.006	0.436	0
Potato skin—oven baked	56	1.220	0.029	13.20	9.8	1.080	0.035	0.034	1.130	0
Potato + peel— microwaved	30	0.692	0.028	6.83	3.1	0.350	0.034	0.009	0.660	0
Peeled potato—boiled	24	0.485	0.029	5.67	2.1	0.088	0.028	0.005	0.426	0
French fries—oven heated	63	0.980	2.480	9.64	2.3	0.380	0.035	0.009	0.567	0
French fries—frozen— vegetable oil	90	1.140	4.690	11.20	5.7	0.215	0.050	0.008	0.567	0
Cottage-fried potatoes	62	0.975	2.320	9.64	2.8	0.425	0.034	0.009	0.567	0
Hash-brown potatoes	30	0.343	1.980	3.02	1.1	0.115	0.010	0.003	0.567	0
Mashed potatoes prep/ milk	22	0.548	0.166	4.98	7.4	0.077	0.025	0.011	0.405	0.5
Mashed potatoes—milk & margarine	30	0.533	1.200	4.74	7.3	0.074	0.024	0.014	0.405	0.5
Potato pancakes	88	1.730	4.700	9.85	7.8	0.451	0.039	0.035	0.563	34.7
Potatoes au gratin mix	26	0.653	1.170	3.65	23.5	0.090	0.006	0.023	0.487	1.4
Scalloped potatoes— recipe	24	0.813	1.040	3.05	16.2	0.163	0.020	0.026	0.289	3.4
Potato chips	148	1.590	10.000	14.70	7.0	0.339	0.040	0.006	1.360	0
Potato flour	100	2.260	0.226	22.60	9.3	4.880	0.119	0.040	0.317	0
Pumpkin—canned	10	0.311	0.080	2.28	7.4	0.394	0.007	0.015	0.519	0
Red radishes	4	0.170	0.151	1.01	5.7	0.082	0.001	0.013	0.624	0
Rutabaga—cooked cubes	10	0.314	0.053	2.19	12.0	0.133	0.020	0.010	0.434	0
Sauerkraut—canned liquid	5	0.258	0.040	1.21	8.7	0.417	0.006	0.006	0.529	0
Soybeans—mature, raw	37	3.700	1.900	3.17	19.4	0.599	0.096	0.033	0.656	0
Spinach—cooked from fresh	7	0.843	0.074	1.06	38.4	1.010	0.027	0.067	0.702	0
Summer squash—raw slices	6	0.334	0.061	1.23	5.7	0.130	0.018	0.010	0.425	0
Zucchini squash—cooked	5	0.181	0.014	1.11	3.6	0.099	0.012	0.012	0.567	0
Acorn squash—boiled/ mashed	10	0.190	0.023	2.49	7.5	0.159	0.028	0.002	0.680	0
Butternut squash/baked— cube	12	0.256	0.026	2.97	11.6	0.170	0.020	0.005	0.794	0
Spaghetti squash—baked/ boiled	8	0.187	0.073	1.83	6.0	0.095	0.010	0.006	0.794	0
Winter squash—boiled	10	0.319	0.050	2.40	5.2	0.136	0.018	0.006	0.794	0
Sweet potato—baked in skin	29	0.487	0.032	6.89	8.0	0.129	0.020	0.036	0.850	0
Candied sweet potatoes	39	0.246	0.920	7.91	7.3	0.324	0.005	0.012	0.545	0
Tofu (soybean curd)	22	2.290	1.360	0.53	29.7	1.520	0.023	0.015	0.343	0
Tomato—fresh whole	6	0.251	0.060	1.23	2.1	0.136	0.017	0.014	0.415	0
Tomatoes—whole canned	6	0.265	0.070	1.22	7.4	0.171	0.013	0.009	0.298	0

VEGETABLES—continued

	kcal	Protein (g)	Lipid (g)	CHO (g)	Ca (mg)	Fe (mg)	B₁ (mg)	B₂ (mg)	Fiber (g)	Cholesterol (mg)
Tomato sauce—canned	9	0.376	0.047	2.04	3.9	0.218	0.019	0.016	0.425	0
Tomato paste—canned	24	1.070	0.249	5.33	9.9	0.848	0.044	0.054	1.210	0
Tomato juice—canned	5	0.215	0.017	1.20	2.6	0.164	0.013	0.009	0.220	0
Turnip cubes—raw	8	0.255	0.028	1.76	8.5	0.085	0.011	0.009	0.587	0
Mixed vegetables—frozen, cooked	17	0.812	0.043	3.70	7.2	0.232	0.020	0.034	1.120	0
Vegetable juice cocktail	6	0.178	0.026	1.29	3.1	0.119	0.012	0.008	0.178	0
Water chestnuts—raw	30	0.398	0.027	6.77	3.2	0.170	0.040	0.057	0.869	0
Watercress—fresh	3	0.650	0.033	0.37	33.4	0.050	0.025	0.033	0.719	0
White yams—raw	34	0.438	0.049	7.90	8.7	0.153	0.032	0.009	0.822	0

SALAD BAR

	kcal	Protein (g)	Lipid (g)	CHO (g)	Ca (mg)	Fe (mg)	B₁ (mg)	B₂ (mg)	Fiber (g)	Cholesterol (mg)
Alfalfa sprouts	8.59	1.130	0.196	1.070	9.45	0.272	0.021	0.036	1.030	0
Artichoke hearts, marinated	28.00	0.680	2.250	2.180	6.50	0.270	0.010	0.029	1.780	0
Asparagus	6.35	0.867	0.062	1.050	6.35	0.193	0.032	0.035	0.432	0
Avocado	45.70	0.563	4.340	2.100	3.07	0.284	0.030	0.035	2.720	0
Bacon, regular	163.00	8.640	14.000	0.164	2.98	0.482	0.195	0.080	0	23.9
Bean sprouts	8.50	0.861	0.050	1.680	3.82	0.258	0.024	0.035	0.7365	0
Beets	8.67	0.300	0.013	1.900	3.00	0.176	0.009	0.004	0.567	0
Beets, canned, diced	9.00	0.260	0.040	2.040	4.34	0.517	0.003	0.012	0.590	0
Broccoli, raw	7.73	0.844	0.097	1.490	13.50	0.251	0.019	0.034	0.934	0
Cabbage	6.48	0.340	0.049	1.520	13.00	0.162	0.015	0.009	0.680	0
Cabbage, red	7.70	0.393	0.073	1.740	14.60	0.142	0.018	0.009	0.648	0
Carrots, grated	12.40	0.289	0.052	2.880	7.73	0.142	0.027	0.016	0.907	0
Cauliflower	6.80	0.561	0.051	1.390	7.94	0.164	0.022	0.016	0.720	0
Celery	4.54	0.189	0.030	1.030	10.40	0.137	0.009	0.009	0.472	0
Chicken salad	96.70	3.820	8.900	0.469	5.92	0.239	0.012	0.028	0.109	17.3
Crab, cooked	23.90	5.050	0.561	0.140	12.90	0.104	0.012	0.044	0	18.0
Croutons, dry bread cubes	105.00	3.690	1.040	20.500	35.00	1.020	0.099	0.099	0.085	0
Cucumber slices	3.69	0.153	0.037	0.824	3.99	0.079	0.009	0.006	0.329	0
Egg, chopped	40.40	3.520	2.790	0.338	13.80	0.475	0.014	0.133	0	113
Escarole/curly endive	4.82	0.354	0.057	0.953	14.70	0.235	0.023	0.022	0.369	0
Garbanzo/chickpeas, cooked	46.50	2.500	0.735	7.780	13.80	0.819	0.033	0.018	1.920	0
Green pepper, sweet	6.80	0.244	0.130	1.500	1.70	0.357	0.024	0.014	0.454	0
Ham salad	51.50	5.000	3.000	0.880	2.00	0.280	0.244	0.072	0	16
Ham, minced	74.20	4.620	5.860	0.526	2.70	0.216	0.203	0.054	0	20.2
Leeks	17.30	0.425	0.085	4.000	16.70	0.594	0.017	0.008	0.688	0
Lettuce, butterhead	3.69	0.366	0.062	0.658	9.47	0.085	0.017	0.017	0.370	0
Lettuce, iceberg	3.69	0.287	0.054	0.592	5.37	0.142	0.013	0.009	0.370	0
Lettuce, loose leaf	5.11	0.369	0.085	0.992	19.20	0.397	0.014	0.023	0.391	0
Lettuce, Romaine	4.54	0.459	0.057	0.673	10.20	0.312	0.028	0.028	0.482	0
Lobster meat	27.80	5.800	0.168	0.364	17.20	0.111	0.020	0.019	0	20.3

SALAD BAR—*continued*

	kcal	Protein (g)	Lipid (g)	CHO (g)	Ca (mg)	Fe (mg)	B₁ (mg)	B₂ (mg)	Fiber (g)	Cholesterol (mg)
Mushrooms, raw	7.09	0.593	0.119	1.320	1.42	0.352	0.029	0.127	0.508	0
Onions	9.57	0.335	0.074	2.070	7.09	0.105	0.017	0.003	0.454	0
Parmesan cheese, grated	129.00	11.800	8.500	1.060	389.00	0.270	0.013	0.109	0	22.0
Peas, cooked	22.30	1.460	0.078	4.040	6.73	0.443	0.080	0.050	1.280	0
Sesame seed kernels, dried	167.00	7.480	15.500	2.660	37.20	2.210	0.204	0.024	1.950	0
Shrimp, boiled	28.00	5.930	0.306	0	11.00	0.876	0.009	0.009	0	55.3
Spinach, fresh	6.23	0.810	0.099	0.992	28.00	0.770	0.022	0.054	0.947	0
Sunflower seeds, dry	162.00	6.460	14.000	5.320	32.90	1.920	0.650	0.070	1.970	0
Tomatoes	5.51	0.252	0.061	1.230	1.89	0.135	0.017	0.014	0.416	0
Tuna salad	53.00	4.550	2.630	2.670	4.84	0.282	0.009	0.019	0.340	3.73
Turkey meat	41.30	5.270	2.030	0.149	11.40	0.358	0.025	0.064	0	11.9

VARIETY

	kcal	Protein (g)	Lipid (g)	CHO (g)	Ca (mg)	Fe (mg)	B₁ (mg)	B₂ (mg)	Fiber (g)	Cholesterol (mg)
Chips & crackers										
Doritos—nacho flavor	139	2.20	6.79	18.00	17.0	0.399	0.040	0.030	1.10	0
Doritos—taco flavor	140	2.60	6.59	17.60	44.9	0.699	0.080	0.090	1.10	0
Potato chips—sour cream & onion	153	2.40	9.48	14.60	21.0	0.474	0.040	0.055	1.35	1.0
Wheat cracker—thin	124	3.19	4.96	17.70	10.6	1.060	0.142	0.106	1.84	0
Whole wheat crackers	124	3.19	5.32	17.70	10.6	1.850	0.070	0.106	2.94	0
Condiments										
Catsup	30	0.52	0.11	7.17	6.2	0.228	0.026	0.020	0.45	0
Mustard	21	1.34	1.25	1.81	23.8	0.567	0.024	0.057	0.11	0
Soy sauce	14	1.46	0.02	2.40	4.7	0.567	0.014	0.036	0	0
Deli meats										
Bologna—beef	89	3.32	8.04	0.56	3.7	0.394	0.016	0.036	0	16.0
Bratwurst	92	4.05	7.90	0.84	13.8	0.292	0.070	0.064	0	17.8
Keilbasa sausage	88	3.76	7.70	0.61	12.0	0.414	0.064	0.061	0	18.5
Knockwurst sausage	87	3.37	7.88	0.05	2.9	0.258	0.097	0.040	0	16.3
Liverwurst	93	4.00	8.10	0.63	7.9	1.810	0.077	0.291	0	44.1
Pepperoni sausage	140	5.94	12.50	0.80	2.8	0.397	0.09	0.07		9.79
Polish sausage	92	3.99	8.13	0.46	3.0	0.409	0.142	0.042	0	20.0
Salami—beef	72	4.17	5.69	0.70	2.47	0.567	0.036	0.073	0	17.3
Salami—pork & beef	72	3.94	5.70	0.64	3.68	0.755	0.068	0.106	0	18.5
Salami—turkey	55	4.62	3.89	0.15	5.47	0.463	0.029	0.075	0	22.9
Salami—dry—beef & pork	120	6.49	9.75	0.74	2.84	0.425	0.170	0.082	0	22.7
Turkey pastrami	37	5.22	1.75	0.43	2.49	0.403	0.022	0.075	0	14.9
Mexican foods										
Beef taco	75.2	4.94	4.80	3.67	30.9	0.469	0.01	0.049	0.407	16.2
Beef enchilada	69.0	3.09	3.26	3.69	60.2	0.418	0.017	0.039	0.465	8.93
Cheese enchilada	78.0	3.12	4.2	3.78	108.0	0.324	0.015	0.050	0.465	10.2
Chicken enchilada	63.6	3.38	2.48	3.69	60.5	0.359	0.018	0.036	0.465	9.10
Corn tortilla, enriched, regular	61.4	1.89	0.964	12.30	39.7	0.567	0.047	0.028	2.27	0

VARIETY—*continued*

	kcal	Protein (g)	Lipid (g)	CHO (g)	Ca (mg)	Fe (mg)	B₁ (mg)	B₂ (mg)	Fiber (g)	Cholesterol (mg)
Mexican Foods—*continued*										
Corn torilla, enriched, thin	61.0	1.64	0.95	12.30	39.8	0.567	0.046	0.028	2.26	0
Corn tortilla, fried	82.2	2.08	2.84	12.30	39.7	0.567	0.047	0.028	2.27	0
Enchirito	60.4	3.15	2.75	3.31	51.5	0.410	0.015	0.037	0.748	9.18
Flour tortilla	84	2.07	2.15	15.50	17.0	0.440	0.102	0.062	0.800	0
Refried beans, canned	30.3	1.77	0.303	5.24	13.2	0.500	0.014	0.016	2.47	0
Nuts & seeds										
Almonds—dried, chopped	167	5.65	14.80	5.78	75.5	1.040	0.060	0.220	3.36	0
Almonds—whole toasted	167	5.77	14.40	6.48	80.0	1.400	0.037	0.170	3.99	0
Sunflower seeds—dry	162	6.46	14.00	5.32	32.9	1.920	0.650	0.070	1.97	0
Oils & shortening										
Cocoa butter oil	251	0	28.40	0	0	0	0	0	0	0
Corn oil	251	0	28.40	0	0	0.001	0	0	0	0
Cottonseed oil	251	0	28.40	0	0	0	0	0	0	0
Olive oil	251	0	28.40	0	0.1	0.109	0	0	0	0
Palm oil	251	0	28.40	0	0.1	0.003	0	0	0	0
Palm kernel oil	251	0	28.40	0	0	0	0	0	0	0
Peanut oil	251	0	28.40	0	0	0.008	0	0	0	0
Safflower oil	251	0	28.40	0	0	0	0	0	0	0
Sesame oil	250	0	28.40	0	0	0	0	0	0	0
Soybean oil	251	0	28.40	0	0	0.007	0	0	0	0
Sunflower oil	251	0	28.40	0	0	0	0	0	0	0
Walnut oil	251	0	28.40	0	0	0	0	0	0	0
Wheat germ oil	250	0	28.40	0	0	0	0	0	0	0
Vegetable shortening	251	0	28.40	0	0	0	0	0	0	0
Pasta & noodles										
Spaghetti, cooked firm, hot	41	1.42	0.142	8.53	3.1	0.454	0.051	0.028	0.482	0
Spaghetti, cooked tender, hot	31	1.01	0.111	6.48	3.0	0.405	0.04	0.022	0.425	0
Whole wheat spaghetti, cooked	35	1.53	0.113	7.49	4.3	0.244	0.048	0.020	1.040	0
Spaghetti + sauce + cheese, canned	22	0.68	0.227	4.42	4.5	0.318	0.040	0.032	0.284	0.3
Spaghetti + sauce + cheese, homemade	30	1.02	1.02	4.20	9.07	0.260	0.028	0.020	0.284	0.9
Spaghetti + sauce + meat, canned	30	1.36	1.13	4.42	6.01	0.374	0.017	0.020	0.312	2.6
Spaghetti + sauce + meat, homemade	38	2.17	1.37	4.46	14.20	0.423	0.029	0.034	0.314	10.2
Spaghetti sauce, homemade	23	0.77	1.25	2.95	6.70	0.380	0.026	0.017	0.343	0
Spaghetti sauce, canned	31	0.52	1.35	4.52	7.97	0.184	0.016	0.017	0.343	0
Spaghetti meat sauce,	30	1.03	1.30	3.72	4.95	0.385	0.028	0.022	0.193	2.3
Spaghetti sauce, dry, packet	79	1.70	0.28	18.20	48.20	0.765	NA	0.162	0.057	0
Spaghetti sauce + mushrooms, packet	85	2.84	2.55	13.90	113.00	0.510	NA	0.136	0.085	0
Egg noodles, cooked	35	1.17	0.35	6.60	3.19	0.400	0.039	0.023	0.624	8.9

VARIETY—*continued*

	kcal	Protein (g)	Lipid (g)	CHO (g)	Ca (mg)	Fe (mg)	B_1 (mg)	B_2 (mg)	Fiber (g)	Cholesterol (mg)
Pasta & noodles—*continued*										
Chow mein noodles, dry	139	3.72	6.93	16.40	8.82	0.252	0.032	0.019	1.100	3.2
Spinach noodles, dry	108	3.97	1.08	20.20	11.60	1.290	0.278	0.133	1.930	0
Spinach noodles, cooked	32	1.13	0.36	5.97	3.37	0.429	0.043	0.027	0.569	0
Chicken + noodles, recipe	43	2.60	2.13	3.07	3.07	0.278	0.006	0.020	0.142	12.2
Chicken + noodles, frozen	32	2.17	1.30	2.49	15.70	0.393	0.009	0.018	0.022	8.0
Noodles-ramen-beef, cooked	28	0.76	0.94	4.17	NA	NA	NA	NA	0.500	NA
Noodles, ramen, chicken, cooked	25	0.76	0.85	3.63	NA	NA	NA	NA	0.512	NA
Noodles, ramen, oriental	26	0.74	1.07	3.83	NA	NA	NA	NA	0.512	NA
Lasagna, frozen entree	38	2.32	1.71	2.61	34.00	0.343	0.026	0.045	0.194	12.4
Pizza										
Pizza—cheese	69	3.54	2.13	9.21	52.00	0.378	0.080	0.069	0.510	13.2
Pizza—mozzarella	80	7.60	4.67	0.89	207.00	0.076	0.006	0.097	0	15.0
Pizza—Canadian bacon	52	6.82	2.36	0.38	3.00	0.229	0.231	0.055	0	16.3
Pizza—pepperoni	140	5.94	12.50	0.81	2.80	0.397	0.090	0.070	0	9.8
Pizza—onion	10	0.34	0.07	2.07	7.10	1.105	0.017	0.003	0.450	0
Popcorn										
Popcorn—plain, air popped	106	3.50	1.42	21.30	3.50	0.709	0.106	0.035	4.600	0
Popcorn—cooked in oil/salted	142	2.32	7.99	15.50	7.70	0.696	0.026	0.052	3.090	0
Popcorn—syrup-coated	109	1.60	0.81	24.30	1.60	0.405	0.106	0.016	0.810	0
Rice										
Brown—dry	102	2.13	0.54	21.90	9.04	0.510	0.096	0.014	0.965	0
Brown—cooked	34	0.709	0.17	7.23	3.40	0.170	0.026	0.006	0.483	0
White—regular, dry	103	1.90	0.11	22.80	6.74	0.828	0.125	0.009	0.340	0
White—regular, cooked	31	0.567	0.03	6.86	2.84	0.397	0.03	0.003	0.102	0
White—converted, dry	105	2.10	0.15	23.00	17.00	0.828	0.124	0.010	0.624	0
White—converted, cooked	30	0.599	0.02	6.60	5.35	0.227	0.03	0.003	0.180	0
White—instant, dry	106	2.13	0.06	23.40	1.42	1.300	0.125	0.008	0.737	0
White—instant, prepared	31	0.624	0.03	6.86	0.85	0.227	0.037	0.003	0.216	0
Wild—cooked	26	1.02	0.06	5.39	1.42	0.312	0.031	0.045	0.709	0
Rice bran	78	3.77	5.44	14.40	21.50	5.500	0.64	0.070	6.150	0
Rice polish	75	3.43	3.62	16.40	19.40	4.560	0.521	0.051	0.680	0
Salad dressings										
Blue cheese salad dressing	143	1.37	14.80	2.09	22.90	0.057	0.003	0.028	0.020	7.6
Caesar's salad dressing	126	2.66	12.70	0.67	44.40	0.239	0.007	0.025	0.050	33.9
French dressing	150	0.16	16.00	1.81	3.55	0.113	0	0	0.220	0
Italian dressing—low calorie	15	0.02	1.18	1.37	0.59	0.059	0	0	0.080	1.7

VARIETY—*continued*

	kcal	Protein (g)	Lipid (g)	CHO (g)	Ca (mg)	Fe (mg)	B₁ (mg)	B₂ (mg)	Fiber (g)	Cholesterol (mg)
Salad dressings—*continued*										
Mayonnaise	203	0.31	22.60	0.77	5.67	0.168	0.005	0.012	0	16.8
Imitation mayonnaise	66	0	5.67	3.78	0	0	0	0	0	7.6
Ranch salad dressing	104	0.86	10.70	1.31	28.40	0.075	0.010	0.040	0	11.1
Russian salad dressing	140	0.45	14.50	3.00	5.44	0.174	0.014	0.014	0.080	18.4
1000 island dressing	107	0.26	10.10	4.30	3.52	0.170	0.006	0.009	0.060	7.3
1000 island dressing— low calorie	45	0.22	3.00	4.58	3.12	1.174	0.006	0.008	0.340	3.4
Vinegar & oil dressing	124	0	14.20	0	0	0	0	0	0	0
Salads, prepared										
Chicken salad w/celery	97	3.82	8.90	0.47	5.92	0.239	0.012	0.028	0.110	17.3
Cole slaw	20	0.36	0.74	3.52	12.80	0.166	0.019	0.017	0.570	2.3
Egg salad	68	2.91	6.01	0.45	14.50	0.525	0.019	0.070	0	97.4
Ham salad spread	62	2.46	4.39	3.01	2.24	0.168	0.123	0.034	0.030	10.4
Macaroni salad—no cheese	75	0.54	6.66	3.52	5.50	0.229	0.020	0.014	0.270	4.9
Potato salad w/mayo + eggs	41	0.76	2.32	3.16	5.44	0.185	0.022	0.017	0.420	19.3
Tuna salad	53	4.55	2.53	2.67	4.84	0.282	0.009	0.019	0.340	3.7
Waldorf salad	85	0.72	8.33	2.62	8.82	0.196	0.020	0.013	0.720	4.3
Sandwiches										
Avocado & cheese— white	64	2.02	4.00	5.39	43.1	0.418	0.057	0.059	0.98	4.4
Avocado & cheese— whole wheat	62	2.14	3.97	5.24	37.8	0.477	0.047	0.05	1.76	4.3
BLT —whole wheat	68	2.49	3.77	6.45	11.4	0.570	0.077	0.043	1.55	4.1
BLT—white	70	2.30	3.77	6.70	18.2	0.489	0.092	0.055	0.43	4.2
Grilled cheese—wheat	91	4.22	5.37	7.10	87.4	0.565	0.057	0.076	1.59	11.8
Grilled cheese— part WW	95	4.39	5.82	6.59	103.0	0.526	0.067	0.093	0.61	13.3
Grilled cheese—white	97	4.22	5.79	6.88	103.0	0.441	0.068	0.092	0.30	13.3
Chicken salad—wheat	80	3.00	4.25	8.13	14.7	0.679	0.066	0.046	1.88	6.2
Chicken salad—white	85	2.83	4.63	8.05	22.7	0.552	0.080	0.060	0.39	7.1
Corn dog	84	2.55	5.10	6.97	8.7	0.495	0.072	0.043	0.03	9.5
Corned beef & swiss on rye	83	5.26	4.59	4.90	63.8	0.768	0.044	0.078	0.97	16.4
English muffin (egg/ cheese/bacon)	74	3.70	3.70	6.37	40.5	0.637	0.095	0.103	0.32	43.8
Egg salad—wheat	79	2.60	4.56	7.44	17.0	0.744	0.063	0.059	1.67	48.8
Egg salad—soft white	83	2.41	4.90	7.25	24.5	0.636	0.075	0.074	0.30	41.6
Ham—rye bread	59	3.84	2.09	6.10	12.0	0.474	0.182	0.073	1.24	7.1
Ham—whole wheat	59	3.79	2.04	6.84	12.4	0.617	0.164	0.060	1.54	6.1
Ham—soft white	61	3.74	2.08	6.60	18.6	0.504	0.186	0.073	0.29	6.7
Ham & swiss—rye	68	4.65	3.23	5.08	63.5	0.389	0.147	0.079	0.99	10.8
Ham & cheese— wheat	67	4.20	3.23	5.72	40.5	0.527	0.136	0.066	1.27	9.7
Ham & cheese—soft white	69	4.20	3.36	5.43	48.0	0.428	0.152	0.078	0.23	10.6
Ham salad—wheat	75	2.45	4.02	7.83	11.5	0.569	0.104	0.045	1.52	5.6
Ham salad—white	78	2.25	4.26	7.71	17.5	0.454	0.119	0.057	0.28	6.2
Hotdog/frankfurter & bun	87	2.80	5.10	7.04	19.6	0.570	0.095	0.062	0.40	7.6

VARIETY—*continued*

	kcal	Protein (g)	Lipid (g)	CHO (g)	Ca (mg)	Fe (mg)	B_1 (mg)	B_2 (mg)	Fiber (g)	Cholesterol (mg)
Sandwiches—*continued*										
Patty melt—gound beef/rye	91	5.09	6.07	3.96	36.5	0.533	0.040	0.072	0.81	17.1
Peanut butter & jam—whole wheat	92	3.40	3.85	12.30	15.4	0.751	0.070	0.045	2.29	0
Peanut butter & jam—white	98	3.29	4.14	12.80	23.4	0.632	0.085	0.059	0.85	0
Reuben grilled	58	3.43	3.38	3.53	43.6	0.633	0.030	0.052	0.80	10.4
Roast beef—whole wheat	64	4.00	2.52	6.71	12.3	0.760	0.061	0.054	1.53	6.2
Roast beef—white	67	3.97	2.63	6.46	18.5	0.665	0.072	0.066	0.27	6.9
Tuna salad—wheat	72	3.29	3.29	8.03	13.0	0.667	0.057	0.040	1.74	5.5
Tuna salad—white	76	3.18	3.47	7.92	19.6	0.555	0.068	0.052	0.44	6.2
Turkey—whole wheat	62	4.09	2.33	6.67	11.6	0.554	0.056	0.044	1.53	6.0
Turkey—white	64	4.07	2.42	6.41	17.8	0.435	0.066	0.055	0.27	6.7
Turkey & ham—rye	58	3.74	2.12	6.18	12.3	0.743	0.060	0.079	1.23	8.4
Turkey & ham— whole wheat	59	3.71	2.07	6.90	12.6	0.846	0.060	0.064	1.54	7.2
Turkey & ham—white	60	3.65	2.10	6.67	18.8	0.762	0.071	0.078	0.28	8.0
Turkey & ham & cheese on rye	68	4.22	3.46	5.04	44.2	0.616	0.050	0.083	0.99	12.1
Turkey & ham & cheese—wheat	67	4.14	3.25	5.77	40.5	0.716	0.051	0.070	1.27	10.6
Turkey & ham & cheese—white	69	4.13	3.38	5.48	48.3	0.636	0.059	0.082	0.23	11.6
Sauces										
Bordelaise sauce	24	0.33	1.46	1.10	3.80	0.179	0.008	0.010	0.01	3.8
Hot chili sauce, red pepper	5	0.25	0.17	1.10	2.51	0.137	0.003	0.026	2.29	0
Teriyaki sauce	24	1.69	0.09	4.52	6.30	0.488	0.008	0.020	0	0
Seafood										
Anchovy—raw	37	5.78	1.37	0	41.7	0.921	0.016	0.073	0	19.6
Frog legs—raw meat	21	4.65	0.085	0	5.1	0.539	0.040	0.070	0	14.2
Lobster meat— cooked	28	5.80	0.17	0.36	17.2	0.111	0.020	0.019	0	20.3
Scampi—fried in crumbs	69	6.07	3.49	3.26	19.0	0.357	0.037	0.039	0.04	50.2
Shrimp—boiled	28	5.93	0.31	0	11.0	0.876	0.009	0.009	0	55.3
Squid (calamari)— fried in flour	50	5.10	2.12	2.20	11.0	0.287	0.016	0.130	0	73.7
Soups										
Cream of celery	20	0.38	1.27	2.00	9.04	0.141	0.007	0.011	0.09	3.2
Chicken, chunky	20	1.43	0.75	1.95	2.71	0.195	0.010	0.020	0.03	3.4
Chicken + dumpling	23	1.30	1.28	1.39	3.34	0.144	0.004	0.017	0.10	7.6
Chicken gumbo	13	0.60	0.32	1.89	5.53	0.201	0.006	0.009	0.05	0.9
Chicken-noodle— chunky	14	1.50	0.70	0.24	2.84	0.170	0.009	0.020	0.09	2.1
Chili with beans	32	1.62	1.56	3.38	13.20	0.973	0.014	0.030	0.91	4.8
Clam chowder— New England	19	1.08	0.75	1.90	21.40	0.169	0.008	0.027	0.11	2.5
Minestrone—chunky	15	0.60	0.33	2.45	7.20	0.209	0.006	0.014	0.12	0.6
Cream of mushroom	29	0.46	2.15	2.10	7.23	0.119	0.007	0.019	0.06	0.4
Mushroom—barley	14	0.43	0.51	1.69	2.82	0.113	0.006	0.020	0.17	0

VARIETY—continued

	kcal	Protein (g)	Lipid (g)	CHO (g)	Ca (mg)	Fe (mg)	B₁ (mg)	B₂ (mg)	Fiber (g)	Cholesterol (mg)
Soups—continued										
Onion—canned	13	0.87	0.40	1.89	6.10	0.156	0.008	0.006	0.11	0
Oyster stew	14	0.49	0.89	0.94	4.96	0.227	0.005	0.008	0	3.1
Pea—prepared w/milk	27	1.40	0.79	3.59	19.30	0.224	0.017	0.030	0.07	2.0
Cream of potato	17	0.39	0.53	2.59	4.52	0.107	0.008	0.008	0.10	1.5
Split pea + ham	22	1.31	0.47	3.17	3.90	0.253	0.014	0.011	0.19	0.8
Tomato—canned	19	0.47	0.43	3.75	3.05	0.396	0.020	0.011	0.11	0
Tomato-beef-noodle	32	1.00	0.97	4.78	3.95	0.252	0.019	0.020	0.03	0.9
Tomato bisque prepared w/milk	22	0.71	0.75	3.32	21.00	0.099	0.013	0.030	0.01`	2.5
Turkey—chunky	16	1.23	0.53	1.69	6.00	0.229	0.010	0.029	0.12	1.1
Turkey noodle	16	0.88	0.45	1.95	2.60	0.212	0.017	0.014	0.03	1.1
Cream vegetable— dry mix	126	2.27	6.84	14.80	1.42	0.539	1.470	0.127	0.22	1.2
Vegetable	16	0.49	0.45	2.77	4.96	0.249	0.012	0.010	0.37	0
Miscellanous										
Garlic cloves	42	1.80	0.14	9.38	51.30	0.482	0.057	0.030	0.47	0
Gelatin salad/desert	17	0.43	0	3.99	0.50	0.024	0.002	0.002	0.02	0
Quiche lorraine	97	2.09	7.73	4.67	34.00	0.226	0.018	0.052	0.09	45.9
Spinach souffle	45	2.29	3.84	0.59	47.90	0.279	0.019	0.064	0.79	38.4

Part 2

NUTRITIVE VALUES FOR ALCOHOLIC AND NONALCOHOLIC BEVERAGES

The nutritive values for alcoholic and nonalcoholic beverages are expressed in 1-ounce (28.4-g) portions. We have also included the nutritive values for the minerals calcium, iron, magnesium, phosphorus, and potassium and the vitamins thiamine (B₁), riboflavin (B₂), niacin, and cobalamin (B₁₂). The alcoholic beverages contain no cholesterol or fat.

ALCOHOLIC BEVERAGES (1OUNCE)

| | kcal | Protein (g) | CHO (g) | Minerals | | | | | Vitamins | | | |
				Ca (mg)	Fe (mg)	Mg (mg)	P (mg)	K (mg)	B₁ (mg)	B₂ (mg)	Niacin (mg)	B₁₂ (mg)
Beer, regular	12	0.072	1.1	1.4	0.009	1.83	3.50	7.09	0.002	0.007	0.128	0.005
Beer, light	8	0.057	0.4	1.4	0.011	1.42	3.44	5.13	0.003	0.008	0.111	0.002
Brandy	69	0	10.6	2.5	0.012		1.01	1.01	0.002	0.002	0.004	0
Champagne	22	0.043	0.6	1.6	0.093	2.40	1.90	22.60	0	0.003	0.019	0
Dessert wine, dry	36	0.057	1.2	2.3	0.068	2.55	2.55	26.20	0.005	0.005	0.060	0
Dessert wine, sweet	44	0.057	3.3	2.3	0.057	2.55	2.64	26.20	0.005	0.005	0.060	0
Gin, rum, vodka, scotch, whiskey, 80 proof	64	0	0	0	0.010	0	0	1.01	0	0	0	0
Gin, rum, vodka, scotch, whiskey, 86 proof	71	0	0	0	0.012	0	1.16	0.55	0.002	0.002	0.004	0

ALCOHOLIC BEVERAGES (1OUNCE)—*continued*

| | kcal | Protein (g) | CHO (g) | Minerals | | | | | Vitamins | | | |
				Ca (mg)	Fe (mg)	Mg (mg)	P (mg)	K (mg)	B₁ (mg)	B₂ (mg)	Niacin (mg)	B₁₂ (mg)
Gin, rum, vodka, scotch, whiskey, 90 proof	74	0	0	0	0.010	0	0	0.86	0	0	0	0
Sherry, dry	28	0.024	0.3	2.1	0.052	1.96	2.60	17.80	0.002	0.002	0.024	0
Sherry, medium	40	0.066	2.3	2.3	0.071	2.27	1.89	23.60	0.002	0.008	0.035	0
Vermouth, dry	34	0.028	1.6	2.0	0.096	1.42	1.89	11.30	NA	NA	0.011	0
Vermouth, sweet	44	0.014	4.5	1.7	0.099	1.13	1.65	8.50	NA	NA	0.011	0
Wine, dry white	19	0.029	0.2	2.6	0.093	2.62	1.67	17.40	0	0.001	0.019	0
Wine, medium white	19	0.028	0.2	2.5	0.085	3.03	3.84	22.60	0.001	0.001	0.019	0
Wine, red	20	0.055	0.5	2.2	0.122	3.60	3.84	31.50	0.001	0.008	0.023	0.004
Wine, rosé	20	0.055	0.4	2.4	0.108	2.74	4.08	28.10	0.001	0.004	0.020	0.002
Creme de menthe	105	0	11.8	0	0.023	0	0	0	0	0	0.001	0
Bloody mary	22	0.153	0.9	1.9	0.105	2.10	4.02	41.40	0.010	0.006	0.123	0
Bourbon and soda	26	0	0	1.0	0.244	0.24	0.48	0.48	0	0	0.005	0
Daiquiri	52	0	1.9	0.9	0.043	0.47	1.89	6.14	0.004	0.	0.012	0
Manhattan	64	0	0.9	0.5	0.025	0.01	1.99	7.46	0.003	0.001	0.026	0
Martini	63	0	0.1	0.4	0.024	0.40	0.81	5.26	0	0	0.004	0
Pina colada	53	0.120	8.0	2.2	0.062		2.01	20.10	0.008	0.004	0.033	0
Screwdriver	23	0.160	2.5	2.1	0.023	2.26	3.86	43.30	0.018	0.004	0.046	0
Tequila	31	0.099	2.4	1.7	0.077	1.98	2.80	29.30	0.010	0.005	0.054	0
Tom collins	16	0.013	0.4	1.3	NA	0.38	0.12	2.30	0	0	0.004	0
Whiskey sour	42	0	3.7	0.3	0.021	0.26	1.60	5.08	0.003	0.002	0.006	0
Coffee + cream liqueur	93	0.784	5.9	4.2	0.036	0.60	13.90	9.05	0	0.016	0.022	0
Coffee liqueur	95	0	13.3	0.5	0.016	0.54	1.64	8.18	0.001	0.003	0.040	0

NONALCOHOLIC BEVERAGES (1OUNCE)

| | kcal | Protein (g) | CHO (g) | Minerals | | | | | Vitamins | | | |
				Ca (mg)	Fe (mg)	Mg (mg)	P (mg)	K (mg)	B₁ (mg)	B₂ (mg)	Niacin (mg)	B₁₂ (mg)
Hot cocoa with whole milk	25	1.030	2.9	33.8	0.088	6.350	30.60	54.400	0.012	0.049	0.041	0.099
Cocoa mix + water—diet	7	0.561	1.3	13.3	0.110	4.870	19.80	59.800	0.006	0.030	0.024	0
Coffee—brewed	0.2	0.016	0.1	0.5	0.113	1.590	0.32	15.400	0	0.002	0.063	0
Coffee—instant dry powder	1.4	0.016	0.3	0.8	0.019	1.100	2.05	67.70	0	0	0.061	0
Coffee—capuchino	9.2	0.059	1.6	1.0	0.022	1.330	3.84	17.600	0	0	0.048	0
Coffee—Swiss mocha	7.7	0.078	1.3	1.1	0.036	1.360	4.37	17.900	0	0	0.039	0
Coffee whitener— nondairy,	38.5	0.284	3.2	2.6	0.009	0.060	18.20	54.1	0	0	0	0
liquid powder	155	1.360	15.6	6.3	0.326	1.200	120.00	230.0	0	0.047	0	0
Cola beverage, regular	12	0	3.0	0.7	0.009	0.230	3.52	0.306	0	0	0	0
Diet cola—w/aspartame	0	0	0	1.0	0.009	0.319	2.40	0	0.001	0.007	0	0
Club soda	0	0	0	1.4	0.012	0.319	0	0.479	0	0	0	0

NONALCOHOLIC BEVERAGES (1 OUNCE)—*continued*

	kcal	Protein (g)	CHO (g)	Ca (mg)	Fe (mg)	Mg (mg)	P (mg)	K (mg)	B_1 (mg)	B_2 (mg)	Niacin (mg)	B_{12} (mg)
				Minerals					Vitamins			
Cream soda	15	0	3.8	1.5	0.015	0.229	0	0.306	0	0	0	0
Diet soda-avg assorted	0	0	0.0	1.1	0.011	0.200	3.03	0.559	0	0	0	0
Egg nog—commercial	38	1.080	3.8	36.8	0.057	5.250	31.00	46.900	0.010	0.054	0.030	0.127
Five Alive citrus	13	0.135	3.1	1.7	0.021	1.950	2.70	34.000	0.015	0.003	0.060	0
Fruit flavored soda pop	13	0	3.2	1.1	0.020	0.305	0.15	1.520	0	0	0.002	0
Fruit punch drink— canned	13	0.015	3.4	2.1	0.058	0.610	0.31	7.160	0.006	0.006	0.006	0
Gatorade	5	0	1.3	2.8	NA	NA	0	2.840	NA	NA	NA	0
Ginger ale	10	0.008	2.5	0.9	0.051	0.232	0.08	0.387	0	0	0	0
Grape soda carbonated	12	0	3.2	0.9	0.024	0.305	0	0.229	0	0	0	0
Kool-Aid w/ NutraSweet	0	0	0	0	0	0.028	0	0	0	0	0	0
Kool-Aid w/sugar added	12	0	3.0	0	0	0	0	0	0	0	0	0
Lemon-lime soda	12	0	3.0	0.7	0.019	0.154	0.08	0.308	0	0	0.004	0
Lemonade drink from dry	11	0	2.9	7.6	0.016	0.322	3.65	3.540	0	0	0.004	0
Lemonade frozen conc	51	0.078	13.3	1.9	0.205	1.420	2.46	19.200	0.007	0.027	0.020	0
Limeade frozen conc	53	0.052	14.0	1.4	0.029	7.800	1.69	16.800	0.003	0.003	0.028	0
Chocolate milkshake	36	0.962	5.8	32.0	0.088	4.700	28.90	56.800	0.016	0.069	0.046	0.097
Strawberry milkshake	32	0.952	5.4	32.0	0.030	3.600	28.40	51.700	0.013	0.055	0.050	0.088
Vanilla milkshake	32	0.982	5.1	34.5	0.026	3.500	29.00	49.300	0.013	0.052	0.052	0.101
Orange drink/ carbonated	14	0	3.5	1.5	0.018	0.305	0.31	0.686	0	0	0	0
Pepper-type soda	12	0	2.9	0.9	0.010	0.077	3.16	0.154	0	0	0	0
Root beer	12	0.008	3.0	1.5	0.014	0.306	0.15	0.230	0	0	0	0
Pineapple grapefruit drink	13	0.068	3.3	2.0	0.087	1.700	1.59	17.500	0.009	0.005	0.076	0
Pineapple orange drink	14	0.352	3.3	1.5	0.076	1.590	1.13	13.200	0.009	0.005	0.059	0
Tang orange juice crystals	13	0.170	0.06	3.1	4.57	0.002	0.02	0.008	0	0	0	0
Tonic water/Quinine water	10	0	2.5	0.4	0.019	0.077	0	0.077	0	0	0	0
Tea-brewed	0	0.001	0.1	0	0.006	0.796	0.16	10.500	0	0.004	0.012	0
Herbal tea, brewed	0	0	0	0.6	0.022	0.319	0	2.390	0.003	0.001	0	0
Perrier water	0	0	0	3.8	0	0.148	0	0	0	0	0	0
Poland Springs bottled water	0	0	0	0.4	0.001	0.239	0	0	0	0	0	0

Note: Alcoholic beverages contain no fat or cholesterol; light beer contains 0.5 g fiber and regular beer contains 1.2 g fiber per 8 oz. serving. All of the other nonmixed alcoholic beverages have no fiber.

Note: Other nonalcoholic beverages are listed in the sections on fruits and vegetables.

Part 3

NUTRITIVE VALUES FOR SPECIALTY AND FAST-FOOD ITEMS

Nutrient information was kindly provided by the manufacturer or its representative, and is reproduced from their literature. Unlike Parts 1 and 2, nutritive values are not given for 1-ounce portions but for actual amounts of the foods sold commercially. To make a direct comparison of the kcal values and the various nutrients, we recommend that the weight of the food and its nutrients be expressed relative to 1-ounce (28.4-g) portions.

ARBY'S

Food Item	Serving Size (g)	kcal	Protein (g)	Lipid (g)	CHO (g)
Bacon Cheddar Deluxe	225	561	28	34	78
Baked Potato Plain	312	291	8	1	0
Beef 'n Cheddar	190	490	24	21	51
Chicken Breast Sandwich	210	592	28	27	57
Chocolate Shake	300	384	9	11	32
French Fries	71	211	2	8	6
Hot Ham 'n Cheese Sandwich	161	353	26	13	50
Jamocha Shake	305	424	8	10	31
Junior Roast Beef	86	218	12	8	22
King Roast Beef	192	467	27	19	49
Potato Cakes	85	201	2	14	13
Regular Roast Beef	147	353	22	15	32
Super Roast Beef	234	501	25	22	40
Superstuffed Potato Broccoli and Cheddar	340	541	13	22	24
Superstuffed Potato Deluxe	312	648	18	38	72
Superstuffed Potato Mushroom and Cheese	300	506	16	22	21
Superstuffed Potato Taco	425	619	23	27	145
Turkey Deluxe	197	375	24	17	39
Vanilla Shake	250	295	8	10	30

Source: Arby's Inc. Nutritional information provided by Consumer Affairs, Arby's Inc., Atlanta, GA, 1986.

BURGER KING

Food Item	Serving Size (g)	kcal	Pro-tein (g)	Total Carbo-hydrate (g)	Total Lipid (g)	Choles-terol (mg)	Sodium (mg)	Dietary Fiber (g)	Vit A	Vit C	Ca	Fe
Burgers												
Whopper sandwich	270	640	27	45	39	90	870	3	10	15	8	25
Whopper with cheese sandwich	294	730	33	46	46	115	1300	3	15	15	25	25
Double Whopper sandwich	351	870	46	45	56	170	940	3	10	15	8	40
Double Whopper with cheese sandwich	375	960	52	46	63	195	1360	3	15	15	25	40
Whopper Jr. sandwich	168	420	21	29	24	60	570	2	4	8	6	20
Whopper Jr. with cheese sandwich	180	460	23	29	28	75	780	2	8	8	15	20
Hamburger	129	330	20	28	15	55	570	1	2	0	4	15
Cheeseburger	142	380	23	28	19	65	780	1	6	0	15	15
Double cheese-burger	213	600	41	29	36	135	1040	1	8	0	20	25
Double cheese-burger with bacon	221	640	44	29	39	145	1220	1	8	0	20	25
Sandwich/Side Orders												
BK Big Fish sandwich	255	720	25	59	43	60	1090	2	2	2	6	20
BK Broiler Chicken sandwich	248	540	30	41	29	80	480	2	4	10	4	30
Chicken sandwich	229	700	26	54	43	60	1400	2	°	°	10	20
Chicken Tenders (6 piece)	88	250	16	14	12	35	530	2	°	°	°	4
Broiled Chicken salad†	302	200	21	7	10	60	110	3	100	25	15	20
Garden salad†	215	90	6	7	5	15	110	3	110	50	15	6
Side salad†	133	50	3	4	3	5	55	2	50	20	6	2
French fries (medium, salted)	116	400	5	43	20	0	240	3	°	4	°	6
Onion rings	124	310	4	41	14	0	810	5	°	°	°	°
Dutch apple pie	113	310	3	39	15	0	230	2	°	10	°	8
Drinks												
Vanilla shake (medium)	284	310	9	53	7	20	230	1	6	6	30	°
Chocolate shake (medium)	284	310	9	54	7	20	230	3	6	°	20	10
Chocolate shake (medium, syrup added)	341	460	11	87	7	20	300	1	6	6	30	°
Strawberry shake (medium, syrup added)	341	430	9	83	7	20	260	1	6	6	30	°

BURGER KING —*continued*

Food Item	Serving Size (g)	kcal	Pro-tein (g)	Total Carbo-hydrate (g)	Total Lipid (g)	Choles-terol (mg)	Sodium (mg)	Dietary Fiber (g)	Percentage of U.S. RDA*			
									Vit A	Vit C	Ca	Fe
Drinks—continued												
Coca-Cola Classic (medium)	22 (fl oz)	260	0	70	0	0	@	0	°	°	°	°
Diet Coke (medium)	22 (fl oz)	1	0	<1	0	0	@	0	°	°	°	°
Sprite (medium)	22 (fl oz)	260	0	66	0	0	@	0	°	°	°	°
Tropicana orange juice	311	140	2	33	0	0	0	0	0	100	0	0
Coffee	355	5	0	1	0	0	5	0	°	°	°	°
Milk—2% low fat	244	120	8	12	5	20	120	0	10	4	30	°
Breakfast												
Croissan'wich with bacon, egg and cheese	118	350	15	18	24	225	790	<1	8	°	15	10
Croissan'wich with sausage, egg and cheese	159	530	20	21	41	255	1000	<1	8	°	15	15
Croissan'wich with ham, egg and cheese	144	350	18	19	22	230	1390	<1	8	°	15	10
French toast sticks	141	500	4	60	27	0	490	1	°	°	6	15
Hash browns	71	220	2	25	12	0	320	2	10	8	°	2
A.M. Express grape jam	12	30	0	7	0	0	0	0	0	0	0	0
A.M. Express strawberry jam	12	30	0	8	0	0	5	0	0	0	0	0
Condiments/ Toppings												
Processed American cheese	25	90	6	0	8	25	420	0	6	°	15	°
Lettuce	21	0	0	0	0	0	0	0	°	°	°	°
Tomato	28	5	0	1	0	0	0	0	2	8	°	°
Onion	14	5	0	1	0	0	0	0	°	°	°	°
Pickles	14	0	0	0	0	0	140	0	0	0	0	0
Ketchup	14	15	0	4	0	0	180	0	4	°	°	°
Mustard	3	0	0	0	0	0	40	0	0	0	0	0
Mayonnaise	28	210	0	<1	23	20	160	0	°	°	°	°
Tartar sauce	28	180	0	0	19	15	220	0	°	°	°	°
Land O' Lakes whipped classic blend	10	65	0	0	7	0	75	0	8	°	°	°
Bull's Eye barbecue sauce	14	20	0	5	0	0	140	0	°	°	°	2
Bacon bits	3	15	1	0	1	5	0	0	°	°	°	°
Croutons	7	30	<1	4	1	0	75	0	°	°	°	°

BURGER KING —*continued*

Food Item	Serving Size (g)	kcal	Protein (g)	Total Carbohydrate (g)	Total Lipid (g)	Cholesterol (mg)	Sodium (mg)	Dietary Fiber (g)	Percentage of U.S. RDA★			
									Vit A	Vit C	Ca	Fe
Burger King Salad Dressings												
Thousand Island dressing	30	140	0	7	12	15	190	<1	30	°	°	°
French dressing	30	140	0	11	10	0	190	0	15	°	°	°
Ranch dressing	30	180	<1	2	19	10	170	<1	°	°	°	°
Bleu cheese dressing	30	160	2	1	16	30	260	<1	°	°	°	°
Reduced calorie light Italian dressing#	30	15	0	3	0.5	0	50	0	°	°	°	°
Dipping Sauces												
A.M. Express dip	28	80	0	21	0	0	20	0	°	°	°	°
Honey dipping sauce	28	90	0	23	0	0	10	0	°	°	°	°
Ranch dipping sauce	28	170	0	2	17	0	200	0	°	°	°	°
Barbecue dipping sauce	28	35	0	9	0	0	400	0	2	2	°	°
Sweet & sour dipping sauce	28	45	0	11	0	0	50	0	°	°	°	°

Source: From Burger King Corporation, Miami, FL, 1996. For additional information, call 1-800-937-1800.
† = Without dressing   @ = Depends on the water supply   ° = Less than 2% of the U.S. RDA
★ = Values for vitamins A and C and minerals calcium and iron represent percent daily values based on a 2,000 calorie diet   # = Regular Italian dressing—150 calories—16 grams (g) Fat.
— = Negligible.

DAIRY QUEEN

Food Item	Serving Size (g)	Description	kcal	Protein (g)	Lipid (g)	CHO (g)	Ca (mg)	Fe (mg)	Vitamin A (IU)	Vitamin C (mg)	Vitamin B₁ (mg)	Vitamin B₂ (mg)
Banana Split	383		540	9	11	103	—	—	—	—	—	—
Big Brazier	213	deluxe	470	28	24	36	111	5.2	—	<2.5	0.34	0.37
Big Brazier	184	regular	184	27	23	37	113	5.2	—	<2.0	0.37	0.39
Big Brazier	213	w/cheese	553	32	30	38	268	5.2	495	<2.3	0.34	0.53
Blizzard Banana Split	—	regular	763	—	—	—	—	—	—	—	—	—
Blizzard Banana Split	—	large	1333	—	—	—	—	—	—	—	—	—
Blizzard chocolate sandwich cookies	—	regular	600	—	—	—	—	—	—	—	—	—
Blizzard chocolate sandwich cookies	—	large	1050	—	—	—	—	—	—	—	—	—

DAIRY QUEEN—*continued*

Food Item	Serving Size (g)	Description	kcal	Protein (g)	Lipid (g)	CHO (g)	Ca (mg)	Fe (mg)	Vitamin A₁(IU)	Vitamin C (mg)	Vitamin B₁ (mg)	Vitamin B₂ (mg)
Blizzard German chocolate	—	regular	794	—	—	—	—	—	—	—	—	—
Blizzard German chocolate	—	large	1460	—	—	—	—	—	—	—	—	—
Blizzard, Heath	—	regular	824	—	—	—	—	—	—	—	—	—
Blizzard, Heath	—	large	1212	—	—	—	—	—	—	—	—	—
Blizzard, M&M	—	regular	766	—	—	—	—	—	—	—	—	—
Blizzard, M&M	—	large	1154	—	—	—	—	—	—	—	—	—
Brazier cheese dog	113		330	15	19	24	168	1.6	—	—	—	0.18
Brazier chili dog	128		330	13	20	25	86	2.0	—	11.0	0.15	0.23
Brazier dog	99		273	11	15	23	75	1.5	—	11.0	0.12	0.15
Brazier french fries	71	regular	200	2	10	25	tr	0.4	tr	3.6	0.06	tr
Brazier french fries	113	large	320	3	16	40	tr	0.4	tr	4.8	0.09	0.03
Brazier onion rings	85		300	6	17	33	20	0.4	tr	2.4	0.09	tr
Brazier regular	106		260	13	9	28	70	3.5	—	<1.0	0.28	0.26
Brazier w/cheese	121		318	18	14	30	163	3.5	—	<1.2	0.29	0.29
Buster Bar	149		460	10	29	41	—	—	—	—	—	—
Chicken sandwich	220		670	29	41	46	—	—	—	—	—	—
Cone	213	large	340	9	10	57	—	—	—	—	—	—
Cone	142	regular	240	6	7	38	—	—	—	—	—	—
Cone	85	small	140	3	4	22	—	—	—	—	—	—
Dairy Queen Parfait	284		460	10	11	81	300	1.8	400	tr	0.12	0.43
Dilly Bar	85		240	4	15	22	100	0.4	100	tr	0.06	0.17
Dilly Bar	85		210	3	13	21	—	—	—	—	—	—
Dipped, cone	234	large	510	9	24	64	—	—	—	—	—	—
Dipped, cone	156	regular	340	6	16	42	—	—	—	—	—	—
Dipped, cone	92	small	190	3	9	25	—	—	—	—	—	—
Double Delight	255		490	9	20	69	—	—	—	—	—	—
Double hamburger	210		530	36	28	33	—	—	—	—	—	—
Double w/cheese	239		650	43	37	34	—	—	—	—	—	—
Chocolate dipped cone	234	large	450	10	20	58	300	0.4	400	tr	0.12	0.51
Chocolate dipped cone	156	medium	300	7	13	40	200	0.4	300	tr	0.09	0.34
Chocolate dipped cone	78	small	150	3	7	20	100	tr	100	tr	0.03	0.17
Chocolate malt	588	large	840	22	28	125	600	5.4	750	6.0	0.15	0.85
Chocolate malt	418	medium	600	15	20	89	500	3.6	750	3.6	0.12	0.60
Chocolate malt	241	small	340	10	11	51	300	1.8	400	2.4	0.06	0.34
Chocolate sundae	248	large	400	9	9	71	300	1.8	400	tr	0.09	0.43
Chocolate sundae	184	medium	300	6	7	53	200	1.1	300	tr	0.06	0.26

DAIRY QUEEN—*continued*

Food Item	Serving Size (g)	Description	kcal	Protein (g)	Lipid (g)	CHO (g)	Ca (mg)	Fe (mg)	Vitamin A (IU)	Vitamin C (mg)	Vitamin B₁ (mg)	Vitamin B₂ (mg)
Chocolate sundae	106	small	170	4	4	30	100	0.7	100	tr	0.03	0.17
Cone	213	large	340	10	10	52	300	tr	400	tr	0.15	0.43
Cone	142	medium	230	6	7	35	200	tr	300	tr	0.09	0.26
Cone	71	small	110	3	3	18	100	tr	100	tr	0.03	0.14
Float	397		330	6	8	59	200	tr	100	tr	0.12	0.17
Freeze	397		520	11	13	89	300	tr	200	tr	0.15	0.34
Sandwich	60		140	3	4	24	60	0.4	100	tr	0.03	0.14
Fiesta sundae	269		570	9	22	84	200	tr	200	tr	0.23	0.26
Fish sandwich	170		400	20	17	41	60	1.1	tr	tr	0.15	0.26
Fish sandwich w/cheese	177		440	24	21	39	150	0.4	100	tr	0.15	0.26
Float	397		410	5	7	82	—	—	—	—	—	—
Freeze	397		500	9	12	89	—	—	—	—	—	—
French fries	71	regular	200	2	10	25	—	—	—	—	—	—
French fries	113	large	320	3	16	40	—	—	—	—	—	—
Frozen dessert	113		180	4	6	27	—	—	—	—	—	—
Hot dog	100		280	11	16	21	—	—	—	—	—	—
Hot dog w/cheese	114		330	15	21	21	—	—	—	—	—	—
Hot dog w/chili	128		320	13	20	23	—	—	—	—	—	—
Hot Fudge brownie delight	266		600	9	25	85	—	—	—	—	—	—
Malt	588	large	1060	20	25	187	—	—	—	—	—	—
Malt	418	regular	760	14	18	134	—	—	—	—	—	—
Malt	291	small	520	10	13	91	—	—	—	—	—	—
Mr. Misty	439	large	340	0	0	84	—	—	—	—	—	—
Mr. Misty	330	regular	250	0	0	63	—	—	—	—	—	—
Mr. Misty	248	small	190	0	0	48	—	—	—	—	—	—
Mr. Misty float	404		440	6	8	85	200	tr	120	tr	0.12	0.17
Mr. Misty float	411		390	5	7	74	—	—	—	—	—	—
Mr. Misty freeze	411		500	9	12	91	—	—	—	—	—	—
Mr. Misty Kiss	89		70	0	0	17	—	—	—	—	—	—
Onion rings	85		280	4	16	31	—	—	—	—	—	—
Parfait	283		430	8	8	76	—	—	—	—	—	—
Peanut Buster Parfait	305		740	16	34	94	—	—	—	—	—	—
Shake	588	large	990	19	26	168	—	—	—	—	—	—
Shake	418	regular	710	14	19	120	—	—	—	—	—	—
Shake	291	small	490	10	13	82	—	—	—	—	—	—
Single hamburger	148		360	21	16	33	—	—	—	—	—	—
Single w/cheese	162		410	24	20	33	—	—	—	—	—	—
Strawberry shortcake	312		540	10	11	100	—	—	—	—	—	—
Sundae	248	large	440	8	10	78	—	—	—	—	—	—
Sundae	177	regular	310	5	8	56	—	—	—	—	—	—
Sundae	106	small	190	3	4	33	—	—	—	—	—	—
Super Brazier	298		783	53	48	35	282	7.3	—	<3.2	0.39	0.69
Super Brazier chili dog	210		555	23	33	42	158	4.0	—	18.0	0.42	0.48

DAIRY QUEEN—*continued*

Food Item	Serving Size (g)	Description	kcal	Protein (g)	Lipid (g)	CHO (g)	Ca (mg)	Fe (mg)	Vitamin A (IU)	Vitamin C (mg)	Vitamin B₁ (mg)	Vitamin B₂ (mg)
Super Brazier dog	182		518	20	30	41	158	4.3	tr	14.0	0.42	0.44
Super Brazier dog w/cheese	203		593	26	36	43	297	4.4	—	14.0	0.43	0.48
Super hot dog	175		520	17	27	44	—	—	—	—	—	—
Super hot dog w/cheese	196		580	22	34	45	—	—	—	—	—	—
Super hot dog w/chili	218		570	21	32	47	—	—	—	—	—	—
Triple hamburger	272		710	51	45	33	—	—	—	—	—	—
Triple w/cheese	301		820	58	50	34	—	—	—	—	—	—

Source: International Dairy Queen, Inc., Minneapolis, MN, 1982. Nutritional information reviewed and edited by Dr. David J. Aulik in cooperation with Raltech Scientific Services.

JACK IN THE BOX

Menu Item	Serving Size (g)	Calories (per serving)	Protein (g)	Lipid (g)	Carbohydrates (g)	Percentage of U.S. RDA			
						Calcium	Iron	Vitamin A	Vitamin C
Sandwiches									
Beef Gyro	260	620	27	32	55	8	30	4	15
Chicken Fajita Pita	189	290	24	8	29	25	15	10	10
Chicken sandwich	160	400	20	18	38	15	10	4	0
Chicken supreme	245	620	25	36	48	20	15	10	4
Country fried steak sandwich	153	450	14	25	42	6	15	2	8
Fish supreme	245	590	22	32	51	20	20	10	8
Grilled chicken fillet	211	430	29	19	36	15	35	6	10
Smoked chicken cheddar & bacon	223	540	30	30	37	30	15	10	15
Sourdough ranch chicken sandwich	225	490	29	21	45	—	10	—	0
Spicy crispy chicken sandwich	224	560	24	27	55	10	15	4	8
Hamburgers									
Hamburger	97	280	13	11	31	10	15	2	2
Cheeseburger	110	330	16	15	32	20	15	6	2
Double cheeseburger	152	450	24	24	35	25	20	10	0
Jumbo Jack	229	560	26	32	41	10	25	4	10
Jumbo Jack with cheese	242	610	29	36	41	20	30	6	10
Bacon bacon cheeseburger	242	710	35	45	41	25	30	8	15
Grilled sourdough burger	223	670	32	43	39	20	25	15	10
Ultimate cheeseburger	280	830	47	57	33	30	35	15	0
¼ lb. burger	172	510	26	27	39	15	20	6	0
The Colossus burger	272	940	52	60	48	30	35	10	6
Teriyaki Bowls									
Chicken Teriyaki bowl	440	580	28	1.5	115	10	10	110	15
Beef Teriyaki bowl	440	580	28	3	124	15	25	100	10
Soy sauce	9	5	°°	0	°°	0	0	0	0

JACK IN THE BOX—*continued*

Menu Item	Serving Size (g)	Calories (per serving)	Protein (g)	Lipid (g)	Carbo-hydrates (g)	Percentage of U.S. RDA			
						Calcium	Iron	Vitamin A	Vitamin C
Breakfast									
Breakfast Jack	121	300	18	12	30	20	15	8	15
Pancake platter	231	610	15	22	87	10	10	8	10
Sausage crescent	156	580	22	43	28	15	15	10	0
Scrambled egg platter	213	560	18	32	50	15	25	15	15
Scrambled egg pocket	183	430	29	21	31	20	20	20	0
Sourdough breakfast sandwich	147	380	21	20	31	25	20	15	15
Supreme crescent	153	530	23	33	34	15	20	15	20
Hash browns	57	160	1	11	14	0	2	0	10
Country Crock Spread	5	25	0	3	0	0	2	4	0
Grape jelly	14	40	0	0	9	0	0	0	0
Pancake syrup	42	120	0	0	30	0	0	0	0
Salads									
Chef salad	324	320	19	30	9	35	15	90	35
Taco salad	397	470	23	34	30	40	25	30	15
Side salad	111	50	3	7	°°	6	0	60	15
Bleu cheese dressing	70	260	22	°°	14	0	0	0	0
Buttermilk house dressing	70	360	36	°°	8	0	0	0	0
Low calorie Italian dressing	70	25	2	°°	2	0	0	0	0
Thousand Island dressing	70	310	30	°°	12	0	0	0	0
Mexican Food									
Taco	78	190	11	7	15	10	6	0	0
Super taco	126	280	17	12	22	15	10	0	4
Guacamole	25	50	4	°°	3	°	°	2	70
Salsa	28	10	0	0	2	°	°	2	°
Sides & Desserts									
Seasoned curly fries	109	360	5	20	39	2	8	0	8
Small french fries	68	220	3	11	28	0	4	0	30
Regular french fries	109	350	4	17	45	0	6	0	40
Jumbo fries	123	400	5	19	51	0	8	0	45
Onion rings	103	380	5	23	38	2	10	0	4
Sesame breadsticks	16	70	2	2	12	0	0	0	0
Tortilla chips	28	140	2	6	18	0	0	0	0
Hot apple turnover	110	350	3	19	48	0	10	0	15
Cheesecake	99	310	8	18	29	10	2	0	0
Chocolate chip cookie dough cheesecake	102	360	7	18	44	15	6	6	0
Cinamon Churritos	75	330	3	21	34	2	30	0	0
Finger Foods									
Egg rolls-3 piece	165	440	3	24	54	8	15	0	6
Egg rolls-5 piece	285	750	5	41	92	15	20	0	10
Chicken strips (breaded)-4 piece	112	290	25	13	18	0	4	0	0
Chicken strips (breaded)-6 piece	177	450	39	20	28	0	6	0	0
Chicken Taquitos-5 piece	136	350	19	15	34	15	10	4	2
Chicken Taquitos-8 piece	218	560	30	25	54	20	15	8	4
Barbeque sauce	28	45	1	0	11	0	0	0	0
Buttermilk house sauce	25	130	°°	13	3	0	°	0	2
Hot sauce	13	5	°°	0	1	0	0	0	0
Sweet & sour sauce	28	40	°°	0	11	0	0	0	0

JACK IN THE BOX—*continued*

Menu Item	Serving Size (g)	Calories (per serving)	Protein (g)	Lipid (g)	Carbo-hydrates (g)	Percentage of U.S. RDA			
						Calcium	Iron	Vitamin A	Vitamin C
Drinks									
Orange juice	183	80	1	0	20	2	2	8	160
Lowfat milk (2%)	244	120	8	5	12	30	0	10	4
Vanilla milk shake (regular)	304	350	9	7	62	30	0	0	0
Chocolate milk shake (regular)	322	330	11	7	59	35	4	0	0
Strawberry milk shake (regular)	298	330	9	7	60	30	0	0	0
Iced tea (small)	16	0	0	0	0	0	0	0	0
Coffee (small)	8	5	0	0	1	0	0	0	0

Source: Jack In The Box; nutritional information provided by Foodmaker, Inc., San Diego, CA.

KENTUCKY FRIED CHICKEN

Food Item	Serving Size (g)	kcal	Protein (g)	CHO (g)	Lipid (g)	Cholesterol (mg)	Vit A (mg)	Vit C (mg)	Thia (mg)	Ribo (mg)	Nia (mg)	Ca (mg)	Fe (mg)
Original Recipe Chicken													
Wing	55	178	12.2	6.0	11.7	64	<100	<1.0	0.03	0.08	3.7	47.9	1.2
Side breast	90	267	18.8	10.8	16.5	77	<100	<1.0	0.06	0.13	6.9	68.0	1.2
Center breast	115	283	27.5	8.8	15.3	93	<100	<1.0	0.09	0.17	11.5	68.0	1.0
Drumstick	57	146	13.1	4.2	8.5	67	<100	<1.0	0.05	0.12	3.2	21.2	1.1
Thigh	104	294	17.9	11.1	19.7	123	104	<1.0	0.08	0.30	5.5	65.1	1.3
Extra Tasty Crispy Chicken													
Wing	65	254	12.4	9.3	18.6	67	<100	<1.0	0.04	0.06	3.3	17.8	0.6
Side breast	110	343	21.7	14.0	22.3	81	<100	<1.0	0.09	0.10	8.5	30.4	0.8
Center breast	135	342	33.0	11.7	19.7	114	<100	<1.0	0.11	0.13	13.1	33.3	0.8
Drumstick	69	204	13.6	6.1	13.9	71	<100	<1.0	0.06	0.12	3.7	12.9	0.7
Thigh	119	406	20.0	14.4	29.8	129	131	<1.0	0.10	0.21	6.5	49.0	1.2
Kentucky Nuggets	16	46	2.8	2.2	2.9	11.9	<100	<1.0	<0.01	0.03	1.00	2.4	0.1
Barbeque sauce	28.3	35	0.3	7.1	0.6	<1.0	<370	<1.0	<0.01	0.01	0.19	6.1	0.2
Sweet 'n sour	28.3	58	0.1	13.0	0.6	<1.0	<100	<1.0	<.01	0.02	0.04	4.7	0.2
Honey	14.2	49	0.0	12.1	<0.01	<1.0	<100	<1.0	<0.01	0.00	0.04	0.6	0.1
Mustard	28.3	36	0.9	6.1	0.9	<1.0	<100	<1.0	<0.01	0.01	0.16	10.2	0.3
Chicken Littles	47	169	5.7	13.8	10.1	18	<100	<1.0	0.16	0.12	2.2	22.6	1.7
Buttermilk biscuits	65	235	4.5	28.0	11.7	1	<100	<1.0	0.24	0.19	2.6	95.0	1.6
Mashed potatoes w/gravy	98	71	2.4	11.7	1.6	<1	<100	<1.0	<0.01	0.04	1.2	21.8	0.04
French fries	77	244	3.2	31.1	11.9	2	<100	15.7	0.15	0.05	2.0	12.5	0.06
Corn on the cob	143	176	5.1	31.9	3.1	<1	272	2.3	0.14	0.11	1.8	7.2	0.08
Cole slaw	91	119	1.5	13.2	6.6	5	310	21.5	0.03	0.03	0.2	32.8	0.02
Colonel's Chicken sandwich	166	482	20.8	38.6	27.3	47	<100	<1.0	0.38	0.27	11.1	46.1	1.3

Source: Public Affairs Department, KFC Corporation, Louisville, KY.

LONG JOHN SILVER'S

Food Item	Serving Size (g)	Description	kcal	Protein (g)	Lipid (g)	CHO (g)
3 Pc. Nugget dinner		6 chicken nuggets, Fryes, slaw	699	23	45	54
Apple pie	113		280	2	11	43
Barbecue sauce	34		45	0	0	11
Battered shrimp dinner		6 battered shrimp, Fryes, slaw	771	17	45	60
Bleu cheese dressing	45		225	4	23	3
Breaded clams			465	13	25	46
Breaded fish sandwich platter		Fish sandwich, Fryes, slaw	835	30	42	84
Breaded oysters		6 pieces	460	14	19	58
Breaded shrimp platter		Breaded shrimp, Fryes, slaw, 2 hush puppies	962	20	57	93
Cherry pie	113		294	3	11	46
Chicken planks		4 pieces	458	27	23	35
Clam chowder	187		128	7	5	15
Clam dinner		Clams, Fryes, slaw	955	22	58	100
Cole slaw			138	1	8	16
Cole slaw, drained on fork	98		182	1	15	11
Combo salad		4.25 oz. seafood salad, 2 oz salad shrimp, 6 oz lettuce, 2.4 oz tomato, 1 pkg crackers	397	27	29	21
Corn on the cob	150	1 ear	176	5	4	29
Fish & Chicken		1 fish, 2 tender chicken planks, Fryes, slaw	935	36	55	73
Fish & Fryes		3 fish, Fryes	853	43	48	64
Fish & Fryes		2 pc fish, Fryes	651	30	36	53
Fish & More		2 fish, Fryes, slaw, 2 hush puppies	978	34	58	92
Fish w/batter		2 pieces	319	19	19	19
Fish w/batter		3 pieces	477	28	28	28
Four nuggets and Fryes			427	16	24	39
Fryes 85			247	4	12	31
Fryes			275	4	15	32
Honey-Mustard sauce	35		56	—	—	14
Hush Puppies	47	2 pieces	145	3	7	18
Hush Puppies		3 pieces	158	1	7	20
Kitchen–breaded fish (three piece dinner)		3 kitchen breaded fish, Fryes, slaw, 2 hush puppies	940	35	52	84

LONG JOHN SILVER'S — *continued*

Food Item	Serving Size (g)	Description	kcal	Protein (g)	Lipid (g)	CHO (g)
Kitchen–breaded (two piece dinner)		2 kitchen-breaded fish, Fryes, slaw, 2 hush puppies	818	26	46	76
Lemon Meringue pie	99		200	2	6	37
Ocean chef salad		6 oz lettuce, 1.25 oz shrimp, 2 oz seafood blend, 2 tomato wedges, ¾ oz cheese	229	27	8	13
Ocean scallops		6 pieces	257	10	12	27
One fish and Fryes			449	16	24	42
One fish, two nuggets, and Fryes			539	23	30	46
Oyster dinner		6 oysters, Fryes, slaw	789	17	45	78
Pecan pie	113		446	5	22	59
Peg leg w/batter		5 pieces 514	25	33	30	
Pumpkin pie	113		251	4	11	34
Reduced calorie Italian dressing	49		20	0	1	3
Scallop dinner		6 scallops, Fryes,	747	17	45	66
Sea salad dressing	45		220	4	21	5
Seafood platter shrimp, 2 scallops, Fryes, slaw		1 fish, 2 battered	976	29	58	85
Seafood salad		5.6 oz seafood salad, 6 oz lettuce, 2.4 oz tomato	426	19	30	22
Shrimp & Fish dinner		1 fish, 3 battered shrimp, Fryes, slaw, 2 hush puppies	917	27	55	80
Shrimp salad shrimp, 6 oz lettuce, 2.4 oz tomato		4.5 oz salad	203	28	3	16
Shrimp w/batter		5 pieces	269	9	13	31
Sweet-n-sour sauce	30		—	—	—	—
Tartar sauce	30		117	—	11	5
Tender chicken plank dinner		3 chicken planks, Fryes, slaw	885	32	51	72
Tender chicken plank dinner		4 chicken planks, Fryes, slaw	1037	41	59	82
Thousand Island dressing	48		223	—	22	8

LONG JOHN SILVER'S —*continued*

Food Item	Serving Size (g)	Description	kcal	Protein (g)	Lipid (g)	CHO (g)
Three piece fish dinner		3 fish, Fryes, slaw, 2 hush puppies	1180	47	70	93
Treasure chest		2 pc fish, 2 peg legs	467	25	29	27
Two planks and Fryes			551	22	28	51

Source: Long John Silver's Seafood Shoppes; sampling and nutrient analysis conducted independently by the Department of Nutrition and Food Science, University of Kentucky, April 10, 1986.

MCDONALD'S

Menu Item	Serving Size	Calories	Pro-tein (g)	Carbo-hydrates (g)	Total Lipid (g)	Choles-terol (mg)	Sodium (mg)	Dietary Fiber (g)	Percentage of U.S. RDA Vitamin A	Vitamin C	Calcium	Iron
Sandwiches												
Hamburger	160 g	270	12	34	10	30	520	2	2	4	15	15
Cheeseburger	120 g	320	15	35	14	45	750	2	6	4	15	15
Quarter Pounder	172 g	420	23	37	21	70	690	2	4	4	15	25
Quarter Pounder with cheese	200 g	530	28	38	30	95	1160	2	10	4	15	25
McLean deluxe	214 g	350	24	38	12	60	800	3	8	15	15	25
McLean deluxe with cheese	228 g	400	27	39	17	70	1040	3	10	15	15	25
Big Mac	216 g	530	25	47	28	80	960	3	6	4	20	25
Filet-O-Fish	143 g	360	14	40	16	35	690	2	2	°	10	10
McGrilled chicken Classic	189 g	260	24	33	4	45	500	2	4	8	10	10
McChicken sandwich	190 g	510	17	44	30	50	820	2	2	2	15	15
French Fries												
Small French fries	68 g	210	3	26	10	0	135	2	°	15	°	2
Large French fries	147 g	450	6	57	22	0	290	5	°	30	2	6
Super Size French fries	176 g	540	8	68	26	0	350	6	°	35	2	8
Chicken McNuggets/Sauce												
Chicken McNuggets (4 piece)	73 g	200	12	10	12	40	350	0	°	°	°	4
Chicken McNuggets (6 piece)	109 g	300	19	16	18	65	530	0	°	°	2	6
Chicken McNuggets (9 piece)	165 g	450	28	24	27	95	800	0	°	°	2	8
Hot Mustard (1 pkg)	28 g	60	1	7	3.5	5	240	<1	°	°	°	4
Barbeque sauce (1 pkg)	28 g	45	0	10	0	0	250	0	°	6	°	°
Sweet 'n sour sauce (1 pkg)	28 g	50	0	11	0	0	140	0	6	°	°	°
Honey (1 pkg)	14 g	45	0	12	0	0	0	0	°	°	°	°
Honey mustard (1 pkg)	14 g	50	0	3	4.5	10	85	0	°	°	°	°
Salads												
Chef salad	313 g	210	19	9	11	180	730	2	90	35	16	10
Fajita chicken salad	285 g	160	20	9	6	65	400	3	160	50	4	10

MCDONALD'S —*continued*

Menu Item	Serving Size	Calories	Pro-tein (g)	Carbo-hydrate (g)	Total Lipid (g)	Choles-terol (mg)	Sodium (mg)	Dietary Fiber (g)	Percentage of U.S. RDA			
									Vitamin A	Vitamin C	Calcium	Iron
Salads—cont'd												
Garden salad	234 g	80	6	7	4	140	60	2	60	35	6	8
Side salad	139 g	45	3	4	2	70	35	1	50	20	4	4
Croutons (1 pkg)	11 g	50	1	7	1.5	0	125	0	°	°	2	2
Bacon bits (1 pkg)	3 g	15	1	0	1	5	90	0	°	°	°	°
Salad Dressings												
Bleu cheese (1 pkg)	60 g	190	2	8	17	30	650	0	2	°	6	2
Ranch (1 pkg)	60 g	230	1	10	21	20	550	0	°	2	4	°
1000 Island	63 g	190	1	16	13	25	510	1	2	2	2	2
Lite Vinaigrette (1 pkg)	62 g	50	0	9	2	0	240	0	6	6	°	°
Red French reduced calorie (1 pkg)	68 g	160	0	23	8	0	490	0	4	6	°	°
Breakfast												
Egg McMuffin	137 g	290	17	27	13	235	730	1	10	2	15	15
Sausage McMuffin	112 g	360	13	26	23	45	750	1	4	°	15	10
Sausage McMuffin with Egg	163 g	440	19	27	29	255	820	1	10	°	15	15
English muffin	55 g	140	4	25	2	0	220	1	°	°	10	8
Sausage biscuit	119 g	430	10	32	29	35	1130	1	°	°	8	15
Sausage biscuit with egg	170 g	520	16	33	35	245	1220	1	6	°	10	15
Bacon, egg & cheese biscuit	152 g	450	17	33	27	240	1340	1	10	°	10	15
Biscuit	76 g	260	4	32	13	0	840	1	°	°	6	10
Sausage	43 g	170	6	0	16	35	290	0	°	°	°	2
Scrambled eggs (2)	102 g	170	13	1	12	425	190	0	10	°	6	6
Hash browns	53 g	130	1	14	8	0	330	1	°	4	°	2
Hotcakes (plain)	150 g	310	9	53	7	15	610	2	°	°	10	15
Hotcakes (margarine 2 pats & syrup)	222 g	580	9	100	16	15	760	2	8	°	10	15
Cheerios (1 pkg)	19 g	70	2	15	1	0	180	2	15	15	2	25
Wheaties (1 pkg)	23 g	80	2	18	0.5	0	160	2	15	15	4	30
Muffins/Danish												
Fat free apple bran muffin	70 g	170	4	38	0	0	200	1	°	°	4	6
Apple danish	105 g	360	5	51	16	40	290	1	10	°	8	6
Cheese danish	105 g	410	7	47	22	70	340	0	15	°	8	6
Cinnamon Raisin danish	105 g	430	5	56	22	50	280	1	10	°	10	8
Raspberry danish	105 g	400	5	58	16	45	300	1	10	°	8	6
Desserts/Shakes												
Vanilla lowfat frozen yogurt cone	90 g	120	4	24	0.5	5	85	0	°	2	15	2
Strawberry lowfat frozen yogurt sundae	178 g	240	6	51	1	5	115	1	°	2	20	2
Hot caramel lowfat frozen yogurt sundae	182 g	310	7	63	3	5	200	1	2	2	25	°
Hot fudge sundae	179 g	290	8	54	5	5	190	2	°	2	25	4
Nuts (sundaes)	7 g	40	2	2	3.5	0	0	0	°	°	°	°
Baked apple pie	77 g	260	3	34	13	0	200	<1	°	40	2	6
McDonaldland cookies (1 pkg)	56 g	260	4	41	9	0	270	1	°	°	°	10
Vanilla shake—small	414 mL	340	11	62	5	25	220	0	4	6	40	2

MCDONALD'S—*continued*

Menu Item	Serving Size	Calories	Protein (g)	Carbo-hydrate (g)	Total Lipid (g)	Choles-terol (mg)	Sodium (mg)	Dietary Fiber (g)	Percentage of U.S. RDA			
									Vitamin A	Vitamin C	Calcium	Iron
Desserts/Shakes—*continued*												
Chocolate shake—small	414 mL	340	12	64	5	25	300	1	4	6	45	4
Strawberry shake—small	414 mL	340	12	63	5	25	220	0	4	10	40	4
Milk/Juices												
1% lowfat milk (8 fl oz)	1 crtn.	100	8	13	2.5	10	115	0	10	4	30	°
Orange juice (6 fl oz)	177 mL	80	1	20	0	0	20	0	2	90	2	2
Apple juice (6 fl oz)	177 mL	80	0	20	0	0	0	0	°	°	°	2

Source: McDonald's Corporation. Oak Brook, IL 60521. (708) 575-3663. 1996.

° = less than 2% of the U.S. RDA

PIZZA HUT

Food Item (1 slice)	kcal	Protein (g)	Lipid (g)	CHO (g)	Ca (mg)	Fe (mg)	Vitamin A (IU)	Vitamin C (mg)	Vitamin B_1 (mg)	Vitamin B_2 (mg)
Thick 'n' chewy, beef	620	38	20	73	400	7.2	750	<1.2	0.68	0.60
Thick 'n' chewy, cheese	560	34	14	71	500	5.4	1000	<1.2	0.68	0.68
Thick 'n' chewy, pepperoni	560	31	18	68	400	5.4	1250	3.6	0.68	0.68
Thick 'n' chewy, pork	640	36	23	71	400	7.2	750	1.2	0.90	0.77
Thick 'n' chewy, supreme	640	36	22	74	400	7.2	1000	9.0	0.75	0.85
Thick 'n' crispy, beef	490	29	19	51	350	6.3	750	<1.2	0.30	0.60
Thick 'n' crispy, cheese	450	25	15	54	450	4.5	750	<1.2	0.30	0.51
Thick 'n' crispy, pepperoni	430	23	17	45	300	4.5	1000	<1.2	0.30	0.51
Thick 'n' crispy, pork	520	27	23	51	350	6.3	1000	<1.2	0.38	0.68
Thick 'n' crispy, supreme	510	27	21	51	350	7.2	1250	2.4	0.38	0.68

Source: Research 900 and Pizza Hut, Inc., Wichita, KS.

ROY ROGERS

Food Item	Serving Size (g)	kcal	Protein (g)	Lipid (g)	CHO (g)
Apple danish	71	249	4.5	11.6	31.6
Bacon cheeseburger	180	581	32.3	39.2	25.0
Biscuit	63	231	4.4	12.1	26.2
Breakfast crescent sandwich	127	401	13.3	27.3	25.3
Breakfast crescent sandwich w/bacon	133	431	15.4	29.7	25.5
Breakfast crescent sandwich w/ham	165	557	19.8	41.7	25.3
Breakfast crescent sandwich w/sausage	162	449	19.9	29.4	25.9
Breast & wing	196	604	43.5	36.5	25.4

ROY ROGERS—*continued*

Food Item	Serving Size (g)	kcal	Protein (g)	Lipid (g)	CHO (g)
Brownie	64	264	3.3	11.4	37.3
Caramel sundae	145	293	7.0	8.5	51.5
Cheese danish	71	254	4.9	12.2	31.4
Cheeseburger	173	563	29.5	37.3	27.4
Cherry danish	71	271	4.4	14.4	31.7
Chicken breast	144	412	33.0	23.7	16.9
Chocolate shake	319	358	7.9	10.2	61.3
Cole slaw	99	110	1.0	6.9	11.0
Crescent roll	70	287	4.7	17.7	27.2
Egg and biscuit platter	165	394	16.9	26.5	21.9
Egg and biscuit platter w/bacon	173	435	19.7	29.6	22.1
Egg and biscuit platter w/ham	200	442	23.5	28.6	22.5
Egg and biscuit platter w/sausage	203	550	23.4	40.9	21.9
French fries	85	268	3.9	13.5	32.0
Hamburger	143	456	23.8	28.3	65.6
Hot chocolate	8 oz	123	3.0	2.0	22.0
Hot fudge sundae	151	337	6.5	12.5	53.3
Hot topped potato plain	227	211	5.9	0.2	47.9
Hot topped potato w/bacon 'n cheese	248	397	17.1	21.7	33.3
Hot topped potato w/broccoli 'n cheese	312	376	13.7	18.1	39.6
Hot topped potato w/oleo	236	274	5.9	7.3	47.9
Hot topped potato w/sour cream 'n chives	297	408	7.3	20.9	47.6
Hot topped potato w/taco beef 'n cheese	359	463	21.8	21.8	45.0
Large fries	113	357	5.3	18.4	42.7
Large roast beef	182	360	33.9	11.9	29.6
Large roast beef w/cheese	211	467	39.6	20.9	30.3
Leg	53	140	11.5	8.0	5.5
Macaroni	100	186	3.1	10.7	19.4
Milk	8 oz	150	8.0	8.2	11.4
Orange juice	8 oz	99	1.5	0.2	22.8
Orange juice	8 oz	136	2.0	0.3	31.3
Pancake platter (w/syrup, butter)	165	452	7.7	15.2	71.8
Pancake platter (w/syrup, butter) w/bacon	173	493	10.4	18.3	72.0
Pancake platter (w/syrup, butter) w/ham	200	506	14.3	17.3	72.4

ROY ROGERS—*continued*

Food Item	Serving Size (g)	kcal	Protein (g)	Lipid (g)	CHO (g)
Pancake platter (w/syrup, butter) w/sausage	203	608	14.2	29.6	71.8
Potato salad	100	107	2.0	6.1	10.9
Roast beef sandwich	154	317	27.2	10.2	29.1
Roast beef sandwich w/cheese	182	424	32.9	19.2	29.9
RR bar burger	208	611	36.1	39.4	28.0
Salad bar 1,000 Island	2 T	160	NA	16.0	4.0
Salad bar bacon 'n tomato	2 T	136	NA	12.0	6.0
Salad bar bacon bits	1 T	24	4.0	1.0	38.0
Salad bar blue cheese dressing	2 T	150	2.0	16.0	2.0
Salad bar cheddar cheese	¼ cup	112	5.8	9.0	0.8
Salad bar Chinese noodles	¼ cup	55	1.5	2.8	6.5
Salad bar chopped eggs	2 T	55	4.0	4.0	0.7
Salad bar croutons	2 T	132	5.5	0	31.0
Salad bar cucumbers	5–6 slices	4	NA	0	1.0
Salad bar green peas	¼ cup	7	0.5	0	1.2
Salad bar green peppers	2 T	4	0.3	0	1.0
Salad bar lettuce	1 cup	10	NA	0	4.0
Salad bar lo-cal Italian	2 T	70	NA	6.0	2.0
Salad bar macaroni salad	2 T	60	1.0	3.6	6.2
Salad bar mushrooms	¼ cup	5	0.5	0	0.7
Salad bar potato salad	2 T	50	1.0	3.0	5.5
Salad bar ranch	2 T	155	NA	14.0	4.0
Salad bar shredded carrots	¼ cup	12	0.6	0	24.0
Salad bar sliced beets	¼ cup	16	0.5	0	3.8
Salad bar sunflower seeds	2 T	101	4.0	9.0	5.0
Salad bar tomatoes	3 slices	20	0.8	0	4.8
Strawberry shake	312	315	7.6	10.2	49.4
Strawberry shortcake	205	447	10.1	19.2	59.3
Strawberry sundae	142	216	5.7	7.1	33.1
Thigh	98	296	18.4	19.5	11.7
Thigh & leg	151	436	29.9	27.5	17.2
Vanilla shake	306	306	8.0	10.7	45.0
Wing	52	192	10.5	12.8	8.5

Source: Roy Rogers Restaurants, Marriott Corporation, Washington, DC. Nutritional data furnished by Lancaster Laboratories, 1985.

TACO BELL

Food Item	kcal	Protein (g)	Fat (g)	Calories From Lipid	Saturated Fat	Cholesterol (mg)	Na (mg)	Percent U.S. RDA Ca	Percent U.S. RDA Fe
Tacos & Tostadas									
Chicken soft taco	223	14	10	90	4	58	553	6	8
Soft taco	223	12	11	100	5	32	539	5	10
Soft taco supreme	268	13	15	140	8	47	551	8	11
Steak soft taco	217	12	9	80	4	31	569	5	6
Taco	180	10	11	100	5	32	276	8	5
Taco supreme	225	11	15	130	7	47	287	10	6
Tostada	242	9	11	100	4	14	593	17	8
Burritos									
7 layer burrito	485	15	21	190	8	28	1115	25	25
Bean burrito	391	13	12	110	4	5	1138	19	20
Beef burrito	432	22	19	170	8	57	1303	16	22
Big beef burrito supreme	525	25	25	220	11	72	1418	20	25
Burrito supreme	443	18	19	170	9	47	1184	20	21
Chicken burrito	345	17	13	110	5	57	854	14	14
Chicken burrito supreme	520	27	23	200	9	125	1130	15	50
Chili cheese burrito	391	17	18	160	9	47	980	30	17
Combo burrito	412	17	16	140	6	32	1221	17	21
Steak burrito supreme	500	26	23	200	11	75	1350	20	15
Specialty Items									
Beef MexiMelt	262	13	14	130	7	38	711	23	8
Cinnamon twists	139	1	6	50	0	0	189	°	2
Mexican pizza	574	19	38	340	12	50	1003	31	25
Nachos	345	7	18	160	6	9	398	23	4
Nachos BellGrande	633	22	34	300	12	49	952	36	20
Nachos supreme	364	12	18	160	5	17	470	19	15
Pintos 'n cheese	190	9	9	80	4	14	640	15	7
Taco salad	838	31	55	490	16	79	1132	25	34
Side Orders & Condiments									
Green sauce	4	0	0	0	0	0	136	°	°
Guacamole	36	0	3	30	1	0	132	4	°
Hot taco sauce	2	0	0	0	0	0	91	°	°
Milk taco sauce	0	0	0	0	0	0	6	°	°
Nacho cheese sauce	51	2	4	40	2	4	196	6	°
Picante sauce	3	0	0	0	0	0	132	2	0
Pico de Gallo	6	0	0	0	0	0	65	°	°
Ranch dressing	136	1	14	130	3	20	330	2	°
Red sauce	10	0	0	0	0	0	261	°	°
Salsa	27	1	0	0	0	0	709	5	3
Seasoned rice	110	2	3	30	1	5	230	°	8
Sour cream	44	1	4	40	3	15	11	2	°

Source: Taco Bell Corporation, Irvine, CA. 1996.

° = trace

WENDY'S

Food Item	Serving Size (g)	kcal	Protein (g)	CHO (g)	Lipid (g)	Cholesterol (mg)	Vit A (mg)	Vit C (mg)	Thia (mg)	Ribo (mg)	Nia (mg)	Ca (mg)	Fe (mg)
							\multicolumn{7}{Percentage of U.S. RDA}						
Sandwiches													
½ lb. hamburger patty	74	180	19	—	12	65	—	—	4	—	20	—	20
Plain single	126	340	24	30	15	65	—	—	25	20	30	10	30
Single with everything	210	420	25	35	21	70	5	15	25	20	30	10	30
Wendy's Big Classic	260	570	27	47	33	90	10	20	30	25	35	15	35
Jr. Hamburger	111	260	15	33	9	34	2	4	25	20	20	10	20
Jr. cheeseburger	125	310	18	33	13	34	2	4	25	50	20	10	20
Jr. bacon cheeseburger	155	430	22	32	25	50	2	15	30	50	25	10	20
Jr. Swiss deluxe	163	360	18	34	18	40	4	10	25	60	20	20	20
Kids' meal hamburger	104	260	15	32	9	35	2	2	25	20	20	10	20
Kids' meal cheeseburger	116	300	18	33	13	35	2	2	25	50	20	10	20
Grilled chicken fillet	70	100	18	—	3	55	—	—	4	4	35	—	6
Grilled chicken sandwich	175	340	24	36	13	60	2	8	30	25	50	10	20
Chicken breast fillet	99	220	21	11	10	55	—	—	8	8	60	—	70
Chicken sandwich	219	430	26	41	19	60	2	8	30	25	70	10	80
Chicken club sandwich	205	506	30	42	25	70	2	15	35	30	80	10	80
Fish fillet sandwich	170	460	18	42	25	55	2	2	40	35	20	10	15
Kaiser bun	65	200	6	37	3	10	—	—	25	20	10	10	10
White bun	56	160	5	30	3	tr	—	—	20	20	10	10	10
Sandwich Toppings													
American cheese slice	18	70	4	—	6	15	6	—	—	4	—	12	—
Bacon	6	30	2	—	3	5	—	4	4	—	2	—	—
Ketchup	14	17	—	4	—	NA	4	4	—	—	—	—	—
Lettuce	10	1	—	—	—	0	—	—	—	—	—	—	—
Mayonnaise	13	90	—	—	10	10	—	—	—	—	—	—	—
Mustard	5	4	—	—	—	0	—	—	—	—	—	—	—
Onion	10	4	—	—	—	0	—	—	—	—	—	—	—
Pickles	14	2	—	—	—	0	—	—	—	—	—	—	—
Tomatoes	21	4	—	—	—	0	—	6	—	—	—	—	—
Honey mustard	14	71	—	4	6	5	—	—	—	—	—	—	—
Tartar sauce	21	120	—	—	14	15	—	—	15	10	—	—	—
Superbar—Pasta													
Alfredo sauce	56	35	1	5	1	tr	—	—	—	—	—	6	—
Fettucini	56	190	4	27	3	10	—	—	10	6	6	—	6
Garlic toast	18.3	70	2	9	3	tr	4	—	6	2	2	2	2
Pasta medley	56	60	2	9	2	tr	6	15	6	4	4	—	4
Rotini	56	90	3	15	2	tr	—	—	6	4	6	—	4
Spaghetti sauce	56	28	—	7	0	tr	—	—	—	—	—	—	—
Spaghetti meat sauce	56	60	4	8	2	10	4	4	—	2	4	—	4
Garden Spot Salad Bar													
Alfalfa sprouts	28	8	1	1	0	0	—	4	—	2	—	—	—
Applesauce, chunky	28	22	—	6	—	0	—	—	—	—	—	—	—
Bacon bits	14	40	5	—	14	10	—	2	6	4	6	—	—
Bananas	28	26	—	7	—	0	—	4	—	2	—	—	—
Breadsticks	7.5	30	1	5	1	0	—	—	2	2	2	2	2
Broccoli	43	12	1	2	0	0	6	65	2	2	—	2	2
Cantaloupe	57	20	—	5	0	0	20	30	—	—	—	—	—
Carrots	27	12	—	2	0	0	80	4	2	—	—	—	—
Cauliflower	57	14	1	3	0	0	—	70	4	2	2	2	2
Cheddar chips	28	160	3	12	12	5	—	—	2	—	4	6	2
Cheese, shredded (imitation)	28	90	6	1	6	tr	4	—	—	15	—	20	—
Chicken salad	56	120	7	4	8	tr	—	4	—	4	6	—	2
Chives	28	71	6	18	1	0	195	313	15	25	8	25	30
Chow mein noodles	14	74	1	8	4	0	—	—	6	4	4	—	4

WENDY'S—*continued*

| | | | | | | | Percentage of U.S. RDA | | | | | | |
Food Item	Serving Size (g)	kcal	Protein (g)	CHO (g)	Lipid (g)	Cholesterol (mg)	Vit A (mg)	Vit C (mg)	Thia (mg)	Ribo (mg)	Nia (mg)	Ca (mg)	Fe (mg)
Garden Spot Salad Bar—*continued*													
Cole slaw	57	70	—	8	5	5	4	25	—	—	—	2	—
Cottage cheese	105	108	13	3	4	15	6	—	—	10	—	6	—
Croutons	14	60	2	8	3	—	—	—	4	4	4	—	4
Cucumbers	14	2	—	—	0	0	—	—	—	—	—	—	—
Eggs (hard cooked)	20	30	3	—	2	90	4	—	—	6	—	—	—
Garbanzo beans	28	46	3	8	1	0	—	—	2	—	—	—	6
Green peas	28	21	1	4	0	0	4	8	6	2	—	—	2
Green peppers	37	10	—	2	0	0	2	60	2	—	—	—	—
Honeydew melon	57	20	—	5	0	0	—	25	2	—	2	—	—
Jalapeno peppers	14	2	—	—	0	0	—	—	—	—	—	—	—
Lettuce—iceberg	55	8	—	1	0	0	2	4	2	—	—	—	2
Lettuce—romaine	55	9	1	1	0	0	15	20	4	4	—	2	4
Mushrooms	17	4	—	—	0	0	—	—	—	4	4	—	—
Olives, black	28	35	—	2	3	0	—	—	—	—	—	2	4
Oranges	56	26	—	7	0	0	—	50	4	—	—	2	—
Parmesan cheese	28	130	12	1	9	20	6	—	—	6	—	40	—
Parmesan cheese (imitation)	28	80	9	4	3	tr	20	—	—	—	—	50	—
Pasta salad	57	35	2	6	—	0	—	—	—	2	2	—	2
Peaches	57	31	—	8	0	0	2	2	—	—	2	—	—
Pepperoni, sliced	28	140	5	2	12	35	—	—	160	4	10	—	2
Pineapple chunks	100	60	—	16	0	0	—	15	6	—	—	—	2
Potato salad	57	125	—	6	11	10	—	10	2	—	2	—	2
Pudding—butterscotch	57	90	1	11	4	tr	—	—	—	—	—	6	2
Pudding—chocolate	57	90	—	12	4	tr	—	—	2	2	—	15	2
Red onions	9	2	—	—	0	0	—	—	—	—	—	—	—
Red peppers, crushed	28	120	5	15	4	0	200	15	10	15	20	2	15
Seafood salad	56	110	4	7	7	tr	—	2	—	2	—	20	2
Strawberries	56	17	—	4	0	0	—	50	—	2	—	—	—
Sour topping	28	58	—	2	5	0	—	—	—	—	—	—	—
Sunflower seeds & raisins	28	140	5	6	10	0	—	—	30	4	6	2	10
Three bean salad	57	60	1	13	—	—	4	—	—	—	—	—	2
Tomatoes	28	6	—	1	0	0	2	10	—	—	—	—	—
Tuna salad	56	100	8	4	6	tr	—	4	—	4	25	—	2
Turkey ham	28	35	5	—	1	15	—	—	—	4	6	—	4
Watermelon	57	18	—	4	0	0	2	10	4	—	—	—	—
Salad Dressings													
Blue cheese	15	9	—	—	10	10	—	—	—	—	—	—	—
Celery seed	15	70	—	3	6	5	—	—	—	—	—	—	—
French	15	60	—	4	6	0	—	—	—	—	—	—	—
French, sweet red	15	70	—	5	6	0	—	—	—	—	—	—	—
Hidden Valley ranch	15	50	—	—	6	5	—	—	—	—	—	—	—
Italian Caesar	15	80	—	—	9	5	—	—	—	—	—	—	—
Italian, golden	15	45	—	3	4	0	—	—	—	—	—	—	—
Salad oil	28	250	0	0	28	0	—	—	—	—	—	—	—
Thousand island	15	70	—	2	7	5	—	—	—	—	—	—	—
Wine, vinegar	15	2	—	—	0	0	—	—	—	—	—	—	—
Red. Cal. bacon & tomato	15	45	—	3	4	—	—	—	—	—	—	—	—
Reduced calorie Italian	15	25	—	2	2	0	—	—	—	—	—	—	—
Prepared Salads													
Chef salad	331	180	15	10	9	120	110	110	15	25	6	25	15
Garden salad	277	102	7	9	5	0	110	110	10	20	6	20	10
Taco salad	791	660	40	46	37	35	80	80	30	45	25	80	35

WENDY'S—*continued*

Food Item	Serving Size (g)	kcal	Protein (g)	CHO (g)	Lipid (g)	Cholesterol (mg)	Vit A (mg)	Vit C (mg)	Thia (mg)	Ribo (mg)	Nia (mg)	Ca (mg)	Fe (mg)
Superbar—Mexican Fiesta (where available)													
Cheese sauce	56	39	1	5	2	tr	—	—	—	—	—	6	—
Picante sauce	56	18	—	4	—	NA	10	30	2	—	2	—	2
Refried beans	56	70	4	10	3	tr	—	—	4	2	—	2	6
Rice, Spanish	56	70	2	13	1	tr	6	—	45	—	8	4	10
Taco chips	40	260	4	40	10	0	—	—	2	4	—	8	4
Taco meat	56	110	10	4	7	25	—	—	8	6	10	4	10
Taco sauce	28	16	—	3	—	tr	4	2	—	—	—	—	—
Taco shells	11	45	—	6	3	0	—	—	—	—	—	—	—
Tortilla, flour	37	110	3	19	3	NA	—	—	4	2	2	8	2
French fries (small) 3.2 oz°°	91	240	3	33	12	0	—	10	10	2	10	—	4
Chili (regular) 9 oz	255	220	21	23	7	45	15	15	8	10	10	8	35
Cheddar cheese, shredded	28	110	7	1	10	30	10	—	—	6	—	20	—
Sour cream	28	60	1	1	6	10	6	—	—	2	—	4	—
Crispy chicken nuggets (6)	93	280	14	12	20	50	—	—	6	6	30	4	4
Nuggets sauces													
Barbeque	28	50	—	11	—	0	6	—	—	—	—	—	4
Honey	14	45	—	12	—	0	—	—	—	—	—	—	—
Sweet & sour	28	45	—	11	—	0	—	—	—	—	—	—	2
Sweet mustard	28	50	—	9	1	0	—	—	—	—	—	—	—
Hot Stuffed Baked Potatoes													
Plain	250	270	6	63	—	0	—	50	20	6	20	2	20
Bacon & cheese	362	520	20	70	18	20	10	60	35	15	35	8	24
Broccoli & cheese	350	400	8	58	16	tr	14	60	20	10	20	10	15
Cheese	318	420	8	66	15	10	10	50	20	100	20	6	20
Chili & cheese	403	500	15	71	18	25	15	60	20	100	25	8	28
Sour cream & chives	323	500	8	67	23	25	50	75	20	10	20	10	20
Beverages													
Frosty, small°°°	243	400	8	59	14	50	10	—	8	30	2	30	6
Cola, small	8°	100	0	25	0	0	—	—	—	—	—	—	—
Lemon-lime soft drink, small	8°	100	0	24	0	0	—	—	—	—	—	—	—
Diet cola	8°	1	0	—	0	0	—	—	—	—	—	—	—
Coffee	6°	2	0	—	0	0	—	—	—	—	—	—	—
Decaf coffee	6°	2	0	—	0	0	—	—	—	—	—	—	—
Hot chocolate	6°	110	2	22	1	tr	—	—	—	8	—	6	2
Lemonade	8°	90	0	24	0	0	—	15	—	4	—	—	2
Choc milk	8°	160	7	24	5	15	15	4	6	20	—	25	4
Milk, 2%	8°	110	8	11	4	20	10	4	6	20	—	30	—
Tea (hot or ice)	6°	1	0	0	0	0	—	—	—	—	—	—	—
Chocolate chip cookie	64	275	3	40	13	15	2	—	8	8	6	2	8

Source: Consumer Relations, Wendy's International, Dublin, OH.

°Fluid ounces.

°°To determine nutritional information for a large order of Fries, multiply figures by 1.3; Biggie Fries, multiply by 1.87; large Chili, multiply by 1.5; 9-piece Nuggets, multiply by 1.5; 20-piece Nuggets, multiply by 3.3.

°°°To determine nutritional information for a medium Frosty, multiply figures by 1.3; large Frosty, multiply by 1.7. For medium soft drink, multiply by 1.5; large soft drink, multiply by 2. For Biggie soft drink, multiply by 3.5.

APPENDIX B

Energy Expenditure in Household, Occupational, Recreational, and Sports Activities[a,b]

HOW TO USE APPENDIX B

Refer to the column that comes closest to your present body mass. Multiply the number in this column by the number of minutes you spend in an activity. Suppose that an individual weighing 80.0 kg (176 lb) spends 45 minutes working out with free weights. To determine the energy cost of participation, multiply the caloric value per minute (6.8 kcal) by 45 to obtain the 45-minute gross expenditure of 306 kcal. If the same individual does aerobic dance for 60 minutes, the gross (value includes resting energy expenditure) energy expended would be calculated as 7.8 kcal × 60 minutes, or 468 kcal.

---

[a] All values for energy expenditure expressed in kilocalories per minute.

[b] Copyright © 1999, 2004 by Frank I. Katch, Victor L. Katch, and William D. McArdle, and Fitness Technologies, Inc., 5043 Via Lara Land, Santa Barbara, CA, 93111. No part of this appendix may be reproduced in any manner without written permission from the copyright holders.

YOUR BODY WEIGHT

Activity	kg lb	47 104	50 110	53 117	56 123	59 130	62 137	65 143	68 150
Archery		3.1	3.3	3.4	3.6	3.8	4.0	4.2	4.4
Backpacking									
without load		5.7	6.1	6.4	6.8	7.1	7.5	7.9	8.2
with 11 pound load		6.1	6.5	6.8	7.2	7.6	8.0	8.4	8.8
with 22 pound load		6.6	7.0	7.4	7.8	8.3	8.7	9.1	9.5
with 44 pound load		7.0	7.4	7.8	8.2	8.7	9.1	9.6	10.0
Badminton									
leisure		4.6	4.9	5.1	5.4	5.7	6.0	6.3	6.6
tournament		7.0	7.3	7.7	8.1	8.6	9.0	9.4	9.9
Baking, general (F)		1.6	1.8	1.9	2.0	2.1	2.2	2.3	2.4
Baseball									
fielder		2.8	3.0	3.2	3.4	3.6	3.8	4.0	4.1
pitcher		4.2	4.5	4.8	5.0	5.3	5.6	5.9	6.2
Basketball									
competition		7.1	7.4	7.9	8.3	8.7	9.2	9.6	10.1
practice		6.5	6.9	7.3	7.7	8.1	8.6	9.0	9.4
Baton twirling		6.3	6.8	7.3	7.6	8.1	8.5	8.9	9.3
Billiards ("pool")		2.0	2.1	2.2	2.4	2.5	2.6	2.7	2.9
Bookbinding		1.8	1.9	2.0	2.1	2.2	2.4	2.5	2.6
Bowling		4.4	4.8	5.2	5.4	5.7	6.0	6.3	6.6
Boxing									
in ring, match		10.4	11.1	11.8	12.4	13.1	13.8	14.4	15.1
sparring, practice		6.5	6.9	7.3	7.7	8.1	8.6	9.0	9.4
Calisthenics, warm-ups		3.4	3.7	4.0	4.2	4.4	4.7	4.9	5.1
Canoeing									
leisure (2.5 mph)		2.1	2.2	2.3	2.5	2.6	2.7	2.9	3.0
racing ("fast")		4.8	5.2	5.5	5.8	6.1	6.4	6.7	7.0
Car washing		3.3	3.5	3.7	3.9	4.1	4.3	4.5	4.8
Card playing		1.2	1.3	1.3	1.4	1.5	1.6	1.6	1.7
Carpentry, general		2.4	2.6	2.8	2.9	3.1	3.2	3.4	3.5
Carpet sweeping (F)		2.2	2.3	2.4	2.5	2.7	2.8	2.9	3.1
Carpet sweeping (M)		2.3	2.4	2.5	2.7	2.8	3.0	3.1	3.3
Circuit resistance training									
Free weights		4.0	4.3	4.5	4.8	5.0	5.3	5.5	5.8
Hydra-Fitness		6.2	6.6	7.0	7.4	7.8	8.2	8.6	9.0
Nautilus		4.3	4.6	4.9	5.2	5.5	5.8	6.0	6.3
Universal		5.3	5.8	6.2	6.5	6.9	7.2	7.5	7.9
Cleaning (F)		2.9	3.1	3.3	3.5	3.7	3.8	4.0	4.2
Cleaning (M)		2.7	2.9	3.1	3.2	3.4	3.6	3.8	3.9
Coal mining									
drilling coal, rock		4.4	4.7	5.0	5.3	5.5	5.8	6.1	6.4
erecting supports		4.1	4.4	4.7	4.9	5.2	5.5	5.7	6.0
shoveling coal		5.1	5.4	5.7	6.0	6.4	6.7	7.0	7.3
Cooking (F)		2.1	2.3	2.4	2.5	2.7	2.8	2.9	3.1
Cooking (M)		2.3	2.4	2.5	2.7	2.8	3.0	3.1	3.3
Cricket									
batting		3.9	4.2	4.4	4.6	4.9	5.1	5.4	5.6
bowling		4.2	4.5	4.8	5.0	5.3	5.6	5.9	6.1
fielding		3.7	3.9	4.1	4.3	4.8	4.8	5.0	5.3

Note: Symbols (M) and (F) denote experiments for males and females, respectively.

| 71 | 74 | 77 | 80 | 83 | 86 | 89 | 92 | 95 | 98 |
157	163	170	176	183	190	196	203	209	216
4.6	4.8	5.0	5.2	5.4	5.6	5.8	6.0	6.2	6.4
8.6	9.0	9.3	9.7	10.0	10.4	10.8	11.1	11.5	11.9
9.2	9.5	9.9	10.3	10.7	11.1	11.5	11.9	12.3	12.6
9.9	10.4	10.8	11.2	11.6	12.0	12.5	12.9	13.3	13.7
10.4	10.9	11.3	11.8	12.2	12.6	13.1	13.5	14.0	14.4
6.9	7.2	7.5	7.8	8.1	8.3	8.6	8.9	9.2	9.5
10.4	10.8	11.2	11.6	12.1	12.5	12.9	13.4	13.8	14.3
2.5	2.6	2.7	2.8	2.9	3.0	3.1	3.2	3.3	3.4
4.3	4.5	4.7	4.9	5.1	5.2	5.4	5.6	5.8	6.0
6.4	6.7	7.0	7.2	7.5	7.8	8.0	8.3	8.6	8.9
10.5	10.9	11.4	11.8	12.3	12.7	13.1	13.6	14.0	14.5
9.8	10.2	10.6	11.0	11.5	11.9	12.3	12.7	13.1	13.5
9.5	9.7	9.9	10.1	10.4	10.6	10.8	11.0	11.2	11.4
3.0	3.1	3.2	3.4	3.5	3.6	3.7	3.9	4.0	4.1
2.7	2.8	2.9	3.0	3.2	3.3	3.4	3.5	3.6	3.7
6.9	7.2	7.5	7.7	8.1	8.4	8.6	8.9	9.2	9.5
15.8	16.4	17.1	17.8	18.4	19.1	19.8	20.4	21.1	21.8
9.8	10.2	10.6	11.0	11.5	11.9	12.3	12.7	13.1	13.5
5.3	5.5	5.8	6.0	6.2	6.5	6.7	6.9	7.1	7.3
3.1	3.3	3.4	3.5	3.7	3.8	3.9	4.0	4.2	4.3
7.3	7.6	7.9	8.2	8.5	8.9	9.2	9.5	9.8	10.1
5.0	5.2	5.5	5.7	5.7	5.9	6.1	6.3	6.5	6.9
1.8	1.9	1.9	2.0	2.1	2.2	2.2	2.3	2.4	2.5
3.7	3.8	4.0	4.2	4.3	4.5	4.6	4.8	4.9	5.1
3.2	3.3	3.5	3.6	3.7	3.9	4.0	4.1	4.3	4.4
3.4	3.6	3.7	3.8	4.0	4.1	4.3	4.4	4.6	4.7
6.1	6.3	6.6	6.8	7.1	7.4	7.6	7.9	8.1	8.4
9.4	9.7	10.2	10.5	10.9	11.4	11.7	12.1	12.5	12.9
6.6	6.8	7.1	7.4	7.7	8.0	8.2	8.5	8.8	9.1
8.3	8.6	8.9	9.3	9.6	10.0	10.3	10.7	11.0	11.4
4.4	4.6	4.8	5.0	5.1	5.3	5.5	5.7	5.9	6.1
4.1	4.3	4.5	4.6	4.8	5.0	5.2	5.3	5.5	5.7
6.7	7.0	7.2	7.5	7.8	8.1	8.4	8.6	8.9	9.2
6.2	6.5	6.8	7.0	7.3	7.6	7.8	8.1	8.4	8.6
7.7	8.0	8.3	8.6	9.0	9.3	9.6	9.9	10.3	10.6
3.2	3.3	3.5	3.6	3.7	3.9	4.0	4.1	4.3	4.4
3.4	3.6	3.7	3.8	4.0	4.1	4.3	4.4	4.6	4.7
5.9	6.1	6.4	6.6	6.9	7.1	7.4	7.6	7.9	8.1
6.4	6.7	6.9	7.2	7.5	7.7	8.0	8.3	8.6	8.8
5.6	5.9	6.2	6.5	6.8	7.1	7.4	7.7	8.0	8.3

YOUR BODY WEIGHT—*continued*

Activity	kg lb	47 104	50 110	53 117	56 123	59 130	62 137	65 143	68 150
Croquet		2.8	3.0	3.1	3.3	3.5	3.7	3.8	4.0
Cycling									
leisure, 5.5 mph		3.0	3.2	3.4	3.6	3.8	4.0	4.2	4.4
leisure, 9.4 mph		4.8	5.0	5.3	5.6	5.9	6.2	6.5	6.8
racing, fast		8.0	8.5	9.0	9.5	10.0	10.5	11.0	11.5
Dancing									
aerobic, easy		4.3	4.8	5.2	5.6	5.9	6.2	6.4	6.7
aerobic, medium		4.8	5.2	5.5	5.8	6.1	6.4	6.7	7.0
aerobic, intense		6.3	6.7	7.1	7.5	7.9	8.3	8.7	9.2
ballroom		2.4	2.6	2.7	2.9	3.0	3.2	3.3	3.5
choreographed		5.0	5.2	5.5	5.8	6.1	6.4	6.7	7.0
"twist," "lambada"		8.0	8.4	8.9	9.4	9.9	10.4	10.9	11.4
modern		3.4	3.6	3.8	4.0	4.3	4.5	4.7	4.9
Digging trenches		6.8	7.3	7.7	8.1	8.6	9.0	9.4	9.9
Drawing (standing)		1.7	1.8	1.9	2.0	2.1	2.2	2.3	2.4
Eating (sitting)		1.1	1.2	1.2	1.3	1.4	1.4	1.5	1.6
Electrical work		2.7	2.9	3.1	3.2	3.4	3.6	3.8	3.9
Farming									
barn cleaning		6.3	6.8	7.2	7.6	8.0	8.4	8.8	9.2
driving harvester		1.9	2.0	2.1	2.2	2.4	2.5	2.6	2.7
driving tractor		1.8	1.9	2.0	2.1	2.2	2.3	2.4	2.5
feeding cattle		4.2	4.3	4.5	4.8	5.0	5.3	5.5	5.8
feeding animals		3.1	3.3	3.4	3.6	3.8	4.0	4.2	4.4
forking straw bales		6.7	6.9	7.3	7.7	8.1	8.6	9.0	9.4
milking by hand		2.5	2.7	2.9	3.0	3.2	3.3	3.5	3.7
milking by machine		1.1	1.2	1.2	1.3	1.4	1.4	1.5	1.6
shoveling grain		4.2	4.3	4.5	4.8	5.0	5.3	5.5	5.8
Fencing									
competition		7.2	7.6	8.1	8.5	9.0	9.4	9.9	10.8
practice		3.6	3.9	4.2	4.4	4.6	4.9	5.1	5.3
Field hockey		6.5	6.7	7.1	7.5	7.9	8.3	8.7	9.1
Fishing		3.0	3.1	3.3	3.5	3.7	3.8	4.0	4.2
Food shopping (F)		3.0	3.1	3.3	3.5	3.7	3.8	4.0	4.2
Football, competition		6.2	6.6	7.0	7.4	7.8	8.2	8.6	9.0
Forestry									
ax chopping, fast		14.0	14.9	15.7	16.6	17.5	18.4	19.3	20.2
ax chopping, slow		4.0	4.3	4.5	4.8	5.0	5.3	5.5	5.8
barking trees		5.8	6.2	6.5	6.9	7.3	7.6	8.0	8.4
carrying logs		8.7	9.3	9.9	10.4	11.0	11.5	12.1	12.6
felling trees		6.2	6.6	7.0	7.4	7.8	8.2	8.6	9.0
hoeing		4.2	4.6	4.8	5.1	5.4	5.6	5.9	6.2
planting by hand		5.1	5.5	5.8	6.1	6.4	6.8	7.1	7.4
sawing by hand		5.7	6.1	6.5	6.8	7.2	7.6	7.9	8.3
sawing, power		3.5	3.8	4.0	4.2	4.4	4.7	4.9	5.1
stacking firewood		4.2	4.4	4.7	4.9	5.2	5.5	5.7	6.0
trimming trees		6.1	6.5	6.8	7.2	7.6	8.0	8.4	8.8
weeding		3.4	3.6	3.8	4.0	4.2	4.5	4.7	4.9
Frisbee		4.7	5.0	5.3	5.5	5.9	6.2	6.4	6.8
Furriery		3.9	4.2	4.4	4.6	4.9	5.1	5.4	5.6

71	74	77	80	83	86	89	92	95	98
157	163	170	176	183	190	196	203	209	216
4.2	4.4	4.5	4.7	4.9	5.1	5.3	5.4	5.6	5.8
4.5	4.7	4.9	5.1	5.3	5.5	5.7	5.9	6.1	6.3
7.1	7.4	7.7	8.0	8.3	8.6	8.9	9.2	9.5	9.8
12.0	12.5	13.0	13.5	14.0	14.5	15.0	15.5	16.1	16.6
6.9	7.2	7.5	7.8	8.1	8.4	8.8	9.1	9.4	9.7
7.3	7.6	7.9	8.2	8.5	8.9	9.2	9.5	9.8	10.1
9.6	10.0	10.4	10.8	11.2	11.6	12.0	12.4	12.8	13.2
3.6	3.8	3.9	4.1	4.2	4.4	4.5	4.7	4.8	5.0
7.3	7.6	7.9	8.2	8.5	8.9	9.2	9.5	9.8	10.1
11.9	12.4	12.9	13.4	13.9	14.4	15.0	15.5	16.0	16.5
5.1	5.3	5.6	5.8	6.0	6.2	6.4	6.7	6.9	7.1
10.3	10.7	11.2	11.6	12.0	12.5	12.9	13.3	13.8	14.2
2.6	2.7	2.8	2.9	3.0	3.1	3.2	3.3	3.4	3.5
1.6	1.7	1.8	1.8	1.9	2.0	2.0	2.1	2.2	2.3
4.1	4.3	4.5	4.6	4.8	5.0	5.2	5.3	5.5	5.7
9.6	10.0	10.4	10.8	11.2	11.6	12.0	12.4	12.8	13.2
2.8	3.0	3.1	3.2	3.3	3.4	3.6	3.7	3.8	3.9
2.6	2.7	2.8	3.0	3.1	3.2	3.3	3.4	3.5	3.6
6.0	6.3	6.5	6.8	7.1	7.3	7.6	7.8	8.1	8.3
4.6	4.8	5.0	5.2	5.4	5.6	5.8	6.0	6.2	6.4
9.8	10.2	10.6	11.0	11.5	11.9	12.3	12.7	13.1	13.5
3.8	4.0	4.2	4.3	4.5	4.6	4.8	5.0	5.1	5.3
1.6	1.7	1.8	1.8	1.9	2.0	2.0	2.1	2.2	2.3
6.0	6.3	6.5	6.8	7.1	7.3	7.6	7.8	8.1	8.3
11.2	11.7	12.1	12.6	13.1	13.5	14.0	14.4	14.9	15.5
5.6	5.8	6.1	6.3	6.5	6.8	7.0	7.2	7.4	7.7
9.5	9.9	10.3	10.7	11.1	11.5	11.9	12.3	12.7	13.1
4.4	4.6	4.8	5.0	5.1	5.3	5.5	5.7	5.9	6.1
4.4	4.6	4.8	5.0	5.1	5.3	5.5	5.7	5.9	6.1
9.4	9.8	10.2	10.6	11.0	11.4	11.7	12.1	12.5	12.9
21.1	22.0	22.9	23.8	24.7	25.5	26.4	27.3	28.2	29.1
6.0	6.3	6.5	6.8	7.1	7.3	7.6	7.8	8.1	8.3
8.7	9.1	9.5	9.8	10.2	10.6	10.9	11.3	11.7	12.1
13.2	13.8	14.3	14.9	15.4	16.0	16.6	17.1	17.7	18.2
9.4	9.8	10.2	10.6	11.0	11.4	11.7	12.1	12.5	12.9
6.5	6.7	7.0	7.3	7.6	7.8	8.1	8.4	8.6	8.9
7.7	8.1	8.4	8.7	9.0	9.4	9.7	10.0	10.4	10.7
8.7	9.0	9.4	9.8	10.1	10.5	10.9	11.2	11.6	12.0
5.3	5.6	5.8	6.0	6.2	6.5	6.7	6.9	7.1	7.4
6.2	6.5	6.8	7.0	7.3	7.6	7.8	8.1	8.4	8.6
9.2	9.5	9.9	10.3	10.7	11.1	11.5	11.9	12.3	12.6
5.1	5.3	5.5	5.8	6.0	6.2	6.4	6.6	6.8	7.1
7.1	7.4	7.7	8.0	8.2	8.5	8.8	9.1	9.4	9.7
5.9	6.1	6.4	6.6	6.9	7.1	7.4	7.6	7.9	8.1

YOUR BODY WEIGHT—*continued*

Activity	kg lb	47 104	50 110	53 117	56 123	59 130	62 137	65 143	68 150
Gardening									
digging		5.9	6.3	6.7	7.1	7.4	7.8	8.2	8.6
hedging		3.3	3.9	4.1	4.3	4.5	4.8	5.0	5.2
mowing		5.3	5.6	5.9	6.3	6.6	6.9	7.3	7.6
raking		2.5	2.7	2.9	3.0	3.2	3.3	3.5	3.7
Golf		4.0	4.3	4.5	4.8	5.0	5.3	5.5	5.8
Gymnastics		3.0	3.3	3.5	3.7	3.9	4.1	4.3	4.5
Handball		6.9	7.2	7.7	8.1	8.5	9.0	9.4	9.8
orse-grooming		6.0	6.4	6.8	7.2	7.6	7.9	8.3	8.7
Horseback riding									
galloping		6.4	6.9	7.3	7.7	8.1	8.5	8.9	9.3
trotting		5.2	5.5	5.8	6.2	6.5	6.8	7.2	7.5
walking		1.9	2.1	2.2	2.3	2.4	2.5	2.7	2.8
Horseshoes		3.3	3.4	3.5	3.7	3.9	4.1	4.3	4.5
Housework									
mopping floors		2.8	3.1	3.3	3.5	3.7	3.8	4.0	4.2
dusting		3.0	3.3	3.4	3.6	3.8	4.0	4.2	4.4
laundry		3.1	3.4	3.5	3.7	3.9	4.1	4.3	4.5
washing windows		3.2	3.5	3.6	3.8	4.0	4.2	4.4	4.6
vacuuming		3.0	3.3	3.4	3.6	3.8	4.0	4.2	4.4
Hunting		4.1	4.4	4.7	4.9	5.2	5.5	5.7	6.0
Ice hockey		7.4	7.7	8.2	8.6	9.1	9.6	10.0	10.5
Ironing clothes		1.6	1.7	1.7	1.8	1.9	2.0	2.1	2.2
Judo		9.2	9.8	10.3	10.9	11.5	12.1	12.7	13.3
Jumping rope									
70 per min		7.6	8.1	8.6	9.1	9.6	10.0	10.5	11.0
80 per min		7.7	8.2	8.7	9.2	9.7	10.2	10.7	11.2
125 per min		8.3	8.9	9.4	9.9	10.4	11.0	11.5	12.0
145 per min		9.3	9.9	10.4	11.0	11.6	12.2	12.8	13.4
Karate		9.5	9.8	10.3	10.9	11.5	12.1	12.7	13.3
Kendo		9.3	9.7	10.2	10.8	11.4	12.0	12.6	13.2
Knitting, sewing		1.1	1.1	1.2	1.2	1.3	1.4	1.4	1.5
Lacrosse		7.0	7.4	7.9	8.3	8.7	9.2	9.6	10.1
Locksmith		2.8	2.9	3.0	3.2	3.4	3.5	3.7	3.9
Lying at ease		1.0	1.1	1.2	1.2	1.3	1.4	1.4	1.5
Machine-tooling									
machining		2.3	2.4	2.5	2.7	2.8	3.0	3.1	3.3
operating lathe		2.5	2.6	2.8	2.9	3.1	3.2	3.4	3.5
operating punch press		4.2	4.4	4.7	4.9	5.2	5.5	5.7	6.0
tapping and drilling		3.2	3.3	3.4	3.6	3.8	4.0	4.2	4.4
welding		2.4	2.6	2.8	2.9	3.1	3.2	3.4	3.5
working sheet metal		2.3	2.4	2.5	2.7	2.8	3.0	3.1	3.3
Marching, rapid		6.7	7.1	7.5	8.0	8.4	8.8	9.2	9.7
Mountain climbing		7.4	7.9	8.4	8.9	9.4	9.9	10.3	10.8
Motorcycle riding		6.5	6.9	7.3	7.7	8.1	8.5	8.9	9.3

| 71 | 74 | 77 | 80 | 83 | 86 | 89 | 92 | 95 | 98 |
157	163	170	176	183	190	196	203	209	216
8.9	9.3	9.7	10.1	10.5	10.8	11.2	11.6	12.0	12.3
5.5	5.7	5.9	6.2	6.4	6.6	6.9	7.1	7.3	7.5
8.0	8.3	8.6	9.0	9.3	9.6	10.0	10.3	10.6	11.0
3.8	4.0	4.2	4.3	4.5	4.6	4.8	5.0	5.1	5.3
6.0	6.3	6.5	6.8	7.1	7.3	7.6	7.8	8.1	8.3
4.7	4.9	5.1	5.3	5.5	5.7	5.9	6.1	6.3	6.5
10.3	10.7	11.2	11.5	12.0	12.5	12.9	13.3	13.7	14.2
9.1	9.5	9.9	10.2	10.6	11.0	11.4	11.8	12.2	12.5
9.7	10.1	10.6	11.0	11.4	11.8	12.2	12.6	13.0	13.4
7.8	8.1	8.5	8.8	9.1	9.5	9.8	10.1	10.5	10.8
2.9	3.0	3.2	3.3	3.4	3.5	3.6	3.8	3.9	4.0
4.7	4.9	5.1	5.3	5.5	5.7	5.9	6.1	6.3	6.5
4.4	4.6	4.8	5.0	5.2	5.4	5.6	5.8	6.0	6.2
4.6	4.7	4.9	5.1	5.3	5.5	5.7	5.9	6.1	6.3
4.7	4.9	5.1	5.3	5.5	5.7	5.9	6.1	6.3	6.5
4.8	5.0	5.2	5.4	5.6	5.8	6.0	6.2	6.4	6.6
4.6	4.8	5.0	5.2	5.4	5.6	5.8	6.0	6.2	6.4
6.2	6.5	6.7	7.0	7.2	7.5	7.8	8.0	8.2	8.5
11.0	11.5	12.0	12.5	13.1	13.6	14.1	14.6	15.1	15.7
2.3	2.4	2.5	2.6	2.7	2.8	2.9	3.0	3.1	3.2
13.8	14.4	15.0	15.6	16.2	16.8	17.4	17.9	18.5	19.1
11.5	12.0	12.5	13.0	13.4	13.9	14.4	14.9	15.4	15.9
11.6	12.1	12.6	13.1	13.6	14.1	14.6	14.6	15.6	16.1
12.6	13.1	13.6	14.2	14.7	15.2	15.8	16.3	16.8	17.3
14.0	14.6	15.2	15.8	16.4	16.9	17.5	18.1	18.7	19.3
13.8	14.4	15.0	15.6	16.2	16.8	17.4	17.9	18.5	19.1
13.7	14.3	14.9	15.5	16.1	16.7	17.3	17.8	18.4	19.0
1.6	1.6	1.7	1.8	1.8	1.9	2.0	2.0	2.1	2.2
10.4	10.7	11.0	11.2	11.5	11.8	12.1	12.4	12.7	13.0
4.0	4.2	4.4	4.6	4.7	4.9	5.1	5.2	5.4	5.6
1.6	1.6	1.7	1.8	1.8	1.9	2.0	2.0	2.1	2.2
3.4	3.6	3.7	3.8	4.0	4.1	4.3	4.4	4.6	4.7
3.7	3.8	4.0	4.2	4.3	4.5	4.6	4.8	4.9	5.1
6.2	6.5	6.8	7.0	7.3	7.6	7.8	8.1	8.4	8.6
4.6	4.8	5.0	5.2	5.4	5.6	5.8	6.0	6.2	6.4
3.7	3.8	4.0	4.2	4.3	4.5	4.6	4.8	4.9	5.1
3.4	3.6	3.7	3.8	4.0	4.1	4.3	4.4	4.6	4.7
10.1	10.5	10.9	11.4	11.8	12.2	12.6	13.1	13.5	13.9
11.3	11.7	12.2	12.7	13.2	13.7	14.1	14.6	15.0	15.6
9.7	10.1	10.5	10.9	11.3	11.7	12.1	12.5	12.9	13.3

YOUR BODY WEIGHT—*continued*

Activity	kg lb	47 104	50 110	53 117	56 123	59 130	62 137	65 143	68 150
Music playing									
accordion (sitting)		1.5	1.6	1.7	1.8	1.9	2.0	2.1	2.2
cello (sitting)		2.0	2.1	2.2	2.3	2.4	2.5	2.7	2.8
conducting		1.9	2.0	2.1	2.2	2.3	2.4	2.5	2.7
drums (sitting)		3.1	3.3	3.5	3.7	3.9	4.1	4.3	4.5
flute (sitting)		1.7	1.8	1.9	2.0	2.1	2.2	2.3	2.4
horn (sitting)		1.4	1.5	1.5	1.6	1.7	1.8	1.9	2.0
organ (sitting)		2.6	2.7	2.8	3.0	3.1	3.3	3.4	3.6
piano (sitting)		1.9	2.0	2.1	2.2	2.4	2.5	2.6	2.7
trumpet (standing)		1.5	1.6	1.6	1.7	1.8	1.9	2.0	2.1
violin (sitting)		2.2	2.3	2.4	2.5	2.7	2.8	2.9	3.1
woodwind (sitting)		1.5	1.6	1.7	1.8	1.9	2.0	2.1	2.2
Paddleball		8.5	8.9	9.4	10.0	10.5	11.0	11.6	12.1
Paddle tennis		8.4	8.6	9.1	9.6	10.1	10.7	11.1	11.7
Painting									
inside projects		1.6	1.7	1.8	1.9	2.0	2.1	2.2	2.3
outside projects		3.7	3.9	4.1	4.3	4.5	4.8	5.0	5.2
scraping		3.1	3.2	3.3	3.5	3.7	3.9	4.1	4.3
Planting seedings		3.3	3.5	3.7	3.9	4.1	4.3	4.6	4.8
Plastering		3.7	3.9	4.1	4.4	4.6	4.8	5.1	5.3
Printing press work		1.7	1.8	1.9	2.0	2.1	2.2	2.3	2.4
Racquetball		8.4	8.9	9.4	10.0	10.5	11.0	11.6	12.1
Roller skating, leisure		5.3	5.8	6.2	6.5	6.9	7.3	7.3	8.0
Rope jumping									
110 rpm		6.7	7.1	7.5	7.9	8.4	8.8	9.2	9.7
120 rpm		6.4	6.8	7.3	7.7	8.1	8.5	8.9	9.3
130 rpm		6.0	6.4	6.8	7.1	7.5	7.7	8.3	8.7
Rowing									
machine, moderate		5.7	6.0	6.3	6.7	7.0	7.4	7.7	8.1
machine, race pace		8.6	8.9	9.4	10.0	10.5	11.0	11.6	12.1
skull, leisure		4.7	5.0	5.3	5.5	5.9	6.2	6.4	6.8
skull, race pace		8.7	8.9	9.4	10.0	10.5	11.0	11.6	12.1
Running, cross-country		7.8	8.2	8.6	9.1	9.6	10.1	10.6	11.1
Running, on flat surface									
11 min, 30 s per mile		6.3	6.8	7.2	7.6	8.0	8.4	8.8	9.2
9 min per mile		9.1	9.7	10.2	10.8	11.4	12.0	12.5	13.1
8 min per mile		9.8	10.8	11.3	11.9	12.5	13.1	13.6	14.2
7 min per mile		10.7	12.2	12.7	13.3	13.9	14.5	15.0	15.6
6 min per mile		11.8	13.9	14.4	15.0	15.6	16.2	16.7	17.3
5 min, 30 s per mile		13.6	14.5	15.3	16.2	17.1	17.9	18.8	19.7
Sailing, leisure		2.1	2.2	2.3	2.5	2.6	2.7	2.9	3.0
Scrubbing floors		5.1	5.5	5.8	6.1	6.4	6.8	7.1	7.4
Scuba diving		10.9	11.2	11.5	11.8	12.1	12.4	12.7	13.0
Shoe repair, general		2.2	2.3	2.4	2.5	2.7	2.8	2.9	3.1
Sitting quietly		1.0	1.1	1.1	1.2	1.2	1.3	1.4	1.4
Skateboarding		5.6	5.8	6.2	6.5	6.9	7.2	7.5	7.9
Skiing, hard snow									
level, moderate speed		5.6	6.0	6.3	6.7	7.0	7.4	7.7	8.1
level, walking speed		6.7	7.2	7.6	8.0	8.4	8.9	9.3	9.7
uphill, "fast" speed		12.9	13.7	14.5	15.3	16.2	17.0	17.8	18.6

| 71 | 74 | 77 | 80 | 83 | 86 | 89 | 92 | 95 | 98 |
157	163	170	176	183	190	196	203	209	216
2.3	2.4	2.5	2.6	2.7	2.8	2.8	2.9	3.0	3.1
2.9	3.0	3.2	3.3	3.4	3.5	3.6	3.8	3.9	4.0
2.8	2.9	3.0	3.1	3.2	3.4	3.5	3.6	3.7	3.8
4.7	4.9	5.1	5.3	5.5	5.7	5.9	6.1	6.3	6.6
2.5	2.6	2.7	2.8	2.9	3.0	3.1	3.2	3.3	3.4
2.1	2.1	2.2	2.3	2.4	2.5	2.6	2.7	2.8	2.8
3.8	3.9	4.1	4.2	4.4	4.6	4.7	4.9	5.0	5.2
2.8	3.0	3.1	3.2	3.3	3.4	3.6	3.7	3.8	3.9
2.2	2.3	2.4	2.5	2.6	2.7	2.8	2.9	2.9	3.0
3.2	3.3	3.5	3.6	3.7	3.9	4.0	4.1	4.3	4.4
2.3	2.4	2.5	2.6	2.7	2.8	2.8	2.9	3.0	3.1
12.6	13.2	13.7	14.2	14.8	15.3	15.8	16.4	16.9	17.4
12.2	12.7	13.2	13.7	14.2	14.2	15.2	15.8	16.3	16.8
2.4	2.5	2.6	2.7	2.8	2.9	3.0	3.1	3.2	3.3
5.5	5.7	5.9	6.2	6.4	6.6	6.9	7.1	7.3	7.5
4.5	4.7	4.9	5.0	5.2	5.4	5.6	5.8	6.0	6.2
5.0	5.2	5.4	5.6	5.8	6.0	6.2	6.4	6.7	6.9
5.5	5.8	6.0	6.2	6.5	6.7	6.9	7.2	7.4	7.6
2.5	2.6	2.7	2.8	2.9	3.0	3.1	3.2	3.3	3.4
12.6	13.2	13.7	14.2	14.8	15.3	15.8	16.4	16.9	17.4
8.3	8.6	9.0	9.3	9.7	10.1	10.4	10.8	11.1	11.4
10.1	10.5	10.5	11.3	11.8	12.2	12.6	13.1	13.5	13.9
9.8	10.1	10.6	10.9	11.4	11.8	12.2	12.6	13.0	13.4
9.1	9.4	9.8	10.2	10.6	11.0	11.3	11.7	12.1	12.5
8.5	8.9	9.3	9.7	10.1	10.6	11.1	11.6	12.1	12.6
12.6	13.2	13.7	14.2	14.8	15.3	15.8	16.4	16.9	17.4
7.2	7.6	8.0	8.4	8.8	9.2	9.6	10.0	10.4	10.8
12.6	13.2	13.7	14.2	14.8	15.3	15.8	16.4	16.9	17.4
11.6	12.1	12.6	13.0	13.5	14.0	14.5	15.0	15.5	16.0
9.6	10.0	10.5	10.9	11.3	11.7	12.1	12.5	12.9	13.3
13.7	14.3	14.9	15.4	16.0	16.6	17.2	17.8	18.3	18.9
14.8	15.4	16.0	16.5	17.1	17.7	18.3	18.9	19.4	20.0
16.2	16.8	17.4	17.9	18.5	19.1	19.7	20.3	20.8	21.4
17.9	18.5	19.1	19.6	20.2	20.8	21.4	22.0	22.5	23.1
20.5	21.4	22.3	23.1	24.0	24.9	25.7	26.6	27.5	28.3
3.1	3.3	3.4	3.5	3.7	3.8	3.9	4.1	4.2	4.3
7.7	8.1	8.4	8.7	9.0	9.4	9.7	10.0	10.4	10.7
13.3	13.6	13.9	14.2	14.5	14.8	15.1	15.4	15.7	16.0
3.2	3.3	3.5	3.6	3.7	3.9	4.0	4.1	4.3	4.4
1.5	1.6	1.6	1.7	1.7	1.8	1.9	1.9	2.0	2.1
8.3	8.6	8.9	9.3	9.6	10.0	10.3	10.7	11.0	11.4
8.4	8.8	9.2	9.5	9.9	10.2	10.6	10.9	11.3	11.7
10.2	10.6	11.0	11.4	11.9	12.3	12.7	13.2	13.6	14.0
19.5	20.3	21.1	21.9	22.7	23.6	24.4	25.2	26.0	26.9

YOUR BODY WEIGHT—*continued*

Activity	kg / lb	47 / 104	50 / 110	53 / 117	56 / 123	59 / 130	62 / 137	65 / 143	68 / 150
Skiing, soft snow									
leisure (F)		4.6	4.9	5.2	5.5	5.8	6.1	6.4	6.7
leisure (M)		5.2	5.6	5.9	6.2	6.5	6.9	7.2	7.5
Skindiving									
considerable motion		13.0	13.8	14.6	15.5	16.3	17.1	17.9	18.8
moderate motion		9.7	10.3	10.9	11.5	12.2	12.8	13.4	14.0
Snorkeling		4.3	4.6	4.9	5.2	5.5	5.8	6.0	6.3
Snowshoeing, soft snow		7.8	8.3	8.8	9.3	9.8	10.3	10.8	11.3
Snowmobiling		3.4	3.7	4.0	4.2	4.4	4.7	4.9	5.1
Soccer		6.5	6.8	7.3	7.7	8.1	8.5	8.9	9.3
Softball		3.3	3.5	3.7	3.9	4.1	4.3	4.5	4.7
Squash		10.0	10.6	11.2	11.9	12.5	13.1	13.8	14.4
Standing quietly (M)		1.3	1.4	1.4	1.5	1.6	1.7	1.8	1.8
Steel mill, working in									
fettling		4.3	4.5	4.7	5.0	5.3	5.5	5.8	6.1
forging		4.7	5.0	5.3	5.6	5.9	6.2	6.5	6.8
hand rolling		6.4	6.9	7.3	7.7	8.1	8.5	8.9	9.3
merchant mill rolling		6.8	7.3	7.7	8.1	8.6	9.0	9.4	9.9
removing slag		8.4	8.9	9.4	10.0	10.5	11.0	11.6	12.1
tending furnace		5.9	6.3	6.7	7.1	7.4	7.8	8.2	8.6
tipping molds		4.3	4.6	4.9	5.2	5.4	5.7	6.0	6.3
Surfing		3.9	4.1	4.3	4.5	4.8	5.0	5.3	5.5
Stock clerking		2.5	2.7	2.9	3.0	3.2	3.3	3.5	3.7
Swimming, fitness swims									
back stroke		7.9	8.5	9.0	9.5	10.0	10.5	11.0	11.5
breast stroke		7.6	8.1	8.6	9.1	9.6	10.0	10.5	11.0
butterfly			8.6	9.1	9.6	10.1	10.7	11.1	11.7
crawl, fast		7.3	7.8	8.3	8.7	9.2	9.7	10.1	10.6
crawl, slow		6.0	6.4	6.8	7.2	7.6	7.9	8.3	8.7
side stroke		5.7	6.1	6.5	6.8	7.2	7.6	7.9	8.3
treading, fast		8.0	8.5	9.0	9.5	10.0	10.5	11.1	11.6
treading, normal		2.9	3.1	3.3	3.5	3.7	3.8	4.0	4.2
Table tennis (ping pong)		3.2	3.4	3.6	3.8	4.0	4.2	4.4	4.6
Tailoring									
cutting		2.0	2.1	2.2	2.3	2.4	2.5	2.7	2.8
hand-sewing		1.5	1.6	1.7	1.8	1.9	2.0	2.1	2.2
machine-sewing		2.2	2.3	2.4	2.5	2.7	2.8	2.9	3.1
pressing		2.9	3.1	3.3	3.5	3.7	3.8	4.0	4.2
Tennis									
competition		6.9	7.3	7.8	8.2	8.7	9.1	9.5	9.9
recreational		5.1	5.5	5.8	6.1	6.4	6.8	7.1	7.4
Typing									
electric (computer)		1.3	1.4	1.4	1.5	1.6	1.7	1.8	1.8
manual		1.5	1.6	1.6	1.7	1.8	1.9	2.0	2.1
Volleyball									
competition		5.9	7.3	7.8	8.2	8.7	9.1	9.5	10.0
recreational		2.4	2.5	2.7	2.8	3.0	3.1	3.3	3.4

| 71 | 74 | 77 | 80 | 83 | 86 | 89 | 92 | 95 | 98 |
157	163	170	176	183	190	196	203	209	216
7.0	7.3	7.5	7.8	8.1	8.4	8.7	9.0	9.3	9.6
7.9	8.2	8.5	8.9	9.2	9.5	9.9	10.2	10.5	10.9
19.6	20.4	21.3	22.1	22.9	23.7	24.6	25.4	26.2	27.0
14.6	15.2	15.9	16.5	17.1	17.7	18.3	19.0	19.6	20.2
6.6	6.8	7.1	7.4	7.7	8.0	8.2	8.5	8.8	9.1
11.8	12.3	12.8	13.3	13.8	14.3	14.8	15.3	15.8	16.3
5.3	5.5	5.8	6.0	6.2	6.5	6.7	6.9	7.1	7.3
9.8	10.1	10.6	10.9	11.4	11.8	12.2	12.6	13.0	13.4
4.9	5.1	5.3	5.5	5.7	5.9	6.1	6.3	6.5	6.7
15.1	15.7	16.3	17.0	17.6	18.2	18.9	19.5	20.1	20.8
1.9	2.0	2.1	2.2	2.2	2.3	2.4	2.5	2.6	2.6
6.3	6.6	6.9	7.1	7.4	7.7	7.9	8.2	8.5	8.7
7.1	7.4	7.7	8.0	8.3	8.6	8.9	9.2	9.5	9.8
9.7	10.1	10.6	11.0	11.4	11.8	12.2	12.6	13.0	13.4
10.3	10.7	11.2	11.6	12.0	12.5	12.9	13.3	13.8	14.2
12.6	13.2	13.7	14.2	14.8	15.3	15.8	16.4	16.9	17.4
8.9	9.3	9.7	10.1	10.5	10.8	11.2	11.6	12.0	12.3
6.5	6.8	7.1	7.4	7.6	7.9	8.2	8.5	8.7	9.0
5.7	6.0	6.3	6.5	6.8	7.0	7.2	7.4	7.6	7.9
3.8	4.0	4.2	4.3	4.5	4.6	4.8	5.0	5.1	5.3
12.0	12.5	13.0	13.5	14.0	14.5	15.0	15.5	16.1	16.6
11.5	12.0	12.5	13.0	13.4	13.9	14.4	14.9	15.4	15.9
12.2	12.7	13.2	13.7	14.2	14.2	15.2	15.8	16.3	16.8
11.1	11.5	12.0	12.5	12.9	13.4	13.9	14.4	14.8	15.3
9.1	9.5	9.9	10.2	10.6	11.0	11.4	11.8	12.2	12.5
8.7	9.0	9.4	9.8	10.1	10.5	10.9	11.2	11.6	12.0
12.1	12.6	13.1	13.6	14.1	14.6	15.1	15.6	16.2	16.7
4.4	4.6	4.8	5.0	5.1	5.3	5.5	5.7	5.9	6.1
4.8	5.0	5.2	5.4	5.6	5.8	6.1	6.3	6.5	6.7
2.9	3.0	3.2	3.3	3.4	3.5	3.6	3.8	3.9	4.0
2.3	2.4	2.5	2.6	2.7	2.8	2.8	2.9	3.0	3.1
3.2	3.3	3.5	3.6	3.7	3.9	4.0	4.1	4.3	4.4
4.4	4.6	4.8	5.0	5.1	5.3	5.5	5.7	5.9	6.1
10.2	10.6	11.1	11.5	11.9	12.4	12.8	13.2	13.7	14.1
7.7	8.1	8.4	8.7	9.0	9.4	9.7	10.0	10.4	10.7
1.9	2.0	2.1	2.2	2.2	2.3	2.4	2.5	2.6	2.6
2.2	2.3	2.4	2.5	2.6	2.7	2.8	2.9	2.9	3.0
3.6	3.7	3.9	4.0	4.2	4.3	4.5	4.6	4.8	4.9
10.5	10.9	11.4	11.8	12.3	12.7	13.1	13.6	14.0	14.5

YOUR BODY WEIGHT—*continued*

Activity	kg lb	47 104	50 110	53 117	56 123	59 130	62 137	65 143	68 150
Walking, leisure outdoors									
asphalt road		3.8	4.0	4.2	4.5	4.7	5.0	5.2	5.4
fields and hillsides		3.9	4.1	4.3	4.6	4.8	5.1	5.3	5.6
grass track		3.8	4.1	4.3	4.5	4.8	5.0	5.3	5.5
plowed field		3.6	3.9	4.1	4.3	4.5	4.8	5.0	5.2
Walking, treadmill level									
2.0 mph		2.4	2.6	2.8	3.0	3.1	3.3	3.4	3.6
2.5 mph		3.0	3.2	3.4	3.6	3.8	4.0	4.2	4.4
3.0 mph		3.6	3.8	4.0	4.2	4.4	4.6	4.8	5.0
3.5 mph		4.0	4.3	4.6	4.8	5.1	5.3	5.6	6.1
4.0 mph		4.6	4.9	5.2	5.4	5.7	6.0	6.3	6.6
Wallpapering		2.3	2.4	2.5	2.7	2.8	3.0	3.1	3.3
Water polo, recreation		7.0	7.4	7.7	8.1	8.5	8.9	9.3	9.7
Water polo, competition		9.4	9.9	10.4	11.0	11.5	12.0	12.5	13.1
Water-skiing		5.6	6.0	6.4	6.7	7.1	7.5	7.8	8.2
Watch repairing		1.2	1.3	1.3	1.4	1.5	1.6	1.6	1.7
Whitewater rafting, recreational		4.1	4.4	4.6	4.9	5.2	5.4	5.7	6.0
Window cleaning		2.9	3.0	3.1	3.3	3.5	3.7	3.8	4.0
Wind surfing		3.3	3.5	3.7	3.9	4.1	4.3	4.6	4.8
Wrestling, competition		9.1	9.7	10.3	10.8	11.4	12.0	12.6	13.2
Writing (sitting)		1.4	1.5	1.5	1.6	1.7	1.8	1.9	2.0
Yoga		2.9	3.1	3.3	3.5	3.7	3.8	4.0	4.2

| 71 | 74 | 77 | 80 | 83 | 86 | 89 | 92 | 95 | 98 |
157	163	170	176	183	190	196	203	209	216
5.7	5.9	6.2	6.4	6.6	6.9	7.1	7.4	7.6	7.8
5.8	6.1	6.3	6.6	6.8	7.1	7.3	7.5	7.8	8.0
5.8	6.0	6.2	6.5	6.7	7.0	7.2	7.5	7.7	7.9
5.5	5.7	5.9	6.2	6.4	6.6	6.9	7.1	7.3	7.5
3.7	3.9	4.1	4.2	4.4	4.5	4.7	4.9	5.0	5.2
4.5	4.7	4.9	5.1	5.3	5.5	5.7	5.9	6.1	6.3
5.3	5.5	5.7	5.9	6.2	6.5	6.7	6.9	7.1	7.3
6.1	6.4	6.6	6.9	7.1	7.4	7.7	7.9	8.2	8.4
6.9	7.2	7.5	7.8	8.1	8.4	8.7	8.9	9.2	9.5
3.4	3.6	3.7	3.8	4.0	4.1	4.3	4.4	4.6	4.7
10.1	10.5	10.9	11.3	11.7	12.1	12.5	12.9	13.3	13.7
13.6	14.1	14.7	15.2	15.7	16.3	16.8	17.3	17.9	18.4
8.7	9.1	9.4	9.8	10.1	10.5	10.9	11.2	11.6	12.0
1.8	1.9	1.9	2.0	2.1	2.2	2.2	2.3	2.4	2.5
6.2	6.5	6.7	7.0	7.3	7.5	7.8	8.1	8.3	8.6
4.2	4.4	4.5	4.7	4.9	5.1	5.3	5.4	5.6	5.8
5.0	5.2	5.4	5.6	5.8	6.0	6.2	6.4	6.7	6.9
13.8	14.3	14.9	15.5	16.1	16.7	17.2	17.8	18.4	19.0
2.1	2.1	2.2	2.3	2.4	2.5	2.6	2.7	2.8	2.8
4.4	4.6	4.8	5.0	5.1	5.3	5.5	5.7	5.9	6.1

Assessment of Energy and Nutrient Intake: Three-Day Dietary Survey

The three-day dietary survey represents a relatively simple yet accurate method to determine the nutritional quality and total calories of food consumed daily. The key to successfully accomplish these goals requires a daily log of food intake for three days that represent your normal eating pattern (including at least one weekend).

Experiments have shown that calculations of caloric intake made from records of daily food consumption are usually within 10% of the number of calories actually consumed. For example, suppose a bomb calorimeter determined that your daily food intake equaled 2130 kcal. If you kept a three-day dietary history and estimated your calorie intake, the daily value would likely be within 10% of the actual value (1920 and 2350 kcal).

Use four items to measure food: (1) plastic ruler, (2) standard measuring cup, (3) measuring spoons, and (4) balance or weighing scale. Use the Nutritionist Pro™ CD that comes with this text, Appendix A, or consult one of several sources that list the nutritional content of foods including: Pennington JAT, Douglass JP. Bowes & Church's food values of portions commonly used. 18th ed. Baltimore: Lippincott Williams & Wilkins, 2005. You may also wish to consult the following URL: http://nat.crgq.com/mainnat.html.

Measure or weight each of the food items in your diet. This represents the only reliable way to obtain an accurate estimate of the size of a food portion. Be sure to do the following:

- List specific types, brands, and method of preparation.

Example	List as:
Milk	8 fl oz, 2% milk
1/2 chicken breast	3 oz breast, baked, without skin
Margarine	1 tsp. Fleishmann's Light Margarine

- Use these guidelines to estimate cooked portion sizes for these food categories:

  Meat and Fish
  Measure the portion of meat or fish by thickness, length, and width, or record weight on the scale.

  Vegetables, Potatoes, Rice, Cereals, Salads
  Measure the portion in a measuring cup or record weight on the scale.

  Cream or Sugar Added to Coffee or Tea
  Measure with measuring spoons before adding to the drink, or record weight on the scale.

  Fluids and Bottled Drinks
  Check the labels for volume or empty the container into the measuring cup. If you weigh the fluid, be sure to subtract the weight of the cup or glass. Sugar-free soft drinks usually have kcal values listed on their labels.

  Cookies, Cakes, Pies
  Measure the diameter and thickness with a ruler, or weigh on the scale. Evaluate frosting or sauces separately.

  Fruits
  Cut them in half before eating and measure the diameters, or weight them on the scale. For fruits that must be peeled or have rinds or cores, be sure to subtract the weight of the non-edible portion from the total weight of the food. Do this for items such as oranges, apples, and bananas.

Jam, Salad Dressing, Catsup, Mayonnaise
Measure the condiment with the measuring spoon or weigh the portion on the scale.

Record all the foods you consume using the blank 3-day food logs on the pages of this appendix. We encourage you to keep the sheets with you and record the pertinent information about the foods as you consume them.

DIRECTIONS FOR COMPUTING YOUR THREE-DAY DIETARY SURVEY

Step 1. Prepare a table (similar to Table C.1) indicating the intake of food items during a day. Include the amount (g or oz); caloric value; and carbohydrate, lipid, and protein content; the minerals Ca and Fe; and vitamins C, B1 (thiamine), and B2 (riboflavin); fiber; and cholesterol.

Step 2. List each food you consume for breakfast, lunch, dinner, between-meal eating, and snacks. Include food items that are used in preparing the meal (e.g., butter, oils, margarine, bread crumbs, egg coating, etc.).

Step 3. Weigh, measure or approximate the size of each portion of food that you eat. Record these values on your daily record chart (e.g., 3 oz of salad oil, 1/8 piece of 8″ diameter apple pie, etc.).

Step 4. Record your daily calorie and nutrient intake on a chart similar to Table C.1, which was recorded for a 21-year-old college student. Record the daily totals for the caloric and nutrient headings on the "Daily and Average Daily Summary Chart" (Table C.2). When you've completed your three-day survey, compute the three-day total by adding up the values for days 1, 2, and 3; then divide by 3 to determine the daily average of each nutrient category.

Step 5. Using each of the average daily nutrient values, calculate the percentage of the RDA consumed for that particular nutrient and graph your results as shown in Figure C.1 An example for calculating the percentage of the RDA is shown in Table C.3, along with the specific RDA values for men and women.

Step 6. Be as accurate and honest as possible. Do not include unusual or atypical days in your dietary survey (e.g., days that you are sick, special occasions such as birthdays, or eating out at restaurants unless that is normal for you).

Step 7. Remember that the protein RDA equals 0.8 g protein per kilogram of body mass (1 kg = 2.2 lb).

Step 8. Compute the percentage of your total calories supplied from carbohydrate, lipid, and protein.

> *For example, if total average daily caloric intake is 2450 kcal per day, and 1600 kcal are from carbohydrates, the daily percentage of total calories from carbohydrates equals:*
> *1600 ÷ 2450 × 100 = 65%*

Step 9. While there is no specific RDA for lipid or carbohydrate, a prudent recommendation is that lipid should not exceed more than 30% of your total caloric intake; for active men and women, carbohydrates should be approximately 60% of the total calories ingested. Thus, in computing the percentage of "RDA" for graphing purposes in Figure C.1, you should assume that:

a. "RDA" for lipid equals 30% of total calories
b. "RDA" for carbohydrate equals 60% of total calories

> *For example, if 50% of your average daily calories comes from lipid, you are taking in 167% of the recommended value ("RDA") for this nutrient: [50% divided by 30% (recommended percentage) × 100 = 167%]*

Step 10. As was the case for lipid and carbohydrate, no RDA exists for average daily caloric intake. Any recommendation for energy intake must consider body fat level and current daily energy expenditure. However, average values for daily caloric intake have been published for the typical young adult and equal about 2100 kcal for young women and 3000 kcal for young men. Thus, for graphing purposes in Figure C.1, you can evaluate your average daily caloric intake against the "average" values for your sex and age.

> *For example, if you are a 20-year-old female and you consume an average of 2400 kcal daily, your energy intake would equal 114% of the average ("RDA") for your age and sex. [2400 kcal divided by 2100 kcal (average) × 100 = 114%]. This does not mean that you need to go on a diet and reduce food intake to bring you in line with the average U.S. value. To the contrary, your higher-than-average caloric intake may be required to power your active lifestyle that contributes to maintaining a desirable body mass and body composition.*

If you eat a food item not listed in Appendix A, try to make an intelligent guess as to its composition and amount consumed. It is better to overestimate the amount of food consumed than to underestimate or to make no estimation at all. If you go to a restaurant for dinner, or to a friend's house where it may be inappropriate to measure the food, then omit this day from the counting procedure and resume record keeping the following day.

Record-keeping for 3 days is extremely important so an accurate appraisal can be made of the average daily energy and nutrient intake. **Be sure to record everything you eat.** If you are not completely honest, you are wasting your time. Most people find it easier to keep accurate records if they record food items while preparing a meal or immediately afterwards when eating snack items.

Table C.1   **SAMPLE ONE-DAY CALORIC AND NUTRIENT INTAKE FOR A 21-YEAR-OLD COLLEGE STUDENT**

Food Item	Amount	kcal	Protein (g)	CHO (g)	Lipid (g)	Ca (mg)	Fe (mg)	Fiber (g)	Cholesterol (mg)	Thiam[a] (mg)	Ribofl[a] (mg)
Breakfast											
Eggs, hard boiled	2 (2 oz ea)	160	14.1	1.4	11.2	55.2	1.9	0.0	452	0.06	0.53
Orange juice	8 oz	104	0.9	86.4	0.5	72.4	0.8	0.9	0.0	0.20	0.06
Corn flakes	1 cup/1 oz	110	2.3	24.4	0.5	1.0	1.8	0.6	0.0	0.37	0.42
Skim milk	8 oz	80	7.8	10.6	0.6	279.2	0.1	0.0	3.7	0.08	0.32
Snack											
None											
Lunch											
Tuna fish (oil pack)	2 oz	112	16.5	0.0	68.0	7.8	0.8	0.0	10.0	0.02	0.06
White bread (toast)	2 pieces	168	5.3	31.4	2.5	81.2	1.8	1.3	0.0	0.24	0.21
Mayonnaise	1 oz	203	0.3	0.8	22.6	5.7	0.2	0.0	16.8	0.01	0.01
Skim milk	8 oz	80	7.8	10.6	0.6	279.2	0.1	0.0	3.7	0.08	0.32
Plums	4 (2 oz ea)	128	1.8	29.5	1.4	10.3	0.2	4.4	0.0	0.10	0.22
Snack											
Chocolate milkshake	8 oz	288	7.7	46.4	8.4	256	0.7	0.3	29.6	0.13	0.55
Dinner											
Sirloin steak, lean	8 oz	456	64.8	0.0	20.2	18.6	5.8	0.0	173.6	0.21	0.47
French fries, veg. oil	6 oz	540	6.8	67.2	28.1	34.2	1.3	3.4	0.0	0.30	0.05
Cole slaw	4 oz	80	1.4	14.1	3.0	51.2	0.7	2.3	9.2	0.08	0.07
Italian bread	2 oz	156	5.1	32.0	1.0	9.4	1.5	0.9	0.0	0.23	0.13
Light beer	8 oz	96	0.6	8.8	0.0	11.2	0.1	0.5	0.0	0.02	0.06
Snack											
Yogurt, whole milk	6 oz	102	5.9	7.9	5.5	205.8	0.1	0.0	22.1	0.05	0.24
Daily Total		**2863**	**149.1**	**371.5**	**174.1**	**1378.4**	**17.2**	**14.6**	**720.7**	**2.18**	**3.72**

[a] Thiam, thiamin; Ribofl, riboflavin.

Table C.2 **DAILY AND AVERAGE SUMMARY CHART OF THE INTAKE OF CALORIES AND SPECIFIC FOOD NUTRIENTS**

Day	kcal	Protein[a] (g)	Lipid[a] (g)	CHO[a] (g)	Ca (mg)	Fe (mg)	Thiamine (mg)	Riboflavin (mg)	Fiber (g)	Cholesterol (mg)
#1										
#2										
#3										
Three-day total										
Average Daily Value[b]										

[a] Use the following caloric transformations to convert your average daily grams of carbohydrate (CHO), lipid, and protein to average daily calories:

1 g CHO = 4 kcal

1 g Lipid = 9 kcal

1 g Protein = 4 kcal

[b] Use the Average Daily Value to determine the percentage of the RDA for your graph. See Table 1 for sample calculations. Figure C.1 shows a bar graph for the nutrient values as a percentage of the average or recommended value for each item.

Table C.3 **RDA VALUES FOR SELECTED NUTRIENTS INCLUDING SAMPLE COMPUTATIONS FOR DERIVING THE PERCENTAGE OF RDA FROM YOUR DIETARY SURVEY. VALUES LISTED IN TABLE C.1 ARE 100% VALUES FOR GRAPHING YOUR DIETARY SURVEY**

					Men			
Age	kcal[a]	Protein (g/kg)	Ca (mg)	Fe (mg)	Thiamine (mg)	Riboflavin (mg)	Fiber[a] (g)	Cholesterol[a] (mg)
19–22	3000	0.8	1000	8	1.2	1.3	38	300
23–50	2700	0.8	1000	8	1.2	1.3	38	300

					Women			
Age	kcal[a]	Protein (g/kg)	Ca (mg)	Fe (mg)	Thiamine (mg)	Riboflavin (mg)	Fiber[a] (g)	Cholesterol[a] (mg)
19–22	2100	0.8	1000	18	1.1	1.1	25	300
23–50	2000	0.8	1000	18	1.1	1.1	25	300

Source: Recommended Dietary Allowances, Revised 1989, Washington, DC: Food and Nutrition Board, National Academy of Sciences-National Research Council, 1989.

[a] No RDA exists for daily caloric intake or for the intake of fiber or cholesterol. Values for caloric intake represent an average for adult Americans, while fiber and cholesterol values are recommended as being prudent for maintaining good health.

How to determine the percentage of the RDA from your dietary survey

Example #1: Percentage of RDA for protein for a 70-kg
person
  Daily protein intake = 68 g
  RDA = (70 kg × 0.8 g/kg) = 56 g
  % of RDA = 56/68 × 100 = 121%

Example #2: Percentage of RDA for iron (female)
  Daily iron intake = 7.5 mg
  RDA = 15 mg
  % of RDA = 7.5/15 × 100 = 50%

Figure C.1
Example of a bar graph to illustrate the food and nutrient intake expressed as a percentage of recommended values.

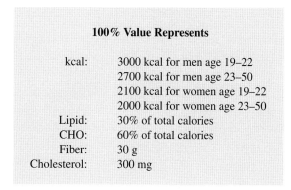

	100% Value Represents
kcal:	3000 kcal for men age 19–22
	2700 kcal for men age 23–50
	2100 kcal for women age 19–22
	2000 kcal for women age 23–50
Lipid:	30% of total calories
CHO:	60% of total calories
Fiber:	30 g
Cholesterol:	300 mg

Sample Food Record

Time	Place	Amount	Description (including preparation)	Comments/Questions
8 AM	Home	3/4 cup	Kellogg's Corn Flakes	Breakfast
		1/2 cup	Skim milk	
		1 large	Orange	
		8 fl. oz.	Coffee, black	
		2 tsp	White sugar	
11:30 AM	Away	1/2 cup	Tuna, water packed	Lunch
		2 Tbls	Mayonnaise, light	
		2 slices	White bread	
		1 cup	Campbell's tomato soup	
		4 rounds	Melba toast (crackers)	
		1 oz.	Potato chips, Lay's	
		1 piece	Apple pie	
3:00 PM	Away	1 large	Apple, red delicious	Snack
6:00 PM	Home	4 oz.	Chicken breast, baked, no skin	Dinner
		1 medium	Baked potato, flesh and skin	
		3 tsp	Light margarine	
		1 cup	Broccoli, steamed, plain	
		1 cup	Salad lettuce, romaine	
		3 whole	Cherry tomatoes	
		5 slices	Cucumber	1/4 inch each
		2 Tbls	Ranch dressing, regular	
		2 cups	Water	
8:30 PM	Home	3 cups	Popcorn, air popped, plain	Snack
		12 oz. can	Orange soda, regular	
		1	Donut, chocolate	Dunkin Donuts
10:00 PM		2 cups	Ice cream, chocolate	Rich but good
10:45 PM		4 oz.	Chocolate bar, regular	Hershey's
11:10 PM		1 large	Apple, Macintosh	
11:30 PM		6 oz.	Apple cider	Hot
11:35 PM		1 small	Cookie, chocolate chip	

3-Day Food Record				Day 1
Time	Place	Amount	Description (including preparation)	Comments/Questions

3-Day Food Record				Day 2
Time	Place	Amount	Description (including preparation)	Comments/Questions

3-Day Food Record				Day 3
Time	**Place**	**Amount**	**Description** (including preparation)	**Comments/Questions**

APPENDIX D

Body Composition Assessment[a]

This appendix contains the age- and sex-specific equations to predict body fat percentage based on three girth measurements. There are four charts, one each for young and older men and women. In our experience, it is important to calibrate the tape measure prior to its use. Use a meter stick as the standard and check the markings on the cloth tape at 10-cm increments. A cloth tape is preferred over a metal one because little skin compression occurs when applying a cloth tape to the skin's surface at a relatively constant tension.

To use the charts, measure the three girths at the sites indicated in Figure 13.11, which shows the anatomic landmarks. The specific equation to predict percentage body fat with its corresponding constant is presented at the bottom of each of the four charts (Charts 2 to 5).

CHART 1
BODY SITES MEASURED BY THE CIRCUMFERENCE METHOD

Age (years)	Sex	Site Measured		
		A	B	C
18–26	M	Right upper arm	Abdomen	Right forearm
	F	Abdomen	Right thigh	Right forearm
27–50	M	Buttocks	Abdomen	Right forearm
	F	Abdomen	Right thigh	Right calf

CHART 2
CONVERSION CONSTANTS TO PREDICT PERCENTAGE BODY FAT FOR YOUNG MEN

Upper Arm			Abdomen			Forearm		
in	cm	Constant A	in	cm	Constant B	in	cm	Constant C
7.00	17.78	25.91	21.00	53.34	27.56	7.00	17.78	38.01
7.25	18.41	26.83	21.25	53.97	27.88	7.25	18.41	39.37
7.50	19.05	27.76	21.50	54.61	28.21	7.50	19.05	40.72
7.75	19.68	28.68	21.75	55.24	28.54	7.75	19.68	42.08
8.00	20.32	29.61	22.00	55.88	28.87	8.00	20.32	43.44
8.25	20.95	30.53	22.25	56.51	29.20	8.25	20.95	44.80
8.50	21.59	31.46	22.50	57.15	29.52	8.50	21.59	46.15
8.75	22.22	32.38	22.75	57.78	29.85	8.75	22.22	47.51
9.00	22.86	33.31	23.00	58.42	30.18	9.00	22.86	48.87
9.25	23.49	34.24	23.25	59.05	30.51	9.25	23.49	50.23
9.50	24.13	35.16	23.50	59.69	30.84	9.50	24.13	51.58
9.75	24.76	36.09	23.75	60.32	31.16	9.75	24.76	52.94
10.00	25.40	37.01	24.00	60.96	31.49	10.00	25.40	54.30
10.25	26.03	37.94	24.25	61.59	31.82	10.25	26.03	55.65
10.50	26.67	38.86	24.50	62.23	32.15	10.50	26.67	57.01

CHART 2—*continued*

Upper Arm			Abdomen			Forearm		
in	*cm*	*Constant A*	*in*	*cm*	*Constant B*	*in*	*cm*	*Constant C*
10.75	27.30	39.79	24.75	62.86	32.48	10.75	27.30	58.37
11.00	27.94	40.71	25.00	63.50	32.80	11.00	27.94	59.73
11.25	28.57	41.64	25.25	64.13	33.13	11.25	28.57	61.08
11.50	29.21	42.56	25.50	64.77	33.46	11.50	29.21	62.44
11.75	29.84	43.49	25.75	65.40	33.79	11.75	29.84	63.80
12.00	30.48	44.41	26.00	66.04	34.12	12.00	30.48	65.16
12.25	31.11	45.34	26.25	66.67	34.44	12.25	31.11	66.51
12.50	31.75	46.26	26.50	67.31	34.77	12.50	31.75	67.87
12.75	32.38	47.19	26.75	67.94	35.10	12.75	32.38	69.23
13.00	33.02	48.11	27.00	68.58	35.43	13.00	33.02	70.59
13.25	33.65	49.04	27.25	69.21	35.76	13.25	33.65	71.94
13.50	34.29	49.96	27.50	69.85	36.09	13.50	34.29	73.30
13.75	34.92	50.89	27.75	70.48	36.41	13.75	34.92	74.66
14.00	35.56	51.82	28.00	71.12	36.74	14.00	35.56	76.02
14.25	36.19	52.74	28.25	71.75	37.07	14.25	36.19	77.37
14.50	36.83	53.67	28.50	72.39	37.40	14.50	36.83	78.73
14.75	37.46	54.59	28.75	73.02	37.73	14.75	37.46	80.09
15.00	38.10	55.52	29.00	73.66	38.05	15.00	38.10	81.45
15.25	38.73	56.44	29.25	74.29	38.38	15.25	38.73	82.80
15.50	39.37	57.37	29.50	74.93	38.71	15.50	39.37	84.16
15.75	40.00	58.29	29.75	75.56	39.04	15.75	40.00	85.52
16.00	40.64	59.22	30.00	76.20	39.37	16.00	40.64	86.88
16.25	41.27	60.14	30.25	76.83	39.69	16.25	41.27	88.23
16.50	41.91	61.07	30.50	77.47	40.02	16.50	41.91	89.59
16.75	42.54	61.99	30.75	78.10	40.35	16.75	42.54	90.95
17.00	43.18	62.92	31.00	78.74	40.68	17.00	43.18	92.31
17.25	43.81	63.84	31.25	79.37	41.01	17.25	43.81	93.66
17.50	44.45	64.77	31.50	80.01	41.33	17.50	44.45	95.02
17.75	45.08	65.69	31.75	80.64	41.66	17.75	45.08	96.38
18.00	45.72	66.62	32.00	81.28	41.99	18.00	45.72	97.74
18.25	46.35	67.54	32.25	81.91	42.32	18.25	46.35	99.09
18.50	46.99	68.47	32.50	82.55	42.65	18.50	46.99	100.45
18.75	47.62	69.40	32.75	83.18	42.97	18.75	47.62	101.81
19.00	48.26	70.32	33.00	83.82	43.30	19.00	48.26	103.17
19.25	48.89	71.25	33.25	84.45	43.63	19.25	48.89	104.52
19.50	49.53	72.17	33.50	85.09	43.96	19.50	49.53	105.88
19.75	50.16	73.10	33.75	85.72	44.29	19.75	50.16	107.24
20.00	50.80	74.02	34.00	86.36	44.61	20.00	50.80	108.60
20.25	51.43	74.95	34.25	86.99	44.94	20.25	51.43	109.95
20.50	52.07	75.87	34.50	87.63	45.27	20.50	52.07	111.31
20.75	52.70	76.80	34.75	88.26	45.60	20.75	52.70	112.67
21.00	53.34	77.72	35.00	88.90	45.93	21.00	53.34	114.02
21.25	53.97	78.65	35.25	89.53	46.25	21.25	53.97	115.38
21.50	54.61	79.57	35.50	90.17	46.58	21.50	54.61	116.74
21.75	55.24	80.50	35.75	90.80	46.91	21.75	55.24	118.10
22.00	55.88	81.42	36.00	91.44	47.24	22.00	55.88	119.45
			36.25	92.07	47.57			
			36.50	92.71	47.89			
			36.75	93.34	48.22			
			37.00	93.98	48.55			
			37.25	94.61	48.88			
			37.50	95.25	49.21			
			37.75	95.88	49.54			

CHART 2—*continued*

Upper Arm			Abdomen			Forearm		
in	*cm*	*Constant A*	*in*	*cm*	*Constant B*	*in*	*cm*	*Constant C*
			38.00	96.52	49.86			
			38.25	97.15	50.19			
			38.50	97.79	50.52			
			38.75	98.42	50.85			
			39.00	99.06	51.18			
			39.25	99.69	51.50			
			39.50	100.33	51.83			
			39.75	100.96	52.16			
			40.00	101.60	52.49			
			40.25	102.23	52.82			
			40.50	102.87	53.14			
			40.75	103.50	53.47			
			41.00	104.14	53.80			
			41.25	104.77	54.13			
			41.50	105.41	54.46			
			41.75	106.04	54.78			
			42.00	106.68	55.11			

Note: Percent Fat = Constant A + Constant B − Constant C − 10.2

CHART 3
CONVERSION CONSTANTS TO PREDICT PERCENTAGE BODY FAT FOR OLDER MEN

Buttocks			Abdomen			Forearm		
in	*cm*	*Constant A*	*in*	*cm*	*Constant B*	*in*	*cm*	*Constant C*
28.00	71.12	29.34	25.50	64.77	22.84	7.00	17.78	21.01
28.25	71.75	29.60	25.75	65.40	23.06	7.25	18.41	21.76
28.50	72.39	29.87	26.00	66.04	23.29	7.50	19.05	22.52
28.75	73.02	30.13	26.25	66.67	23.51	7.75	19.68	23.26
29.00	73.66	30.39	26.50	67.31	23.73	8.00	20.32	24.02
29.25	74.29	30.65	26.75	67.94	23.96	8.25	20.95	24.76
29.50	74.93	30.92	27.00	68.58	24.18	8.50	21.59	25.52
29.75	75.56	31.18	27.25	69.21	24.40	8.75	22.22	26.26
30.00	76.20	31.44	27.50	69.85	24.63	9.00	22.86	27.02
30.25	76.83	31.70	27.75	70.48	24.85	9.25	23.49	27.76
30.50	77.47	31.96	28.00	71.12	25.08	9.50	24.13	28.52
30.75	78.10	32.22	28.25	71.75	25.29	9.75	24.76	29.26
31.00	78.74	32.49	28.50	72.39	25.52	10.00	25.40	30.02
31.25	79.37	32.75	28.75	73.02	25.75	10.25	26.03	30.76
31.50	80.01	33.01	29.00	73.66	25.97	10.50	26.67	31.52
31.75	80.64	33.27	29.25	74.29	26.19	10.75	27.30	32.27
32.00	81.28	33.54	29.50	74.93	26.42	11.00	27.94	33.02
32.25	81.91	33.80	29.75	75.56	26.64	11.25	28.57	33.77
32.50	82.55	34.06	30.00	76.20	26.87	11.50	29.21	34.52
32.75	83.18	34.32	30.25	76.83	27.09	11.75	29.84	35.27
33.00	83.82	34.58	30.50	77.47	27.32	12.00	30.48	36.02
33.25	84.45	34.84	30.75	78.10	27.54	12.25	31.11	36.77
33.50	85.09	35.11	31.00	78.74	27.76	12.50	31.75	37.53

CHART 3— *continued*

Buttocks			Abdomen			Forearm		
in	*cm*	*Constant A*	*in*	*cm*	*Constant B*	*in*	*cm*	*Constant C*
33.75	85.72	35.37	31.25	79.37	27.98	12.75	32.38	38.27
34.00	86.36	35.63	31.50	80.01	28.21	13.00	33.02	39.03
34.25	86.99	35.89	31.75	80.64	28.43	13.25	33.65	39.77
34.50	87.63	36.16	32.00	81.28	28.66	13.50	34.29	40.53
34.75	88.26	36.42	32.25	81.91	28.88	13.75	34.92	41.27
35.00	88.90	36.68	32.50	82.55	29.11	14.00	35.56	42.03
35.25	89.53	36.94	32.75	83.18	29.33	14.25	36.19	42.77
35.50	90.17	37.20	33.00	83.82	29.55	14.50	36.83	43.53
35.75	90.80	37.46	33.25	84.45	29.78	14.75	37.46	44.27
36.00	91.44	37.73	33.50	85.09	30.00	15.00	38.10	45.03
36.25	92.07	37.99	33.75	85.72	30.22	15.25	38.73	45.77
36.50	92.71	38.25	34.00	86.36	30.45	15.50	39.37	46.53
36.75	93.34	38.51	34.25	86.99	30.67	15.75	40.00	47.28
37.00	93.98	38.78	34.50	87.63	30.89	16.00	40.64	48.03
37.25	94.61	39.04	34.75	88.26	31.12	16.25	41.27	48.78
37.50	95.25	39.30	35.00	88.90	31.35	16.50	41.91	49.53
37.75	95.88	39.56	35.25	89.53	31.57	16.75	42.54	50.28
38.00	96.52	39.82	35.50	90.17	31.79	17.00	43.18	51.03
38.25	97.15	40.08	35.75	90.80	32.02	17.25	43.81	51.78
38.50	97.79	40.35	36.00	91.44	32.24	17.50	44.45	52.54
38.75	98.42	40.61	36.25	92.07	32.46	17.75	45.08	53.28
39.00	99.06	40.87	36.50	92.71	32.69	18.00	45.72	54.04
39.25	99.69	41.13	36.75	93.34	32.91	18.25	46.35	54.78
39.50	100.33	41.39	37.00	93.98	33.14			
39.75	100.96	41.66	37.25	94.61	33.36			
40.00	101.60	41.92	37.50	95.25	33.58			
40.25	102.23	42.18	37.75	95.88	33.81			
40.50	102.87	42.44	38.00	96.52	34.03			
40.75	103.50	42.70	38.25	97.15	34.26			
41.00	104.14	42.97	38.50	97.79	34.48			
41.25	104.77	43.23	38.75	98.42	34.70			
41.50	105.41	43.49	39.00	99.06	34.93			
41.75	106.04	43.75	39.25	99.69	35.15			
42.00	106.68	44.02	39.50	100.33	35.38			
42.25	107.31	44.28	39.75	100.96	35.59			
42.50	107.95	44.54	40.00	101.60	35.82			
42.75	108.58	44.80	40.25	102.23	36.05			
43.00	109.22	45.06	40.50	102.87	36.27			
43.25	109.85	45.32	40.75	103.50	36.49			
43.50	110.49	45.59	41.00	104.14	36.72			
43.75	111.12	45.85	41.25	104.77	36.94			
44.00	111.76	46.12	41.50	105.41	37.17			
44.25	112.39	46.37	41.75	106.04	37.39			
44.50	113.03	46.64	42.00	106.68	37.62			
44.75	113.66	46.89	42.25	107.31	37.87			
45.00	114.30	47.16	42.50	107.95	38.06			
45.25	114.93	47.42	42.75	108.58	38.28			
45.50	115.57	47.68	43.00	109.22	38.51			
45.75	116.20	47.94	43.25	109.85	38.73			
46.00	116.84	48.21	43.50	110.49	38.96			
46.25	117.47	48.47	43.75	111.12	39.18			
46.50	118.11	48.73	44.00	111.76	39.41			
46.75	118.74	48.99	44.25	112.39	39.63			

CHART 3—*continued*

Buttocks			Abdomen			Forearm		
in	*cm*	*Constant A*	*in*	*cm*	*Constant B*	*in*	*cm*	*Constant C*
47.00	119.38	49.26	44.50	113.03	39.85			
47.25	120.01	49.52	44.75	113.66	40.08			
47.50	120.65	49.78	45.00	114.30	40.30			
47.75	121.28	50.04						
48.00	121.92	50.30						
48.25	122.55	50.56						
48.50	123.19	50.83						
48.75	123.82	51.09						
49.00	124.46	51.35						

Note: Percent Fat = Constant A + Constant B − Constant C − 15.0

CHART 4
CONVERSION CONSTANTS TO PREDICT PERCENTAGE BODY FAT FOR YOUNG WOMEN

Abdomen			Thigh			Forearm		
in	*cm*	*Constant A*	*in*	*cm*	*Constant B*	*in*	*cm*	*Constant C*
20.00	50.80	26.74	14.00	35.56	29.13	6.00	15.24	25.86
20.25	51.43	27.07	14.25	36.19	29.65	6.25	15.87	26.94
20.50	52.07	27.41	14.50	36.83	30.17	6.50	16.51	28.02
20.75	52.70	27.74	14.75	37.46	30.69	6.75	17.14	29.10
21.00	53.34	28.07	15.00	38.10	31.21	7.00	17.78	30.17
21.25	53.97	28.41	15.25	38.73	31.73	7.25	18.41	31.25
21.50	54.61	28.74	15.50	39.37	32.25	7.50	19.05	32.33
21.75	55.24	29.08	15.75	40.00	32.77	7.75	19.68	33.41
22.00	55.88	29.41	16.00	40.64	33.29	8.00	20.32	34.48
22.25	56.51	29.74	16.25	41.27	33.81	8.25	20.95	35.56
22.50	57.15	30.08	16.50	41.91	34.33	8.50	21.59	36.64
22.75	57.78	30.41	16.75	42.54	34.85	8.75	22.22	37.72
23.00	58.42	30.75	17.00	43.18	35.37	9.00	22.86	38.79
23.25	59.05	31.08	17.25	43.81	35.89	9.25	23.49	39.87
23.50	59.69	31.42	17.50	44.45	36.41	9.50	24.13	40.95
23.75	60.32	31.75	17.75	45.08	36.93	9.75	24.76	42.03
24.00	60.96	32.08	18.00	45.72	37.45	10.00	25.40	43.10
24.25	61.59	32.42	18.25	46.35	37.97	10.25	26.03	44.18
24.50	62.23	32.75	18.50	46.99	38.49	10.50	26.67	45.26
24.75	62.86	33.09	18.75	47.62	39.01	10.75	27.30	46.34
25.00	63.50	33.42	19.00	48.26	39.53	11.00	27.94	47.41
25.25	64.13	33.76	19.25	48.89	40.05	11.25	28.57	48.49
25.50	64.77	34.09	19.50	49.53	40.57	11.50	29.21	49.57
25.75	65.40	34.42	19.75	50.16	41.09	11.75	29.84	50.65
26.00	66.04	34.76	20.00	50.80	41.61	12.00	30.48	51.73
26.25	66.67	35.09	20.25	51.43	42.13	12.25	31.11	52.80
26.50	67.31	35.43	20.50	52.07	42.65	12.50	31.75	53.88
26.75	67.94	35.76	20.75	52.70	43.17	12.75	32.38	54.96
27.00	68.58	36.10	21.00	53.34	43.69	13.00	33.02	56.04
27.25	69.21	36.43	21.25	53.97	44.21	13.25	33.65	57.11
27.50	69.85	36.76	21.50	54.61	44.73	13.50	34.29	58.19

CHART 4— *continued*

Abdomen			Thigh			Forearm		
in	*cm*	*Constant A*	*in*	*cm*	*Constant B*	*in*	*cm*	*Constant C*
27.75	70.48	37.10	21.75	55.24	45.25	13.75	34.92	59.27
28.00	71.12	37.43	22.00	55.88	45.77	14.00	35.56	60.35
28.25	71.75	37.77	22.25	56.51	46.29	14.25	36.19	61.42
28.50	72.39	38.10	22.50	57.15	46.81	14.50	36.83	62.50
28.75	73.02	38.43	22.75	57.78	47.33	14.75	37.46	63.58
29.00	73.66	38.77	23.00	58.42	47.85	15.00	38.10	64.66
29.25	74.29	39.10	23.25	59.05	48.37	15.25	38.73	65.73
29.50	74.93	39.44	23.50	59.69	48.89	15.50	39.37	66.81
29.75	75.56	39.77	23.75	60.32	49.41	15.75	40.00	67.89
30.00	76.20	40.11	24.00	60.96	49.93	16.00	40.64	68.97
30.25	76.83	40.44	24.25	61.59	50.45	16.25	41.27	70.04
30.50	77.47	40.77	24.50	62.23	50.97	16.50	41.91	71.12
30.75	78.10	41.11	24.75	62.86	51.49	16.75	42.54	72.20
31.00	78.74	41.44	25.00	63.50	52.01	17.00	43.18	73.28
31.25	79.37	41.78	25.25	64.13	52.53	17.25	43.81	74.36
31.50	80.01	42.11	25.50	64.77	53.05	17.50	44.45	75.43
31.75	80.64	42.45	25.75	65.40	53.57	17.75	45.08	76.51
32.00	81.28	42.78	26.00	66.04	54.09	18.00	45.72	77.59
32.25	81.91	43.11	26.25	66.67	54.61	18.25	46.35	78.67
32.50	82.55	43.45	26.50	67.31	55.13	18.50	46.99	79.74
32.75	83.18	43.78	26.75	67.94	55.65	18.75	47.62	80.82
33.00	83.82	44.12	27.00	68.58	56.17	19.00	48.26	81.90
33.25	84.45	44.45	27.25	69.21	56.69	19.25	48.89	82.98
33.50	85.09	44.78	27.50	69.85	57.21	19.50	49.53	84.05
33.75	85.72	45.12	27.75	70.48	57.73	19.75	50.16	85.13
34.00	86.36	45.45	28.00	71.12	58.26	20.00	50.80	86.21
34.25	86.99	45.79	28.25	71.75	58.78			
34.50	87.63	46.12	28.50	72.39	59.30			
34.75	88.26	46.46	38.75	73.02	59.82			
35.00	88.90	46.79	29.00	73.66	60.34			
35.25	89.53	47.12	29.25	74.29	60.86			
35.50	90.17	47.46	29.50	74.93	61.38			
35.75	90.80	47.79	29.75	75.56	61.90			
36.00	91.44	48.13	30.00	76.20	62.42			
36.25	92.07	48.46	30.25	76.83	62.94			
36.50	92.71	48.80	30.50	77.47	63.46			
36.75	93.34	49.13	30.75	78.10	63.98			
37.00	93.98	49.46	31.00	78.74	64.50			
37.25	94.61	49.80	31.25	79.37	65.02			
37.50	95.25	50.13	31.50	80.01	65.54			
37.75	95.88	50.47	31.75	80.64	66.06			
38.00	96.52	50.80	32.00	81.28	66.58			
38.25	97.15	51.13	32.25	81.91	67.10			
38.50	97.79	51.47	32.50	82.55	67.62			
38.75	98.42	51.80	32.75	83.18	68.14			
39.00	99.06	52.14	33.00	83.82	68.66			
39.25	99.69	52.47	33.25	84.45	69.18			
39.50	100.33	52.81	33.50	85.09	69.70			
39.75	100.96	53.14	33.75	85.72	70.22			
40.00	101.60	53.47	34.00	86.36	70.74			

Note: Percent Fat = Constant A + Constant B – Constant C – 19.6

CHART 5
CONVERSION CONSTANTS TO PREDICT PERCENTAGE BODY FAT FOR OLDER WOMEN

Abdomen			Thigh			Forearm		
in	*cm*	*Constant A*	*in*	*cm*	*Constant B*	*in*	*cm*	*Constant C*
25.00	63.50	29.69	14.00	35.56	17.31	10.00	25.40	14.46
25.25	64.13	29.98	14.25	36.19	17.62	10.25	26.03	14.82
25.50	64.77	30.28	14.50	36.83	17.93	10.50	26.67	15.18
25.75	65.40	30.58	14.75	37.46	18.24	10.75	27.30	15.54
26.00	66.04	30.87	15.00	38.10	18.55	11.00	27.94	15.91
26.25	66.67	31.17	15.25	38.73	18.86	11.25	28.57	16.27
26.50	67.31	31.47	15.50	39.37	19.17	11.50	29.21	16.63
26.75	67.94	31.76	15.75	40.00	19.47	11.75	29.84	16.99
27.00	68.58	32.06	16.00	40.64	19.78	12.00	30.48	17.35
27.25	69.21	32.36	16.25	41.27	20.09	12.25	31.11	17.71
27.50	69.85	32.65	16.50	41.91	20.40	12.50	31.75	18.08
27.75	70.48	32.95	16.75	42.54	20.71	12.75	32.38	18.44
28.00	71.12	33.25	17.00	43.18	21.02	13.00	33.02	18.80
28.25	71.75	33.55	17.25	43.81	21.33	13.25	33.65	19.16
28.50	72.39	33.84	17.50	44.45	21.64	13.50	34.29	19.52
28.75	73.02	34.14	17.75	45.08	21.95	13.75	34.92	19.88
29.00	73.66	34.44	18.00	45.72	22.26	14.00	35.56	20.24
29.25	74.29	34.73	18.25	46.35	22.57	14.25	36.19	20.61
29.50	74.93	35.03	18.50	46.99	22.87	14.50	36.83	20.97
29.75	75.56	35.33	18.75	47.62	23.18	14.75	37.46	21.33
30.00	76.20	35.62	19.00	38.26	23.49	15.00	38.10	21.69
30.25	76.83	35.92	19.25	48.89	23.80	15.25	38.73	22.05
30.50	77.47	36.22	19.50	49.53	24.11	15.50	39.37	22.41
30.75	78.10	36.51	19.75	50.16	24.42	15.75	40.00	22.77
31.00	78.74	36.81	20.00	50.80	24.73	16.00	40.64	23.14
31.25	79.37	37.11	20.25	51.43	25.04	16.25	41.27	23.50
31.50	80.01	37.40	20.50	52.07	25.35	16.50	41.91	23.86
31.75	80.64	37.70	20.75	52.70	25.66	16.75	42.54	24.22
32.00	81.28	38.00	21.00	53.34	25.97	17.00	43.18	24.58
32.25	81.91	38.30	21.25	53.97	26.28	17.25	43.81	24.94
32.50	82.55	38.59	21.50	54.61	26.58	17.50	44.45	25.31
32.75	83.18	38.89	21.75	55.24	26.89	17.75	45.08	25.67
33.00	83.82	39.19	22.00	55.88	27.20	18.00	45.72	26.03
33.25	84.45	39.48	22.25	56.51	27.51	18.25	46.35	26.39
33.50	85.09	39.78	22.50	57.15	27.82	18.50	46.99	26.75
33.75	85.72	40.08	22.75	57.78	28.13	18.75	47.62	27.11
34.00	86.36	40.37	23.00	58.42	28.44	19.00	48.26	27.47
34.25	86.99	40.67	23.25	59.05	28.75	19.25	48.89	27.84
34.50	87.63	40.97	23.50	59.69	29.06	19.50	49.53	28.20
34.75	88.26	41.26	23.75	60.32	29.37	19.75	50.16	28.56
35.00	88.90	41.56	24.00	60.96	29.68	20.00	50.80	28.92
35.25	89.53	41.86	24.25	61.59	29.98	20.25	51.43	29.28
35.50	90.17	42.15	24.50	62.23	30.29	20.50	52.07	29.64
35.75	90.80	42.45	24.75	62.86	30.60	20.75	52.70	30.00
36.00	91.44	42.75	25.00	63.50	30.91	21.00	53.34	30.37
36.25	92.07	43.05	25.25	64.13	31.22	21.25	53.97	30.73
36.50	92.71	43.34	25.50	64.77	31.53	21.50	54.61	31.09
36.75	93.35	43.64	25.75	65.40	31.84	21.75	55.24	31.45
37.00	93.98	43.94	26.00	66.04	32.15	22.00	55.88	31.81
37.25	94.62	44.23	26.25	66.67	32.46	22.25	56.51	32.17
37.50	95.25	44.53	26.50	67.31	32.77	22.50	57.15	32.54

CHART 5—*continued*

Abdomen			Thigh			Forearm		
in	*cm*	*Constant A*	*in*	*cm*	*Constant B*	*in*	*cm*	*Constant C*
37.75	95.89	44.83	26.75	67.94	33.08	22.75	57.78	32.90
38.00	96.52	45.12	27.00	68.58	33.38	23.00	58.42	33.26
38.25	97.16	45.42	27.25	69.21	33.69	23.25	59.05	33.62
38.50	97.79	45.72	27.50	69.85	34.00	23.50	59.69	33.98
38.75	98.43	46.01	27.75	70.48	34.31	23.75	60.32	34.34
39.00	99.06	46.31	28.00	71.12	34.62	24.00	60.96	34.70
39.25	99.70	46.61	28.25	71.75	34.93	24.25	61.59	35.07
39.50	100.33	46.90	28.50	72.39	35.24	24.50	62.23	35.43
39.75	100.97	47.20	28.75	73.02	35.55	24.75	62.86	35.79
40.00	101.60	47.50	29.00	73.66	35.86	25.00	63.50	36.15
40.25	101.24	47.79	29.25	74.29	36.17			
40.50	102.87	48.09	29.50	74.93	36.48			
40.75	103.51	48.39	29.75	75.56	36.79			
41.00	104.14	48.69	30.00	76.20	37.09			
41.25	104.78	48.98	30.25	76.83	37.40			
41.50	105.41	49.28	30.50	77.47	37.71			
41.75	106.05	49.58	30.75	78.10	38.02			
42.00	106.68	49.87	31.00	78.74	38.33			
42.25	107.32	50.17	31.25	79.37	38.64			
42.50	107.95	50.47	31.50	80.01	38.95			
42.75	108.59	50.76	31.75	80.64	39.26			
43.00	109.22	51.06	32.00	81.28	39.57			
43.25	109.86	51.36	32.25	81.91	39.88			
43.50	110.49	51.65	32.50	82.55	40.19			
43.75	111.13	51.95	32.75	83.18	40.49			
44.00	111.76	52.25	33.00	83.82	40.80			
44.25	112.40	52.54	33.25	84.45	41.11			
44.50	113.03	52.84	33.50	85.09	41.42			
44.75	113.67	53.14	33.75	85.72	41.73			
45.00	114.30	53.44	34.00	86.36	42.04			

Note: Percentage Fat = Constant A + Constant B – Constant C – 18.4

Body Composition Characteristics of Athletes in Different Sports[a,b]

Sport	Sex	N	Age (y)	Stature (cm)	Mass (kg)	Body Fat (%)	Reference Number
Ballet							
	F	34	21.9	168.0	54.4	16.9	3
			±4.3	±6.8	±6.0	±4.7	
Baseball and softball							
Baseball	M		27.4	183.1	88.0	12.6	39
Softball	F	14	22.6	167.1	59.6	19.1	41
			±4.1	±6.1	±5.8	±5.0	
Basketball	F	49	19.3	176.5	66.8	19.2	34
			±1.4	±8.8	±6.7	±4.6	
	M	10	20.9	194.3	87.5	10.5	27
			±1.3	±10.2	±7.2	±3.8	
Biathlon	F	9	25.1	165.9	59.0	15.0	2
			±5.3	±7.1	±7.1	±2.2	
Bicycling	M	11	22.2	176.4	68.5	10.5	40
			±3.6	±7.1	±6.4	±2.4	
Field events							
Decathlon	M	3	22.5	186.3	84.1	8.4	40
			±2.2	±1.4	±9.2	±5.1	
Pentathlon	F	9	21.5	175.4	65.4	11.0	15
			±3.1	±3.0	±5.7	±3.3	
Throwing	F	9	18.8	173.9	80.8	27.0	38
			±3.0	±6.9	±21.1	±8.4	
Discus	M	7	28.3	186.1	104.7	16.4	6
			±5.0	±2.6	±13.2	±4.3	
Shot	M	5	27.0	188.2	112.5	16.5	6
			±3.9	±3.6	±7.3	±4.3	
Jumping	F	13	17.4	173.6	57.1	12.9	33
			±0.9	±8.0	±6.0	±2.5	
	M	16	17.6	181.7	69.2	8.5	33
			±0.8	±6.1	±7.2	±2.1	
Hammer, elite	M	10	24.8	187.3	104.2	15.1	20
			±3.2	±3.1	±9.1	±4.2	
Shotput, elite	M	10	23.5	187.0	112.3	14.8	20
			±4.2	±4.0	±6.2	±3.4	
Discus, elite	M	10	23.5	191.7	108.2	13.2	20
			±4.5	±4.7	±6.9	±4.6	
Javelin, elite	M	10	21.9	186.0	90.6	8.5	20
			±3.7	±5.1	±6.1	±3.2	

continued

Sport	Sex	N	Age (y)	Stature (cm)	Mass (kg)	Body Fat (%)	Reference Number
Field hockey	F	13	19.8 ±1.4	159.8 ±5.5	58.1 ±6.6	21.3 ±7.2	31
Football							
Defensive backs, Pro	M	26	24.5 ±3.2	182.5 ±4.5	84.8 ±5.2	9.6 ±4.2	37
College	M	15		178.3	77.3	11.5	18
College	M	12		179.9	83.1	8.8	
College	M	15		183.0	83.7	9.6	
Pro, current	M	26		182.5	84.8	9.6	
Pro, older	M	25		183.0	91.2	10.7	
Offensive backs and wide receivers, Pro	M	40	24.7 ±3.0	183.8 ±4.1	90.7 ±8.4	9.4 ±4.0	37
College	M	15		179.7	79.8	12.4	36
College	M	29		181.8	84.1	9.5	18
College	M	18		185.6	86.1	9.9	
Pro, current	M	40		183.8	90.7	9.4	
Pro, older	M	25		183.0	91.7	10.0	
Line backers, Pro	M	28	24.2 ±2.4	188.6 ±2.9	102.2 ±6.3	14.0 ±4.6	37
College	M	7		180.1	87.2	13.4	36
College	M	17		186.1	97.1	13.1	18
College	M	17		185.6	98.8	13.2	
Pro, current	M	28		188.6	102.2	14.0	
Offensive line, Pro	M	38	24.7 ±3.2	193.0 ±3.5	112.6 ±6.8	15.6 ±3.8	37
College	M	13		186.0	99.2	19.1	36
College	M	23		187.5	107.6	19.5	18
College	M	25		191.1	106.5	15.3	
Pro, current	M	38		193.0	112.6	15.6	
Defensive line, Pro	M	32	25.7 ±3.4	192.4 ±6.5	117.1 ±10.3	18.2 ±5.4	37
College	M	15		186.6	97.8	18.5	36
College	M	8		188.8	114.3	19.5	18
College	M	13		191.1	109.3	14.7	
Pro, current	M	32		192.4	117.1	18.2	
Pro, older	M	25		185.7	97.1	14.0	
Quarterbacks, Pro	M	16	24.1 ±2.7	185.0 ±5.4	90.1 ±11.3	14.4 ±6.5	37
Total Team							
College	M	65		182.5	88.0	15.0	36
College	M	91		184.9	97.3	13.9	18
College	M	88		186.6	96.6	11.4	
Pro, current	M	164		188.1	101.5	13.4	
Pro, older	M	25		183.1	91.2	10.4	
Dallas-Jets	M	107		188.2	100.4	12.6	
Gymnastics							
	F	44	19.4 ±1.1	160.6 ±4.4	53.7 ±5.9	15.3 ±4.0	30
	F	97	15.7 ±1.1	162.4 ±5.6	54.0 ±6.5	8.2	5
	M	19		168.7 ±6.7	65.8 ±4.3	6.5 ±2.4	32
Lacrosse	F	17	24.4 ±4.5	166.3 ±7.5	60.6 ±7.3	19.3 ±5.7	41
	M	26	26.7 ±4.2	177.6 ±5.5	74.0 ±8.6	12.3 ±4.3	40
Orienteering	M	7	25.9 ±8.5	176.2 ±6.8	64.7 ±5.0	10.7 ±2.9	40

Sport	Sex	N	Age (y)	Stature (cm)	Mass (kg)	Body Fat (%)	Reference Number
Racket sports							
Badminton	F	6	23.0	167.7	61.5	21.0	41
			±5.3	±2.5	±2.6	±2.1	
	M	7	24.5	180.0	71.2	12.8	40
			±3.6	±5.2	±5.6	±3.1	
Tennis	F	7	21.3	164.7	59.6	22.4	31
			±0.9	±4.2	±4.6	±2.0	
	M	9		179.1	73.8	11.3	32
				±4.5	±7.3	±5.2	
Squash	M	9	22.6	177.5	71.9	11.2	40
			±6.8	±4.1	±8.3	±3.7	
Rowers	M	18	20.6	185.8	86.3	12.2	13
			±1.9	±2.2	±6.4	±4.1	
Skating							
Ice hockey	M	27	24.9	182.9	85.6	9.2	1
			±3.6	±6.1	±7.1	±4.6	
Speed skating	F	9	19.7	165.0	61.2	16.5	23
			±3.0	±6.0	±6.9	±4.1	
	M	6	22.2	178.0	73.3	7.4	23
			±4.1	±7.1	±7.1	±2.5	
Skiing							
(Nordic)	F	5	23.5	164.5	56.9	16.1	29
			±4.7	±3.3	±1.1	±1.6	
Alpine	F	6	19.6	165.0	63.6	16.6	35
	F	5	20.2	164.7	60.1	18.5	12
	M	8	19.8	173.0	72.6	6.5	35
	M	5	21.2	175.5	73.0	7.2	12
	M	11	22.8	179.0	71.8	7.2	29
			±1.9	±5.0	±5.4	±1.9	
Soccer	F	11	22.1	164.9	61.2	22.0	41
			±4.1	±5.6	±8.6	±6.8	
	M	19		176.8	72.4	9.5	32
				±6.6	±8.9	±4.9	
Swimming	F	9	13.5	164.5	53.3	17.2	19
			±0.9	±7.4	±5.3	±3.6	
	F	13	16.4	168.8	57.9	15.6	
			±0.9	±7.1	±5.5	±4.0	
	F	19	19.2	169.6	56.0	16.1	
			±0.8	±4.7	±3.1	±3.7	
	M	27		178.3	71.0	8.8	32
				±6.4	±5.9	±3.2	
Channel swimmers	M	11	38.2	173.8	87.5	22.4	24
			±10.2	±7.4	±10.4	±7.5	
Track events							
Distance runners	F	15	27	161.0	47.2	14.3	8
				±4.0	±4.6	±3.3	
	M	20		177.0	63.1	4.7	22
				±6.0	±4.8	±3.1	
Masters and competitors	M	11	40–49	180.7	63.1	4.7	21
		5	50–59	174.2	67.2	10.9	
		6	60–69	175.4	67.1	11.3	
		3	70.8	175.6	66.7	13.6	

continued

Sport	Sex	N	Age (y)	Stature (cm)	Mass (kg)	Body Fat (%)	Reference Number
Masters and competitors *(continued)*							
Sprinters and hurdlers	F	8	15.8 ±2.7	166.5 ±9.3	54.0 ±8.4	10.9 ±3.6	38
	M	5	28.4 ±0.1	179.9 ±0.7	66.8 ±0.9	8.3 ±5.2	40
Walkers	F	4	24.9 ±6.3	163.4 ±3.9	51.7 ±4.8	18.1 ±4.4	41
	M	3	20.3 ±2.0	178.4 ±2.1	66.1 ±1.8	7.3 ±1.3	40
Triathlon	F	16	24.2 ±4.3	162.1 ±6.3	55.2 ±4.6	16.5 ±1.4	16
	M	14	36.0 ±9.9	176.4 ±8.6	73.3 ±8.6	12.5 ±5.9	17
	M	8	29.6 ±2.6	180.0 ±2.4	73.9 ±2.1	7.9 ±0.5	26
Volleyball	F	14	21.6 ±0.8	178.3 ±4.2	70.5 ±5.5	17.9 ±3.6	25
	M	11	20.9 ±3.7	185.3 ±10.2	78.3 ±12.0	9.8 ±2.9	40
Weight lifting and body building							
Power lift	F	10	25.2 ±6.0	164.6 ±3.7	68.6 ±3.6	21.5 ±1.3	10
	M	13	24.8 ±1.6	173.5 ±2.8	80.8 ±3.2	9.1 ±1.2	11
Body builders	F	10	30.4 ±8.2	165.2 ±5.6	56.5 ±0.9	13.5 ±1.5	10
	F	10	27.0	160.8	53.8	13.2	7
	M	16	28.0 ±1.8	175.1 ±1.7	86.2 ±3.1	12.5 ±3.4	4
	M	18	27.8 ±1.8	177.1 ±1.1	82.4 ±1.0	9.3 ±0.8	11
	M	14	31.6 ±6.7	170.8 ±5.6	83.8 ±9.2	10.9 ±2.4	14
Wrestling[c]							
Adult	M	37	19.6 ±1.34	174.6 ±7.0	74.8 ±12.2	8.8 ±4.1	28
Adolescent	M	409	16.2 ±1.0	171.0 ±7.1	63.2 ±10.0	11.0 ±4.0	9
Sumo (seki-tori)	M	37	21.1 ±3.6	178.9 ±5.2	115.9 ±27.4	26.1 ±6.4	14

[a] Values reported as means ± SD.

[b] Modified from Sinning, W.E.: Body composition in athletes. In *Human Body Composition*. Roche, A.F., et al. (eds): Human Kinetics, Champaign, IL, 1996.

[c] Note: consult our web page (http://www.lww.com/mkk) for the recent NCAA policy about minimal wrestling weight certification.

References

1. Agre, J.C., et al.: Professional ice hockey players: Physiologic, anthropometric, and musculoskeletal characteristics. *Arch. Phys. Med. Rehab.,* 69: 188, 1988.

2. Bacharach, D.W., et al.: Relationship of blood urea nitrogen to training intensity of elite female biathlon skiers. *J. Strength Cond. Res.* 10: 105, 1996.

3. Calabrese, L.H., et al.: Menstrual abnormalities, nutrition patterns, and body composition in female classical ballet dancers. *Phys. Sportsmed.* 11: 86, 1983.

4. Cordain, L., et al.: Variability of body composition assessment in men exhibiting extreme muscular hypertrophy. *J. Strength Cond. Res.* 9: 85, 1995.

5. Eckerson, J.M., et al.: Validity of bioelectrical impedence equations for estimating fat-free weight in high school female gymnasts, *Med. Sci. Exerc. Sports,* 29: 962, 1997.

6. Fahey, T.D., et al.: Body composition and VO2max of exceptional weight trained athletes. *J. Appl. Physiol.,* 39: 559, 1975.

7. Freedson, P.F., et al.: Physique, body composition, and psychological characteristics of competitive female body builders. *Phys. Sportsmed.,* 11: 85, 1983.

8. Graves, J.E., et al.: Body composition of elite female distance runners. *Int. J. Sports Med.* 8: 96, 1987.

9. Housh, T.J., et al.: Validity of anthropometric estimations of body composition in high school wrestlers. *Res. Q. Exerc. Sport,* 60: 239, 1989.

10. Johnson, G.O., et al.: A physiological profile comparison of female body builders and power lifters. *J. Sports Med. Phys. Fitness,* 30: 361, 1990.

11. Katch, V.L., et al.: Muscular development and lean body weight in body builders and weight lifters. *Med. Sci. Sports,* 12: 340, 1980.

12. Katch, F.I.: Body composition of elite male and female alpine skiers. Unpublished data. University of Massachusetts, 1998.

13. Katch, F.I.: Physiological characteristics of lightweight and heavyweight male collegiate rowers. Unpublished data. University of Massachusetts, 1999.

14. Kondo, M., et al.: Upper limit of fat-free mass in humans: a study on Japanese Sumo wrestlers. *Am. J. Human Biol.* 6: 613, 1994.

15. Krahenbuhl, G.S., et al.: Characteristics of national and world class female pentathletes. *Med. Sci. Sports,* 11, 20–23, 1979.

16. Leake, C.N., & Carter, J.E.: Comparison of body composition and somatotype of trained female triathletes. *J. Sports Sci.,* 9: 125, 1991.

17. Lofton, M., et al.: Peak physiological function and performance of recreational triathletes. *J. Sports Med. Phys. Fitness,* 28: 330, 1988.

18. McArdle, W.D., et al.: *Exercise Physiology.* 5th edition. Lippincott Williams & Wilkins, Baltimore. 2001, p. 807.

19. Meleski, B.W., et al.: Size, physique and body composition of competitive female swimmers 11 through 20 years of age. *Human Biol.,* 54: 609, 1982.

20. Morrow, J.R., et al.: Anthropometric strength, and performance characteristics of American world class throwers. *J. Sports Med. Phys. Fitness* 22: 73, 1982.

21. Pollock, M.L., et al.: Physiological characteristics of champion American track athletes 40 to 75 years of age. *J. Gerontol.,* 29: 645, 1974.

22. Pollock M.L., et al.: Body composition of elite class distance runners. Ann. *New York Acad Sci.,* 301: 361, 1977.

23. Pollock, M.L., et al.: Comparison of male and female speedskating candidates. In D.M. Landers (ed.), *Sports and Elite Performance* Champaign, IL: Human Kinetics, pp. 143–152.

24. Pugh, L.G., et al.: A physiological study of channel swimming. *Clin. Sci.,* 19: 257, 1955.

25. Puhl, J., et al.: Physical and physiological characteristics of elite volleyball players. *Res. Q. Exerc Sport,* 53: 257, 1982.

26. Rowbottom, D.G., et al.: Training adaptation and biological changes among well-trained male triathletes. *Med. Sci. Sports Exerc.,* 29: 1233, 1997.

27. Siders, W.A., et al.: Effects of participation in a collegiate sport season on body composition. *J. Sports Med. Phys. Fitness,* 31: 571, 1991.

28. Sinning, W.E.: Body composition assessment of college wrestlers. *Med. Sci. Sports,* 6: 139, 1974.

29. Sinning, W.E., et al.: Body composition and somatotype of male and female Nordic skiers. *Res. Q.,* 48: 741–749, 1977.

30. Sinning, W.E.: Anthropometric estimation of body density, fat, and lean body weight in women gymnasts. *Med. Sci. Sports,* 10: 243, 1978.

31. Sinning, W.E., and Wilson, J.R.: Validity of "generalized" equations for body composition analysis in women athletes. *Res. Q. Exerc. Sports;* 55: 153, 1984.

32. Sinning, W.E., et al.: Validity of generalized equations for body composition analysis in male athletes. *Med. Sci. Sports Exerc.,* 17: 124, 1985.

33. Thorland, W.G., et al.: Body composition and somatotype characteristics of junior olympic athletes. *Med. Sci. Sports Exerc.,* 13, 332, 1981.

34. Walsh, F.K., et al.: Estimation of body composition of female intercollegiate basketball players. *Phys. Sportsmed.,* 12: 74, 1984.

35. White, A., Johnson, S.: Physiological comparison of international, national, and regional alpine skiers. *Int. J. Sports Med.,* 12: 374, 1991.

36. Wickkiser, J.D., and Kelly, J.M. The body composition of a college football team. *Med. Sci. Sports.,* 7: 199, 1975.

37. Wilmore, J.H., et al.: Football pro's strengths and CV weaknesses charted. *Phys. Sportsmed.,* 4: 45, 1976.

38. Wilmore, J.H., et al.: Body physique and composition of the female distance runner. *Ann. New York Acad. Sci.,* 301: 764, 1977.

39. Wilmore, J.H.: Body composition in sport and exercise: Directions for future research. *Med. Sci. Sports Exerc.,* 15: 21, 1983.

40. Withers, R.T., et al.: Relative body fat and anthropometric prediction of body density of male athletes. *Eur. J. Appl. Physiol.,* 56: 191, 1987.

41. Withers, R.T., et al.: Relative body fat and anthropometric prediction of body density of female athletes. *Eur. J. Appl. Physiol.,* 56: 169, 1987.

Three-Day Physical Activity Log

A three-day log of physical activities provides a relatively simple yet accurate way to assess average daily energy expenditure.

Step 1: Review Table 1 which provides an example of a daily physical activity log for one of your textbook authors. Note that the list includes mostly typical activities of daily living.

Step 2: Record your daily physical activities on each of the log entry forms for three typical days. Be specific for the beginning and ending times of activity; round off to the nearest minute.

Step 3: Consolidate the information from the three log entry forms (Step 2) to the Master Log in Table 2. If you devote more than 120 minutes to one of the recreational and sports activities, check the 120 minute box. For typical household activities, list activities by minutes and hours.

Step 4: Determine your basal metabolic rate (BMR) in $kcal \cdot h^{-1}$ as follows:

Men

$$BMR\ (kcal \cdot h^{-1}) = 38\ kcal \cdot m^2 \cdot h^{-1} \times surface\ area^a\ (m^2)$$

Women

$$BMR\ (kcal \cdot h^{-1}) = 35\ kcal \cdot m^2 \cdot h^{-1} \times surface\ area^a\ (m^2)$$

Example of BMR Calculations
Data: Male
Age, 40y

Stature, 182 cm (72 in.)
Body mass, 86.4 kg (190 lb)
Body surface area = $2.08\ m^2$
$kcal \cdot m^2 \cdot h^{-1} = 38.0$

Calculations

a. $kcal \cdot h^{-1} = 38.0 \times 2.08 = 79.0$
b. $kcal \cdot min^{-1} = 79.0 \div 60 = 1.3$

Step 5: Determine energy expenditure $(kcal \cdot min^{-1})$ for each of the activities in the Master Log (Table 2). Use Appendix B to determine caloric expenditure per minute. The values represent gross values plus resting. If an activity is not included, list one most similar to yours. The bottom of the Daily Log form includes a box to record daily total kcal.

Step 6: Multiply energy expenditure for each activity by the number of minutes of participation.

Step 7: Sum the total energy expenditure for each activity, including the value for sleep, to arrive at your TOTAL daily energy expenditure.

Step 8: Repeat Steps 5–7 for Days 2 and 3. Calculate average daily calorie by summing the total calories expended for three days and divide by 3.

Total energy expenditure (kcal) = Day 1 kcal + Day 2 kcal + Day 3 kcal

= ___ kcal + ___ kcal + ___ kcal

Average daily energy expenditure = Total kcal ÷ 3

= _____ kcal ÷ 3

---

^{a} Compute body surface area (BSA, m^2) as: Body mass, $kg^{0.425} \times$ stature, $cm^{0.725} \times 0.007184$
Example: Body Mass = 162 lb (73.5 kg); stature = 5'9" (175.3 cm)
BSA, $m^2 = 73.5^{0.425} \times 175.3^{0.725} \times 0.007184$
$= 6.210 \times 42.332 \times 0.007184$
$= 1.89$

Table 1. **EXAMPLE OF DAILY PHYSICAL ACTIVITY LOG. [COLUMN 5 LISTS ACTIVITIES SIMILAR TO THOSE IN COLUMN 1.]**

Activity	Begin Time	End Time	Total Minutes	Similar Activity[a]	kcal·min⁻¹	Total kcal
Wake, bathroom use	6:45AM	6:53AM	8	Standing quietly	2.3	18.4
Go back to bed	6:53	7:30	38	BMR	1.3	48.1
Eat breakfast	7:30	7:50	10	Eating, sitting	2.0	40.0
Use bathroom	7:50	8:00	10	Standing quietly	2.3	23.0
Dress	8:00	8:06	6	Standing quietly	2.3	13.8
Drive to school	8:06	8:17	11	Sitting quietly	2.0	22.0
Walk to office	8:17	8:25	8	Walking, normal pace	6.9	55.8
Work in office, pick up mail	8:25	10:00	95	Writing, sitting	2.5	237.5
Up/down stairs	10:00	10:10	10	11 min 30 sec pace	11.7	117.0
Work in office	10:10	12:10PM	120	Writing, sitting	2.5	300.0
Go to locker	12:10PM	12:12	2	Walking, normal pace	6.9	13.8
Get dressed	12:12	12:16	4	Standing quietly	2.3	9.2
Walk to track	12:16	12:20	4	Walk, normal pace	6.9	27.6
Wait for friend	12:20	12:30	10	Standing quietly	2.3	23.0
Run to park, back	12:30	2:00	90	8-min mile pace	17.2	1553.0
Walk to locker	2:00	2:04	4	Walk, normal pace	6.9	27.6
Shower, dress	2:04	2:20	16	Quiet standing	2.3	36.8
Walk to office	2:20	2:24	4	Walk, normal pace	6.9	27.6
Meeting/lunch	2:24	3:00	36	Eating, sitting	2.0	72.0
Work in office	3:00	5:05	125	Writing, sitting	2.5	312.5
Walk to library	5:05	5:12	7	Walk, normal pace	6.9	48.3
Work in library	5:12	6:05	53	Writing, sitting	2.5	132.5
Walk to dean	6:05	6:10	5	Walk, normal pace	6.9	34.5
Meeting, dean	6:10	6:35	25	Writing, sitting	2.5	62.5
Walk to office	6:35	6:43	8	Walk, normal pace	6.9	55.2
Walk to car	6:43	6:51	8	Walk, normal pace	6.9	55.2
Drive home	6:51	7:03	12	Sitting quietly	1.8	21.6
Change clothes	7:03	7:07	4	Standing quietly	2.3	9.2
Wash-up	7:07	7:11	4	Standing quietly	2.3	9.2
Cook dinner	7:11	8:00	49	Cooking	4.1	200.9
Watch TV	8:00	8:30	30	Sitting quietly	1.8	54.0
Eat dinner	8:30	9:00	30	Eating, sitting	2.0	60.0
Mail letter	9:00	9:05	5	Walk, normal pace	6.9	34.5
Listen to stereo	9:05	9:30	25	Sitting quietly	1.8	45.0
Watch TV	9:30	10:30	60	Sitting quietly	1.8	108.0
Wash-up	10:30	10:38	8	Standing quietly	2.3	18.4
Read in bed	10:38	11:15	37	Lying at ease	1.9	70.3

DAILY TOTAL = 4583

[a] When you cannot match a specific activity with a table value in Appendix B (or the activity in the Diet and Physical Activity CD-ROM), select a similar activity and base the kcal value on that activity.

Day 1.   Physical Activity Log

Activity	Begin Time	End Time	Total Minutes	Similar Activity	$kcal \cdot min^{-1}$	Total kcal

DAILY TOTAL =

Day 2.   Physical Activity Log

Activity	Begin Time	End Time	Total Minutes	Similar Activity	$kcal \cdot min^{-1}$	Total kcal

DAILY TOTAL =

Day 3.   Physical Activity Log

Activity	Begin Time	End Time	Total Minutes	Similar Activity	$kcal \cdot min^{-1}$	Total kcal

DAILY TOTAL =

Table 2.　**MASTER LOG OF PHYSICAL ACTIVITY**

Activity	Day			Minutes												Kcal
	1	2	3	0–10	10–20	20–30	30–40	40–50	50–60	60–70	70–80	80–90	90–100	100–110	110–120	
Aerobics	☐	☐	☐	☐	☐	☐	☐	☐	☐	☐	☐	☐	☐	☐	☐	___
Basketball	☐	☐	☐	☐	☐	☐	☐	☐	☐	☐	☐	☐	☐	☐	☐	___
Fitness Center	☐	☐	☐	☐	☐	☐	☐	☐	☐	☐	☐	☐	☐	☐	☐	___
Rowing Machine	☐	☐	☐	☐	☐	☐	☐	☐	☐	☐	☐	☐	☐	☐	☐	___
Stair Master	☐	☐	☐	☐	☐	☐	☐	☐	☐	☐	☐	☐	☐	☐	☐	___
Stationary Bike	☐	☐	☐	☐	☐	☐	☐	☐	☐	☐	☐	☐	☐	☐	☐	___
Treadmill	☐	☐	☐	☐	☐	☐	☐	☐	☐	☐	☐	☐	☐	☐	☐	___
Weight Lifting	☐	☐	☐	☐	☐	☐	☐	☐	☐	☐	☐	☐	☐	☐	☐	___
_____	☐	☐	☐	☐	☐	☐	☐	☐	☐	☐	☐	☐	☐	☐	☐	___
_____	☐	☐	☐	☐	☐	☐	☐	☐	☐	☐	☐	☐	☐	☐	☐	___
_____	☐	☐	☐	☐	☐	☐	☐	☐	☐	☐	☐	☐	☐	☐	☐	___
_____	☐	☐	☐	☐	☐	☐	☐	☐	☐	☐	☐	☐	☐	☐	☐	___
Cycling	☐	☐	☐	☐	☐	☐	☐	☐	☐	☐	☐	☐	☐	☐	☐	___
Field Hockey	☐	☐	☐	☐	☐	☐	☐	☐	☐	☐	☐	☐	☐	☐	☐	___
Hiking	☐	☐	☐	☐	☐	☐	☐	☐	☐	☐	☐	☐	☐	☐	☐	___
Jogging/Running	☐	☐	☐	☐	☐	☐	☐	☐	☐	☐	☐	☐	☐	☐	☐	___
Soccer	☐	☐	☐	☐	☐	☐	☐	☐	☐	☐	☐	☐	☐	☐	☐	___
Softball	☐	☐	☐	☐	☐	☐	☐	☐	☐	☐	☐	☐	☐	☐	☐	___
Swimming	☐	☐	☐	☐	☐	☐	☐	☐	☐	☐	☐	☐	☐	☐	☐	___
Racket Sports	☐	☐	☐	☐	☐	☐	☐	☐	☐	☐	☐	☐	☐	☐	☐	___
Martial Arts	☐	☐	☐	☐	☐	☐	☐	☐	☐	☐	☐	☐	☐	☐	☐	___
_____	☐	☐	☐	☐	☐	☐	☐	☐	☐	☐	☐	☐	☐	☐	☐	___
_____	☐	☐	☐	☐	☐	☐	☐	☐	☐	☐	☐	☐	☐	☐	☐	___
_____	☐	☐	☐	☐	☐	☐	☐	☐	☐	☐	☐	☐	☐	☐	☐	___
_____	☐	☐	☐	☐	☐	☐	☐	☐	☐	☐	☐	☐	☐	☐	☐	___
	☐	☐	☐													

Activity	Day			Minutes						Hours								Kcal
	1	2	3	0–10	10–20	20–30	30–40	40–50	50–60	1	2	3	4	5	6	7	8	
Sleep	☐	☐	☐	☐	☐	☐	☐	☐	☐	☐	☐	☐	☐	☐	☐	☐	☐	___
Walking	☐	☐	☐	☐	☐	☐	☐	☐	☐	☐	☐	☐	☐	☐	☐	☐	☐	___
Resting	☐	☐	☐	☐	☐	☐	☐	☐	☐	☐	☐	☐	☐	☐	☐	☐	☐	___
Personal Hygiene	☐	☐	☐	☐	☐	☐	☐	☐	☐	☐	☐	☐	☐	☐	☐	☐	☐	___
Watch TV	☐	☐	☐	☐	☐	☐	☐	☐	☐	☐	☐	☐	☐	☐	☐	☐	☐	___
Attend Class	☐	☐	☐	☐	☐	☐	☐	☐	☐	☐	☐	☐	☐	☐	☐	☐	☐	___
Homework	☐	☐	☐	☐	☐	☐	☐	☐	☐	☐	☐	☐	☐	☐	☐	☐	☐	___
Computer	☐	☐	☐	☐	☐	☐	☐	☐	☐	☐	☐	☐	☐	☐	☐	☐	☐	___
Eating	☐	☐	☐	☐	☐	☐	☐	☐	☐	☐	☐	☐	☐	☐	☐	☐	☐	___
_____	☐	☐	☐	☐	☐	☐	☐	☐	☐	☐	☐	☐	☐	☐	☐	☐	☐	___
_____	☐	☐	☐	☐	☐	☐	☐	☐	☐	☐	☐	☐	☐	☐	☐	☐	☐	___
_____	☐	☐	☐	☐	☐	☐	☐	☐	☐	☐	☐	☐	☐	☐	☐	☐	☐	___
_____	☐	☐	☐	☐	☐	☐	☐	☐	☐	☐	☐	☐	☐	☐	☐	☐	☐	___

INDEX

Page numbers in *italics* indicate figures. Page numbers ending in "t" indicate tables. Page numbers ending in *B* indicate boxed material.